Clinical Imaging of the Small Intestine

Second Edition

Springer
*New York
Berlin
Heidelberg
Barcelona
Hong Kong
London
Milan
Paris
Singapore
Tokyo*

Dean D.T. Maglinte
Department of Radiology
Indiana University School of
Medicine and Methodist
Hospital of Indiana
Indianapolis, IN

Hans Herlinger
Department of Radiology
University of Pennsylvania
Medical Center
Philadelphia, PA

Bernard A. Birnbaum
Department of Radiology
University of Pennsylvania
Medical Center
Philadelphia, PA

Editors

Clinical Imaging of the Small Intestine

Second Edition

Foreword by Emil J. Balthazar, M.D.

With 591 Illustrations in 1178 Parts

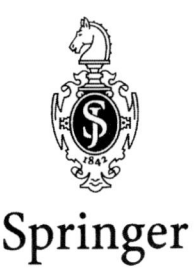

Springer

Hans Herlinger, M.D., Department of Radiology, University of Pennsylvania Medical Center, 3400 Spruce Street, Philadelphia, PA 19104, USA

Dean D. T. Maglinte, M.D., Department of Radiology, Indiana University School of Medicine, Methodist Hospital of Indiana, Indianapolis, IN 46206, USA

Bernard A. Birnbaum, M.D., Department of Radiology, University of Pennsylvania Medical Center, Philadelphia, PA 19104, USA

Library of Congress Cataloging-in-Publication Data
Herlinger, Hans, 1915-
Clinical imaging of the small intestine / Hans Herlinger,
Dean Maglinte, Bernard Birnbaum—2nd ed.
  p. cm.
  Rev. ed. of Clinical radiology of the small intestine. 1989.
  Includes bibliographical references and index.
  ISBN 0-387-95388-4 (softcover : alk. paper)
  1. Intestine, Small—Imaging. I. Maglinte, Dean D. T.
II. Birnbaum, Bernard. III. Herlinger, Hans, 1915-Clinical radiology
of the small intestine. IV. Title.
RC804.D52 H47 1998
616.3′40754—ddc21   98-16317
                                                        CIP

Printed on acid-free paper.

Previously published under the title: *Clinical Radiology of the Small Intestine*, Copyright 1989 by W.B. Saunders Company.

First softcover printing, 2001.

© 1999 Springer-Verlag New York, Inc.
All rights reserved. This work may not be translated or copied in whole or in part without the written permission of the publisher (Springer-Verlag New York, Inc., 175 Fifth Avenue, New York, NY 10010, USA), except for brief excerpts in connection with reviews or scholarly analysis. Use in connection with any form of information storage and retrieval, electronic adaptation, computer software, or by similar or dissimilar methodology now known or hereafter developed is forbidden.
The use of general descriptive names, trade names, trademarks, etc., in this publication, even if the former are not especially identified, is not to be taken as a sign that such names, as understood by the Trade Marks and Merchandise Marks Act, may accordingly be used freely by anyone.
While the advice and information in this book are believed to be true and accurate at the date of going to press, neither the authors nor the editors nor the publisher can accept any legal responsibility for any errors or omissions that may be made. The publisher makes no warranty, express or implied, with respect to the material contained herein.

Production coordinated by WordCrafters Editorial Services, Inc., and managed by Lesley Poliner; manufacturing supervised by Thomas King.
Typeset by MATRIX Publishing Services, Inc., York, PA.
Printed and bound by Maple-Vail Book Manufacturing Group, York, PA.
Printed in the United States of America.

9 8 7 6 5 4 3 2 1

ISBN 0-387-95388-4   SPIN 10856770

Springer-Verlag New York Berlin Heidelberg
A member of BertelsmannSpringer Science+Business Media GmbH

*To the memory of my wife, Betty,
her love and her courage.*

Hans Herlinger

*To my wife, Eleanor,
for her unfailing support and understanding
over the many years of long working hours
both at the hospital and at home.*

Dean D.T. Maglinte

*To my wife, Maj,
whose patience and understanding made it possible;
and to the memory of my parents,
William and Bernice Birnbaum*

Bernard A. Birnbaum

Foreword to the Second Edition

Nova ex Veteris

The publication of the second edition of *Clinical Imaging of the Small Intestine* is cause for celebration. We celebrate not only the scientific achievement of its authors, but we remember and recognize the contribution made by our predecessors to the development of medicine, which has made this book possible.

To understand the progress in medicine in the second half of the twentieth century, one must pay homage to the philosophical contributions made in the few centuries known as the Age of Enlightenment or the Age of Reason. The deplorable condition of the "art of healing" as late as the middle of the eighteenth century was sarcastically characterized by Voltaire: "The role of the physician is to entertain the patient while the body takes care of the disease." Concepts that we are all familiar and comfortable with, such as the relationship between cause and effect, etiology and disease, the need for evidence or proof, reliance on scientific experiments and clinical research, and analysis and debate are by and large products of the nineteenth century. They are based, however, on philosophical concepts formulated earlier, in the seventeenth and eighteenth centuries.

Francis Bacon (1561–1626) proposed the theory of scientific knowledge based on observations and experiments, called the *inductive method*. René Descartes (1596–1650) discarded the authoritarian system and promoted a belief in universal doubt: "Only one thing cannot be doubted: doubt itself." Two centuries later (circa 1880), Friedrich Nietzsche introduced the concept of objectivity. Since the truth is a matter of perspective, truth can be achieved only by the synchronized efforts of many eyes: "The more different eyes we can use to observe one thing, the more complete will our concept be."

The field of gastroenterology began as a clinical branch of internal medicine based on experiments and novel observations of the physiology of the intestinal tract and of the digestive process. Early practitioners included Claude Bernard (1813–1878), considered the founder of experimental gastroenterology; Ivan Pavlov (1849–1936), recipient of the Nobel Prize for his work on the physiology of the digestive system; and Walter Cannon (1871–1945), pioneer researcher who used fluoroscopy to study the physiology of the intestinal tract. As in other fields of medicine, the patient's history, an elaborate physical examination, and a few rudimentary laboratory tests were the only available tools of clinical evaluation. Objective parameters of investigation were lacking. At the beginning of this century, confirmation of clinical diagnosis could be made only at the time of exploratory laparotomy of postmortem examination.

Technological progress achieved in the twentieth century has promoted the rapid development of tests and procedures that can objectively evaluate patients and confirm or disprove the working clinical diagnosis in most instances. Gradually, clinical gastroenterology has been transformed into a reliable science rather than a subjective art.

Many factors have facilitated this progress, most of them beyond the scope of this Foreword. An important milestone was Roentgen's discovery of x-rays, with its clinical application in gastroenterology and the development of fiberoptic endoscopy.

Objective assessment of the small bowel has been and, to a certain degree, still is the challenge of gastroenterology. The very long (20 to 22 feet) small intestine crowded into a small space, with its tortuous mobile and overlapping coils, has been difficult to examine. Flexible endoscopy can reach only its proximal and distal segments. Thus, the evaluation of intestinal morphology has remained in the domain of radiology.

For many years the only means to visualize the small intestine was the barium meal follow-through examination. One of the most convincing proponents of this method, using large amounts of barium, was Richard Marshak, whose strong personality, power of persuasion, controversial statements, lectures, and two monographs on the radiology of the small bowel propelled his field of investigation into the forefront of gastroenterology.

Further improvements were achieved with the introduction of the intubation method called the small bowel enema or enteroclysis. Developed in Europe, used and popularized by J. L. Sellink, its main promoter, enteroclysis was introduced in the United States with modifications and several improvements by Hans Herlinger and Dean Maglinte. Although more cumbersome to perform, enteroclysis offers distinct advantages over the follow-through method in its ability to reliably and exquisitely visualize the intestinal mucosa and actively challenge the distensibility of the small intestine. For his tireless work and seminal contributions, Hans Herlinger has been awarded the Cannon Medal of the Society of Gastrointestinal Radiologists.

More recent advances utilizing sonography, MRI, and particularly CT abdominal imaging have enhanced our ability to evaluate the small bowel. For the last twenty years, CT has been used extensively to assess bowel wall thickness, the attached mesentery, as well as the adjacent intra-abdominal structures and organs. We have reached the end of a long chain of events that have placed small bowel imaging among the most important objective methods of investigation of the small intestine.

The extensively revised second edition of this comprehensive monograph incorporates all the substantive progress made in the last ten years in the field of enterology. Several chapters, including "Computed Tomography of the Small Bowel," "Magnetic Resonance Imaging for Small-Bowel-Related Diagnosis," "Physiology and Pathophysiology," "The Small Bowel in Immunology," "Angiography and Interventional Radiology," are completely new. Other chapters have been thoroughly revised and expanded. References have been updated and many new high-resolution images have been incorporated into the text.

The current volume is not only a state-of-the-art expression of the advances made in intestinal imaging. Its review of the physiology, pathophysiology, immunology, and pathology of the small intestine, together with the well described clinical features of numerous entities, will prepare the reader to properly interpret imaging findings. As stated by Louis Pasteur, "Chance favors the prepared man." This volume can be used as a practical clinical guide or as a reliable reference textbook. I will cherish it as a constant reminder and as a paradigm of modern scientific reasoning at the end of the twentieth century.

Finally, while congratulating the authors, I must confess to a feeling of ambivalence. On one hand, I feel a sense of admiration and pride for the efforts and contributions of so many researchers and educators responsible for the advances made in the radiology of the gastrointestinal tract. On the other hand, I feel a sense of nostalgia and regret for the accelerated pace of development of medicine, which is bound to render accomplishments of a lifetime obsolete or irrelevant within the next generation. In the words of the Greek philosopher Heraclitus, "There is nothing permanent except change."

EMIL J. BALTHAZAR, M.D.

Foreword to the First Edition

For most of the 50 years since I graduated from medical school, the small intestine has remained *terra incognita*, defying the depredations of gastroenterologists. Endoscopists, who nowadays are so comfortable in the esophagus, stomach, and duodenum, have to be content with glimpses of the small intestine about the ligament of Treitz; working from the nether end, they are barred by the ileocecal valve from peering too far into the ileum. Clinicians largely see the small intestine through a glass darkly rather than face to face.

This new book serves not only as a compendium of what is known about how to spread images of the small intestine out for all to see, but it also serves as a road map for future exploration. In its chapters, we learn how enteroclysis, sonography, computed tomography, and more can unfold the sinuous and shining coils of the small intestine. After reading this book, clinicians and radiologists will have learned how to explore the small intestine and how to get the best of what the "imager" can do.

Still, I hope the small bowel will not be studied in every patient. Current preoccupation with ordering an old-fashioned, follow-through study of the small intestine leads to too many bored radiologists—and to unnecessary radiation exposure for their patients. So many physicians believe that ordering such a study is an adequate way to exclude small intestinal disease that, in a frenzy of completeness, they order an "upper GI with small bowel follow-through" almost routinely, thinking that they are learning something about the gut—or at least "ruling out" small bowel disease. As the editors of this text cannily observe, this routine approach to excluding small bowel disease seems to work largely because small bowel disease is so rare. It is rather like testing for porphyria in every patient with an irritable bowel syndrome; you could throw all the urines down the sink and still remain almost 100% accurate.

The small bowel deserves the radiologist's enthusiastic study *only* when the clinician really expects to find something there. That is not often, and it is not easy. Indeed, the recognition of small bowel disorders has often seemed a triumph of the human spirit over adversity. Its great length and coils account in part for the way in which the small intestine hides its secrets, and its suppleness allows it to tolerate disease processes for some time without producing symptoms. Four symptoms finally tell its tale: (1) colic, (2) diarrhea, (3) malabsorption, and (4) bleeding.

Colic is usually recurrent and spasmodic with relaxation every 2 to 3 minutes, and the pain often centers around the umbilicus. Diarrhea from a small intestinal cause is less likely to have the urgency of colonic diarrhea. Malabsorption offers fewer clues; weight loss and foul stools are the classic ones. The practitioner must remember that steatorrhea is only a symptom of a disease, not of itself a diagnosis. Often the radiologist must pinpoint the cause. This is also true of bleeding that often tends to be so occult that anemia is its first sign. The first step in finding a small bowel lesion is, therefore, to think about it. When the first sign is intestinal obstruction, the clinician usually turns quickly to a radiologist for advice, but it is dismaying how often the small bowel is still neglected as a source of recurrent gastrointestinal bleeding or other abdominal complaints.

The small intestine is a vast storehouse of hormones, largely from the integrating cells of the foregut, those nerveless emissaries of the central nervous system. Ultimately, the symptoms of which the patient complains are the net result of abnormalities of absorption, secretion, and motility. I suspect, however, that over the next decade, physicians will realize how much enterochromaffin-like cells contribute to the symptoms of small bowel origin.

Curiously, the small intestine is the site of the only disorders that require specific dietary control: celiac sprue and lactose intolerance. For the rest of the gut, nonspecific diets will do. That is fitting enough, for the small intestine is crucial to life. People can thrive without a colon, may live comfortably without an esophagus or a stomach, but cannot live without a small intestine, parenteral nutrition aside. Liver and pancreas may be transplanted, but the small intestine, so far, cannot be replaced. We get only one chance with it.

This book by Drs. Herlinger and Maglinte serves as a monumental market of small bowel disease. It is a fitting heir to Ross Golden's classic and Marshak and Lindner's sequel. Nothing of which I am aware has quite the breadth and capacity of this remarkable achievement. All radiologists will want to own one and to study it; gastroenterologists and surgeons will do more for their patients if they understand how the radiologists and other imagers must proceed. The book records and advances all that is currently known about the study of the small bowel. I am grateful for having had the chance to write this foreword because reading the book has made me a wiser gastroenterologist.

HOWARD SPIRO

Preface

Ten years have elapsed since we conceived and put together the first edition of this book on small bowel radiology. At that time we stressed the need to combine state-of-the-art barium studies with the increasingly important imaging technology. The roles of CT, ultrasound, and MRI have expanded greatly and many of the former indications for barium examinations have moved into imaging. To underscore the relevance of this trend, we have modified the title of the book to incorporate the term *imaging* and have been fortunate to add Dr. Bernard Birnbaum to the editorship. Unchanged, however, is our philosophy that diagnostic radiology can be effective only if it incorporates into the interpretation of images an understanding of the clinical background and the pathophysiology related to each patient referred to us.

A number of changes have been made in this second edition. Seven of the first edition chapters have been omitted and four chapters originally concerned with double-contrast barium work have been combined into a single chapter. New chapters have been added dealing with MRI, immunedeficiency diseases, postsurgical small bowel, and the differential diagnosis of small bowel diseases with radiologic–pathologic explanation. Several new contributors have generously accepted our invitation to join in the new edition. We wish to express our sincere gratitude to several contributors to the first edition who are now no longer among the authorship. And we express our very sincere gratitude to our new publishers, Springer-Verlag of New York.

This is also our opportunity to express our gratitude to so many who have made it possible to reach the point of completion of this book. Physicians and surgeons at the University of Pennsylvania have referred to us cases of great interest and have always helped with follow-up information. Ever-helpful advice in matters of gastrointestinal pathology was provided by Dr. Beth Furth of the University of Pennsylvania. We are also grateful to gastroenterological and surgical colleagues at the Methodist Hospital in Indianapolis, especially Dr. Randall Strate for his expertise and cooperation in matters concerning gastrointestinal pathology. Technologists—too numerous to mention by name—have provided the vast material that has formed the basis for the pictorial and scientific content of the book. Indefatigable and very able secretaries, including Fran Shaul in Indianapolis and Cheryn Jarvis of the University of Pennsylvania, spent countless hours transforming the text into a format acceptable to our publishers.

We have been fortunate to have worked in this stimulating environment, aided and advised by so many colleagues and friends.

HANS HERLINGER
DEAN D.T. MAGLINTE
BERNARD A. BIRNBAUM

Contents

Foreword to the Second Edition vii
Foreword to the First Edition ix
Preface xi
Contributors xv

Part 1 Introduction

1 Anatomy of the Small Intestine 3
  HANS HERLINGER

2 Physiology and Pathophysiology 13
  JOYANN A. KROSER, DALE R. BACHWICH, and DAVID C. METZ

3 The Small Bowel in Immunology 29
  THOMAS JUDGE

Part 2 Imaging Techniques

4 Barium for the Small Bowel: Historical Aspects 41
  HANS HERLINGER and DEAN D.T. MAGLINTE

5 Plain Film Radiography of the Small Bowel 47
  DEAN D.T. MAGLINTE and HANS HERLINGER

6 The Small Bowel Follow-Through and Its Modifications 81
  DEAN D.T. MAGLINTE and HANS HERLINGER

7 Enteroclysis: Technique and Variations 95
  HANS HERLINGER and DEAN D.T. MAGLINTE with TSUNEYOSI YAO

8 Sonography of the Small Bowel and Related Structures 125
  MICHEL RIOUX

9 Computed Tomography of the Small Bowel: Technique and Principles
  of Interpretation 153
  BERNARD A. BIRNBAUM

10 Magnetic Resonance Imaging for Small-Bowel-Related Diagnosis: Contrast Agents and
   MR Angiographic Techniques 167
   EVAN S. SIEGELMAN and PABLO R. ROS

11	Scintigraphy	187
	CHRISTOPHER F. SCHULTZ, ABASS ALAVI, and GARY R. LICHTENSTEIN	
12	Angiography and Interventional Radiology	203
	JAMES E. JACKSON and DAVID J. ALLISON	
13	Enteroscopy	223
	LEWIS R. FELDER and J. S. BARKIN	
14	Congenital and Developmental Anomalies of the Small Bowel in Adolescents and Adults	227
	DEAN D.T. MAGLINTE and GEORGE S. BISSET III	
15	Crohn's Disease	259
	FREDERICK M. KELVIN and HANS HERLINGER	
16	Parasitic and Bacterial Inflammatory Diseases	291
	HANS HERLINGER	
17	Immune Deficiency Diseases	309
	HANS HERLINGER	
18	Malabsorption States	331
	HANS HERLINGER and DAVID C. METZ	
19	Small Bowel Neoplasms	377
	DEAN D.T. MAGLINTE and HANS HERLINGER	
20	Vascular Disorders of the Small Intestine	439
	JILL E. JACOBS, BERNARD A. BIRNBAUM, and DEAN D.T. MAGLINTE	
21	Small Bowel Obstruction	467
	BERNARD A. BIRNBAUM and DEAN D.T. MAGLINTE	
22	Postsurgical Small Bowel	507
	JOHN C. LAPPAS and WILLIAM L. CAMPBELL	
23	Differential Diagnosis of Small Intestinal Abnormalities with Radiologic-Pathologic Explanation	527
	STEPHEN E. RUBESIN and EMMA E. FURTH	
	Index	567

Contributors

ABASS ALAVI, M.D.
Department of Radiology
University of Pennsylvania Medical Center
3400 Spruce Street
Philadelphia, PA 19104, USA

DAVID J. ALLISON, F.R.C.R.
Department of Imaging
Imperial College of Science, Technology and Medicine
Hammersmith Hospital
Du Cane Road
London, W12 0HS
England

DALE R. BACHWICH, M. D.
Division of Gastroenterology
University of Pennsylvania School of Medicine
3400 Spruce Street
Philadelphia, PA 19104, USA

JAMIE S. BARKIN, M.D., F.A.C.G., M.A.C.G.
Division of Gastroenterology
University of Miami, School of Medicine
4300 Alton Road
Miami, FL 33140-2849, USA

BERNARD A. BIRNBAUM, M.D.
Department of Radiology
University of Pennsylvania Medical Center
3400 Spruce Street
Philadelphia, PA 19104, USA

GEORGE S. BISSET, M.D.
Department of Pediatric Radiology
Duke University Center
Box 3808
Durham, NC 27710, USA

WILLIAM L. CAMPBELL, M.D.
Chief, Gastrointestinal Radiology
University of Pittsburgh Medical Center
200 Lothrop
Pittsburgh, PA 15213, USA

LEWIS R. FELDER, M.D.
Division of Gastroenterology
University of Miami, School of Medicine
Mt. Sinai Medical Center
Miami, FL 33140, USA

EMMA E. FURTH, M.D.
Department of Pathology and Laboratory Medicine
University of Pennsylvania Medical Center
3400 Spruce Street
Philadelphia, PA 19104, USA

HANS HERLINGER, M.D., F.R.C.R.
Department of Radiology
University of Pennsylvania Medical Center
3400 Spruce Street
Philadelphia, PA 19104, USA

JAMES E. JACKSON, F.R.C.R.
Department of Imaging
Hammersmith Hospital
Du Cane Road
London, W12 0HS
England

JILL E. JACOBS, M.D.
Department of Radiology
University of Pennsylvania Medical Center
3400 Spruce Street
Philadelphia, PA 19104, USA

THOMAS JUDGE, M.D.
Department of Medicine
Division of Gastroenterology
University of Pennsylvania Medical Center
3400 Spruce Street
Philadelphia, PA 19104, USA

FREDERICK M. KELVIN, M.D., F.R.C.R.
Department of Radiology
Methodist Hospital of Indiana and
Indiana University School of Medicine
1701 North Senate Boulevard
Indianapolis, IN 46206, USA

JOYANNE A. KROSER, M.D.
Division of Gastroenterology
University of Pennsylvania Health System
Presbyterian Medical Center
54 N. 39th Street
Philadelphia, PA 19104, USA

JOHN C. LAPPAS, M.D.
Department of Radiology
Indiana University School of Medicine
Wishard Memorial Hospital
Indianapolis, IN 46202, USA

GARY R. LICHTENSTEIN, M.D.
Department of Medicine
Division of Gastroenterology
University of Pennsylvania Medical Center
3400 Spruce Street
Philadelphia, PA 19104, USA

DEAN D.T. MAGLINTE, M.D.
Department of Radiology
Methodist Hospital of Indiana and
 Indiana University School of Medicine
1701 North Senate Boulevard
Indianapolis, IN 46206, USA

DAVID C. METZ., M.D.
Department of Medicine
Division of Gastroenterology
University of Pennsylvania School of Medicine
3400 Spruce Street
Philadelphia, PA 19104, USA

MICHAEL RIOUX, M.D.
University Laval/CHUQ
Department of Radiology
Pavilion Saint-Francois d Assise
10, Rue de L Espinay
Quebec, Canada GIL 3L5

PABLO R. ROS, M. D., F.A.C.R.
Department of Radiology
Harvard Medical School
Brigham Women s Hospital
75 Francis Street
Boston, MA 02115, USA

STEPHEN E. RUBESIN, M.D.
Department of Radiology
University of Pennsylvania Medical Center
3400 Spruce Street
Philadelphia, PA 19104, USA

CHRISTOPHER F. SCHULTZ, M.D.
Department of Medicine
Division of Gastroenterology
University of Pennsylvania Medical Center
3400 Spruce Street
Philadelphia, PA 19104, USA

EVAN S. SIEGELMAN, M.D.
Department of Radiology
University of Pennsylvania Medical Center
3400 Spruce Street
Philadelphia, PA 19104, USA

TSUNEYOSI YAO, M.D.
Chikushi Hospital
Fukuoka University
377-1 Ohaza-Zokumyoin
Chikushino-shi
Fukuoka, 818
Japan

Part 1

Introduction

Anatomy of the Small Intestine

Hans Herlinger

Chapter Contents

Length of Small Bowel
The Mesentery
Distribution of Loops
Bowel Wall
Small Bowel Folds
Villi
Superior Mesenteric Artery
The Enteric Nervous System

The following description of small intestinal anatomy mostly relates to barium radiology. Anatomic features as they are elicited by sonography, computed tomography (CT), and magnetic resonance imaging (MRI) are briefly mentioned but are more fully described in Chapters 8, 9, and 10.

Length of Small Bowel

The mesenteric small intestine is the least accessible portion of the alimentary tract. Anatomists have defined the jejunum as the upper two fifths of the mesenteric small intestine and the ileum as the remaining three fifths. The small bowel is a tube of unpredictable length, usually reported to have a mean length of 20 ft (6.38 m); the range of length (also measured at autopsy) was 4.88 to 7.85 m.[1] Small bowel length is slightly greater in men than in women and significantly greater in the obese compared to patients of normal body weight.[2] Radiologic measurements of length are imprecise because of loop superimposition.[3]

The Mesentery

The jejunum and ileum are suspended by their mesentery, the root of which measures only 6 to 7 in and extends from the duodenojejunal flexure at the left of the L-2 vertebra obliquely caudad to the ileocecal junction. Its pleated intestinal border fans out to anchor the entire length of the small bowel.[4] The distance between the root of the mesentery and its intestinal margin is greatest (up to 25 cm) at and above the midintestinal level, thus ensuring considerable mobility within the abdomen.[4]

The mesentery is composed of two layers of parietal peritoneum that derive from the posterior abdominal wall and surround bowel loops as their serosal layer. The root of the mesentery encloses a narrow bare area that forms part of the anterior pararenal space of the retroperitoneum. Vessels, nerves, lymphatics, and fat extend from the bare area to occupy the subperitoneal space within the mesentery, which forms an important bidirectional link between bowel within the peritoneal cavity and the structures of the retroperitoneum.[5–7] The root of the small bowel mesentery can also establish continuity between the upper and lower abdomen.[8] It is relevant to note that the subperitoneal fat layer is significantly thicker at the level of the ileum than of the jejunum.[9] In consequence, loop separation due to mesenteric fat hypertrophy most noticeably displaces loops of ileum.

The margin of attachment of the mesentery to the small intestine is known as the mesenteric border.[4] It can be identified as the concave border of small bowel loops, best shown when the lumen is distended. The convex border, facing away from the axis of the mesentery, constitutes the antimesenteric border. Identification of the borders, when involved by disease, can be of differential diagnostic value.[4]

Demonstration by Cross-Sectional Imaging

The normal peritoneum covering the small bowel mesentery is usually not visible by CT, but the neurovascular bundles that are enclosed by it are easily identified because they are surrounded by mesenteric fat [Fig. 1-1(a)]. In the presence of ascites, sonography can clearly demonstrate the outline of mesenteric folds [Fig. 1-1(b)]. MRI depicts the mesentery by outlining its vascular component [Fig. 1-1(c)]. Mesenteric lymph nodes are normally not seen or seen only as small (>5 mm) linear or nodular soft tissue densities.[10] Adenopathy may be recognized when a few nodes exceed 15 mm in size or when there is an increased number of smaller nodes. The omentum may be identified in cross section as it extends inferiorly from the transverse colon, draping over the ventral aspect of small bowel loops, but its differentiation from these structures may not be possible in patients with insufficient intra-abdominal fat.

Distribution of Loops

The small bowel occupies the inframesocolic space of the peritoneal cavity. The right portion of this space can extend into the pelvic cavity, and it is not unusual for ileal loops to have prolapsed into the pelvis, especially after hysterectomy. The undulating small bowel loops have considerable mobility within the inframesocolic space, except for segments closer to the points of mesenteric attachment at the ends of the mesenteric root. The jejunum generally occupies the left upper and midportions and the ileum the right mid and

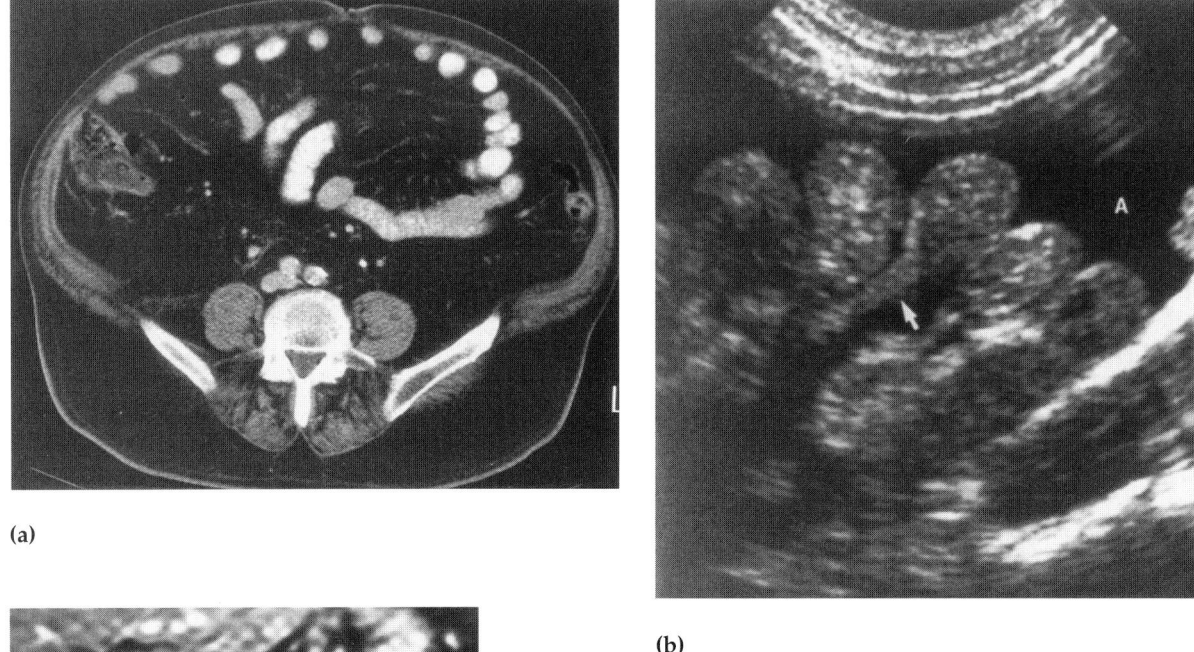

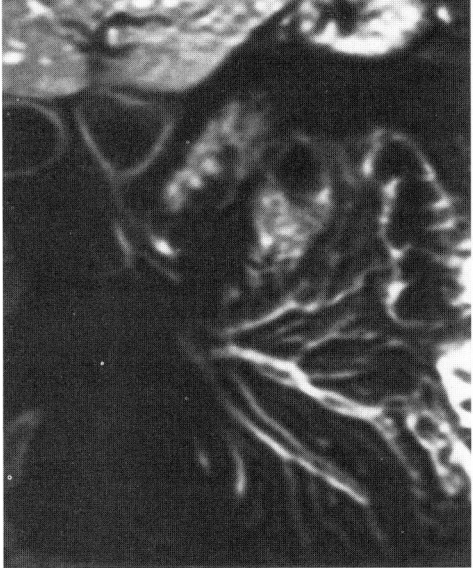

Fig. 1-1. Demonstration of the mesentery by cross-sectional imaging. (a) CT scan through the midabdomen shows normal vascular structures within the mesentery, outlined by mesenteric fat. (b) Ultrasound scan of normal mesenteric folds (arrow) outlined by ascitic fluid (A). (Courtesy of Amorino Vecchioli, MD, Rome.) (c) MRI demonstration of normal artery branching within the mesentery.

lower portions of the abdominal cavity (Fig. 1-2). Upper jejunal loops are folded in the left upper abdomen, usually showing an almost vertical course. One or two distal jejunal loops cross the spine to the right side and continue there as the ileum. Most of the ileum occupies the area above the pelvic inlet. The terminal ileum is usually directed cephalad and to the right. Jejunal loops are generally more anteriorly located in the abdomen than are loops of ileum.

Individual loops normally present gentle curves, their limbs in closer apposition. Fluoroscopic palpation elicits two important features of normality: mobility and pliability. Mobile loops can be displaced from their position by gentle manual pressure. Pliability implies a change of shape and diameter in response to palpation and change in position.

Bowel Wall

There is a gradual but significant change in structure by which segments of jejunum can be distinguished from ileum by radiology or at laparotomy. For this reason, there can be only an arbitrary level of demarcation between jejunum and ileum.

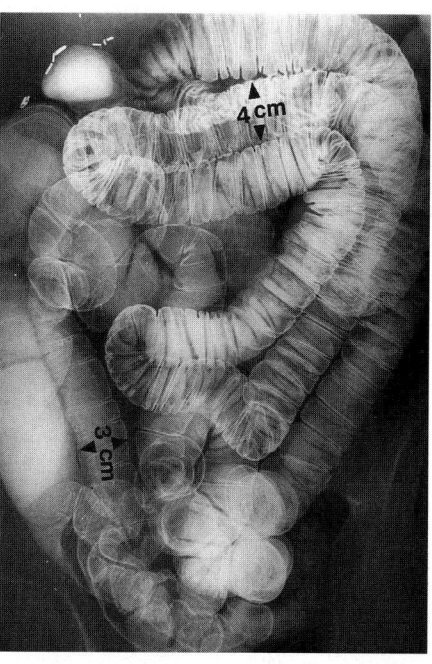

Fig. 1-3. Double contrast enteroclysis, normal appearance. Overview film at the end of examination shows gradually decreasing lumen diameter from the proximal jejunum at 4 cm, to the midileum at 3 cm.

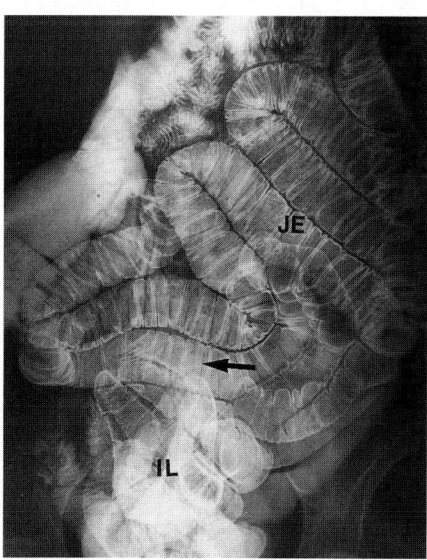

Fig. 1-2. Location of jejunal and ileal loops in the inframesocolic space of the peritoneal cavity.
Jejunal loops (JE) are generally located in the left upper abdomen. A still jejunum-like bowel segment crosses to the right (arrow) to merge into the distal two thirds of the small intestine, the ileum. Ileal loops mostly occupy the right side of the abdomen, tend to crowd into the inferior abdomen (IL), and may extend into the pelvic inlet.

The lumen diameter decreases gradually from the jejunum in the direction of the distal ileum. Normal values for lumen caliber vary with the examination technique. During enteroclysis, a method characterized by lumen distention, lumen diameter is considered abnormal if it exceeds 4.5 cm in the upper jejunum or 3 cm in the ileum (Fig. 1-3). In the follow-through examination the lumen should not exceed 3.5 cm in the jejunum or 2.5 cm in the ileum.[11] The same upper limits for normality generally apply also to the demonstration by CT, MRI, and ultrasonography.

Wall thickness, as demonstrated by pneumoperitoneum, measures between 1 and 2 mm. The wall of the jejunum is slightly thicker than that of the ileum. Double-contrast enteroclysis has given the same reading [Figs. 1-4 (a), (b)]. To measure wall thickness by enteroclysis, the barium-coated mucosal surfaces of two adjacent bowel loops need to remain in parallel for about 4 cm; the distance between them then equals their combined wall thicknesses. Measured in this way, individual wall thickness is about 2 mm in the jejunum and 1 mm in the ileum. Sonographic measurements are reported to be slightly higher. The normal intestinal wall thickness as obtained by CT is considered to be less than 3 to 4 mm. The bowel wall or the mucosal folds may appear spuriously thickened if

6 • 1. Anatomy of the Small Intestine

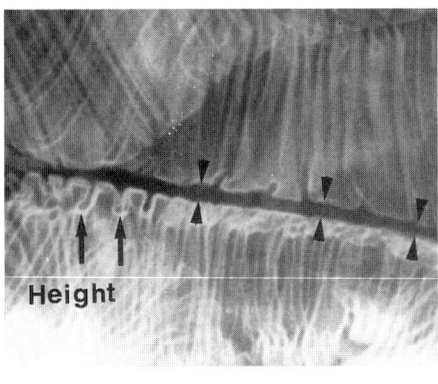

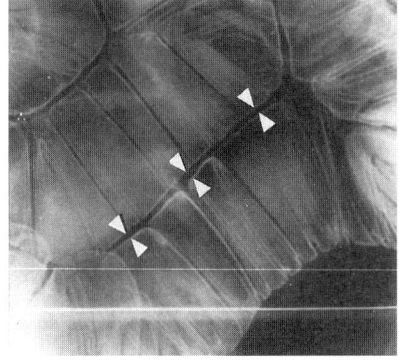

Fig. 1-4. Enteroclysis demonstration of the combined wall thickness of two adjacent and parallel bowel loops (between arrow heads).
(a) Jejunum (arrows also indicate height of jejunal folds). (b) Wall thickness of ileum, about half that of jejunum.

the lumen is not distended. Furthermore, bowel wall thickness can be accurately measured only when the lumen is clearly defined, by either intraluminal gas or opacifying fluid.

Mucosa

The small bowel is essentially a multilayered tube (Fig. 1-5). In adults, the height of villi should amount to at least three times the depth of the crypts. The mucosa lining the lumen shows three distinct layers. The epithelium next to the lumen lines the villi and crypts and is composed of a single layer of cells with digestive and absorptive functions. These cells should be tall and uniform and aligned in neat rows along a thin basement membrane. The nuclei should be uniform, small relative to the cytoplasm, and basally oriented. Intraepithelial T lymphocytes (IEL) are normally found in mainly basal position between epithelial cells,

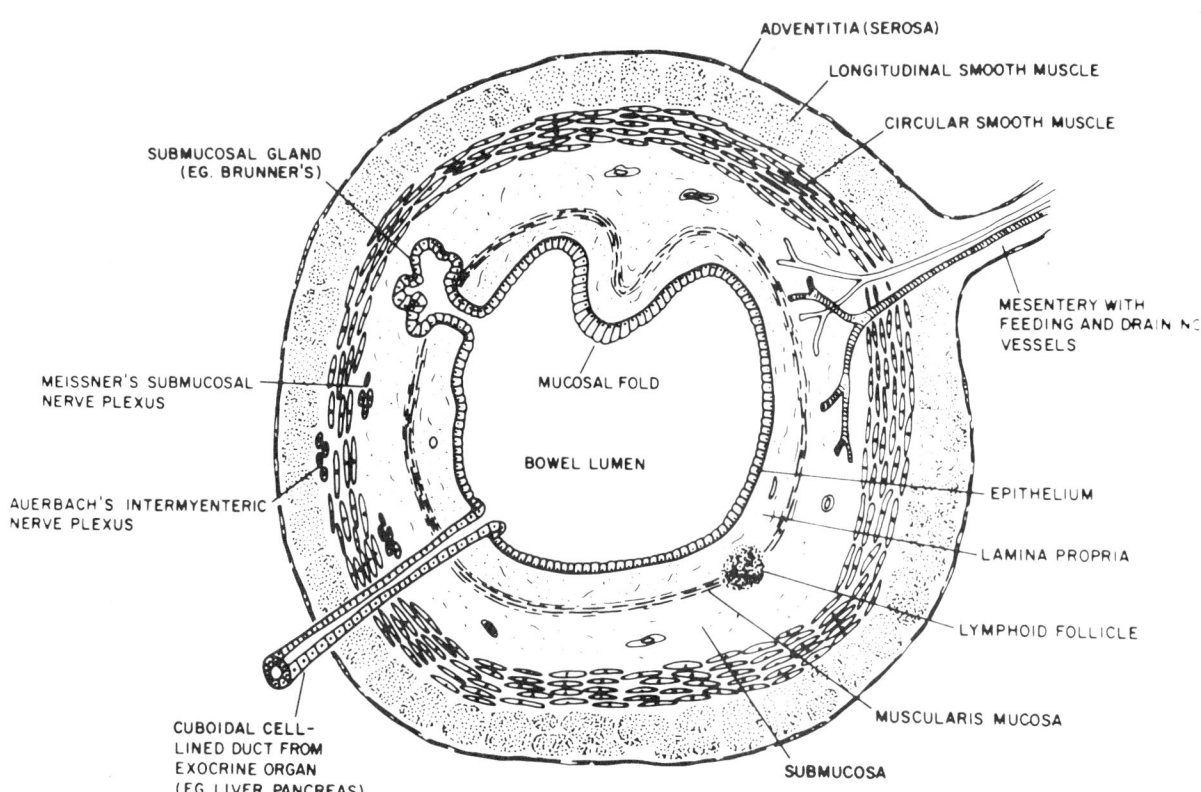

Fig. 1-5. Schematic cross section of the small bowel wall showing its major constituents. (Courtesy of J. E. Lichtenstein, MD.)

about 12 to 35 IELs per 100 cells of villous epithelium. These T cells are 85% suppressor/cytotoxic and 15% helper/inducer phenotypes. The luminal surfaces of the absorptive epithelial cells are amplified 40-fold by fingerlike microvilli that form the brush border. A continuous membrane, a filamentous-appearing glycoprotein coat, covers the microvilli and is firmly anchored to their surfaces.[9] Microvilli participate in absorption as well as in digestive processes (see Chapter 2). Goblet cells and few enterochromaffin cells are distributed among the absorptive cells. Undifferentiated cells predominate in the crypts; their purpose is the constant renewal of the surface epithelium with its rapid turnover. Important among the crypt cells are a variety of enterochromaffin cells that produce hormones and peptides, including gastrin, secretin, somatostatin, motilin, vasoactive intestinal peptide, and serotonin. Deep in the proliferative zone in the crypts are Paneth cells, their function the secretion of bioactive molecules with microbicidal activities.[12]

The second layer of the mucosa is the lamina propria, which extends as the core into each villus and surrounds each crypt. It is composed of loose connective tissue and contains many cell types, including plasma cells, lymphocytes, mast cells, macrophages, and eosinophils. Neutrophils are normally not identified outside capillaries. The lamina propria contains an important part of the intestinal immune system (see Chapter 3).

The third and deepest layer of the mucosa is a thin band of smooth muscle, the muscularis mucosae. It is only a few cells thick and separates the mucosa from the submucosa.

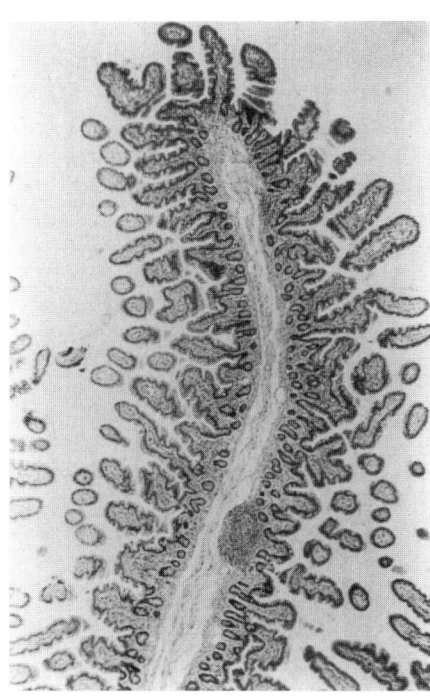

Fig. 1-7. Low-power photomicrograph of a normal jejunal fold.
Height of such folds is about 5 to 6 mm and width, about 1 to 2.5 mm, including the covering villi. Note the thin, fibrovascular submucosal core extending into the fold and the lymphoid follicle bridging the muscularis mucosae along the right edge of the fold (H&E original magnification × 400). (Courtesy of J. E. Lichtenstein, MD.)

Submucosa

The submucosa is the main connective tissue supporting substrate for the mucosa. The submucosa contains the main vascular and lymphatic channels and nerve plexuses. Meissner's autonomic nerve plexus is situated in its deeper portion adjacent to the muscularis propria. In the proximal duodenum, Brunner's glands fill much of the submucosa.

Lymphoid follicles are found scattered throughout the gut, being most numerous in the terminal ileum. They are aggregates of lymphocytes with germinal centers. Lymphoid follicles are principal sites for the maturation of plasma cells, which, in turn, are associated with immunoglobulin production. These follicles are located along the muscularis mucosae and may extend into both the lamina propria and superficial submucosa. Usually the lymphoid follicles are submerged in the detail of the mucosal villi and are not evident radiologically, unless enlarged. Larger and flatter lymphocyte aggregates, composed of many individual follicles, are called Peyer's patches and are

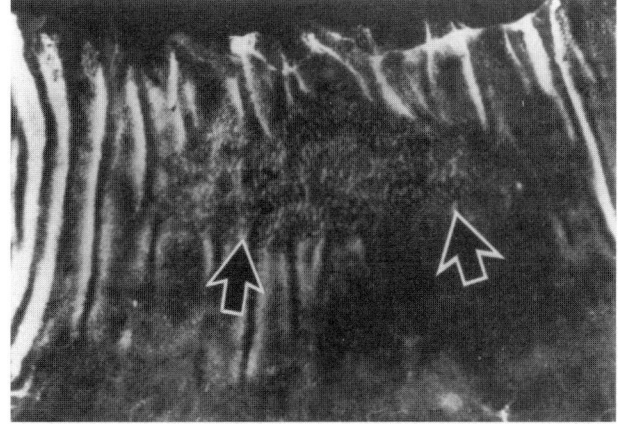

Fig. 1-6. Radiograph of a fixed surgical specimen.
A Peyer's patch at the antimesenteric border of the midileum presents a coarse surface pattern that interrupts Kerckring's folds (arrows). (Courtesy of K. Ushio K, MD.)

more numerous in the distal ileum but do also occur more proximally.[13] They measure up to 1 in in length, are oval, and are mostly found along the antimesenteric border (Fig. 1-6). Peyer's patches are usually not seen with ordinary roentgen techniques but can be identified by specimen radiography. Peyer's patches increase in number from birth to puberty and later begin to involute, but they do not disappear.

Muscularis and Serosa

The main muscle wall of the bowel, the muscularis propria, is made up of an outer longitudinal and an inner circular layer. Auerbach's autonomic nerve plexus is mostly located between the two layers. Meissner's nerve plexus is located between the circular layer and the muscularis mucosae.

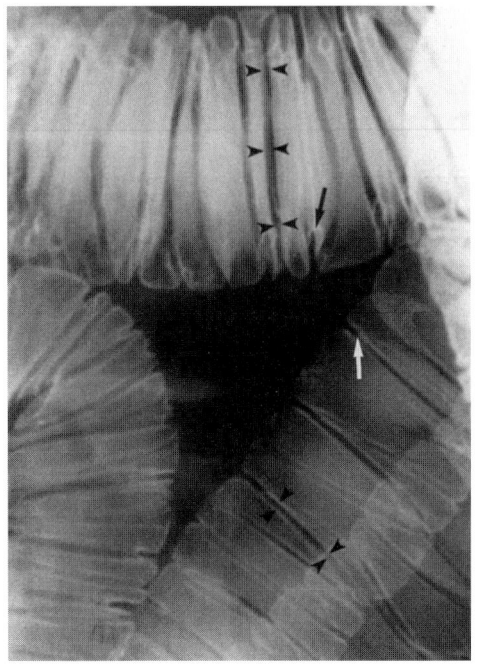

(a)

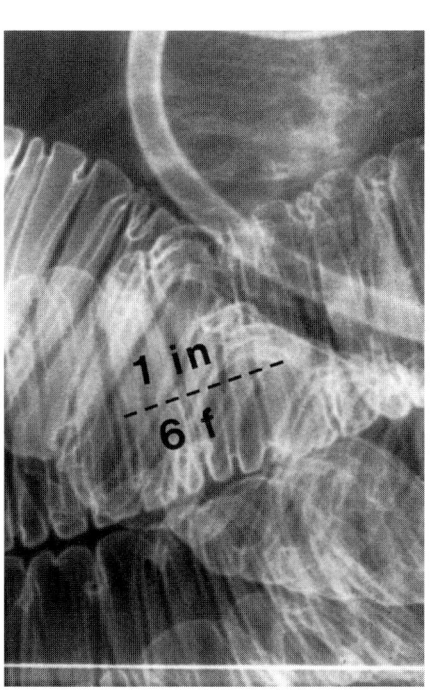

(b)

Fig. 1-8. Images of enteroclysis in double contrast phase. (a) Comparison of fold thicknesses in jejunum above and ileum below (between arrow heads). Comparative height of jejunal and ileal folds is indicated by arrows. (b) Fold density proximal jejunum. There are six folds over 1 in long. (c) Fold density in distal ileum. Three folds are seen over length of 1 in.

(c)

Adventitia is the general term for the outer covering of the bowel. Except for the retroperitoneal portion of the duodenum, this consists of a peritoneal covering called the serosa and a thin mesenchymal connective tissue, the subserosa.

Small Bowel Folds

The normal small bowel folds are fixed crescentic bands that extend round the antimesenteric aspect of the bowel to fade close to the mesenteric border. These valvulae conniventes or Kerckring's folds consist of full-thickness mucosa supported by a core of fibrovascular submucosa (Fig. 1-7). The folds start to appear in the second part of the duodenum and become most prominent in the proximal jejunum. Jejunal folds are normally wider and taller than those in the ileum. They are spaced a few millimeters apart, becoming further apart in the ileum. The changing pattern of normal folds through the length of the small intestine can be accurately documented by enteroclysis.[11]

Jejunal folds, measured during lumen distention, are normally up to 2 mm in width, and ileal folds are about 1 mm wide [Fig. 1-8(a)]. In the lumen distended state, normal folds are seen to extend across the lumen with straight and parallel surfaces. Fold height that is 3 to 8 mm in the jejunum reduces gradually to about 2 mm in the ileum [Figs. 1-4(a), 1-8(a)]. During lumen distention, there are normally 4 to 7 folds per inch in the proximal jejunum [Fig. 1-8(b)] and 2 to 4 folds per inch in the distal ileum [Fig. 1-8(c)].[14] In the terminal ileum, folds may be well developed or almost absent (Fig. 1-9).

Generally, the appearance of the folds will vary with the technique used for their radiologic demonstration. The tone of the bowel wall also influences the appearance of the folds. A feathery pattern (Fig. 1-10) is produced by the collapsed small intestine. In the jejunum the folds are not obliterated even with pronounced distention, whereas in the ileum the folds are more likely to become obliterated.[14]

Villi

Each villus contains a core of lamina propria that contains the vascular supply (Fig. 1-11). A small arteriole extends through each villus and reaches its tip, where it branches out like a fountain of capillaries to supply the epithelium. A similar pattern applies to the venous return. Often a single blind-ending lymphatic channel extends out of the center of each villus to communicate with the submucosal lymphatic plexus. Normal villi are usually at or just below our limits of roentgen definition.[15] Important factors for their X-ray demonstration are a high-definition radiographic system and a barium suspension of medium viscosity and high density. Villi appear as submillimeter, fin-

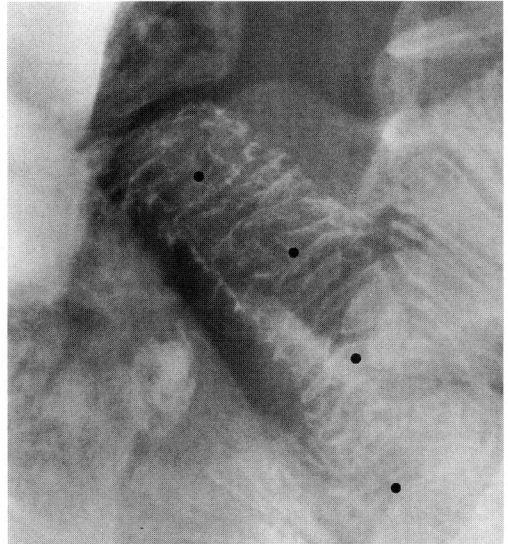
(a)

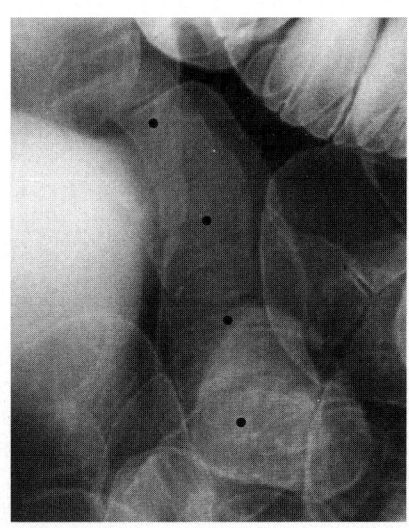
(b)

Fig. 1-9. Normal terminal ileum (dots) as shown by double-contrast enteroclysis.
Fold patterns are unpredictable. (a) Crowded normal folds. (b) Widely spaced normal folds.

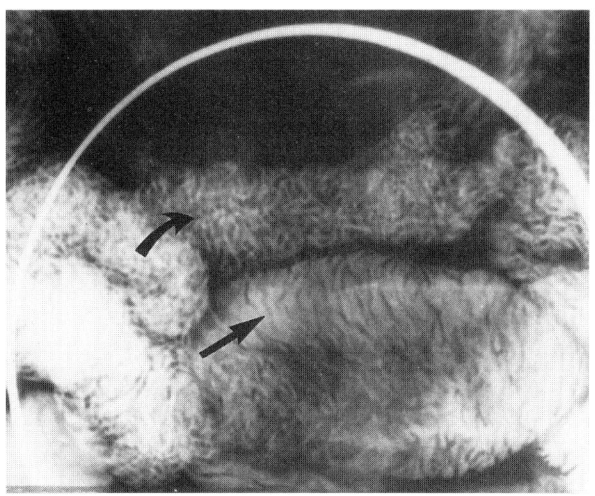

Fig. 1-10. Barium follow-through demonstrates a collapsed bowel segment with a feathery pattern of folds (curved arrow) and a slightly wider segment with barely recognizable fold characteristics (straight arrow).

jejunum and much shorter and submerged in mesenteric fat near the distal ileum. Vasa recta usually divide into anterior and posterior branches that penetrate the muscularis and merge into an extensively anastomotic arteriolar plexus in the submucosa. Further arterial branches, the vasa brevia, arise from the marginal artery and enter directly into the mesenteric border. A recent report[16] of studies carried out on adult cadavers found the vasa recta derived submucosal vascular plexuses to intercommunicate freely, while the ileal vasa brevia plexuses behaved as end arteries. Generally, out of the submucosal vascular plexus the mucosa receives about 75% of the blood, leaving most of the remainder for the muscularis. Single arterioles supply a villus or several crypts. Venules gerlike soft tissue projections into the barium layer, imparting a "salt-and-pepper" appearance when seen en face. In profile view on the sides of folds, villi may appear as punctate intermediate densities protruding into the opaque barium coating (Fig. 1-12).[15]

Superior Mesenteric Artery

The superior mesenteric artery (SMA) arises from the anterior aspect of the aorta at the level of the first lumbar vertebra. Part or all of the hepatic arterial supply may arise from the proximal SMA. Rarely, the SMA takes origin from the celiac axis. The SMA courses in an anteroinferior direction and gives rise to the inferior pancreaticoduodenal artery and the middle colic artery. It then enters the subperitoneal space of the small bowel mesentery where jejunal and ileal branches arise from its left side. The ileocolic artery virtually represents the termination of the SMA (Fig. 1-13).

About 12 or more jejunal and ileal branches fan out within the mesentery and form interconnecting arcades. The number of arcades varies from one to five, with the largest number found in the mid to distal portions of the small bowel. The most distal arcades interconnect to form a marginal continuum that can serve as a useful collateral channel between duodenum and colon. The marginal arterial channel gives rise to the vasa recta, which are 5 to 6 cm long in the

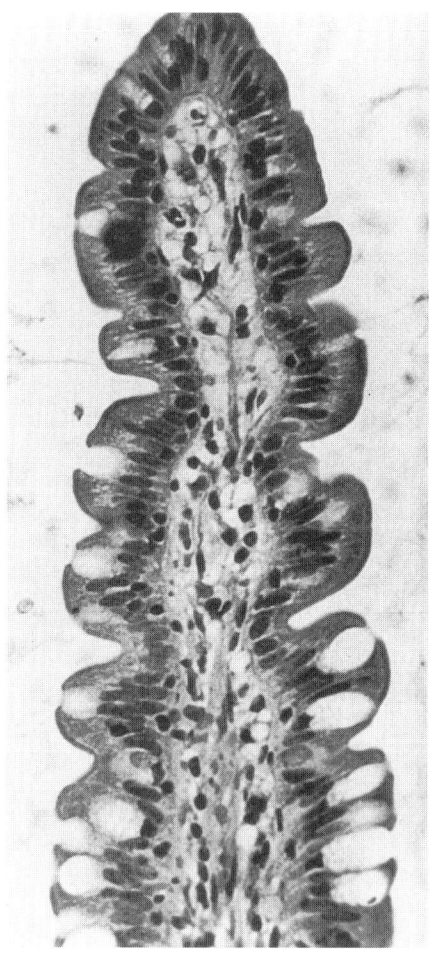

Fig. 1-11. High-power photomicrograph of a single, normal small bowel villus.
Its core is composed entirely of lamina propria. Normally arranged individual cell nuclei are clearly demonstrated. Blood and lymphatic capillaries (lacteals) are not strikingly distinguished unless distended (H&E original magnification × 400). (Courtesy of J. E. Lichtenstein, MD.)

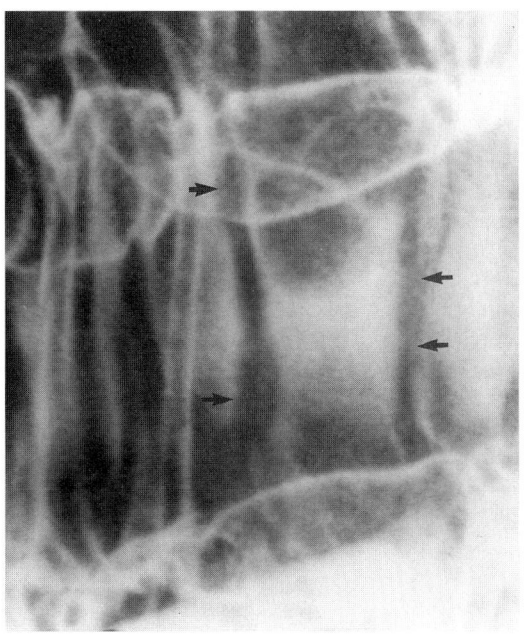

Fig. 1-12. Normal villi are occasionally visible at enteroclysis.
The slightly magnified view gives the impression of a "salt and pepper" surface pattern. On the side of folds it is possible to identify tiny filling defects in the barium coating (arrows).

return to a submucosal venous plexus. Further venous return parallels the pattern of the arteries.[17]

The various collateral vascular connections, jejunoileal arcades, the marginal vessel, and the extensive submucosal plexuses are important pathways in SMA branch occlusions and in the interventional management of bleeding.

Mucosal lymphatics drain into a submucosal lymphatic plexus from which penetrating lymphatics reach a subserosal plexus. Valved chyliferous ducts up to 1 mm in diameter extend through the mesentery and converge on lymph nodes at the mesenteric root. Lymph draining the small bowel is changed from clear to milky white during fat absorption. From preaortic superior mesenteric lymph nodes the lymph reaches the cisterna chyli, a retroperitoneal, retroaortic structure underneath the diaphragm.[17]

The Enteric Nervous System

More recent understanding of the myenteric and submucosal nerve plexuses of the gut and of their ramifications has led to regarding this entity as a remote part of the central nervous system, with which it communicates through sympathetic and parasympathetic afferent and efferent neurons (see Chapter 2).[18]

References

1. Underhill BML. Intestinal length in man. *Br Med J.* 1955;2:1243–1246.
2. Backman L, Hallberg D. Small-intestinal length: an intraoperative study in obesity. *Acta Chir Scand.* 1974;140: 57–63.
3. Fanucci A, Cerro P, Fraracci L, Letto F. Small bowel length measured by radiography. *Gastrointest Radiol.* 1984;9:349–351.
4. Meyers MA. Clinical involvement of mesenteric and antimesenteric borders of small bowel loops. Parts I and II. *Gastrointest Radiol.* 1976;1:41–58.
5. Oliphant M, Berne AS, Meyers MA. Spread of disease via the subperitoneal space: the small bowel mesentery. *Abdom Imaging.* 1993;18:109–116.
6. Oliphant M, Berne AS, Meyers MA. Bidirectional spread of disease via the subperitoneal space: the lower abdomen and left pelvis. *Abdom Imaging.* 1993;18:117–125.
7. Oliphant M, Berne AS, Meyers MA. Direct spread of subperitoneal disease into solid organs: radiologic diagnosis. *Abdom Imaging.* 1995;20:141–147.
8. Oliphant M, Berne AS, Meyers MA. The subperitoneal space of the abdomen and pelvis: planes of continuity. perspective. *AJR.* 1996;167:1433–1439.
9. Silverman PM, Kelvin FM, Korobkin M, Dunnick NR. Computed tomography of the normal mesentery. *AJR.* 1984;143:953–957.
10. Trier JS, Winter HS. Anatomy, embryology and developmental abnormalities of the small bowel and colon.

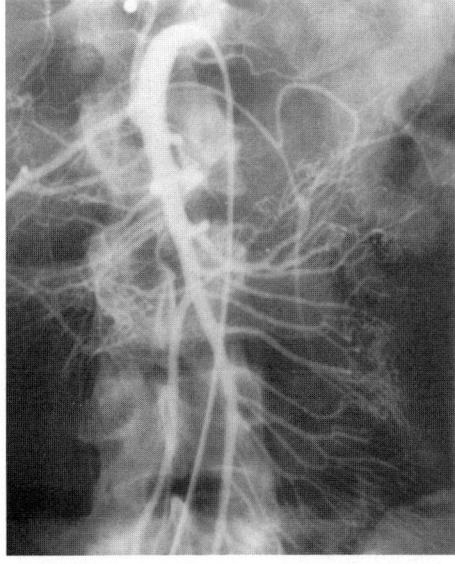

Fig. 1-13. Normal superior mesenteric arteriogram.
Note left-sided origin and course of jejunal and ileal arteries, their arcades (mostly ileal), and their final arborization.

In: Sleisenger MH, Fordtran JS, eds. *Gastrointestinal Disease*. 4th ed. Philadelphia, Pa: WB Saunders Co; 1989: 991–1002.
11. Herlinger H. Small bowel. In: Laufer I, Levine MS, eds. *Double Contrast Gastrointestinal Radiology with Endoscopic Correlation*. Philadelphia, Pa: WB Saunders Co; 1992:363–422.
12. Quellette AJ. Paneth cells and innate immunity in the crypt microenvironment. *Gastroenterology*. 1997;113: 1779–1784.
13. Ushio K, Yamada T, Itibashi M, Hirota T, Ichikawa H. Roentgenologic specimen study of Peyer's patches in the jejunum and proximal ileum. In: Herlinger H, Megibow AJ, eds. *Gastrointestinal Radiology Reviews 1988/89*, Vol I. New York, NY: Marcel Dekker; 1988:1–13.
14. Herlinger H, Maglinte DDT. Jejunal fold separation in adult celiac disease: relevance of enteroclysis. *Radiology*. 1986;158:605–611.
15. Gelfand DW, Ott DL. Radiographic demonstration of small intestinal villi on routine clinical studies. *Gastrointest Radiol*. 1981;2:21–26.
16. Anthony A, Pounder RE, Wakefield AJ, et al. Mesenteric marginal ulceration in Crohn's disease: correlation with vascular anatomy and critically perfused sites. *Gut*. 1997;40(suppl 1):A24.
17. Gannon B. The vascular and lymphatic drainage. In: Whitehead R, ed. *Gastrointestinal and Oesophageal Pathology*. 2nd ed. Edinburgh: Churchill Livingstone; 1995:157–171.
18. Goyal RK, Hirano I. The enteric nervous system. *N Eng J Med*. 1996;334:1106–1114.

Physiology and Pathophysiology

Joyann A. Kroser, Dale R. Bachwich, and David C. Metz

Chapter Contents

Normal Physiology
Differentiation of Absorptive Function
Integration of Function
Principles of Digestive and Absorptive Physiology
Digestion and Absorption of Specific Nutrients
Motor Function of the Small Intestine
Pathophysiology
Secretory Diarrhea
Maldigestion and Malabsorption
Inflammatory Diseases
Motor Disorders of the Small Intestine

Normal Physiology

The small intestine undergoes a constant self-renewal of its mucosal surface due to many intricate developmental mechanisms that maintain functional and structural integrity. It plays a vital role in the digestion, absorption, and assimilation of nutrients as well as the balance of fluids and electrolytes. This chapter will first review the normal physiology of digestion, absorption, and motor function of the small intestine and then address major pathophysiologic mechanisms that may affect small intestinal function leading to clinical disease states.

Differentiation of Absorptive Function

Embryology

The small intestine is initially lined by simple cuboidal epithelium. By the 8th week of gestation, the epithelium is stratified and a basement membrane is formed. This cellular proliferation temporarily occludes the lumen, which is recanalized by the 10th week. By the 12th week simple columnar epithelium is again present. Villi form first in the proximal intestine during the 9th week of gestation and successively develop distally. Crypt formation begins in the 10th to 12th weeks of gestation and also occurs in a proximal to distal sequence. The entire process is complete by the end of the 14th week of gestation.[1]

As gestation continues, the intestinal tube develops different layers that serve specific needs. The four cell types found within the intestinal epithelium are absorptive columnar, goblet, enteroendocrine, and Paneth cells. There appears to be a common stem cell in the middle to high part of the crypt that gives rise to each of these epithelial cell types, which are responsible for the mucosal functions of absorption and secretion. Absorptive cells migrate up the villus and secretory cells migrate into the crypts. The villi are low permeability sites for digestion and absorption of nutrients, minerals, and electrolytes. Conversely, crypts represent highly permeable areas for active secretion of electrolytes and water (Fig. 2-1).[2] Cell turnover occurs over a 3- to 5-day period after which mature cells slough off into the lumen. The intestinal tube is initially surrounded by a layer of mesoderm that ultimately forms additional wall layers corresponding to the submucosa, the dual-layered muscularis propria for motility, and the serosa for support. Although the structural features of the small intestine are well developed by the end of the second trimester, functional maturation continues throughout fetal gestation and into postnatal life.[3]

Intrinsic Enteric Nervous System

The enteric nervous system is a network of neurons in the gastrointestinal tract that constitutes the "brain of the gut" and can function independently of the central nervous system. This system controls motility, ex-

---

The authors wish to thank Mr Jason Schmoyer for designing and producing the figures for this chapter.

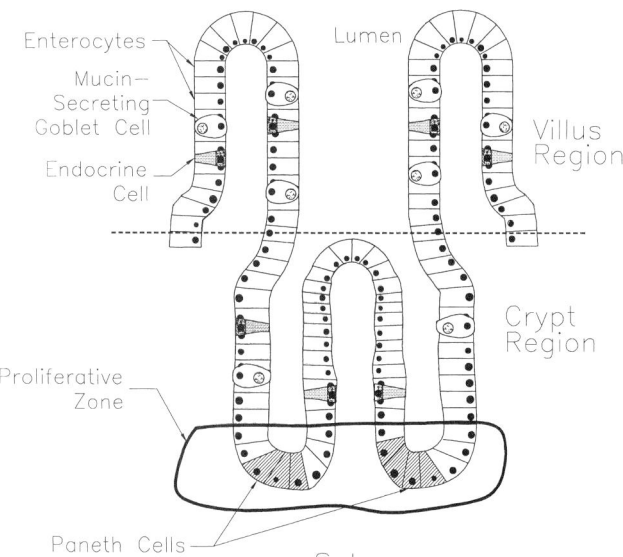

Fig. 2-1. Epithelial cells of the intestinal mucosa.
There are functional differences between crypt and villus regions. In the villus region, brush border hydrolases are abundantly expressed, nutrient transport is high, permeability is low, and there is net absorption. In the crypt region, brush border hydrolases are minimally expressed, nutrient transport is low, permeability is high, and there is net secretion. See text for further details.

tine where it plays an important role in secretory control. Additionally, this plexus innervates the muscularis mucosa, intestinal endocrine cells, and submucosal blood vessels.

The chemical mediators of the enteric nervous system were initially thought to be limited to neurotransmitters such as acetylcholine and serotonin. Subsequent research has led to the identification of purines (eg, adenosine triphosphate [ATP]), amino acids (eg, gamma amino butyric acid [GABA]), and peptides (eg, vasoactive intestinal polypeptide [VIP]) as additional mediator classes.[6] Currently, more than 20 candidate neurotransmitters have been identified in enteric neurons, and most neurons contain several of them.

ocrine and endocrine secretions, and microcirculation of the gastrointestinal tract. It is also involved in regulating immune and inflammatory processes. The enteric nervous system is primarily derived from cells of the vagal segment of the neural crest that migrate to the cranial portion of the gut and subsequently move caudally to populate the entire gastrointestinal tract.

The enteric nervous system, like the spinal cord, contains at least 100 million neurons.[4] Communication with the central nervous system occurs via sympathetic and parasympathetic afferent and efferent neurons in an area now known as the central autonomic neural network (Fig. 2-2).[5] In the enteric nervous system, the nerve-cell bodies are grouped into small ganglia that are connected by bundles of nerve processes forming two major plexi, the myenteric (Auerbach's) plexus and the submucosal (Meissner's) plexus. The myenteric plexus lies between the longitudinal and circular layers of muscle and extends the entire length of the gut. It primarily provides motor innervation to the two muscle layers and secretomotor innervation to the mucosa. The submucosal plexus, located between the circular muscle layer and the muscularis mucosae, is best developed in the small intes-

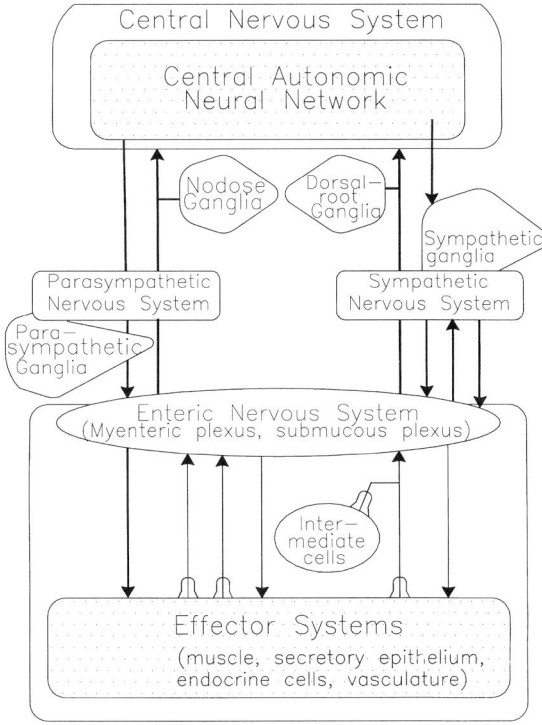

Fig. 2-2. Innervation of the gastrointestinal tract.
The enteric nervous system (ENS) is an independently functioning network of neural plexuses in the gastrointestinal tract. Parasympathetic and sympathetic nerves connect the ENS to the central autonomic neural network in the central nervous system. The cell bodies of the primary vagal and primary splanchnic afferent neurons are located in the nodose ganglia and the dorsal-root ganglia, respectively. The symbol (⌒) represents afferent nerve endings, and the arrows indicate the direction of neural transmission. Adapted from Goyal and Hirano,[5] with permission. Copyright 1996 Massachusetts Medical Society. All rights reserved.

Extrinsic Enteric Nervous System

Although the enteric nervous system can function independently of the central nervous system, the latter has an important role in coordinating the diverse functions of the enteric nervous system (Fig. 2-2). The vagus nerves contain parasympathetic motor pathways that control the motor and secretomotor functions of the small intestine. These cholinergic excitatory preganglionic neurons connect with small clusters of select myenteric neurons in the small intestine that may serve as pattern generators. There are much richer connections more proximally in the esophagus and stomach and distally in the sigmoid and rectum than in the small intestine.[7] These differences reflect the fact that the central nervous system exerts less direct control on the function of the small intestine.

The sympathetic innervation of the small intestine consists of adrenergic postganglionic fibers with cell bodies in the prevertebral ganglia.[8] These efferent neurons have at least four different targets in the gut: secretomotor neurons containing VIP, presynaptic cholinergic nerve endings, submucosal blood vessels, and gastrointestinal sphincters. There are no adrenergic nerve-cell bodies in the enteric plexuses.[9]

Neurons that carry sensory information from the enteric nervous system to the central nervous system are termed primary afferent neurons. Small intestinal afferents are carried in the vagus and splanchnic nerves. Vagal afferent neurons in the smooth-muscle layer are sensitive to mechanical distention of the gut. They have very low thresholds and convey information about motor activity of the gut. Additional vagal afferent neurons in the mucosa are sensitive to luminal concentrations of glucose, amino acids, or long-chain fatty acids, whereas others respond to a wide variety of chemical and mechanical stimuli.[10]

Splanchnic afferent neurons have their endings in the wall of the intestine and their cell bodies in dorsal root ganglia. These are multimodal nociceptive neurons that respond to high-intensity mechanical, thermal, and chemical stimuli that damage or threaten tissue. The neurotransmitters calcitonin gene-related peptide (cGRP) and substance P may be important in the activation of nociceptive afferent neurons in conditions such as irritable bowel syndrome, intestinal ischemia, and inflammatory bowel disease.[11] Splanchnic primary afferent neurons can also act directly on nearby gastrointestinal effector systems. Via long bifurcated processes they are able to stimulate collateral axonal limbs that cause the release of neurotransmitters. This ability comes into play during submucosal vasodilatation, duodenal secretion of bicarbonate, and mast-cell degranulation.[12]

Integration of Function

The control of complex physiologic functions, including effective responses to varied environmental and physiologic conditions, requires the coordinated efforts of many tissues and cell types. Essential to these efforts is efficient communication among specialized cells in different locations. Intercellular communication is particularly important in the gastrointestinal tract since this system is large, complex, and responsible for a wide variety of functions.

Cells use a variety of chemical messengers to communicate, including hormones, neurotransmitters, cytokines, and growth factors. Requisite to effective intercellular communication are well-ordered mechanisms for producing, distributing, and receiving the molecular signals. Several different mechanisms are used for each of these processes, allowing for a rich array of communication patterns (Fig. 2-3).

Endocrine communication is defined as communication by means of blood-borne messengers.[13] The term "hormone" refers specifically to compounds released into the bloodstream by endocrine cells that act on effector cells located at some distance away. Bloodstream release allows hormones to exert their effects over a wider area. Like transmitters generally, hormones can be divided into two groups: those that bind to cell surface receptors and those that act via intracellular receptors. Surface active hormones include peptides such as secretin, cholecystokinin (CCK), and gastrin. Steroids and steroidlike compounds comprise the second group.

Paracrine communication occurs between individual cells or groups of cells in close proximity to each other.[14] Chemical transmitters released by the paracrine cell bind to specific receptors on neighboring cells.[15] The region of transmitter distribution is relatively small, limited by diffusion during biological life of the signaling compound. Thus rapidly degraded or volatile compounds such as nitric oxide would exert their effects over a narrower region than small, diffusible, and relatively more stable compounds such as adenosine.

Neurocrine communication is a third form of communication. In many ways, neurocrine communication is a specialized paracrine method, with transition occurring in a small extracellular space. Neurocrine communication combines cell specificity with the capacity to transmit signals to effector cells rapidly and over a long distance. Transmitters stored in granules in the nerve terminal are released in response to an action potential emanating from the cell body. Neurocrine communication facilitates regulation of functions

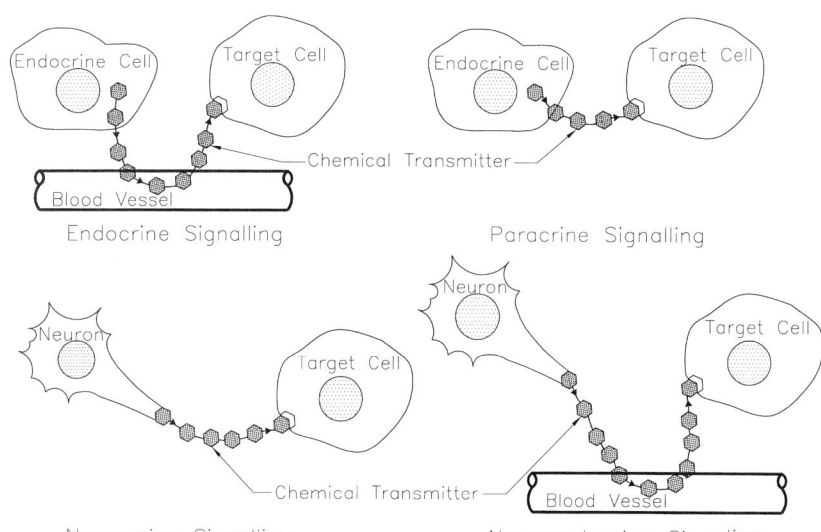

Fig. 2-3. Modes of intercellular communication, illustrating endocrine, paracrine, neurocrine, and neuroendocrine mechanisms. See text for further details.

that must be coordinated in space as well as time, such as peristalsis, alterations in blood flow, and segmental control of absorption and secretion.[16]

Additional mechanisms of cellular communication have been described.[17] *Neuroendocrine* communication is a specialized form of endocrine communication whereby neurons release chemical transmitters directly into the bloodstream. *Autocrine* communication is a specialized paracrine mechanism whereby a cell regulates itself. Within the gastrointestinal tract, a *luminal* communication mechanism allows compounds present in food or colonic bacteria, or secretions of the stomach or salivary glands, to regulate mucosal cell function. Examples of luminal communication include regulation of peristaltic and secretory function by duodenal and jejunal pH, stimulation of mucosal growth by salivary growth factors, and control of colonic blood flow and mucosal absorption by bacterial adenosine.

Since the discovery of secretin in 1902, the number of putative gastrointestinal regulatory substances has rapidly increased, especially over the past 10 to 15 years. More than 50 gastrointestinal peptides have now been identified.[18] Many of these peptide messengers have been classified into the four principal functional groups (as discussed above), according to their cellular location and the manner of delivery from storage sites to target cells (Table 2-1). Based on their amino acid sequences, several peptide messengers have been categorized into a variety of families. These include the gastrin/cholecystokinin family, the secretin/glucagon/vasoactive intestinal polypeptide (VIP)/pituitary adenylyl cyclase–activating polypeptide (PACAP)/peptide histidine methionine (PHM) family, the pancreatic polypeptide/neuropeptide Y/peptide YY family, the opioids/enkephalins/endorphins family, and the tachykinin/bombesin families. Several other peptides, including insulin, somatostatin, calcitonin, motilin, neurotensin, galanin, and thyrotropin-releasing hormone (TRH), have unique structures, distinct from any of the known peptide families.[19,20]

Because of their profound and wide-ranging effects on the gastrointestinal system, several peptide messengers (or analogues of native peptides) have been used in a number of clinical settings. For example, glucagon is used for the short-term management of motility disorders during endoscopic and radiological procedures because of its ability to inhibit gastrointestinal motility. The long-acting somatostatin analogue octreotide also has clinical utility in small intestinal disease.[21] Octreotide is used to control diarrhea and flushing in patients with hypersecretory states such as metastatic carcinoid and VIP-secreting tumors (VIPomas) by inhibiting hormone secretion by these endocrine tumors. Other possible mechanisms of antidiarrheal action by octreotide include stimulating absorption and nonpropulsive contractions and inhibiting secretion and propulsive contractions. It is also useful in the setting of AIDS-related diarrhea because it directly inhibits intestinal secretion induced by peptide 5, a fragment of the integral transmembrane glycoprotein (gp41) of human immunodeficiency virus.[22] Lastly, octreotide is becoming the drug of choice in the management of variceal bleeding by virtue of its ability to reduce splanchnic blood flow and reduce portal venous pressures without significant deleterious side effects.

Table 2-1. Physiologic actions of gastrointestinal peptides

Peptide	Endocrine	Paracrine	Neurocrine	Primary actions
Somatostatin	•	•	•	↓ Acid secretion ↓ Pancreatic function
Gastrin	•	•		↑ Acid secretion ↑ Tissue proliferation
CCK	•		•	↑ Pancreatic secretion ↑ Gallbladder contraction
Secretin	•			↑ Pancreatic secretion
Glucagon	•			↓ Intestinal motility
VIP			•	↑ Pancreatic secretion
Motilin	•			↑ Intestinal motility
Neurotensin	•		•	↓ Acid secretion ↓ Gastric motility
PP	•	•		↓ Pancreatic secretion
Galanin			•	↑ Plasma glucose ↑ Fundus contraction
Opioids			•	↓ Intestinal transit
PYY	•	•	•	↓ Pancreatic function
NPY			•	↑ Vasoconstriction
Substance P			•	↑ Smooth muscle contraction
GRP			•	↑ Gastrin release
Pancreastatin			•	↓ Islet somatostatin release
Peptide HM			•	↑ Pancreatic secretion
Enteroglucagon	•			↑ Tissue proliferation

Principles of Digestive and Absorptive Physiology

General Concepts

Food assimilation takes place primarily in the small intestine and is aided by anatomical modifications that increase the luminal surface area, namely, valvulae conniventes, villi, and microvilli. The microvilli are prominent on the apical surface of columnar epithelial cells or enterocytes and occur to a lesser degree on goblet cells. Collectively the microvillus region comprises the brush border. Several cell types make up the intestinal epithelium. Enterocytes function in digestion, absorption, and secretion. Goblet cells secrete mucus. Paneth cells secrete defensins that act in an antimicrobial fashion.[23]

Several important general concepts relate to the functional and structural differences between villi and crypts. In general, cells proliferate at the bottom of the crypt, mature as they migrate to villus regions, and slough off in 3 to 5 days. Villi are the sites for nutrient digestion and for absorption of nutrients, minerals, and electrolytes. Permeability to passive diffusion is low in this region. Crypts are the sites for active secretion of water and electrolytes. Permeability is high in these regions, allowing for water to follow secretion of electrolytes. Paneth cells are located in the crypts (Fig. 2-1).

There are also regional differences in small bowel function. Permeability decreases from proximal to distal. Regional specialization with regard to nutrient, electrolyte, and mineral absorption exists. For example, calcium, iron, and copper are absorbed in the

Table 2-2. Daily intestinal fluid balance and ionic constituents

	Duodenum	Jejunum	Ileum
Flow rate (L/day)	9	3	1
[Na$^+$] (mEq/L)	60	140	140
[K$^+$] (mEq/L)	15	6	8
[Cl$^-$] (mEq/L)	60	100	60
[HCO$_3^-$] (mEq/L)	15	30	70
Osmolality	Variable	Isotonic	Isotonic

[Na$^+$] = sodium concentration; [K$^+$] = potassium concentration; [Cl$^-$] = chloride concentration; [HCO$_3^-$] = bicarbonate concentration
Source: Data from Fine, Krejs, and Fordtran[58]

proximal small intestine, while bile salts and the fat-soluble vitamins (A, D, E, K) are absorbed in the distal small bowel. There is bulk flow of water and electrolytes high in the proximal bowel. The maximal capacity of the small bowel to absorb a balanced electrolyte solution amounts to 18 L per day. However, in a typical 24-hour period for an adult eating three meals, the daily volume of fluid passing through the duodenum is 9 L (3.5 L dietary and salivary, 2.5 L gastric, 2.0 L pancreatic, 1.0 L biliary) and traversing the ileocecal valve is approximately 1 to 1.5 L. Therefore the small bowel absorbs approximately 8 L of fluid per day and empties 1.0 to 2.0 L into the colon (Table 2-2).

Water movement across the intestinal epithelial cell is a passive event that follows the osmotic gradient. This osmotic gradient across the intestinal epithelial cell is created by solute transport. Intestinal transport is a bidirectional phenomenon. Movement from the mucosal side to the serosal side is defined as absorption. Opposite movement is defined as secretion. Absorption of sodium cations in the jejunum is coupled to glucose and amino acids while in the ileum sodium is absorbed via a sodium/hydrogen exchanger (Fig. 2-4). Absorption of chloride anions is passive in the jejunum but coupled with bicarbonate exchange in the ileum and colon. Absorption of bicarbonate is linked to hydrogen ion secretion in both the small and large intestine (Fig. 2-4). Lastly, absorption of potassium cations is a passive process at all levels.[24]

Secretory mechanisms in the small intestine center on the chloride (Cl$^-$) ion. At the cellular level, the Na$^+$, K$^+$, Cl$^-$ cotransporter on the basolateral membrane serves as the Cl$^-$ uptake step, with the Na$^+$, K$^+$ ATPase pump providing the driving force and recycling the Na$^+$ (Fig. 2-5). Excess K$^+$ is recycled by way of K$^+$ channels on the basolateral membrane, and the chloride exits by way of a Cl$^-$ channel on the apical membrane. Regulation of the Cl$^-$ secretory process is at the level of the Cl$^-$ channels and/or K$^+$ channels. Sodium ions follow for electrical neutrality, and water follows passively.[25]

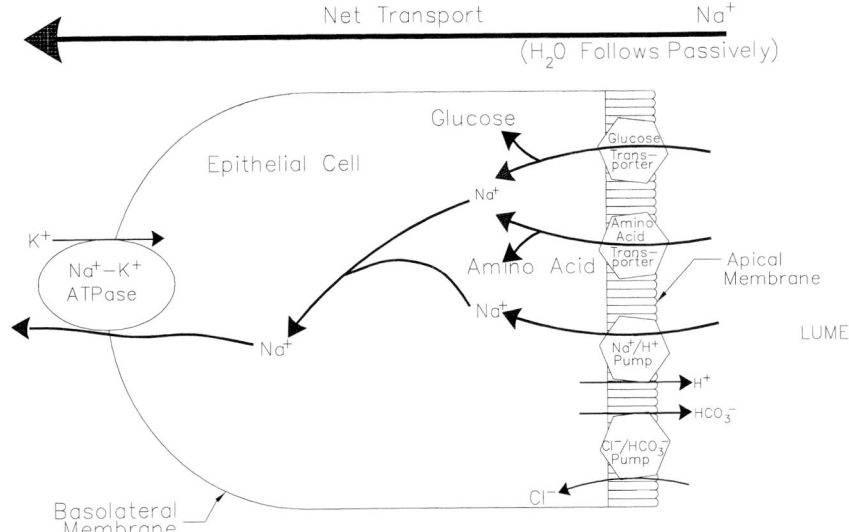

Fig. 2-4. Mechanisms of normal electrolyte transport in the small intestine.
There is net uptake of Na$^+$ from the lumen leading to fluid absorption. See text for further details.

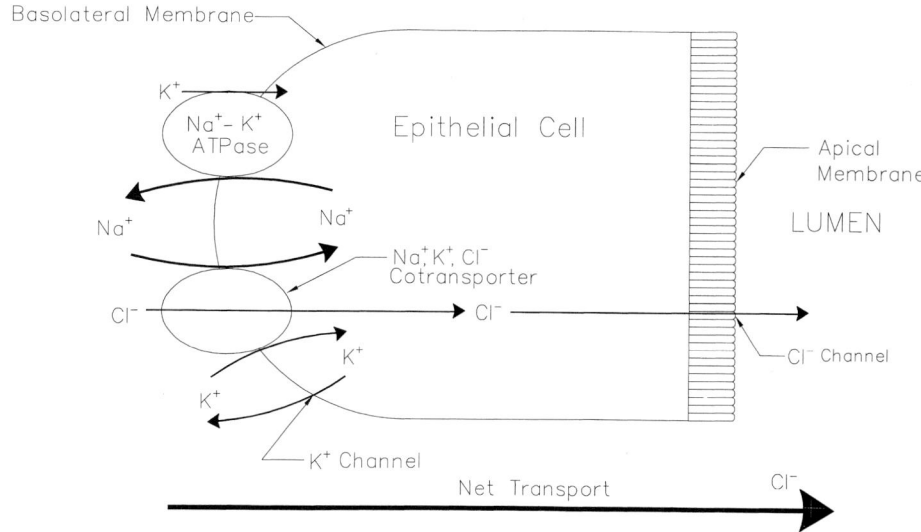

Fig. 2-5. Mechanisms of chloride secretion in the small intestine. When transport into the lumen exceeds uptake (see Fig. 2-4), net loss of fluid results, ie, secretory diarrhea.

Digestion and Absorption of Specific Nutrients

Carbohydrates

Luminal digestion of starch begins in the mouth with the action of salivary amylase and ends in the small intestine through the action of pancreatic amylase. Products of amylase action on starch and other major dietary sugars are hydrolyzed by brush border carbohydrases. Several brush border enzymes hydrolyze more than one substrate. Maltase, sucrase, and iso-maltase hydrolyze maltose and maltotriose to glucose. Sucrase, lactase, and trehalase break down sucrose, lactose, and trehalose, respectively. There is a large disaccharidase reserve in the small intestine, so that the rate-limiting step in sugar assimilation is not digestion but absorption of free hexoses following hydrolysis. Under normal circumstances the major portion of sugar assimilation is complete in the proximal jejunum.[26–28]

Glucose absorption from the intestine occurs by passive as well as active processes (Fig. 2-6). Fructose is transported by facilitated diffusion. Glucose and galactose are absorbed actively via a Na^+-dependent common carrier system. Energy input (ATP) drives

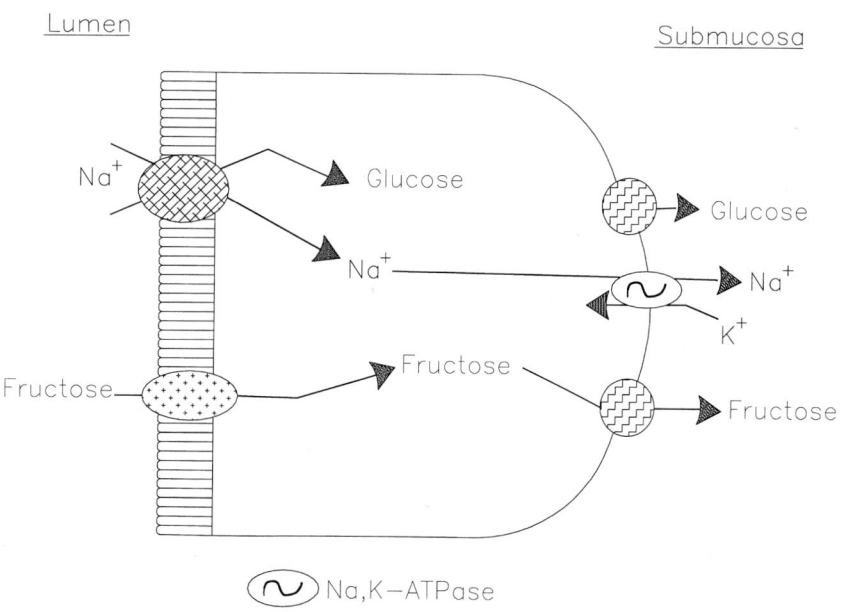

Fig. 2-6. Monosaccharide transport by enterocytes. Sugars such as sucrose, maltose, or lactose are hydrolysed to monosaccharides by villus brush border enzymes such as sucrase, maltase, and lactase. The monosaccharides are rapidly absorbed by specific transport pathways. See text for further details.

the sodium pump and maintains a Na$^+$ gradient favoring glucose entry. The exit of glucose from the cytosol into the intracellular space is due to a sodium-independent carrier on the basolateral membrane.[27,28]

Protein

Protein digestion begins in the stomach with the action of pepsin. Pepsin is an endopeptidase with a specificity for peptide bonds involving aromatic L-amino acids. Pepsin activity terminates when the gastric contents mix with alkaline pancreatic juice in the small intestine. Food in the intestine stimulates the release of secretin and CCK, which in turn cause the pancreas to release pancreatic proteases into the duodenum as inactive precursors. Trypsinogen is activated by enterokinase, an enzyme located in the brush border of duodenal enterocytes. Once formed, active trypsin autocatalytically activates trypsinogen. Trypsin also activates other peptide precursors from the pancreas (Fig. 2-7).[29]

Membrane digestion and absorption are closely related phenomena in protein assimilation.[30] L-isomers of amino acids are absorbed by carrier-mediated mechanisms. There are several different carrier systems for amino acid absorption. There is a separate carrier system for small peptides and for free amino acids. These two systems exist and work in parallel (Fig. 2-8).[31,32]

Lipids

Dietary lipids including phospholipids, sterols, and triglycerides enter epithelial cells by a sequence of

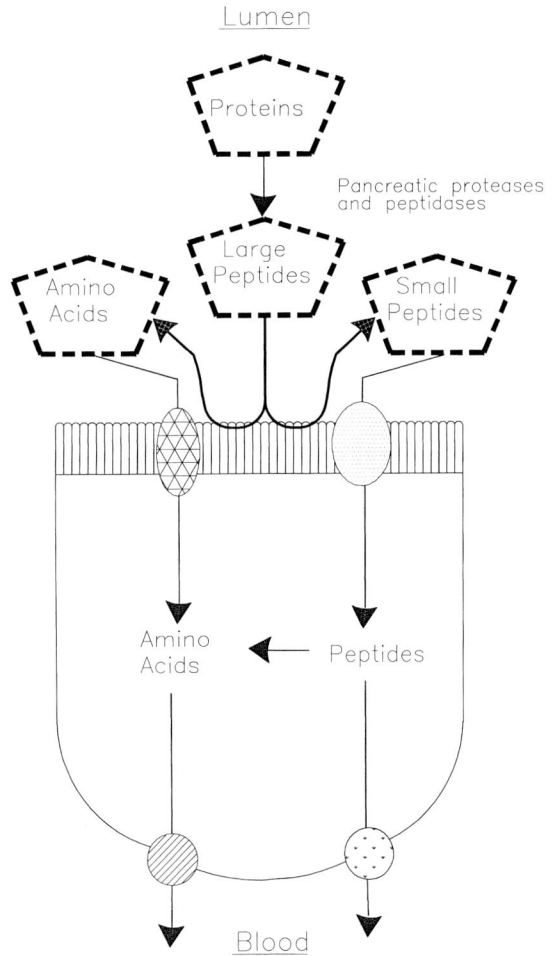

Fig. 2-8. Protein digestion and absorption.
Protein digestion takes place in the intestinal lumen, at the brush border of the intestinal mucosa, and in the cytoplasm of enterocytes. See text for further details.

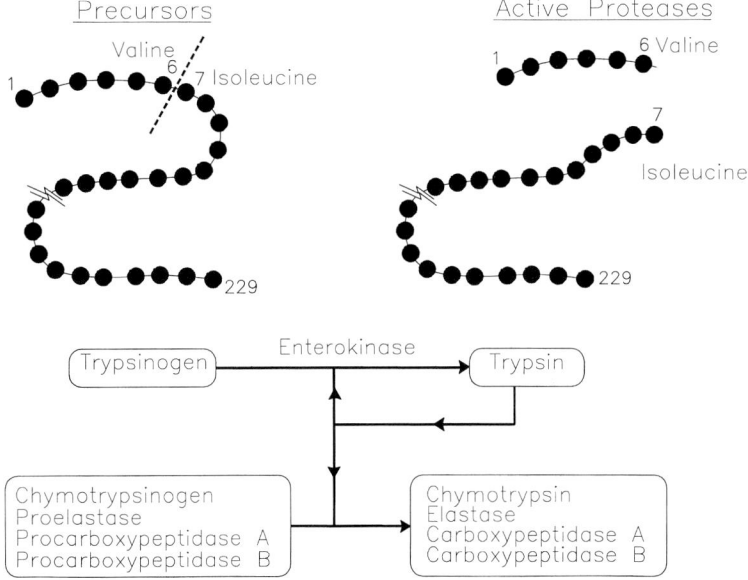

Fig. 2-7. Activation of pancreatic proteolytic enzymes. See text for further details.

chemical and physical events that render water-insoluble molecules capable of being absorbed by passive diffusion. The process depends on four major events: 1) secretion of bile and various lipases, 2) emulsification, 3) enzymatic hydrolysis of ester linkages, and 4) the solubilization of lipolytic products within bile salt micelles.[33]

The release of fat into the small intestine is controlled by CCK, which also stimulates the release of pancreatic lipase and gallbladder contraction. Bile salts that are released into the duodenum emulsify fat droplets and thereby increase the surface area of lipids in preparation for hydrolysis. Pancreatic lipases include the lipase-colipase complex, phospholipase A_2 (PA_2), and cholesterol esterase (CE). Colipase prevents the inactivation of lipase by bile salts. Lipase is secreted in large excess and rapidly hydrolyzes triglycerides. It cleaves the 1 and 3 ester linkages, yielding free fatty acids and 2–monoglycerides (Fig. 2-9). Bile salts and phospholipids form mixed micelles that become substrates for PA_2.[34] Pancreatic cholesterol esterase hydrolyzes not only cholesterol esters but also the esters of vitamins A and D, as well as those of glycerides. Thus the end-products of enzyme digestion by lipase, PA_2 and CE are 2-monoglycerides and fatty acids, lysophospholipids and fatty acids, and cholesterol and fatty acids, respectively.

When their intraluminal concentration reaches a critical level, bile salt monomers form water-soluble aggregates called micelles. The water-insoluble monoglycerides, fatty acids, cholesterol, and fat-soluble vitamins are solubilized within the hydrophobic center of the micelle. Micellar formation is important since it enhances diffusion of poorly soluble dietary lipids through the unstirred aqueous layer overlying the enterocytes. Monoglycerides and free fatty acids are absorbed by enterocytes and resynthesized into di- and triglycerides primarily by monoglyceride acylation. Water-soluble medium and short chain fatty acids and dietary cholesterol (absorbed in an unchanged form) leave the cell within chylomicrons, which traverse the basement membrane and enter lymph vessels.[35]

Specific Trace Elements and Vitamins[36]

The primary site for divalent cation absorption is the duodenum and proximal jejunum. Heme iron is more rapidly absorbed than non-heme iron.[37] Calcium absorption is regulated by vitamin D. Absorption of water-soluble vitamins is predominantly passive and carrier-mediated. Folic polyglutamate is hydrolyzed to monoglutamate and absorbed in the jejunum. Cobalamin (vitamin B_{12}) is released from food by gastric acid and pepsin. After separation from R protein in the duodenum it binds to intrinsic factor released from gastric parietal cells. Intrinsic factor facilitates B_{12} absorption primarily in the distal ileum. The absorption of the fat-soluble vitamins (A, D, E, K) parallels that of fats with which they solubilize.

Motor Function of the Small Intestine

Smooth-muscle cells of the small intestine generate their own intrinsic myoelectric activity. This activity can be separated into slow waves (basic electrical rhythm) and spike potentials (action potentials, spike bursts). Intracellular recordings show that slow waves consist of two electrical events: 1) an initial upstroke potential and 2) a plateau potential. Spike potentials usually occur during the plateau phase of the slow wave. When the sum of the plateau potential and the superimposed spike potential reaches a threshold value, the contractile process is activated by electromechanical coupling.[38]

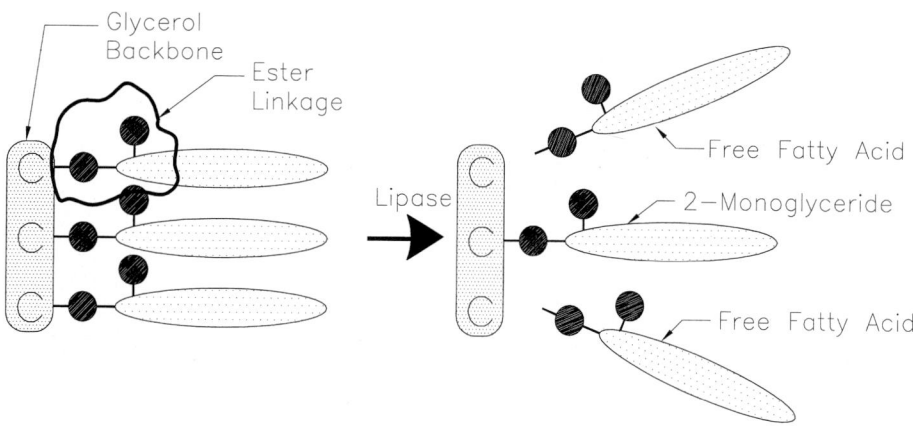

Fig. 2-9. Role of lipase in fat digestion.
Once lipase is bound to the micelle, it hydrolyses triglyceride to monoglyceride and fatty acid. These products are much more soluble in the micelle.

Slow waves originate in the longitudinal smooth-muscle layer, are calcium-dependent, determine the location and frequency of both spike potentials and contractions, and are responsible for the direction of propagation. Slow wave frequency varies at different sites. Slow waves are conducted to adjacent muscle cells via gap junctions, which can affect slow wave frequency and contraction of adjacent cells via electrical coupling (pacemaker effect). Spike potentials are calcium-dependent, produce influx of external calcium or release of internal calcium that initiates contractions, occur only near the peak of the slow wave, and determine the magnitude of the contractile response.[39]

Myoelectric activity varies in different regions of the small intestine.[40] For example, the slow wave frequency in the duodenum is 12 cycles per minute compared to 8 cycles per minute in the distal ileum. Also, in contrast to the stomach, the small intestine is characterized by a series of pacemakers throughout its length. Each pacemaker regulates a short segment of the small intestine no more than 10 cm in length. The effect that any contraction has on intestinal contents depends on the state of the musculature above and below the point of the contraction. If a contraction is not coordinated with activity above and below, intestinal contents are displaced both proximally and distally during the contraction and may flow back during the period of relaxation. This would serve to mix and locally circulate the contents. Such contractions appear to divide the bowel into segments, from which the term segmentation arises (Fig. 2-10, right).

The small intestine is also capable of eliciting a highly coordinated contractile response that is propulsive in function. When an area of bowel is stimulated, the bowel responds with contraction proximal and relaxation distal to the point of stimulation. These events tend to move the material in a distal direction, and they can happen sequentially to propel a bolus the entire length of the gut (Fig. 2-10, left). This peristaltic response, first described by Bayliss and Starling, is known as the law of the intestines.[41] Often it is invoked to explain how material normally is propelled through the small bowel. Recently, however, its importance in healthy individuals has been downgraded.

Not only are there differences in individual contractions of the small intestine, there are also different patterns of contractions.[42] Motor activity in the small intestine can be divided into two general categories: fasting (interdigestive, inter-meal) and fed (postprandial) (Fig. 2-11). Each type of myoelectric and motor activity is characterized by a typical pattern. During fasting, migrating myoelectric and motor (ie motility) complexes have been observed and called MMCs. MMCs typically begin in the stomach. Once initiated, MMCs typically propagate from the point of origin over the entire length of the stomach and small intestine. When an MMC arrives at the terminal ileum, another MMC is initiated. The fasting period begins when the first MMC is observed after a meal. The interval between MMCs varies normally between 84 and 144 minutes.[43] The duration of the fed period is defined as the time from meal ingestion to the initial MMC and varies with meal composition. For human subjects who eat a normal mixed meal, the fed state is approximately 210 minutes. Some investigators have speculated that MMCs are due to the release of motilin; others, however, have questioned whether the MMCs actually cause the release of motilin from the small bowel mucosa. Szurszewski and Code suggested that the MMCs function was to propel indigestible and waste material out of the proximal gastrointestinal tract into the colon. Thus, they coined the term "interdigestive housekeeper" to describe this phenomenon.[44] Administration of a number of agents

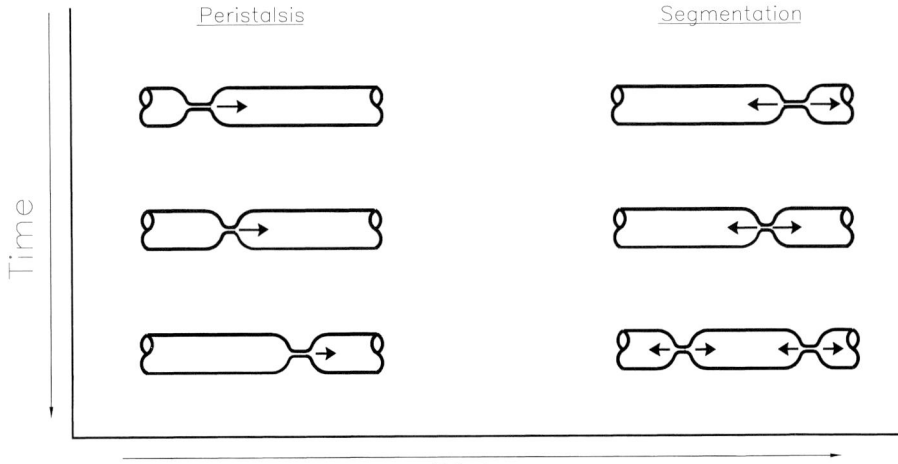

Fig. 2-10. Peristalsis versus segmentation.
Intestinal contractions may be localized or propagated. Propagated (peristaltic) contractions propel the luminal contents forward. Localized (segmented) contractions serve to mix the luminal contents.

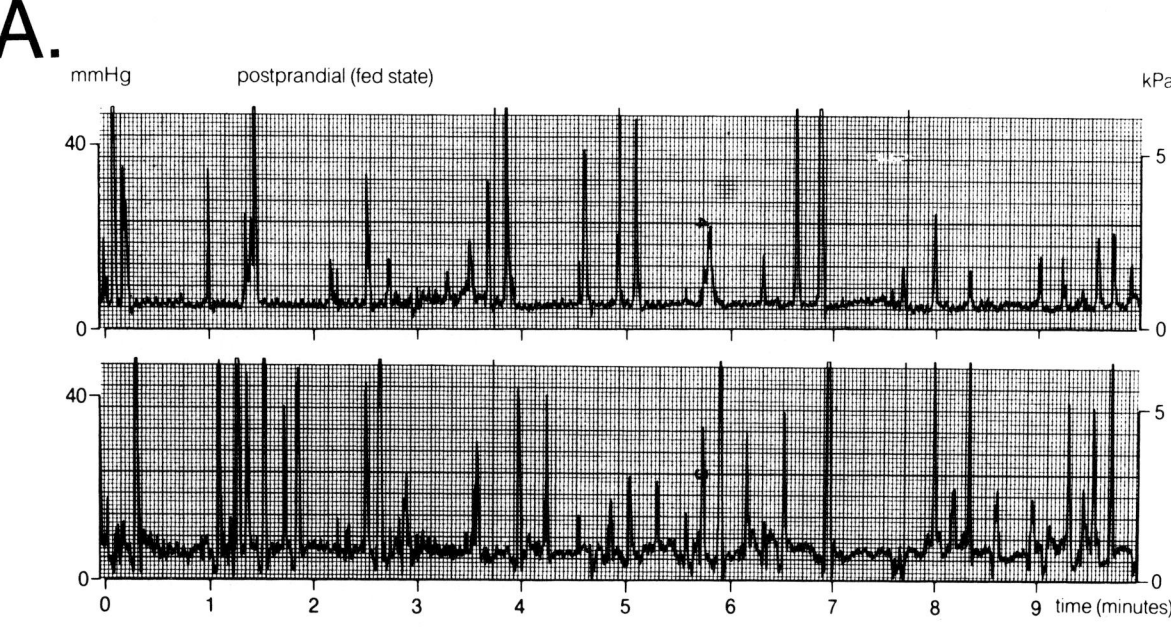

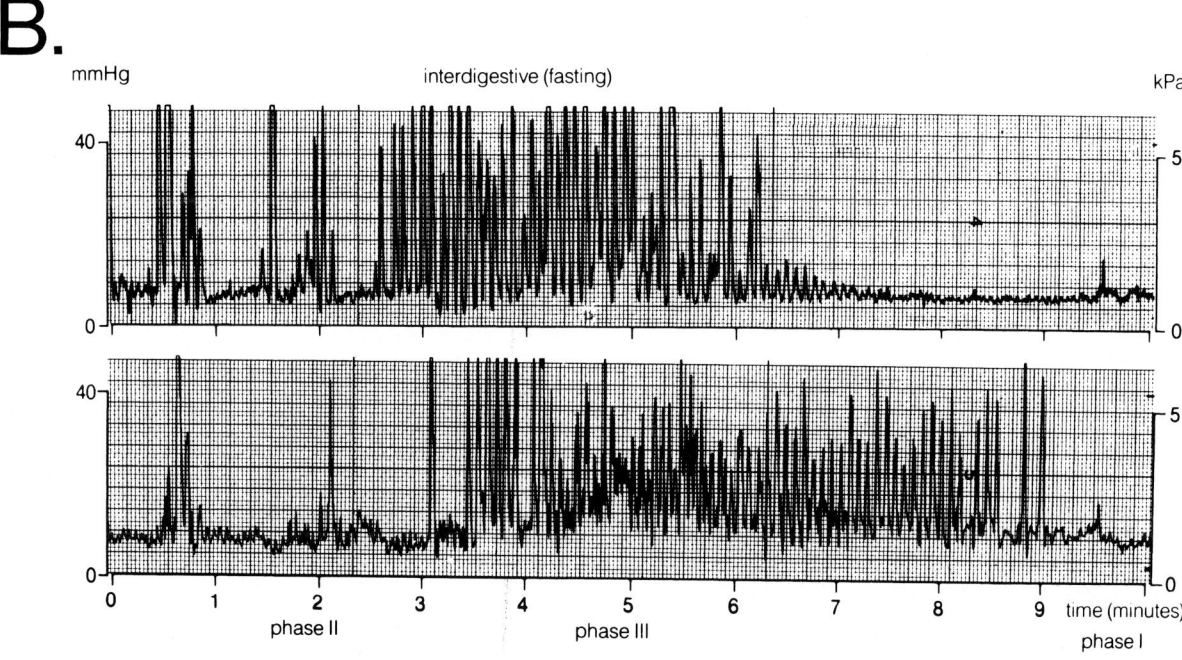

Fig. 2-11. Fed versus fasting pattern.
The postprandial (fed) pattern as shown in part A is characterized by irregular contractions with a relatively low amplitude. The interdigestive (fasting) pattern as shown in part B exhibits strong contractions at maximum frequency. (Adapted with permission from Smout A, Akkermans L. The small intestine. In: *Normal and Disturbed Motility of the Gastrointestinal Tract*. Hampshire, England: Wrightson Biomedical Publishing; 1992:134–135.)

including morphine, erythromycin, octreotide, metoclopramide, cisapride, and intraduodenal methysergide has been reported to stimulate MMC-like activity in the small intestine.[45,46] Interestingly, the solid and liquid foods that empty into the small intestine during the fed period are propagated all the way to the terminal ileum during the fed and not the fasting period. Thus, the propulsive force that carries the bulk of digestible and absorbable nutrients seems to be the noncyclical myoelectric and motor activity that characterizes small intestinal electromechanical activity during the fed period.[47]

Pathophysiology

Given that the main functions of the small intestine are secretion, absorption, digestion, and motility, one can see that most pathophysiologic disorders of the small intestine manifest themselves as secretory diarrhea, malabsorption, maldigestion, motility abnormalities, or inflammatory conditions. The following section reviews pertinent examples within each pathophysiologic category.

Secretory Diarrhea[48]

Active chloride secretion is the basic mechanism leading to secretory diarrhea. There are many known stimuli for intestinal secretion including toxins, peptides, and derivatives of arachidonic acid. These substances exert their action through intracellular mediators that stimulate active chloride secretion. One of the most important intracellular mediators is cyclic AMP (cAMP). Increased cellular cAMP stimulates chloride secretion by crypt cells and inhibits the neutral NaCl absorptive mechanism of surface or villous cells. *Vibrio cholerae* produces a toxin that works via this mediator to produce dramatic secretory diarrhea.[49]

Important causes for secretory diarrhea are either exogenous or endogenous. Some examples of exogenous sources of secretory diarrhea include 1) laxatives (phenolthalein, anthraquinones, senna, ricinoleic acid, and bisacodyl), 2) medications (diuretics, theophylline, cholinergic agents, and prostaglandins), 3) toxins (heavy metals, organophosphates, seafood toxins, plant toxins, caffeine, ethanol, and preformed bacterial toxins [eg, *Vibrio cholera*, toxigenic *E coli*, and *Staph aureus*]) and 4) gut allergies without histologic change. Endogenous causes can be congenital or more commonly acquired. Important examples of acquired endogenous causes of secretory diarrhea include endogenous laxatives (eg, bile acids and long chain fatty acids) and hormone-producing tumors (VIPoma, gastrinoma, mastocytosis).

Maldigestion[50] and Malabsorption[51]

A comprehensive review of malabsorptive disorders is discussed in Chapter 18. In general, the diseases that manifest as malabsorption or maldigestion can be divided into three broad, often overlapping categories: 1) intraluminal maldigestion, 2) mucosal malabsorption, and 3) postmucosal conditions. Broad pathophysiologic concepts related to malabsorption and maldigestion will be reviewed here using bacterial overgrowth as a protypical example.

Intestinal peristalsis and gastric acid secretion normally prevent excessive proliferation of bacteria in the proximal small intestine. Its contents usually include less than 10^5 bacteria per ml. Any condition that induces stasis in the intestine can predispose to bacterial overgrowth by enteric flora that normally resides in the more distal intestine. Some causes of bacterial overgrowth are listed in Table 2-3.

Intraluminal bacterial overgrowth results primarily in intraluminal maldigestion; however, mucosal lesions induced by bacterial products and altered intraluminal bile acids may impair mucosal absorption as well. Malabsorption in intestinal bacterial overgrowth can occur by at least three mechanisms. First, bacterial overgrowth interferes with intraluminal fat digestion, resulting in steatorrhea. In bacterial overgrowth, bile salts are deconjugated to free bile acids by hydrolytic bacterial enzymes. Free bile acids are more lipid soluble than are conjugated bile salts and are readily absorbed by passive diffusion in the upper small bowel, resulting in intraluminal bile salt deficiency. A second effect of bacterial overgrowth is the binding and uptake of vitamin B_{12} by the bacteria in

Table 2-3. Selected causes of bacterial overgrowth

Motor abnormalities
   Scleroderma
   Amyloidosis
   Pseudo-obstruction
   Vagotomy
   Diabetes with visceral neuropathy (rare)

Structural abnormalities
   Diverticuli
   Strictures
      Crohn's disease
      Ischemic disease
      Radiation enteritis
   Adhesions causing partial obstruction
   Afferent loop stasis after Billroth II gastrectomy
   Fistulas
      Gastrocolic
      Jejunocolic
      Jejunoileal

Hypo- or achlorhydria
   Pernicious anemia
      Vagotomy or gastric resection

Hypo- or agammaglobulinemia

Source: Trier[51]

the proximal intestine, which reduces its availability for normal absorption in the distal ileum. Finally, bacteria and their products can also directly damage the intestinal mucosa, thus damaging the brush border on intestinal absorptive cells. Deconjugated bile acids may also contribute to the observed mucosal damage.

Inflammatory Diseases[52]

Conditions that cause inflammatory diarrhea are usually associated with a damaged intestinal epithelial lining. Proteases, oxygen radicals, and toxic cytokines work together with complement activation and activation of killer lymphocytes to damage the epithelium and cause ulcerations. Noxious stimuli activate white blood cells to release inflammatory mediators that cause intestinal secretion. The clinical manifestations of these intestinal responses include secretory diarrhea, exudation with protein-losing enteropathy, bleeding, and malabsorption. This is a protective response overall as it washes out and expels antigens and microorganisms from the gut.

Infections are the most common cause of inflammatory diarrhea. T-lymphocyte activation of the immune system has been demonstrated as a fundamental cause of villus atrophy and crypt hyperplasia,

Table 2-4. Causes of secondary chronic intestinal pseudo-obstruction

Myopathic
    Collagen vascular diseases: scleroderma, dermatomyositis, lupus
    Muscular dystrophies: myotonic dystrophy, Duchenne's muscular atrophy
    Amyloidosis

Neuropathies
    Chagas' disease
    Hirschsprung's disease
    Parkinson's disease
    Ganglioneuroma of the intestine
    Carcinomatosis
    Diabetes mellitus
    Amyloidosis

Endocrinopathies
    Myxedema
    Hypoparathyroidism
    Pheochromocytoma

Electrolyte imbalances
    Hypokalemia
    Hypocalcemia
    Hypomagnesemia

Pharmacologic agents
    Phenothiazines
    Tricyclic antidepressants
    Narcotic analgesics
    Anti-parkinsonian medications
    Ephedrine
    Clonidine

Miscellaneous
    Nontropical sprue
    Jejunal diverticulosis
    Jejunoileal bypass
    Paraneoplastic syndrome
    Eosinophilic gastroenteritis
    Cathartic colon
    Psychosis
    Porphyria
    Radiation enteritis

Source: Schuffler et al.[56]

which is commonly seen in small intestinal infections of various types. Other causes of diarrheas due to brush border or enterocyte damage or death include autoimmune disorders (eg, graft-versus-host disease), hypersensitivity reactions (eg, food allergy, celiac sprue, eosinophilic gastroenteritis), chemotherapeutic agents, radiation therapy, and idiopathic inflammatory conditions such as Crohn's disease and lymphocytic or collagenous colitis. Clinically this group of diarrheal disorders always exhibits mucosal damage, which can be detected endoscopically or with barium radiographs.

Motor Disorders of the Small Intestine

Motor disorders that delay small intestinal transit time can be divided into two general categories: myopathy and neuropathy. In myopathies, the amplitudes of contractions are reduced markedly during both the fasting and fed periods. The cyclical and propagative aspects of the MMCs remain normal. In addition, the conversion from fasting to fed motility patterns remains intact. In contrast, patients with neuropathic disorders demonstrate a variety of patterns. The amplitudes of contractions are usually preserved; however, MMCs originate in the mid-small intestine rather than in the stomach; they may be simultaneous rather than propagative; they may be high in amplitude and/or simultaneous (clustered contraction); there may be high amplitude spastic contractions at a single recording site; contractions may propagate in a retrograde rather than an antegrade direction.[53] Finally, the normal conversion from the fasting to the fed pattern after meal ingestion may be disrupted. The ability to clearly document the differences between myopathy and neuropathy has been compromised by the limited availability of tissue for adequate pathologic examination of the muscles and nerves as well as the paucity of pathologists skilled in differentiating gastrointestinal myopathy from neuropathy. Ultimately, it may be found that the majority of patients have mixed disorders, ie, neuromyopathies.[54]

Major etiologies of delayed small intestinal transit include pregnancy, bacterial overgrowth syndromes, certain functional disorders (small intestinal constipation), and chronic intestinal pseudo-obstruction (CIP). CIP is a syndrome, caused by a severe disorder in gastrointestinal motility, in which the patient has signs and symptoms of intestinal obstruction without a detectable mechanical obstructing lesion.[55] Not only the small intestine, but also the colon, esophagus, and stomach may be involved. Primary (idiopathic) CIP encompasses familial visceral myopathy, familial visceral neuropathy, sporadic visceral myopathy, sporadic visceral neuropathy, and hollow visceral myopathy.[56] Etiologies for secondary CIP are more common and are represented in Table 2-4.

Important causes of rapid small intestinal transit are listed in Table 2-5. Noninvasive bacteria increase small bowel transit by increasing migrating action po-

Table 2-5. Causes of rapid small bowel transit

Infectious diarrheas

    Noninvasive bacteria: ↑ Migrating Action Potential Complexes (MAPC)
        Vibrio cholera
        Shigella dysenteria
        Clostridium perfringens
        Clostridium difficile
        Enterotoxigenic *E coli*

    Invasive bacteria: ↑ Rapid Burst Action Potential (RBAP)
        Shigella flexneri
        Enteroinvasive *E coli*

    Mixed disorder: ↑ MAPCs and ↑ RBAPs
        Shigella dysenteriae I, 3818-T (invasive and toxin-producing)
        Trichinella spiralis

Castor oil (ricinoleic acid): ↑ MAPCs

Radiation enteritis

Functional gastrointestinal disorders: Variable changes in transit time

Source: Fisher[59]

tential complexes. Ricinoleic acid also works by this mechanism. Invasive bacteria increase rapid burst action potentials to effect a change in overall transit time. As noted in Table 2-5, *Shigella* and *Trichinella* act via both mechanisms. As for functional gastrointestinal disorders, small bowel transit time has not been studied carefully in gastroduodenal motor disorders or subtypes of irritable bowel syndrome with predominantly diarrhea. It may be rapid in some cases and slow in others.[57]

References

1. Grand RJ, Watkins JB, Torti FM. Development of the human gastrointestinal tract: a review. *Gastroenterology*. 1976;50:790–801.
2. Cheng H, Leblond CP. Origin, differentiation and renewal of the four main epithelial cell types in the mouse small intestine, V: unitarian theory of the origin of the four epithelial cell types. *Am J Anat*. 1974;141:537–548.
3. Rubin D. Small intestine: anatomy and structural anomalies. In: Yamada T, ed. *Textbook of Gastroenterology, 1*. Philadelphia, Pa: JB Lippincott Co; 1991:1555–1576.
4. Costa M, Brookes SJ. The enteric nervous system. *Am J Gastroenterol*. 1994;89:S129–S137.
5. Goyal RK, Hirano I. The enteric nervous system. *N Engl J Med*. 1996;334:1106–1115.
6. Gershon MD. The enteric nervous system. *Annu Rev Neurosci*. 1981;4:227–240.
7. Gershon MD, Kirchgessner AL, Wade PR. Functional anatomy of the enteric nervous system. In: Johnson LR, ed. *Physiology of the Gastrointestinal Tract*. New York, NY: Raven Press; 1994:381–422.
8. Llewellyn-Smith IJ, Furness JB, O'Brien PE, et al. Noradrenergic nerves in human small intestine: distribution and ultrastructure. *Gastroenterology*. 1984;87:513–521.
9. Furness JB, Bornstein JC. The enteric nervous system and its extrinsic connections. In: Yamada T, ed. *Textbook of Gastroenterology, 1*. Philadelphia, Pa: JB Lippincott Co; 1995:2–24.
10. Lundgren O, Svanvik J, Jivegard L. Enteric nervous system, I: physiology and pathophysiology of the intestinal tract. *Dig Dis Sci*. 1989;34:264–283.
11. Mayer EA, Raybould HE. Role of visceral afferent mechanisms in functional bowel disorders. *Gastroenterology*. 1990;99:1688–1700.
12. Gabella G. Structure of muscles and nerves in the gastrointestinal tract. In: Johnson LR, ed. *Physiology of the Gastrointestinal Tract*. New York, NY: Raven Press; 1994:751–794.
13. Antonson DL. Anatomy and physiology of the small and large intestine. In: Wyllie R, Hyams JS, eds. *Pediatric Gastrointestinal Disease: Pathophysiology, Diagnosis, Management*. Philadelphia, Pa: WB Saunders Co; 1993:145–156.
14. Larsson LI, Goltermann N, De Magistris L, et al. Somatostatin cell processes as pathways for paracrine secretion. *Science*. 1979;205:1393–1401.
15. Dockray GJ. Physiology of enteric neuropeptides. In: Johnson LR, ed. *Physiology of the Gastrointestinal Tract, 1*. New York, NY: Raven Press; 1994:169–174.
16. Makhlouf GM. Neural and hormonal regulation of function in the gut. *Hosp Pract*. 1990;25:79–90.
17. Berridge MJ. The molecular basis of communication within the cell. *Sci Am*. 1985;253:142–152.
18. Dockray GJ. Physiology of enteric neuropeptides. In: Johnson LR, ed. *Physiology of the Gastrointestinal Tract, 1*. New York, NY: Raven Press; 1994:41–52.
19. Taylor IL. Pancreatic polypeptide family: pancreatic polypeptide, neuropeptide Y, and peptide YY. In: Makhlouf GM, ed. *Handbook of Physiology*. Bethesda, Md: American Physiological Society; 1989:475–482.
20. Makhlouf GM. Enteric neuropeptides: role in neuromuscular activity of the gut. *Trends Pharmacol Sci*. 1985;6:214–220.
21. Gorden P, Comi RJ, Maton PN, et al. NIH conference: somatostatin and somatostatin analog (SMS 201–955) in treatment of hormone-secreting tumors of the pituitary and gastrointestinal tract and non-neoplastic diseases of the gut. *Ann Intern Med*. 1989;110:35–42.
22. Gaginella TS, O'Dorisio TM, Fassler JE, et al. Treatment of endocrine and nonendocrine secretory diarrheal states with Sandostatin. *Metabolism*. 1990;39:172–175.
23. Fawcett DW. The intestines. In: Fawcett DW, Bloom W, eds. *A Textbook of Histology*. Philadelphia, Pa: WB Saunders Co; 1986:53–67.
24. Barrett K, Dhamasathaphorn K. Secretion and absorption: small intestine and colon. In: Yamada T, ed. *Textbook of Gastroenterology, 1*. Philadelphia, Pa: JB Lippincott Co; 1991:268–279.
25. Field M, Rao MC, Chang EB. Intestinal electrolyte transport and diarrheal disease. *N Engl J Med*. 1989;321:800–806.
26. Gray GM. Starch digestion and absorption in nonruminants. *J Nutr*. 1992;122:172–178.
27. Rumessen JJ. Fructose and related food carbohydrates: sources, intake, absorption, and clinical implications. *Scand J Gastroenterol*. 1992;27:819–825.
28. Traber PG. Carbohydrate assimilation. In: Yamada T, ed. *Textbook of Gastroenterology, 1*. Philadelphia, Pa: JB Lippincott Co; 1995:405–427.
29. Ahnen DJ. Protein digestion and assimilation. In: Yamada T, ed. *Textbook of Gastroenterology, 1*. Philadelphia, Pa: JB Lippincott Co; 1995:456–466.
30. Freeman HJ, Sleisenger MH, Kim YS. Human protein digestion and absorption: normal mechanisms and protein-energy malnutrition. *Clin Gastroenterol*. 1983;12:357–370.
31. Gardner MG. Absorption of intact peptides—studies on transport of protein digests and dipeptides across rat small intestine in vitro. *Q J Exp Physiol*. 1982;67:629–635.
32. Chung YC, Kim YS, Shadchehr A, et al. Protein digestion and absorption in human small intestine. *Gastroenterology*. 1979;76:1415–1420.
33. Davidson NO, Magun AM. Intestinal lipid absorption. In: Yamada T, ed. *Textbook of Gastroenterology, 1*. Philadelphia, Pa: JB Lippincott Co; 1995:428–452.

34. Borgstrom B. The importance of phospholipids, pancreatic phospholipase A_2 and fatty acid for the digestion of dietary fat. *Gastroenterology.* 1980;78:954–962.
35. Shiau YF. Mechanisms of intestinal fat absorption. *Am J Physiol.* 1981;240:G1–G9.
36. Schron CM. Vitamins and minerals. In: Yamada T, ed. *Textbook of Gastroenterology, 1.* Philadelphia, Pa: JB Lippincott Co; 1995:467–484.
37. Finch CA, Huebers H. Perspectives in iron metabolism. *N Engl J Med.* 1982;306:1520–1527.
38. Sarna SK, Otterson MF. Gastrointestinal motility: some basic concepts. *Pharmacology.* 1988;36(Suppl 1):7–15.
39. Thompson DG, Wingate DL, Archer L, et al. Normal patterns of human upper small bowel motor activity recorded by prolonged radiotelemetry. *Gut.* 1980;21:500–509.
40. Malagelada JR, Robertson JS, Brown ML, et al. Intestinal transit of solid and liquid components of a meal in health. *Gastroenterology.* 1984;87:1255–1262.
41. Bayliss WM, Starling EH. The movements and innervation of the small intestine. *J Physiol (Lond).* 1899;24:99–104.
42. Kellow JE, Borody TJ, Phillips SF, et al. Human interdigestive motility: variations in patterns from esopahgus to colon. *Gastroenterology.* 1986;91:386–392.
43. Husebye E, Skar V, Aalen OO, et al. Digital ambulatory manometry of the small intestine in healthy adults: estimates of variation within and between individuals and statistical management of incomplete MMC periods. *Dig Dis Sci.* 1990;35:1057–1069.
44. Code CF, Schlegel JF. The gastrointestinal housekeeper. In: Daniel EE, ed. *Gastrointestinal Motility.* Vancouver, BC: Mitchell Press; 1974:631–649.
45. Valori RM, Kumar D, Wingate DL. Effects of different types of stress and of "prokinetic" drugs on the control of the fasting motor complex in humans. *Gastroenterology.* 1986;90:1890–1897.
46. Reynolds JC, Putnam PE. Prokinetic agents. *Gastroenterol Clin North Am.* 1992;21:567–596.
47. Kachel G, Ruppin H, Hagel J, et al. Human intestinal motor activity and transport: effects of a synthetic opiate. *Gastroenterology.* 1986;90:85–92.
48. Phillips SF. Diarrhea. a current view of pathophysiology. *Gastroenterology.* 1972;63:495–506.
49. Powell D. New paradigms for the pathophysiology of infectious diarrhea. *Gastroenterology.* 1994;106:1705–1715.
50. Riley SA, Turnberg LA. Maldigestion and malabsorption. In: Sleisenger MH, Fordtran JS, eds. *Gastrointestinal Disease.* Philadelphia, Pa: WB Saunders Co; 1993:1009–1027.
51. Trier JS. Intestinal malabsorption: differentiation of cause. *Hosp Pract.* 1988;23:195–211.
52. Powell DW. Approach to the adult patient with diarrhea. In: Yamada T, ed. *Textbook of Gastroenterology, 2.* Philadelphia, Pa: JB Lippincott Co; 1995:813–863.
53. Camilleri M, Vassallo M. Small intestinal motility and transit in disease. *Baillieres Clin Gastroenterol.* 1991;5:431–451.
54. Krishnamurthy S, Schuffler MD. Pathology of neuromuscular disorders of the small intestine and colon. *Gastroenterology.* 1987;93:610–639.
55. Hirsh EH, Bradenburg D, Hersh T, et al. Chronic intestinal pseudoobstruction. *J Clin Gastroenterol.* 1981;3:247–255.
56. Schuffler MD, Rohrmann CA, Chaffer RG, et al. Chronic intestinal pseudoobstruction: a report of 27 cases and review of the literature. *Medicine.* 1981;60:173–177.
57. Quigley EMM. Intestinal manometry: technical advances, clinical limitations. *Dig Dis Sci.* 1992;37:10–13.
58. Fine KD, Krejs GJ, Fordtran JS. Diarrhea. In: Sleisenger MH, Fordtran JS, eds. *Gastrointestinal Disease: Pathophysiology, Diagnosis, Management.* Philadelphia, Pa: WB Saunders Co; 1989:293.
59. Fisher RS. Motor function of the stomach and small intestine in health and disease. Presented at the American Gastroenterological Association Fall Postgraduate Course; 8 September 1995; Philadelphia, Pa.

The Small Bowel in Immunology

Thomas Judge

Chapter Contents

Introduction
Components of the Gastrointestinal Immune Function
The Integrated Immune Response

Introduction

The gastrointestinal (GI) tract plays an important role in the body's immune responses to both foreign antigens and potential pathogens. The very large mucosal surface of the GI tract is exposed to great numbers of microorganisms and antigens such as food particles and the metabolic byproducts of the normal intestinal flora. The immune function within the GI tract involves a variety of cellular and humoral components that interact to generate a coordinated defense. The intestinal mucosal immune system has evolved to function, in part, independently of blood-borne immune mechanisms. A related consequence of continued antigenic challenge has been the evolution of immune-mediated mechanisms to limit inflammatory responses that might otherwise be deleterious.

Components of the Gastrointestinal Immune Function

The Epithelial Barrier

Immunity within the gastrointestinal tract consists of three interdependent components: 1) an epithelial barrier, 2) humoral substances, and 3) cellular immune mechanisms. The gastrointestinal epithelium strictly regulates exposure of the underlying tissues of the GI tract to the multiple foreign antigens present in the lumen at any time (Fig. 3-1). Tight junctions between the apical regions of adjacent epithelial cells impede free movement of antigens and microorganisms into the lamina propria of the GI mucosa. The barrier function of the epithelium is significantly assisted by the mucous layer, which covers the epithelium and limits access to the surface of the lining cells. This mucous layer also serves as the medium into which various humoral elements such as antibodies and complement components are secreted by the adjacent mucosa. In addition, digestive enzymes and bile salts within the lumen create a formidable environment for any potential pathogen. The importance of the epithelial tight junction in controlling immune responses to foreign antigens has recently been demonstrated in animal models featuring defective interepithelial interactions.[1] Mice with defective expression of N-cadherin (a molecule critical to the formation and maintenance of epithelial tight junctions) by the crypt compartment of the epithelium develop severe inflammatory reactions unless raised in a germ-free environment. Selective disruption of epithelial tight junctions within the villous tip does not cause marked inflammation, suggesting that the GI barrier function is more critical for mucosal protection at particular sites. The location of Paneth cells, which secrete antibacterial products within the crypt compartment of the mucosa, also emphasizes the importance of the epithelium in the establishment of an effective barrier against potential pathogens.[2,3] Epithelial cells lining the gastrointestinal lumen also secrete a variety of cytokines that regulate the responses of cellular elements of the immune system, thus emphasizing the dynamic nature of this barrier function.[4–6] The interrelationship between the epithelium and the immune response is further demonstrated by the presence of specialized epithelial cells, known as microfold or M cells, which have evolved to selectively adsorb large molecules and some microorganisms and transport them to underlying lymphoid tissue. As a result of these M cells, luminal contents may be monitored for potential pathogens while maintaining the integrity of the barrier.

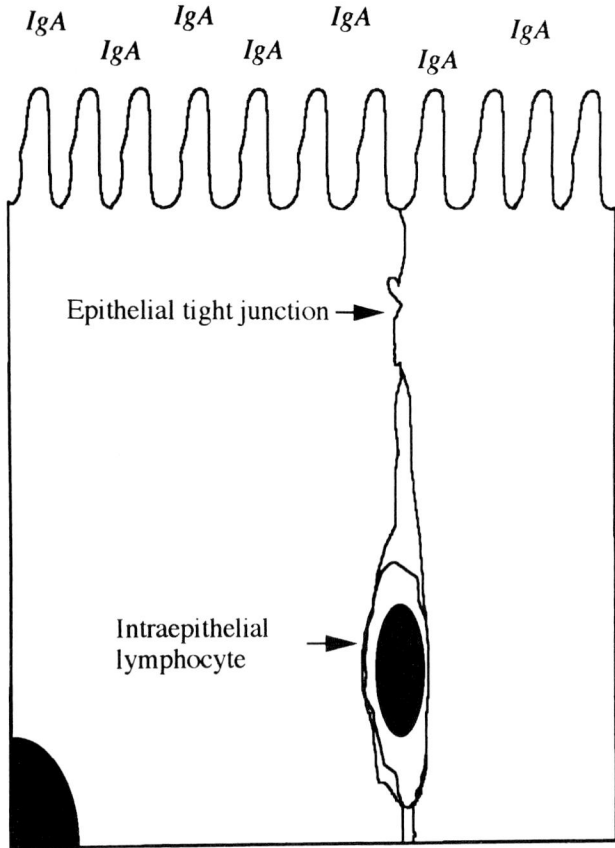

Fig. 3-1. Schematic representation of the epithelial barrier.
The principal components of this barrier include the epithelial cell, the epithelial tight junctions at the apical membranes of adjacent cells, and the mucous layer coating the apical brush border in which secretory IgA molecules, complement components, and proteolytic enzymes reside. Intraepithelial lymphocytes are typically found in small numbers (4 to 5 per small intestinal villus) located along the basolateral membranes of epithelial cells.

Humoral Immunity

The humoral components of the immune response within the gastrointestinal tract include antibodies, complement components, and a variety of reactive compounds such as plasma proteases, kinins, and prostagladins, as well as cytokines.[7–10] The gastrointestinal mucosa is the largest producer of antibodies in the body, secreting vast amounts daily into the gastrointestinal lumen. In contrast to the systemic humoral response, which is characterized by the production of IgG, antibodies produced by the GI tract consist primarily of IgA and IgM isotypes. Secretion of dimeric IgA is the principal protective immune mechanism for the gastrointestinal tract.[11–13] Intestinal antibodies are produced from plasma cells residing in the lamina propria. Antibodies consist of four covalently bound peptide molecules (two light chains, two heavy chains) that combine to form a single molecule with two antigen recognition sites and a single constant region (Fig. 3-2). The antigen recognition and binding site (Fab), a unique three-dimensional structure dictated by the peptide sequences of the variable regions of both the light and heavy chains of the antibody, binds to specific regions or epitopes present on large molecules or microorganisms. The biological behavior of antibodies (ie, complement-fixation, opsonization) is dictated by the characteristics of the Fc portion of the antibody molecule, composed exclusively of the constant regions of the heavy chains. Intestinal plasma cells may generate either monomeric or dimeric IgA molecules. Dimeric IgA results from polymerization of two IgA molecules in combination with a J (joining) chain produced by the plasma cell. The J chain allows polymerization of as many as five IgM molecules. The J chain also binds to the transmembrane form of secretory component present on the basal surface of intestinal epithelial cells and initiates a process of endocytosis and transcellular transport of the IgA-secretory component complex within endosomal vesicles and subsequent secretion of this complex from the apical membrane of the epithelial cell into the lumen (Fig. 3-3). Secretory component present on biliary epithelium also permits secretion of polymeric IgA and IgM antibodies into the bile.[12] Maintenance of the IgA-secretory complex within the lumen protects secreted IgA from premature degradation by bacteria and digestive enzymes. Secretory IgA provides protection against bacteria, viruses, and toxins present in the lumen by inhibiting bacterial adherence to epithelial cells and neutralizing viral particles and macromolecules.[13] In addition, IgA complexes with bacterial toxins and luminal antigens reduce the exposure of the surface epithelium to damage and protect the gut from invasion when the mucosal barrier is disrupted by disease.

Cell-Mediated Immunity

The cellular component of gastrointestinal immunity consists of cells responsible for both innate and acquired immune responses. Innate immunity does not require prior exposure to foreign antigens or microorganisms in order to activate a response. In contrast, more specific and coordinated immune responses result from the activation of lymphocytes, the principal mediators of acquired immunity.

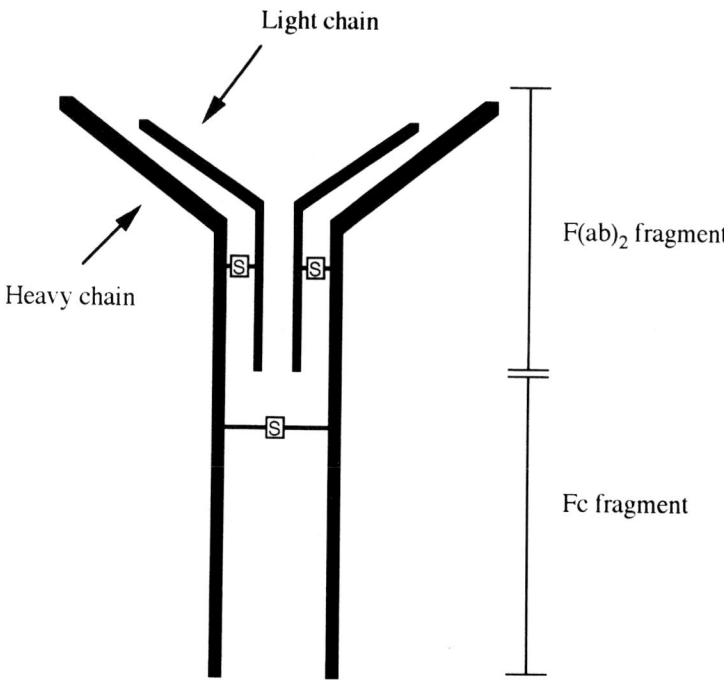

Fig. 3-2. Representation of an immunoglobulin (Ig) molecule composed of two Ig light chains and two Ig heavy chains linked by three intermolecular disulfide bonds (—S—).
Five major classes of immunoglobulin exist in humans based on the heavy chain present in the molecule (IgM, IgG, IgA, IgE, and IgD). The antigen recognition site (Fab) is formed by the variable regions of both the light and heavy chains. Following primary stimulation of the naive B cell, DNA encoding peptides within the Fab site undergo hypermutation with preferential clonal expansion of those B cells with high-affinity interaction with the antigen. The Fc fragment dictates the biological activity of immunoglobulin, containing sites for binding to Fc receptors on mast cells and monocytes, activation of complement, and ligation to the J chain (in the case of IgA and IgM).

Innate Immunity

Mast cells, granulocytes, macrophages, and natural killer cells within the GI mucosa form the basis for an innate immune response to antigenic challenge. Macrophages and mast cells within the GI mucosa are particularly important in developing immune responses. Mucosal mast cells are characterized by several features that distinguish these cells from mast cells located in other connective tissues of the body.[14] Although both types of mast cells are present in the intestine, mucosal mast cells release chondroitin sulfate rather than heparin upon activation, bind IgE at reduced levels, and reside in close proximity to nerves of the gut that modulate the release of vasoactive substances from the mast cells. Increased vascular permeability and vasodilation induced by the activated mast cell allow entry into the mucosa of circulating humoral factors such as complement factors, antibodies, coagulation proteins, and components of the kallikrein-kinin pathway. Concomitant release of chemoattractant factors by the mast cells as well as the secretion of cytokines such as interleukin-1, tumor necrosis factor, and g-interferon by macrophages lead to recruitment of neutrophils, eosinophils, and lymphocytes into areas of ongoing inflammation. Granulocytes play a principal role as effector cells directed against intestinal pathogens and are a hallmark of acute inflammatory responses in the gut. Neutrophils rapidly adhere to intestinal endothelium, migrate to sites of inflammation in response to inflammatory mediators such as C5a and leukotriene B_4, and begin to engulf and degrade the microorganisms or cellular toxins initiating the inflammatory reaction. The release of potent proteolytic substances and toxic oxygen-free radicals generated by granulocytes and macrophages to kill infectious agents often overwhelms the limited stores of antioxidants and proteinase inhibitors within the mucosa and may be responsible for significant tissue injury in the setting of extensive inflammation. Apoptosis of epithelial cells in response to oxygen metabolites and inflammatory cytokines and continued migration of granulocytes through the epithelial barrier into the lumen lead to the altered intestinal permeability present in inflammatory disorders of the intestine.[15] Expansion of the

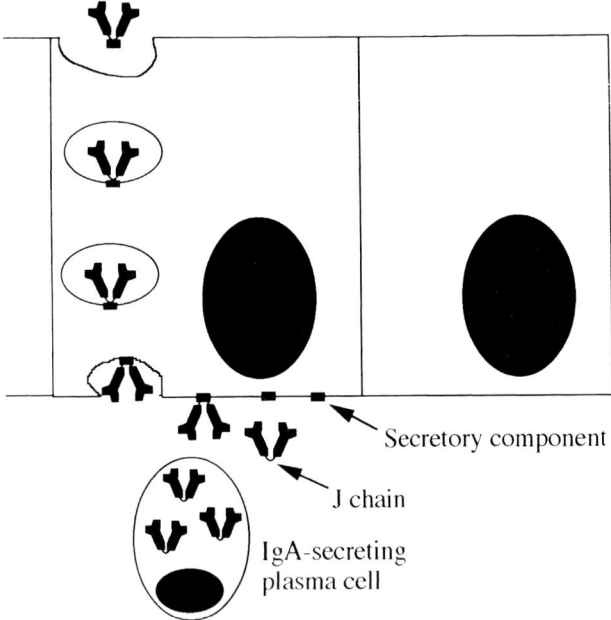

Fig. 3-3. Schematic representation of secretory IgA formation and transport across the intestinal epithelium. Secretory component produced by the epithelial cells combines with dimeric IgA secreted by the plasma cells in the lamina propria along the basolateral surface of the epithelial cell. The secretory IgA complex undergoes endocytosis and is transported across the epithelial cell and released into the lumen. Within the lumen, secretory IgA binds and neutralizes bacteria, viral particles, and potential toxins, thus reducing the amount of free antigen in contact with the apical surface of the epithelial cells.

mucosal eosinophil population is a prominent feature of parasitic infection, and release of degradative enzymes from eosinophilic granules appears to be particularly important in innate immunity to these pathogens.[16]

Acquired Immunity

Acquired immunity results from the formation of antibodies and effector cells derived from precursor lymphocytes. The principal function of acquired immunity is the generation of vast numbers of lymphocytes capable of initiating "memory" responses upon restimulation with antigen. In contrast to primary immune responses, which are slow and frequently ineffective due to the relatively few lymphocytes that recognize any particular antigen, secondary immune responses occur quite briskly on rechallenge with antigen. These responses are generally more effective due to the enhanced numbers of clonally derived lymphocytes that respond to antigen and to qualitative differences in the functional capacities of the more terminally differentiated lymphocytes present at the time of rechallenge. There are two forms of lymphocytes: B lymphocytes, which are responsible for antibody production, and T lymphocytes, which coordinate and effect cell-mediated immune responses. B lymphocytes arise from stem cells in the bone marrow and complete their initial development in this site. During bone marrow maturation, immunoglobulin gene rearrangement occurs, which results in the formation of surface immunoglobulin receptors presented on the surfaces of the virgin B lymphocytes as they enter the systemic circulation. As shown in Fig. 3-4, activation of these virgin B cells within the mucosa results in the expansion and terminal differentiation of these cells into plasma cells, which secrete high-affinity IgA antibodies. T lymphocytes also arise from pleuripotential stem cells within the bone marrow. However, following early differentiation toward the lymphocyte lineage, pre–T cells leave the marrow and migrate to the thymus to complete development [Fig. 3-5(a)]. Within the thymus, immature T cells rapidly proliferate and undergo random rearrangement of the T-cell receptor genes. T lymphocytes recognize antigens in complex with cell surface proteins encoded by genes in the major histocompatibility complex (MHC). During thymic development, immature T cells undergo selection during which potentially autoreactive T cells are eliminated (negative selection), while those T cells capable of recognizing antigens presented in complex with self-MHC molecules (positive selection) are retained. There are two classes of mature T cells which may be identified by the expression of cell surface proteins: $CD4^+$ T cells [Fig. 3-5(b)], which recognize antigen complexed to MHC class II molecules (expressed primarily by "professional" antigen presenting cells [APCs] such as dendritic cells, macrophages, and activated B cells), and $CD8^+$ T cells, which recognize antigen complexed to MHC class I molecules (present on all nucleated cells in the body). Functionally, $CD4^+$ T cells typically respond to exogenous antigens engulfed by APCs and release large amounts of cytokines to help B-cell development or amplify cell-mediated responses. $CD8^+$ T cells generally recognize endogenous antigens such as viral particles and intracellular pathogens. Following activation, $CD8^+$ T cells differentiate into cytotoxic T cells, which then eliminate infected cells. After completion of T-cell maturation within the thymus, naive T cells circulate to secondary lymphoid tissues throughout the body.

Gut-Associated Lymphoid Tissue

Secondary lymphoid tissue with the gastrointestinal mucosa, also known as gut-associated lymphoid tis-

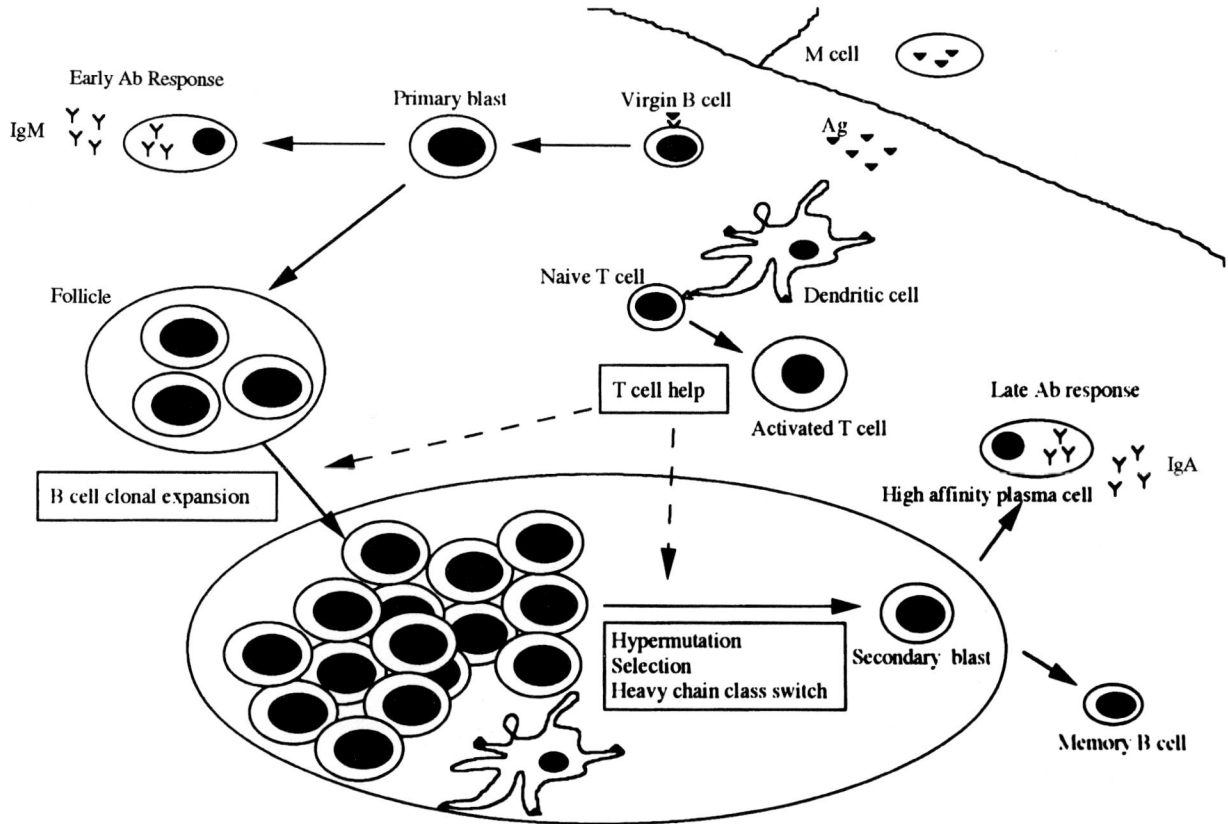

Fig. 3-4. Activation of virgin B cells within the mucosa follows engagement of the Ig surface receptor by antigen presented by epithelial M cells.
This results in the formation of a primary B-cell blast, which may either differentiate into primary plasma cells secreting low-affinity IgM antibodies (early Ab response) or enter a germinal center within a mucosal lymphoid follicle or mesenteric lymph node. Supported by cell-to-cell interactions and by cytokines secreted by helper T cells, the B-cell blasts undergo clonal expansion, hypermutation of the antigen recognition portion of the immunoglobulin gene, and continued differentiation of those B-cell clones that have high-affinity interactions with antigen. The majority of these high-affinity clones develop into secondary plasma cells, which reenter the mucosa and secrete IgA antibodies (late Ab response). A smaller number of these high-affinity B cells differentiate into memory B cells, which recirculate to mucosal surfaces and lymph nodes throughout the body.

sue (GALT), provides the structural basis for acquired immunity within the intestine. This tissue consists of both aggregated and nonaggregated groups of hematopoietic cells associated with all gastrointestinal organs. GALT forms one subsegment of the larger mucosa-associated lymphoid tissue (MALT), which provides immune support to other mucosal surface tissues including the respiratory and urogenital systems.

Lymphoid Aggregates

Aggregated lymphoid tissue within the intestine consists of lymphoid follicles and mesenteric lymph nodes. Lymphoid follicles are found throughout the small intestine in mice but are concentrated in the distal ileum of humans, where they are frequently grouped in clusters known as Peyer's patches. In humans, as many as 1000 individual Peyer's patches may be seen in the distal ileum. Epithelium overlying lymphoid follicles form domelike structures consisting of M cells that translocate antigen across the epithelial barrier, where they may undergo phagocytosis by antigen-presenting cells such as macrophages and dendritic cells situated directly under the M cells.[17] The lymphoid follicles consist largely of a germinal center containing rapidly proliferating activated B-cell clones surrounded by a mixture of T cells, macrophages, and dendritic cells. The mesenteric lymph nodes make up the remainder of the aggregated lymphoid tissue in the gut. Lymphocytes activated in the intestine migrate through afferent lymphatic vessels into the

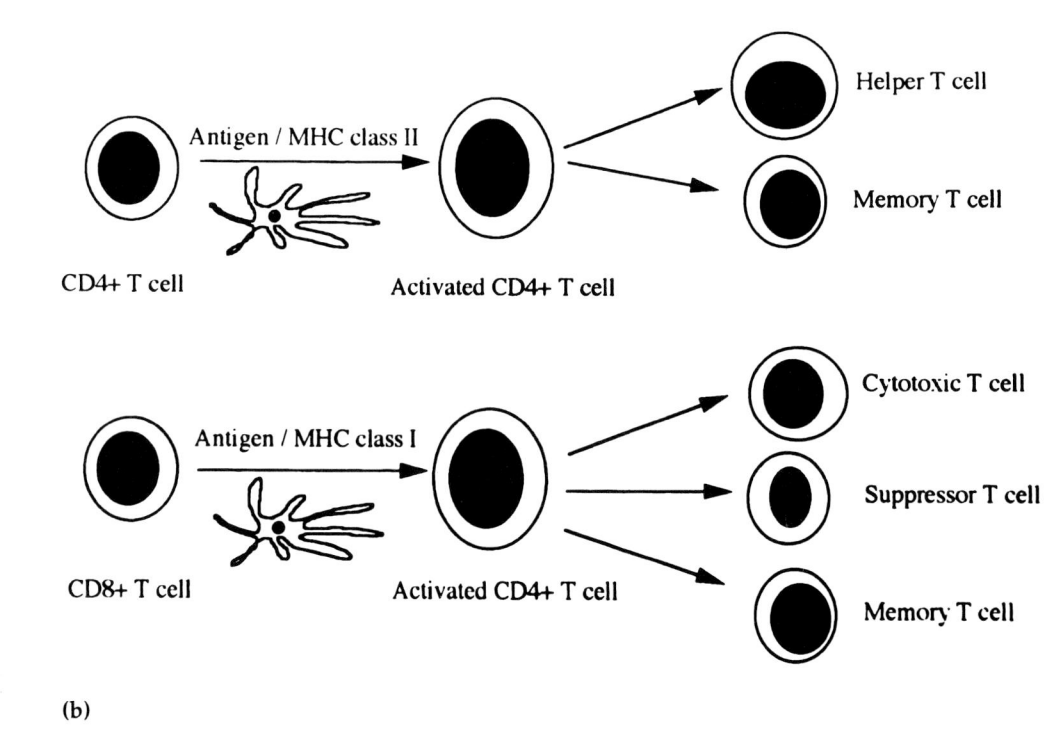

Fig. 3-5. Schematic representation of T-lymphocyte development.
(a) Primary T-lymphocyte development occurs within the thymus following engraftment of lymphocyte precursor cells in the cortex. Immature T cells undergo enormous expansion within the cortex during which time the T-cell receptor (TCR) gene segments rearrange and T-cell accessory molecules, CD4 and CD8, are expressed on the surface membrane. Thymocytes that successfully produce a functional TCR are rigorously selected to eliminate potentially autoreactive T cells (negative selection) while ensuring the ability of these cells to recognize self-MHC molecules (positive selection). Surviving T cells, expressing either CD4 or CD8, complete maturation within the medulla of the thymus and subsequently circulate to secondary lymphoid tissues throughout the body. (b) Activation of naive T cells within secondary lymphoid tissue occurs upon contact with specific antigen combined with either MHC class I or class II molecules on the surface of antigen-presenting cells (APCs). These APCs also provide important costimulatory signals to the T cells, thus limiting inappropriate activation of T cells within the mucosa. Following activation, T cells clonally expand and differentiate into either cytotoxic T cells, suppressor cells, or cytokine-secreting cells (helper T cells). Small numbers of activated T cells differentiate into memory cells, which recirculate throughout the body to allow rapid immune responses upon rechallenge with antigen.

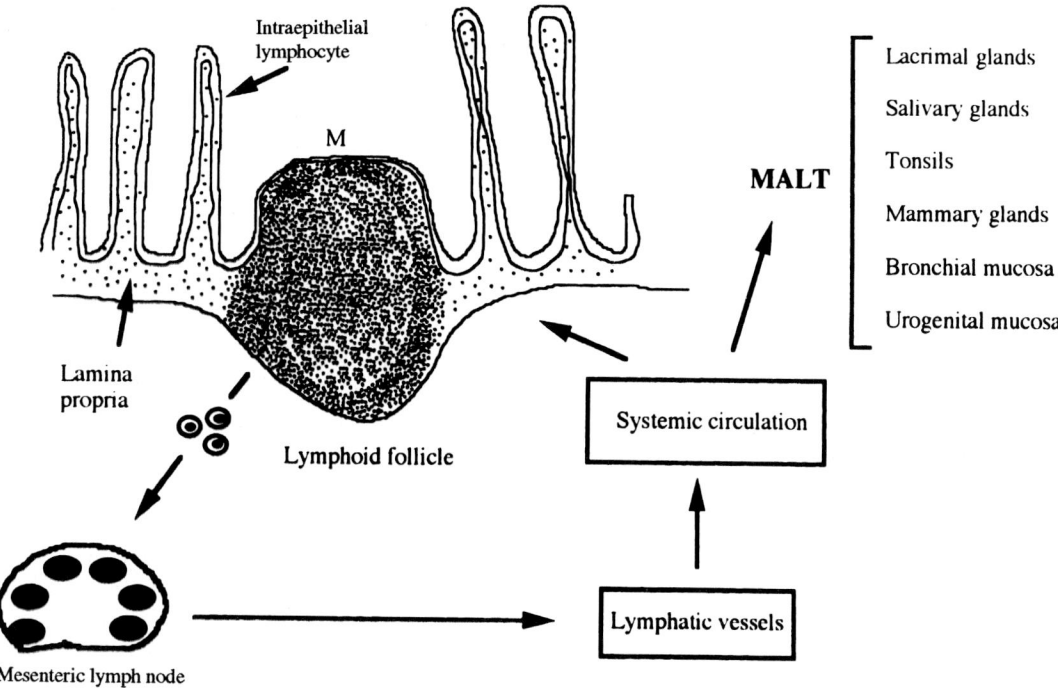

Fig. 3-6. Gut-associated lymphoid tissue.
Translocation of antigen across M cells overlying lymphoid follicles results in activation and migration of lymphocytes first to the regional lymph nodes and subsequently through the lymphatics to the systemic circulation. Integrin molecules on the surface of mucosal lymphocytes recognize specific homing receptors on endothelial cells lining vessels within the mucosal tissues throughout the body and allow reentry of differentiated lymphocytes and memory cells to these tissues. Within the intestine, specific homing selectins direct lymphocytes to either the lamina propria or the epithelium.

mesenteric lymph nodes, where they continue to expand and differentiate into effector T and B cells. During this maturation within the mesenteric lymph nodes, many B cells undergo further rearrangement of their genomic DNA encoding immunoglobulin, resulting in the replacement of the μ heavy chain gene with the α heavy chain gene, a process known as "class switching." Class switching requires the interaction of helper T cells with the developing B cells and genetic abnormalities. Following maturation, mature T cells and B cells exit the mesenteric lymph nodes, enter the systemic circulation via the thoracic duct, and subsequently reenter the intestinal mucosa (Fig. 3-6).

Nonaggregated Lymphoid Tissue

The majority of gut-associated lymphoid cells exist within the lamina propria of the intestine. Circulating lymphoid cells derived from the mesenteric lymph nodes are selectively targeted to the gastrointestinal mucosal tissues through interactions between ligands expressed on the surface of the lymphocytes and their counter-receptors expressed by endothelial cells in the mucosa.[18–20] Similar homing receptors present on endothelial cells in the mucosa of the lacrimal glands, salivary glands, mammary glands, bronchi, and urogenital tissues permit entry of lymphocytes initially activated and differentiated within the aggregated lymphoid tissues of the gut, thus extending protection to all mucosal surfaces. These endothelial markers are upregulated by inflammatory mediators enabling increased lymphocyte migration into regions of active inflammation. Plasma cells derived from terminally differentiated B lymphocytes are the principal lymphoid cells within the lamina propria and are responsible for the secretion of mucosal antibodies. Mature T lymphocytes exist in several forms in the gut. A small population of differentiated T cells mediate cell-directed cytotoxicity against infected intestinal cells. In contrast to cytotoxic T-cell precursors derived from the spleen or peripheral blood, lamina propria T cells exhibit very restricted cell-mediated cytotoxicity, thus limiting indirect damage to the surrounding tissues.[21] A second population of T cells consists of $CD4^+$ helper cells that regulate cell-mediated immune responses through the secretion of various cytokines.[22] Cytokines derived from these cells not only support T-cell and B-cell functions but also promote the proliferation of mast cells, granulocytes, and macrophages by their effects on bone marrow precursors. In addition, activation of macrophages by T-cell-associated cytokines stimulates granuloma formation in clinical situations associated with poor antigen clearance. A unique population of intestinal T cells consists of intraepithelial lymphocytes (IELs). These T cells, which are predominantly CD8$^+$, migrate between epithelial cells in response to specific cell surface integrins and appear to mediate cytotoxic responses, although their precise role in intestinal defense remains uncertain. Certain diseases such as celiac sprue and parasitic infections are characterized by expansion in the numbers of IELs present in the intestinal villi.[23,24] Interestingly, the IEL compartment in humans also contains small numbers of lymphocytes expressing distinct T-cell receptors ($\gamma\lambda$ T cells). The role of these particular lymphocytes in intestinal immune function is presently the subject of intense investigation.

The Integrated Immune Response

When antigens in the gut lumen reach the surface of the dome of Peyer's patches, they encounter M cells (Fig. 3-6). M cells are characterized by a lack of microvilli, a poorly developed glycocalyx, and an absence of lysosomes. Macromolecules and even entire viral particles may be endocytosed by the M cell and transported intact to the basal membrane, where they are released.[25] These molecules are phagocytosed by dendritic cells and macrophages which then present the processed antigen to naive T cells or memory T cells. This initiates T-cell clonal expansion and differentiation in the lymphoid follicles and mesenteric lymph nodes (Fig. 3-4). Translocated antigen directly stimulates virgin B cells in the lymphoid follicles, and these cells migrate into the germinal centers and undergo clonal proliferation and subsequent Ig class switching with the assistance of cytokines such as IL-4 secreted by helper CD4$^+$ T cells (Fig. 3-6). Terminally differentiated plasma cells then migrate to the lamina propria where high-affinity secretory IgA is produced and transported into the lumen. The generation of significant amounts of secretory IgA as a result of intestinal immune stimulation has made oral vaccination particularly valuable in immunization strategies directed against enteric pathogens such as poliomyelitis and cholera.[26]

In contrast to normal intestinal immunity, disruption of the gastrointestinal barrier by bacterial or viral infection results in the marked activation of both humoral and cellular immune mechanisms.[27] The immediate inflammatory response is effected by mast cells and macrophages, which release inflammatory mediators and chemoattractant factors. Macrophages and dendritic cells also migrate to the mesenteric lymph nodes, where antigenic material derived from the invading microorganisms is presented to lymphocytes. Granulocytes and activated macrophages enter the sites of inflammation, destroy the pathogens, and remove the antigenic debris. Antibodies and cytokines derived from activated lymphocytes potentiate the impact of these effector cells by opsonizing bacteria and eliminating infected cells or parasites. Removal of antigenic stimuli from the site of inflammation normally leads to a downregulation of the immune response as the levels of inflammatory mediators and cytokines are reduced. Epithelial growth factors such as trefoil proteins rapidly restore the epithelial barrier, while secretion of newly derived high-affinity IgA antibodies reduces the antigen load present in the lumen. Within the mucosa itself, cytotoxic T cells directly eliminate effector cells at the conclusion of the immune reaction. Restoration of intestinal mucosal integrity is also accompanied by circulation of memory lymphocytes to other mucosal surfaces. Ineffective clearance of pathogens or a loss in these normal counter-regulatory mechanisms may give rise to persistent intestinal inflammation associated with disease.

References

1. Hermiston ML, Gordon JI. Inflammatory bowel disease and adenomas in mice expressing a dominant negative N-cadherin. *Science*. 1995;270:1203–1207.
2. Umesaki Y, Okada Y, Imaoka A, Setoyama H, Matsumoto S. Interactions between epithelial cells and bacteria, normal and pathogenic. *Science*. 1997;276:964–965.
3. Mahida YR, Rose F, Chan WC. Antimicrobial peptides in the gastrointestinal tract. *Gut*. 1997;41:161–163.
4. Shanahan F. A gut reaction: lymphoepithelial communication in the intestine. *Science*. 1997;275:1897–1898.
5. Wang J, Whetsell M, Klein JR. Local hormone networks and intestinal T cell homeostasis. *Science*. 1997;275:1937–1939.
6. Tlaskalova-Hogenova H, Farre-Castany MA, Stepankova R, et al. The gut as a lymphoepithelial organ: the role of intestinal epithelial cells in mucosal immunity. *Folia Microbiol*. 1995;40:385–391.
7. Fiocchi C. Cytokines and intestinal inflammation. *Transplant Proc*. 1996;28:2442–2443.
8. MacDermott RP. Alterations of the mucosal immune system in inflammatory bowel disease. *J Gastroenterol*. 1996;31:907–916.
9. Strober W, Kelsall B, Fuss I, et al. Reciprocal IFN-gamma and TGF-beta responses regulate the occurrence of mucosal inflammation. *Immunol Today*. 1997;18:61–64.

10. Wallace JL. Cooperative modulation of gastrointestinal mucosal defense by prostaglandins and nitric oxide. *Clin Invest Med*. 1996;19:346–351.
11. Childers NK, Bruce MG, McGhee JR. Molecular mechanisms of immunoglobulin A defense. *Annu Rev Microbiol*. 1989;43:503–536.
12. Tamaru T, Brown WR. IgA antibodies in rat bile inhibit cholera toxin-induced secretion in ileal loops in situ. *Immunology*. 1985;55:579–583.
13. Williams RC, Gibbons RJ. Inhibition of bacterial adherence by secretory immunoglobulin A: a mechanism of antigen disposal. *Science*. 1972;177:697–699.
14. Bienenstock J, Denburg J, Scicchitano R, et al. Role of neuropeptides, nerves, and mast cells in intestinal immunity and physiology. *Monogr Allergy*. 1988;24:134–143.
15. Parkos CA, Colgan SP, Liang TW, et al. CD47 mediates post-adhesive events required for neutrophil migration across polarized intestinal epithelia. *J Cell Biol*. 1996;132:437–450.
16. Gleich GG, Adolphson CR. The eosinophilic leukocyte structure and function. *Adv Immunol*. 1986;39:177–253.
17. Siebers A, Finlay BB. M cells and the pathogenesis of mucosal and systemic infections. *Trends in Microbiol*. 1996;4:22–29.
18. Kantele JM, Arvilommi H, Kontiainen S, et al. Mucosally activated circulating human B cells in diarrhea express homing receptors directing them back to the gut. *Gastroenterology*. 1996;110:1061–1067.
19. Halstensen TS, Lien B, Kilshaw PJ, et al. Distribution of beta 7 integrins in human intestinal mucosa and organized gut-associated lymphoid tissue. *Immunology*. 1996;89:227–237.
20. Huleatt JW, Lefrancois L. Beta 2 integrins and ICAM-1 are involved in establishment of the intestinal mucosal T cell compartment. *Immunity*. 1996;5:263–273.
21. MacDermott R. Isolation and characterization of cytotoxic effector cells and antibody producing cells from human intestine. *Acta Chir Scand*. 1985;525 (suppl): 25–43.
22. Abreu-Martin MT, Targan SR. Regulation of immune responses of the intestinal mucosa. *Crit Rev Immunol*. 1996;16:277–309.
23. Jenkins D, Goodall A, Scott BB. T-lymphocyte populations in normal and coeliac small intestinal mucosa defined by monoclonal antibodies. *Gut*. 1986;27:1330–1332.
24. Halstensen TS, Scott H, Brandtzaeg P. Intraepithelial T cells of TcR g/d$^+$ CD8$^-$ and Vd1/Jd1$^+$ phenotypes are increased in coeliac disease. *Scand J Immunol*. 1989;30: 665–671.
25. Mayer L, So LP, Yio XY, et al. Antigen trafficking in the intestine. *Ann N Y Acad Sci*. 1996;778:28–35.
26. Yamamoto M, Vancott JL, Okahashi N, et al. The role of Th1 and Th2 cells for mucosal IgA responses. *Ann N Y Acad Sci*. 1996;778:64–71.
27. Reyes VE, Ye G, Ogra PL, et al. Antigen presentation of mucosal pathogens: the players and the rules. *Int Arch Allergy Immunol*. 1997;112:103–114.

Part 2

Imaging Techniques

Barium for the Small Bowel
Historical Aspects

Hans Herlinger and Dean D.T. Maglinte

Dante, when ascending the mountain of purgatory, having reached a high terrace, said to his conductor: "All men are delighted to look back."

Chapter Contents

Early Contributors to Small Bowel Radiology
Intubation Studies
Clinical Application
The Small Bowel Meal
Enteroclysis or the Small Bowel Enema
The "Dedicated" Small Bowel Meal
Other Barium-Based Methods
CT Enteroclysis (CT-E)

Early Contributors to Small Bowel Radiology

The application of radiologic techniques to the study of the small intestine began to interest physicians very early in the history of clinical roentgenology. Although most of his work dealt with the "facultas expultrix" of the stomach, Cannon in 1898 also reported on small bowel activity that he had studied fluoroscopically on cats.[1] Rieder, in Germany, using subnitrate of bismuth as contrast medium, reported gross anatomy and function throughout the gastrointestinal tract.[2] Only 6 years after the discovery of X-rays, Williams published the first textbook of clinical roentgenology, which included a consideration of the small intestine in its 658 pages.[3] In 1904, Cannon[4] described the use of barium sulfate in studies that attempted to distinguish functional from mechanical disorders of the stomach and intestine. Hulst described his method of skiagraphy of the stomach and intestine in a report dated 1905.[5] It was not until 1910 when, with the report by Bachem and Günther,[6] the potentially toxic bismuth nitrate was generally replaced by barium sulfate.

Lewis Gregory Cole, a fiery, innovative radiologist and prolific writer on matters gastrointestinal, described the radiographic appearances of the mucosa of the small bowel in 1911[7] and claimed to have been the first to perform systematic serial examinations of the small bowel. The normal anatomy of the small intestine, the distribution of its coils, and the changing appearance of its folds were carefully observed and described by Morse and Cole[8] and by Forssell.[9] Morse and Cole stressed that "roentgenographic examinations must be made at intervals which will show the various parts of the small intestine when they are best filled."

Intubation Studies

Prior to the introduction and clinical acceptance of cholecystography, a diagnosis of gallstones largely depended on the demonstration of crystals in bile aspirated through tubes introduced into the duodenum.[10] Cole,[7] who considered the radiologic demonstration of the duodenum adversely affected by the only intermittent passage of barium through the pylorus, used a modified Einhorn tube with side ports above an inflatable balloon. He introduced the tube into the distal duodenum and inflated its balloon to inject barium to outline an obstructed and distended proximal duodenum. However, the obturation was incomplete and contrast material flowed into the jejunum to give us the first published illustration of a small bowel enema, unintended though it was. Utilization of a duodenal tube to produce air double contrast was first reported by Pribram and Kleiber—a method they called pneumoduodenography.[11] Two years later, Pesquera[12] was the first to report the use of enteroclysis for the diagnosis of tuberculous enteritis. It took another 10 years for larger series of intubation studies of the small bowel to be reported. Ghelew and Mengis[13] infused thorium and water, Gershon-Cohen and Shay[14] barium and air. In a presentation to the Philadelphia

Roentgen Ray Society dated March 2, 1939, Gershon-Cohen included the following remarks, which are valid to the present day: "technique depends upon intubation of the duodenum and has the shortcomings inherent in this procedure. The ease and rapidity in which the entire small intestinal tract may be visualized more than compensates for this handicap. Errors of diagnosis incident upon incomplete filling of the intestines and the poor timing of serial examinations of a progress meal are avoided."

Clinical Application

The diagnosis of tuberculous ileocolitis had generally been the focus of attention of early investigators of the small intestine. In 1929, Soper[15] also described the diagnosis of asymptomatic diverticula, adhesive obstruction, and carcinoma metastases. He claimed to have diagnosed two cases of small bowel adenocarcinoma 20 years before. According to Rigler and Weiner,[16] an abdominal compression device to avoid exposure to the hands by direct radiation was in general use by Holzknecht and the Vienna School of Radiology but was then not available in the United States. The description of regional ileitis by Crohn and his colleagues in 1932[17] greatly increased interest in small bowel radiography. In this connection, Goldfarb, a radiologist associated in practice with Crohn, reported a more standardized method for small bowel radiography.[18] He recognized a variety of small bowel pathologies and organized his findings in a detailed table that included obstruction by several intrinsic and extrinsic lesions, hernias, and inflammatory disease including tuberculosis, Meckel's diverticulitis, and regional ileitis. Goldfarb's work has laid down the basic principles for the understanding of the radiologic features of the inflammatory process subsequently known as Crohn's disease. This early work was developed further by the extensive studies and many classic publications by Marshak.[19]

The Small Bowel Meal

Golden[20] and Pendergrass and his colleagues[21] have made highly significant contributions with their methods for the detailed examination of the jejunum and ileum using barium sulfate USP suspended in water. Both investigators were interested in normal appearances, in morphologic changes in disease, and in small bowel physiology as affected by food, emotions, and systemic disease. According to Golden, optimization of the technique of the examination depended on a radiologist approaching it with interest and care. Golden favored the use of smaller quantities of barium (up to 2 oz in water) to avoid overdistention and overlapping of loops. But Marshak[19] advised using 16 to 20 oz of barium suspension to obtain more complete and continuous filling of loops, thus requiring fewer films yet producing a more sensitive examination.

The introduction of nonflocculating barium suspensions in the 1950s made possible further improvements of examination quality. Ardran and his colleagues[22] were foremost in appreciating the importance of this development, which made it possible to produce greater intestinal mucosal detail. The full potential of the small bowel meal in its clinical diagnostic application was clearly set out by Marshak and Lindner in their classic monograph *Radiology of the Small Intestine*.[23]

Methods to accelerate small bowel transit were also investigated. Earlier reports had recommended the use of ice-cold normal saline to follow the barium mixture[24] or a right lateral recumbent position for patients to achieve more rapid gastric emptying and more uniform filling of the small intestine.[25] Transit-accelerating agents were then introduced. Neostigmine, cholecystokinin, ceruletide, metoclopramide, and the addition of Gastrografin (diatrizoate meglumine; Bristo-Meyers Squibb, Princeton, NJ) to barium suspensions were tested and reported.[26-33]

Enteroclysis or the Small Bowel Enema

The limitations of the oral small bowel meal have been recognized by several investigators. There has long been an awareness of having to choose between an oral method more acceptable to the patient and an intubation method that is less acceptable, yet more likely to be diagnostically rewarding. As mentioned earlier, it was Gershon-Cohen who expressed this dilemma in clearest terms.[14] Several larger series of intubation studies were published in the 1940s and 1950s.[34-38] The introduction of the Bilbao-Dotter tube in 1967 gave radiologists a tube that could be readily maneuvered[39] into the small bowel. However, problems associated with difficulty of reproducing the high quality that can be achieved have restricted the more widespread use of enteroclysis, especially in the United States.

The appearance of Sellink's book *Radiological Atlas of Common Diseases of the Small Bowel* changed the climate for enteroclysis, and its use became widespread.[40] Reflecting the significant influence of Sellink's books and other publications is the fact that, in some parts of Europe, enteroclysis is still known as "the Sellink." On the basis of a method first introduced by Trickey and coworkers,[41] Herlinger[42] described the modified and standardized method of the methylcellulose double-contrast small bowel enema. Enteroclysis was further popularized when the 1979 meeting of the Society of Gastrointestinal Radiologists conferred award paper of the year status to a presentation by Maglinte on the use of enteroclysis in the preoperative diagnosis of Meckel's diverticulum, a heretofore difficult lesion to show by radiography.[43] Nolan, working in Oxford, became a convincing protagonist of the widespread use of single contrast enteroclysis in the United Kingdom.[44]

Modifications of the original Bilbao-Dotter tube further facilitated the small bowel enema technique. Sellink lengthened the tube,[45] Herlinger[42] changed it into an endhole catheter, Nolan[44] decreased its diameter to reduce nasopharyngeal irritation, and Maglinte[46] added a balloon to its tip to reduce duodenogastric reflux. Several modifications of the methylcellulose technique were reported.[47,48] Others preferred the use of air double contrast,[49,50] a method that had been developed and perfected in Japan.[51,52] The response of the small bowel to variations of the infusion flow rate was the theme of Oudkirk's thesis, presented to the University of Leiden.[53] The use of mechanical devices for infusion during enteroclysis has made it possible to measure flow rate and has rendered the examination more reproducible.[54-56]

The "Dedicated" Small Bowel Meal

Differing significantly from the mainly "overhead" film-based standard follow-through method, the "dedicated" meal relies largely on meticulous fluoroscopy and can be regarded an alternative technique to enteroclysis.[57] The importance of this essential difference between the two methods was emphasized by Maglinte, who drew attention to the number of lesions missed by the former technique.[58,59]

Other Barium-Based Methods

Several other techniques have been reported. Miller, refluxing barium from the colon, could produce a good-quality demonstration of much of the small bowel.[60] A more detailed evaluation of the distal ileum was achieved by administering barium orally and introducing air rectally when barium had reached the right side of the colon.[61] Fraser and Preston described the use of orally administered effervescents to follow the ingestion of barium and to produce a transradiant pattern in the small bowel.[62]

CT Enteroclysis (CT-E)

A number of centers are evaluating the enteroclysis-like effect of CT following naso- or orojejunal intubation and infusion of water-soluble contrast as described by Bender et al.[63] Others are also using a diluted barium suspension or methylcellulose solution.

References

1. Cannon WB. The movements of the stomach studied by means of the roentgen rays. *Am J Physiol*. 1898;1:369–382.
2. Rieder H. Radiologische Untersuchungen des Magens und Darmens beim lebenden Menschen. *München Med Wschr*. 1904;51:1548.
3. Williams FH. *The Roentgen Rays in Medicine and Surgery*. New York, NY: Macmillan Publishing Co; 1901.
4. Cannon WB. The passage of different food-stuffs from the stomach and through the small intestine. *Am J Physiol*. 1904;12:387–418.
5. Hulst H. Skiagraphy of the stomach and intestines. *Physicians and Surgeons* (Detroit and Ann Arbor) 1905; 77:391–411.
6. Bachem C, Günther H. Barium sulfate as a shadow-forming contrast agent in röntgenologic examinations. *Zeitschrift f Röntg*. 1910;12:369–376.
7. Cole LG. Artificial dilatation of the duodenum for radiographic examination. *AJR*. 1911;3:204.
8. Morse RW, Cole LG. The anatomy of the normal small intestine as observed roentgenographically. *Radiology*. 1927;8:149.
9. Forssel G. Studies of the mechanism of movement of the mucous membrane of the digestive tract. *AJR*. 1923;10:81.
10. Einhorn M. *The Duodenal Tube and Its Possibilities*. 2nd ed. Philadelphia, Pa: FA Davis Co; 1926.
11. Pribram BO, Kleiber N. Ein neuer Weg zur röntgenologischen Darstellung des Duodenums (Pneumo-duodenum). *Forstschr Geb Röntgenstr*. 1927;36:739.
12. Pesquera GS. Method for direct visualization of lesions in the small intestine. *AJR*. 1929;22:254–257.
13. Ghelew B, Mengis O. Mise en evidence de l'intestin grêle par une nouvelle technique radiologique. *Presse Med*. 1938;46:444–445.
14. Gershon-Cohen J, Shay H. Barium enteroclysis method

for direct immediate examination of the small intestine by single and double contrast technique. *AJR*. 1939;42: 456–458.
15. Soper HW. Carcinoma and other lesions of the small bowel. *JAMA*. 1929;92:286–291.
16. Rigler LG, Weiner M. History of roentgenology of the gastrointestinal tract. In: Margulis AR, Burhenne AJ, eds. *Alimentary Tract Roentgenology*. 2nd ed. St. Louis, Mo: CV Mosby Co; 1973:14–15.
17. Crohn BB, Ginzburg L, Oppenheimer GD. Regional ileitis: a pathological and clinical entity. *JAMA*. 1932;99:1323–1328.
18. Goldfarb SJ. Roentgen diagnosis of lesions of the small intestine. *NY State J Med*. 1934;34:500–505.
19. Marshak RH, Wolf BS. Chronic ulcerative granulomatous jejunitis and ileojejunitis. *AJR*. 1953;70:93–112.
20. Golden R. The small intestine and diarrhea. *AJR*. 1936;36:892–901.
21. Pendergrass EP, Ravdin IS, Johnston CB, Hodes PJ. Studies of the small intestine: the effect of foods and various pathological states on the gastric emptying and the small intestinal pattern. *Radiology*. 1936;26:651–662.
22. Ardran GM, French JM, Mucklow EH. Relationship of the nature of the opaque medium to small intestine radiograph pattern. *Br J Radiol*. 1950;23:697–702.
23. Marshak RH, Lindner AE. *Radiology of the Small Intestine*. Philadelphia, Pa: WB Saunders Co; 1970.
24. Weintraub S, Williams RG. A rapid method of roentgenologic examination of the small intestine. *AJR*. 1949;61:45–55.
25. Nice CM. Roentgenographic pattern and motility in small bowel studies. *Radiology*. 1963;80:39–45.
26. Howarth FH, Cockel R, Roper BW, Hawkins CF. The effect of metoclopramide upon gastric motility and its value in barium progress meals. *Clin Radiol*. 1969;20: 294–300.
27. Kreel L. The use of oral metoclopramide in the barium meal and follow-through examination. *Br J Radiol*. 1970;43:31–35.
28. Parker JG, Beneventano TC. Acceleration of the small bowel contrast study by cholecystokinin. *Gastroenterology*. 1970;58:679–684.
29. Rosenquist CJ. Methods of acceleration of small intestinal radiographic examination. *West J Med*. 1975;122:320.
30. Kreel L. Pharmacoradiology in barium examination with special reference to glucagon. *Br J Radiol*. 1975;48:691–703.
31. Efsing Ho, Lindroth B. Small bowel examination after injection of cholecystokinin. *Clin Radiol*. 1980;31:225–226.
32. Novak D. Acceleration of the small intestine contrast study by ceruletide. *Gastrointest Radiol*. 1980;5:61–65.
33. Robbins AH, Wetzner SM, Landy MD. Ceruletide-assisted examination of the small bowel. *AJR*. 1980;134: 343–347.
34. Schatzki R. Small bowel enema. *AJR*. 1943;50:743–751.
35. Lura, A. Radiology of the small intestine. IV. Enema of the small intestine with special emphasis on the diagnosis of tumors. *Br J Radiol*. 1951;24:264–270.
36. Pygott F, Street DF, Schellshear MF, Rhodes CJ. Radiological investigation of the small intestine by small bowel enema technique. *Gut*. 1960;1:366–370.
37. Wissenberg P. Rontgenundersogelse af tyndtarm efter indhaeldning af knotrast gennem duodenalsonde. *Mord Med*. 1942;16:3433–3436.
38. Scott-Harden WG. Examination of the small bowel. In: McLaren JW, ed. *Modern Trends in Diagnostic Radiology*. London, England: Butterworth; 1960:84–87.
39. Bilbao MK, Firsche LH, Dotter CT, Roesch J. Hypotonic duodenography. *Radiology*. 1967;89:438–443.
40. Sellink JL. *Radiological Atlas of Common Diseases of the Small Bowel*. Leiden, the Netherlands: HE Stenfert Kroese BV; 1976.
41. Trickey SE, Halls J, Hodson CJ. A further development of the small bowel enema. *J Roy Soc Med*. 1963;56: 1070–1073.
42. Herlinger H. A modified technique for the double contrast small bowel enema. *Gastrointest Radiol*. 1978;3: 201–207.
43. Maglinte DD, Elmore MF, Isenberg M, Dolan PA. Meckel diverticulum radiologic demonstration by enteroclysis. *AJR*. 1980;134:925–932.
44. Nolan DJ. *Radiological Atlas of Gastrointestinal Disease*. New York, NY: John Wiley & Sons; 1984.
45. Sellink JL. *Examination of the Small Bowel by Means of Duodenal Intubation*. Leiden, the Netherlands: HE Stenfert Kroese BV; 1971.
46. Maglinte DDT. Balloon enteroclysis catheter. *AJR*. 1984;143:761–762.
47. Antes G, Lissner S. Double contrast small bowel examination with barium and methylcellulose: results in 300 cases. *Radiology*. 1983;148:37–40.
48. Maglinte DDT, Miller RE, Lappas JC, et al. The biphasic enteroclysis. *Appl Radiol*. 1985;14:39–44.
49. Ekberg O. Double contrast examination of the small bowel. *Gastrointest Radiol*. 1977;1:349–353.
50. Pajewski M, Eschar J, Manor A. Visualization of the small intestine by double contrast. *Clin Radiol*. 1975;26: 491–493.
51. Nakamur Y, et al. X-ray examination of the small intestine by means of duodenal intubation—double contrast study of the small bowel. *Stom Intest*. 1974;9:1461–1469.
52. Kobayashi N. X-ray examination of the small intestine—double contrast methods by duodenal intubation. *Stom Intest*. 1976;11:157–165.
53. Oudkirk M. *Infusion Rate in Enteroclysis Examination*. Leiden, the Netherlands: Leiden University; 1981. Thesis.
54. Maglinte DDT, Burney FT, Miller RE. Technical factors for a more rapid enteroclysis. *AJR*. 1982;138:558–591.
55. Abu-Yousef NM, Benson CA, Lu CH, Franken EA. Enteroclysis aided by an electric pump. *Radiology*. 1983;147:268–269.
56. Maglinte DDT, Miller RE. A comparison of pumps used for enteroclysis. *Radiology*. 1984;152:815.
57. Herlinger H, Lintott DJ. Standard examination of the small bowel. In: Margulis AR, Burhenne HJ, eds. *Alimentary Tract Radiology*. 3rd ed. St. Louis, Mo: CV Mosby Co; 1983:907–914.
58. Maglinte DDT, Burney BT, Miller RE. Lesions missed on

small bowel follow-through: analysis and recommendations. *Radiology.* 1982;144:737–739.
59. Maglinte DDT, Lappas JC, Kelvin FM, Chernish SM. Small bowel radiography: how, when and why? *Radiology.* 1987;163:297–305.
60. Miller RE. Complete reflux small bowel examination. *Radiology.* 1965;84:457–463.
61. Kellett MJ, Zboralske FF, Margulis AR. Per oral pneumocolon examination of the ileocecal region. *Gastrointest Radiol.* 1977;1:361–365.
62. Fraser GM, Preston PG. The small bowel barium follow-through enhanced with an oral effervescent agent. *Clin Radiol.* 1983;34:673–679.
63. Bender GN, Timmons JH, Williard WC, Carter J. Computed tomographic enteroclysis: one methodology. *Invest Radiol.* 1996;31:43–49.

Plain Film Radiography of the Small Bowel

5

Dean D.T. Maglinte and Hans Herlinger

Chapter Contents

Relevance of Plain Abdominal Radiography
Technical Considerations
Essentials of Interpretation
Normal Intestinal Gas Pattern
Distribution of Small Bowel Gas in Obstruction
Level of Small Bowel Obstruction
Significance of Specific Plain Film Intestinal Patterns
Plain Film Determination of Severity of Obstruction
Plain Film Findings in Strangulating Obstruction
Small Bowel in the Immediate Postoperative Period
Pneumoperitoneum Secondary to Small Bowel Perforation
Pneumatosis Cystoides Intestinalis
Enterolithiasis
Foreign Bodies in the Small Bowel

Relevance of Plain Abdominal Radiography

In spite of advances in imaging, plain film examination has remained the first radiologic investigation to follow clinical evaluation of acute abdominal diseases, particularly those presenting with possible obstruction.[1] It is readily available, noninvasive, and inexpensive, and requires only a low level of patient cooperation.[2] Although a specific and correct interpretation may be difficult at times, sufficiently useful information is frequently obtained that influences the sequencing of subsequent imaging investigations. Plain film examination can be most useful in patients suspected of having bowel obstruction, perforation, ischemia, or biliary or urinary calculi, or those with significant abdominal tenderness. It is least contributory as a screening study in patients with mild or nonspecific symptoms.[3,4] Unfortunately, although it has a modest sensitivity in some acute abdominal conditions (ie, obstruction or perforation), it has a low specificity. Low grades of obstruction or perforation with small amount of gas are not ruled out by abdominal plain films. Interpretation of the plain films is strongly influenced by the experience and perceptiveness of the observer.[5] Since symptoms of small bowel disease are often intermittent, information is more likely to be obtained when the examination is done during a symptomatic period. Occasionally, the radiologic findings may be those of an acute abdomen even though the clinical presentation is indeterminate. Inversely, clinical signs may be severe yet the radiographic findings uncertain.[6]

Imaging modalities (ultrasound, CT, and MRI) are adjuncts to plain film radiography, particularly in patients with small bowel obstruction. A carefully taken history and physical examination remain the mainstay in the evaluation of the acute abdomen. Currently there is lack of agreement whether unenhanced helical CT, ultrasound, or plain film radiography should be the initial radiologic study in patients who present with acute abdominal pain.[7,8] Economic considerations and local expertise will be significant factors in influencing decision making.

This chapter will describe basic principles of interpretation of normal and abnormal intestinal gas patterns, and the role of the plain film as diagnostic triage in patients with suspected intestinal obstruction.

Technical Considerations

Intubation and suction are widely used in acute abdominal disorders, especially in small bowel obstruction. Whenever possible, suction should be avoided before plain film examination, as it may eliminate important diagnostic clues. If a tube has already been introduced, the radiologist should be informed of the approximate amount of any fluid aspirated. The urinary bladder should be emptied before the examination, since a distended bladder may be mistaken for fluid in the pelvis or for fluid-filled loops of small bowel.

The *acute abdominal series* for patients with possible small bowel obstruction or visceral perforation should consist of a supine and an erect abdominal radiograph and an erect chest film, and these should be done in this sequence to promote the rise of gas to the diaphragm. In critically ill or immobile patients the series should comprise a supine abdomen, a left lateral decubitus view of the abdomen, and a supine view of the chest.[6,7] In such cases, it may further promote the rise of gas to keep the patient in left lateral decubitus position for several minutes before proceeding to the chest film. Prolonged left lateral decubitus positioning may allow gas to rise out of the lesser sac to increase the accumulation beneath the iliac crest or over the right margin of the liver.[9] Collimated, low kilovoltage films will improve the visualization of free air or of gas in abscesses, pneumatosis intestinalis, and the biliary or portal tracts (Fig. 5-1). It is important that the abdominal radiograph include the inferior pubic rami, as some important etiologic clues may be detected there (Fig. 5-2). Assessment of the diaphragmatic regions is optimally done by the chest radiograph.

The *supine anteroposterior radiograph* of the abdomen is the mainstay in the plain film examination for small bowel disorders. Assessment of the series should start with the supine abdominal radiograph. It has been claimed to permit the diagnosis of most acute abdominal conditions.[9,10] The supine film allows gas distribution and caliber of bowel loops to be determined and will show soft tissue masses (Fig. 5-3). Subtle signs of free intraperitoneal gas are also diagnosed in this view (see section on pneumoperitoneum secondary to small bowel perforation). Normal fat lines can be identified and, if found obliterated, may indicate the presence of fluid or inflammatory exudate. With correct interpretation of the supine abdominal radiograph, the erect radiograph only rarely adds materially to the diagnosis.

The *erect abdominal radiograph*, however, can increase confidence in the diagnosis of intra-abdominal pathology, especially important to the less experienced observer. Frimann-Dahl believed that the upright or lateral decubitus film can give a clearer evidence of an abnormality and, in a few cases of obstruction, that the results of a supine film may be completely negative, whereas the erect film may be diagnostic.[6] Although some reports have claimed that the erect abdominal radiograph made no contribution to the management of many patients with acute abdominal conditions,[10,11] this view (or the left lateral decubitus radiograph) is helpful in patients with suspected bowel obstruction, mainly to assess the proportion of gas and fluid in the distended small bowel (Fig. 5-4).[12] On a supine abdominal radiograph when the small bowel contains an increase of intraluminal fluid, the valvulae conniventes may appear falsely thickened. The true width of the walls and thickness of the valvulae are accurately evaluated by the upright radiograph.[7] Findings in the upright and decubitus views have been able to distinguish high-grade or complete from low-grade obstruction.[13] Both abdominal plain films are, therefore, important to serve the triage to additional radiological work-up of patients with suspected small bowel obstruction.

The *chest radiograph* is an important part of the acute abdominal series because of the frequency with which active chest disease can simulate abdominal conditions.[14] The erect posteroanterior (PA) chest radiograph is also the best position to show the presence of a small pneumoperitoneum. Small gas collections between the liver and diaphragm are penetrated obliquely by the divergent X-ray beam of an erect abdominal radiograph but are projected in an almost true tangent on a chest film. It was shown in a recent report that the lateral chest radiograph could allow visualization of subdiaphragmatic free air that was not identified in the frontal view.[15] This finding is most likely to occur if air localizes in a more anterior or medial position and cannot rise over the liver or the gastric fundus, possibly owing to adhesions from prior inflammation or surgery. The central X-ray beam of the anteroposterior (AP) or PA erect film may then cross the long axis of the air collection. In the lateral projection, the central beam may pass through the length of the collection, thus increasing its density dif-

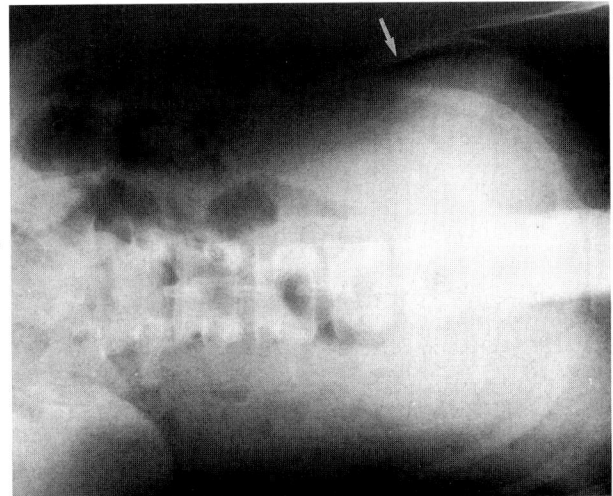

Fig. 5-1. Free air secondary to small bowel perforation (arrow) demonstrated by low kilovoltage radiography in the left lateral decubitus position.
The lateral edge of the liver and the lateral abdominal wall should be clearly shown on this view.

Fig. 5-2. Inferior pubic rami as lower anatomical boundary for positioning in abdominal radiography.
(a) Note gas (arrowhead) superimposed on right obturator foramen, allowing early diagnosis of incarcerated obturator hernia in an elderly female with abdominal pain. Mild to moderate small bowel dilatation is present. Gas is still seen in the cecum (C). (b) Increased soft tissue density and gas (arrowhead) are noted superimposed below inferior ramus of right pubic bone in another patient with right inguinal hernia who presented with lower abdominal pain.

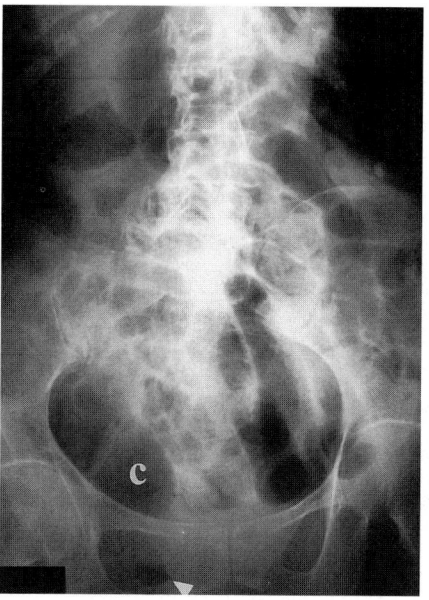
(a)

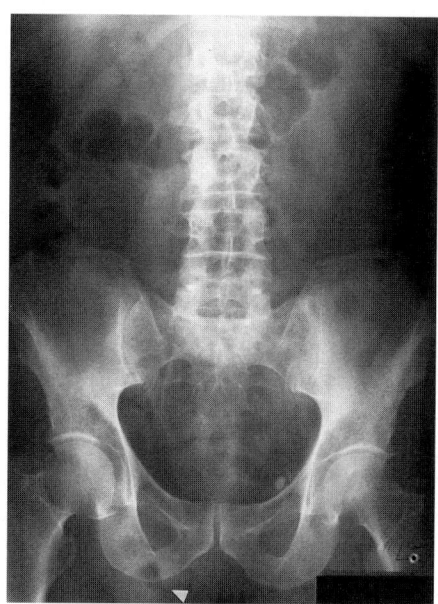
(b)

ference against superimposed soft tissue. A lateral chest radiograph should therefore be added when uncertainty exists over the presence of free air in either the erect chest or the erect abdominal radiograph (Fig. 5-5).

Pleural effusion following abdominal surgery is likely to be due to a subphrenic abscess and is better demonstrated on chest X-rays.[16] Particularly in elderly patients, an acute abdomen may be complicated by cardiac failure or aspiration into bronchi.

The *left lateral decubitus film* needs to be distinguished from the *left lateral view of the abdomen*. In both these views the patient lies on his or her left side. However, the former projection has been found more

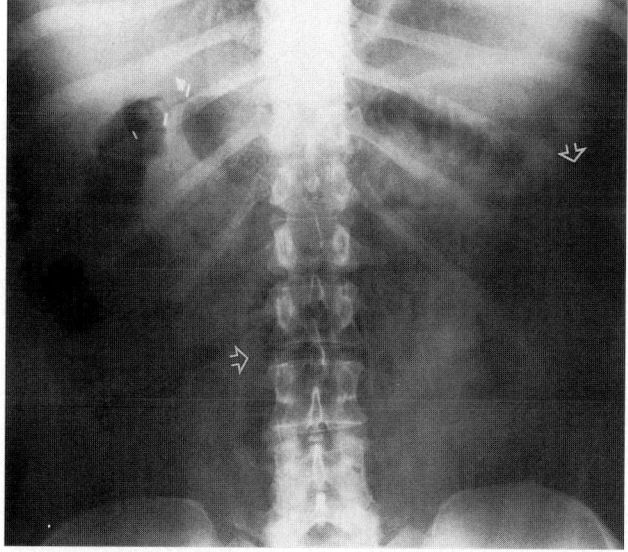
(a)

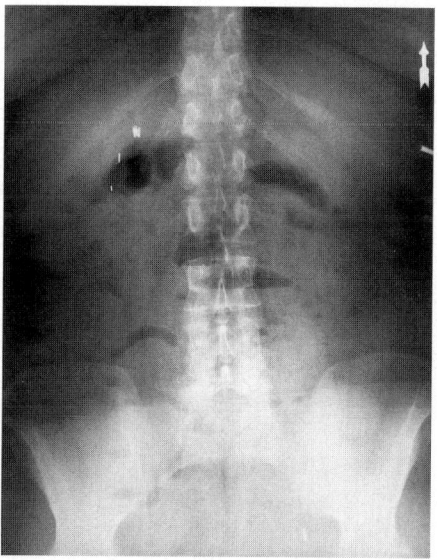
(b)

Fig. 5-3. Value of erect abdominal radiography in suspected small bowel obstruction.
(a) Supine abdominal radiograph shows fluid-filled loops of small bowel in mid and left hemiabdomen (arrows), which may be subtle to less experienced observers. (b) Upright radiograph allows confident diagnosis of predominantly fluid-filled loops of small bowel in obese patient found at surgery to have tight adhesive band obstruction in distal small bowel.

50 • 5. Plain Film Radiography of the Small Bowel

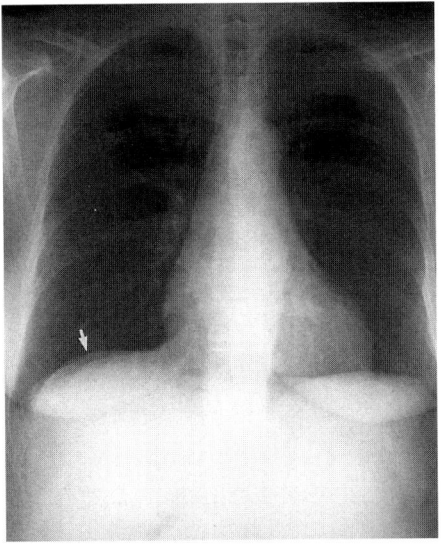

(a)

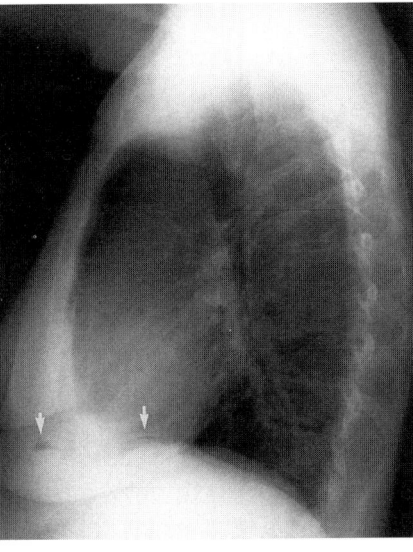

(b)

Fig. 5-4. Value of erect lateral chest radiograph for demonstration of subtle pneumoperitoneum.
(a) Posteroanterior chest radiograph shows questionable subdiaphragmatic lucency on right side (arrow) in patient with unremarkable abdominal radiographs. (b) Lateral chest radiograph shows small subdiaphragmatic gas collection (arrows) unequivocal for free air. Surgery disclosed perforated small bowel from impacted chicken bone in the distal ileum.

accurate in demonstrating free gas than an erect chest film (96% versus 85%)[17] and will also optimally demonstrate gas from a gastroduodenal perforation, or a gas-filled, distended duodenal loop in acute pancreatitis or cholecystitis.[7] The *left lateral abdomen view*, on the other hand, which is obtained with the vertical X-ray beam traversing the lateral dimension of the abdomen, is primarily centered on the rectum. It

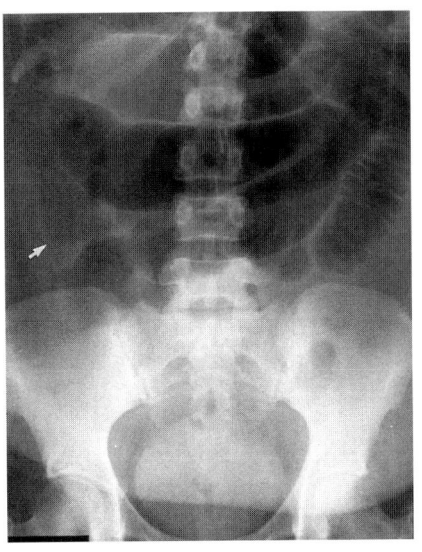

(a)

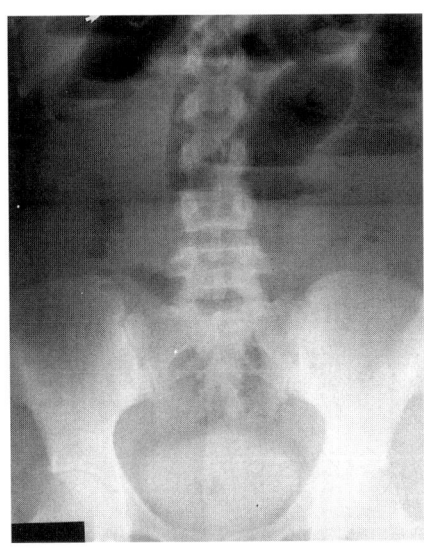

(b)

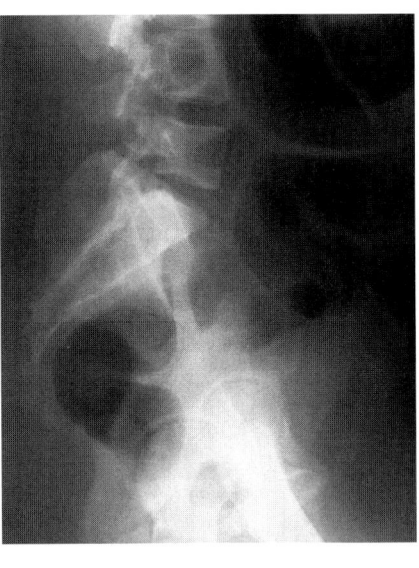

(c)

Fig. 5-5. The left lateral abdomen projection in the differentiation of nonobstructive ileus from distal colonic obstruction.
(a) Supine abdominal radiograph 9 days following hysterectomy, bilateral salpingo-oophorectomy, and lysis of pelvic adhesions shows marked dilatation of small bowel with gas and fluid in ascending colon (arrow) but no appreciable gas in sigmoid. A small amount of gas is seen in rectal ampulla. (b) Upright radiograph shows air-fluid levels in markedly distended small bowel. Note small amount of gas showing interhaustral fold in hepatic flexure (arrow). The pattern could easily be misinterpreted as postoperative small bowel obstruction. (c) A lateral abdominal radiograph exposed after 5 minutes with the patient in the left lateral position shows gas in the rectosigmoid, allowing for a confident diagnosis of severe postoperative ileus. The findings resolved with long tube and rectal tube decompression.

is an additional useful projection when there is difficulty in differentiating a distal colonic obstruction from adynamic neuromuscular dysfunction or pseudo-obstruction indicated on prior supine and erect views.[18] This important position allows air to fill the rectosigmoid, indicating absence of obstruction (Fig. 5-6). The left lateral abdomen view is technically easier to perform than the left lateral decubitus view. It is the simplest and most helpful plain film view for differentiation of distal colonic obstruction from nonobstructing ileus. Immediate addition of this view to the full abdominal series in a suitable setting can prevent needless performance of contrast enemas or computerized tomography to confirm a diagnosis of postoperative or nonobstructive colonic ileus.

Abdominal radiographs required for acute abdominal disorders should be obtained in the X-ray department whenever possible, as portable radiographs are of lower quality. Portable abdominal radiographs suffice, however, for assessing the position of tubes and catheters.

The acute abdominal series should be monitored by a radiologist for adequacy of technique and for the possible and immediate need for additional views to clarify questionable observations. Prompt interpretation of findings is desirable.

Essentials of Interpretation

In the plain film interpretation of intestinal disorders, a systematic approach to the sequence of anatomical assessment should be adopted to obtain the maximum diagnostic information. In the patient with an acute abdomen, the intestinal gas pattern in general should be assessed first. This is followed by a search for extraluminal gas and the evaluation of the chest radiograph. Any abnormal gas collection or distribution should be explained. The soft tissue structures of the peritoneal cavity, retroperitoneum, pelvis, and abdominal wall are then analyzed, and a search for extraluminal fluid collections should be done. A search for abdominal calcifications and assessment of the visible bone structures completes the plain film examination. When digital radiographic systems are used, the different structures assessed should be highlighted appropriately.

The most useful natural contrast material for the gastrointestinal tract is its gas content. The presence of

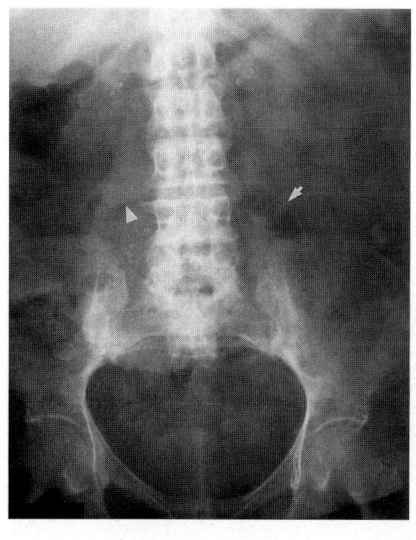
(a)

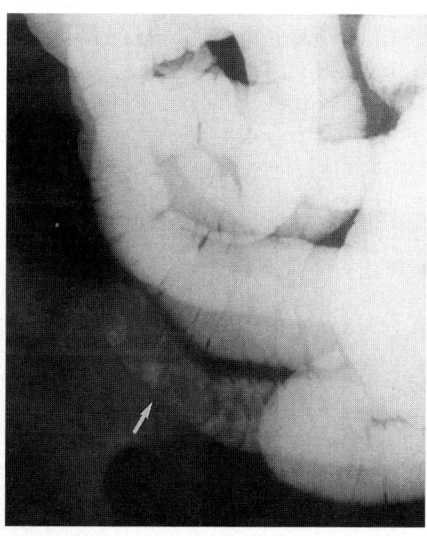
(b)

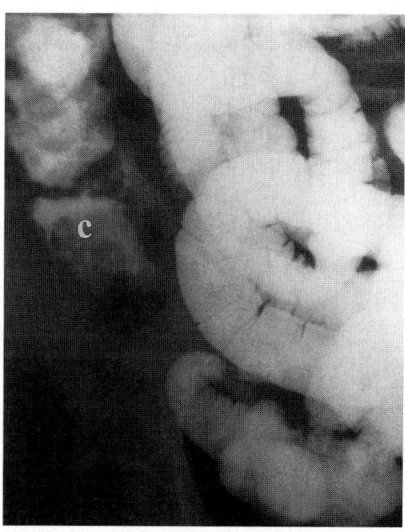
(c)

Fig. 5-6. Stasis of gas in small bowel secondary to medication-related decrease of intestinal peristalsis. The patient was on antidepressants and analgesics.
(a) Supine abdominal radiograph of a 66-year-old obese chronic renal patient with a history of a recent ventral herniorrhaphy who presented with intermittent abdominal pain, nausea, and vomiting suspicious for intestinal obstruction. A few scattered nondistended small bowel loops are noted (arrow). The ends of the gas-filled loops are tapered. Note fluid-filled nondistended (arrowhead) small bowel. (b) Early enteroclysis radiograph shows retained food material in distal ileum (arrow). (c) Late enteroclysis radiograph shows the retained debris in the distal ileum pushed to the right colon and the absence of mechanical obstruction. (C = cecum).

fat in the subcutaneous tissue, mesentery, retroperitoneum, and pelvis permits the recognition of the outline of soft tissue structures in the peritoneal and retroperitoneal areas. The demonstration of the different structures contained in the abdominal radiograph is aided by differential attenuation of the X-ray beam in the patient. The reader is referred to recent descriptions of normal abdominal plain film anatomy, soft tissue abnormalities, and calcifications.[19–21]. A thorough knowledge of these subjects together with an understanding of the significance of the various intestinal gas patterns is important for a comprehensive interpretation of the plain film of the abdomen.

Normal Intestinal Gas Pattern

Gas in the intestines comes from three sources: swallowed air, bacterial synthesis, and diffusion from blood.[22] Most of the bowel gas is the result of swallowed air, predominantly nitrogen. Gas derived from the various secretions in the course of the digestive process is mostly carbon dioxide, which remains in solution and is absorbed into the bloodstream. Additional gas, particularly in the colon, is formed by the action of other bacteria. Extraneous gases and nitrogen are not readily absorbed and may persist for a considerable time in the lumen of the gastrointestinal tract. In most normal adults, the transit time through the small bowel is sufficiently rapid to prevent swallowed air from accumulating in small bowel loops, so that these loops are usually barely visible on plain films. Any larger amount of gas in the mesenteric segment of the small bowel needs to be explained.

The distribution of gas in the intestinal tract is determined by the patient's position and the quantity of intestinal gas present. In normal adults the intestinal tract usually contains less than 200 ml of gas. In the supine position swallowed air reaches the body and antrum of the stomach and, pyloric sphincter permitting, usually continues into the small bowel. Gas tends to accumulate in anteriorly placed segments of intestine (jejunum rather than ileum), but more often the transverse and sigmoid colon. Gas is also frequently found in the rectum (Fig. 5-3). Should exit of fluid and gas be restricted, their accumulation is more likely to occur in the stomach and the colon.

It is common to see within the length of the small bowel many small, irregularly shaped collections of gas distributed apparently at random, particularly in more nervous patients who swallow air. Almost all recumbent patients, particularly those with abdominal pain, swallow air that progresses through the bowel to reach the colon. Gas is usually present in the small intestine of hospitalized patients who have no gastrointestinal pathology. Decreased intestinal peristalsis as a result of medications, bed rest, or changed eating patterns is common in hospitalized patients who may then show moderate amounts of fluid and air in normal small bowel. Gas-filled small bowel segments, usually tapered at both ends, are seen in nonobstructed patients under these circumstances (Fig. 5-7). The caliber of the normal small bowel is rarely above 2.5 cm, and the nondistended valvulae conniventes, when seen, appear relatively thick.

The observations of Frimann-Dahl on the pertinence of air-fluid levels to distinguish ileus from mechanical obstruction were not borne out in later literature. Many studies have demonstrated the relative nonspecificity and insensitivity of these signs.[23,24] Air-fluid levels should be recognized as an abnormal finding that can accompany an adynamic ileus or a mechanical obstruction. A more recent study has shown that the presence of differential air-fluid levels together with a mean air-fluid level width greater than 25 mm is predictive of a higher grade of small bowel obstruction, information of value in the additional work-up of such patients.[13]

However, there are many causes for the presence of small bowel fluid levels; their number, distribution, and length will not always help to distinguish obstruction from paralytic ileus. Air and fluid levels (usually less than 2.5 cm in width) are also seen in normal patients following the administration of cleansing enemas or ingestion of cathartics or carbonated beverages, and in patients with gastroenteritis, hypokalemia, uremia, mesenteric thrombosis, jejunal diverticulosis, and peritoneal irritation (Fig. 5-8). This

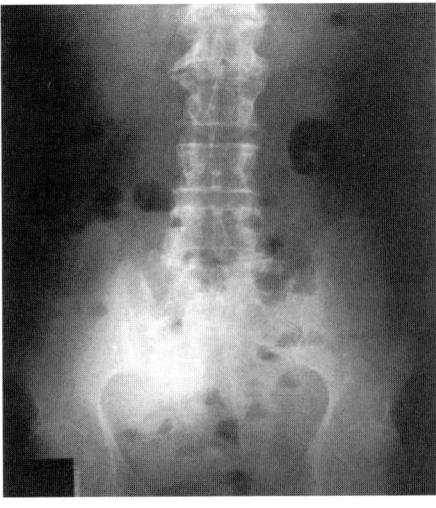

Fig. 5-7. Multiple short air-fluid levels in nondilated small bowel loops in a patient with acute gastroenteritis.

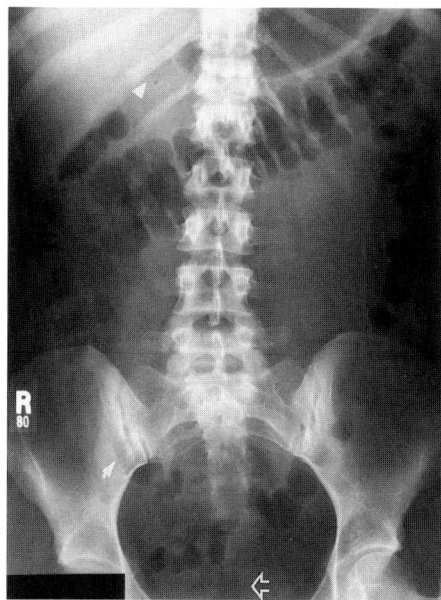

Fig. 5-8. Normal intestinal gas distribution.
Gas outlines stomach and colon of normal caliber. Except for a small amount of gas in nondistended duodenal cap (arrowhead) and distal ileum (arrow) there is no gas in the small bowel. Interhaustral folds are apparent in the transverse colon. A small amount of gas is present in the rectal vault (open arrow). Inherent contrast provided by fat allows delineation of soft tissue planes.

pattern had been labeled "hyperdynamic ileus" in the past,[6] a contradictory term. Small bowel stasis appears to be an appropriate and noncommittal term.[2,25]

The ability to distinguish gas- and fluid-containing loops of small bowel from loops of large intestine is fundamental to the analysis of abdominal films. This distinction is made by their location and anatomic features. Demonstration of the valvulae conniventes, which are seen as circular white lines running across the gas-distended lumen, is a reliable means of identifying small intestine. Gas-filled ileal loops usually have no detectable valvulae. Enough gas is usually present in peripherally located parts of the colon for haustra to be identified. The presence of fecal material further identifies it as a colonic segment [Fig. 5-6(b)]. The sigmoid colon is often devoid of haustration and tends to share its position with that of the ileum; therefore, differentiation may occasionally be difficult.

The haustra of the colon tend to be 2 to 3 mm wide and occur at intervals of 2 to 3 cm, whereas the circular folds of the small bowel are 1 to 2 mm in width and are 1 to 3 mm apart. The extension of folds across the entire width of the bowel lumen may not be a helpful point of distinction. The locations of the loops can be more important distinguishing features. The caliber of the normal colon varies from 3 to 8 cm, with the largest diameter found in the cecum. The normal small bowel width should not exceed 2.5 cm on plain films.

Distribution of Small Bowel Gas in Obstruction

Interobserver Variations

The interpretation of intestinal gas patterns in patients with small bowel obstruction varies considerably.[26] The lack of a definition of various terms used in describing these gas patterns has caused interpretive confusion affecting clinical significance. The term "nonspecific abdominal gas pattern" has entered the clinical and radiologic literature without any hint of its precise meaning. Emergency physicians frequently use the term "nonspecific abdominal gas pattern" in their preliminary interpretations when, in fact, they mean that the bowel gas pattern is normal.[5] A recent survey of community-based teaching hospital radiologists showed that 70% of the radiologists used this term;[27] 65% of these radiologists considered this to mean "normal or probably normal," 22% defined it as "cannot tell if normal or abnormal," and 13% thought the term to imply "abnormal but cannot tell if due to mechanical obstruction or adynamic ileus." Of the referring physicians who received the report in the same survey, 44% thought it to mean "normal," 51% "normal or abnormal," and 5% "abnormal, representing either mechanical obstruction or adynamic ileus." Some did not know what the term meant. Although several communications have called for the abandonment of the term "nonspecific abdominal gas pattern,"[9,27,28] the term continues to be used. A recent editorial[29] has suggested that the use of this term continues because an intestinal gas pattern exists that is neither normal nor fits the categories of probably or definitely obstructed.[30] Gammill and Nice considered this pattern to mean ileus, the small bowel being unable to push fluid along.[25] Indeed, the word "ileus" means stasis and does not differentiate between mechanical and nonmechanical causes. We suggest that the terms "small bowel stasis" or "abnormal but nonspecific," when used, be followed by a recommendation for further radiologic work-up, including a repeat plain film of the abdomen after 24 hours.

Definition of the Gas Patterns

To prevent imprecise or poorly understood reports of plain film examinations, a definition of the various intestinal gas patterns is an essential requirement.[29,30] 1) *Normal intestinal gas pattern* is defined as either an absence of small intestinal gas (without abnormal increase in abdominal density or loss of soft tissue planes) or the presence of gas in up to four variably shaped small intestinal loops that measure less than 2.5 cm in diameter. In addition, there should be a normal gas and/or fecal distribution in a nondistended colon (Fig. 5-8). 2) *Mild small bowel stasis* (an abnormal but nonspecific pattern) should describe images with

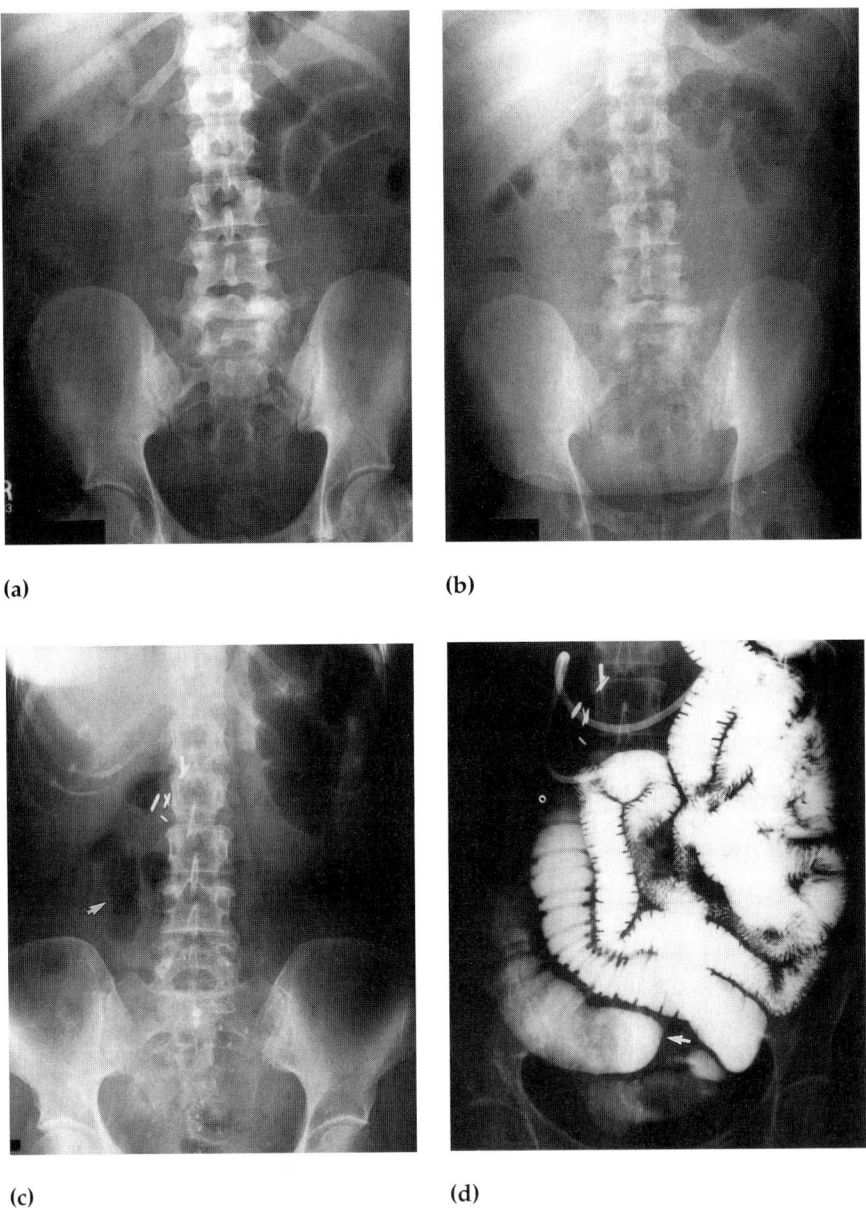

Fig. 5-9. **Small bowel stasis or abnormal but nonspecific small intestinal gas patterns: variable causes.**
(a/b) Supine and upright (b) abdominal radiograph in a patient with abdominal and back pain show slightly dilated loops of small bowel with air-fluid levels. Subsequent urography showed right hydronephrosis due to a calculus at the ureterovesical junction. The abnormal bowel gas pattern represented focal small bowel stasis secondary to renal colic. (c) Supine abdominal radiograph of a patient with acute abdominal pain and distention shows slightly dilated gas-filled small bowel in right hemiabdomen (arrow). Comparison of psoas margins suggests slight increase of density on the right due to fluid-filled loops. No upright radiograph was obtained. (d) Enteroclysis done the next day shows high-grade partial adhesive band obstruction in a pelvic segment of ileum (arrow); confirmed at surgery.

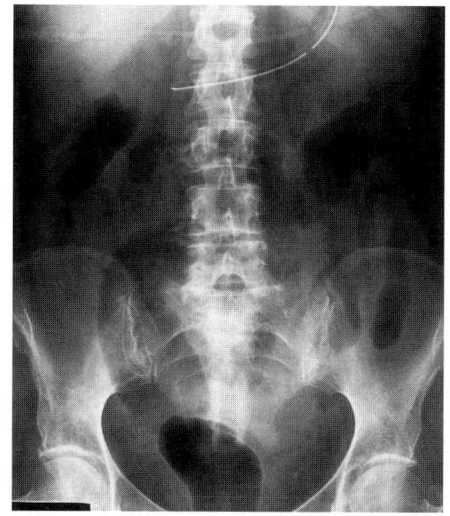 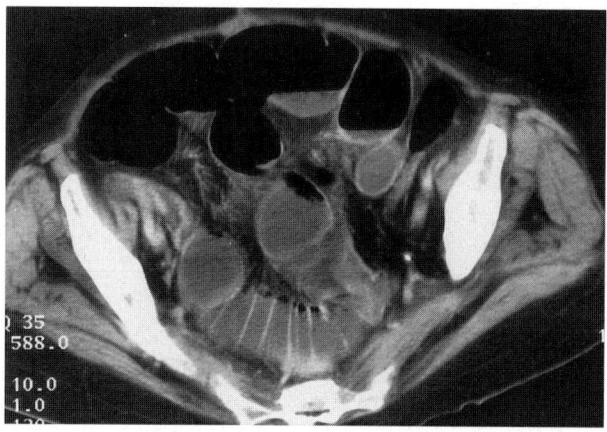

Fig. 5-10. Probable small bowel obstruction pattern.
(a) Supine abdominal radiograph in a middle-aged female with a history of prior surgery for colon malignancy who presented with acute abdominal pain shows moderate gaseous distention of multiple loop of small bowel with gas still present in multiple segments of colon. Nasogastric tube was introduced because of vomiting. (b) CT performed shows findings consistent with distal mechanical small bowel obstruction. No mass was noted. Surgery confirmed adhesive obstruction.

single or multiple loops of borderline or slightly dilated small intestine (2.5 to 3 cm in diameter) and with three or more air/fluid levels on upright or decubitus films. There should be no disproportionate distention of the small intestine relative to the gas- or feces-containing colon. Some of the patients in this category have low-grade obstruction and are difficult to diagnose clinically. Others may have reflex or reactive ileus secondary to a variety of processes, eg, trauma, pancreatitis, or urinary tract calculus. In some patients the pattern may relate to medication-induced hypoperistalsis and to air swallowing. This borderline pattern inevitably causes difficulty in interpretation (Fig. 5-9).
3) *Probable small bowel obstruction pattern* is defined as consisting of unequivocally dilated, multiple gas- and/or fluid-filled loops of small intestine with a moderate amount of colonic gas, but in which the degree of small bowel distention relative to the colon is insufficient to make a definite diagnosis (Fig. 5-10). 4) *Definite small bowel obstruction pattern* is defined as abnormal and clearly disproportionate gas and/or fluid distention of small bowel relative to the colon (or to other segments of small intestine). Air-fluid levels are evident and the diagnosis of small bowel obstruction is considered unequivocal (Fig. 5-11).

Application of Plain Film Findings

Based on the acknowledged limitations of plain film examinations,[30] on the value of CT in the emergency situation,[31–35] and on the problem-solving ability of enteroclysis in the subacute or chronic setting,[36,37] an algorithm has been proposed for additional imaging in the work-up of patients with suspected intestinal obstruction (see Chapter 21). This algorithm is intended to expedite diagnosis and decrease the cost of the work-up of patients with suspected intestinal obstruction in whom the plain film examination was the starting point in the radiologist's involvement.

Plain film findings in small bowel obstructions differ from those in colorectal obstructions. A dilated colon usually measures more than 8 cm in the cecum and 5.5 cm in other segments, whereas distended small intestinal loops may measure up to 5 cm in width. Although differentiation is possible in most patients, diagnostic problems may occur and should be resolved by CT in the acute setting and by enteroclysis or CT enteroclysis in the subacute or chronic situation.

The most common causes of small intestinal obstruction (75% of all cases) are adhesions due to previous surgery; this applies to countries with a high incidence of elective surgery where strangulated hernias are now the cause of only 8% of obstructions. In underdeveloped countries hernias still remain the most frequent cause. The etiology of obstruction may occasionally be suggested by the plain film examination (Fig. 5-12).

In small bowel obstruction, 12 to 24 hours after the onset of symptoms, radiographic findings show an almost 100% correlation with the clinical impression. Obstruction can occasionally be diagnosed radiologi-

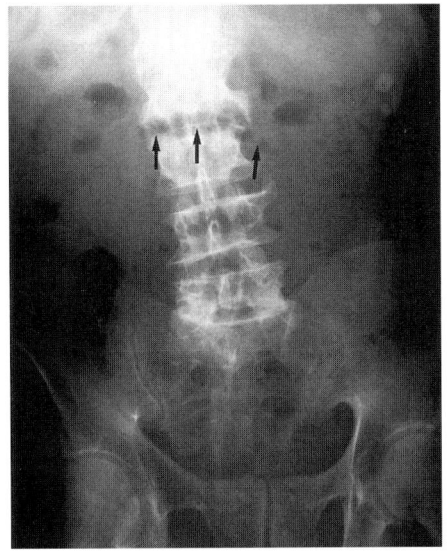
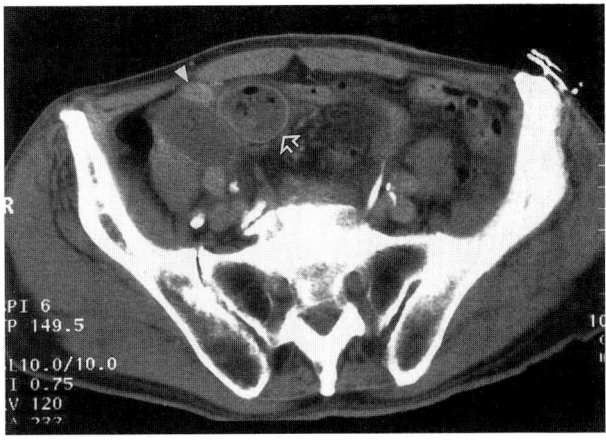

Fig. 5-11. Unequivocal small bowel obstruction pattern.
(a) Upright abdominal radiograph of an elderly male with acute abdominal pain shows a "string of pearls" pattern (arrows) suggesting dilated fluid-filled loops of small bowel with a small amount of gas. (b) CT demonstrates obstruction with the transition point in the right lower quadrant without evidence of a mass or inflammatory process. Surgery confirmed adhesive obstruction. Arrowhead points to normal or collapsed bowel adjacent to markedly dilated, fluid-filled loops with few bubbles of gas (arrow).

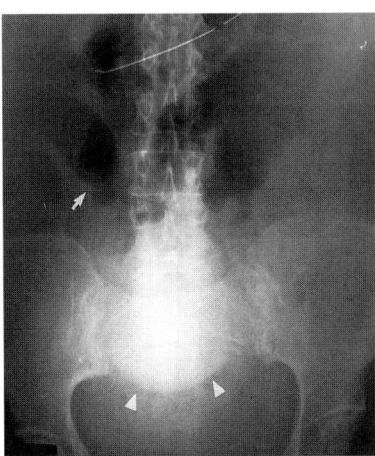

Fig. 5-12. Plain film demonstration of etiology of obstruction.
Strangulated small bowel obstruction secondary to an incarcerated umbilical hernia. Multiple dilated loops of small bowel, some with thickened walls (arrow), and an almost empty colon are consistent with mechanical small bowel obstruction. The "incomplete rim sign" (arrowheads) support the diagnosis of an umbilical hernia.

cally before it is possible to make the diagnosis clinically. Dilated segments of small bowel are usually recognizable 3 to 5 hours from the start of a complete obstruction. Small bowel distention may be minimal if obstruction is incomplete or if the radiographic examination is done very soon after the onset of symptoms. When the development of such an obstruction is followed by plain abdominal images, an initial nonspecific pattern progresses to the probable and then to the unequivocal pattern of a small bowel obstruction, provided there has been no intervention. Small bowel loops that are predominantly fluid-filled, with little or no visible gas, occur in some 6% of small bowel obstructions. They are shown radiographically as spherical, oval, or lobulated soft tissue densities (Fig. 5-13). Small amounts of gas in fluid-filled loops may be trapped between valvulae conniventes on erect or decubitus views to produce a "string of pearls" appearance, a finding seldom found in adynamic ileus [Figs. 5-14 and 5-11(a)]. Such predominantly fluid-filled loops may not be suspected clinically, since the "tinkling bowel sounds" usually indicative of obstructed bowel require larger amounts of gas and may not be heard. A diagnosis based on radiologic findings can avoid undue delay of appropriate management.[38]

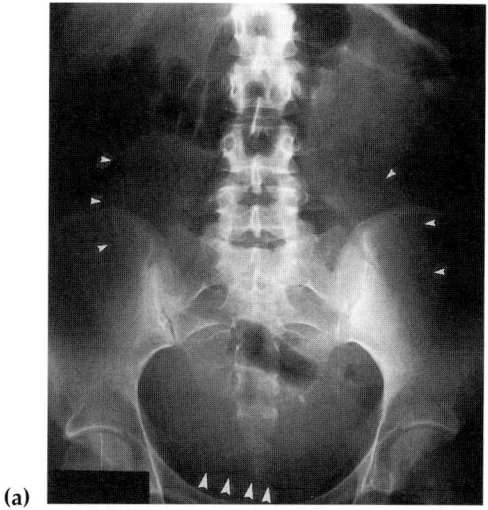
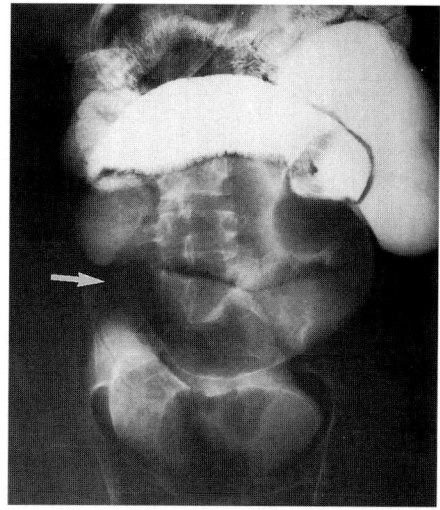

Fig. 5-13. Lobulated soft tissue density secondary to fluid-filled loops of distended small bowel.
(a) Supine abdominal radiograph of a patient who presented with symptoms of small bowel obstruction shows a large pelvic soft tissue density simulating a distended urinary bladder. On close scrutiny, the superior margin of the urinary bladder can be seen (lower arrowheads), flattened by the fluid-filled pelvic ileum. Lobulated soft tissue densities (upper arrowheads) are seen on both sides of the lower abdomen, blending with the pelvic soft tissue density. This finding, the "pseudotumor" sign as also seen in strangulated obstruction, is produced by fixed fluid-filled loops of small bowel. (b) At enteroclysis, the pelvic mass and the lobulated soft tissue densities were shown to be due to markedly distended, fluid-filled loops of small bowel, obstructed by a tight Crohn's stricture (arrow).

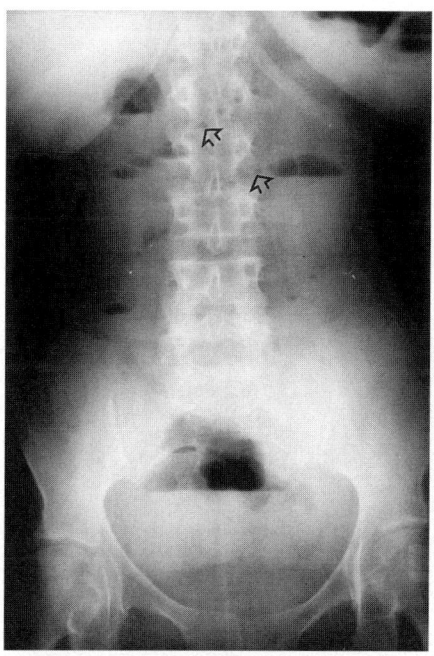

Fig. 5-14. "String of pearls" sign (arrows).
Upright abdominal radiograph shows predominantly fluid-filled loops of dilated small bowel and small amounts of gas trapped between valvulae conniventes in a patient with hemorrhagic intestinal infarct.

Level of Small Bowel Obstruction

An accurate radiologic diagnosis of the site of obstruction depends on the demonstration of lumen dilatation above loops with normal or reduced caliber. The radiologic findings vary with the site of obstruction and the time elapsed from the onset of symptoms. In general, plain film determination of the exact level of obstruction is not reliable.[30]

In proximal small bowel obstruction, gas is often regurgitated into the stomach; the plain film diagnosis can become difficult if only little gas remains in the proximal small bowel. Proximal obstruction should be suspected when valvulae, contrasted by fluid and little air, are seen in a distended jejunum (Fig. 5-15). If enough gas is present in the obstructed segment, distended gas-filled jejunum and fluid levels are formed high in the abdomen (Fig. 5-16). However, exact localization may be difficult because mid small bowel obstruction may show similar findings as gas tends to collect in left anteriorly and superiorly situated jejunal loops (Fig. 5-17). Numerous distended loops indicate a distal obstruction of longer duration. The dilated loops are arranged in a craniad and left directed pattern, corresponding to the inclination of mesenteric root (Fig. 5-18). Occasionally, such dilated loops may be seen high under the left hemidiaphragm, positioned in front of the transverse colon, or displaced by a low abdominal mass, or pregnancy. The identification of the prestenotic loop, more hoop-shaped and distended than the others, can facilitate the localizing of the site of obstruction. As a rule, the point of obstruction is further distal than the most distal fluid level or most distended loop shown (Fig. 5-19).

Significance of Specific Plain Film Intestinal Patterns

It is possible to approach the radiologic diagnosis of intestinal distention by plain film radiography in a practical, pattern-based manner.[9] The plain film findings and their significance can be grouped according to predominant features.

1. *Stepladder or hairpin loops of small bowel without fluid levels in the colon.* This pattern is usually unequivocal for mechanical small bowel obstruction, usually high-grade and subacute. The more common location is the distal small bowel. Loops tend to form part of a circle, and in the erect view each end of a segment is limited by a fluid level (Fig. 5-20). A fluid level in one limb of the loop may be at a different height

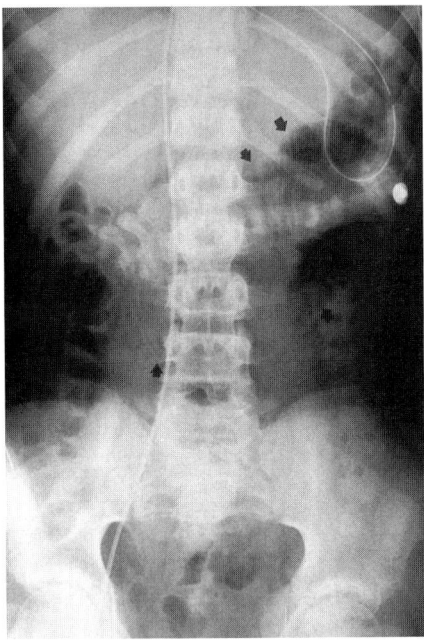

Fig. 5-15. **Proximal small bowel obstruction.**
Distended proximal small bowel with stretched valvulae (the "stretched fold sign," arrows). The location of the dilated segment and absence of other dilated folds suggest a proximal jejunal obstruction. At surgery, a tight stricture was found at the site of prior atresia surgery.

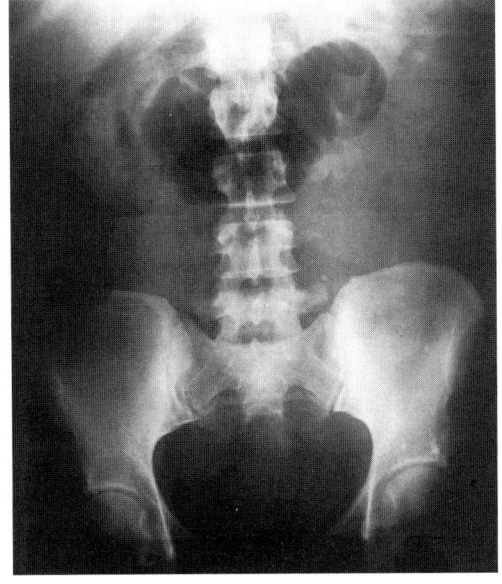
(a)

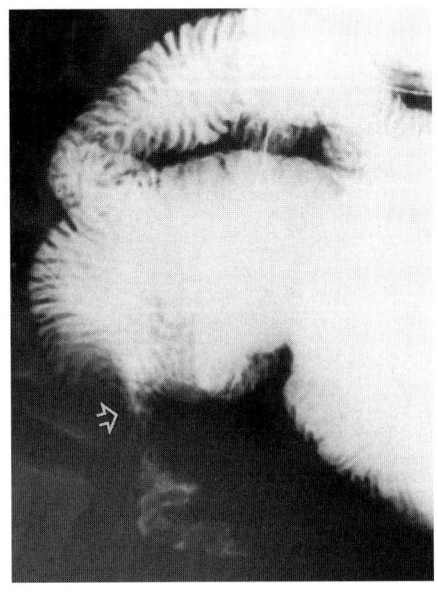
(b)

Fig. 5-16. **Distended gas filled jejunum in high small bowel obstruction.**
(a) Supine abdominal radiograph shows gas-filled distended jejunum in mid upper abdomen, suggesting proximal obstruction. (b) Enteroclysis shows volvulus involving distal jejunum (arrow). At surgery, an adhesive band was found serving as a fulcrum for the jejunal twist.

Fig. 5-17. Mid small bowel obstruction.
(a) The supine abdominal radiograph shows a markedly dilated loop of small bowel in the upper abdomen, suggesting proximal jejunal obstruction. (b) Upright abdominal radiograph shows the dilated loop high in the left upper quadrant. The presence of fluid-filled segments with air-fluid levels in the lower abdomen indicates that the obstruction may not be proximal. Surgery confirmed tight adhesive band obstruction at mid ileal level.

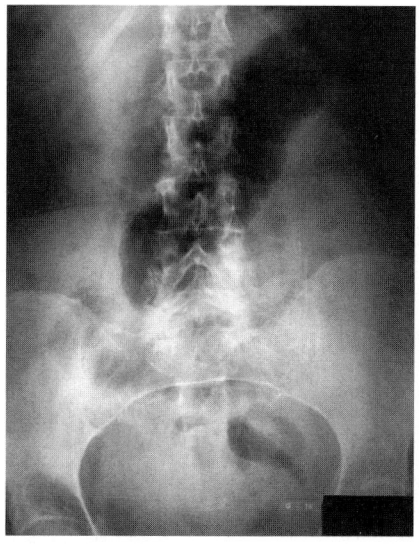 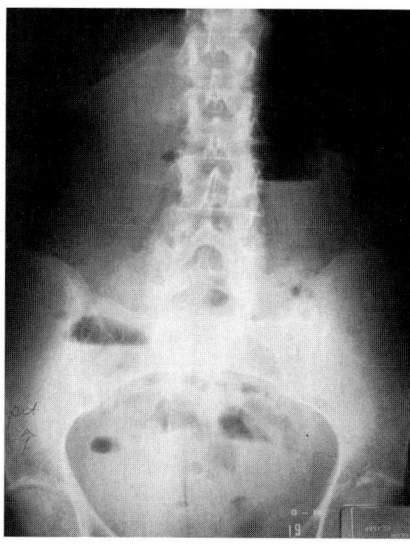

(a)   (b)

from that in the other limb. This observation, however, will not always differentiate mechanical obstruction from adynamic ileus.

Occasionally this pattern may be due to functional obstruction, ie, the stasis of bowel contents above a segment of nonpropulsive bowel that acts as an obstruction (Fig. 5-21). This pattern may be found in conditions such as scleroderma, amyloidosis, vascular disease, and nonstenotic local inflammatory diseases.

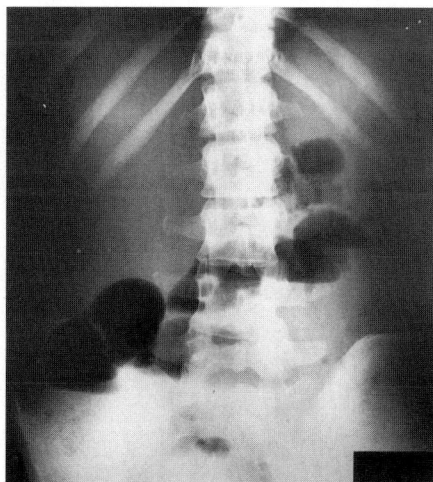

Fig. 5-18. Distal small bowel obstruction.
Note the oblique arrangements of dilated loops corresponding to the direction of the mesenteric root. The presence of many dilated loops with air-fluid levels points to a distal obstruction.

Early postoperative abdominal states may produce this pattern (Fig. 5-5). Moderate amounts of colon gas and feces without fluid levels are frequently seen in cases of early or incomplete obstruction.

Attention should be directed toward the estimation of the wall thickness of dilated small bowel loops. The soft-tissue shadow between two adjacent gas-filled loops can represent the combined thickness of the two bowel walls. Normally a distended segment should have a wall thickness of less than 2 mm. Occasionally the thickness of the wall of a single segment can be more accurately measured when outlined between luminal gas and serosal fat. An increased wall thickness is an important sign that an obstruction is no longer uncomplicated. Increased peristaltic movements of loops proximal to an obstruction, as indicated on serial films, favor a radiologic diagnosis of simple obstruction.

It is usually known clinically when a strangulated external hernia is the cause of obstruction. In obese patients, however, this cause may be overlooked. A careful search for evidence of a hernia should be part of the plain film evaluation (Fig. 5-2). The mere presence of a hernia does not mean that it is the cause of obstruction, unless a dilated loop is demonstrated terminating at the hernial orifice (Fig. 5-12).

2. *Mild to moderately dilated small bowel with some fluid levels.* The radiologic significance of this appearance is indeterminate. This is the so-called abnormal but nonspecific intestinal gas pattern. Only follow-up films, clinical progress, or additional imaging methods will differentiate obstructive from adynamic ileus or from a variant of normality. Correlation with the

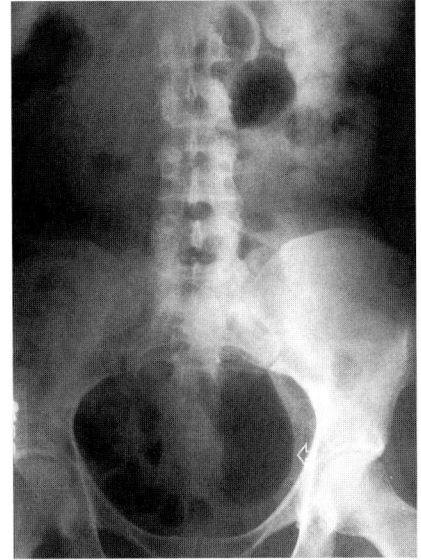 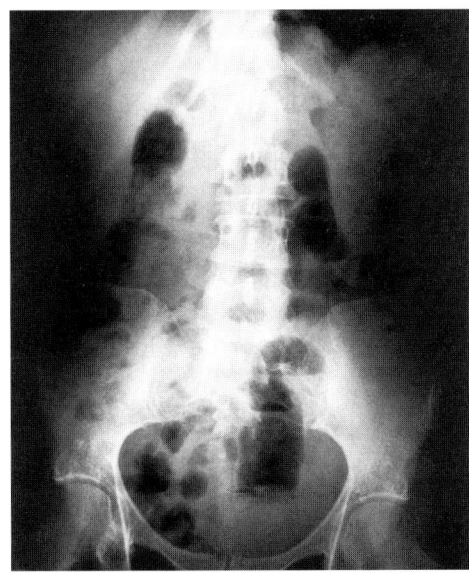

Fig. 5-19. The prestenotic loop.
(a) The prestenotic loop (arrow) is often more distended than other loops and indicates the approximate level of obstruction. (b) In the upright position, the prestenotic loop is more hoop-shaped or has a longer fluid level. Tight adhesive band obstruction, as indicated by the prestenotic loop, was confirmed by enteroclysis.

clinical history is helpful. There is a tendency for the less experienced radiologist to report small bowel obstruction too frequently. Clinical credence is often given to such reports even in the absence of positive symptoms, since it is accepted that radiologic findings can precede clinical evidence. When presented with an indeterminate small bowel gas pattern, it is wiser for the radiologist to recommend a 24-hour follow-up film or, should an early diagnosis be required, to suggest additional imaging (Figs. 5-9, 5-10).

3. *Obstructive small bowel pattern plus fluid in the right colon.* This pattern can be due to strangulating ob-

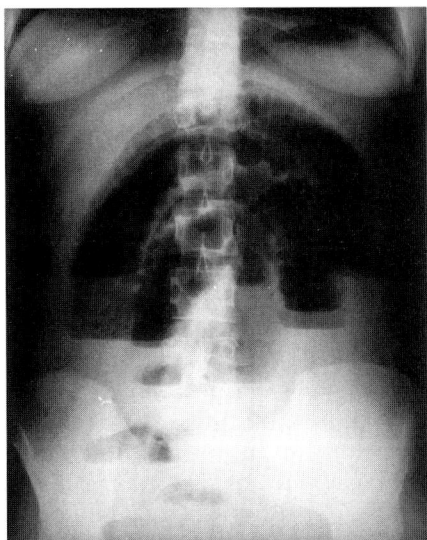 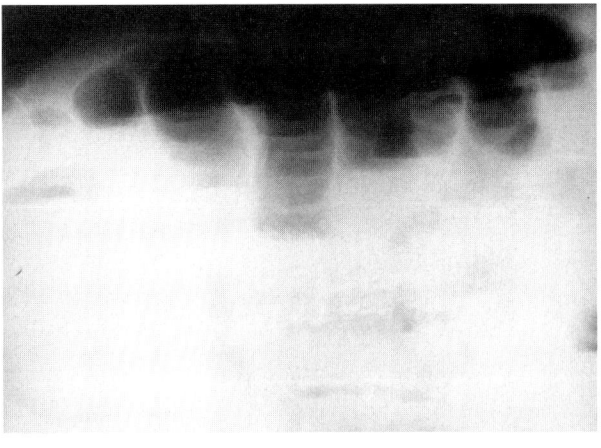

Fig. 5-20. Mechanical small bowel obstruction.
Upright abdominal radiograph showing hairpin loops. Note collapsed airless colon. This pattern is characteristic of simple mechanical obstruction.

Fig. 5-21. Functional or pseudo-obstruction pattern.
Air-fluid levels of different heights are noted on left lateral decubitus abdominal radiogram of a patient who presented with abdominal pain and distention. Surgery did not reveal a point of obstruction. The patient had been on ganglion blocking agents for hypertension.

struction (see below), right-sided inflammatory disease (eg, appendicitis, Crohn's disease), or a right-sided colon obstruction. Air/fluid levels are seen in the small bowel, and there is increase of soft-tissue density in the right lower abdomen. The latter change is due to fluid in a distended cecum or to an abscess in the right lower quadrant. This pattern can be resolved readily by CT (Fig. 5-22). An appendiceal abscess may present as small bowel obstruction when a loop of ileum adheres to the wall of the abscess. This may be identified as a soft-tissue mass, sometimes containing gas, indenting the cecum. In a recent study,[39] functional small bowel obstruction was the most important plain radiographic finding in cases of perforated appendicitis and in some cases of impending perforation.

Small bowel obstruction is a common complication of Crohn's disease, but an etiologic basis for the obstruction may be difficult to determine on the plain film. Occasionally thickened, fixed loops of pelvic segments of ileum can be identified, allowing the diagnosis of inflammatory bowel disease (Fig. 5-23).

4. *Distention and air-fluid levels in small bowel and right colon with a moderately distended gas-filled cecum.* This pattern is suggestive of colon obstruction, with an incompetent ileocecal valve allowing reflux into the small bowel. The plain film findings can change significantly with time and radiologic method. Multiple projections, including both decubitus and left lateral abdomen views, may be needed to detect right-sided colon distention that may be masked when fluid-filled. Follow-up abdominal radiographs may show a change in the gas distribution and will clarify the level of obstruction so that a more appropriate examination (colon enema or CT) can be done (Fig. 5-24).

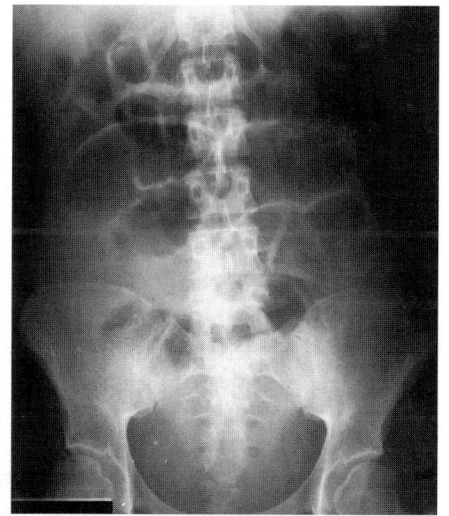
(a)

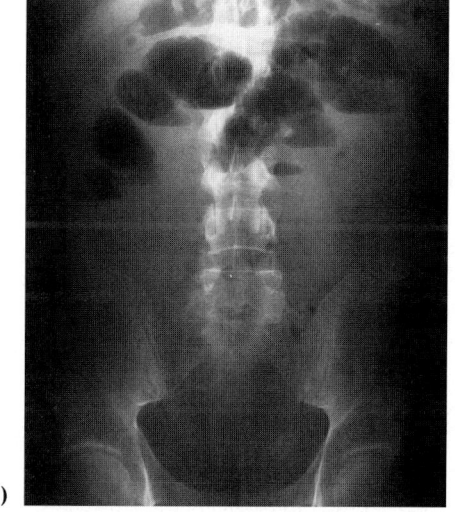
(b)

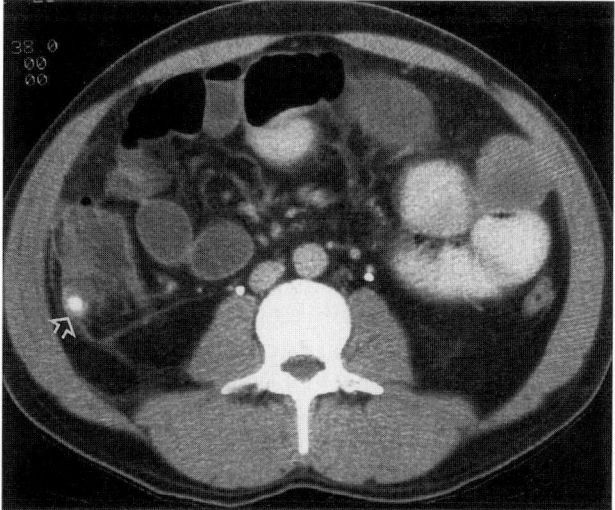
(c)

Fig. 5-22. Obstructive small bowel pattern plus fluid-filled cecum.
(a) Supine abdominal radiograph shows distended gas-filled small bowel as well as increased soft tissue density in right lower abdomen. (b) Upright abdominal radiograph is very suggestive of mechanical small bowel obstruction. (c) CT shows an appendiceal abscess in the right lower quadrant. An appendicolith (arrow) not appreciated on the abdominal radiographs is present. Note fluid-filled distended small bowel.

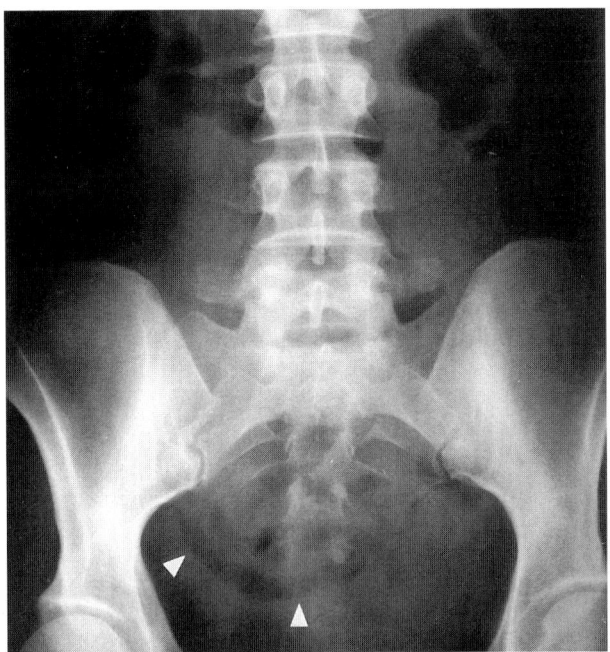 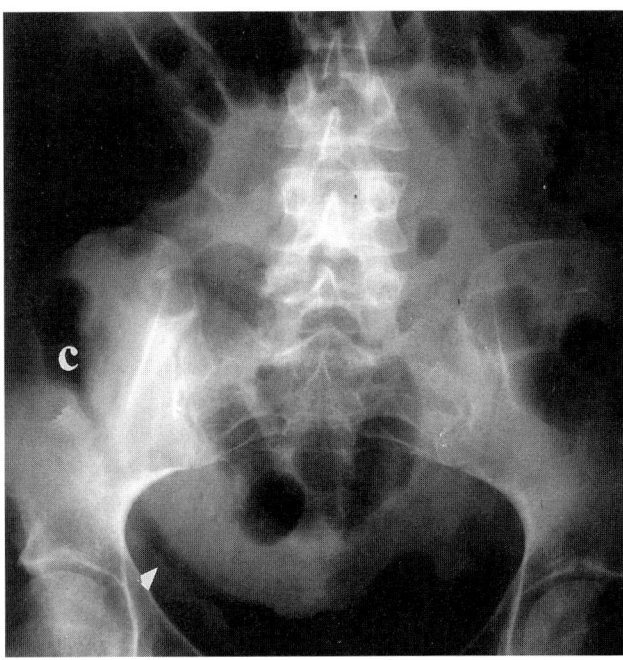

(a) (b)

Fig. 5-23. A patient with chronic Crohn's disease who presented clinically with obstruction.
(a) The supine abdominal radiograph shows long and narrow, fixed and featureless tubular gas shadows (arrowheads) in the course of the distal ileum, favoring a diagnosis of Crohn's disease. (b) Another patient with more severe Crohn's disease shows a longer narrowed segment of distal ileum (arrowheads), more widely separated from other small bowel. (C = diseased cecum.)

5. *Uniformly distended small bowel, colon, and stomach.* This pattern is typical of adynamic ileus (Fig. 5-25). The usual clinical background is a patient with a history of recent surgery or trauma, electrolyte imbalance, or medication causing decreased intestinal motility. This finding should be differentiated from a low colonic obstruction. A left lateral abdominal view (left side down vertical beam) may show continuity of gas through the descending colon, into the sigmoid and rectum.[18] Prone as well as right and left side down decubitus views (horizontal beam) may demonstrate that gas can rise into the rectum in a patient with adynamic ileus. However, the left lateral abdomen view suffices in most instances and is easier to perform in an elderly or a critically ill patient (Fig. 5-5). A barium enema or CT needs to be done only in questionable cases (Fig. 5-26).

Impending cecal perforation complicating adynamic ileus should be considered when the cecum is distended out of proportion to the rest of the colon and small bowel. Evidence for intramural cecal gas and edema should be sought on images of optimal quality taken in several projections.

6. *The "gasless" abdomen.* This pattern suggests a large amount of fluid in the bowel that may be difficult to appreciate if films are of suboptimal quality. When a small amount of gas is present, one sees the "string of pearls" or the "stretched fold" sign (Figs. 5-14, 5-15). The association of this pattern with closed loop obstruction or with mesenteric vascular occlusion (see subsequent discussion) is well known. More fluid than gas may be found in an ileus of any of the following etiologies: 1) in a patient in whom swallowed air has not yet reached the dilated loops (early obstruction), 2) in a stoic patient who does not swallow air, and 3) in a patient too weak to swallow. There may also be a paucity of gas without fluid in severe vomiting of any etiology, eg, high obstruction, pancreatitis, and gastroenteritis.

7. *Bowel distention, gas in biliary tree, ectopic gallstone.* Gallstone ileus is the most insidious and diagnostically difficult form of intestinal obstruction and carries a mortality rate five times higher than that of adhesive obstructions. The diagnosis is usually a matter for the radiologist and is often suspected or made on the basis of the plain film examination. Gallstone ileus accounts for 1% to 3% of all small bowel obstructions but may be found in as many as 24% of patients over 70 years old, the majority being women.[40]

Though specific radiologic signs are absent in about half the patients, a diagnosis of gallstone ileus must be

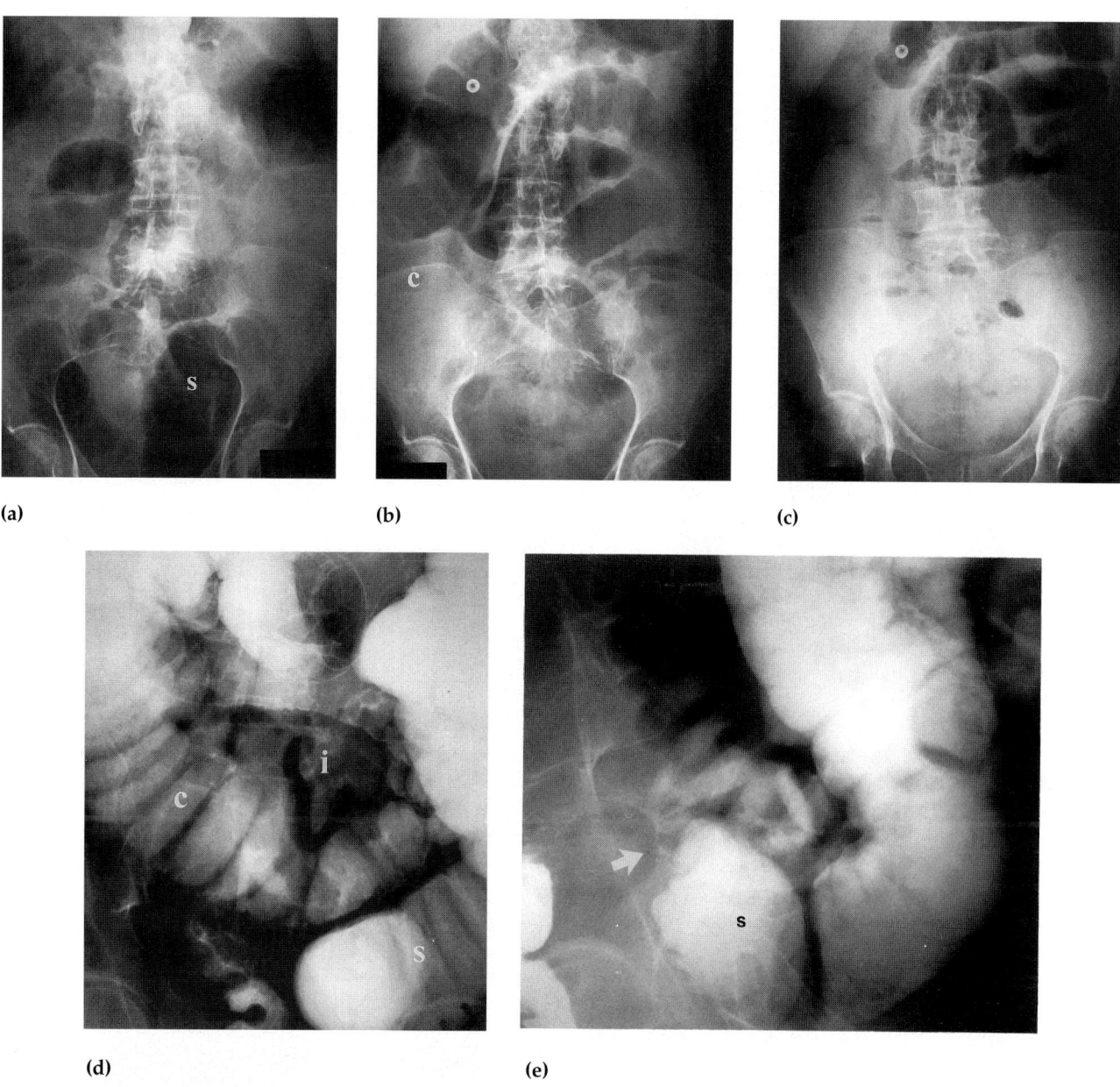

Fig. 5-24. Influence of a patulous ileocecal valve on the plain film gas pattern.
(a) Initial supine abdominal radiograph of an elderly female, referred from a nursing home with an acute abdomen, shows dilated loops of small bowel and colon. Gas is present in a dilated sigmoid (S). Interpreted as consistent with an adynamic ileus. (b) Supine abdominal radiograph done the next day was interpreted as increased colonic gas, suggesting improvement. Note a slight further distention of small bowel. The dilated, fluid-filled sigmoid and right colon (C) were not appreciated on the supine view. (c) Upright abdominal radiograph done on the third day because of high clinical suspicion of small bowel obstruction. Absence of gas in the colon; multiple dilated loops of small bowel with air-fluid levels. High-grade distal mechanical small bowel obstruction. Decompression and enteroclysis suggested. (d) Delayed radiograph of the enteroclysis shows uniform dilatation of entire small bowel to terminal ileum (I). Small bowel obstruction ruled out, obstruction of sigmoid colon (S) is indicated. (C = ascending colon.) (e) Lateral radiograph of (d) shows a tight stricture (arrow) in the distal sigmoid (S), secondary to diverticular disease. Barium should be followed to the rectum if a dilated terminal ileum is seen during a study for small bowel obstruction. This case illustrates the vagaries of plain film patterns often associated with an incompetent ileocecal valve. A more appropriate work-up would have been a barium enema after film (a).

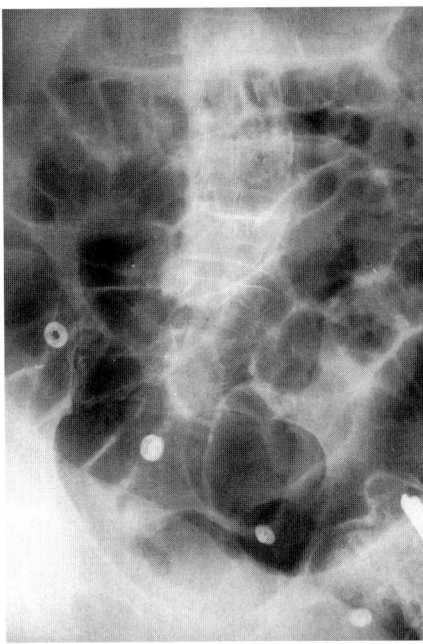

Fig. 5-25. Supine abdominal radiograph of a nursing home patient with abdominal distention shows diffused distention of stomach, small bowel, and colon typical of adynamic ileus.

suspected an any elderly female presenting with features of small bowel obstruction. Rigler's triad of hoop-shaped, dilated small bowel loops; air in the biliary tree; and a gallstone in an ectopic location is as valid now as in 1941.[41] Gas in the biliary tree or in the gallbladder is seen in almost two thirds of these patients (Fig. 5-27). However, gas can normally be seen in the biliary tree of patients with prior Oddi sphincterotomy or after choledochoenteric anastomoses. The clinical history aids proper interpretation. The ectopic gallstone is identified in less than half the patients and may be missed if insufficiently calcified or if overlying the sacrum (Fig. 5-28). The site of obturation is usually the distal ileum (Fig. 5-29), less often the proximal ileum or distal jejunum. Barium studies can identify a cholecystoduodenal communication. Currently, CT is the simplest method of diagnosing gallstone ileus[42] by

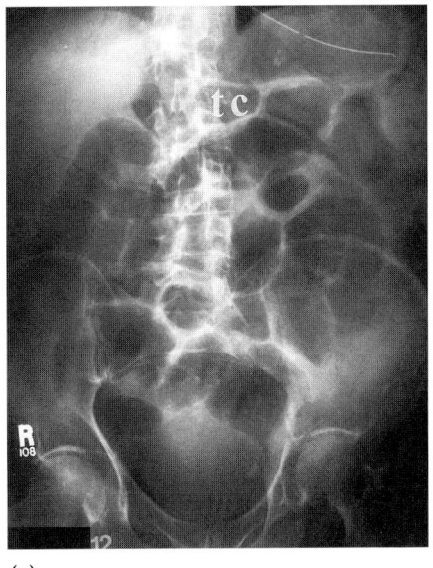

(a)

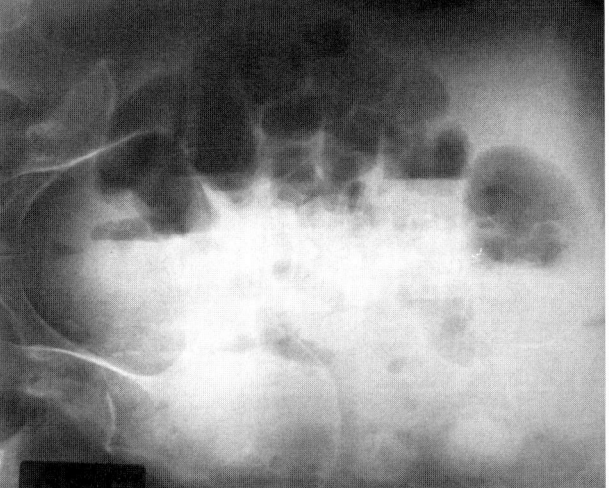

(b)

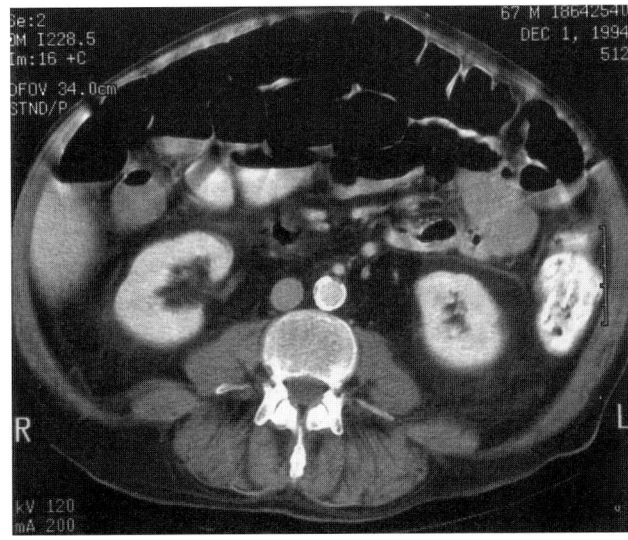

(c)

Fig. 5-26. Adynamic ileus secondary to hypothyroidism. (a) Supine abdominal radiograph of a 67-year-old man with known hypothyroidism who presented with abdominal pain shows distended gas-filled small bowel. Gas in transverse colon (TC) is difficult to appreciate. (b) Left decubitus abdominal radiograph shows air-fluid levels in small bowel suspicious for small bowel obstruction. (c) CT section at level of kidneys shows gas-distended small bowel and colon. The rectum (not shown) was also distended.

Fig. 5-27. Obstructive small bowel gas pattern and air in biliary tree in two patients.
(a) Gas outlining dilated right and left hepatic ducts and the small bowel allows a diagnosis of gallstone ileus without demonstration of an ectopic gallstone. (b) A small amount of gas in the biliary tree (arrow) coupled with the finding of dilated small bowel suggests gallstone ileus. Note residual stone in the gallbladder.

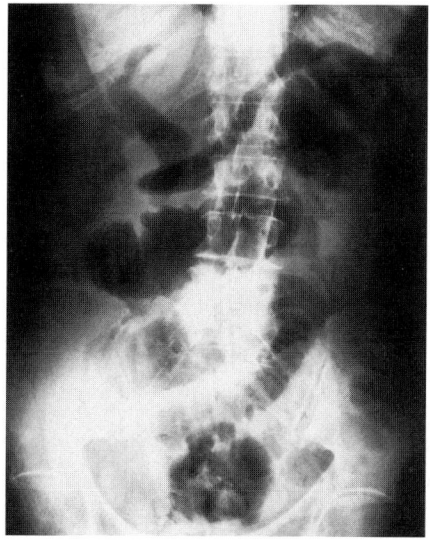
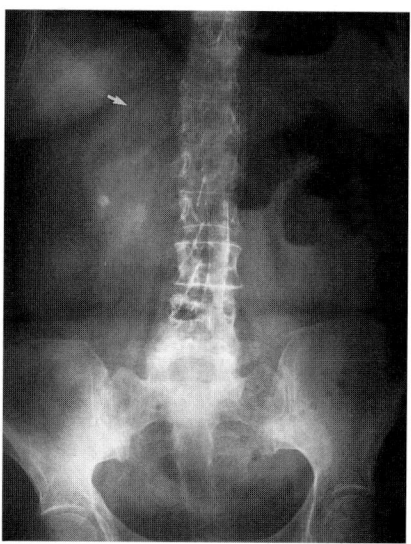

(a)   (b)

also outlining stones not visible on plain films. The obturation obstruction caused by the ectopic gallstone (usually >2 cm) is readily shown by CT (Fig. 5-30) and can also be demonstrated by ultrasound.

The operative mortality is high, though it has been reduced from 57.4% in the period during 1925 to 1940 to 16.3% during 1971 to 1980. Heightened radiologic awareness of the diagnosis and improved surgery are considered responsible for the reduction.

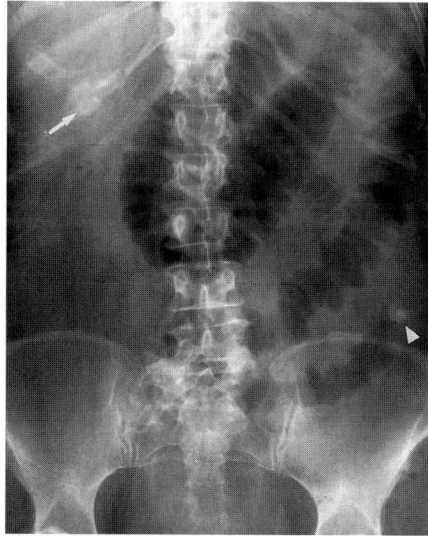

Fig. 5-28. Supine abdominal radiograph shows one large lamellated gallstone in the right upper quadrant (arrow) and another in the left lower quadrant (arrowhead). The fold thickening proximal to the gallstone is due to retained fluid in obstructed small bowel.

Ascribing a precise clinical significance to intestinal gas patterns based on the plain film appearances may be difficult; it requires interpreter experience and close correlation with the history and clinical findings.[37] The plain film examination can serve as the triage point for additional diagnostic work-up (see Chapter 21) in the subacute or chronic situation. In the work-up of the acute abdomen, current literature recommends that the plain film be followed by CT.[2] This is of considerable importance in the acute setting, since intestinal obstruction is only one of the more common differential diagnoses in a patient with acute abdominal pain.[43]

Plain Film Determination of Severity of Obstruction

The use of enteroclysis has allowed an objective and reproducible method of grading the severity of small bowel obstruction.[30,32] The current recommendation to use plain film examination as triage for additional work-up in the nonacute setting[43] rests on the ability of plain films to distinguish high-grade (or complete) from low-grade or absence of obstruction. The recommendations state that if plain films suggest high-grade obstruction and no surgery is planned, CT would be the imaging modality of choice. On the other hand, if the plain films suggest low-grade small bowel obstruction or are normal, enteroclysis (or CT enteroclysis) is preferred.

A recent study has shown that findings on erect or decubitus abdominal radiographs may allow distinction of severity of small bowel obstruction on plain

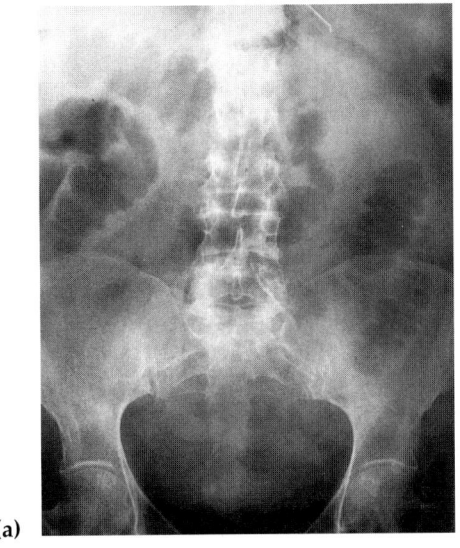
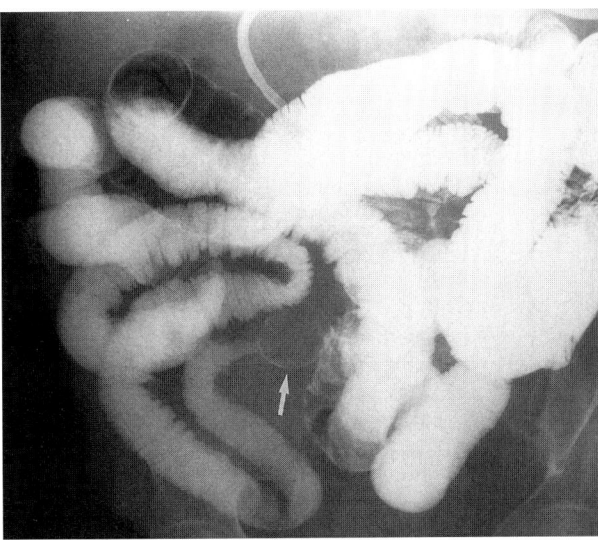
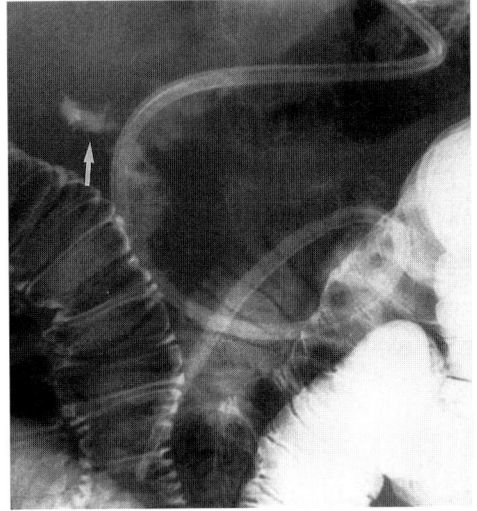

Fig. 5-29. Demonstration of site of gallstone obstruction. (a) Supine abdominal radiograph in an elderly female with acute abdominal pain shows findings consistent with small bowel obstruction. No air in biliary tree or ectopic gallstone is noted. (b) Enteroclysis done following long tube decompression shows an ovoid defect (arrow) producing complete obstruction in distal ileum. A large gallstone was found at surgery. (c) Delayed radiograph shows barium having entered through the cholecystoduodenal communication (arrow). If no fistula is shown by reflux, the enteroclysis tube should be withdrawn into the duodenum and contrast injected there to outline the fistula.

film.[13] Of 27 radiographic signs studied, two plain film findings were found to be most predictive of a higher grade of obstruction. These are the presence of a differential air-fluid level height and the presence of a mean air/fluid level width greater than 25 mm. When both signs are present, there is an 86% chance that the patient has a complete or high-grade small bowel obstruction. On the other hand, when both signs are absent, there is an 83% chance that the patient has a low-grade small bowel obstruction or no obstruction. Unfortunately, in 38% of patients only one of the two signs was present, making the plain film sign evaluation "indeterminate," although still compatible with a higher-grade small bowel obstruction. In these patients, the authors suggest that any additional workup should be based on the clinical findings or the history.[13] Anecdotally, experienced radiologists have used the "string of beads" finding to indicate a predominantly fluid-filled small bowel, hence a higher grade of obstruction. This sign showed a predictive value of 39% for high-grade obstruction in this study.[13]

Plain Film Findings in Strangulating Obstruction

Strangulation implies interference with the intestinal blood supply in an obstruction that need not be complete. Obstruction is frequently of the closed loop type, ie, the closure of the lumen at two ends of the same loop of bowel, including its mesentery. Strangulation has a striking effect on mortality rate. In one series, the mortality rate for simple obstruction was 5% and that for strangulated obstruction 30%.[44] Unfortunately, simple mechanical obstruction cannot be

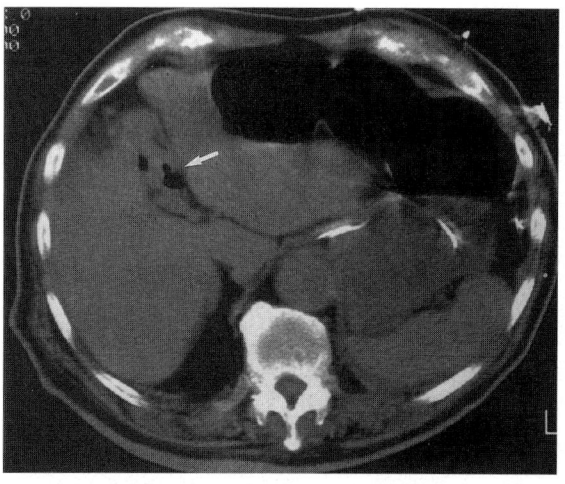
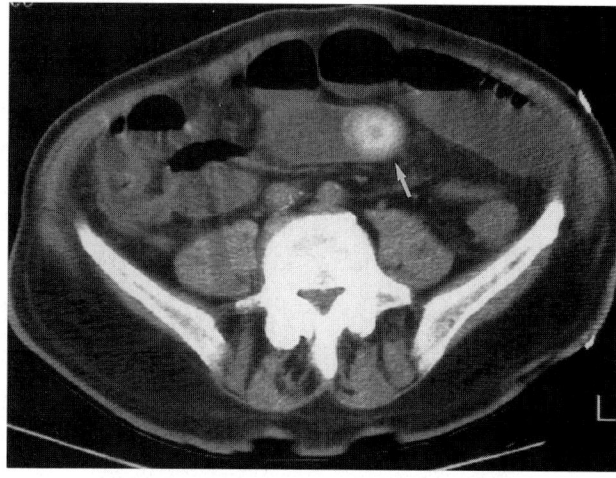

Fig. 5-30. CT diagnosis of gallstone ileus.
(a) CT section at level of liver shows gas in biliary tree (arrow) in an elderly man admitted for possible diverticulitis. (b) CT section just below level of iliac crest shows a lamellated gallstone (arrow) and fluid-filled distended small bowel proximal to the obstructing gallstone.

reliably differentiated from strangulated obstruction on the basis of clinical, laboratory, and plain film findings.[45–50]

Among the common causes of strangulation are incarcerated hernia and volvulus. As the venous pressure is lower than the arterial, veins are obstructed first, and there is often extravasation of blood into the lumen. If the lumen is not blocked completely, gas may enter it from above. The plain film diagnosis is difficult. The indirect signs of strangulating obstruction are as follows:

1. *Intramural gas.* If necrosis develops, gas may be found within the wall of the involved bowel. Crescentic, linear, ringlike, or semicircular gas collections are noted outside the gas-filled lumen of the bowel, separated from it by a stripe of greater density representing the bowel wall (Fig. 5-31).[51,52] Infrequently, gas may enter the mesenteric venous system and then extend into the portal vein.

2. *Pseudotumor sign.* A fluid-filled incarcerated loop may appear as a tumorlike density with a convex or polycyclical outline. This "pseudotumor" may indent adjacent gas-containing loops (Fig. 5-32). In the upright or lateral decubitus position only few fluid levels are seen within the fluid-distended bowel loop, including the "string of pearls" sign.[6,53,54] However, this sign can also be seen in a simple mechanical obstruction associated with dilated, fluid-filled bowel loops.

3. *Reduced small bowel activity* indicated on successive abdominal films obtained in the identical position at 5-minute intervals.[55] This simple method has been superceded by more precise investigation, eg, real-time ultrasound and CT.

4. *Loss of valvular pattern.* In simple obstruction, jejunal distention does not obliterate the folds. When the blood supply of a closed loop obstruction has been compromised, the folds tend to disappear and the margins of the gas-outlined loops become smooth. These signs are of value only if it has been possible to identify the loop as jejunum, since distal ileal folds normally disappear when distended (Fig. 5-33).

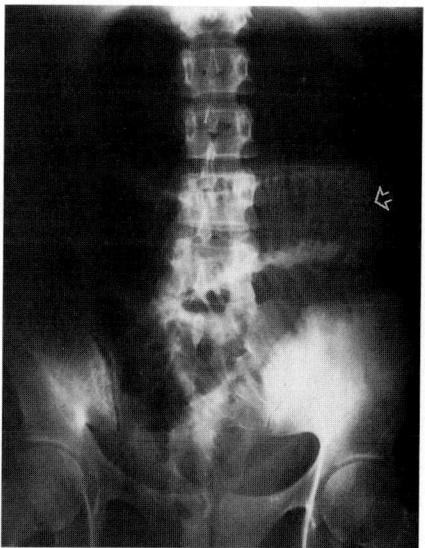

Fig. 5-31. Intramural gas.
Rounded lucencies are noted in a loop of small bowel in the left hemiabdomen (arrow) corresponding to pneumatosis in an infarcted loop of small bowel secondary to closed loop obstruction.

68 • 5. Plain Film Radiography of the Small Bowel

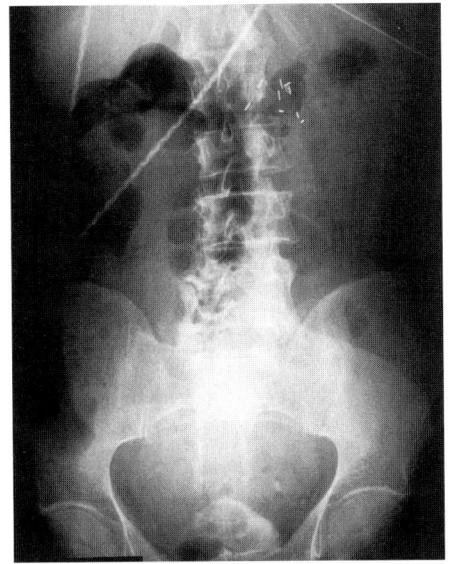 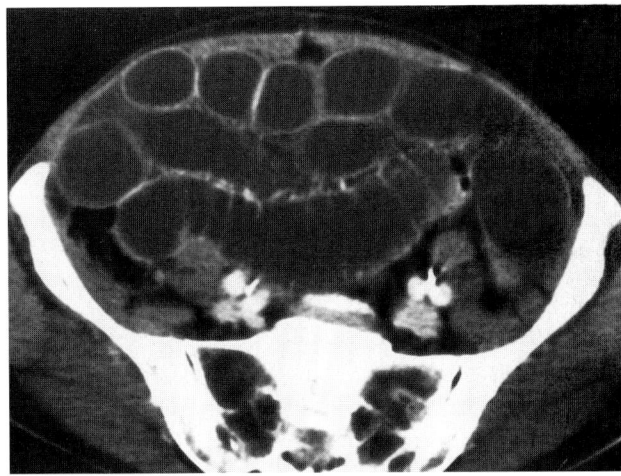

(a) (b)

Fig. 5-32. Pseudotumor sign.
(a) Supine abdominal radiograph in an elderly patient with closed small bowel loop obstruction by extensive adhesions. Note the paucity of gas and the large soft tissue density in the right hemiabdomen and pelvis, displacing right colon gas laterally and superiorly, ie, a pseudotumor. (b) Abdominal computed tomography shows the soft tissue mass to be caused by fluid-filled and dilated loops of small bowel.

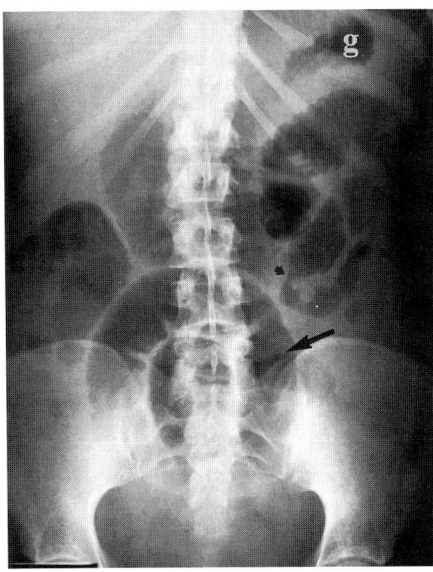

Fig. 5-33. Unreliablilty of loss of valvulae pattern.
Note the dilated loop of jejunum in the left upper abdomen below the gastric shadow (g). It continues into a narrowed segment (arrow). Below is a loop of dilated bowel with effaced folds (long arrow), thought to be possibly strangulated jejunum. At surgery the site of obstruction was confirmed but the involved bowel was ileum. There was no evidence of strangulation. Loss of valvulae pattern is significant only if it involves jejunum.

5. *Peritonitis with fluid* in the peritoneal cavity, which may give the appearance of thickening of the bowel wall. This may be caused by inflammatory changes within the wall, by exudate on its serosal surface, or by fluid between loops (Fig. 5-34). Shifting fluid densities may be demonstrated when radiographs are obtained in multiple positions of the patient.

6. *Coffee bean configuration.* During the early stage of strangulation, the roentgen signs may be indistinguishable from those of simple obstruction. Later, gas and fluid trapped within an obstructed loop may outline two short, side-by-side segments of distended bowel, separated by a soft-tissue space that represents their thickened walls. This has been termed "coffee bean configuration." Gas-distended bowel proximal to the obstructed loop can obscure this sign. The "coffee bean" sign is, therefore, best seen in jejunal obstructions when vomiting has reduced gas accumulation proximally.

7. *Long air/fluid levels.* On the erect film each loop appears flattened and does not show a "hoop shape." The maximum length of these levels exceeds by at least 2 cm the greatest diameter of identical loops measured on the recumbent film.[6,38]

8. *Fixation of loops.* This is shown as lack of alteration of the position of loops between films taken supine and erect (Fig. 5-35) or compared with follow-up films.[6,53]

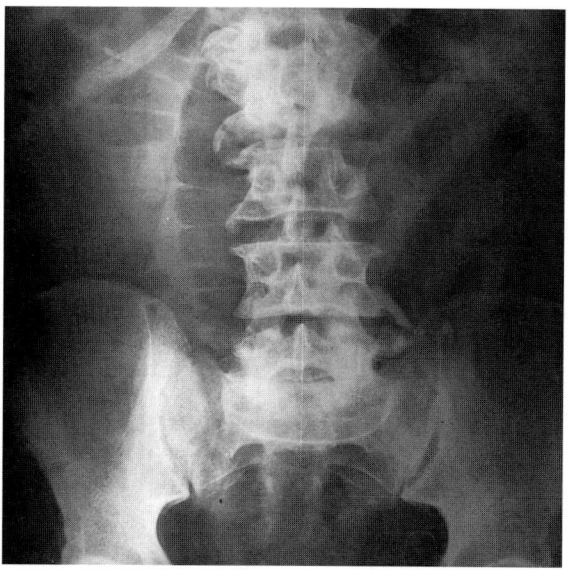 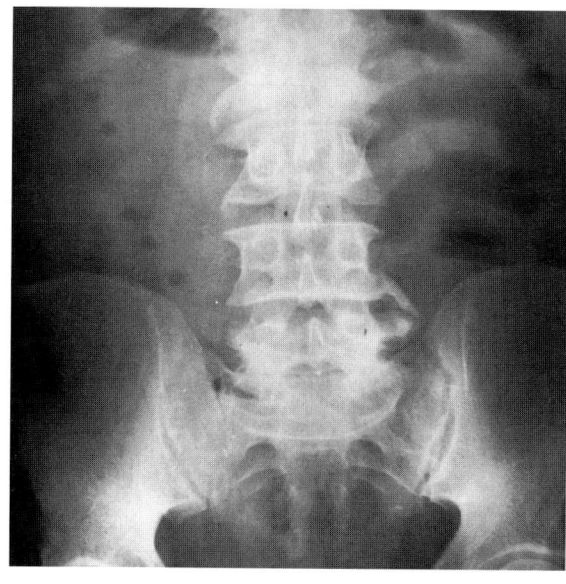

Fig. 5-34. Gangrene of ileum secondary to volvulus.
(a) Supine abdominal radiograph showing thick-walled loops of small bowel in the left abdomen. Note the marked separation between rigid appearing bowel loops. (b) Upright abdominal radiograph shows a fixed position of the loops in the left hemiabdomen, also "string of pearls" in the right hemiabdomen. At autopsy, there was extensive gangrene without obstruction of major vessels. (Courtesy of the College of Physicians: Philadelphia General Hospital X-Ray Teaching File; Philadelphia.)

9. *Rigid narrow loop.* The strangulated loop shows a narrow, gas-outlined lumen with an irregularly serrated contour due to edema of the bowel wall. This configuration does not change between films taken in several positions of the patient.[56]

10. *Relatively gasless abdomen.* As noted previously, the relative absence of small intestinal gas and the predominance of fluid in patients clinically suspected of small intestinal obstruction should arouse the radiologist's suspicion of strangulation (Fig. 5-36).[53]

11. *Persistence of fecal material in the right colon.* The prolonged presence of bubbly appearing fecal matter in the right colon in association with gas-distended loops of small bowel should cause the radiologist to become suspicious of strangulation. In simple obstructions, initially seen right colonic fecal residue is soon cleared.[57]

Relevance of Above Signs of Strangulation

Lack of activity of a small bowel loop, shown on repeated supine films taken at 5-minute intervals or demonstrated by real-time ultrasonography, are the only frequently seen sign of strangulation (58% of cases) and show statistically significant discrimination against simple obstruction. Other signs, such as predominant distention of a single segment, the pseudotumor sign, and evidence of loop fixation, show a marginally increased incidence in strangulation but are infrequently demonstrated. The most specific signs, a narrow rigid loop and evidence of intramural gas (Fig. 5-37) are rare. The other signs mentioned occur with greater frequency but demonstrate an almost equal incidence in simple small bowel obstruction.[55]

Numerous aspects of the patient's history, physical examination, and laboratory findings have been analyzed to determine their correlation with strangulation obstruction. Of clinical features reviewed in 52 cases of strangulation obstruction, abdominal tenderness was found in 82%, a pulse rate above 100/min in 78%, leukocytosis of >10,000 cells/mm^3 in 63%, constant abdominal pain in 61%, a temperature >99.6°F in 55%, a hernia or mass in 32%, and guarding in 29%. All patients with strangulation obstruction had two or more of these signs.[58] Another report found that strangulation obstruction showed a positive correlation with a patient age of more than 70 years, a white blood cell count of >18,000 cells/mm^3, feculent vomiting, and decreased bowel sounds.[46] Shock, hypothermia, rectal bleeding, and abdominal rigidity

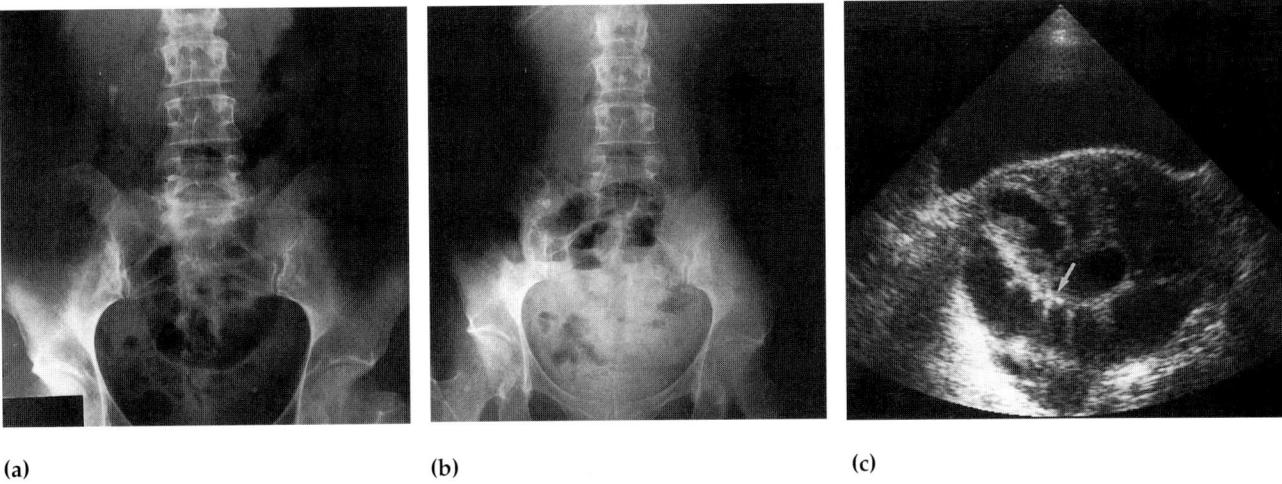

Fig. 5-35. Fixation of loops.
(a) Supine abdominal radiograph shows dilated loops of small bowel in the upper pelvis. (b) Upright radiograph shows the slightly dilated, gas- and fluid-filled loops to be fixed in the pelvic region. (c) Sonography followed abdominal radiography because of a possible pelvic mass found on clinical examination. No pelvic mass is seen. There are dilated fluid-filled, fixed loops of small bowel behind the urinary bladder and uterus. Note the prominent valvulae pattern ("keyboard sign") in a dilated, fixed loop (arrow). The keyboard sign represents valvulae conniventes in a loop of jejunum and indicates fold thickening in a dilated segment. The dilated loops were aperistaltic as shown by real-time evaluation. At surgery, volvulus with infarction of the distal ileum was found.

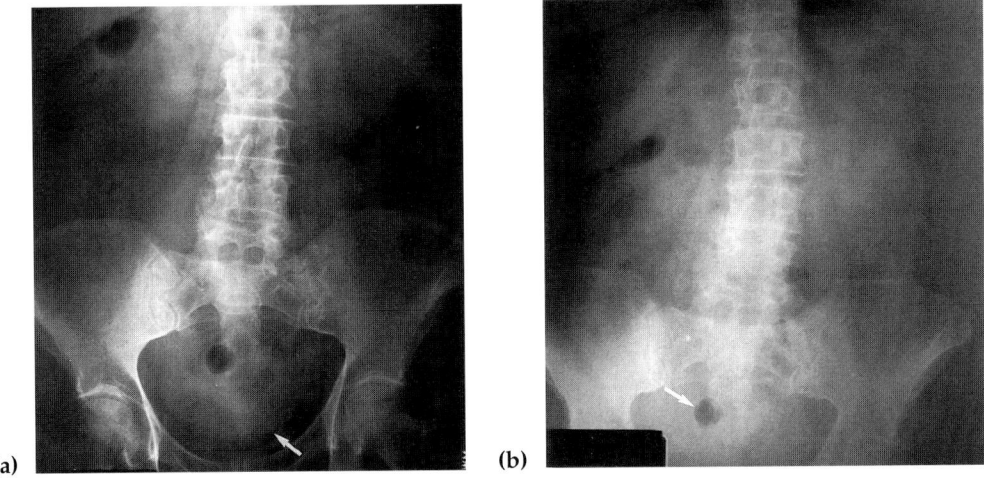

Fig. 5-36. Gasless abdomen.
(a) Supine abdominal radiograph shows a virtually gas-free abdomen with only a few scattered gas collections in seemingly nondilated small bowel loops. Note soft tissue density in the pelvis (pseudotumor sign) (arrow). The colon is empty. (b) The upright abdominal radiograph shows short air-fluid levels in the right upper quadrant. A fixed pelvic loop of ileum has not changed its position compared with the supine film (arrow). The threshold of suspicion for strangulated small bowel obstruction or ischemia should be lowered when such a pattern is observed in an elderly patient with an acute abdomen. CT can be a valuable adjunct. At surgery, there was extensive small bowel infarction secondary to mesenteric venous thrombosis.

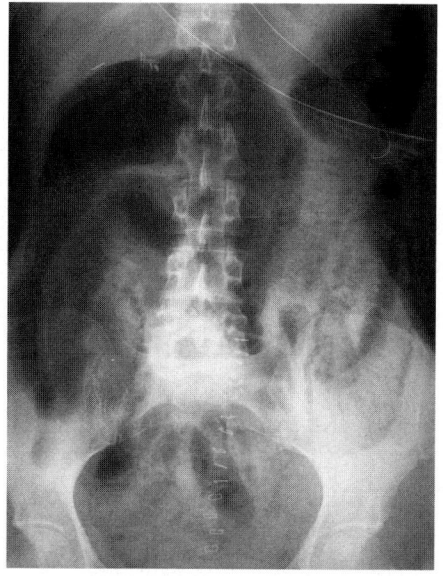 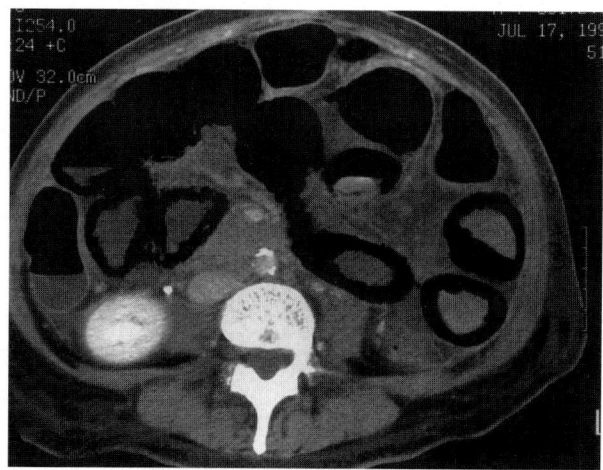

Fig. 5-37. Intramural gas in intestinal infarction.
(a) Supine abdominal radiograph in a hypertensive patient who recently underwent small bowel resection for infarction shows rounded, linear, and speckled intramural gas in small bowel indicating infarction. (b) CT shows diffuse mural gas in small bowel.

were good indicators of strangulation obstruction.[59] These signs, however, indicated an advanced stage of strangulation.

In patients with any of the above physical examination and laboratory findings, CT scans should be done regardless of the plain film findings. This may lead to a more precise, earlier radiologic diagnosis of strangulation.[60,61]

Mesenteric Vascular Disease: Plain Film Findings

In elderly patients who present with an acute abdomen, in diabetics, or in those with a history of cardiovascular or collagen vascular diseases, the possibility of mesenteric vascular disease should be a primary consideration.

Plain abdominal radiographs remain important for the diagnosis of several causes of abdominal pain but are of little value in the confirmation of an acute mesenteric ischemia. Completely normal plain film findings have been reported in more than 25% of patients with mesenteric ischemia.[62] Plain film findings have already been described under the subheading of strangulation obstruction.

In mesenteric venous thrombosis, plain abdominal radiographs may show dilated and gas-filled loops of intestine with pronounced wall thickening and mucosal irregularity. An edematous bowel segment may appear as a gas-containing structure, straight or gradually curving because of wall thickening and not changing in shape between erect and decubitus views.[56] Thumbprinting may be identified along the mesenteric margin of a distended loop. The plain film, however, may also appear "benign," yet CT scans may show extensive abnormalities (Fig. 5-38).

Small Bowel in the Immediate Postoperative Period

The plain film pattern of an adynamic ileus has already been described. Though abdominal surgery is the most frequent cause of intestinal atony, there can be several other associated conditions.[63–65]

Unless further complicating factors exist, small bowel contractions return within a few hours of a laparotomy.[63] Gastric stasis, however, can be more prolonged and is compounded by increased air swallowing. Atony of the colon persists for 1 to 2 days, at times longer. Swallowed air passes out of the distended stomach and is moved into the atonic colon, which it increasingly distends. This almost "physiologic" postoperative ileus rarely lasts for more than 48 hours. More severe degrees, affecting the entire intestinal tract, are likely to follow laparotomies for mechanical

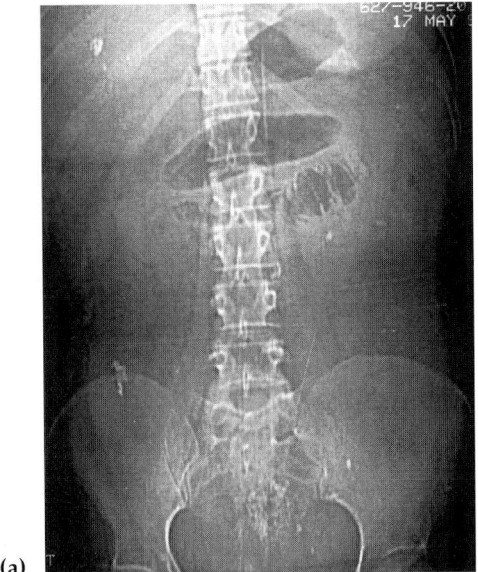 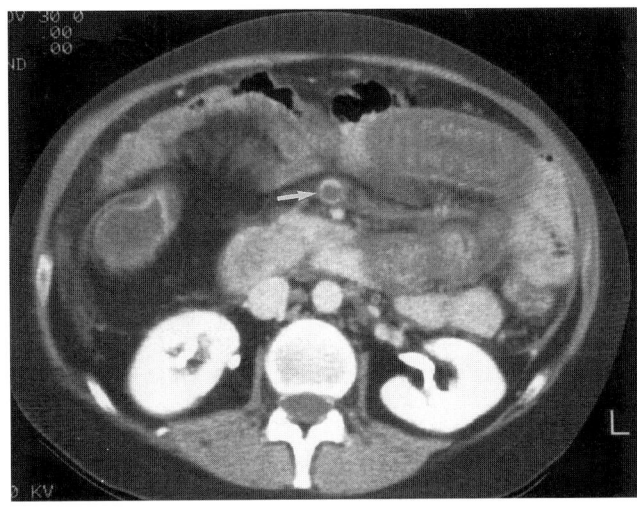

Fig. 5-38. Unreliability of plain film in mesenteric vascular disease.
(a) Supine abdominal radiograph in a 48-year-old female with known Crohn's disease presenting with severe abdominal pain shows a dilated loop of small bowel in upper midabdomen but is otherwise unremarkable. (b) CT shows diffuse edema of loops of small bowel and thrombus in superior mesenteric vein (arrow). Small rounded gas collection in left upper abdomen is intraluminal gas.

obstruction and may be termed "paralytic" or "neurogenic" ileus.[64]

Between 2 and 5 days, especially following pelvic surgery, the small bowel and colon may show plain film findings that resemble mechanical obstruction (Fig. 5-5). Motor inhibition of the pelvic small intestine secondary to manipulation at surgery or local inflammation may act as a temporary block to intestinal transport. This will improve spontaneously within a few days, aided by nasogastric suction. Persistence of decreased activity and distention beyond 5 days postoperatively should lead to a search for additional responsible factors, such as an intra-abdominal abscess or electrolyte imbalance. Identification of long segments of gas-distended small bowel with fluid levels more than 5 to 6 days after surgery should be viewed with suspicion, as these findings can reflect early mechanical obstruction. Rearrangement of such gas shadows, as shown by serial films, is taken as evidence of peristalsis and favors postoperative obstruction.[66] If the patient has vomited, a normal small bowel gas pattern may be found, even with partial obstruction. Whenever the question of small bowel obstruction arises and is not answered by plain films or by clinical evaluation, or if signs of sepsis or pancreatitis develop, CT examination is advised.[37] Enteroclysis or CT enteroclysis should be used only if additional management questions are left unanswered.[2]

Pneumoperitoneum Secondary to Small Bowel Perforation

Free air is demonstrated by plain films in only 18% of patients with spontaneous nontraumatic small bowel perforation.[67] Perforation secondary to blunt trauma results in a recognizable pneumoperitoneum in less than 50% of patients.[68,69] This is explained by the fact that small bowel normally contains very little air and that perforations are rapidly sealed by the omentum. This rapid "walling off" of perforations is induced by a local, transmural inflammatory process.[70] In some instances, eg, in cases of foreign body perforation, small bowel obstruction may be the only plain film finding. In a series dealing with pelvic trauma, small bowel perforation was the most commonly associated visceral lesion,[71] with an obstructive pattern as the only plain film evidence. Gas-containing diverticula may rupture from abdominal trauma, and some gas may escape into the peritoneal cavity.

In the diagnosis of pneumoperitoneum secondary to small bowel perforation, radiologists should search for subtle signs of small amounts of gas. As little as 1 to 2 ml of free air can be detected on erect chest and left decubitus radiographs of the abdomen.[72] Because many sick patients can not undergo the sequences of erect views, the plain film detection of free air in the supine position has been emphasized.[73–79]

Cho and Baker[80] have divided the supine film signs of free intraperitoneal air into three groups: 1) bowel-related signs, 2) anterior peritoneal ligament signs, and 3) right upper quadrant signs. The bowel-related signs include: A) *"Rigler's or bas-relief sign,"* the plain film demonstration of a bowel wall by the simultaneous presence of bowel gas within and free air on the outside. A further bowel-related feature is B) the *"triangle sign,"* caused by small amounts of gas trapped among three adjacent loops of bowel or between two loops of bowel and the parietal peritoneum. Among anterior peritoneal ligament signs are C) the *falciform ligament sign,* which is an obliquely oriented linear shadow that bisects the ovoid upper peritoneal cavity. This has been likened to a football, with the falciform ligament as the central ace.[81] Further anterior peritoneal ligament signs are D) the *urachus sign,* an elongated tubular or slightly triangular density located between the umbilicus and the bladder, and E) the *lateral umbilical ligament sign,* an inverted "V" formed by the lateral umbilical ligaments (or medial umbilical folds) outlined by free air as they descend inferiorly and laterally. The right upper quadrant signs include: F) the *hyperlucent liver sign,* describing the pneumoperitoneal replacement of the brightness of the hepatic shadow; G) the *hepatic edge sign,* the medial portion of the inferior edge of the liver seen as a well-defined linear shadow with its long axis directed superomedially and outlined by free air in the anterior peritoneal cavity; and H) the *fissure for ligamentum teres sign,*[79] a sharply defined vertically oriented slitlike or oblong lucency in the region of the porta hepatis. When larger amounts of free air are present, the extrahepatic segment of the ligamentum teres can also be visualized.[82] I) *Morison's pouch sign* refers to free air in the superior extension of the posterior subhepatic space and is seen as a crescentic or triangular lucency located right and medially below the 11th rib. J) The *anterior superior oval* is applied to a single or multiple ovoid lucencies overlying the liver, usually on its medial aspect. Recently described is K) the *diaphragmatic muscle slip sign,* depicting two or three arcuate, air-outlined long costal muscle bundles on the under surface of the right diaphragm.[83]

Most of the above signs are seen only when moderate to massive amounts of free air are present in the anterior peritoneal cavity. Since little air is liberated from perforation of the small bowel, signs produced by subtle amounts of free air such as the "triangle sign" and "fissure for ligamentum teres sign" should be sought. The place to look for evidence of free air in the recumbent patient is the right upper quadrant. An air collection of a few milliliters can be detected (Fig. 5-39).

The current practice of performing CT scans first or immediately after plain film examination in many emergent abdominal situations makes it possible to identify smaller amounts of extraluminal gas. The threshold for diagnosing small bowel perforation should be low when a small extraluminal gas is seen adjacent to a fluid-filled dilated loop of small bowel or to a focal extraluminal fluid collection in the mesentery. In one report, CT demonstrated free air in all patients (100%), whereas the erect chest film could identify air in only 3 of 11 patients (27%) who had an air collection less than 13 mm in diameter.[84] Using the "lung window," CT can best visualize small amounts of air in the midabdomen and over the anterior surface of the liver. Numerous tiny pockets of air trapped in recesses of the peritoneal and extraperitoneal cavities are also best shown by CT.

Pneumatosis Cystoides Intestinalis

This is an uncommon condition characterized by the presence of multiple gas-filled cysts within the wall of any part of the gastrointestinal tract. It is usually first diagnosed by plain film radiography or by CT. Mayer coined the term "pneumatosis cystoides intestinorum" in 1825, but the disease was first described in the 18th century by duVernai in France and John Hunter in England. Pneumatosis intestinalis occurs more fre-

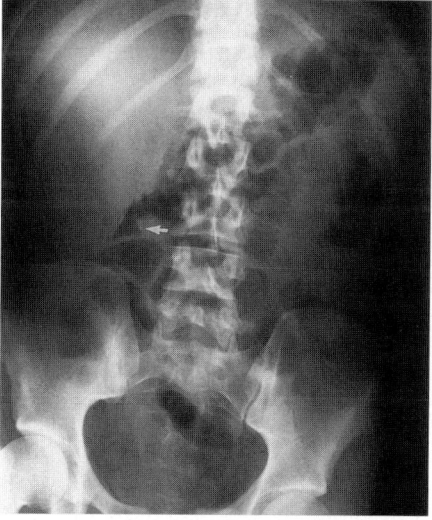

Fig. 5-39. "Triangle sign" in minimal pneumoperitoneum.
Triangular gas collection (arrow) is seen in right upper quadrant in a case of foreign body perforation of distal small bowel.

quently in the small bowel, but large bowel involvement is increasingly reported.[85–87]

Pathogenesis

The gas collections in the intestinal wall can be found in the subserosa, mucosa, and submucosa, the muscular layer being least affected.[87] The gas collections range in size from a few millimeters to several centimeters and are predominantly found on the mesenteric border. The cysts are lined by flat cells that resemble endothelium; they do not contain fluid.

Several explanations have been suggested for the formation of the gas collections:[85–95] 1) A mechanical theory postulates that gas may be forced into the bowel wall by several mechanisms.[85,86] These may be associated with an ulcer in the intestinal mucosa, direct injury during endoscopic procedures, enteric tube placement, or blunt abdominal trauma. Small bowel obstruction with its increased intraluminal pressure and increase of intraluminal gas may lead to penetration through minute mucosal defects. Increased pulmonary pressure with alveolar rupture and dissection of gas through the mediastinum and along the great vessels into the retroperitoneum and then through the subperitoneal space of the mesentery into the bowel wall is a likely explanation in cases of chronic obstructive airway disease and in cystic fibrosis.[91–93] 2) A bacterial theory is supported by the cysts containing hydrogen, a product of bacterial metabolism and not of mammalian cells.[94] However, the absence of an inflammatory reaction around the cysts and the rarity of peritonitis being associated with a pneumoperitoneum are against a bacterial cause of pneumatosis intestinalis.[95] Yet, breath hydrogen measurement in patients with intestinal pneumatosis exceeds that in normals or disease controls,[96] and cyst shrinkage has been reported followed treatment with metronidazole.[97] A direct communication between the cysts and the lumen of the bowel has never been demonstrated.[98] The persistence of the cysts suggests that they are replenished at a rate that equals or exceeds the rate of absorption. Hyperbaric oxygen therapy is based on the principle of alternating the balance between diffusion of gases into and out of the cysts, thus favoring their absorption.[98–100]

Clinical Considerations

In the majority of cases, pneumatosis intestinalis is an incidental finding. Symptoms attributed to this condition include diarrhea, rectal bleeding, large amounts of flatus, colicky abdominal pain, and mucous discharge per rectum.[87] There is a fulminant form, which accompanies necrotizing enterocolitis in infants. Pneumatosis intestinalis secondary to bowel ischemia or gangrene, although rarely "cystoides" in its radiologic appearance, has also been included among the pneumaroses. Asymptomatic pneumoperitoneum without evidence of peritonitis has been frequently reported and should be managed conservatively.[101,102]

Radiology

Although more recent experience has indicated that CT is more sensitive than plain film examination in the diagnosis of pneumatosis intestinalis,[102,103] the initial diagnosis is usually made by plain film examination.

Plain film findings are characteristic (Fig. 5-40).[90] The gas collections appear as round or ovoid lucencies, 0.5 to 3.0 cm in diameter, and may be clustered like bunches of grapes along the margins of the bowel involved, at times the colon.[80,104] This may simulate polypoid lesions on barium enema examinations if the radiolucency of the protrusions is not recognized. In pneumatosis usually associated with bowel ischemia (secondary pneumatosis), the gas collections are pre-

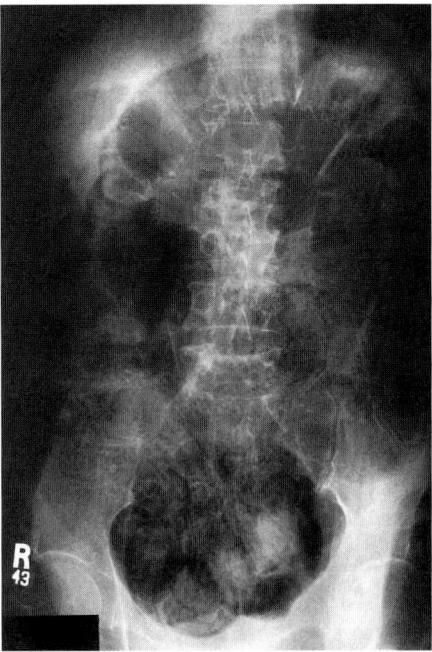

Fig. 5-40. Pneumatosis intestinalis in an elderly patient with known scleroderma.
The cystic and linear accumulations of mural gas follow the contour of the small bowel and impart a characteristic plain film appearance.

dominantly linear, paralleling the lumen, but they can be somewhat bubbly, circumferential, or amorphous and are usually associated with linear streaks, clearly different from the larger, well-defined gas cysts of the primary form. Although the two types of pneumatosis can be readily distinguished from one another by radiology, attributing clinical significance to their difference does not always hold true,[102] and the radiologic appearance is not a predictor of the severity of the condition.[103–107] The presence or absence of pneumoperitoneum does not affect the clinical significance of the pneumatosis. Development of pneumoperitoneum probably depends on the layer of the bowel wall involved by the gas cysts and is more likely to occur when they are located in the subserosa. Gas entry into the portal system in conjunction with secondary pneumatosis, usually of the linear variety, carries a serious connotation. This combination is frequently seen in necrotizing enterocolitis of infants or in bowel infarction of adults. Yet, there have been reports of portal vein gas in association with a benign pneumatosis.[103]

Pneumatosis is seen on CT as collections of gas in the periphery of the bowel loops. This is shown to best advantage by using lung window settings. Bubbles of gas trapped in stool or in diverticula or within mostly fluid-filled small bowel loops can mimic the appearance of pneumatosis.[80] The absence of air-fluid or air-contrast levels and a distribution that includes the dependent wall of bowel loops favors the diagnosis of pneumatosis.[107]

Pneumatosis has been well shown by ultrasound, both in the bowel wall and within the portal system (see Chapter 8).

Enterolithiasis

A bezoar or enterolith in the small intestine is a rare condition. The detection of enteroliths on abdominal imaging studies is an indication of underlying functional or structural abnormalities in the intestinal tract, and of the likely need for surgical relief.[108]

Enteroliths can be separated into two types: 1) false enteroliths that are of exoenteric origin and include fecaliths and bezoars; and 2) true enteroliths that form within the small intestine. Bezoars are classified according to the materials of which they are composed: phytobezoars, trichobezoars, lactobezoars, and medication bezoars (cholestyramine, sucralfate, calcium phosphate, nifedipine, sodium polystyrene sulfonate and aluminum hydroxide gel).[109] Bezoars may also form when large doses of nonabsorbable aluminum hydroxide are administered to patients with little bowel motility or with renal failure and dialysis associated desiccation of intestinal contents.[110] Bezoars may form if nonabsorbable antacids are associated with H_2 blockers, reduced acid secretion, and delayed gastric emptying.[111] Patients with impaired gastric emptying (diabetics, prior vagotomy) are at increased risk for bezoar formation. Although gastric bezoars have traditionally been removed surgically, nonsurgical treatment alternatives are available. These include endoscopic manipulation and fragmentation, enzymatic digestion using cellulase, and dissolution by sodium bicarbonate, to produce fragments that can pass into the small bowel, where they may become a nidus for enterolith formation.[112]

True enteroliths are subdivided into those containing mainly biliary constituents, usually formed in the duodenum or jejunum, and those composed mainly of mineral salts, usually calcium carbonate or oxalate and deposited in the more alkaline environment of the ileum.[112] Enteroliths of the former type are radiolucent, those of the latter type are radio-opaque.[113]

Enteroliths form in areas of stasis, mostly diverticula, and above strictures. Since Meckel's diverticulum is the most frequently encountered diverticulum of the small bowel, it is not surprising that it has been the site of most of the enteroliths reported in the literature (see Chapter 14).

Radiology

Radiopaque enteroliths tend to be laminated and can be identified on plain films (Fig. 5-41). They range in size from 1 to 5 cm and can be single or multiple.[108] Bezoars that are radiolucent or faintly opaque conform to the shape of the small-bowel. Other bezoars may manifest as mottled densities difficult to differentiate from fecal debris, although their location in the small bowel and associated plain film findings of obstruction should suggest their presence. Barium filling the interstices of some bezoars produces a mottled appearance similar to that of a villous tumor. However, small bezoars and other foreign bodies may be seen to be mobile, which will exclude a neoplasm.

Small bowel bezoar can be demonstrated ultrasonographically (see Chapter 8). CT not only will demonstrate an enterolith but will give additional insight into any associated abnormality such as a Meckel's diverticulitis or Crohn's disease and will also indicate the site of the usually associated small bowel obstruction.[112,114–116]

The radiographic differential diagnosis of enterolith is lengthy and includes many extraintestinal

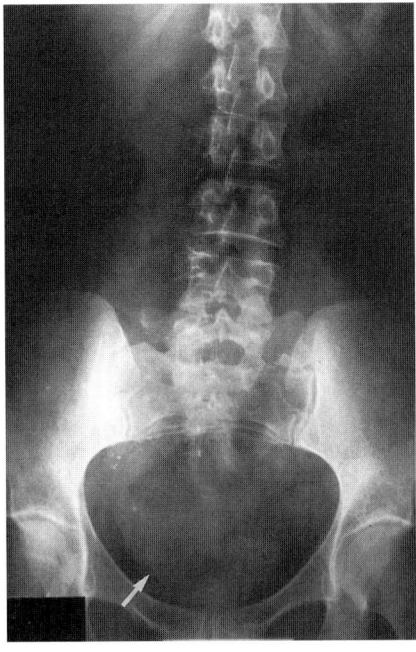
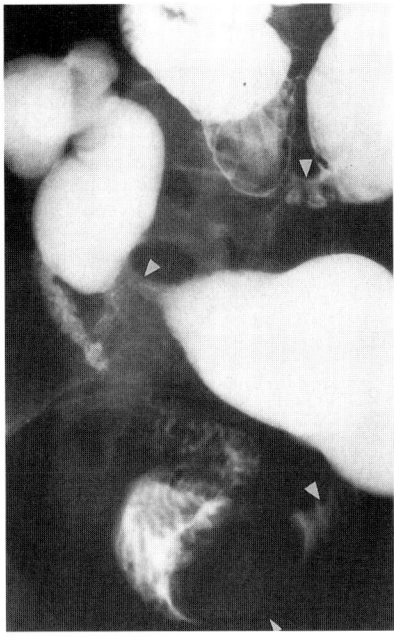

Fig. 5-41. Enterolith in stenosing Crohn's disease.
(a) Supine abdominal radiograph in a patient with Crohn's disease and symptoms of obstruction shows a faintly laminated rounded density (arrow) in right hemipelvis. (b) Enteroclysis shows multiple segmental Crohn's strictures with intervening dilatations (arrowheads). The enterolith (arrow) is in a dilated pelvic segment.

(a) (b)

entities.[113,116,117] Small bowel enteroliths are frequently misinterpreted as biliary or urinary calculi or as innocuous concretions in the peritoneal or extraperitoneal spaces. A solitary stone in a Meckel's diverticulum may be difficult to distinguish from an appendicolith or urinary tract calculus. The considerable mobility of an enterolith in a Meckel's diverticulum is an important differentiating point. The presence of a stone in Meckel's diverticulum leads to its obstruction, inflammation, or perforation (see Chapter 14). Identification of an enterolith in the pelvis or lower abdomen of a patient with known Crohn's disease indicates its formation proximal to a stricture.[115] The association of biliary lithogenesis with Crohn's disease may very occasionally cause gallstone passage to be obstructed by a segment of stenotic ileal disease.[118] Enterolithiasis can also be a late sequela of intestinal tuberculosis with stricture formation[119] or may complicate a blind pouch syndrome.[120]

Miscellaneous rare conditions presenting with calcification of the small bowel or its mesentery include mesenteric cysts, especially of a chylous type, and calcium deposits in mesenteric fat necrosis. Widespread amorphous calcifications, characterizing the spread of ovarian cystadenocarcinoma through the peritoneal cavity, or the even more unusual psammomatous bodies from a spreading papillary cystadenocarcinoma of the ovary deserve brief mention.

Foreign Bodies in the Small Bowel

Once a swallowed foreign body has passed through the pylorus, it will eventually make it through the small bowel also. In spite of the numerous convolutions of the small bowel, damage to the bowel wall is

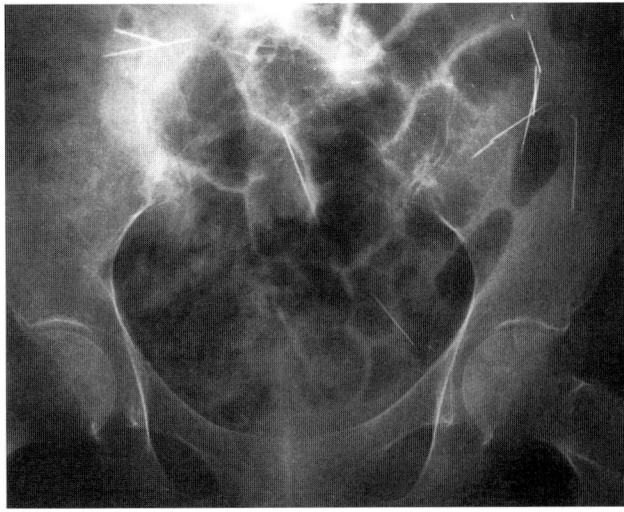

Fig. 5-42. Ten needles were recovered at surgery from the small intestine of this seamstress who habitually held needles between her teeth during work.

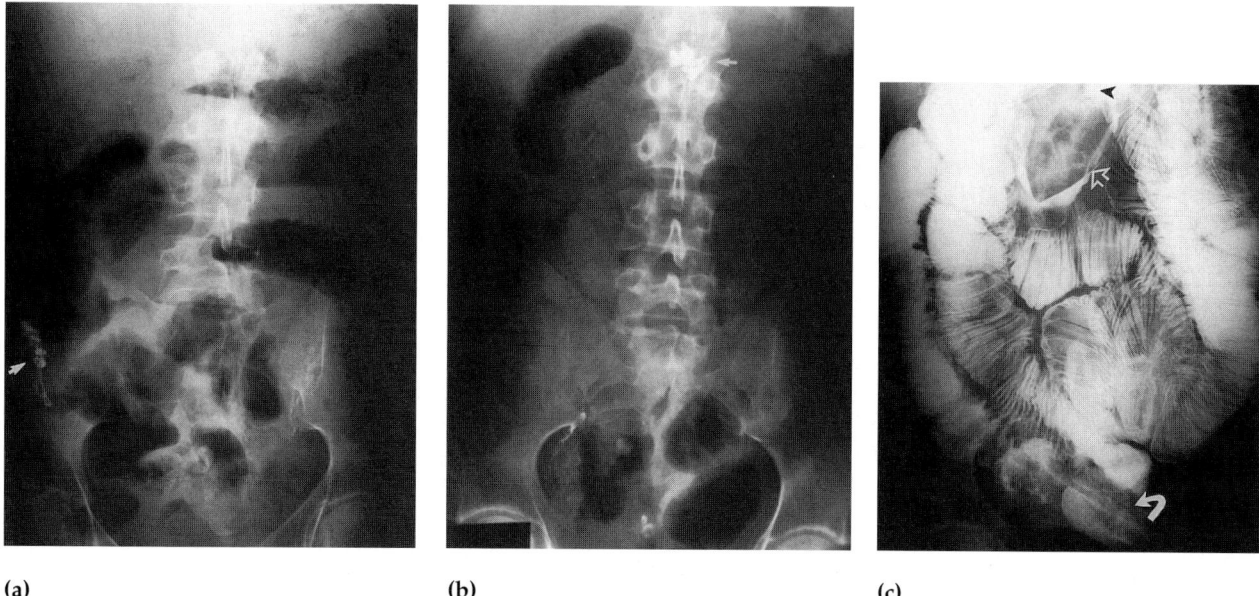

(a) (b) (c)

Fig. 5-43. Foreign bodies in the small intestine. A 29-year-old schizophrenic complained of vomiting and anemia. Stools were positive for occult blood.
(a) Abdominal radiograph shows multiple distended loops of small bowel consistent with distal mechanical obstruction. Also noted is a bracelet in the right lower abdomen (arrow) and foreign material in the pelvis. (b) Follow-up radiographs show limited progress of the bracelet, now in the epigastrium (arrow), and persistent distention of small bowel loops. (c) Enteroclysis demonstrates obstruction of further progress of bracelet (arrowhead) by a diamond-shaped foreign body (open arrow) impacted at a stricture. Inferiorly, tubular foreign bodies (curved arrow) are lodged in the ileum. At surgery, the bracelet was found proximal to a sponge obstructed by a benign stricture. The dilated inferior bowel segment was ulcerated and contained vaginal tampons fixed by adhesions.

uncommon, even with sharp foreign bodies. Only a small percentage (3.3%) of foreign bodies lodge in the small bowel compared with the esophagus (68%), stomach (11.6%), and colon (11.6%).[121] There may be delay of foreign body passage through the ileocecal valve.

Ingested foreign bodies are more likely to be found in patients from psychiatric hospitals[122] and in infants and children. Some foreign materials, such as bags of heroin, packages of cocaine, and marijuana-filled balloons, are deliberately swallowed for concealment from legal authorities.[123–125] Plain films of the abdomen are the usual method of their verification at airports. Most nondigestible food substances pass readily through the small bowel unless an obstructing lesion is present.[126] Frequently found, usually in edentulous patients, is the prune pit, which tends to become calcified.[127] The persimmon fruit can be a nucleus for repeated bezoar formation, a fairly frequent finding in Israel.

Radiology

Serial plain film radiography usually suffices to determine whether a foreign body is advancing or stationary. Long or sharply pointed objects may become lodged and will require laparotomy for their removal (Fig. 5-42). Diagnosis of small bowel perforation by a radiolucent toothpick can be done by expert ultrasonography (Fig. 8-43) (see Chapter 8).

Contrast examination or cross-section imaging are warranted when symptoms of obstruction are present or when patients have increasing anemia (Fig. 5-43). Ingested prune pits have a characteristic configuration on contrast study with tapering pointed ends and a radiolucent, striated center.

References

1. Maglinte DDT, Reyes BL, Harmon BH, et al. Reliability and role of plain film radiography and CT in the diagnosis of small-bowel obstruction. *AJR*. 1996;167: 1451–1455.
2. Maglinte DDT, Balthazar EJ, Kelvin FM, Megibow AJ. The role of radiology in the diagnosis of small-bowel obstruction. *AJR*. 1997;168:1171–1180.
3. Brewer RJ, Golden GT, Hitch DC, et al. Abdominal pain: an analysis of 1000 consecutive cases in a univer-

sity hospital emergency room. *Am Surg.* 1976;131:219–244.
4. Eisenberg RL, Heineken P, Hedgcock MW, et al. Evaluation of plain abdominal radiographs in the diagnosis of abdominal pain. *Ann Surg.* 1983;197:464–469.
5. Suh RS, Maglinte DDT, Lavonas EJ, et al. Emergency abdominal radiography discrepancies of preliminary and final interpretation and management relevance. *Emerg Radiol.* 1995;2:1–4.
6. Frimann-Dahl J. *Roentgen Examination in Acute Abdominal Diseases.* 3rd ed. Springfield, Ill: Charles C Thomas Publisher; 1974.
7. Mindelzun RE, Jeffrey RB. Unenhanced helical CT for evaluating acute abdominal pain: a little more cost, a lot more information. *Radiology.* 1997;205:43–45.
8. Baker SR. Unenhanced helical versus plain abdominal radiography: a dissenting opinion. *Radiology.* 1997;205:45–47.
9. Mindelzun RE, McCort JJ. Acute abdomen. In: Margulies AR, Burhenne JH, eds. *Alimentary Tract Radiology.* 4th ed. St Louis, Mo: CV Mosby Co; 1989:333.
10. Mirvis SE, Young JWR, Keramati B, et al. Plain film evaluation of patients with abdominal pain: are three radiographs necessary? *AJR.* 1986;147:501–503.
11. Field S. Plain films: the acute abdomen. *Clin Gastroenterol.* 1984;13:3–40.
12. Simpson A, Sanderman D, Nixon SJ, et al. The value of the erect abdominal radiograph in the diagnosis of intestinal obstruction. *Clin Radiol.* 1985;36:41–42.
13. Reyes BL, Lappas JC, Maglinte DDT, Hanna M. Plain film findings in patients with suspected small-bowel obstruction: relevance to triage for additional work-up. Presented at the 27th Annual Meeting and Postgraduate Course, Society Gastrointestinal Radiologists, February 22–27, 1998; Rancho Mirage, Calif.
14. Miller RE. The technical approach to the acute abdomen. *Semin Roentgenol.* 1973;8:267–279.
15. Woodring JH, Heiser MJ. Detection of pneumoperitoneum on chest radiographs: comparison of upright lateral and posteroanterior projections. *AJR.* 1995;165:45–47.
16. Sanders RC. Postoperative pleural effusion and subphrenic abscess. *Clin Radiol.* 1970;21:308–312.
17. Roh JJ, Thompson JS, Harned RK, Hodgson P. Value of pneumoperitoneum in the diagnosis of visceral perforation. *Am J Surg.* 1983;146:830–833.
18. Laufer I. Left lateral view in the plain film assessment of abdominal distention. *Radiology.* 1976;119:265–269.
19. Williams SM. Abdominal plain film: technique and normal anatomy. In: Gore R, Levine M, Laufer I, eds. *Textbook of Gastrointestinal Radiology, I.* Philadelphia, Pa: WB Saunders Co; 1994:152–168.
20. Messmer JM. Abdominal plain film: gas and soft tissue abnormalities. In: Gore R, Levine M, Laufer I, eds. *Textbook of Gastrointestinal Radiology, I.* Philadelphia, Pa: WB Saunders Co; 1994:169–192.
21. Baker SR. Abdominal plain film: abdominal calcifications. In: Gore R, Levine M, Laufer I, eds. *Textbook of Gastrointestinal Radiology, I.* Philadelphia, Pa: WB Saunders Co, 1994:193–200.
22. Levitt MD, Bond JH Jr. Volume, composition and source of intestinal gas. *Gastroenterology.* 1970;59:921–929.
23. Bryk D, Wolf BS. A radiological evaluation of small-bowel activity in the acute abdomen. *Crit Rev Diagn Imaging.* 1977;10:99–128.
24. Harlow CL, Stears RLG, Zeligman BE, Archer PG. Diagnosis of bowel obstruction on plain abdominal radiographs: significance of air-fluid levels at differential heights in the same loop of bowel. *AJR.* 1993;161:291–295.
25. Gammill SL, Nice CM Jr. Air fluid levels, their occurrence in normal patients and their role in the analysis of ileus. *Surgery.* 1972;71:771–780.
26. Markus JB, Somers S, Slobodan FF, et al. Interobserver variation in the interpretation of abdominal radiographs. *Radiology.* 1989;171:69–71.
27. Patel NH, Lauber PR. The meaning of a nonspecific abdominal gas pattern. *Acad Radiol* 1995;2:667–669.
28. Bohrer SP. Nonspecific gas pattern (letter to the editor). *Radiology.* 1989;173:283.
29. Maglinte DDT. Nonspecific abdominal gas pattern: an interpretation whose time is gone. *Emerg Radiol.* 1996;3:93–95.
30. Shrake PD, Rex DK, Lappas JC, Maglinte DDT. Radiographic evaluation of suspected small-bowel obstruction. *Am J Gastroenterol.* 1991;86:175–178.
31. Megibow AJ, Balthazar EJ, Cho KC, et al. Bowel obstruction: evaluation with CT. *Radiology.* 1991;180:313–318.
32. Maglinte DDT, Gage S, Harmon B, et al. Obstruction of the small intestine: accuracy and role of CT in diagnosis. *Radiology.* 1993;186:61–64.
33. Gazelle GS, Goldberg MA, Wittenberg J, et al. Efficacy of CT in distinguishing small-bowel obstruction from other causes of small-bowel dilatation. *AJR.* 1994;162:43–47.
34. Balthazar EJ. CT of small-bowel obstruction. *AJR.* 1994;162:255–261.
35. Taourel PG, Fabre JM, Pradel JA, et al. Value of CT in diagnosis and management of patients with suspected acute small-bowel obstruction. *AJR.* 1995;165:1187–1192.
36. Maglinte DDT, Peterson LA, Vahey TN, et al. Enteroclysis in partial small-bowel obstruction. *Am J Surg.* 1984;147:325–329.
37. Maglinte DDT, Herlinger H, Turner WW, Kelvin FM. Radiologic management of small-bowel obstruction: a practical approach. *Emerg Radiol.* 1994;1:138–149.
38. Gough NR. Strangulating adhesive small-bowel obstruction with normal radiographs. *Br J Surg.* 1978;65:431–434.
39. Phillpot JW, Swischuk LE, John SD. Appendicitis in the era of ultrasound: are plain radiographs still useful? *Emerg Radiol.* 1997;4:68–71.
40. Hudspeth AS, McGuirt WF. Gallstone ileus, a continuing surgical problem. *Arch Surg.* 1970;100:668–672.
41. Rigler LG, Bormen CN, Noble JF. Gallstone obstruction: pathogenesis and roentgen manifestations. *JAMA.* 1941;77:1753.
42. Grumbach K, Levine MS, Wexler JA. Gallstone ileus di-

agnosed by computed tomography. *J Comput Assist Tomogr* 1986;10:146–148.
43. Siewert B, Raptopoulos V. CT of the acute abdomen: findings and impact on diagnosis and treatment. *AJR.* 1994;163:1317–1324.
44. Kaltiala EH, Lenkkeri H, Lapmu TK. Mechanical intestinal obstruction, an analysis of 577 cases. *Ann Chir Gynaecol Fenniae* 1972;61:87–93.
45. Brolin RE, Krasna MJ, Mast BA. Use of tubes and radiographs in the management of small-bowel obstruction. *Ann Surg.* 1987;206:126–133.
46. Bizer LS, Leibling RW, Delany HM, Gliedman ML. Small-bowel obstruction: the role of nonoperative treatment in simple intestinal obstruction and predictive criteria for strangulation. *Surgery.* 1981;89:407–413.
47. Sarr MG, Bulkley GB, Zuidema GD. Preoperative recognition of intestinal strangulation obstruction: prospective evaluation of diagnostic capability. *Am J Surg.* 1983;145:176–182.
48. Barnett WO, Petro AB, Williamson JW. A current appraisal of problems with gangrenous bowel. *Ann Surg.* 1976;183:653–659.
49. Leffall LD, Syphax B. Clinical aids in strangulation intestinal obstruction. *Am J Surg.* 1970;120:756–759.
50. Nadrowski LF. Pathophysiology and current treatments of intestinal obstruction. *Rev Surg.* 1974;31:381–407.
51. Rigler LG, Pogue WL. Roentgen signs of intestinal necrosis. *AJR.* 1965;94:402.
52. Schorr S. Small intestinal intramural gas. *Radiology.* 1963;81:285.
53. Mellins HZ, Rigler LG. The roentgen findings in strangulating obstructions of the small intestine. *AJR.* 1954;71:404–416.
54. Williams JL. Fluid filled loops in intestinal obstruction. *AJR.* 1962;88:677–686.
55. Bryk D. Functional evaluation of small-bowel obstruction by successive abdominal roentgenograms. *AJR.* 1972;116:262–275.
56. Schauffer IA, Ferris EJ. The mass sign in primary volvulus of the small intestine in adults. *AJR.* 1965;94:374.
57. Nelson SW, Eggleston W. Findings on plain roentgenograms of the abdomen associated with mesenteric vascular occlusion with a possible new sign of mesenteric venous thrombosis. *AJR.* 1960;83:86–89.
58. Schmidt AG. Roentgen signs in strangulating obstructions of small intestine. *Radiology.* 1965;85:698.
59. Leffall LD, Quander J, Syphax B. Strangulation intestinal obstruction. *Arch Surg.* 1965;91:592–596.
60. Shatila AH, Chamberlain BE, Webb WR. Current status of diagnosis and management of strangulation obstruction of the small-bowel. *Am J Surg.* 1976;132:299–303.
61. Mathis J, Zelenek ME, Staab EV. CT detection of bowel infarction. *Comput Radiol.* 1985;9:177–179.
62. Federle MP, Chun G, Jeffrey RB, Raylor R. Computed tomographic findings in bowel infarction. *AJR.* 1984;142:91–95.
63. Smerud MJ, Daniel-Johnson C, Stephens DH. Diagnosis of bowel infarction: a comparison of plain films and CT scans in 23 cases. *AJR.* 1990;154:99–103.
64. Rothnie NG, Harper RAK, Cathpole BN. Early postoperative gastrointestinal activity. *Lancet* 1963;2:64–67.
65. Smith J, Kelly KA, Weinshilboum RM. Pathophysiology of postoperative ileus. *Arch Surg.* 1977;112:203–209.
66. Ellis H. Acute intestinal obstruction. In: Maingot R, ed. *Abdominal Operations*, 7th ed. New York, NY: Appleton-Century-Crofts; 1980.
67. Bryk D, Lehrer S. Successive abdominal roentgenograms: new method of evaluating postoperative small-bowel activity. *Invest Radiol.* 1977;12:520–526.
68. Mischinger HJ, Berger A, Kronberger L, Felbaum C. Spontaneous small-bowel perforation. Rare cause of acute abdomen. *Acta Chir Scand.* 1989;155:593–599.
69. Ting YM, Reuter SR. Hollow viscus injury in blunt abdominal trauma. *AJR.* 1973;119:408–413.
70. Love L. Radiology of abdominal trauma. *JAMA.* 1975;231:1377–1380.
71. Maglinte DDT, Taylor SD, Ng AC. Gastrointestinal perforation by chicken bones. *Radiology.* 1979;130:597–599.
72. Moore JR. Pelvic fractures: associated intestinal and mesenteric lesions. *Can J Surg.* 1966;9:253–261.
73. Miller RE, Nelson SW. The roentgenologic demonstration of tiny amounts of free intraperitoneal gas: experimental and clinical studies. *AJR.* 1971;112:574–585.
74. Rigler LG. Spontaneous pneumoperitoneaum. A roentgen sign found in the supine patient. *Radiology.* 1941;37:604–607.
75. Jelaso DV, Schultz EH Jr. The urachus—An aid to the diagnosis of pneumoperitoneum. *Radiology.* 1969;92:295–298.
76. Weiner CI, Diaconis JN, Dennis JM. The "inverted V": a new sign of pneumoperitoneum. *Radiology.* 1973;107:47–48.
77. Menuck L, Siemers PT. Pneumoperitoneum: importance of right upper quadrant features. *AJR.* 1976;127:753–756.
78. Cho KC, Baker SR, Thornhill BA, et al. Supine film diagnosis of pneumoperitoneum: new observations in the right upper quadrant. *Radiology.* 1988;169:405.
79. Levine MS, Scheiner JD, Rubesin SE, et al. Diagnosis of pneumoperitoneum on supine abdominal radiographs. *AJR.* 1991;156:731–735.
80. Cho KC, Baker SR. Air in the fissure for the ligamentum teres: new sign of intraperitoneal air on plain radiographs. *Radiology.* 1991;178:489–492.
81. Cho KC, Baker SR. Extraluminal air—diagnosis and significance. In: Balthazar EJ, ed. *Imaging the Acute Abdomen. Radiol Clin North Am.* 1994;32:829–844.
82. Miller RE. The "football sign" in neonatal perforated viscus. *Am J Dis Child.* 1962;104:311.
83. Cho KC, Baker S. Visualization of the extrahepatic segment of the ligamentum teres: a new sign of free air on plain films. *Radiology.* 1997;202:651–654.
84. Cho KC, Baker S. Depiction of diaphragmatic muscle slips on supine plain radiographs: sign of pneumoperitoneum. *Radiology.* 1997;203:431–433.
85. Stapakis JC, Thickman D. Diagnosis of pneumoperi-

86. Koss LG. Abdominal gas cysts (pneumatosis cystoides intestinorum hominis). *Arch Pathol.* 1952;53:523–549.
87. Galandiuk S, Fazio VW. Pneumatosis cystoides intestinalis. A review of the literature. *Dis Colon Rectum.* 1986;29:358–363.
88. Shallal JA, Van Heerden JA, Bartholomew LG, Cain JC. Pneumatosis cystoides intestinalis. *Mayo Clin Proc.* 1974;49:180–184.
89. Ecker JA, Williams RG, Clay KL. Pneumatosis cystoides intestinalis—bulbous emphysema of the intestine: a review of the literature. *Am J Gastroenterol.* 1971;56:125–136.
90. Ghahremani GG, Port RB, Beachley MC. Pneumatosis coli in Crohn's disease. *Am J Dig Dis.* 1974;19:315–323.
91. Nelson SW. Extraluminal gas collections due to diseases of the gastrointestinal tract. *AJR.* 1972;155:225–248.
92. Smith BH, Welter LH. Pneumatosis intestinalis. *Am J Clin Pathol.* 1967;48:455–465.
93. Elliott GB, Elliott KA. The roentgenologic pathology of so-called pneumatosis cystoides intestinalis. *AJR Radium Ther Nucl Med.* 1963;98:720–729.
94. Hernanz-Schulman M, Kirkpatrick J Jr, Schwachmann H, et al. Pneumatosis intestinalis in cystic fibrosis. *Radiology.* 1986;160:497–499.
95. Hughes DT, Gordon KC, Swann JC, Bolt GL. Pneumatosis cystoides intestinalis. *Gut.* 1966;7:553–557.
96. Goodall RJR. Pneumatosis coli: report of two cases. *Dis Colon Rectum.* 1978;21:61–65.
97. Gillon J, Tadesse K, Logan RF, et al. Breath hydrogen in pneumatosis cystoides intestinalis. *Gut.* 1979;20:1008.
98. Ellis BW. Symptomatic treatment of primary pneumatosis coli with metronidazole. *Ann Surg.* 1978;187:245.
99. Forgacs P, Wright PH, Wyatt AP. Treatment of intestinal gas cysts by oxygen breathing. *Lancet.* 1973;1:579–582.
100. Holt S, Gilmour HM, Buist TAS, Marwick K, Heading RC. High flow oxygen therapy for pneumatosis coli. *Gut.* 1979;20:493–498.
101. Masterson JS, Fratkin BL, Osler TR, Trapp WG. Treatment of pneumatosis cystoides intestinalis with hyperbaric oxygen. *Ann Surg.* 1978;187:245–247.
102. Broecker BH, Moore EE. Pneumoperitoneum due to pneumatosis cystoides intestinalis in idiopathic megacolon. *JAMA.* 1977;237:1963.
103. Caudill JL, Rose BS. The role of computed tomography in the evaluation of pneumatosis intestinalis. *J Clin Gastroenterol.* 1987;9:223–226.
104. Lund EC, Han SY, Holley HC, Berland LC. Intestinal ischemia: comparison of plain radiographic and computed tomographic findings. *Radiographics.* 1988;8:1083–1108.
105. Feczko PJ, Mezwa DG, Farah MC, White BD. Clinical significance of pneumatosis of the bowel wall. *Radiographics.* 1992;12:1069–1078.
106. Rice RP, Thompson WM, Gedgaudas RK. The diagnosis and significance of extraluminal gas in the abdomen. *Radiol Clin North Am.* 1982;20:819–837.
107. Knechtle SJ, Davidoff AM, Rice RP. Pneumatosis intestinalis: surgical management and clinical outcome. *Ann Surg.* 1990;212:160–165.
108. Kelvin FM, Korobkin M, Ranch RF, et al. Computed tomography of pneumatosis intestinalis. *J Comput Assist Tomogr.* 1984;8:276–280.
109. Paige ML, Ghahremani GG, Brosnan JJ. Laminated radioopaque enteroliths: diagnostic clues to intestinal pathology. *Am J Gastroenterol.* 1987;82:432–437.
110. Tatekawa Y, Nakatani K, Ishii H, et al. Small obstruction caused by a medication bezoar: report of a case. *Surg Today.* 1996;26:68–70.
111. Townsend CM, Remmers AR, Sarles HE. Intestinal obstruction from medication bezoars in patients with renal failure. *N Engl J Med.* 1973;288:1058–1059.
112. Burruss GL, Van Voorst SJ, Crawford AJ. Small-bowel obstruction from an antacid bezoar: a ranitidine-antacid interaction? *South Med J.* 1986;79:917–918.
113. Rumley TO, Hocking PH, King CE. Small-bowel obstruction secondary to enzymatic digestion of a gastric bezoar. *Gastroenterology.* 1983;84:627–629.
114. Brettner A, Euphrad E. Radiological significance of primary enterolithiasis. *Radiology.* 1970;94:283–288.
115. Macari M, Panicek DM. CT findings in acute necrotizing Meckel diverticulitis due to obstructing enterolith. *J Comput Assist Tomogr.* 1995;19:808–810.
116. Schut JM, Mallens WMC. Calcified enteroliths in regional enteritis. *Diagn Imaging Clin Med.* 1986;55:146–150.
117. Nigogosyan M, Dolinskas C. Case report. CT demonstration of inflamed Meckel's diverticulum. *J Comput Assist Tomogr.* 1990;14:140–142.
118. Shapiro JH, Rubenstein B, Jacobson HG, Poppel MA. Enteroliths in the small intestine. *AJR.* 1956;75:343–348.
119. Senofsky GM, Stabile BE. Gallstone ileus associated with Crohn's disease. *Surgery.* 1990;108:114–117.
120. Chawla S, Bery K, Indra KJ. Enterolithiasis complicating intestinal tuberculosis. *Clin Radiol.* 1966;17:274–279.
121. Gin FM, Maglinte DDT, Chua GT. Enterolith in a blind pouch (blind pouch syndrome secondary to side-to-side enteroanastomosis). *Radiographics.* 1993;13:965–967.
122. Bloom RR, Nakano PH, Gray SW, Skandalakis JE. Foreign bodies of the gastrointestinal tract. *Am Surg.* 1986;52:618–621.
123. Roake G, Subramanyan K, Patterson M. Ingested foreign bodies in mentally disturbed patients. *South Med J.* 1983;76:1125–1127.
124. Dunne JW. Drug smuggling by internal bodily concealment. *Med J Aust.* 1983;2:436–439.
125. McCarron MM, Wood JD. The cocaine "body packer" syndrome. *JAMA.* 1983;250:1417–1420.
126. Dassel PM, Punjabi E. Ingested marijuana filled balloons. *Gastroenterology.* 1979;76:166–169.
127. Price JE, Michael SL, Morgenstern L. Fruit pit obstruction. "The propitious pit." *Arch Surg.* 1976;111:773–775.

The Small Bowel Follow-Through and Its Modifications

Dean D.T. Maglinte and Hans Herlinger

Chapter Contents

"Requiem" for the "Conventional" Follow-Through
Alternative Techniques
The Fluoroscopic Small Bowel Follow-Through
Modifications of the Fluoroscopic SBFT
Limitations and Indications of the Fluoroscopic SBFT
Conclusion

"Requiem" for the "Conventional" Follow-Through

Small bowel diseases frequently present with nonspecific abdominal symptoms. Although the small bowel represents 75% of the length and 90% of the mucosal surface of the intestinal tract, its incidence of disease is low. Clinically effective diagnostic screening for possible small bowel disease requires methods of examination that can provide documentation of small structural abnormalities or reliable evidence of normality.[1] Because of current limitations of enteroscopy (limited availability and low level of interest), barium examination has retained primary responsibility for the diagnostic assessment of the small bowel mucosa.[2]

At present, the "conventional" small bowel follow-through (SBFT) examination is routine in most radiology departments. Among its weaknesses is the fact that it may commence with a double-contrast upper gastrointestinal (GI) study, even in patients without symptoms of upper GI tract disease. A further dose of lower-density barium is then administered and successive overhead (overcouch) films are used to monitor progress. The appearance of barium in the cecum becomes an indication for fluoroscopy to demonstrate the terminal ileum ("spot the TI"). The various overhead films are inspected, and fluoroscopy is carried out if it is thought that an abnormality has been demonstrated. Because of its crowded location in the peritoneal cavity, multiple segments of the small bowel cannot be adequately delineated with this form of SBFT. A large multi-institutional prospective study (the National Cooperative Crohn's Disease Study) showed inadequate definition of the proximal ileum in 35%, of the distal ileum in 32%, and of the jejunum in 24% of patients.[3] Garvey et al[4] showed poor radiographic visualization of the proximal ileum in 28% of 133 consecutive patients having a small bowel barium follow-through. This is a significant proportion of patients with incompletely delineated segments. The experience of any physician active in this field includes several examples of lesions that were not detected by inspection of the overhead radiographs.[5,6] We have reported 45 such conventional studies that missed 48 significant lesions that were later demonstrated by enteroclysis.[7] However, because of the simplicity of this flawed technique, many clinicians order it almost routinely, "thinking that they are learning something about the gut—or at least ruling out small-bowel disease."[8] There should be no doubt at all that the so-called "conventional" small bowel follow-through fails to apply the same principles of diagnostic care that are the rule in virtually all other areas of radiology, and must be abandoned.[9]

Alternative Techniques

A very accurate alternative technique would be enteroclysis, which, by the direct infusion of contrast into the small bowel, bypasses the pyloric sphincter to be able to challenge the distensibility and fixation of individual segments of small bowel. Furthermore, the hypotonia induced by this controlled infusion produces hypotonia and allows improved demonstration of mild strictures and adhesions and the detection of small nodules.[2] However, many radiology departments do not have the personnel and resources that can be committed to the efficient performance of enteroclysis.[10] Added problems are the increased cost and radiation exposure and the discomfort to the patient.[11–14] The need for conscious sedation in many patients requires a hospital-based radiology practice and further adds to the cost. Experience has also shown that enteroclysis is not a procedure diagnostic radiologists can adequately perform merely because they have done other barium examinations, just as enteroscopy is not a procedure for all endoscopists who have done gastric or colonic endoscopies.[15] Since enteroclysis is, therefore, unlikely to deal with all or most of the diagnostic problems of the small bowel, it follows that the "conventional" follow-through must be modified to avoid those significant false-negative and false-positive error rates.[6,7]

First of all, it is necessary to face the inherent limitations of any follow-through examination.[7] These are: 1) the slow and intermittent emptying of the stomach, which should serve as the main pump to fill the small bowel with contrast, 2) the unpredictable transit through the small bowel, with the possibility of flocculation occurring, 3) the problem of detecting lesser strictures, smaller nodules, or masses in a contracted bowel wall, and 4) the difficulty in determining mobility and pliability of the bowel with very limited use of fluoroscopy and compression. A properly performed "dedicated" SBFT can deal with most but not all of the above limitations but cannot equal the accuracy of enteroclysis. However, its clinical relevance can be significantly improved, particularly in situations where the diagnosis or exclusion of disease of the more distal ileum is a primary clinical concern (eg, endoscopically diagnosed inflammatory bowel disease of the colon).

This chapter will now describe practical aspects and general principles for the "dedicated" or "fluoroscopic" SBFT as well as various modifications of the procedure.

The Fluoroscopic Small Bowel Follow-Through

Aspects of Patient Preparation

Preliminary cleansing of the colon has no appreciable effect on small bowel transit and quality of examination.[4,16] Cleansing enemas as administered for the colon (for a barium enema) should not be done, as they push debris back into the distal ileum. An abbreviated form of preparation is suggested by some authors.[17,18] One recommended preparation[17] is a normal breakfast on the day before the examination. At noon the patient takes a bottle of magnesium citrate followed by a glass of water and then by a glass of clear fluid every hour until bedtime. No solid food is allowed for the rest of the day. At 4 pm the patient takes two biscodyl tablets (Dulcolax, Boehringer, Ingelheim, Germany) with sufficient water. Other authors merely administer a colon-active laxative in the afternoon before the study—for example, three or four tablets of biscodyl (Dulcolax)—and have the patient abstain from food and drink from 8 pm.[18] The limited preparation clears the right colon of fecal debris and fluid, which becomes important should a peroral pneumocolon be required during the follow-through.

Patients who are insulin-dependent diabetics are asked to take a can of Ensure (Ross) at lunch and supper and half a can as an evening snack. They are told to continue with their normal insulin routine except for the morning of the study, when only half the insulin dose is taken. Patients on other medications are asked to take them up to 2 hours before the small bowel examination. However, all iron-containing medications should be stopped at least 2 days before the examination.

Principles Related to Transit Acceleration

Acceleration of barium transit through the small intestine has three purposes: 1) to lower the incidence of degradation of the barium suspension, 2) to improve lumen distention of the small bowel, and 3) to render the examination less burdensome to the radiology department and the patient.[18]

Barium suspensions tend to deteriorate if exposed to the small bowel luminal milieu for too long. This deterioration can occur within the wide range of normal transit time (15 minutes to 3 hours) even in persons without small bowel disease. Degradation can produce a spectrum of changes, from a mere flaky appearance of the suspension to a fully developed flocculation. Either change will adversely affect the coating ability of barium, producing grades of nonadherence to the mucosa. It is the aim of the follow-through to achieve uniform filling of the entire mesenteric small bowel with a barium suspension that is capable of demonstrating mucosal detail.

The time taken for the transit of barium from ingestion to its entry into the colon can be influenced at two stages of the examination: 1) at the outflow of contrast from the stomach and 2) during its passage through the small bowel.

Outflow from the Stomach

The ingestion of a larger amount (400 to 600 ml)[19–21] of barium or of a colder (5°C) barium suspension,[22] or of both in combination,[23] has been shown to accelerate outflow and shorten transit. A right-sided decubitus position of the patient after ingestion can speed gastric emptying further but is not required when 500 ml or more barium suspension has been given to form a constant sump against the pylorus in the sitting position.[24]

Metoclopramide is a drug with strong gastrokinetic action due to its cholinergic effect.[25–27] It increases the resting muscle tension in the gastric fundus and the size of the peristaltic contractions in the antrum. Outflow is further aided by associated relaxation of the pylorus.

Accelerated Passage Through the Small Bowel

Peristaltic activity in the small intestine is initiated as a response to intraluminal boluses that activate mechanoreceptors by pressure against the bowel wall.[28] More rapid gastric emptying of a larger amount of barium, therefore, can produce or intensify aborally propagated waves of contraction. In this way, accelerated outflow from the stomach directly influences the speed of transit through the small bowel. Because of activation of the mechanoreceptors, there is little associated increase in luminal distention.

Meglumine diatrizoate (Gastrografin, Bristol-Myers Squibb, Princeton, NJ), 10 ml, added to the barium suspension has been reported to cause significant acceleration of transit without obvious osmosis and image deterioration.[29] Its mode of action remains unclear. The addition of only partially absorbed sorbitol to barium in concentrations at or above 2% speeds transit through the small bowel, owing to its osmotic effect. In consequence, image quality is somewhat impaired. Neostigmine, a synthetic anticholinesterase, given by subcutaneous injection, accelerates gastric and small bowel transit but has a number of side effects and contraindications.[30] It is only rarely used.

Metoclopramide (Reglan; Robins, Richmond, Va), in addition to its gastrokinetic function, also exerts a prokinetic effect in the small intestine. It increases the amplitude of ring contractions that involve longer segments of bowel, rendering the sweeping action more effective. Increased resting tension is associated with a decreased lumen diameter and mostly affects the proximal gut. Metoclopramide is usually administered as 1 to 2 tablets (10 mg each) or as a slow intravenous injection of 10 mg in a 2-ml vial. Absorption from the gut requires up to 30 minutes to reach maximum serum level, though with a somewhat variable bioavailability.[27] The intravenous injection acts within 3 minutes and is effective for about 1 hour. The dose for children is 0.1 mg/kg of body weight. Anticholinergic drugs and glucagon inhibit or abolish the action of metoclopramide. It appears to be less effective in the elderly. Complications from a single dose are very rare. Dystonic reactions have been reported. Contraindications to the use of metoclopramide are perforation, high-grade mechanical obstruction, and major gastrointestinal bleeding. It should not be used in patients with pheochromocytoma or together with phenothiazines.

Cholecystokinin and its synthetic decapeptide *ceruletide* have virtually identical effects on the gastrointestinal tract. They produce pylorospasm, delay gastric emptying, inhibit proximal duodenal motility, and markedly increase peristalsis of the jejunum, ileum, and colon.[31] Ceruletide should be administered by intramuscular injection (0.3 $\mu g/kg$) and only after a sufficient amount of barium has entered the jejunum. Dilution with an equal quantity of water prevents pain at the site of injection. The mean duration of ceruletide-assisted small bowel examinations, from the time of the injection, has been reported to be 10 to 20 minutes, compared with 45 to 80 minutes for controls.[32,33] Ceruletide is currently not available in the United States.

The *combined use* of metoclopramide and ceruletide has been tested.[34] The gastrokinetic effect of intravenous metoclopramide produced earlier barium filling of the jejunum, and ceruletide could be injected sooner. The combined examination was completed within 30 minutes in 62% of 50 patients, with a mean duration of 29.3 minutes. When only metoclopramide was given to a further 50 patients, the corresponding figures were 50% and 37.6 minutes. Without drugs they were 14% and 69.1 minutes. Ceruletide produces significant lumen reduction and vigorous peristalsis, especially of the ileum. Longitudinally arranged folds in contracted segments could still be assessed for shape and thickness of folds. Loops tended to be elevated out of the pelvis to become more accessible to compression. The examination of the majority of patients could be completed during a single occupancy of a radiographic room.[34]

Drugs Delaying Transit

Anticholinergics have a profound relaxant effect on the small bowel. Transit can be inordinately delayed, and flaccid loops are difficult to assess accurately. Hyoscine-N-butyl bromide (Buscopan) is shorter acting and has a less pronounced delaying effect on the small bowel.[30] Its use should be discontinued for a few hours before a small bowel meal. Diphenoxylate (Lomotil) impairs small bowel motility and causes luminal distention and fluid increase. It should not be used 24 hours before the examination. Morphine, codeine, and atropine also produce small bowel atony and should not be given to patients for at least 6 hours before the examination. Increasing the dose of metoclopramide intravenously will usually restore peristalsis.

Types of Barium Suitable for the SBFT

A 40 to 50% wt/vol suspension of barium specifically formulated for the small bowel is used.[10] Such factory-prepared liquid suspensions are convenient and satisfactory. These can be Entrobar (Lafayette Pharmacol, Lafayette, Ind) or Entero-H diluted with an equal quantity of water (E-Z-EM Co, Westbury, NY). The barium should not contain sorbitol, which is hyperosmolar and in higher concentration causes diarrhea and in lower concentration reduces the crispness of the barium-outlined mucosal folds.

Compression Devices

Abdominal compression is an integral part of the fluoroscopic SBFT. Most fluoroscopic X-ray tables incorporate a compression cone that can conveniently be moved in whenever needed. Other compression devices include the F spoon, the Mayo spoon, and an inflatable balloon compression device, all excellent for different situations.[17,35] A rolled-up towel taped into a cylinder shape 9 in. long and 3 to 4 in. in diameter is useful. The Malmö technique uses a rolled and taped firm cloth cylinder 3 ft long and 3 to 4 inches in diameter for use with the patient prone; it is positioned transversely under the upper abdomen and slowly pulled down.[17]

Technique of the Fluoroscopic (or Dedicated) SBFT

If desirable, a promotility agent (usually metoclopramide) should have been given by mouth some 20 minutes before starting the examination.

A preliminary plain film of the abdomen may be useful if there is a history of abdominal surgery, in a patient with possible bowel obstruction, or when there have been recent radiological studies using contrast materials. This film should be seen by the radiologist before starting the examination.

This examination should not be preceded by a double-contrast gastroduodenal study. An "in passing" single-contrast examination of the esophagus, stomach, and duodenum may be done, provided the patient's upper gastrointestinal tract has not been examined recently.[36] For this limited "in passing" study, the erect patient drinks 300 ml of the recommended barium suspension, and any required images are exposed. The patient then returns to the waiting area, sits down, and slowly sips the remaining 200 to 300 ml of the barium. Without the need for an upper GI investigation, the patient should sip the entire 500 to 600 ml of the barium suspension, while sitting comfortably.[36]

The first small bowel fluoroscopic session is done 15 to 20 minutes after ingestion of the barium suspension. In this and subsequent radiologist-conducted sessions all opacified bowel loops should be fluoroscopically studied during graded compression and in optimally rotated positions of the patient. Spot images are taken as needed. An overhead film may be added but is best left till later. Subsequent fluoroscopic sessions follow at 20- to 30-minute intervals, as judged by the progress of the barium column. To improve the sensitivity of the examination, fluoroscopy and compression radiography should be done at least two or three times during the course of the follow-through examination,[7] to be continued until the colon is reached (Fig. 6-1).

Proximal loops of jejunum are best viewed with the patient supine and turned to the right. All bowel loops must be separated from one another by compression and should be imaged when filled with barium as well as when somewhat flattened by grades of compression, always in some degree of patient rotation. Overcompression results in anatomical distortion and should be avoided. This is continued until the terminal ileum has been studied and recorded on a spot image. Overhead views of the abdomen, with the patient prone, may be taken at intervals after the fluoroscopic sessions but are usually not critical to the result of the examination. It is during fluoroscopy that normality or pathology of the bowel segments is ascertained. However, a final prone overhead image of the entire abdomen should be done, mainly for the purpose of orientation (Fig. 6-2).

When examined for unexplained abdominal pain, spot films during a Valsalva maneuver in the lateral position can be of value to identify anterior abdominal wall hernias in obese patients in whom a clinical diagnosis may have been missed. Upright radiographs with appropriate obliquity should also be done to demonstrate reducible groin hernias.[37]

The emphasis of this form of the SBFT is on fluoroscopy, fluoroscopic spot filming, and compression, not on overhead radiography. Attention must also be directed to a study of the mobility and pliability of all small bowel loops during compression.[36] Mobility implies displacement of bowel loops by compression, pliability their change of outline when compressed.

The success of the fluoroscopic SBFT depends on close supervision throughout the procedure by an interested radiologist. The multiple fluoroscopic ses-

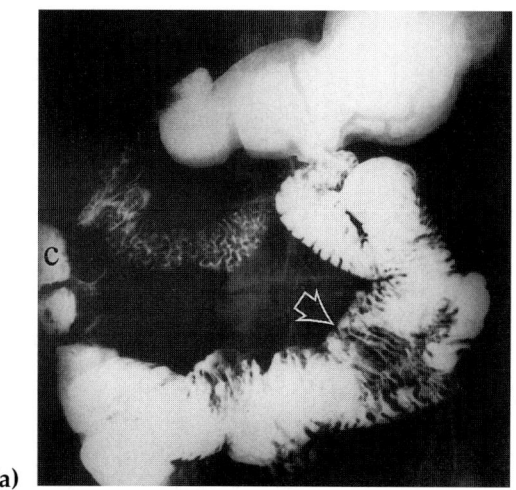 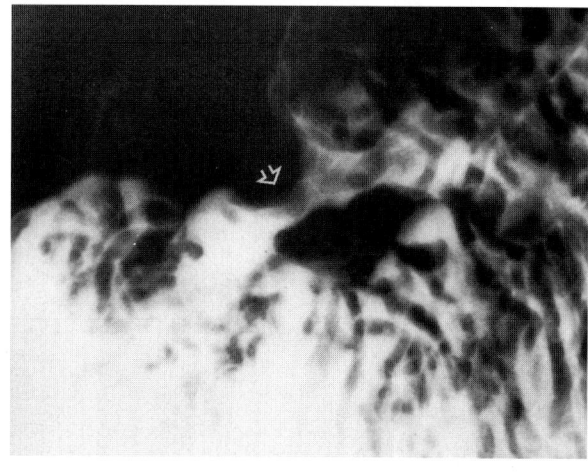

Fig. 6-1. Patient with short bowel syndrome secondary to multiple resections because of Crohn's disease.
(a) Prone overhead radiograph 15 to 20 minutes after ingestion of contrast shows no obvious abnormality. (Arrow points to likely area of compression view shown below.) The right colon (C) has been reached and subsequent radiographs revealed no abnormality in this area. (b) Compression radiograph with patient turned right obtained during fluoroscopy (after A) reveals a jejunal stricture (arrow) with absent folds and without ulceration or features of obstruction. Although the distensibility of each segment is not challenged as it would be by enteroclysis, the fluoroscopic small bowel follow-through is a worthwhile examination when done meticulously.

sions, the nonreliance on full-size overhead radiographs of the abdomen, and the adoption of modifications (to be described below) to improve visualization of questionable segments distinguish the modern dedicated small bowel follow-through from the inadequate "conventional" small-bowel follow-through examination.[2]

Modifications of the Fluoroscopic SBFT

The Peroral Pneumocolon

This technique is indicated whenever the distal ileum cannot be evaluated adequately during peroral examinations because of poor filling, a low-lying pelvic cecum, or pelvic adhesions. It is particularly useful in patients suspected of having inflammatory bowel disease and in those with ileocolic anastomoses.[38–40] Peroral pneumocolon has occasionally been used to improve distal small bowel detail during enteroclysis when not enough barium or too much methylcellulose had been administered.[41] A clean colon is advantageous. It reduces artifacts caused by the reflux of stool content into the distal small bowel. It also appears to reduce patient discomfort during the insufflation of gas or carbon dioxide; the gas passage round a clean colon is associated with less distention.

The examination is performed after barium filling of the right side of the colon during a dedicated small bowel follow-through. Glucagon (1.0 mg IV) is given to facilitate reflux of air or carbon dioxide through the ileocecal valve, to reduce patient discomfort during insufflation and to induce small bowel hypotonia.[42,43]

A large Foley catheter (26F or 28F) or a rectal tube for barium enema is introduced into the rectum and gas insufflation can begin. If necessary, a balloon may have to be inflated and gently retracted to occlude the anal canal. By gravity-related positioning, the air or carbon dioxide is advanced into the right colon and cecum. Overdistention of the cecum should be avoided. To direct the air through the valve, it may help to have the patient turn to the left into a semiprone position. As the administered glucagon ensures persistent distention of the ileocecal region, the rectal tube may be removed as soon as sufficient air has entered the ileum in order to diminish patient discomfort. Supine and oblique spot images are then taken with compression. This technique achieves excellent distention of the distal ileum and can produce exquisite double-contrast detail to distinguish clearly a pathologic from a normal appearance (Fig. 6-3). It may also be of value in double-contrast imaging of the right colon, provided bowel preparation has been adequate. There is a failure rate of less than 10%, when gas cannot be induced to reflux through the ileocecal valve.

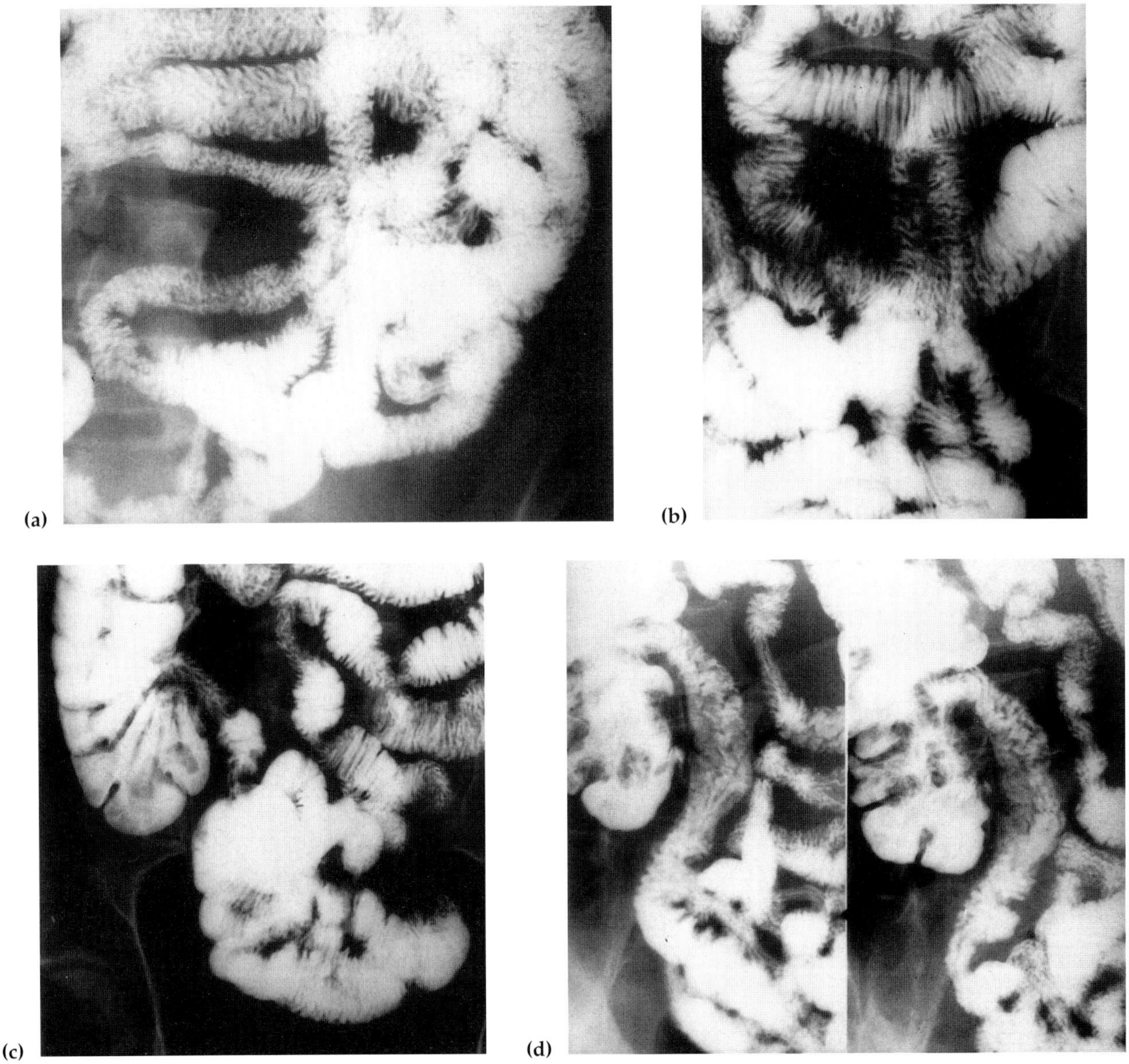

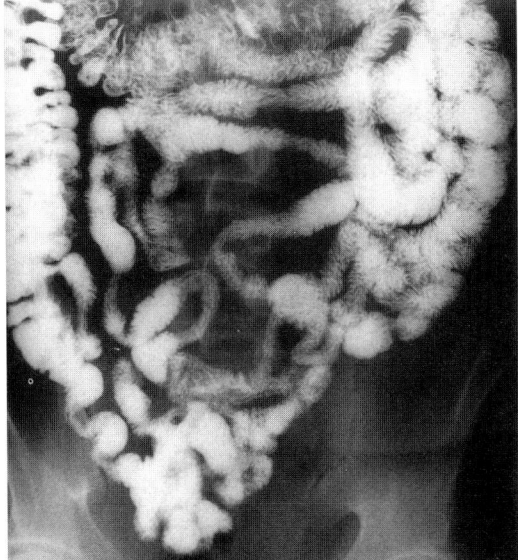

Fig. 6-2. The fluoroscopic small bowel follow-through.
(a) Compression radiograph of jejunum 10 to 15 minutes after ingestion of 500 ml of contrast material. Metoclopramide had been given before. (b, c) Compression radiographs of upper and lower pelvic segments of ileum done at 30 minutes show contrast having reached colon and reveal no abnormality. (d) Additional compression radiograph shows better distention of the terminal ileum. The use of the accelerating agent resulted in a faster examination with improved definition of folds. (e) A final overhead radiograph with the patient prone was obtained for anatomic orientation, mainly for the referring clinician. All areas appear to be normal; however, there is lumen contraction throughout the small bowel.

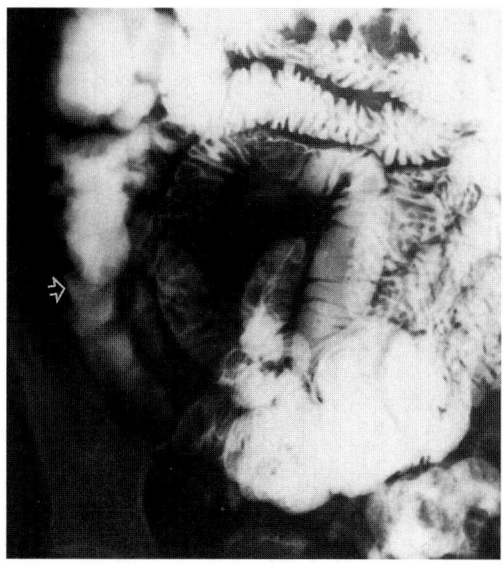 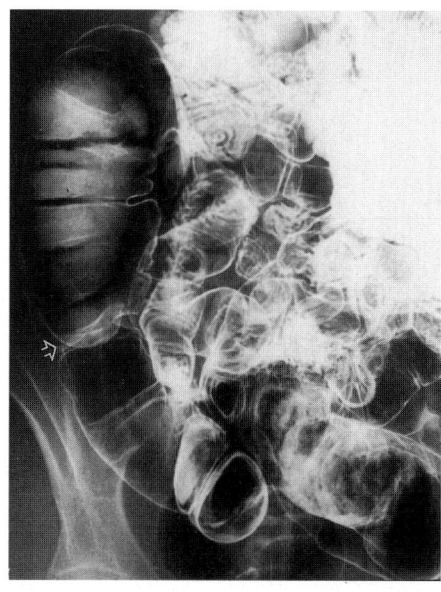

Fig. 6-3. Peroral pneumocolon in the demonstration of an ileocolic anastomosis and neoterminal ileum in a patient with suspected recurrence of Crohn's disease.
(a) Compression radiograph of ileoascending colon (arrow) does not demonstrate diagnostic features. (b) Following insufflation of gas per rectum, the normality of the ileoascending colon anastomosis (arrow) and of the mucosal pattern of the distal ileum are clearly defined. (Note the fecal debris distended sigmoid elevating pelvic segment of ileum.)

Per Ileostomy Pneumoileum

This modification is done in conjunction with a dedicated small bowel follow-through to improve distention and fold visualization of the prestomal and pelvic loops of ileum. When barium starts to exit the ileostomy, an injection of 0.5 mg of glucagon is given intravenously to abolish peristalsis, which would be intensified by introducing air. This also decreases patient discomfort. This results in satisfactory double-contrast examination of the distal small bowel in most instances.

A small Foley balloon catheter (16F or 18F) is used. The balloon can prevent reflux out of the stoma, and its use is safe provided certain precautions are observed. The purpose of the balloon is not to occlude the bowel lumen but to act as a seal from within against the usually narrower and nondistensible opening through the fascia. The balloon should, therefore, be positioned well inside the ileostomy, away from the stoma. The balloon should then be inflated by the radiologist under fluoroscopic control with 2 to 3 ml of air, merely enough to produce resistance to its gentle withdrawal. If needed, a further inflation by 1.0 ml aliquots of air can be made until occlusion is attained. However, a total amount of 5.0 ml of air should not be exceeded. A balloon should never be inflated if there is any bleeding from the stoma and it should be stopped if the patient feels any discomfort. Mild traction on the catheter by the radiologist or technologist during air inflation prevents contrast leakage. Enough air can be introduced to opacify the distal and more central bowel segments, as long as the patient can tolerate it without discomfort. Following compression spot imaging of the pelvic and more proximal segments of ileum in double contrast, the balloon is deflated and the catheter removed during fluoroscopy. As the gas and contrast rush out, the prestomal segment can be imaged again in oblique or lateral positions (Fig. 6-4).

Small Bowel Fistulography

The small bowel origin of fistulae can be indicated by the often considerable output of thin, alkaline fluid and by the history of usually recent surgery or of inflammatory bowel disease, mostly Crohn's. The purpose of radiology is to determine the site of origin of the fistula, its length, and complexity. A fluoroscopic barium follow-through or, preferably an enteroclysis (always with an opaque marker over the orifice of the fistula), may already have demonstrated its origin and underlying pathology but may not have provided enough information regarding the fistula itself.

A preliminary plain film in two projections can be helpful and may demonstrate a foreign body, eg, a

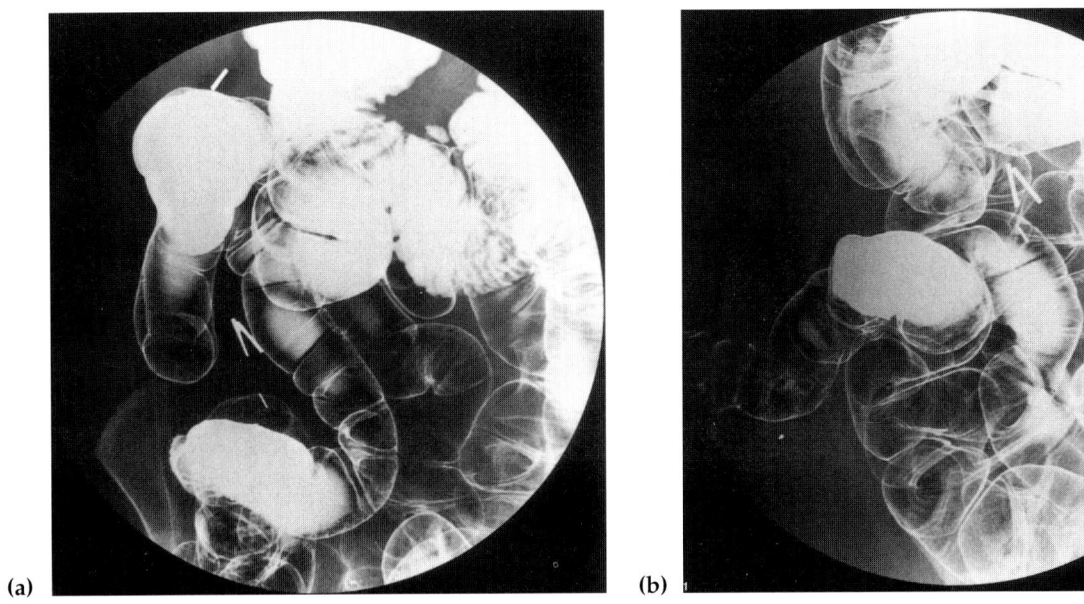

Fig. 6-4. Per ileostomy pneumoileum.
(a) Spot image of air double contrast in distal ileum shows good distention and excellent delineation of folds. (b) Spot image including normal prestomal ileum in steep oblique position just prior to removal of catheter.

sponge. A soft catheter of suitable diameter is then gently introduced. Pressure applied at the opening of the fistula is needed to reduce reflux of contrast material. This can be done by the finger of a cooperative patient, by a sponge clamped in a long forceps and held by the radiologist, or by the application of a prosthetic foam (Q7-4290, Dow Corning Corp, Midland, Mich). Water-soluble contrast should be injected at least at first, but may have to be followed by a low-viscosity barium suspension to depict more accurately the small bowel changes at the origin of the fistula and details of the course of the fistula itself. Important is a final image of the fistula taken in best projection the moment the catheter has been removed.

Gas-Enhanced Double-Contrast SBFT

This modification can improve delineation of the folds of any portion of the small bowel, including the pelvic and distal ileum. When the barium column reaches the cecum, an effervescent agent is given to generate a total of 750 to 1000 ml of gas (eg, two packets of E-Z gas, E-Z-EM Co, Westbury, NY) or Baros (Mallinckrodt, St. Louis, Mo). The patient is then placed in a left lateral or left posterior oblique position with a slight Trendelenburg tilt to allow gas to enter the duodenum and small bowel. The patient then assumes a supine position, still in Trendelenburg tilt. In many instances, gas reaches the distal ileum in 8 to 10 minutes. Radiographs of the small bowel with mild compression are obtained in the supine or oblique positions.

For the imaging of the distal ileum this technique is generally not as reliable as the peroral pneumocolon nor does it approach its image quality. However, more proximal bowel segments are often shown in better detail (Fig. 6-5). In one series, small bowel double contrast was obtained in 43% of patients, with improved luminal distention claimed in 96% and separation of loops possible in 85% (Fig. 6-6).[44]

In our experience, satisfactory visualization of all segments of the small bowel has been inconsistent with this technique.[10] Patients with slow transit (more than 1 hour in reaching the cecum) or with fluid in the distal small bowel do not usually show satisfactory gas-enhanced double contrast. Patients with delayed gastric emptying may have severe abdominal pain from the additional gas. Patients with incompetent lower esophageal sphincters may vomit following gas administration. In these situations the peroral pneumocolon is better tolerated, but does not serve quite the same purpose.

SBFT After Double-Contrast Upper Gastrointestinal Examination

This sequence of studies is undesirable for several reasons: 1) There is an excessive difference in concentration and viscosity (240% wt/vol against 40 to 50%

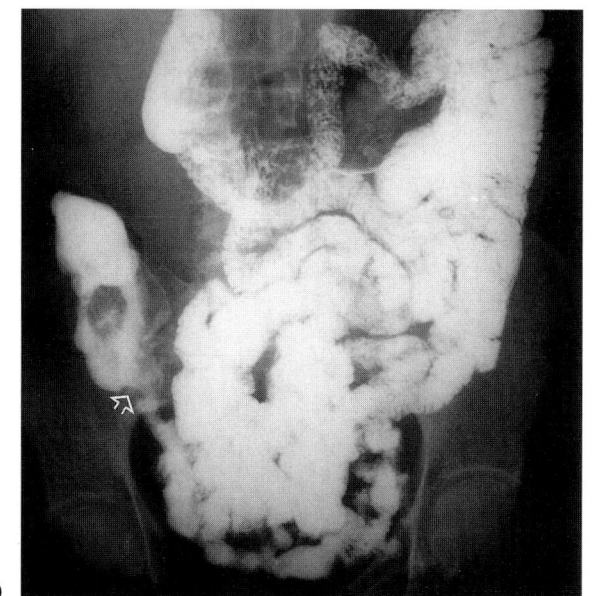 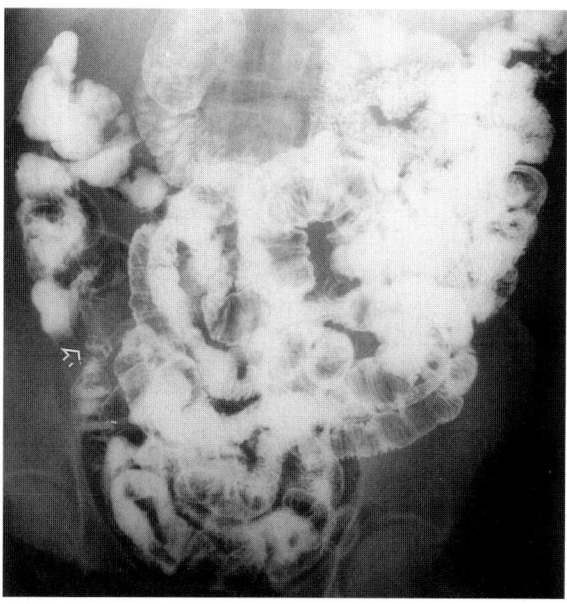

(a) (b)

Fig. 6-5. Gas-enhanced peroral double-contrast follow-through.
(a) Overhead radiograph obtained at 30 minutes and before gas ingestion shows contrast in the cecum and ascending colon. The folds of the pelvic segments and distal ileum (arrow) are poorly defined. (b) Eight minutes after ingestion of two packets of gas-producing crystals, gas is seen throughout the small bowel and cecum. The folds are better defined in both the pelvic segments and terminal ileum (arrow). Note extent of double contrast produced by this method.

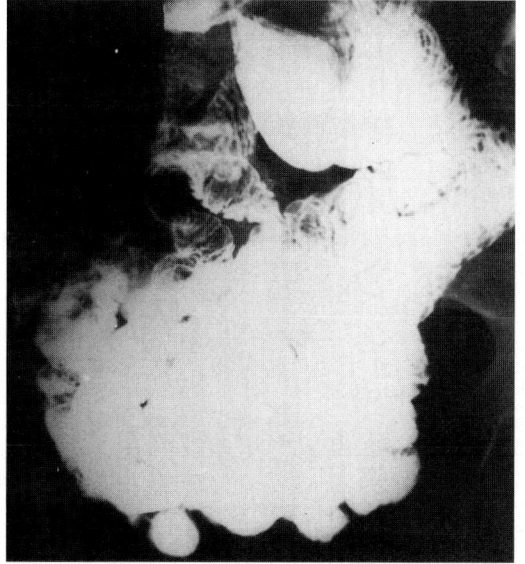 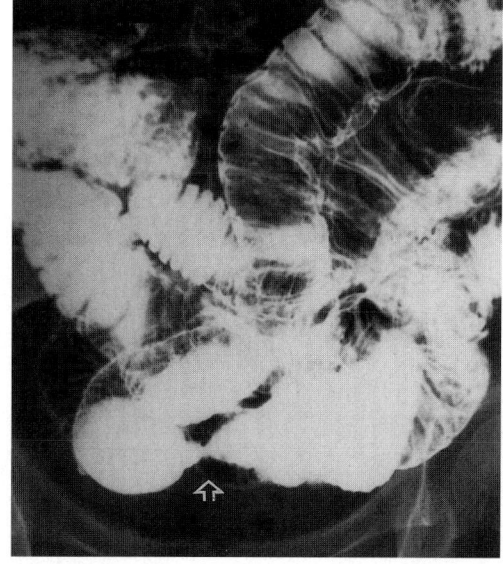

(a) (b)

Fig. 6-6. Gas-enhanced double-contrast follow-through.
(a) Prone overhead radiograph obtained in a patient with a history of radiation for carcinoma of the cervix shows featureless contrast-filled small bowel. Barium has appeared in the cecum. (b) Following ingestion of a gas-producing mixture, a supine radiograph of a pelvic segment of ileum shows a radiation stricture (arrow) not seen before. This underutilized modification of the follow-through can clarify appearances in pelvic loops of ileum. (Courtesy of G. M. Fraser, MD)

wt/vol) between the barium suspensions used in double-contrast study of the upper gastrointestinal tract and those suitable for small bowel passage. These suspensions do not readily mix and may remain largely separate by the time they reach the ileum. 2) The leading, heavier and denser barium suspension for the upper gastrointestinal study tends to sink into pelvic loops of ileum and may produce a "white" lower abdomen that defies transradiation. Suboptimal visualization of folds is likely.

If information regarding the distal ileum is the only concern, this form of examination can be salvaged by a peroral pneumocolon (Fig. 6-7). Other segments, however, are inadequately assessed. This should be understood by referring clinicians so that an interpretation of normality of the entire small intestine is not assumed when only the distal ileum can be clearly shown. We have attempted to improve this combination of examinations by giving the patient, after the double-contrast upper GI study, 100 ml of a 50% to 70% wt/vol barium mixture followed by 600 ml of a 0.5% methylcellulose solution. In spite of the high-density barium mixture used for the double-contrast examination, visualization of small bowel folds was adequate provided that the patient could ingest the 600 ml of methylcellulose in one setting. However, we favor the use of the peroral pneumocolon modification over the other techniques available to improve visualization of the distal ileum because of its ability to achieve at least partial lumen distention.

The "See-Through" Small Bowel Examination

This method of examination has been proposed to overcome the disadvantages of combining the double-contrast upper gastrointestinal examination and the small bowel follow-through. In this technique, the small bowel is examined first using a 13% wt/vol proprietary barium methylcellulose mixture (Entero Vu, E-Z-EM Co, Westbury, NY). The patient ingests 600 ml of the mixture during 10 to 15 minutes. Prone overhead radiographs are taken at 20-minute intervals until the cecum is reached. A double-contrast upper gastrointestinal examination is then performed.[45]

This method of examination has been claimed to be superior to the "conventional" follow-through in bowel loop and fold visualization because of the transradiancy property of methylcellulose.[46] No large series has been published to verify these claims.

We recommend two or more fluoroscopic sessions using compression during the course of the examination. Compression should be "light," as the low density of the barium suspension and its methylcellulose content easily disperse the barium coating. Although distensibility of the bowel wall is not challenged, improved visualization of folds, particularly of the jejunum, is an advantage (Fig. 6-8).

It has been suggested[45,47] that a double-contrast upper gastrointestinal examination can be done at the end of the small bowel see-through study if it is considered necessary for the two examinations to be car-

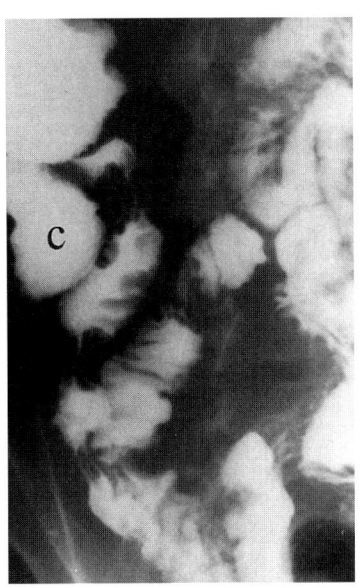
(a)

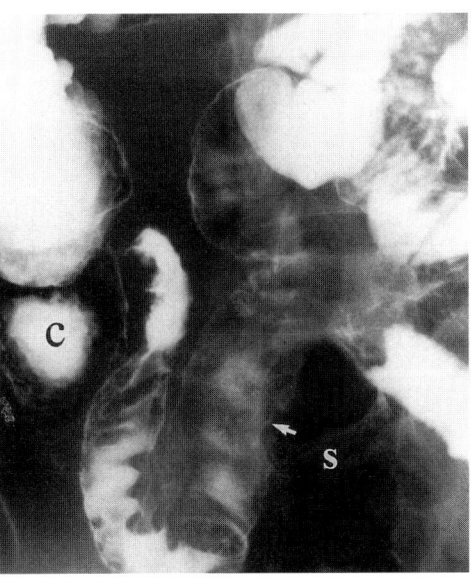
(b)

Fig. 6-7. Peroral pneumocolon in the diagnosis of distal small bowel Crohn's disease. Patient with endoscopically diagnosed Crohn's colitis.
(a) Compression radiograph of distal ileum during a follow-through that was preceded by a double-contrast upper GI study. Mild fold thickening was suspected but the barium mixture was too dense for adequate assessment of folds. (C = cecum.) (b) A peroral pneumocolon provides unequivocal findings of aphthous ulcers (arrow) to a segment with multiple ulcers not shown on (A). The distended sigmoid (S) elevates the distal ileum out of pelvis.

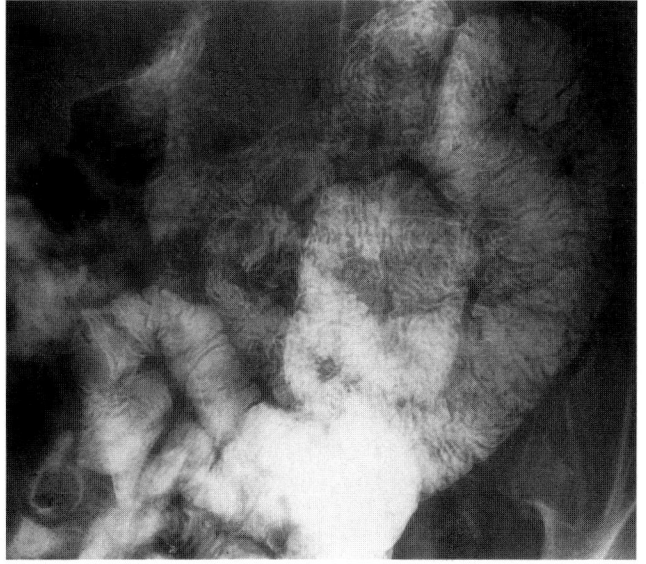 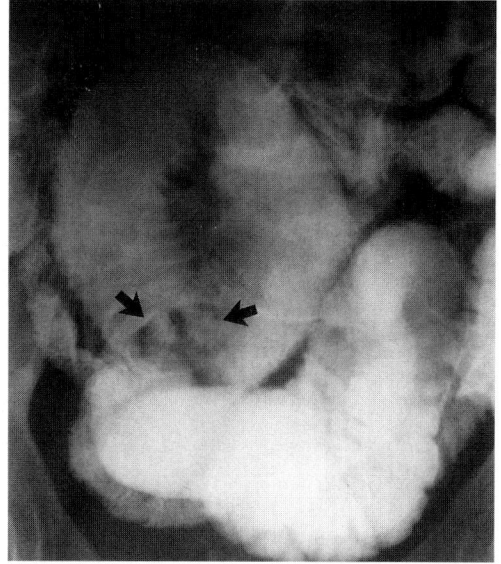

Fig. 6-8. The see-through SBFT.
(a) Early prone radiograph following ingestion of barium mixture containing methylcellulose shows good distention and delineation of folds of proximal small bowel. Note, however, increasing density of pelvic segments not uncommonly seen in patients with pelvic adhesions and asthenic habitus. (Courtesy of Barbara E. Taylor, MD.) (b) Barium/methylcellulose suspension outlines an ileal carcinoid with its typical desmoplastic effect on mucosal folds (arrows). (Courtesy of T. Stephen Kilcheski, MD.)

ried out in the same session. A problem of this sequencing, however, could be an accumulation of barium in the transverse colon, obscuring the stomach, together with impaired gastric coating caused by likely residual fluid in the stomachs of most patients.

Limitations and Indications of the Fluoroscopic SBFT

A significant limitation of the fluoroscopic follow-through is that drug-induced transit acceleration is inevitably associated with narrowing of the bowel lumen. In consequence, mucosal folds appear somewhat crowded and are often difficult to assess, regardless of the type of barium mixture used. A spurious appearance of nodularity may be produced by the overlap of loops with crowded folds. Furthermore, this technique cannot test the distensibility of the lumen and may miss segments with early mural infiltration, minimal obstruction, or small nodules.

The dedicated fluoroscopic follow-through adequately demonstrates longer small bowel segments with nondistensible walls such as those in radiation enteropathy, ischemia, and more advanced Crohn's disease. If combined with a pneumocolon, it is the peroral method of choice for the investigation of the distal ileum. This supplementary procedure is most valuable in questionable distal ileal inflammatory disease (Fig. 6-7). The "see-through" barium and the gas-enhanced double-contrast modifications improve fold visualization of more proximal segments and of pelvic segments in patients without pelvic adhesions but cannot provide the same degree of lumen distention of the distal ileum as is produced by the pneumocolon technique.

Concerning the combining of upper GI and small bowel studies in the same session, it is our belief that it is best to perform the gastroduodenal study with small bowel type barium in single contrast, with very adequate mucosal relief and compression techniques, and then to continue with the fluoroscopic small bowel follow-through.[10,17]

Conclusion

Small bowel radiography starts with careful selection of patients by knowledgeable clinicians.[48,49] Clinically effective imaging of the small bowel should be able to diagnose small structural lesions and provide reliable assurance of morphologic normality.[1,9,10] Although the performance of biphasic enteroclysis increases the diagnostic yield of the contrast examination,[5,6] a meticulously conducted fluoroscopic follow-through examination, augmented by some of the modifications described, can be an eminently worthwhile procedure in selected clinical situations. It should be a reasonable alternative where resources for a properly performed enteroclysis are not available. As in all radiologic examinations, a high technical standard should be maintained. If unequivocal small bowel normality has not been assured, enteroclysis ought to be performed in patients in whom small bowel disease is suspected.

References

1. Maglinte DDT, Herlinger H. Small-bowel radiography: an overview. *Dig Dis Sci.* 1984;29:1057–1059.
2. Maglinte DDT, Kelvin FM, O'Connor K, et al. Current status of small-bowel radiography. *Abdom Imaging.* 1996;21:247–257.
3. Goldberg HI, Caruthers SB Jr, Nelson JA, et al. Radiographic findings of the National Cooperative Crohn's Disease Study. *Gastroenterology.* 1979;77:925–937.
4. Garvey DJ, de Lacey G, Wilkins RA. Preliminary colon cleansing for small-bowel examinations: results and implications of a prospective survey. *Clin Radiol.* 1985;36:503–506.
5. Gurian L, Jendrzewski S, Katon RR, et al. Small-bowel enema: an underutilized method of small-bowel examination. *Dig Dis Sci.* 1982;27:1101–1108.
6. Maglinte DDT, Hall R, Miller RE, Chernish SM. Detection of surgical lesions of the small-bowel by enteroclysis. *Am J Surg.* 1984;127:225–229.
7. Maglinte DDT, Burney BT, Miller RE. Lesions missed on small-bowel follow-through: analysis and recommendations. *Radiology.* 1982;144:737–739.
8. Spiro H. Foreword. In: Herlinger H, Maglinte D, eds. *Clinical Radiology of the Small Intestine.* Philadelphia, Pa: WB Saunders Co; 1989.
9. Herlinger H. Why not enteroclysis? *J Clin Gastroenterol.* 1982;4:277–283.
10. Maglinte DDT, Lappas JC, Kelvin FM, et al. Small-bowel radiography: how, when and why? *Radiology.* 1987;163:297–305.
11. Ott DJ, Chen YM, Gelfand DW, et al. Detailed peroral small-bowel examination vs enteroclysis. Part 1: expenditures and radiation exposure. *Radiology.* 1985;155:29–34.
12. Salomonowitz E. Radiation dose of double contrast and single contrast examinations. In: Herlinger H, Maglinte D, eds. *Clinical Radiology of the Small Intestine.* Philadelphia, Pa: WB Saunders Co; 1989:147–150.
13. Thoeni RF, Gould RG. Enteroclysis and small-bowel series: comparison of radiation dose and examination time. *Radiology.* 1991;178:659–662.
14. Hart D, Haggett PJ, Boardman P, et al. Patient radiation doses from enteroclysis examinations. *Br J Radiol.* 1994;67:997–1000.
15. Maglinte DDT, Lappas JC. Sedation for enteroclysis using oral diazepam (letter/reply). *AJR.* 1996;167:1591.
16. Richards DG, Stevenson GW. Laxatives prior to small-bowel follow-through: are they necessary for a rapid and good-quality examination? *Gastrointest Radiol.* 1990;15:66–68.
17. Somers S, Stevenson GW. The small-bowel: anatomy and nontube examinations. In: Freeny PC, Stevenson GW, eds. *Margulis and Burhennes Alimentary Tract Radiology.* 5th ed. St. Louis, Mo: CV Mosby Co, 1994:512–532.
18. Herlinger H. Barium examinations. In: Gore R, Levine M, Laufer I, eds. *Textbook of Gastrointestinal Radiology.* Philadelphia, Pa: WB Saunders Co; 1994:766–772.
19. Kim SK. Small intestine transit time in the normal small-bowel study. *AJR.* 1968;104:522–524.
20. Weltz GA. Der Kranke Duenndarm im Roentgenbild. *ROFO.* 1937;55:20.
21. Marshak RH, Lindner AE. *Radiology of the Small Intestine.* 2nd ed. Philadelphia, Pa: WB Saunders Co; 1976.
22. Gershon-Cohen J, Shay H, Fels SS. The relation of meal temperature to gastric motility and secretion. *AJR.* 1940;43:237.
23. Brun B, Hegedus V. Radiology of the small intestine with large amounts of cold contrast medium. *Acta Radiol.* 1980;21:65–70.
24. Lintott DJ. The small-bowel follow-through: time to sit up (letter). *Clin Radiol.* 1995;50:133.
25. Kreel L. The use of oral metoclopramide in the barium meal and follow-through examination. *Br J Radiol.* 1970;43:31–35.
26. Kreel L. The use of metoclopramide in radiology. *Postgrad Med J.* July 1973;42–45.
27. Schulze-Delrieu K. Metoclopramide. In: Koch-Weser J, ed. *Drug Therapy. N Engl J Med.* 1981;305:28–33.
28. Wood JD. Physiology of the enteric nervous system. In: Johnson CR, ed. *Physiology of the Gastrointestinal Tract.* New York, NY: Raven Press; 1981:1–37.
29. Goldstein HM, Poole GJ, Rosenquist CJ, et al. Comparison of methods for acceleration of small intestinal radiographic examination. *Radiology.* 1971;98:519–523.
30. Kreel L. Review article: pharmacoradiology in barium examinations with special reference to glucagon. *Br J Radiol.* 1975;48:691–703.
31. Efsing HO, Lindroth B. Small-bowel examinations after injection of cholecystokinin. *Clin Radiol.* 1980;31:225–226.
32. Thompson WM, Halvorsen RA, Shaw M, et al. Evaluation of intramuscular ceruletide for shortening small-bowel transit time. *Gastrointest Radiol.* 1982;7:141–147.
33. Sargent EN, Halls JM, Colletti P, Wieier M. Efficacy and tolerance of ceruletide in radiography of the small intestine. *Radiology.* 1980;136:57–60.
34. Grumbach K, Herlinger H, Laufer I, Levine MS. Metoclopramide-ceruletide assisted small-bowel examination. *ROFO.* 1988;149:47–51.
35. Herlinger H, Lintott DJ. Standard examination of the small-bowel. In: Margulis AR, Burhenne HJ, eds. *Ali-*

mentary Tract Radiology. 3rd ed. St. Louis, Mo: CV Mosby Co; 1983:907–914.
36. Scholz FJ. Manual compression device for fluoroscopy. *Radiology*. 1989;170:564–565.
37. Maglinte DDT, Miller RE, Lappas JC. Radiologic diagnosis of occult incisional hernias of the small intestine. *AJR*. 1984;142:931–932.
38. Kellett MJ, Zboralske FF, Margulis AR. Peroral pneumocolon examination of the ileocecal region. *Gastrointest Radiol*. 1977;1:361–365.
39. Kelvin FM, Gedgaudas RK, Thompson WM, Rice RP. The peroral pneumocolon: its role in evaluating the terminal ileum. *AJR*. 1982;139:115–121.
40. Kressel HY, Evers KA, Glick SA, et al. The peroral pneumocolon examination: technique and indications. *Radiology*. 1982;144:414–416.
41. Fitzgerald EJ, Thompson GT, Somers SS, Franc SS. Pneumocolon as an aid to small-bowel studies. *Clin Radiol*. 1985;36:633–637.
42. Violon D, Steppe R, Potvelig AR. Improved retrograde ileography with glucagon. *AJR*. 1981;136:833–834.
43. Monsein LH, Halpert RD, Harrid ED, Feczko P. Retrograde ileography: value of glucagon. *Radiology*. 1986;161:558–559.
44. Fraser GM, Preston PG. The small-bowel barium follow-through enhanced with an oral effervescent agent. *Clin Radiol*. 1983;34:673–679.
45. Fitch D. The small-bowel see-through: an improved method of radiographic small-bowel visualization. *Can J Med Radiation Tech*. 1995;26:167–171.
46. Bourana A, Bourdon F. Improving the image quality of the dedicated single contrast small-bowel study by modifying the contrast medium. Presented at the 1994 Scientific Program of the Radiology Society of North America.
47. Bret P, Cuche C, Schmutz G. *Radiology of the Small Intestine*. New York, NY: Springer-Verlag; 1989:8–9.
48. Rabe FE, Becker GJ, Besozzi MJ, Miller RE. Efficacy of the small bowel examinations. *Radiology*. 1981;140:47–50.
49. Fried AM, Poulos A, Hayfield DR. The effectiveness of the incidental small bowel series. *Radiology*. 1981;140:45–46.

Enteroclysis
Technique and Variations

Hans Herlinger and Dean D.T. Maglinte with Tsuneyosi Yao

Chapter Contents

Advantages of Enteroclysis
Disadvantages of Enteroclysis
Digital Fluoroscopy for Enteroclysis

The development of intubation-based barium studies of the small intestine derived from a realization of the inherent limitations of the standard follow-through examination. To quote Pesquera (1929), the problems facing barium when passing through the small intestine include, "the irregularity of its action, its motility, and the flaky distribution that the mestrum assumes in this position of the gastrointestinal tract. . . ."[1] Some of these problems have been overcome by improvements to barium suspensions and to the technique of the follow-through examination (see Chapter 6).

Advantages of Enteroclysis

Intubation bypasses the regulatory action of the pylorus so that contrast fluid can be administered at a required rate. More rapid through-flow reduces the time of exposure of the barium to the adverse environment of the small intestine.

A larger amount and greater rate of inflow challenge the distensibility of the bowel lumen. Conditions restricting distention (eg, adhesive bands, fixation by tumor, annular lesions) are revealed in this way. Small sinus tracts or fistulae are opacified.

Adjustments to the rate of inflow control the speed of transit and can ensure a gradual filling and uniform distention of successive loops. Adequate distention straightens folds for a more accurate assessment of normality or subtle disease.

The entire small bowel can be demonstrated in a distended state at the end of the infusions. All loops can be studied fluoroscopically, by spot images, and by angled views.

The examination can usually be done in a single session of 20 to 30 minutes. Continued supervision by the radiologist is an essential and desirable component of the method.

Disadvantages of Enteroclysis

Intubation is a requirement. The unpleasantness of tube insertion can be mitigated by conscious sedation (see later).

Radiation: The mean skin entry dose of 123 mGy for enteroclysis is higher than the entry dose of 84 mGy for the barium follow-through. However, the mean completion time of enteroclysis is about half that of the follow-through.[2]

Digital Fluoroscopy for Enteroclysis

Digital fluoroscopy with digital imaging offer significant advantages over X-ray film-based methods. Rapid image taking at the right moment and rapid sequencing when needed are part of this advantage. Even more important is the ability to take magnification images as needed, to compare preceding images with an actual appearance, and in this way to demonstrate the presence of an unchanging outline or verify response to peristalsis or compression.

An important advantage is the postfluoroscopic manipulation of the recorded images. Selected images can be magnified, inverted, or edge-enhanced, or changes made to their contrast and brightness values. Reports can be rendered more meaningful when accompanied by hard-copy images, possibly adorned with arrows and explanations.

Fluoroscopy during enteroclysis, digital or otherwise, has the following purposes and limitations: 1) to control the rate of infusions, 2) to determine the most appropriate projection and degree of compression for spot images, and 3) to use compression by gloved hand or a compression device to test mobility and pliability of bowel loops. 4) In addition, most abnormalities that can be recognized at fluoroscopy can be seen in the single-contrast phase of the enteroclysis and should be recorded. Finer surface detail, which is optimally imaged in the double-contrast or intermediate phases and may not be fully appreciated during fluoroscopy, should be recorded and can be improved at the work station.

This chapter will describe enteroclysis in the following order:

1. Patient preparation
2. Catheters and infusions
3. Intubation
4. Single-contrast enteroclysis
5. Enteroclysis using methylcellulose as double-contrast agent
6. Biphasic enteroclysis
7. Modifications of the enteroclysis
8. Air double-contrast enteroclysis

Patient Preparation

Dietary

As far as possible the small intestine should be free of food and ingested fluid. A barium enema–type preparation is unnecessary. Magnesium citrate should be avoided. It generally suffices to abstain from food and fluid intake from the evening before the morning's examination. It is also useful to have a fairly empty right colon. To achieve this we suggest taking three bisacodyl (Dulcolax) tablets with two glasses of water on the afternoon before the examination. Laxatives are not indicated or needed in patients with inflammatory bowel disease.

Drugs

Peristalsis-inhibiting medications, such as morphine or Demerol, should be avoided from the evening before the enteroclysis. Metoclopramide, two tablets (each 10 mg), may be given to the patient about 20 minutes before the examination or intravenously to precede conscious sedation. It speeds transgastric intubation and improves progress through the small bowel. Repeated doses of metoclopramide are contraindicated for patients with high-grade small bowel obstruction, but a single intravenous dose of 10 to 20 mg aids transgastric and transduodenal passage of enteroclysis/decompression tubes without complications.[3]

Sedation

Enteroclysis can be performed with only surface anesthesia in the majority of patients. Generally transnasal intubation is better tolerated by patients who warn the radiologist that gagging is a problem for them. For enteroclysis only a low level of drowsy/arousable sedation is justified. But even this requires nurse-assisted patient monitoring throughout the sedation, using pulse oximetry, pulse, and blood pressure recordings. Midazolam, a mainly anxiolytic drug, and diazepam are the generally preferred medication and may be administered by slow intravenous injection of 1 to 5 mg, titrated according to effect. Higher doses of diazepam are needed in some patients. Midazolam may have to be combined with Fentanyl for more adequate sedative-analgesic effect.[4]

Catheters and Infusions

The senior author uses an enteroclysis catheter set produced by E-Z-EM Co (Westbury, NY), F13 × 135 cm with silicone balloon and eight side holes beyond it; a 0.065-inch Teflon-coated guide wire has torque control characteristics. Before use both the guide wire and inside of the catheter should be well lubricated with food-grade silicone spray. An alternative is Maglinte's balloon catheter F13 × 160 cm, with a tapered tip supplied with torque wire with both straight and angled tip, supplied by Cook (MDEC, Bloomington, Ind).[5]

For easier intubation there is Nolan's F10 × 135 cm catheter without balloon (Cook, Europe).[6] Three different types of F10 catheters are manufactured by E. Merck Ltd.[7]

Mostly for use in children (and some adults) is a thinner, softer catheter from Guerbet GmBH (POB 1240, 65838 Sulzbach/Taunus, Germany), F8 × 150 cm, endhole through metal tip, with flexible wire and adapter.[8]

Maglinte's multipurpose triluminal catheter,[9] F14 × 155 cm, with torque cable and adapter is ideal for nasogastric drainage and, if indicated, can be advanced for enteroclysis to the proximal jejunum and for long tube small bowel decompression in patients with small bowel obstruction (MDEC, Cook, Bloomington, Ind) (see Chapter 21 on small bowel obstruction).

Infusions

Barium 80% wt/vol Entero-h by E-Z-EM Co is the preferred suspension used in Herlinger's double-contrast-emphasized form of enteroclysis.[10] The biphasic technique advocated by Maglinte prefers a 50% wt/vol suspension, Entrobar, by Lafayette Pharmaceuticals

(Lafayette, Ind). A similar barium suspension (Miscropaque Flüssig) is used by Antes.[11] Methylcellulose (MC) is presently supplied as Entrocel (Lafayette Pharmaceuticals), 500 ml of a concentrate to which we add 1400 ml of water to obtain a 0.5% solution of MC.

Barium suspensions can be infused using 50-ml syringes or by a peristaltic pump (eg, Minipump, Renal Systems Inc, Minneapolis, Minn).[12] The methylcellulose solution has been infused by gravity, by injection, but most reliably and conveniently by the peristaltic pump.

Intubation

Preparing the Catheter

The guide wire should be introduced to the tip of the catheter, ascertaining at the same time that both have been well lubricated with silicon spray. A fairly abrupt, at least 90 degree, bend of the guide wire tip is shaped while it is inside the catheter. The opposite free end of the wire is then sharply bent for later tip turning. This bend should be about 2 in beyond the catheter to allow for some degree of catheter stretching. The wire is then withdrawn about 3 in from the catheter tip, ready for insertion through the anesthetized nose or mouth.

A guiding principle applies to tube passages through flexures in which one of the limbs is fixed in position, the other being movable. This is to turn the patient in the direction that will cause the movable portion of a flexure to shift sideways to widen the flexure for easier tube transit. For the upper duodenal flexure, turning the patient to the left shifts stomach and mobile postbulbar duodenum away from the retroperitoneally fixed descending duodenum. Equally, turning the patient well to the left moves the mobile jejunum left and anteriorly to widen the duodenojejunal flexure. This cannot apply to the entirely retroperitoneal distal duodenal flexure where manual pressure may be required to assist tube passage through it. Turning the patient to the right also makes it easy to move a tube out of a deep fundal recess into the body of the stomach, because the shifting of the stomach to the right almost eliminates the depth of the fundal recess.

Transnasal Introduction of the Catheter

With the patient supine or sitting upright, 2 to 3 ml of 2% lidocaine jelly (Copley Pharmaceuticals, Canton, Mass) is slowly introduced into the more open nostril. This nostril is then occluded by light pressure of the patient's finger to continue the local action of the anesthetic for a few minutes. A further 1 ml is then introduced and the patient is asked to sniff and swallow. Further anesthesia to the throat is rarely required.

The outer surface of distal part of the already prepared catheter/guide wire combination should be lubricated with lidocaine gel. With the patient's neck hyperextended, the catheter, held between thumb and index finger, is gently introduced into the anesthetized nostril, its slightly curved tip directed downward. Should resistance be met during introduction, the catheter is pulled back slightly, the tip redirected and gently reintroduced. If these steps fail, the other nostril is used. Normally a mild resistance is felt when the posterior wall of the nasopharynx has been reached and passed. At this point, after about 5 in of the tube has been introduced, the patient's neck is flexed toward the chest, and the catheter is gently advanced while the patient swallows. This maneuver directs the catheter tip posteriorly and into the esophagus. In patients who have to remain supine during catheter insertion, placement of pillows can assist head positioning. Fluoroscopic monitoring of the catheter position should be done whenever there is any resistance to its passage into and through the esophagus. At no time should the tube be forced against resistance. Once the stomach is believed to have been reached, the patient is turned supine (if initially sitting upright) for further tube advancement under fluoroscopic guidance.

It has been claimed that the transnasal route allows faster intubation and is preferred over peroral passage by patients who have undergone both forms of insertion.[12] The transnasal route should always be used in uncooperative, more heavily sedated, or psychotic patients and in children.

Peroral Intubation

The throat should be sprayed at most three times with Hurricaine, a 20% benzocaine anesthetic spray (Beutlich Pharmaceuticals, Waukegan, Ill), making sure that the posterior wall of the oropharynx is included. The peroral approach is ideally performed with the patient sitting upright but can be done in the supine position. The previously prepared catheter/guide wire combination (distal 3 in without wire) is placed on the middle of the tongue, with the patient's neck well flexed, is introduced fairly briskly during a swallow and, provided no resistance is met, is taken as far as the estimated entry into the stomach. The patient then lies down for further tube manipulation. Alternatively, after the tube has entered the esophagus, the patient may be asked to lie down on the right side, which will often cause the tube to pass directly into the body of the stomach.

Transgastric Catheter Passage (Transnasal/Oral Introduction)

Fluoroscopy is now required. With the patient supine, the catheter may have just reached the lower end of the esophagus, may have curled into the fundal recess, or may already be found in the body of the stomach. For the catheter to exit from the fundal recess the patient needs only to be turned on the right side, the tube pulled back to the cardia and then reinserted (Fig. 7-1). If there is a need to help with the advance towards the pylorus, gloved hand pressure against the greater curvature would do this. In all this, the guide wire should be kept 2 to 3 inches away from the catheter tip.

The catheter has now reached the prepyloric area. Turning the patient toward the left not only opens the upper duodenal flexure, but also promotes brief air entry into the duodenal bulb (Fig. 7-2). Advance through the pylorus should not be rushed; a short wait in the right position can result in almost effortless advance of the tube into the bulb. In a patient premedicated with 20 mg of metoclopramide the catheter will generally pass through the stomach more rapidly and will move sooner through the relaxed pylorus. Occasionally, injection of 20 ml of air into the main lumen aids in the transpyloric tube passage.

In some cases the guide wire may never have to leave the stomach; in others it should be held at the upper or lower duodenal flexure with the tube advancing over it. Occasionally it is taken further to stiffen the more duodenal sweep and help tube transit through the duodenojejunal flexure with the patient in left lateral/semiprone position. Once the tube has reached as far as intended or accepted, the balloon should be slowly inflated with 15 to 20 ml of air. Occasionally a patient complains of acute pain at this moment. The withdrawal of a very few milliliters of air will stop the pain with equal suddenness. If

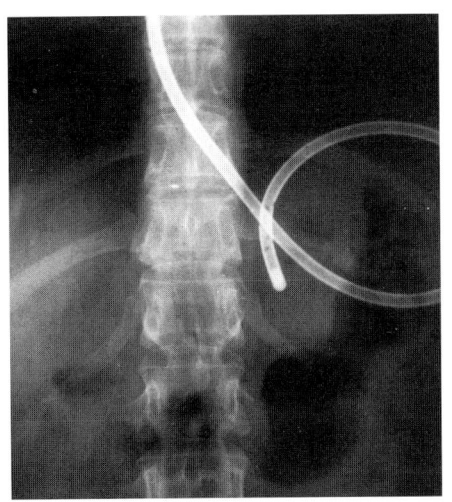

(a)

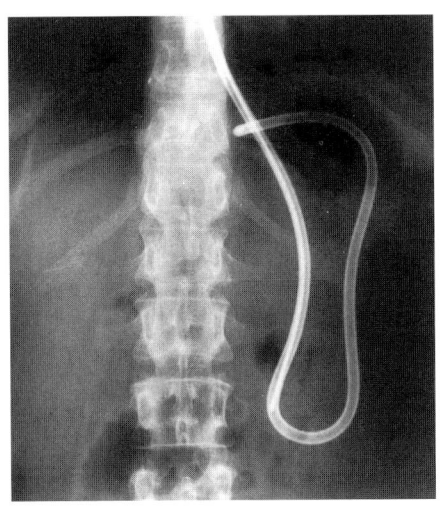

(b)

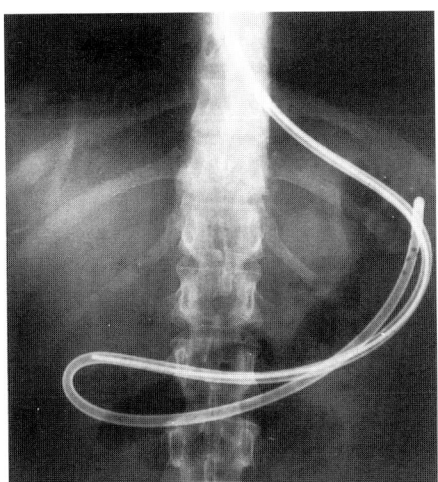

(c)

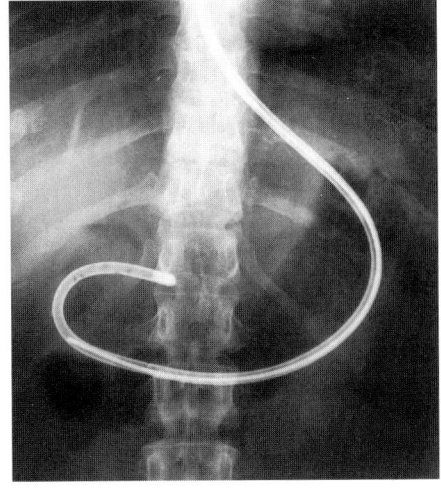

(d)

Fig. 7-1. Enteroclysis tube was introduced into the esophagus with patient seated at the side of the X-ray table. Patient now recumbent. (a) Tube is found coiled in the fundus of the stomach. (b) The wire is gradually advanced while the tube is carefully withdrawn—the "double-back maneuver." (c) Further advance into antrum; tube now to be withdrawn more rapidly over the wire. (d) Image just before final double-back; forward flipping of tube tip is imminent.

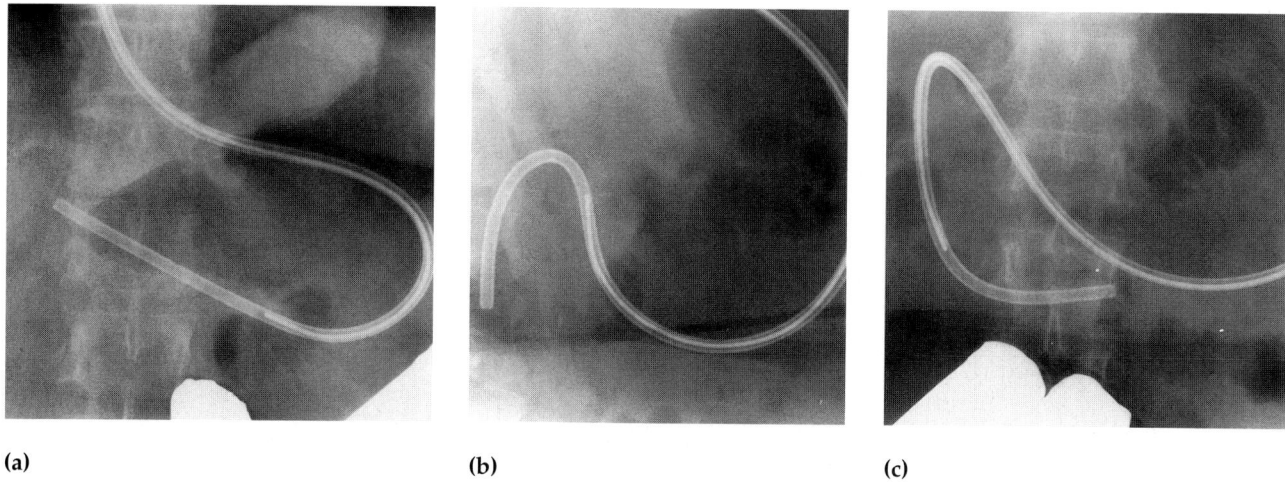

Fig. 7-2. Simple way of taking tube from stomach into duodenum.
(a) Tip of tube probably near pylorus. (b) Patient was turned left, duodenum identified, slow passage into descending duodenum. (c) Manual pressure aids tip of tube round inferior duodenal flexure.

needed at a later stage, the balloon can be topped up again.

Problems of Intubation

As the tip points, so goes the tube as it is advances. We can never predict the exact shape of the stomach/duodenum combination (Fig. 7-3), the level of the duodenojejunal flexure, nor its direction (more often left forward than right forward). If the tube takes an unexpected turn, as long as it does not buckle (ie, fold sharply with occlusion of lumen), it is better to let the catheter continue into this direction and test inject (barium or air) if in doubt. It is a mistake to spend too much time and cause too much discomfort to the patient by persevering unduly in efforts to get the tube into the jejunum. If it does not succeed with two or three attempts one should stop trying and inflate the balloon in the ascending duodenum just beyond the crossing superior mesenteric vessels.

Tube Buckled in Esophagus

This is more likely to occur when the wire has been pulled back too far during introduction (Fig. 7-4). The diameter of the esophagus is not sufficient for a double-back maneuver. It is best to advance the buckled tube into the stomach and there double-back by withdrawing the tube gradually while at the same time trying to advance the wire.[13] This will invariably straighten the tube, which, however, once buckled will tend to buckle again. Such tubes have to be advanced carefully, at times with the wire fairly close to the tip, just beyond the recognizable postbuckling scar.

Large, Fixed Hiatus Hernia

Such a hernia is probably recognized as soon as fluoroscopy reaches it. The tube is held up and, if made to advance, may circumnavigate the hernia without exiting from it. The simplest way of dealing with this obstacle is to inject barium or air and, with the right turned patient supine again, direct the barium round the hernia to outline the exit through the diaphragm (Fig. 7-5). Once the way is identified, the catheter, with the guide wire not too far from the tip, is advanced round the hernia to follow the road map into the abdomen. Actually, it is quite easy.

Tube Entry into Pylorus Difficult

It may be necessary to withdraw the wire, inject air, and observe the antropyloric and duodenal bulb areas, as there may be abnormal angulation or distortion related to ulcer disease (Fig. 7-6). If necessary, barium can be used to outline the anatomy.

Tube Coiled in Gastric Fundus, Antrum, or Duodenum

This presents a very small problem which is remedied by correctly turning the patient, possibly combined with a simplified version of the "double-back" maneuver (Fig. 7-7). The wire is then reintroduced, at times after reshaping the tip in accordance with the shown anatomy. Occasionally, the tube coils back in the antrum, yet initially simulates a successful duodenal intubation (Fig. 7-8). The gastric position of the tube should be suspected when the tube points to the left and extends parallel to the line of the greater cur-

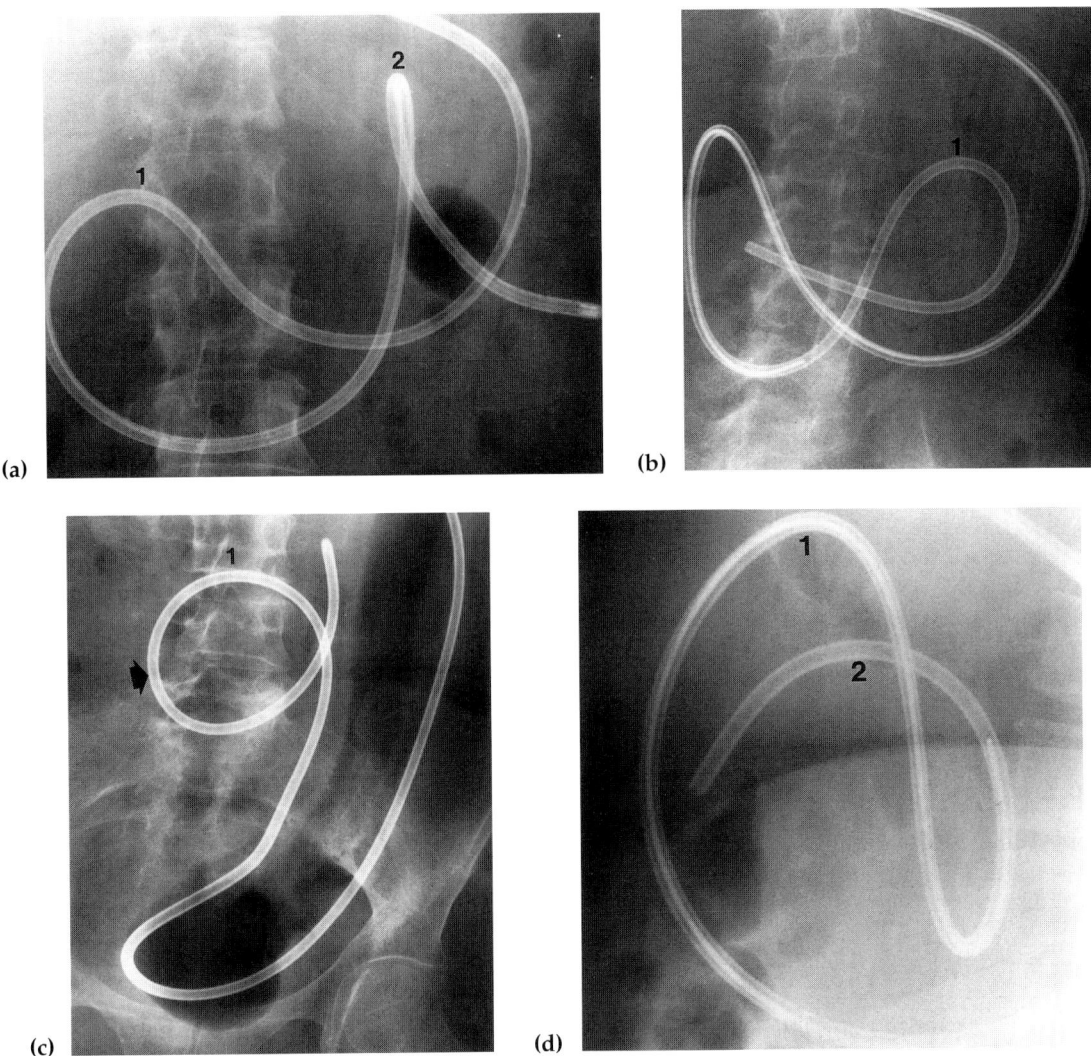

Fig. 7-3. A few of the varied shapes of the gastroduodenal combination.
(a) The most often found pattern. (b) Duodenojejunal flexure in normal position but jejunum exits to right. (c) Ptosed, elongated stomach, levels of entry into duodenum and of duodenal sweep in normal positions. (d) Patient turned right, entry into duodenum well above level of duodenojejunal flexure; jejunum exits to the right. (1 = level of pylorus; 2 = duodenojejunal flexure.)

vature. It is also possible for the tube to appear to have doubled back in the stomach and yet to have advanced into the duodenum (Fig. 7-9). These distinctions can be a problem only if the patient is left lying flat on the table. When the patient is turned left, there can never be any doubt over the gastric or duodenal position of the tube.

Duodenojejunal Flexure

This passage can be difficult and, as just mentioned, is not always mandatory. Once turned as already suggested, the patient can assist tube advance by deep breathing and an occasional convincing cough (Fig. 7-10). If this fails, one can only try again with the patient supine or turned somewhat to the right. And then one just gives up!

Tube Arrested at an Unexpected Level

This could be in the descending duodenum, possibly having entered a diverticulum or come up against a tumor. It could be at a point outside the usual course or even in the lower cervical area. In these and similar situations, the wire needs to be removed and air or a few milliliters of barium injected. This will show the cause of the problem and the way to bypass it (Fig. 7-11).

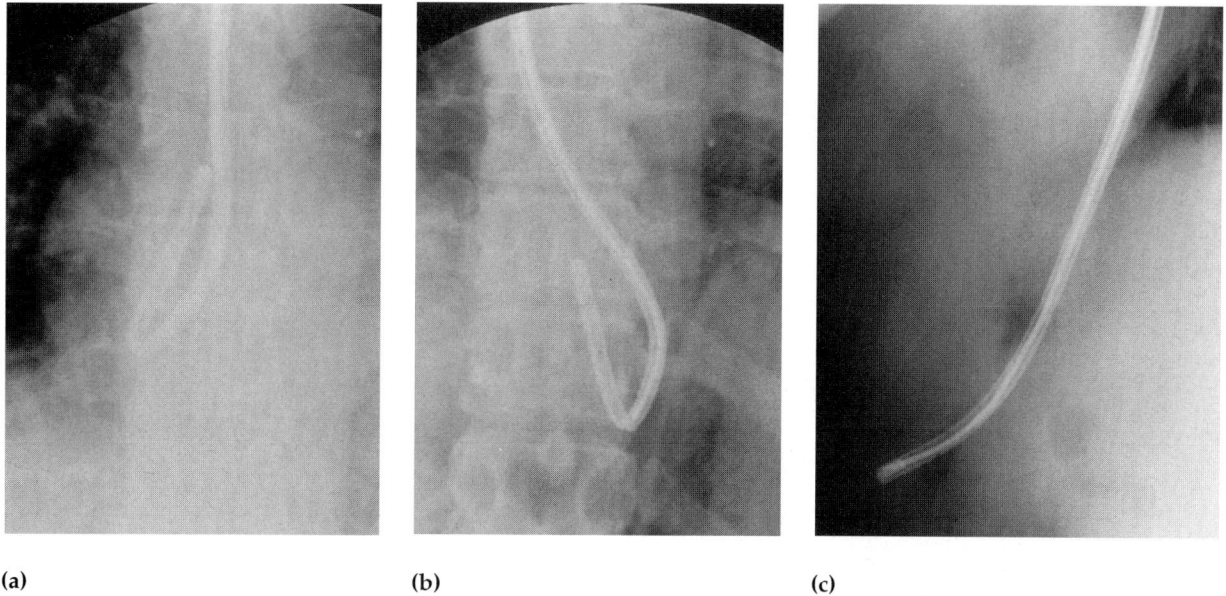

Fig. 7-4. The tube has buckled in the esophagus.
(a) Buckled tube, guide wire (arrow) at point of buckling. (b) Buckled tube continues its passage into stomach. (c) With sufficient space there, a "double-back maneuver" was done.

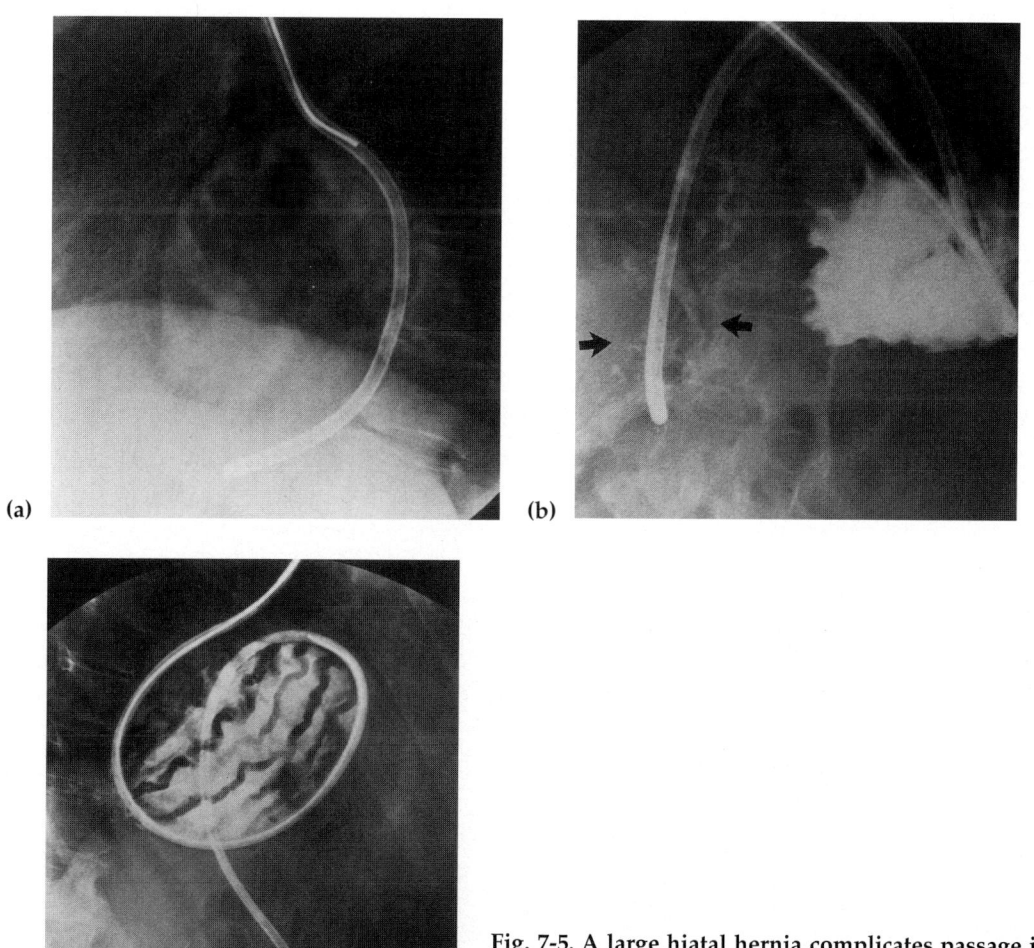

Fig. 7-5. A large hiatal hernia complicates passage into stomach.
(a) The large hernia was noted; attempts to pass through failed. (b) Barium was injected and the patient turned to coat the exit (arrows). (c) Passage through the hiatus was then no problem.

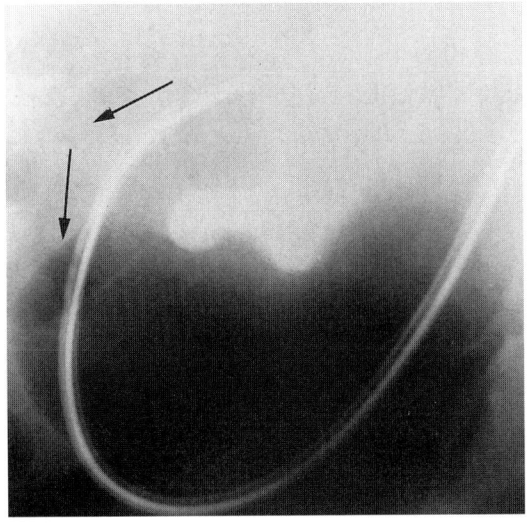

Fig. 7-6. After repeatedly failing to enter the pyloric channel, the wire was removed and air injected. The antrum is deformed and there is sharp angulation against the descending duodenum (arrows).

History of Gastric Surgery or of Other Upper GI Problems

There is need to review any previous upper GI studies and/or see more detailed surgical notes. A plain film of the abdomen may help (Fig. 7-12). However, in the absence of all this, the best way to aid intubation is for the patient to swallow the metoclopramide tablets with half an ounce of barium suspension instead of water, which should leave enough barium coating on the mucosa to guide the subsequent intubation.

Single-Contrast Enteroclysis

Sellink's Technique

In a 1981 article Sellink and Rosenbusch summarized their accumulated experience with enteroclysis.[14] The wt/vol percentages of the barium suspensions depended on the patient's size and varied between 42% and 28%.

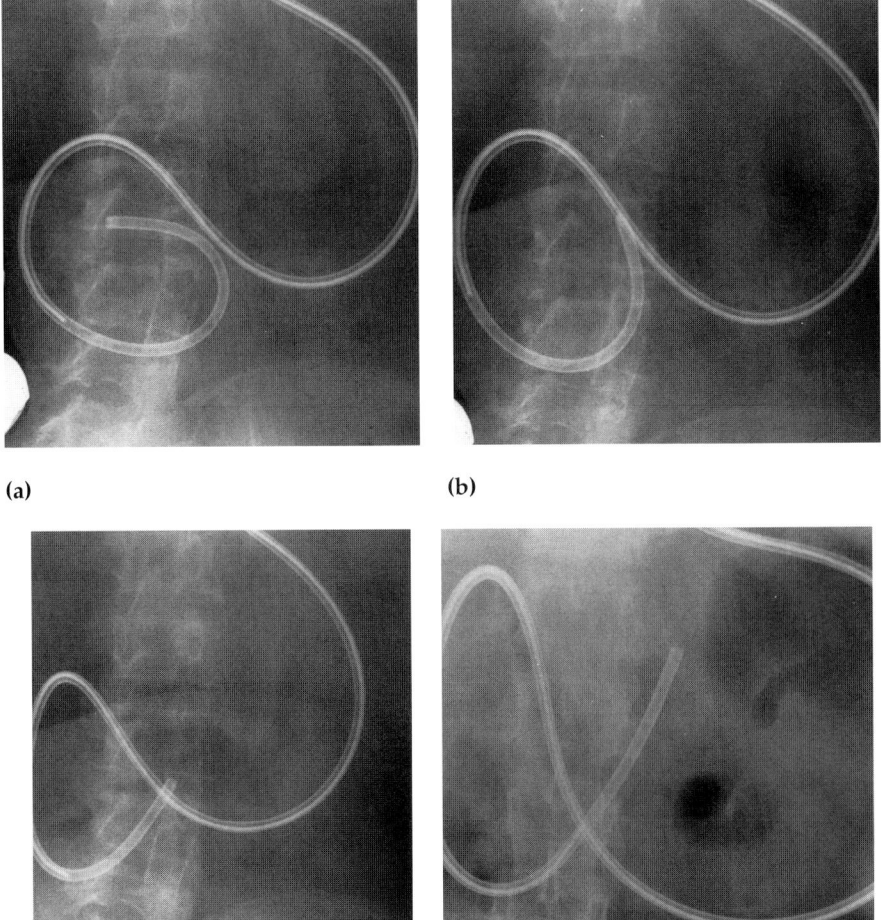

Fig. 7-7. Minor problem when trying to advance in the duodenum. (a) Tube coils within duodenum. (b) Simple "double-back maneuver" advances wire while slightly withdrawing tube. (c) Tube now correctly lined up in direction of duodenojejunal flexure. (d) Tube now close to flexure.

Nolan's Technique

In a very recent report[15] the single-contrast examination and its indications and results are reviewed. An F10 catheter is now used for duodenal intubation. He follows closely Sellink's method, insisting on a clean colon and administering about 1000 ml of dilute barium with imaging at high kilovoltages. The combination of narrower tubing taken only as far as the duodenum and the fairly rapid infusion of barium have shortened the examination time and have rendered enteroclysis more patient acceptable. This is an excellent method for routine enteroclysis. However, lumen distention without methylcellulose appears to be suboptimal. This has been made clear in the fact that this single-contrast method has mostly failed to diagnose celiac disease.[16]

Enteroclysis with Methylcellulose

Is Double Contrast Desirable?

As in every other part of the gastrointestinal tract, double contrast produces the best attainable degree of mucosal surface detail. Enteroclysis with methylcellulose achieves best possible lumen distention, to reveal areas of lumen restriction and test for abnormal fold separation. However, there is no need to complete full double-contrast development in every patient. In some cases the single-contrast phase will be diagnostic; in others intermediate phases will provide the full answer. For more routine use of enteroclysis we, there-

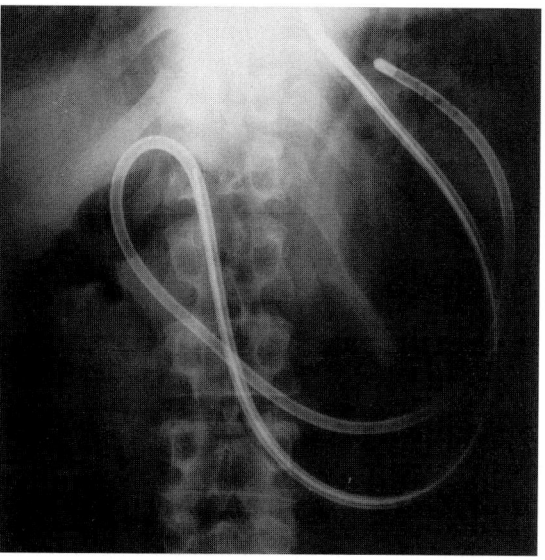

Fig. 7-8. There was the false impression that the catheter had turned into the duodenal sweep. However, the tube has doubled back into the gastric fundus.

The rate of infusion of the barium is considered optimal at 75 ml/min; in patients with hypermotility the flow rate is increased to even 150 ml/min, after barium has reached the cecum. The usual quantity of barium suspension infused is about 700 ml but may be as high as 1500 ml in cases with hypotonic small bowel. Air or water is suggested as a possible double-contrast agent.

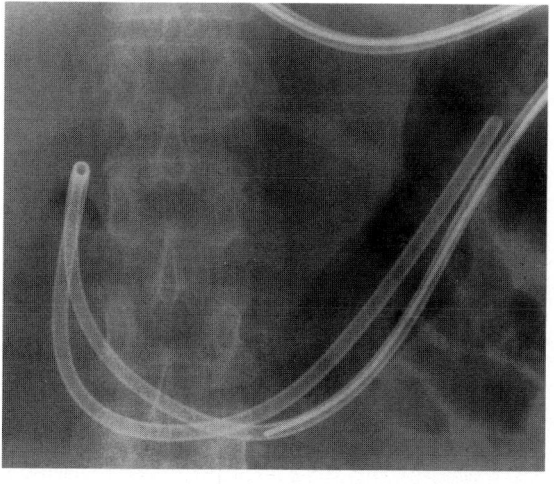

(a)

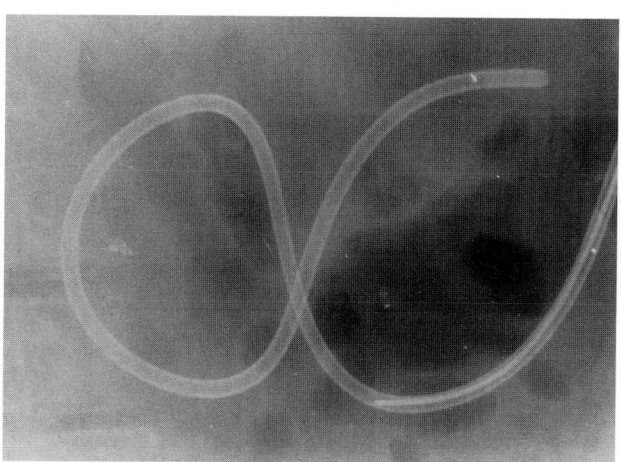

(b)

Fig. 7-9. One should never judge tube position without turning patient.
(a) Patient supine; here false impression of tube having doubled back into the stomach. (b) This time, patient was turned left, which made it clear that the tube was in best normal position.

104 • 7. Enteroclysis: Technique and Variations

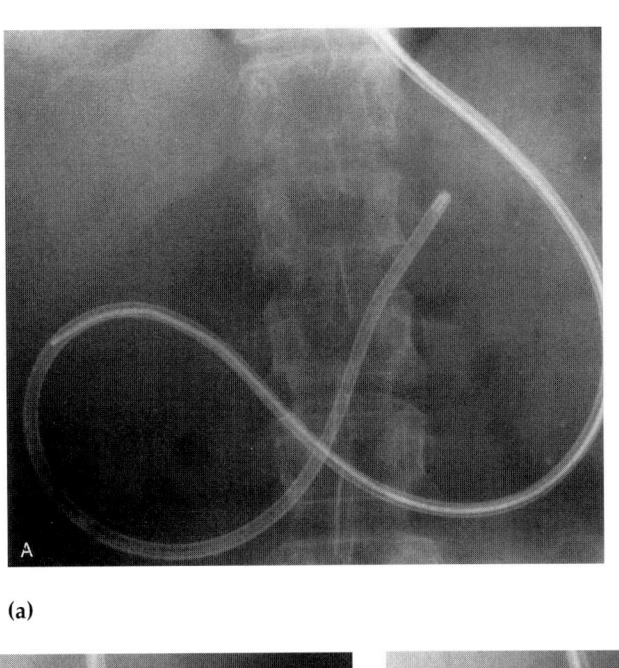
(a)

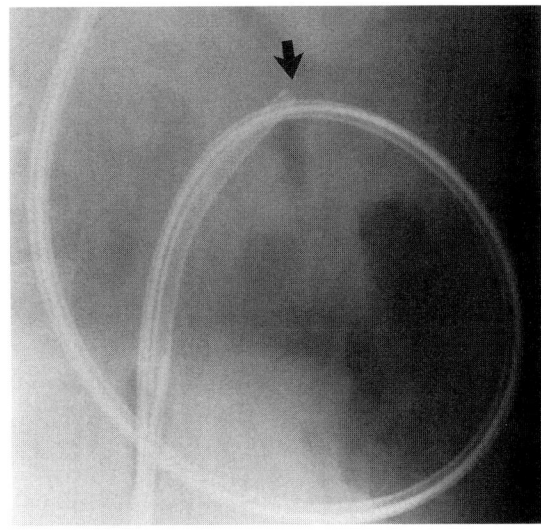
(b)

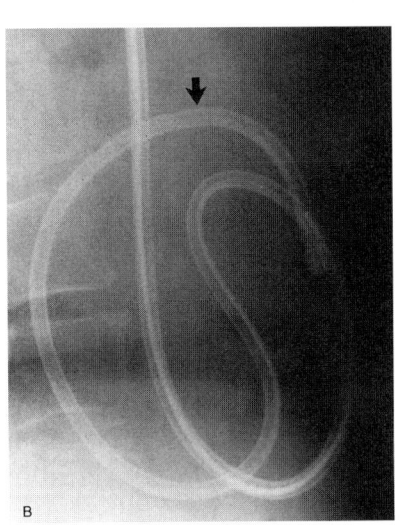
(c)

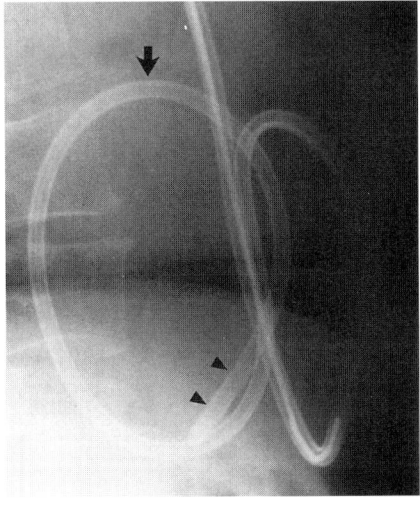
(d)

Fig. 7-10. Successful passage through a normal duodenojejunal flexure.
(a) Catheter tip close to flexure. (b) Patient turned left semiprone; confirms tube position at flexure. (c) A few deep breaths and one or two coughs help tube to pass through. (d) Tube now advances further and balloon may be inflated (arrow to flexure, arrowheads to tip of tube).

fore, recommend a less time-consuming, more purpose-of-examination-related approach to enteroclysis, terminating the procedure at the point of diagnosis.

Why Methycellulose as Double-Contrast Agent?

Air has inherent advantages as a double-contrast agent against barium suspensions. A liquid phase like barium cannot intermix with a gaseous phase, and the density difference between the two is maximal (see later). The air double-contrast enteroclysis, however, has generally not been successful in our hands and with our patients. Though we will use it in selected cases, we prefer the routine use of MC even though a number of potential problems exist and need to be avoided, if double contrast is the aim of the examination.

Action of methylcellulose after barium. 1) It propels the barium column through the small intestine and into the right colon; 2) It optimally dilates the lumen of the entire small bowel and straightens the valvulae conniventes for their accurate assessment; 3) The lumen-filling solution of 0.5% MC sustains the high-density barium lining of the mucosa to produce a double-contrast effect lasting 20 to 30 minutes;[8,10,11] 4) The translucency of bowel loops in double contrast makes it possible to identify mucosal detail in areas where two or more bowel loops overlap (Fig. 7-13).

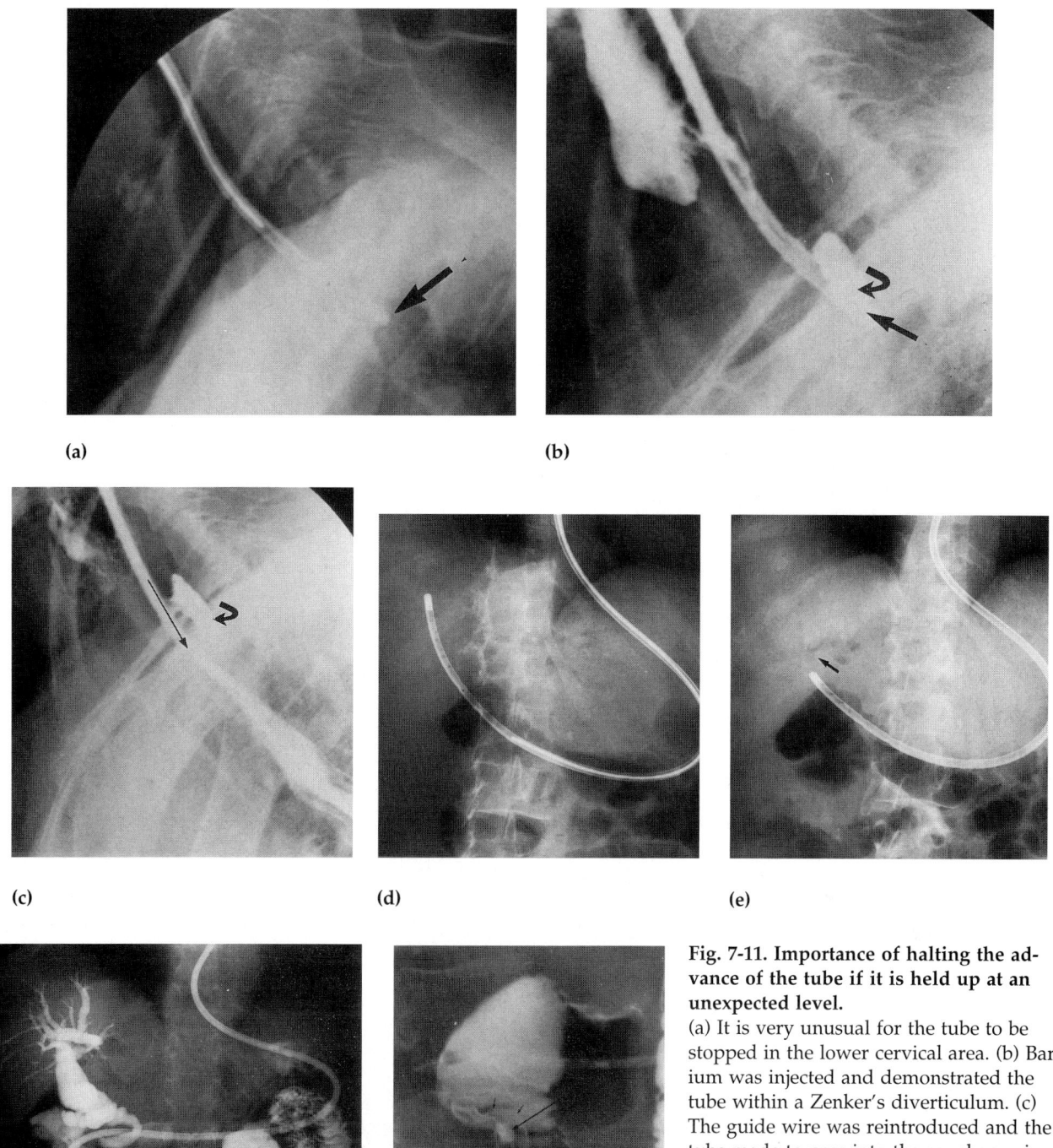

Fig. 7-11. Importance of halting the advance of the tube if it is held up at an unexpected level.

(a) It is very unusual for the tube to be stopped in the lower cervical area. (b) Barium was injected and demonstrated the tube within a Zenker's diverticulum. (c) The guide wire was reintroduced and the tube made to pass into the esophagus in front of the diverticulum. (Arrow = end of tube; curved arrow = Zenker; long arrow = catheter passing anterior to diverticulum.) (d) In another patient, tube held up with its tip projected high over the liver. (e) Tube pulled back and air injected; bile duct outlined (arrow). (f) Tube into duodenum, barium infused, unexpected prior choledochoduodenostomy. Enteroclysis then proceeded normally. (g) Tube led up at upper duodenal flexure with patient turned to the left. Barium injected; a protruding ulcerated leiomyoma revealed (small arrows = surface of tumor, long arrow = ulcer).

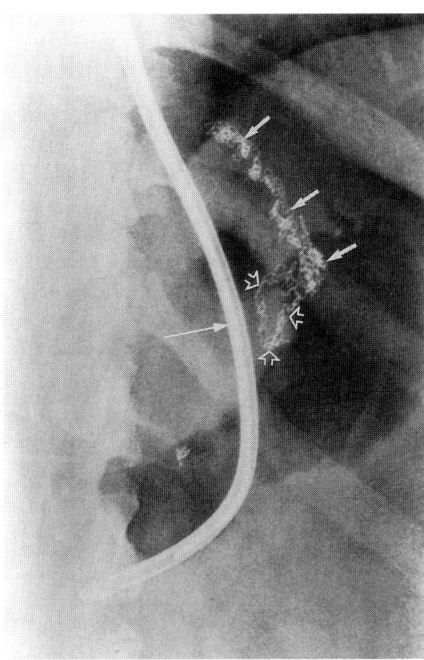

Fig. 7-12. Female patient, 35 years old, with history of vertical banded gastroplasty for morbid obesity. Enteroclysis done to rule out small bowel origin of intermittent bleeding. A plain film of the abdomen depicted the suture landmarks, important for damage-free intubation. This image, with the catheter in place, demonstrates these landmarks. The vertical segment extends medial to the vertical line of clips (small arrows); the circular suture line (open arrows) indicates the level of the horizontal banding (long arrow) that restricts the exit from the vertical segment above. The catheter had to be passed out of the vertical segment medial to the circular suture. No cause for the bleeding was demonstrated.

Diffusion of Barium into Methylcellulose

To achieve satisfactory double contrast (if desired) there should be only minimal diffusion between the two liquids. This depends on the following: 1) Compatibility between MC and the barium suspension used. The two barium suspensions mentioned earlier are highly compatible. 2) Aspects of technique. In the static situation of a slide test, there is total absence of diffusion between MC and suitable barium. In the realistic environment of the small bowel lumen, however, a static barium coating of the mucosa is exposed to a flowing MC solution. Even under the best conditions, this will produce some washing away of barium by the MC and a gradually caudad increase of contamination of the MC with barium. This normally acceptable diminution of double contrast can be accentuated, if mixing of the two substances is promoted by vigorous abdominal compression or even by abrupt movement or coughing of the patient (Fig 7-14). With good compatibility and careful technique, satisfactory double contrast can be obtained throughout the small bowel in almost 90% of examinations.

Introduction of Barium

Adjustment of rate of flow during infusion. Frequent adjustment is essential if uniform distention of the entire small bowel is to be achieved. Such adjustment needs to be based on an understanding of the response of the small bowel to different rates of inflow, which implies a response to the degree of distention of the jejunum at the inflow site. With barium injected by means of syringes, the flow rate is frequently altered. The barium suspension should advance into the small bowel as an unbroken column. If it is seen to advance too fast and as broken columns, a more rapid injection rate for a short time will normalize the advance.[17] A too rapid injection overdistends the first segments of jejunum and may completely stop the progress of barium. There usually is return to a normal progress after having stopped injecting for a short time. It may, however, cause persistent overdistention of the proximal jejunum, a not desirable feature. To sum up, flow of barium is highly influenced by the rate of injection; ideally this rate should be slow enough to achieve uninterrupted forward flow, with only brief changes to more rapid inflow to slightly slow down the barium moving through the small bowel. The use of syringes makes it easier to vary the rate of injection as required. When infusing barium by peristaltic pump one should start at a slow rate (eg, 55 ml/min) and only carefully increase it.

Quantity injected. It is best to base the required amount on the habitus of the patient, the purpose of the examination, and a possible finding of retained fluid (Fig. 7-15) or dilated bowel loops. Between 180 and 200 ml suffice in most patients of average build. Larger patients may require up to 250 ml of barium. If the most distal bowel is of primary interest or where even limited colon preparation has been omitted, the amount injected should be increased by 20 to 60 ml. In patients with fluid and/or dilated loops, up to 300 even 400 ml of barium may have to be introduced. It must also be remembered that the overall length of small bowel can vary from 18 to 22 feet! Experience is a good guide for choosing the correct amount. Before experience, we recommend injecting more rather than too little barium.

Infusion of Methycellulose

While injected barium requires peristaltic activity for its progression through the small bowel, MC advance is largely inflow rate depended and eventually pro-

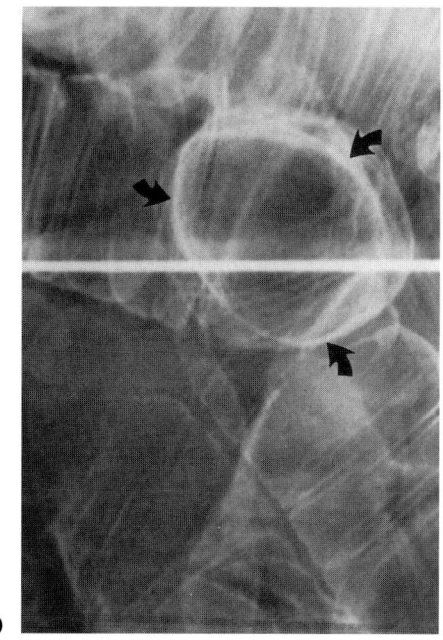 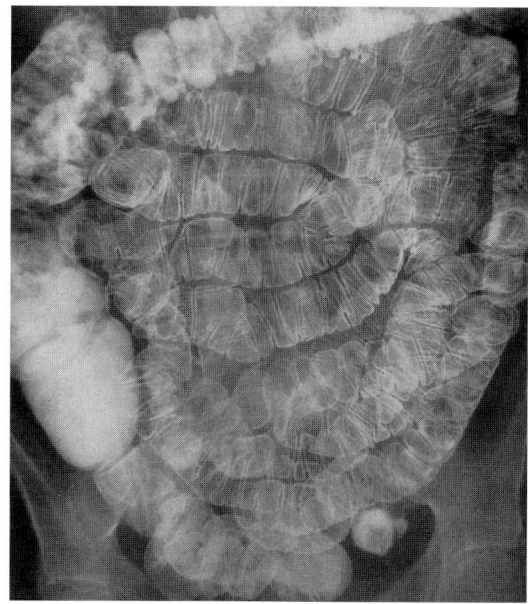

Fig. 7-13. With good technique, barium lining of the mucosa persists.
(a) End-on view of a forward curving segment of mid-small bowel (arrows). It demonstrates the contrast between barium coating the mucosa and the water density of MC solution distending the lumen. (b) Final prone view at end of enteroclysis, at least 15 to 20 minutes from the start of contrast material infusion. Double contrast persists.

duces limited hypotonia throughout the small bowel. As already mentioned, infusion by peristaltic pump is preferred. The rate of infusion of MC should be between 55 and 100 ml/min, occasionally below and rarely above these rates. It is best to start at the low range and increase gradually, usually not exceeding 80 ml/min. Even when using balloon catheters, the

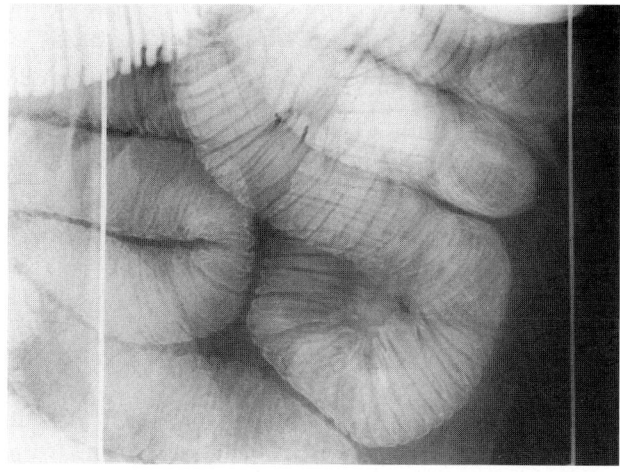 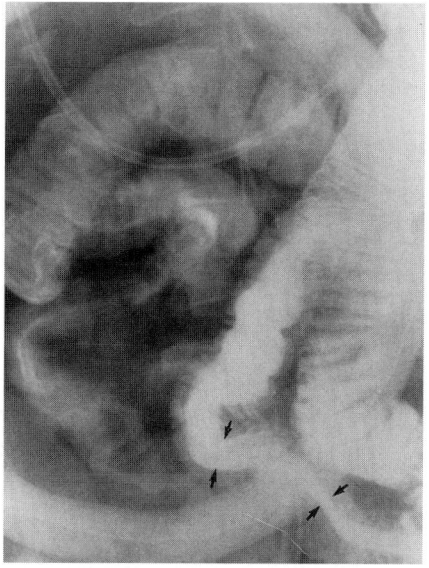

Fig. 7-14. Unintended though acceptable single contrast with distended and translucent bowel loops. This was due to overenthusiastic abdominal compression during the study.

Fig. 7-15. Streaming of injected barium (arrows) at the bottom of fluid-filled moderately distended small bowel loops.
Fluid within bowel would have made an excellent contrast agent for CT and MRI. Enteroclysis requires a greatly increased amount of barium to be infused.

rate is also limited by the need to avoid reflux into duodenum and stomach. A total amount of 1200 to 2000 ml of MC is normally required to extend double contrast or sufficient lumen distention into the terminal ileum.[10]

We suggest having the patient turned toward the left (including the shoulders!) during the first part of the infusion to delay onward flow from the jejunum before it has become distended. It is then time to turn the patient supine to promote MC extension into the ileum.

Fluoroscopy and Imaging—Single-Contrast Phase

The role of the radiologist is to inspect the advancing barium column with intermittent fluoroscopy and keep an eye on possible reflux into the duodenum. The patient, being turned half left during much of the barium injection, is intermittently turned supine for more accurate imaging with abdominal compression. It must be understood that the single-contrast phase continues as the advancing, gradually shorter undiluted barium column, with double-contrast development through its intermediate phases following behind. Some intraluminal filling defects may be appreciated better in single than in double contrast, eg, smaller melanoma metastases and lipomas. During the single-contrast filling of the small bowel lumen, it is of particular value to observe the advancing head of the barium column. Outline abnormalities or extravasations may be readily identified at this stage, and can be studied in greater detail later.

Phase of Developing Double Contrast

The radiologist, in addition to continuing the observation of the advancing single-contrast filled loops, will study the more proximal segments as they gradually distend and become increasingly translucent. As mentioned already, during this phase it is essential to avoid any abrupt compression of the abdomen, or even sudden turns of the patient, as these would increase diffusion between the barium lining of the mucosa and surges of MC flow and would adversely affect double-contrast formation. For the study of bowel loops in changed positions, the patient should be helped to turn or slide slowly.

With the upper and mid small bowel sufficiently distended, returning the patient to supine position may cause a rapid filling of distal and terminal ileum. This is an excellent moment to observe and image these areas in their gradual change to double contrast.

Double-contrast Phase

Double contrast is considered to be fully established when the terminal ileum, at fluoroscopy, is seen to be adequately translucent and sufficiently distended. The instillation of MC is then stopped or reduced to a very slow rate, and it becomes possible to turn the patient more freely and take compression spot films with less constraint.

It is our custom, at this stage, to record again major areas of the small intestine with adequate compression. The proximal and distal jejunum can best be shown with the supine patient turned half right. Turning to the left is usually best for the demonstration of the proximal and midileum, mostly found in the right upper and midabdomen. The distal ileum is imaged supine, with supplementary imaging in unpredictable degrees of obliquity. A lateral or off-lateral view of the pelvis may be required. We may also turn the patient prone and image during compression from underneath by an inflated balloon–equipped paddle. Comparison images taken of selected parts of the small bowel in single and completed double contrast are seen in Fig. 7-16.

A standard overhead film of the whole abdomen is taken with the patient prone and is often followed by another, angled 35 degrees caudad (Fig. 7-17). By this time, barium and MC will have advanced into the colon, where MC may exert a peristalsis-promoting effect.

Technical Problems

Too much barium injected. If significantly more than the recommended amount of barium suspension has been injected, more MC solution will be required to wash the excess into the colon. Though very adequate double contrast can still be produced throughout the small intestine, too much barium will have accumulated in the colon, may obscure intestinal loops, and will increasingly inconvenience the patient. To remedy this, or at times when a correct amount of barium has reached the rectum prematurely, we have always available an empty barium enema bag with all its tubing. The patient is turned right, the tube is inserted into the rectum, and the bag is placed at floor level. The barium/MC outflow can then be adjusted by opening or closing the tubing.

Insufficient barium injected. If this is not realized in good time, the MC solution may overtake the remnant of barium, and distal small bowel loops will be outlined in only faintest contrast. If noted at an earlier stage, it is still possible to interrupt the MC flow and inject a further quantity of barium. As a general principle, it is better to inject more than too little barium at the start of the study.

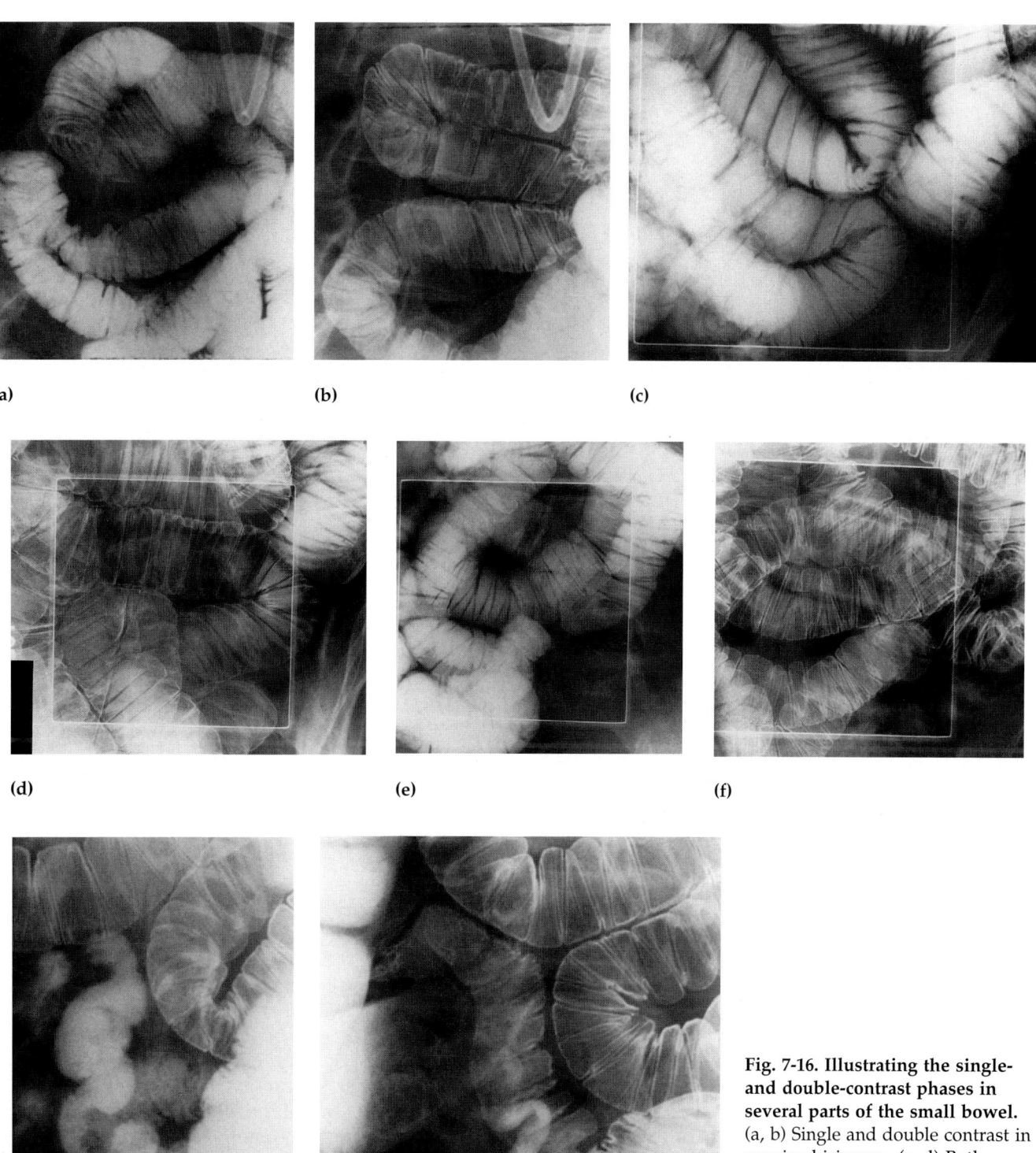

Fig. 7-16. Illustrating the single- and double-contrast phases in several parts of the small bowel. (a, b) Single and double contrast in proximal jejunum. (c, d) Both phases in mid-small bowel. (e, f) Both phases in distal ileum. (g, h) Both phases in the terminal ileum area.

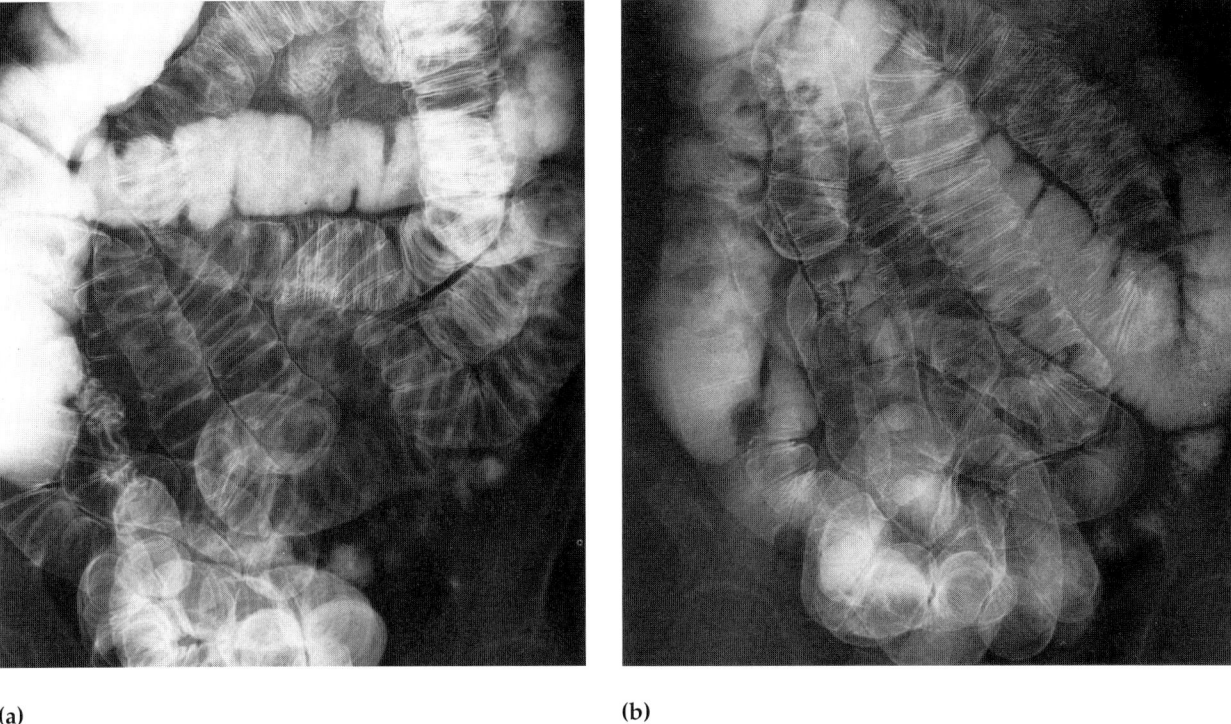

Fig. 7-17. Overhead prone films at end of enteroclysis.
(a) PA view at right angle to table top. (b) Angled view 35 degrees caudad improves demonstration of distal ileum at pelvic inlet.

Distention and double contrast in terminal ileum. Generally, the terminal ileum is the least distended part of the small bowel in enteroclysis. The reason is the usually freely available passage through the ileocecal valve. It is also an area where MC-induced hypotonia is least effective. This can become a not infrequent problem. As long as barium has reached the right colon and MC double contrast is seen close behind the distal ileum, we now resort to an IV injection of glucagon 0.5 mg. With moderate compression in optimal rotation of the patient, it is then possible in most cases to obtain double contrast or distended translucent single-contrast images with very adequate demonstration of mucosal surface detail (Fig. 7-18).

Reflux. Inflatable balloons on F14 catheters have reduced the incidence of reflux. However, reflux can happen even with the balloon distended to its maximum. Such reflux may cause vomiting and possible aspiration. It is important to always be on the lookout for it. If seen, infusion rates have to slow or infusion may have to be halted. The table head should be elevated and the patient turned to the left.

Fecal matter in the distal ileum. It is surprising how often an incompetent ileocecal valve allows fecal material to reflux into the terminal ileum out of a loaded cecum in an unprepared patient. As mentioned previously, if enteroclysis needs to be done in an unprepared patient, a greater than normal amount of barium has to be injected. Its purpose is to clear all refluxed material out of the terminal ileum before useful imaging can take place (Fig. 7-19). It has also been noted that an unprepared patient shows a slower progress of contrast material through the small bowel, not always a disadvantage.

Prolapse of small bowel into the pelvis. It is not unusual for a few loops of ileum to dip into the pelvis. Most of the time it is possible to move them into the abdomen by applying prolonged balloon paddle compression over the suprapubic area, with the patient supine and the head of the table lowered (Fig. 7-20). Only loops fixed by adhesion will resist. In a patient with prior hysterectomy or pelvic exenteresis, several loops tend to occupy the empty space in the pelvis and may adhere. These loops are best imaged in a lateral or off-lateral projection, but only after double contrast has been established (Fig. 7-21). The prone, overhead film angled 35 degrees caudad can be a useful alternative view. A full bladder is not helpful in most cases as it merely causes compression of the usually fixed-in-position loops and increases patient discomfort.

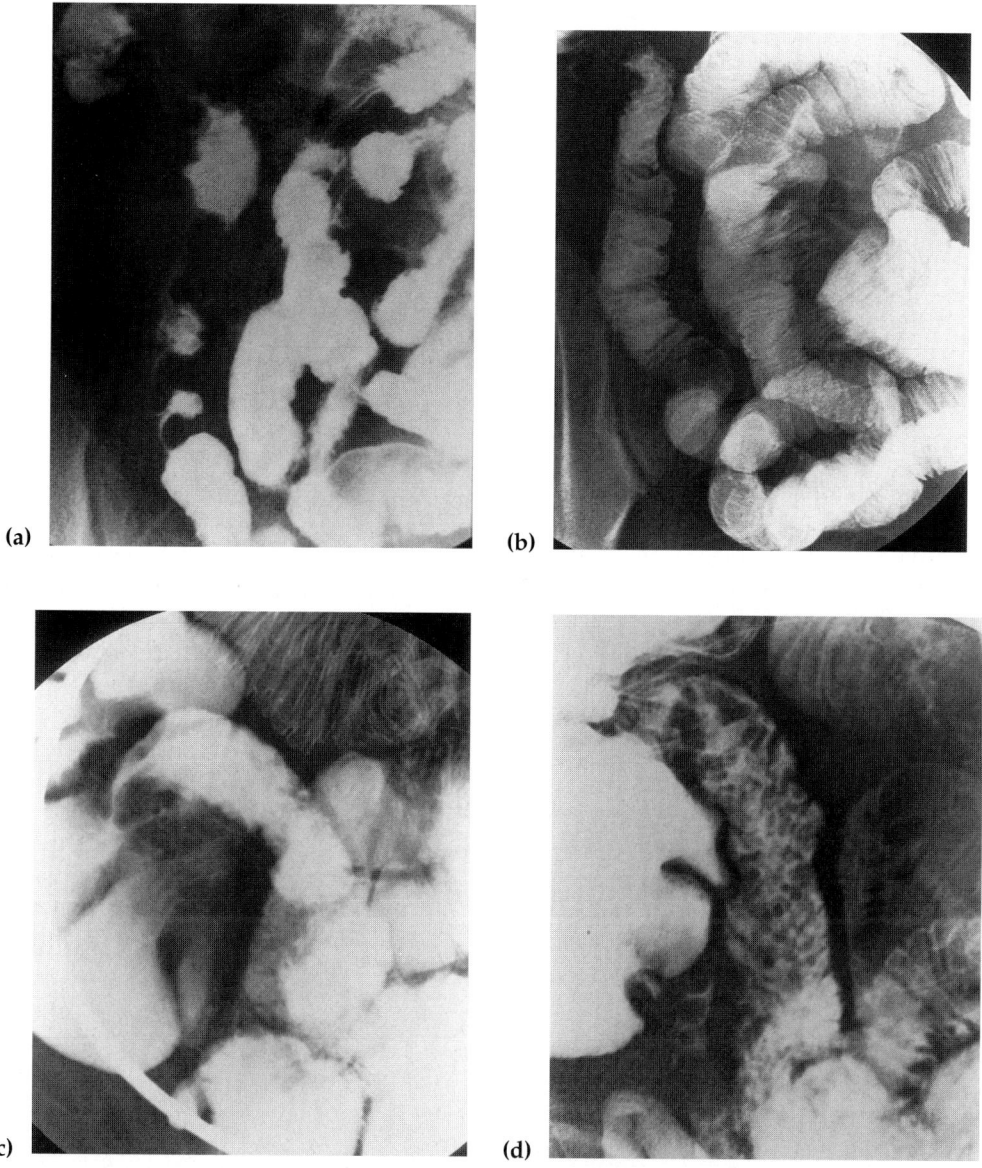

Fig. 7-18. Hastening double contrast and distention of the terminal ileum (TI).
(a) In early single-contrast phase, discontinuous filling. (b) After 0.5 mg of glucagon IV, rapid change to well-distended, transradiant TI but in single contrast. (c) In another patient with known IgA deficiency and celiac disease, diarrhea recurred during careful dieting. Single contrast fails to reveal finer TI detail. (d) After glucagon, adequate TI double contrast demonstrated multiple lymphoid nodular hyperplasia with areas of confluence. Lymphoma was excluded by biopsy/histology. IgA deficiency considered to be the cause of the nodularity.

Biphasic Enteroclysis

This method, popularized by Maglinte et al,[18] uses a 50% wt/vol barium mixture (Entrobar), the amount varying depending on the approximate length of the small bowel (350 to 500 ml). The methylcellulose suspension is similar to Herlinger's methylcellulose primary double-contrast method. The amount and density of barium mixture used in the biphasic enteroclysis technique allow for a completed single-contrast evaluation up to the distal ileum. Evaluation of the distal ileum, particularly for inflammatory bowel disease, is excellent. No additional maneuvers are needed to image the distal ileum. The double-contrast phase allows a second look of all segments of the small bowel in better distention (Fig. 7-22). The use of methylcellulose promotes evacuation of barium and allows performance of other procedures without delay.

112 • 7. Enteroclysis: Technique and Variations

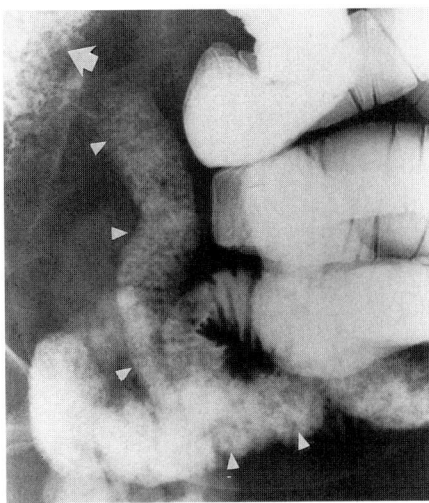

Fig. 7-19. Refluxed colonic contents extend through all of the terminal ileum (arrowheads).
The same material is seen in right colon (arrow). More barium needed to be infused to wash contaminants back into colon.

Modifications of Enteroclysis

Through a Decompression Tube

The ideal scenario is to have used Maglinte's decompression sump/balloon enteroclysis catheter for nasogastric suction instead of the commonly used Salem sump nasogastric tube and then advance it into the jejunum should enteroclysis or long tube decompression be required. However, long established tubes for the decompression of partially obstructed small bowel are still in use, mostly the Miller-Abbott and Cantor tubes. Advantages of using these tubes for enteroclysis are that part of the retained fluid can be drained before contrast material injection and that barium and MC can be delivered closer to the site of obstruction. All these functions are readily performed with the multipurpose triluminal tube.[9] Its use at the initial diagnostic encounter in place of the traditional nasogastric tube diminishes the trauma of multiple intubations[3] (Fig. 7-23). (See also Chapter 21.)

Certain caveats are relevant when using these tubes for enteroclysis: 1) The tubes should have advanced at least 18 in into the jejunum for all side holes to be beyond the ligament of Treitz; however, reflux still remains a possible problem. 2) Long tubes should not be taken too close to the site of obstruction, where spasm-related, misleading artifacts can obscure the true pathology (Fig. 7-24). Even at a higher level in the small bowel, the stiffer, double lumen Miller-Abbott tube can cause bowel segments to go into spasm to assume outline changes that can be mistaken for pathology. Attempts to withdraw the tube may cause painful pleating and shortening of the bowel along the tube, even retrograde intussusception (Fig. 7-25). A decompression tube should be withdrawn only after an in-

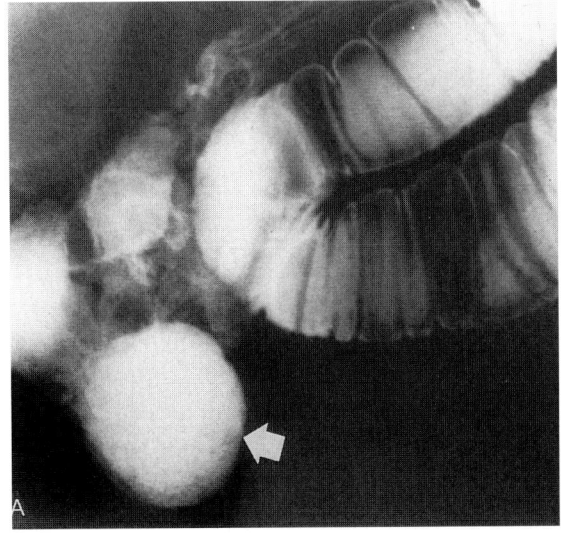
(a)

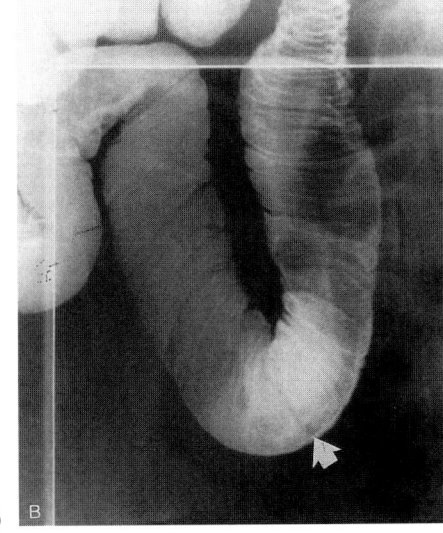
(b)

Fig. 7-20. Trying to move bowel loops out of the pelvis.
(a) Apparently ileal loop fixed in pelvis. Could this be a Meckel? (b) Suprapubic compression with patient in Trendelenberg position had to be applied for 1 to 2 minutes; gradually the now well distended bowel loop emerged, could be compressed, was normal.

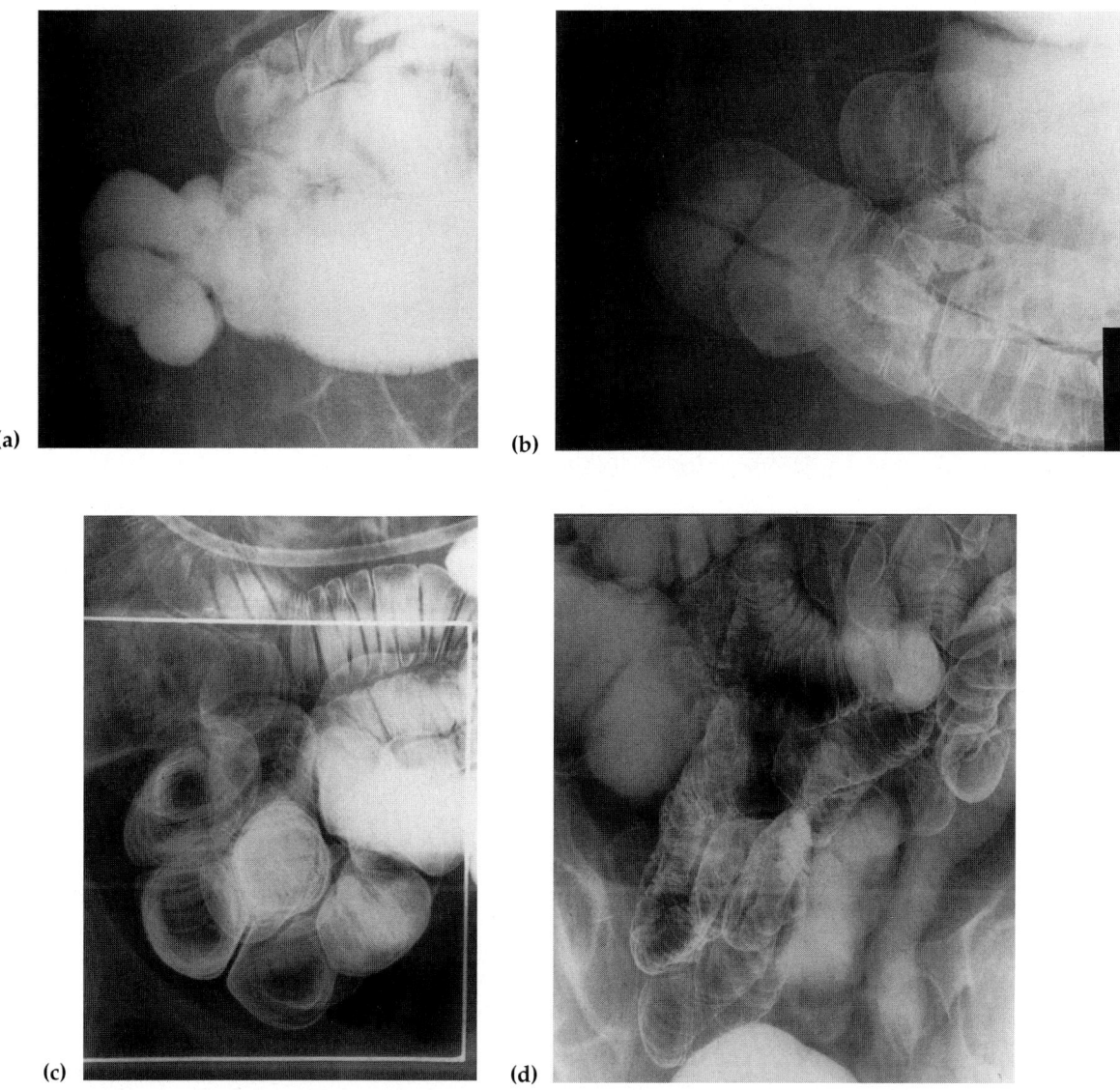

Fig. 7-21. Imaging a loop of ileum prolapsed deep into pelvis.
(a) Lateral view in single contrast; only surface outlines appreciated. (b) Same view after double contrast became established. (c) Anteroposterior view of prolapsed loops in double contrast. (d) Additional view with patient prone, tube angled 35 degrees caudad.

jection of 1.0 to 2.0 mg of glucagon, when it becomes a simple, painless procedure. 3) Occasionally long tubes fail to advance into the jejunum. If enteroclysis is required, we introduce a standard small bowel tube transorally alongside the decompression tube and advance it into the first loop of jejunum (Fig. 7-26). 4) The amount of barium to be injected depends on the distance of the long tube from the level of obstruction, the degree of lumen dilatation, and the amount of retained fluid. As much as 400 ml had to be injected on occasions. 5) In long-standing obstructions or those of high grade it is a mistake to attempt enteroclysis. Barium advance would be very slow and its presence would interfere with surgery or computed tomography (CT). In fact, CT is then the radiologic method of choice (see Chapter 21).

Enteroclysis Combined with Endoscopy

There are clinical situations in which diagnostic benefit can derive from following an endoscopy of the duodenum or proximal jejunum with an enteroclysis.[19] Examples are malabsorption states and unexplained upper gastrointestinal bleeding. Technique, indica-

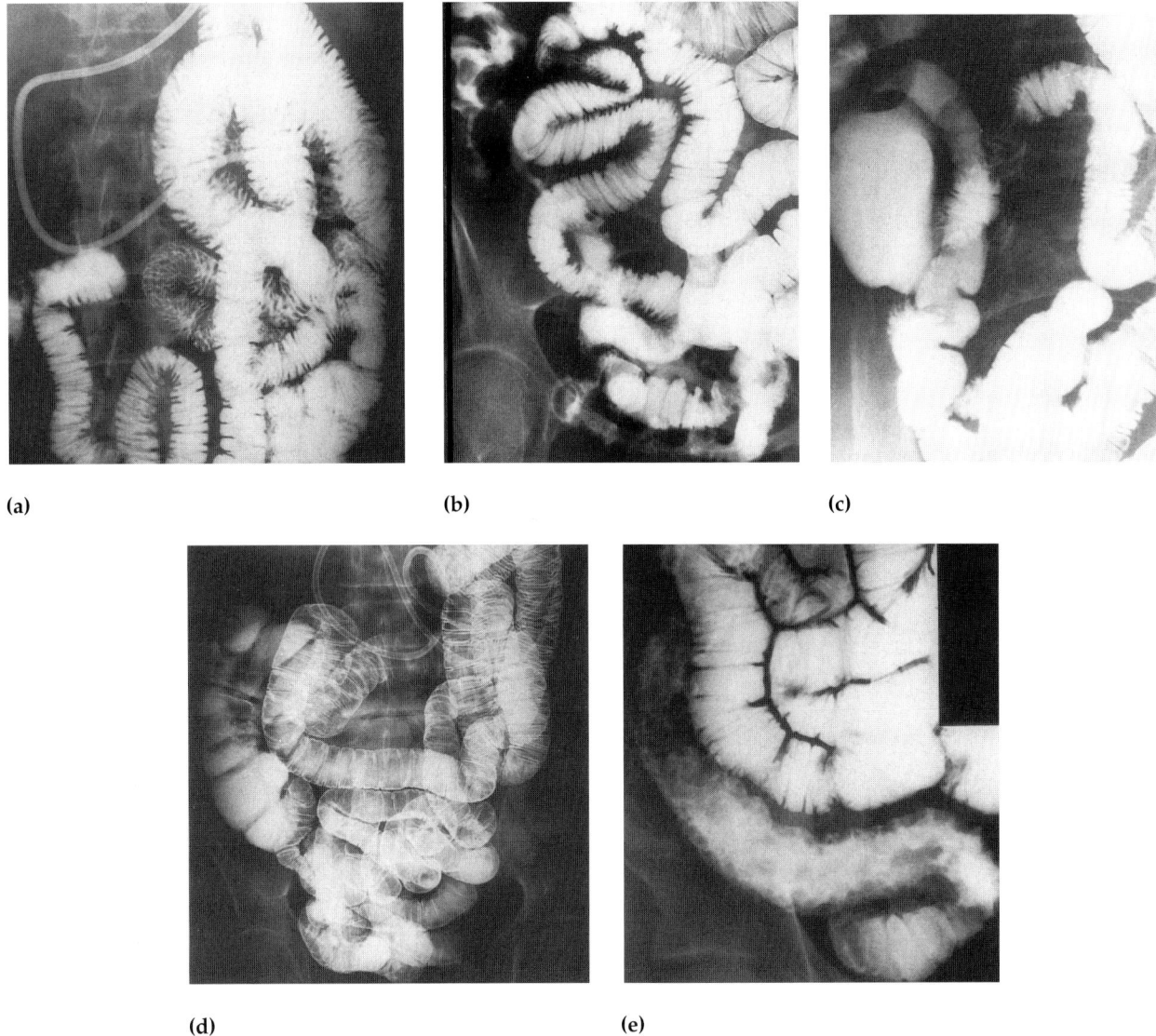

Fig. 7-22. Filming sequence in biphasic enteroclysis using a remote-control fluoroscopic unit.
(a) A compression radiograph is obtained to show the jejunum after 300 ml of 50% wt/vol barium mixture has been infused. (b) Following infusion of a total of 400 to 500 ml of barium and at the start of methylcellulose infusion, angled compression radiograph of proximal ileum in single contrast is obtained. (c) With more methylcellulose infused, angled compression radiograph obtained to show distal ileum to best advantage. (d) Following infusion of 1 L of methylcellulose, an overview (14- × 17-in film) of entire small bowel in double contrast is done. Note uniform distention of entire small bowel without barium in left colon after using an appropriate rate of flow of contrast. Additional compression radiographs with mild compression of other segments are taken as well as a lateral view of pelvic segments of ileum. (e) In another patient, compression radiograph of distal ileum during the single-contrast phase of a biphasic enteroclysis shows a cobblestone pattern of the mucosa due to Crohn's disease.

tions, and results are described in Chapter 13. In a recent report[20] combined examinations were done in 54 patients with a history of obscure bleeding; enteroscopy identified sites for bleeding in 29 of the patients (54%). All endoscopy-negative patients had follow-on enteroclysis, which produced only two additional diagnoses.

Enteroclysis in Malabsorption States

The purpose of radiology in malabsorption states is the most accurate possible delineation of mucosal detail to aid in the often difficult clinical differential diagnosis. However, in patients with steatorrhea and an increased amount of fluid in the small bowel lumen,

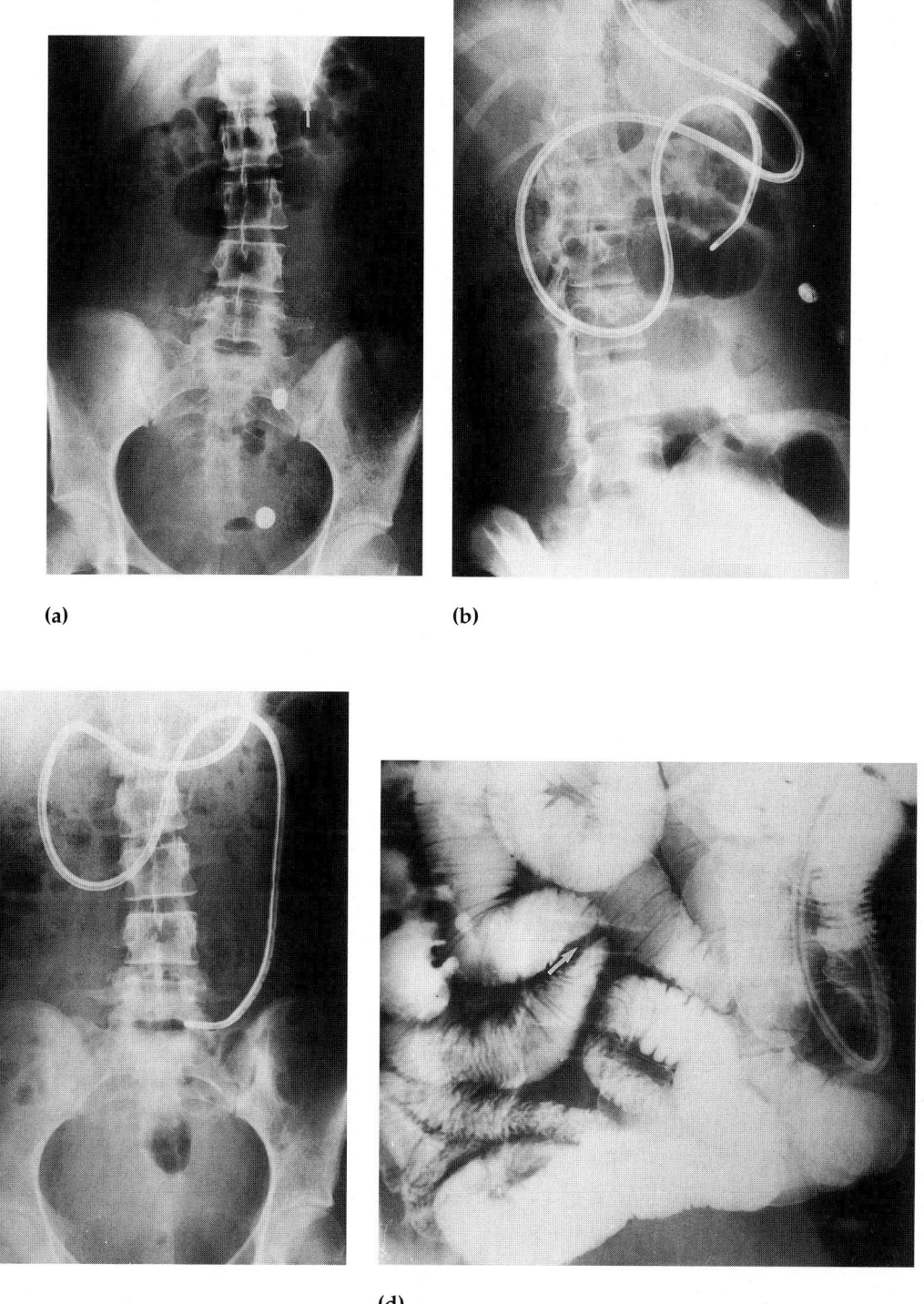

Fig. 7-23. Enteroclysis via multipurpose (decompression/enteroclysis) tube.
(a) Supine abdominal radiograph of teenage patient with symptoms of mechanical small bowel obstruction. Note kinked nasogastric tube in body of stomach (arrow) following failed decompression for 24 hours. A dilated loop of small bowel is seen below transverse colon and patient remains symptomatic. (b) Nasogastric tube replaced by multipurpose tube anchored in proximal jejunum. (c) Follow-up radiograph after 24 hours of intermittent suction shows satisfactory decompression. Relief of symptoms was felt by patient. (d) Enteroclysis done after (c) shows single adhesive band (arrow) causing low-grade partial obstruction. The use of the multipurpose tube simplified performance of enteroclysis and can be used for long tube decompression. It is better tolerated by patients than the 18F nasogastric tubes currently used in most hospitals.

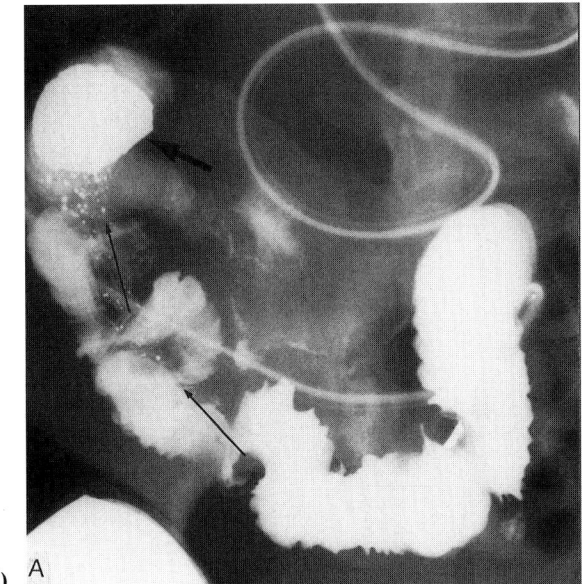 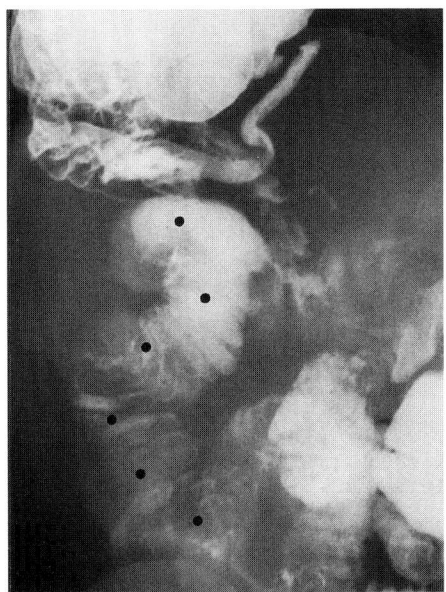

Fig. 7-24. Miller-Abbott tube has advanced into terminal ileum.
(a) Infused barium shows bowel in spasm; this was initially mistaken for ischemic bowel. (Long arrows = tube in terminal ileum; arrow = mercury-filled balloon.) (b) Tube withdrawn after IV glucagon; residual barium showed normality of bowel segment (dots).

barium suspensions may flocculate, and this should be avoided or deferred. For this purpose, enteroclysis is modified by injecting a larger amount of barium (up to 240 ml), followed by a rapid infusion of MC and by very early compression spot imaging of the proximal jejunum, disregarding the possible adverse effect on full double-contrast formation. All other loops of intestine are imaged as soon as they have become sufficiently transradiant. It may also be important to include all of the duodenojejunal flexure (eg, in celiac disease); the balloon of the catheter should, therefore, be inflated close to the ligament of Treitz.

Enteroclysis in Undiagnosed Blood Loss

About 10% of positive findings are made in the duodenum, an area not always covered during upper endoscopy. Chapter 13 reports that 50% of positive enteroscopies have shown a duodenal cause. Enteroclysis is carried out in its normal manner. If no cause for bleeding has been found, the catheter is taken back into the duodenum and the balloon inflated in the duodenal bulb. A double-contrast study of the duodenal sweep is then made, now using air as double-contrast agent. An alternative technique would be not to inflate the balloon of the tube and encourage backflow into the duodenum (Fig. 7-27).

Enteroclysis in Children

An early diagnosis of conditions like Crohn's disease and a malabsorption state is particularly relevant in childhood because of their adverse effect on physical development.

Premedication by an anxiolytic agent is essential. A general anesthetic is only rarely justified. The small bowel tube used has to be significantly smaller; we recommend the F8 tube already mentioned earlier. A barium suspension of 40% wt/vol (Entero-h with an equal amount of water) is infused until most of the small bowel has been outlined. In younger children there is an increased likelihood for rapid flocculation. Spot films should be taken early during the single-contrast phase. Double contrast with MC is used in older children. Reduction of the radiation dose is important. Fluoroscopy should be done in short bursts with critical coning down to minimum field size.

CT Enteroclysis

A limitation of the standard, nonintubation CT technique is that it cannot assess bowel wall distensibility, a most important feature of enteroclysis. On the other hand enteroclysis fails to outline extramural extensions of small bowel diseases or other remote but surgically relevant features. An early report of a tech-

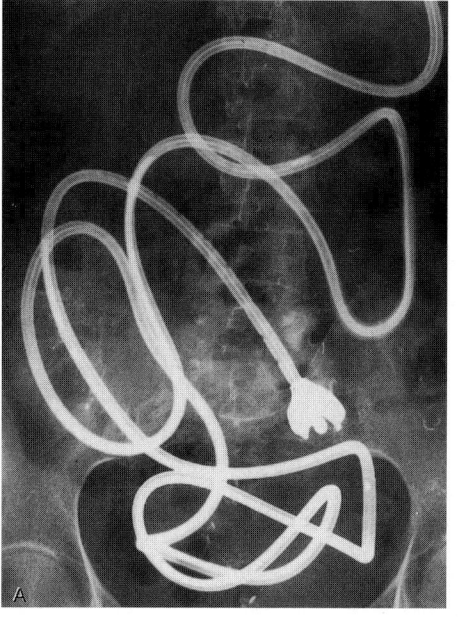
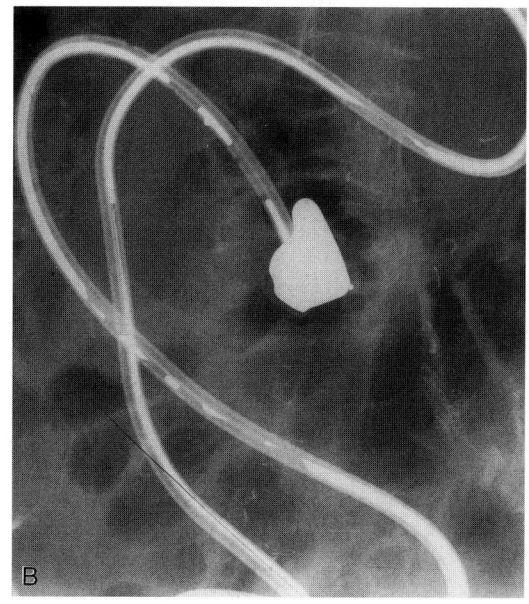
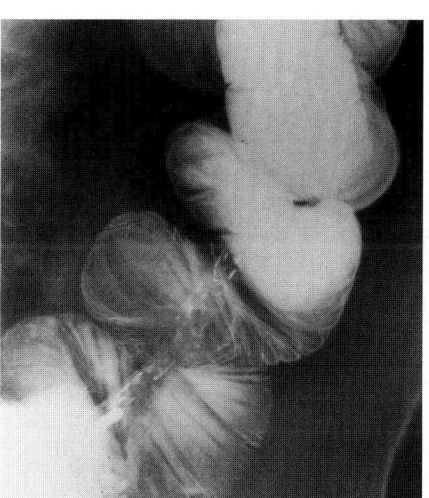
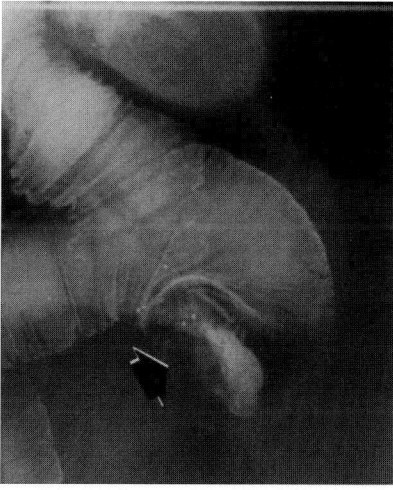

Fig. 7-25. Spasm-related changes during removal of Miller-Abbott tube.
(a) View of tube with its mercury bag in ileum. (b) Withdrawing several feet of tubing had to stop because of pain. The position of the head of the tube has not changed from (a). (c) Concentrating round tube of small bowel in painful spasm explains the reduced length of tubing with the tip still in its original position. (d) Any further withdrawal can lead to retrograde intussusception (arrow). Such stiff tubes should be withdrawn only after injecting 1 to 2 mg glucagon IV!

nique that attempts to add distensibility to other features of CT was named CT-Sellink and appeared in 1992.[21] Bender et al[22] carefully assessed the performance and applications of his technique of CT enteroclysis (CT-E). Water-soluble contrast (hypaque 10 to 15%) was infused via nasojejunal intubation. Under fluoroscopic guidance the advance of the contrast material was observed and recorded. The patient was then transferred to CT where the catheter was hooked up to an enteroclysis pump for continued infusion. CT images were done before and after IV contrast if needed (Fig. 7-28). A further publication[23] compared CT-E with traditional CT in the diagnosis of small bowel obstruction. In partial obstructions CT-E achieved a sensitivity of 89% against only 50% for traditional CT.

A different form of enteroclysis combined with spiral CT (ESCT) has been developed in the Department of Radiology at the University of Vienna, Austria.[24] Methylcellulose solution is infused through a nasojejunal tube to produce sufficient distention throughout the small bowel. Intravenous contrast is injected and the abdomen is scanned in a single breath-hold period. Inflammatory bowel disease, including Crohn's disease (Fig. 7-29), tumors, and obstructions are among the applications of ESCT.

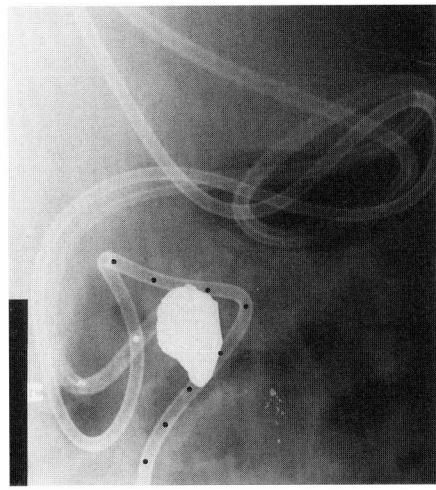

Fig. 7-26. Miller-Abbott tube (dots) did not pass beyond ligament of Treitz. After waiting several days it was easier to pass a small bowel tube alongside and proceed with the enteroclysis.

Small Bowel Biopsy Combined with Enteroclysis

Passing a 180-cm-long endoscopy-type biopsy forceps through the lumen of a 150-cm-long, endhole 14F Madison-2 Cook enteroclysis catheter has obtained multiple mucosal biopsies in 17 patients.[25]

Contraindications to Enteroclysis

Only few contraindications exist: 1) Intubation is inadvisable in a patient with a severe form of reflux esophagitis or with any active specific esophagitis. Intubation would also be contraindicated within 2 weeks of gastric or duodenal surgery. 2) Enteroclysis is inadvisable in patients with complete or high-grade small bowel obstruction and should be avoided in patients with likely bowel infarction. Nor should it be done when a barium enema, an ileostomy enema, or CT would be the more rational approaches to diagnosis. 3) Enteroclysis is not justified in patients who would be adequately served by a fluoroscopic follow-through examination, combined with peroral pneumocolon if indicated.

Complications of Enteroclysis

Major complications are most unlikely. During nearly 35 years of doing enteroclysis we have had only one case in which esophageal perforation was discovered the next day. However, this patient also had esophagoscopy the same day as the enteroclysis, and it was in nobody's interest to assign blame. This patient had severe esophagitis with friable mucosa, and enteroclysis should not have been done.

We are aware of only two reports in the literature of complications during enteroclysis.[26,27] Perforations or mucosal dissections are possibilities, if the guide wire is allowed to either exit from the tip of the tube or to pass through a side hole, which is possible in some types of tubing.

Minor complications are not infrequent. Vomiting due to substantial reflux into the stomach occurs in some 10% of patients when a balloon catheter has not been used, and is infrequent when it is used. Some patients may complain of abdominal fullness or of crampy pain during the infusion of MC. Again we wish to stress the need to monitor reflux, especially in aged and ill patients, and to prevent aspiration of MC solution. Methylcellulose and barium refluxed in the stomach should be aspirated before tube removal.

Air Double-Contrast Enteroclysis

In Japan, the development of double-contrast study of the stomach by Shirakabe et al[28] has significantly raised the detection rate of early gastric cancer.[29]

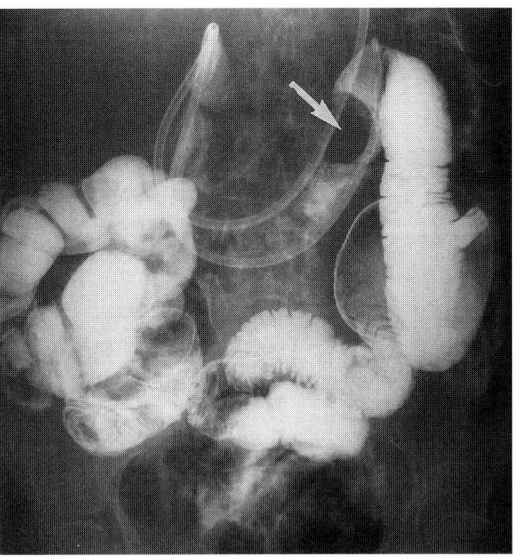

Fig. 7-27. Male patient, referred to enteroclysis for diagnosis of source of intermittent bleeding. Negative upper and lower endoscopies.
Enteroclysis was done without inflation of balloon to promote limited reflux into the duodenum, a frequent site of origin for bleeding. A submucosal type mass effect was demonstrated in the duodenum close to the ligament of Treitz (arrow). At laparotomy an ulcerated leiomyoma was resected.

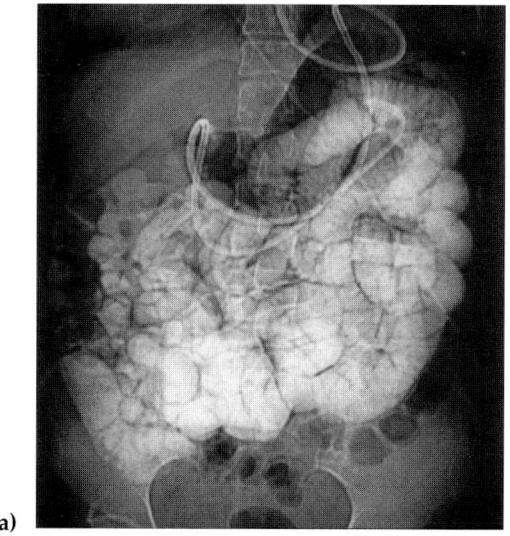 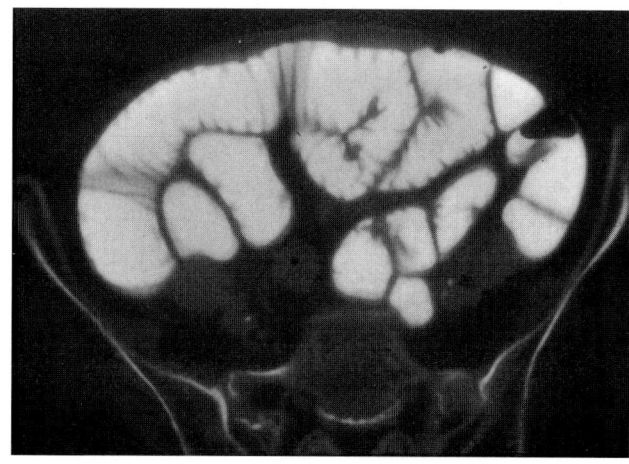

Fig. 7-28. CT enteroclysis.
(a) Digital scout image following infusion of 12% sodium diatrizoate under fluoroscopy. (b) Normal CT-E. Note distention of bowel and good demonstration of folds. The technique combines the advantages of volume challenge on the small bowel with the cross-sectional display of CT. (Courtesy of Greg N. Bender, MD.)

Many researchers have attempted to apply this technique to the small intestine, but with little success. Aware of the availability of tubes for duodenal intubation and of suitable concentrations of barium suspensions,[30] Kobayashi[31] and Yao and his colleagues[32] reported a standardized double-contrast technique for the small intestine. This technique has found wide acceptance in Japan and has contributed to research into small bowel diseases.[33]

However, there remain problems associated with this intricate technique that limit its value as a routine examination.

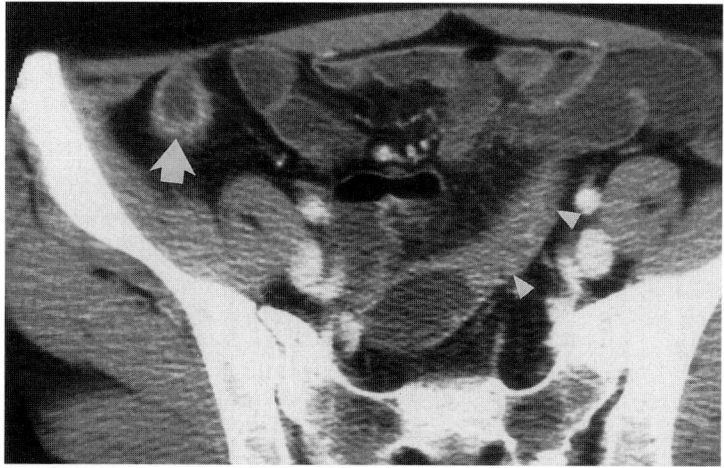 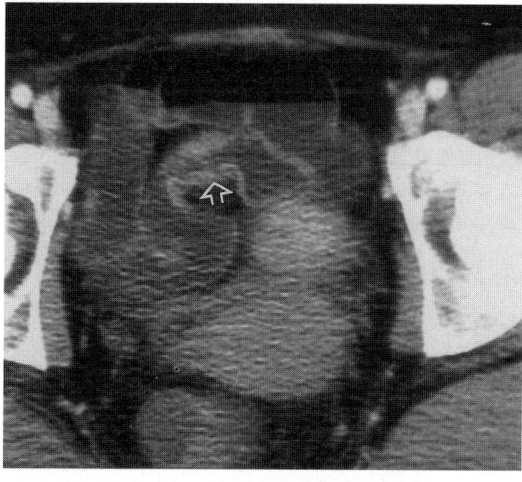

Fig. 7-29. Enteroclysis with spiral CT (ESCT). During methylcellulose infusion CT before and after IV contrast.
(a) Patient with Crohn's disease developing obstructive symptoms. Long strictured segment (arrowheads) with nearby dilated bowel, separate from the known involvement of the terminal ileum (arrow), a skip lesion. (b) In same patient, at a higher level, a short stricture (open arrow) with high-intensity wall thickening, a second short skip lesion. The short stricture was treated by strictureplasty, the long stricture was resected. (Courtesy of E. Schober, MD, and colleagues, Vienna.)

Table 7-1. Sequence of the air double-contrast method

1. **Patient preparation:** Laxatives night before examination
   Nothing by mouth until examination

2. **Intubation:** No pharyngeal anesthesia
   Transnasal intubation with balloon catheter

3. **Infusion of barium:** 70% wt/vol, by syringes, approximately 60 ml/min
   Slowly 150 to 200 ml; when peristalsis stops
   Further 50 to 100 ml to a total 300 to 400 ml

4. **Infusion of air:** Total 800 to 1000 ml; initially 200 ml slowly
   Once barium reaches terminal ileum, 200 ml of air injected several times

5. **Antispasmodic:** With enough air in distal ileum, buscopan IV or IM

6. **Filming:** Light compression, patient different obliquities, separation overlapping loops

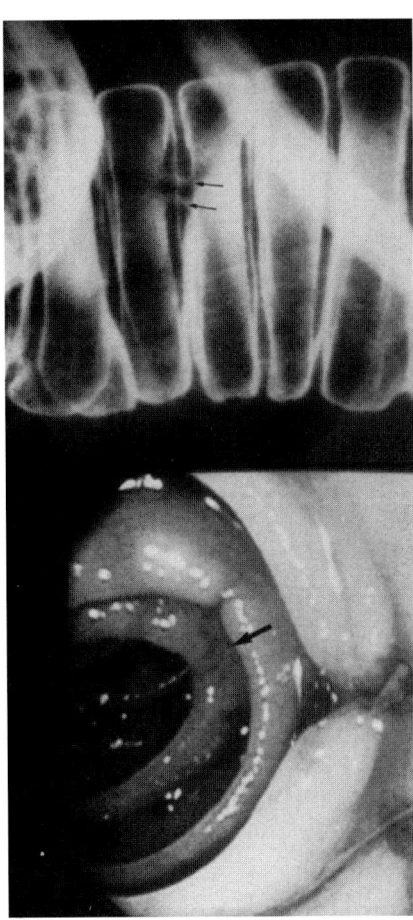

Fig. 7-30. **57-year-old male patient, referred because of melena.**
(a) Double-contrast view shows two abnormal linear shadows intersecting a fold (arrows). (b) Push enteroscopy shows subtle linear ulcerations (arrow). (Further tiny ulcers were shown by double contrast and by enteroscopy.)

Technique of the Air Double-Contrast Examination[34]

The administration of laxatives the night before the examination accelerates transit of barium to the terminal ileum. This is important because air, unlike methylcellulose, cannot actively propel the barium (see Table 7-1).

Air is, therefore, injected only after the barium column has reached the terminal ileum. Very prolonged transit leads to degeneration of the barium, after which optimal double contrast can no longer be obtained. Intermittent administration of the barium helps it to reach the terminal ileum sooner. A duodenal tube with a balloon near its tip helps to prevent reflux of air into the stomach.

Manual compression under fluoroscopic observation should be used to prevent pooling of barium at any point, especially in the left upper abdomen. This is aided by turning and deep breathing of the patient. The total amount of barium ought to be limited to 400 ml, if possible even to 300 ml, in order to demonstrate all the bowel loops in double contrast.

To achieve an even distribution of air throughout the small bowel, an initial 200 ml of air is slowly injected. After observing the distal progress of the air and barium by fluoroscopy, 50 to 100 ml of air is added repeatedly, at the same time appropriately changing the patient's position. When the air reaches the pelvis, double-contrast views of intrapelvic intestinal loops are obtained with the patient in prone position. After adequate double-contrast views of the jejunum and ileum have been recorded, a spasmolytic agent is injected to obtain hypotonicity.

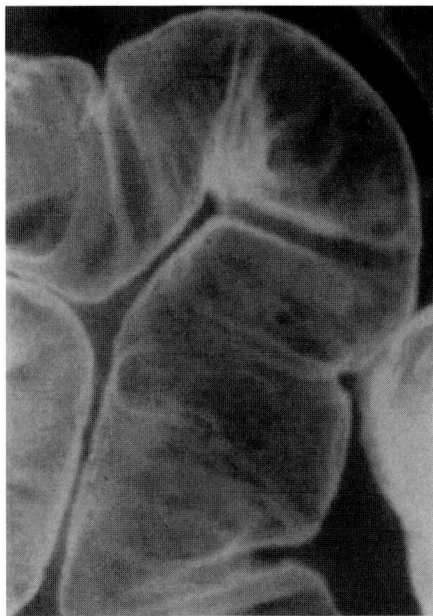

Fig. 7-31. Male patient, 51 years old, with adult T-cell leukemia.
Double-contrast image demonstrates multiple small elevations thought to represent enlarged solitary lymph follicles.

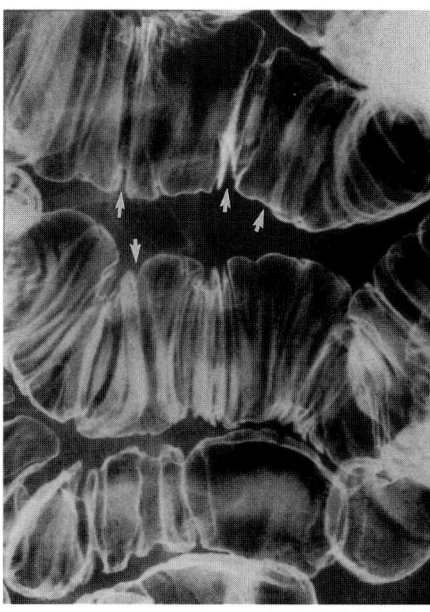

Fig. 7-32. Male patient, 58 years old, with primary amyloidosis showing focal thickening of Kerckring's folds (arrows to some).
This was not recognized during fluoroscopy. (Confirmed histologically.)

To produce radiographs of high quality, suitable obliquity of the patient and light abdominal compression are a requirement for the imaging of the various bowel loops in double contrast. Light compression usually helps to separate superimposed bowel loops.

Advantages of air double-contrast studies. When successful, the examination produces exquisite surface detail. Lesions not recognized under fluoroscopic observation are demonstrated. Examples are tiny lesions (Figs 7-30, 7-31), barely thickened Kerckring's folds (Fig. 7-32), and an abnormal mucosal surface pattern[35] (Fig 7-33). Ulcerations can be demonstrated en face to express disease activity and, at a later time, to evaluate response to treatment [Fig. 7-34 (a), (b)].

Problems in presence of stenoses. In patients with established stenoses transit to the ileum can be delayed for more than one hour and satisfactory double-contrast views cannot be achieved in the usual way. In such cases double-contrast views are taken of the jejunum, and the ileum is left for later. Other patients in whom such a stenosis is known to exist swallow 250 ml of 70% wt/vol of barium and are intubated 2 to 3 hours later, when injection of air can achieve double-contrast views of the ileum. However, in cases with severely stenotic lesions double-contrast studies are not feasible, and alternative techniques are used, such as a barium follow-through or a barium enema.

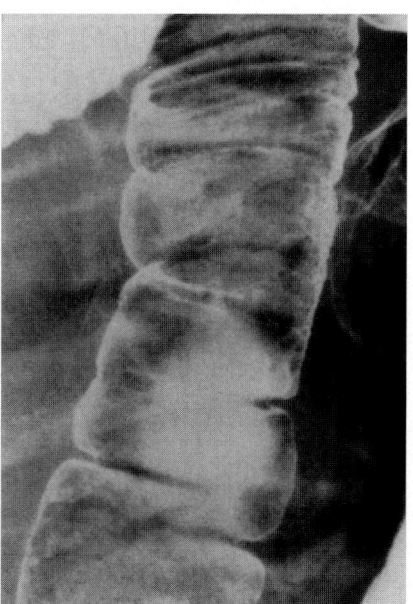

Fig. 7-33. 59-year-old male patient with secondary amyloidosis.
Air double contrast shows irregular outline of folds and a diffuse coarse mucosal pattern with granular elevations into the barium surface coating. Pathology of biopsy specimen confirmed AA amyloid.

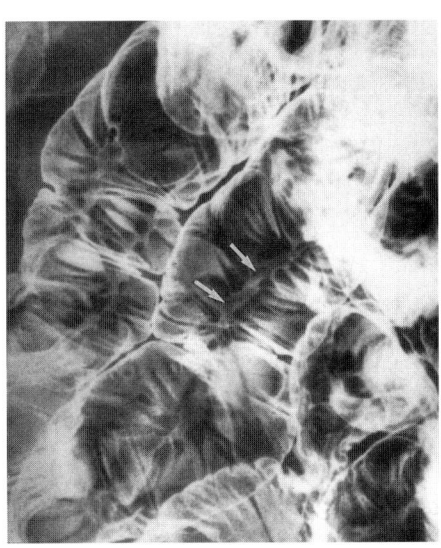
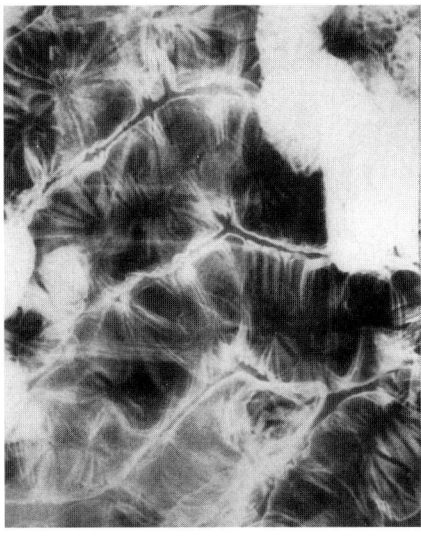

Fig. 7-34. Female patient, aged 41 years, with known Crohn's disease.
(a) Linear mesenteric border ulcers demonstrated en face with typical convergence of thickened folds (arrows to one of the ulcers). (b) After 6 weeks' treatment with an elemental diet, air double contrast could demonstrate healing of most and reduction of other ulcers.

(a)   (b)

References

1. Pesquera GS. Method for direct visualization of lesions in the small intestine. *AJR.* 1929;22:254–257.
2. Thoeni RF, Gould RG. Enteroclysis and small bowel series: comparison of radiation dose and examination time. *Radiology.* 1991;178:659–662.
3. Maglinte DDT, Kelvin FM, Micon LT, et al. Nasointestinal tube for decompression or enteroclysis: experience with 150 patients. *Abdom Imaging.* 1994;19:108–112.
4. Stevenson GW, Malone DE. Sedation and analgesia in abdominal imaging and intervention. Communication to the Society of Gastrointestinal Radiology Meeting; 1998.
5. Maglinte DDT. Balloon enteroclysis catheter. *AJR.* 1984;143:761–762.
6. Traill ZC, Nolan DJ. Technical report: intubation fluoroscopy times using new enteroclysis tube. *Clin Radiol.* 1994;50:339–340.
7. Taverner DS, Odurny A. Enteroclysis—the influence of tube design. *Clin Radiol.* 1994;49:176–178.
8. Antes G, Eggemann F. Problemlose Sondenlegung beim Dünndarm-einlauf (Enteroclysis). *Rontgenpraxis* 1987;40:411.
9. Maglinte DDT, Stevens LH, Hall RC, et al. Dual-purpose tube for enteroclysis and nasogastric-nasoenteric decompression. *Radiology.* 1992;185:281–282.
10. Herlinger H. A modified technique for the double contrast small bowel enema. *Gastrointest Radiol.* 1978;2:397–400.
11. Antes G, Lissner J. Double-contrast small-bowel examination with barium and methylcellulose: results in 300 cases. *Radiology.* 1983;148:33–40.
12. Maglinte DDT, Miller RF. A comparison of pumps used for enteroclysis. *Radiology.* 1984;152:1984.
13. Maglinte DDT, Burney BT, Miller RE. Technical factors for a more rapid enteroclysis. *AJR.* 1982;138:588–591.
14. Sellink JL, Rosenbusch G. Moderne Untersuchungstechnik des Dünndarms oder Die zehn Gebote des Enteroklysmas. *Radiologe.* 1981;21:366–376.
15. Nolan DJ, Traill ZC. The current role of the barium examination of the small intestine. *Clin Radiol.* 1997;52:809–820.
16. Maglinte DDT, Kelvin FM, O'Connor K, et al. Current status of small bowel radiography. *Abdom Imaging.* 1996;21:247–257.
17. Oudkerk M, Rijke AM. The effect of barium infusion rate on the diagnostic value of enteroclysis. *J Med Imaging.* 1988;2:123–125.
18. Maglinte DDT, Lappas JC, Kelvin FM, et al. Small bowel radiography: how, when and why? *Radiology.* 1982;163:297–305.
19. McGovern R, Barkin JS. Enteroscopy and enteroclysis: An improved method for combined procedure. *Gastrointest Radiol.* 1990;15:327–328.
20. Willis JR, Chokshi HR, Zuckerman GR, Aliperti G. Enteroscopy-enteroclysis: experience with a combined endoscopic-radiographic technique. *Gastrointest Endosc.* 1997;45:163–167.
21. Klöppel R, Thiele J, Bosse J. CT-Sellink [in German]. *ROFO.* 1992;156:291–292.
22. Bender GN, Timmons JH, Williard WC, Carter J. Computed tomographic enteroclysis: one methodology. *Invest Radiol.* 1996;31:43–49.
23. Walsh DW, Bender GN, Timmons JH. Comparison of computed tomography—enteroclysis and traditional computed tomography in the setting of suspected partial small bowel obstruction. *Emerg Radiol.* 1998;5:81–88.
24. Schober E, Tujretschek K, Sschina W, Oberhuber G, Moeschl P, Mostbeck GH. Methylcellulose enteroclysis spiral CT in the preoperative assessment of Crohn's disease: radiologic pathologic correlation. Scientific exhibit of the 83rd Assembly and Annual Meeting of the Radi-

ological Society of North America; December 1997; Chicago, Ill; 205:717.
25. Bender GN, Lane JD, Tsuchida A, Clark JA. Small bowel biopsy through an enteroclysis catheter to augment findings at enteroclysis and hypotonic duodenography. *Radiology.* 1994;191:573–575.
26. Diner WC. Duodenal perforation during intubation for small bowel enema study. *Radiology.* 1988;168:39–41.
27. Ginaldi S. Small bowel perforation during enteroclysis. *Gastrointest Radiol.* 1991;16:29–31.
28. Shirakabe H, Nishizawa M, Hayakawa H, et al. X-ray diagnosis of early gastric cancer. *Stom Intest.* 1966; 1:11–24.
29. Maruyama M, Hamada T. Diagnosis of gastric cancer in Japan. In: Freeny PC, Stevenson GW, eds. *Margulis and Burhenne's Alimentary Tract Radiology.* 5th ed. St. Louis, Mo: CV Mosby Co; 1994:399–428.
30. Sellink JL. Examination of small intestine by means of duodenal intubation. Leiden, the Netherlands: HE Steinfert Kroese BV, 1971.
31. Kobayashi S, Nishizawa M, Mizuno K, et al. Double contrast study of the small bowel. *Jpn Clin Radiol.* 1974;19:619.
32. Nakamura Y, Tani K, Yao T, et al. X-ray examination of the small intestine by means of duodenal intubation—double contrast of the small bowel. *Stom Intest.* 1974;9:1461–1469.
33. Tsukasa S, Tokutome K, Iris T, et al. Roentgenographic diagnosis of Crohn's disease of the small intestine. *Stom Intest.* 1978;13:335–349.
34. Yao T. Double-contrast enteroclysis with air. In: Freeny PC, Stevenson GW, eds. *Margulis and Burhenne's Alimentary Tract Radiology.* 5th ed. St Louis, Mo: CV Mosby Co; 1994:548–550.
35. Tada S, Iida M, Yao T, et al. Gastrointestinal amyloidosis: radiologic features by chemical types. *Radiology.* 1994;190:37–42.

Sonography of the Small Bowel and Related Structures

Michel Rioux

Chapter Contents

Introduction
The Sonographer's Approach
Normal Anatomy
Abnormalities of the Peritoneal Cavity, Mesentery, and Omentum
Pathologies of the Small Bowel
Small Bowel Dilatation
Small Bowel Hematoma or Hemorrhage
Inflammatory Conditions
Small Bowel Tumors
Congenital Disorders
Miscellaneous Disorders

Introduction

It would be most unusual for a physician who has taken a patient's history and completed the physical examination not to require investigations to shorten the differential diagnostic possibilities. In view of the increasing patient load, growing social and economic pressures, and delays before hospitalization, it is very important to select an appropriate diagnostic technique. Sonography has emerged as the low-cost, rapidly available imaging method for the abdomen that is without side effects. Furthermore, special patient preparation and contrast material administration, both of which may cause delay, are not needed.

The Sonographer's Approach

A careful history and relevant physical examination are mandatory before scanning is started. An overview of the abdomen is first performed with the use of a 3.5-MHz probe. This overview may indicate an abnormality or an unexplained finding or could be normal in a patient whose physical appearance or laboratory findings suggest an underlying pathology. It is then necessary to proceed to *high resolution sonography* (HRS). This requires scrutiny of the entire abdomen with a 5- or 7.5-MHz linear probe or its equivalent. It requires visualization of the different layers of the bowel wall and a search for abnormal fat.

Scanning is done transversely in 3-in lengths starting below the right lobe of the liver and descending into the right iliac fossa. One then moves upwards to left of the starting position and repeats the scanning verticals until the entire abdomen has been scanned. A pelvic sonogram is always included. A full bladder is useful as it displaces most of the distal small bowel, the sigmoid, and the omentum. If the bladder is empty or if the pelvic organs remain inadequately visualized in spite of a full bladder, the examination may be completed using an endovaginal or even an endorectal probe.

Sonography is mostly done with the patient supine. However, sometimes it is useful to examine the patient on his or her right or left side. This induces displacement of intestinal fluid and air, creating new and possibly more revealing sonographic windows. These different scanning approaches are particularly useful in a patient with ileus of any type.[1]

The sonographer should first identify the starting point in the abdomen. A good way to do this is to search for the right colon or the sigmoid. After the colon has been located, the ileocecal valve and the cecum should be demonstrated [Fig. 8-1(a)] and the distal ileum followed in transverse direction [Fig. 8-1(b)]. If confronted with an unexpected or unexplained sonographic finding, a complementary procedure (computed tomography, barium studies, etc) may be indicated. In an ideal situation the sonographer is in close relationship to CT scanning and can be involved in the patient's CT immediately after the sonogram. In any other patient who is referred for CT scans, skin markers should be applied by the sonographer to indicate the point(s) of maximum interest.

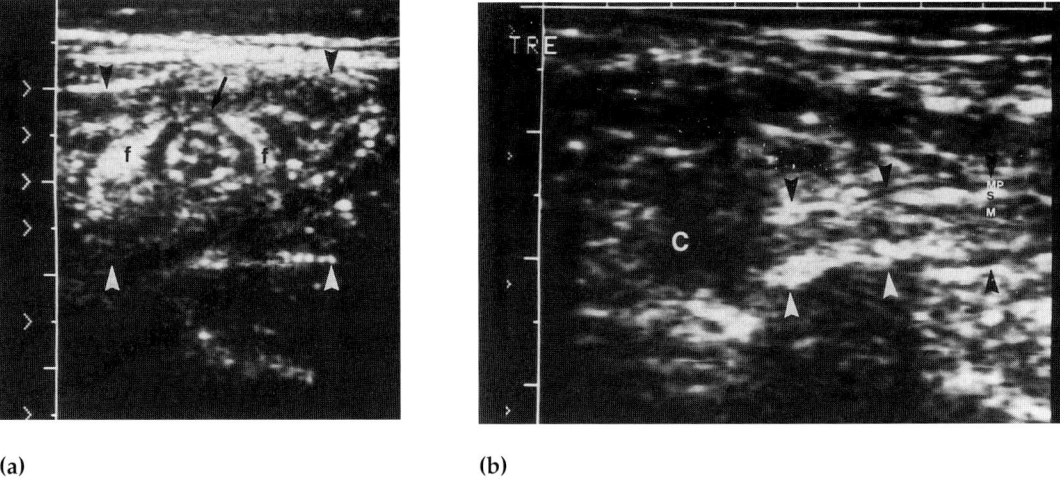

Fig. 8-1. US appearances of a normal ileocecal region.
(a) The longitudinal view of the cecum (between arrowheads) demonstrates the hyperechoic fat (f) of the ileocecal valve. This fat surrounds the typical cross-sectional appearance of the terminal ileum (arrow). (b) In the transverse view of the same region, the longitudinally shown terminal ileum (between arrowheads) extends into the cecum (c). The layers of the ileal wall are distinctive. (MP = hypoechoic muscularis propria, S = hyperechoic submucosa, M = hypoechoic mucosa.)

Normal Anatomy

Abdominal Wall and Peritoneum

Wherever sonography is used one should always scan from superficial to deeper structures. Thus, following the skin with its variable amount of subcutaneous fat, scanning should test the hypoechoic abdominal musculature and its surrounding hyperechoic fat. Study of the peritoneum follows (Fig. 8-2). The parietal peritoneum (PP) is represented by a fixed, thin, continuous, hyperechoic line, which is separated from the identical-looking visceral peritoneum (VP) by a very thin hypoechoic space representing the lubricating layer. The VP slides on the PP during respiration.

Omentum

The omentum can be found between the peritoneum and the small bowel mesentery. It is invisible in children. In adults, it is recognized as a mobile and most superficial structure of the abdominal cavity (Fig. 8-3). Its thickness varies greatly with patient body habitus and so does its location within the abdomen. In addition, although fat is hyperechoic most of the time, a few patients have normal hypoechoic fat.[2] The omentum should be slightly compressible and it should move during respiration.

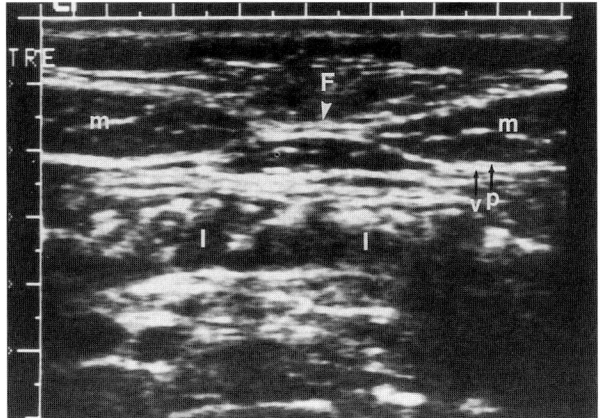

Fig. 8-2. Transverse view of the midline of the abdominal wall.
Underneath the subcutaneous fat (F), the rectus muscles (m) are separated from a fibrous hyperechoic white line (arrowhead) and both layers of the peritoneum (v = visceral, p = parietal). In this case, the omentum is too thin to be visible (l = underlying intestine seen longitudinally).

Small Bowel Mesentery

The mesentery is delineated by the fat that surrounds the mesenteric vessels. At sonography, the mesentery is shown to be composed of multiple mobile folds, which contain fat, mesenteric nodes, and numerous small transsonic vessels. When visible, normal mesenteric nodes are flattened or disk-shaped, have moderate echogenicity, and do not exceed 5 mm in anteroposterior (AP) diameter. The thickness of each mesenteric fold varies with patient body habitus.

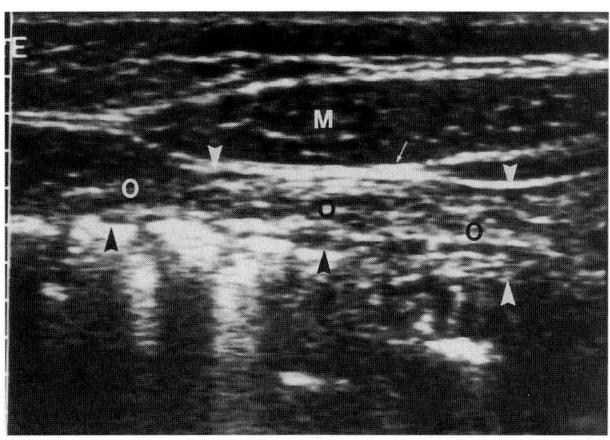

Fig. 8-3. US appearance of a normal omentum.
The transverse view shows the left paramedial abdominal wall, the rectus muscle (m), both peritoneal surfaces (arrow), and the omentum (O). The last is of variable thickness (between arrowheads). Below the omentum, hyperechoic areas represent gas in a bowel segment.

The mesenteric fat is not always homogeneous. In obese patients, a fold of mesentery appears as two layers of peripheral hypoechoic fat with central hyperechoic perivascular fat. The reflecting peritoneal interface between two superimposed folds of mesentery forms a bright hyperechoic line (Fig. 8-4). This stratified appearance, which is continuous to the gut wall, is a sonographic indication of a normal mesentery. Sonographic studies of the mesentery should always include visualization of the proximal portion of the superior mesenteric vein and artery. Their interrelated anatomic positions as well as their permeability should be ascertained. Doppler technology may be used as an additional technique.

Small Bowel

It is usual for the left upper quadrant of the abdomen to be occupied by proximal jejunum (Fig. 8-5), the lower left quadrant by distal jejunum and proximal ileum, the right upper quadrant by more ileum, and the right lower quadrant by the distal ileum. There are frequent normal variations in the location of these segments. However, if a normal relationship between the superior mesenteric artery (SMA) and superior mesenteric vein (SMV) is present, significant variations of small bowel distribution are unlikely.

The small intestine can be likened to a hollow tube. It should therefore be round in the transverse and tubular in the longitudinal view. The lumen diameter changes during peristalsis but should always be less than 3 cm. The wall thickness is also affected by peristalsis and should not exceed 3 mm during relaxation and 5 mm during contraction. The different layers of the wall are often visible and should be imaged (Figs. 8-5, 8-6). The hyperechoic central line represents the interface between the luminal contents and the mucosa. The *mucosa* (M) is hypoechoic and barely visible under normal conditions. The *submucosa* (SM) is hyperechoic because it contains abundant fat and collagenous material. The submucosa is usually the most apparent and easily recognized layer. The *muscularis propria* (MP) is hypoechoic and composed of an outer longitudinal and inner circular layer. Both are separated by a faint linear hyperechoic interface. The outermost hyperechoic layer consists of subserosal fat and the *serosa* (S). The thickness of the wall is measured as the distance between the serosa and the endoluminal interface.[3]

With lumen distention or with compression it is normally possible to reduce the thickness of the submucosal layer. The hyperechogenicity of the submucosa may also be reduced by an increased presence of normal, hypoechoic *lymphoid tissue* (Fig. 8-6). This tends to be a more prominent feature in the terminal ileum of children and young adults.[3]

Abnormalities of the Peritoneal Cavity, Mesentery, and Omentum

Since the ultrasound (US) features of peritoneal, mesenteric, and omental pathologies often overlap,

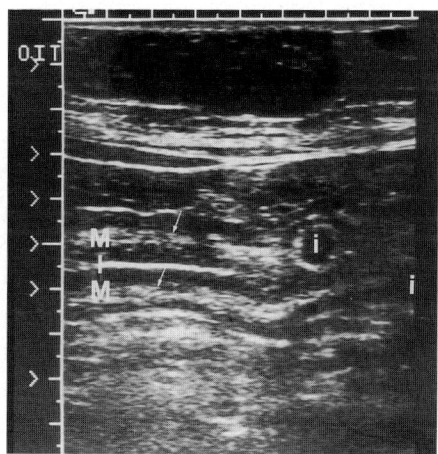

Fig. 8-4. US appearance of normal small bowel mesentery.
Transverse section of two superimposed folds of small bowel mesentery. Every mesenteric fold (M) is composed of hyperechoic perivascular fat (arrows) with hypoechoic fat on either side. A bright hyperechoic line (l) represents the interface caused by the peritoneal lining of each mesenteric fold. (i = bowel seen in transverse view at the end of each mesenteric fold.)

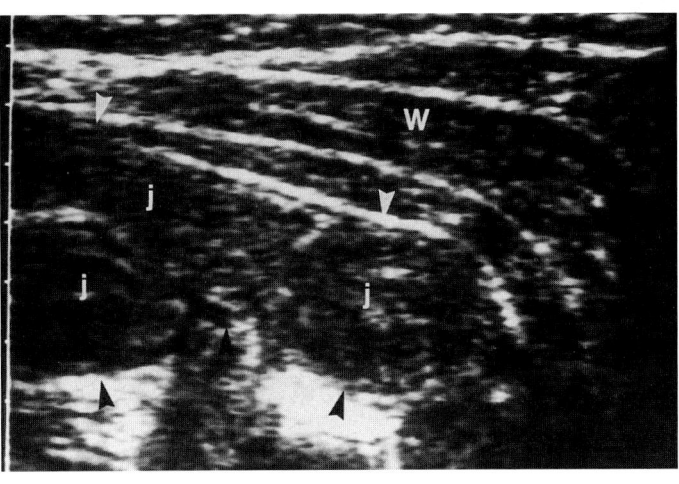
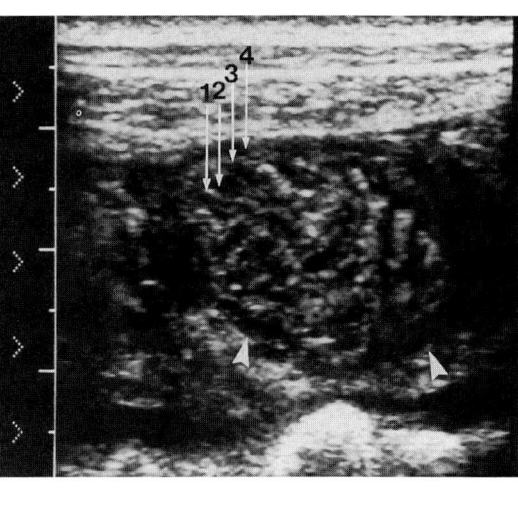

Fig. 8-5. Changed US aspects of jejunal loops when using (a) a 5-Mhz and (b) a 7.5-Mhz transducer. W = wall of abdomen. (a) Behind the left abdominal wall, there are several loops of jejunum (j) (between arrowheads). Many mucosal folds crowd their lumens. (b) High-resolution transverse sonography of a segment of jejunum (arrowheads) outlines numerous mucosal folds and separately identifies the different layers of the bowel walls. (1 = hyperechoic interface between folds; 2 = hypoechoic mucosa; 3 = hyperechoic submucosa; 4 = hypoechoic muscularis proprio.)

they are discussed together. The purpose of sonography is to recognize the abnormality, determine its origin, and narrow its differential diagnosis. Small bowel diseases related to abnormalities of these anatomic regions will be discussed in later sections.

Ascites

Serous ascites is usually echo-free, while *exudative ascites* contains echogenic debris or diffusely distributed or locally deposited particles. However, this distinc-

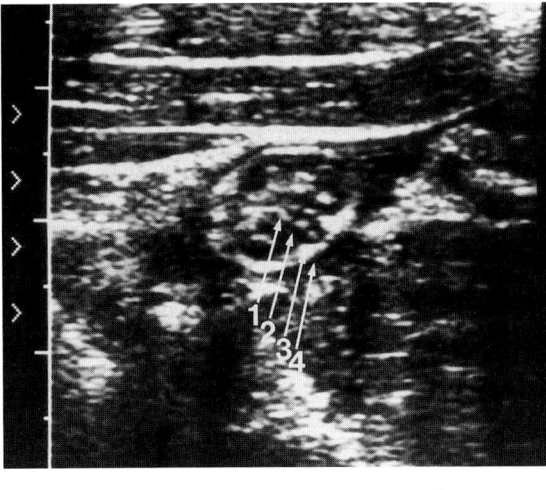
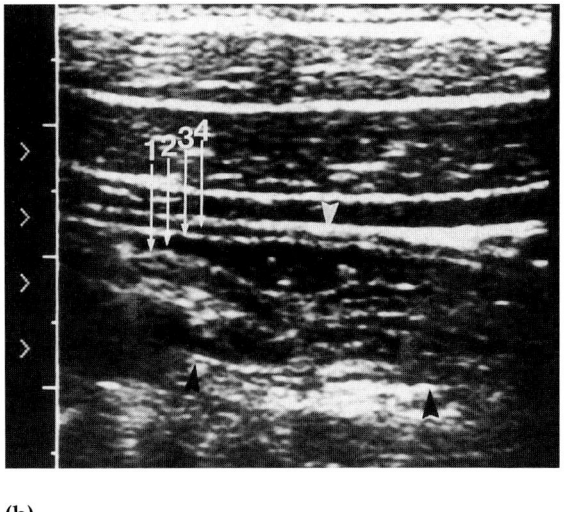

Fig. 8-6. US appearances of the terminal ileum in an asymptomatic child.
(a) Transverse view of the ileum with the characteristic appearance of the layers of the wall. Fewer folds are seen than in the jejunum (see Fig. 8-5). (1 = Hyperechoic interface between folds; 2 = hypoechoic mucosa; 3 = hyper-echoic submucosa [usually the thickest layer]; 4 = hypo-echoic muscularis propria.) (b) Longitudinal view of the same ileum (between arrowheads); a few areas exhibit a thicker hypoechoic mucosal lining (2) and a thinner hyperechoic submucosa (3). This apparent enlargement of the mucosa is due to the presence of underlying hyperplastic lymphoid tissue that is as hypoechoic as the mucosa itself. The sharp delineation between mucosa and submucosa as well as the normal peristalsis favors simple lymphoid hyperplasia.

tion does not always apply since a purely sonolucent ascites may be found in peritonitis, hemoperitoneum, or ascites associated with peritoneal carcinomatosis.

Loculated ascites (because of previous adhesion formation) may not be distinguished from other peritoneal processes, like a hematoma, abscess, lymphocele, pancreatic pseudocyst, or cystic tumor.

Seroma, Abscess, and Biloma

Seromas and abscesses are often encountered after abdominal surgery and should be differentiated from each other. The majority of *seromas* are compressible and painless. Sonographic patterns include single or multiple, sonolucent or hypoechoic, uni- or multiloculated, encapsulated processes with posterior acoustic enhancement. In contrast, an *abscess* is usually painful and delineated by a thick hypoechoic pseudocapsule of variable thickness and without distinct layers. The contents of an abscess show any combination of sonolucent or hypoechoic exudate, echogenic debris (from the bowel wall and/or mesenteric fat), and variable amounts of echogenic gaseous particles (Fig. 8-7). Although seromas and abscesses are usually molded by the shapes of adjacent structures, a "mass effect" can occur with both entities. However, this is usually more impressive with an abscess.

Bilomas present US features that resemble those of a seroma. They are usually located in the vicinity of the porta hepatis. A biloma can also become infected.

Generally, having demonstrated any image that suggests a fluid collection, a fine needle biopsy or drainage under US guidance can further refine the diagnosis.

Pneumoperitoneum

In a supine patient, a pneumoperitoneum is recognized as a reflective, mobile, hyperechoic line anterior to the liver capsule, the omentum, or the small bowel (Fig. 8-8).

Cystic Lesions of the Omentum and Mesentery

Such lesions are readily identified by US. Most are sonolucent with posterior acoustic enhancement. However, their true nature and origin can be difficult to assess. Cystic lesions have recently been classified into five groups[4]: *lymphangioma, enteric duplication, mesenteric cyst, mesothelial cyst,* and *nonpancreatic pseudocyst*. In a further article,[5] a thin-walled cystic lesion without septations was considered most likely to be a mesothelial cyst. The presence of several septa favored a cystic lymphangioma. The presence of thick inner septa suggests a pseudocyst (usually posttraumatic). A thick-walled cyst was compatible with a diagnosis of an enteric duplication cyst.

The presence of echoes in a cystic lesion is nonspecific. It may be seen in normal enteric or *chylous cysts* as well as in a complicated cyst of any origin. The presence of a fluid-fluid level can be observed in a chylous cyst.[6]

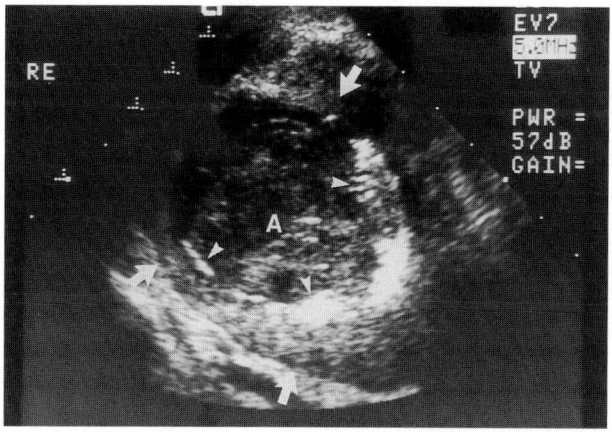
(a)

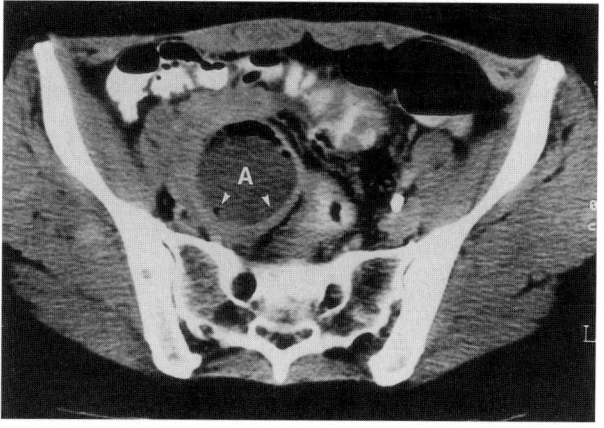
(b)

Fig. 8-7. Postoperative peritoneal abscess (7 days after a gynecologic surgery).
(a) US shows the abscess (A between arrows) to be filled with pus of moderate echogenicity. Hyperechoic gas bubbles (arrowheads) delineate the outer thick wall of the abscess. (b) CT correlation (A = abscess; arrowheads = gas bubbles).

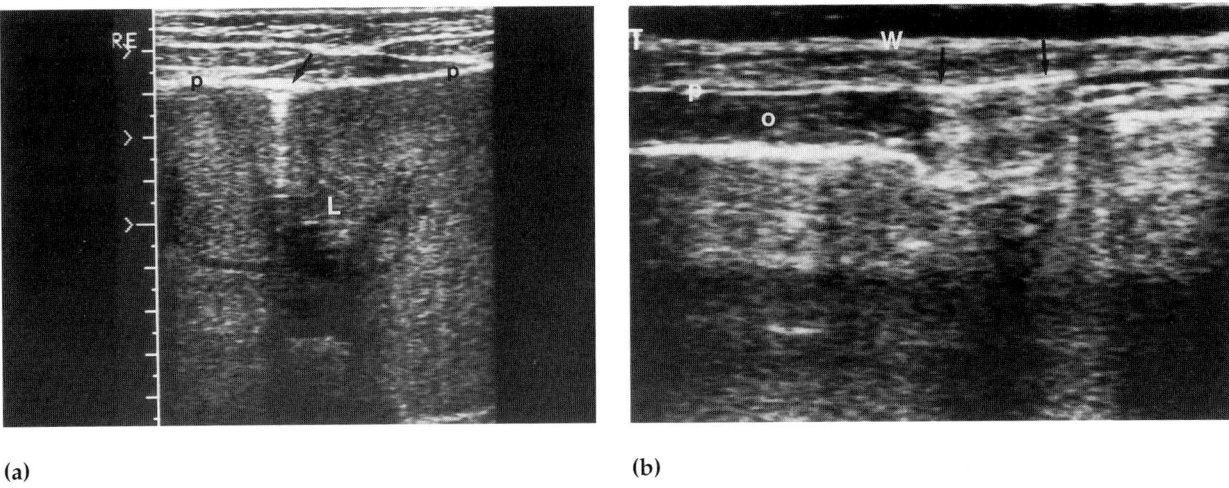

Fig. 8-8. Two different locations of pneumoperitoneum at US.
(a) In front of the liver (L) and behind the peritoneum (p), a small amount of free air (arrow) is observed as a hyperechoic line with its characteristic posterior artifact due to reverberations. (b) Between the abdominal wall (W) and the omentum (O), there is a hyperechoic line (arrows). During respiration, this line slides under the parietal peritoneum (p), confirming that it represents free peritoneal air.

A *pancreatic pseudocyst* may be mesenteric or retroperitoneal in location. Its associated history, the US finding of concomitant pancreatitis, and the demonstration of a thick-walled cyst(s) containing variable amounts of echogenic debris are supportive findings. Cystic tumors such as *cystic mesothelioma, pseudomyxoma peritonei, cystic spindle cell tumor, cystic carcinoid,* and *cystic teratoma* remain difficult to diagnose, short of recognizing the presence of inner mural or septal hypoechoic or echogenic nodules and a thick capsule (Fig. 8-9).

When a mesenteric mass contains calcification, fat, and/or a hyperechoic "hairball," a *teratoma* or an *ectopic ovarian dermoid* is suggested (Fig. 8-10). The pres-

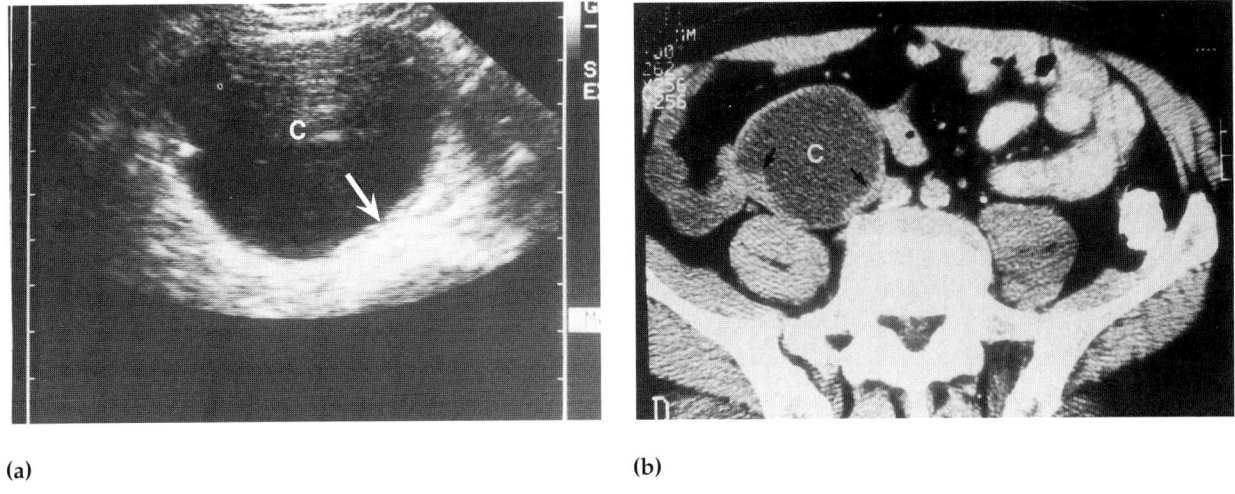

Fig. 8-9. Cystic mass in the mesentery.
(a) In the right lower abdomen, US demonstrates a fixed, well-delineated sonolucent mass (c) with posterior acoustic enhancement and nodularity of the inner surface of its wall (arrows). One mural nodule was partly calcified (upper arrow). At real-time sonography, the mass showed no relation to bowel. (b) A CT transverse section confirmed the cystic mass (c) and the nodularity of its wall (arrows). However, based on CT alone, it is not possible to exclude concomitant gut wall involvement. (Surgery revealed a primary cystic carcinoid tumor of the mesentery.)

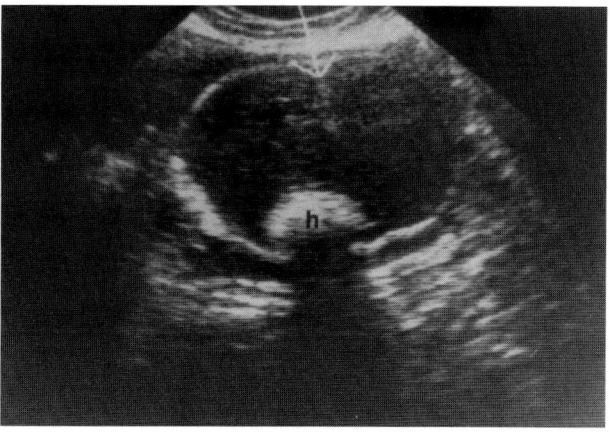 (a)
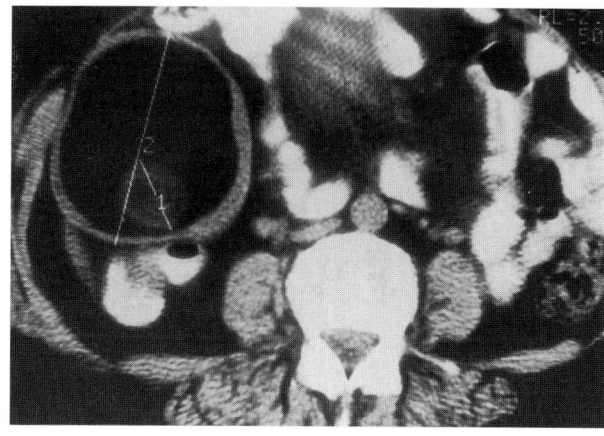 (b)

Fig. 8-10. Ectopic ovarian dermoid.
(a) A thick-walled, cystic, well-delineated mass was found by US below the right lobe of the liver (arrow). It contained a mobile hyperechoic ball (h) that caused posterior acoustic shadowing. It might have been mistaken for a gallbladder with a calculus, but a normal gallbladder was identified near the porta hepatis. (b) A CT scan transverse section outlined a hyperdense hairball (1) within the fat density of an ovarian dermoid (2). The dermoid had been displaced into the right hypochondrium by a huge uterine fibroid.

ence of a cystic mass fixed in the space of Retzius suggests a diagnosis of a *urachal cyst*.

Lymphadenopathies

The most frequently found masses in the small bowel mesentery are *lymphadenopathies*. Their size, number, and location are variable. Most are hypoechoic and nonspecific. A presentation similar to that of anechoic masses is frequently observed in lymphoma, *Mycobacterium avium intracellular* (MAI) infection, and metastatic melanoma.

Mesenteric and Omental Tumors

The finding of a single infiltrating mass in the mesentery or the omentum may represent any primary or secondary tumor, or even an inflammatory or infective process.

A *mesenteric lymphoma* is a frequent finding and may present as a hypoechoic, ill- or well-defined process. Bowel walls are often spared though displaced. The preservation of the hyperechoic perivascular mesenteric fat between surrounding nodes is suggestive of lymphoma, and represents an US feature called "the sandwich sign" (Fig. 8-11).

A *mesenteric desmoid tumor* can be associated with Gardner's syndrome in 13% of cases.[7] It is usually observed as a circumscribed mass with scattered high-level echoes. It is hypervascular at Doppler flow imaging and, unlike a lymphoma, is not associated with enlarged nodes.

Stromal tumors are the most frequent primary solid tumors of the mesentery. Primary mesenteric or omental *sarcomas* are rare and present nonspecific appearances. In our experience, the presence of intratumoral necrosis and the size of the mass are not sufficient criteria for distinguishing a benign from a malignant tumor.

Lipomas of the mesentery are rare. They can be suspected on sonographic grounds when hyperechoic fat is observed within the tumor. Intratumoral fat is less granular than normal mesenteric fat and forms a mass that is surrounded by a thin capsule.

Infectious Diseases

Primary Infection of the Mesentery or Omentum

This is a rare finding and may resemble a tumor. *Actinomycosis* is an interesting rarity as it may present as a single bulky mass with a mixed heterogeneous echotexture and an associated desmoplastic reaction. As the appendix is the most likely site of origin of the actinomycosis, an investigation of its sonographic status should always be included.[8]

Primary and Secondary Mesenteric Panniculitis

Symptoms are no guide to this diagnosis. Sonography shows the mesenteric folds to be drawn together, form-

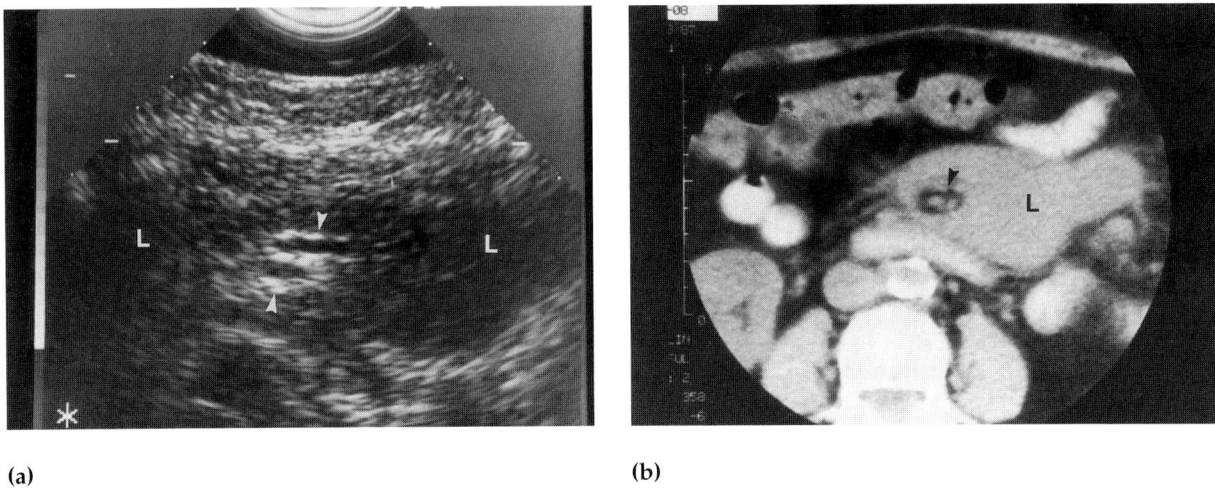

Fig. 8-11. Mesenteric lymphoma with a "sandwich sign."
(a) US transverse scan shows a hypoechoic, ill-defined lymphomatous mass (L) surrounding the mesenteric vessels (arrowheads) with sparing of the perivascular hyperechoic fat, the so-called "sandwich sign." (b) T correlation, scanned through the same level, also shows the classic "sandwich sign" with sparing of the perivascular fat (arrowhead).

ing a firm mass. The echogenicity of the fat is slightly decreased together with a loss or interruption of the normal multiple-layer appearance of the mesentery (Fig. 8-12). The diseased area feels firm and is tender to palpation. Bowel loops are displaced. Primary and secondary mesenteric paniculitis are ultrasonographically similar. In our institution secondary mesenteritis has been found associated with pancreatitis, Crohn's disease, subacute or chronic abscesses, and other conditions. Biopsies are recommended to rule out possible liposarcoma.

Spontaneous Segmental Necrosis or Torsion of the Omentum

This condition may be clinically mistaken for cholecystitis or appendicitis. Characteristically, the painful

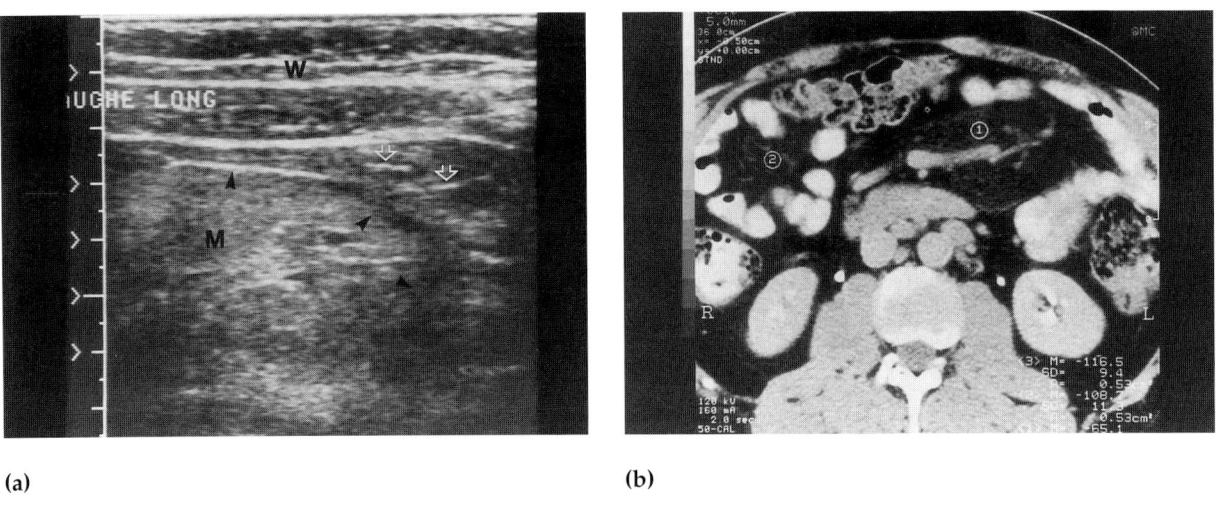

Fig. 8-12. Primary mesenteric paniculitis in a 50-year-old man with chronic abdominal pain.
(a) Longitudinal scan through the root of the mesentery shows a firm, hyperechoic, and relatively homogeneous, elongated mass (M). It is well delineated (arrowheads), contains normal mesenteric vessels, and interrupts the adjacent normal mesenteric outlines (open arrows). There was tenderness to palpation of the abdominal wall (W) at this site. (b) CT demonstrates diffuse infiltration of the mesenteric fat (1), readily distinguished from adjacent normal fat (2) (Fat density: of 1 = 65 HU [Hounsfield units], of 2 = 108 HU). Surgical biopsy confirmed the diagnosis.

area is precisely located by the patient pointing to it. Viewed by ultrasound, the omentum remains hyperechoic. Its normal granular aspect becomes diffusely decreased, a result of edema and hemorrhage and of the multiple interfaces created by the fat lobules with thin and reflective membranes and septa of collagen between them (Fig. 8-13). Abnormal omentum can also be solid and fixed to the anterior peritoneum. It is important to have the patient breathe during scanning, to increase awareness of the subtle changes of the mobility, echogenicity, and granularity of the omentum. Sometimes, hypoechoic areas representing advanced hemorrhagic or necrotic zones are found within the omentum.[9] The omental mass is usually situated medial to the colon, unlike the changes caused by epiploic appendagitis, which are mainly lateral to the colon.[10] An adjacent bowel wall may present a slightly thickened hyperechoic MP layer. This is due either to focal edema or to a fibrotic process attaching the bowel wall to the omentum. Normal small bowel mesentery is displaced posteriorly by the omental mass. As both structures have similar echogenicity, the identification of mesenteric vessels and of normal mesenteric linear interfaces helps to separate ultrasonically the normal mesentery from the diseased omentum.

Pathologies of the Small Bowel

Of increasing importance and widening application is the use of ultrasound in the recognition of the many diseases that can affect the small intestine. Experience in the technique and an understanding of the many forms of the disease-related pathologic anatomy are essential for deriving a maximum of information from this application of sonography.

Small Bowel Dilatation

In the course of an US examination it is not unusual to become aware of distended bowel loops. Dilatation of the small bowel is regarded as significant if the diameter exceeds 3 cm and extends over a length of at least 10 cm. The following ultrasonic observations are relevant:

Peristalsis

Normal waves of contraction and relaxation move bowel contents distally and proximally.[11] These movements of the bowel wall and of its contents can be observed on real-time sonography. Increased peristalsis is suggested by the observation of a more rapid progression with turbulence of the bowel contents.

Identification of the Part That Is Dilated

Transverse scanning of the left colon, right colon, and terminal ileum will determine if the dilatation involves the colon and/or the small bowel. Differentiation of dilated colon from dilated small bowel is made by identifying the location and the course of the dilated

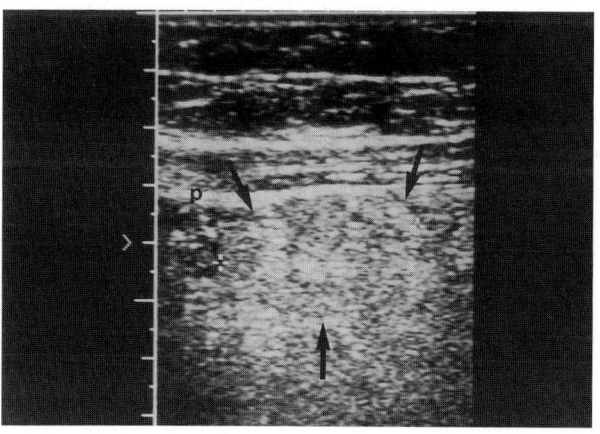
(a)

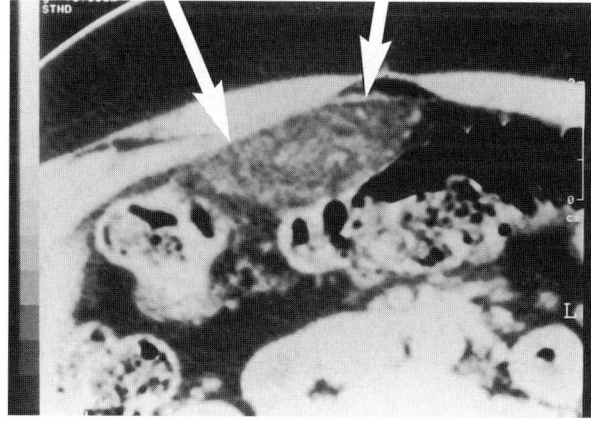
(b)

Fig. 8-13. Spontaneous segmental necrosis of the omentum.
(a) US transverse view of the right abdomen shows a fixed, less granular than normal, hyperechoic omental mass (between arrows). Respiration showed the mass to be attached to the peritoneum (p). (b) CT demonstrates infiltration of the omentum (arrows) with slight thickening of the overlying peritoneum. The mass displaces the transverse colon posteriorly. The diagnosis was confirmed by laparoscopy.

loops and distinguishing valvulae conniventes of the small bowel from the haustra of the colon (Fig. 8-14).[12]

Demonstration of a Possible Transition Zone

A point of transition from dilated to normal or collapsed bowel is the critical finding that suggests an obstruction. Various features observed by US at the transition site will often indicate the cause of an obstruction. The transition site is always akinetic[13] and is often marked by edematous mesenteric fat. Different causes of obstruction are discussed later.

Signs of Possible Strangulation

US features indicating strangulation are discussed below.

Adynamic Ileus

It characteristically involves both the small and large bowel. The degree of distention varies. Peristalsis is rare or totally absent, but needs to be tested in several separate locations. There should be no transition zone, and all bowel walls should be of normal thickness.

A Possible Pitfall

Although the entire intestinal tract is expected to be distended in the diagnosis of adynamic ileus, in some cases the ileum and/or the splenic flexure of the colon are found to be collapsed. This might suggest the presence of a transition zone with collapsed bowel distal to an obstruction. The normal US appearance of the bowel walls and of the surrounding fat and the distention of more distal bowel should help to reaffirm the presence of a paralytic ileus without obstruction. This pitfall has also affected plain film diagnosis and CT imaging of the abdomen.[14]

Small Bowel Obstruction

Obstructions can be divided into simple obstruction and closed-loop obstruction.[14]

Simple Obstruction

This implies lumen reduction at a single small bowel site. Based only on clinical and plain radiographic findings, the diagnosis of obstruction remains uncertain in 20% to 50% of cases.[14] It is suggested that sonography should then be the next diagnostic technique employed. The presence of normal peristalsis in the entire, dilated small bowel is the main criterion on which a diagnosis of simple obstruction can be based. However, it must be remembered that in simple obstructions that have persisted for more than about a week, peristaltic activity can cease in the dilated loops, without this implying a further complication. Furthermore, ascites and thickened bowel walls are also compatible with a simple obstruction.

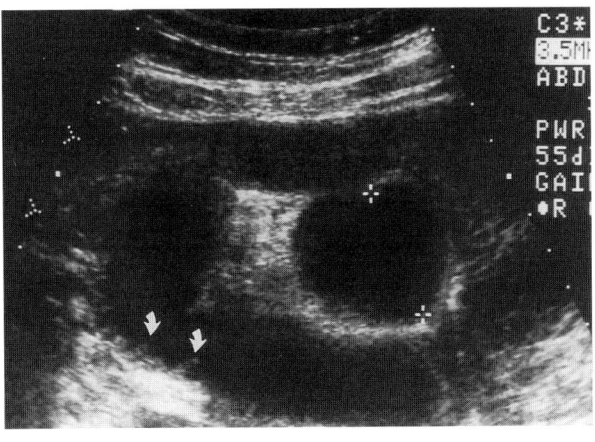

(a)

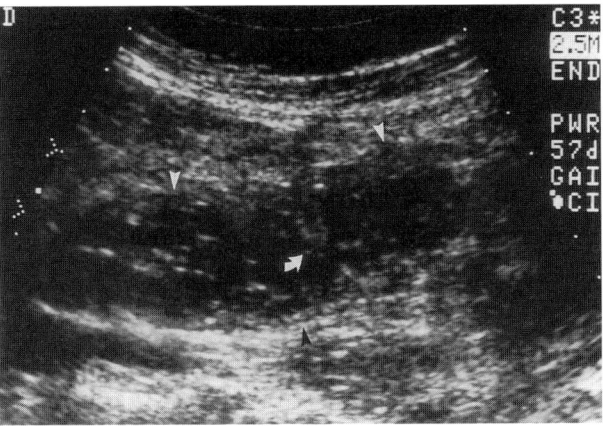

(b)

Fig. 8-14. Which part of the GI tract is being imaged?
(a) Longitudinal and transverse US scans outline multiple loops of fluid-distended jejunum. Their valvulae conniventes are demonstrated (curved arrows) and the bowel walls are normal and thin. The diameter of the lumen measures 3 cm (between crosses). (b) Longitudinal US scan shows the right colon (arrowheads) filled with fluid. A haustral fold (curved arrow) is seen as a thick and incomplete echogenic band perpendicular to the gut lumen. It is easy to distinguish it from a small bowel fold.

The cause of a simple obstruction may be recognized at the transition site, the site where lumen dilatation abruptly changes to lumen reduction. It is generally agreed that, when the site of obstruction can be clearly defined and when there is no other associated ultrasonic abnormality, adhesions may be assumed to be the cause of obstruction. Adhesions have been the cause of obstruction in 50% to 65% of cases.[14,15] In our experience, when the transition site reveals a collapsed segment of bowel with fixed, angulated, or serrated contours, and a localized asymmetric thickening of the hypoechoic muscularis propria layer, a diagnosis of adhesions is strongly suggested (Fig. 8-15). In some cases, adhesive bands could be identified as hypoechoic structures of variable length and thickness (Fig. 8-16).

Closed-Loop Obstruction

A closed loop or incarcerated bowel obstruction exists when a loop of bowel is occluded at two adjacent points along its course. Unlike a simple obstruction, this often leads to strangulation, a life-threatening condition that requires rapid surgical intervention. The closed loop may involve a single loop or a greater length of bowel. At sonography, when a single loop is

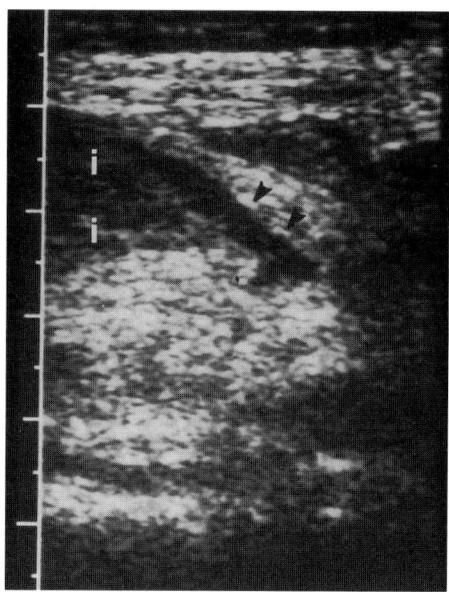

Fig. 8-16. US features of an adhesive band.
The ileum (i) is distorted and presents asymmetric thickening of the MP leading to a hypoechoic linearity (arrowheads). Surgery showed this to represent a fibrous band causing traction and compression of the gut. Strangulation was absent.

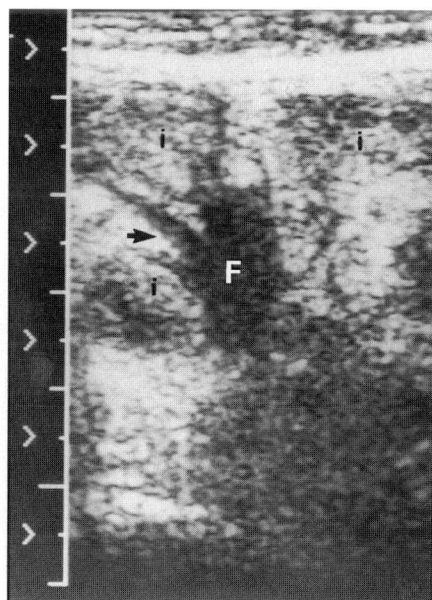

Fig. 8-15. US features of adhesions proved at surgery.
Three segments of distended ileum (I) are seen in transverse sections. A hypoechoic focus corresponding to a fibrous adhesion (F) produces angulation and fixation at the transition site. The hypoechoic focus presents an appearance of asymmetric thickening of the muscularis propria layer (arrow).

involved, it may be seen as a fixed, akinetic, dilated, U-shaped bowel segment (Fig. 8-17). The wall of the bowel may be slightly thickened, suggesting normality, or very thin, which may mean that it is necrotic. As suggested by Balthazar,[14] the closed loop is often filled with fluid while the dilated proximal bowel is largely gas-containing. The adjacent mesenteric fat may be edematous.

Closed-loop obstructions that involve several loops are more difficult to diagnose by US. The radial distribution of incarcerated bowel with mesenteric vessels converging toward the site of obstruction or torsion, as described for CT, is difficult to visualize by ultrasonography.

Strangulation

In the case of any dilated small bowel, strangulation should always be considered a possibility. Strangulation is a frequent complication of closed-loop obstructions that are associated with ischemia. Strangulation can also be a complication of an intussusception, of a hernia, volvulus, a mesenteric vascular occlusion, and of vasculitides forming part of collagenoses; other abnormalities that may lead to vascular strangulation are hypersensitivity reactions to a drug, radiation damage, or even a simple adhesive obstruction.[16,17]

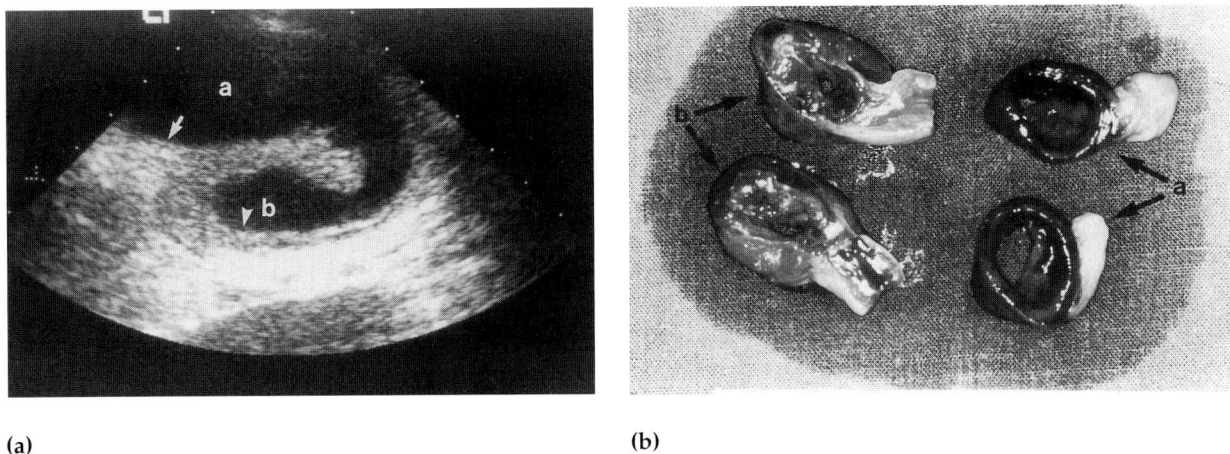

Fig. 8-17. Closed-loop obstruction with strangulation.
(a) US discloses an akinetic, distended loop of ileum in an inverted C-shape. The gut walls appear thin (3 mm) in one segment (a, arrow) and thicker (6 to 8 mm) in another segment (b, arrowhead). Closed-loop obstruction with incarceration was suspected. (b) Cross sections of the gross specimen of the incarcerated loop found at surgery. Segment (a) is collapsed, its wall thin, of a dark color and necrotic. Segment (b) is thick-walled, presents a near normal color, and was shown to be edematous at histology.

Several ultrasonic criteria may suggest the possibility of strangulation: *Aperistalsis* in a dilated bowel loop in the presence of peristaltic activity in dilated small bowel proximal to it. However, peristalsis can persist in a still viable strangulated loop (false-negative diagnosis of strangulation). It is also possible for peristalsis to be missed at the time of sonographic examination (false-positive).

Circumferential wall thickening greater than 5 mm in an akinetic and dilated bowel loop or in a prestenotic distended loop. This sign applies to about 50% of strangulated loops. Conversely, when there is abrupt cessation of arterial blood flow and chemical mediators of inflammation are still absent, the bowel wall, although necrotic, may be unusually thin (Figs. 8-17, 8-18).

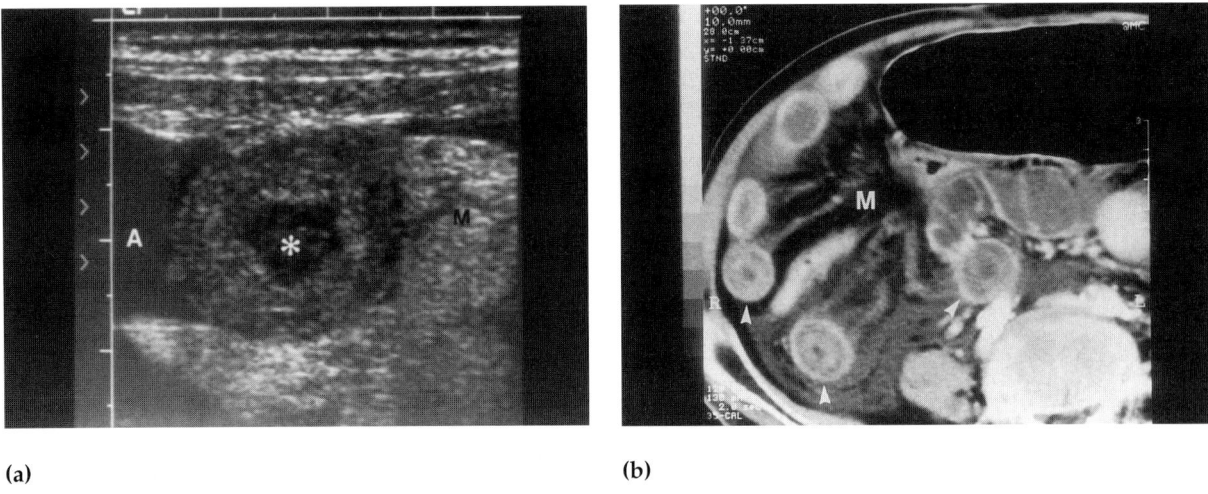

Fig. 8-18. Impaired venous drainage in a closed-loop obstruction.
(a) Transverse US view of a segment of small bowel shows a thick (8 mm) wall of moderate echogenicity with a narrowed lumen (*). Ascites (A) and a hypoechoic mesenteric (M) linear infiltration were demonstrated. (b) Contrast-enhanced CT confirms the wall thickening with a target appearance affecting multiple bowel loops (arrowheads), as well as ascites and mesenteric (M) edema. At surgery, the bowel was initially dark blue in color but recovered to a normal pink color after lysis of adhesions and application of warmth. Arterial flow was still present. The bowel was not resected.

Insufficiently granular mesenteric fat surrounding an akinetic, dilated bowel loop together with sonolucent fluid next to the serosa. However, these changes can be caused by any adjacent inflammatory condition, eg, an abscess.

Rapid accumulation of ascites. This sign is not sufficiently specific and should be used only to support other features of strangulation.

Intestinal pneumatosis and/or portal venous gas. These are the most reliable signs and also apply to CT and plain films. However they are infrequent and represent late changes in bowel ischemia.[18] Pneumatosis is shown as hyperechoic longitudinal or circular foci in the intestinal wall (Fig. 8-19). Portal venous gas may appear as mobile hyperechoic dots within the portal vein or its branches. Beyond the hyperechoic areas there may be reverberations or ring-down artifacts. Pneumatosis can also be unrelated to ischemia, due to chronic obstructive pulmonary disease, intestinal obstruction, peptic ulceration, or steroid administration.

Direct observation of occluded mesenteric vessels. The observation of a hyperechoic calcified atheromatous plaque at the origin of the SMA is a frequent finding in asymptomatic persons.

Absence of Doppler flow in the bowel wall. The considerable difficulty of assessing Doppler sampling in thin walls of dilated bowel in a patient who moves and breathes should not be underestimated.

Conclusion

It follows from the above that an US diagnosis of small bowel strangulation should be based on a combination of the above-mentioned criteria.

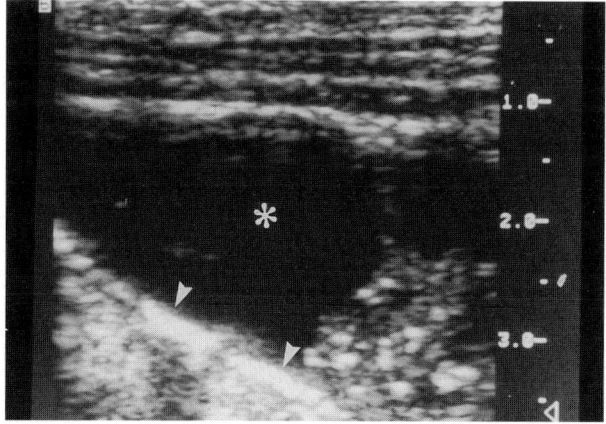

Fig. 8-19. US demonstration of pneumatosis.
In a patient with SMA thrombosis and ischemic bowel, US outlines fluid distended loops (*) with numerous hyperechoic dots (arrowheads) representing air within the posterior bowel wall.

Midgut Malrotation with or Without Volvulus

In the neonate, midgut malrotation is a potentially lethal condition, usually presenting as small bowel obstruction. Malrotation with or without volvulus may also occur in the infant or adult.

At sonography, midgut malrotation is suggested when the SMV is to the left of the SMA. However, this sign is not pathognomonic for midgut malrotation or volvulus. In midgut volvulus, US may show duodenal obstruction associated with thickened bowel loops to the right of the spine and free peritoneal fluid,[19] or an isolated hyperdynamic, pulsating SMA.[20] However, these are indirect US features of midgut volvulus. The "whirl" sign described by Pracros et al[21] directly indicates the anatomic alterations caused by midgut volvulus. At a transverse US scan of the upper abdomen, it is seen as a whirling mass composed of concentric hypoechoic structures within the mesenteric fat caused by a clockwise turning of the involved bowel loops together with their blood vessels around the root of the mesentery. In association with this sign, US criteria suggesting strangulation should be looked for.

Small Bowel Hematoma or Hemorrhage

A compatible history such as trauma, biopsy, hemophilia, anticoagulant therapy, or Henoch-Schönlein purpura will suggest the possibility of this diagnosis.

Trauma-Related Hematoma

An intramural hematoma involves the second and third parts of the duodenum in 70% of patients.[22] Sonography, at an early stage of the hematoma, presents it as a hyperechoic mass asymmetrically encircling the duodenum. Echolucent liquefaction occurs about 96 hours after clotting. Later in its course, the hematoma becomes cystic, sometimes with small residual echogenic clots in its dependent areas.

Hemorrhage Complicating Anticoagulant Therapy

At sonography, ascites and mesenteric edema are usually seen to surround a thick-walled bowel segment. HRS shows the bowel wall to be hyperechoic without recognizable layers. A diminished peristalsis is often preserved. Return to a normal US state is expected to occur within a week after cessation of anticoagulants.

Henoch-Schönlein Syndrome (HSS)

Most patients who have HSS together with abdominal pain show US abnormalities.[23] The small bowel is most frequently involved (Fig. 8-20). US findings are similar to those found in ischemic bowel (see Strangulation section). Hypomotility, dilated loops, ascites, mesenteric adenitis, and abdominal wall hemorrhage may also occur. Rare surgical complications such as intussusception and perforation may develop in 2% to 6% of the patients.[24]

Inflammatory Conditions

Crohn's Disease (CD)

It is generally agreed that a mean delay of 2 to 4 years occurs before CD of the small bowel is diagnosed.[25] Sonography may help to reduce the diagnostic delay by using HRS in patients who present with nonspecific symptoms. US examination of the terminal ileum is particularly easy, fast, and pertinent, since CD involves it in 75% to 85% of cases.[26] At US, the wall of the terminal ileum is more than 5 mm thick and may even be thicker than 2 cm.[27] In uncomplicated CD, the layers of the wall are evenly thickened (Fig. 8-21). The bowel wall feels firm, almost rigid, with absent or reduced peristalsis.

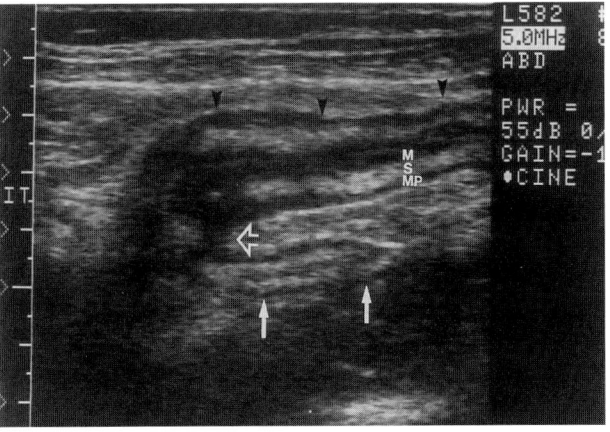

Fig. 8-21. US features of a granulomatous ileitis.
Longitudinal US scan of a segment of ileum (below arrowheads) reveals thickened wall layers. Between the two mucosal surfaces is a hyperechoic line representing the lumen interface. Valvulae conniventes are absent. A hypoechoic fistula (open arrow) emerges from a totally hypoechoic part of the wall and extends to a slightly edematous appendix (above the arrows). (M = mucosa; S = submucosa; MP = muscularis propria.)

The US differentiation of the layers of the bowel wall may persist, or may become partially or completely blurred. This feature relates to the severity and duration of the disease and to the response to medical treatment. In the acute stage of severe disease, the entire wall can become hypoechoic, a result of edema and aggregations of inflammatory cells that extend through the normally hyperechoic submucosa. Later, fibrosis of the bowel wall will produce the same hypoechogenicity. With steroid treatment, however, hyperechoic fat may accumulate in the submucosa.[28] Serositis causes extramural fibrosis indicated by abnormal fixation and angulation of bowel.

Transmural inflammation and fibrosis induce fibrofatty changes in the adjacent mesenteric fat. This development aids the sonographic delineation between possibly normal and transmurally diseased gut. Fibrofatty tissue has moderate US echogenicity and is relatively homogeneous, as it has less granularity than normal fat (Fig. 8-22). In acute CD, the fat may be infiltrated by hypoechoic linear strands of variable length and thickness. These lines represent dissecting inflammatory liponecroses (Fig. 8-23) and, when they derive from a bowel wall ulcer, are probably the precursors of sinus tracts and fistulas.[3] Enlarged mesenteric nodes are frequently found in CD. They are round or oval, and their dimensions vary. At US, they are hypoechoic and homogeneous.

Color Doppler imaging in CD often reveals hyperemia and hypervascularity of the gut wall and mesen-

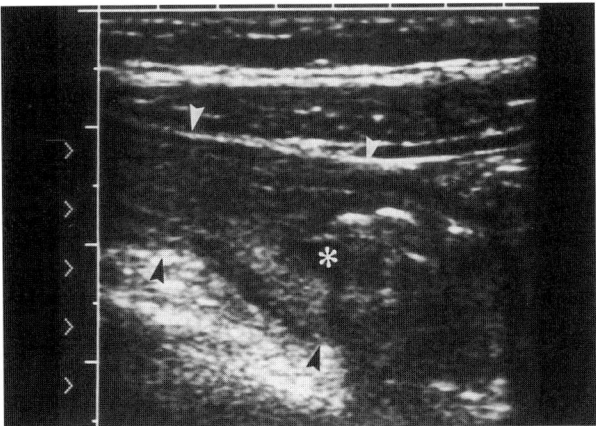

Fig. 8-20. Henoch-Schönlein syndrome in a 14-year-old patient.
The patient complained of abdominal pain. A segment of jejunum (arrowheads) is shown in longitudinal US scans. Bowel walls are thickened and echogenic. Only the hypoechoic muscularis propria layer remained visible in some of the areas. Peristalsis was normal. Fluid was seen in the gut lumen (*). The patient recovered with medical treatment, and US follow-up two weeks later was normal.

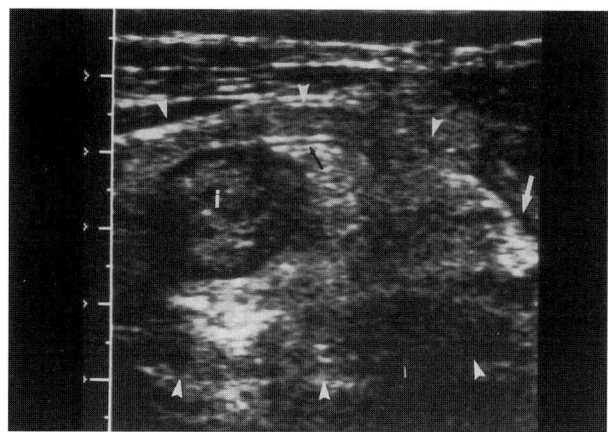

Fig. 8-22. Massive fibrofatty hypertrophy in Crohn's ileitis.
A transverse US view in Crohn's ileitis shows the diseased segment completely surrounded by abnormal, hypertrophied fat (white arrowheads). The abnormal fat is less granular and of lower echogenicity than adjacent normal mesenteric fat (white arrow). A barium study showed the diseased ileum to be widely separated from the rest of the small bowel. An enlarged mesenteric vascular branch is seen entering the gut wall (black arrow).

tery. There continues to be disagreement about whether color Doppler can help to differentiate active from inactive disease.

At US, ulcers may be seen as hyperechoic dots in the inflamed hypoechoic mucosa (Fig. 8-24). These dots represent either interfaces or air in the ulcers. Although the submucosa has becomes thicker due to infiltration by inflammatory cells, edema, and/or fibrosis, the thickness of its hyperechogenic fatty component decreases in the vicinity of ulcerations. When ulcers reach the serosa, the bowel wall near them becomes totally hypoechoic with the loss of its distinctive layers. If the ulcer extends beyond the serosa, the hypoechoic wall is seen to bulge when scanned transversely. When air containing, an ulcer appears as a hyperechoic line crossing the hypoechoic bulge. Such eccentric widening when seen close to a segment with symmetric wall thickening is characteristic of CD, expressing its well-known transaxial differentiation of involvement. Extension of an ulcer beyond the serosa to form a sinus tract or fistula has already been mentioned. These tracts are hypoechoic (see Fig. 8-23), may end abruptly, or may lead into a phlegmon or an abscess. A phlegmon is characterized by an ill-defined, scattered hypoechoic infiltration of the fat, lacking a discernible mass with an identifiable wall. An abscess is usually a cystic or hypoechoic mass with variable wall thickness (Fig. 8-25). Fistulas are a hallmark of CD. They may at times be closed, but even then can be observed at US. They appear as persistent, hypoechoic tracts. Gas or echogenic particles may be intermittently found in them.

In CD, obstruction is usually the result of a stricture or an abscess. A stricture is entirely hypoechoic and of variable length. Spontaneous perforation rarely occurs (1% to 2%) in CD. When a perforation does occur, signs of pneumoperitoneum (see earlier) may be found at US. A perforation is often associated with ascites containing echogenic debris.

In all patients with CD, the sonographer should perform a complete examination of the abdomen to search for complications. Abscesses can be found anywhere, and genitourinary tract complications are reported in 5% to 20% of cases (Fig. 8-26).[29]

Infections

Gastroenteritis

US findings are nonspecific. Multiple, usually hyperperistaltic, fluid-filled loops of intestine are found. A paralytic ileus may be associated with very severe disease.

Mesenteric Adenitis

A few days after a cold or a pharyngitis, a patient may complain of right-sided lower abdominal pain. Sonography may demonstrate hypoechoic lymphoid tissue in the wall of the terminal ileum and a variable number of adjacent hypoechoic, round mesenteric nodes

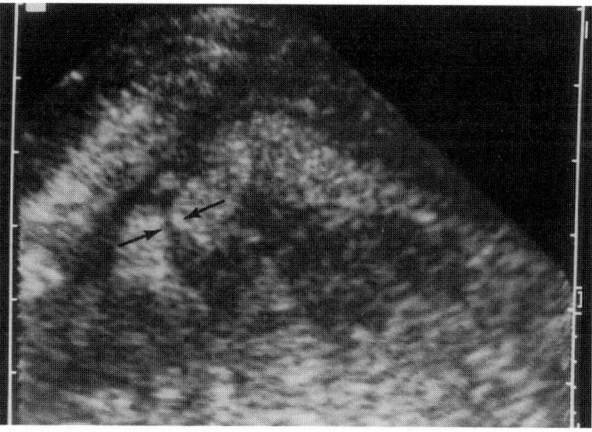

Fig. 8-23. US features of mesenteric liponecrosis.
In the mesenteric fat, adjacent to a Crohn's ileitis (not included in this view), there are multiple hypoechoic linear structures (one of them delineated by arrows). These lines correspond to tracts of liponecrosis considered to be precursors of sinus tracts and fistulas.

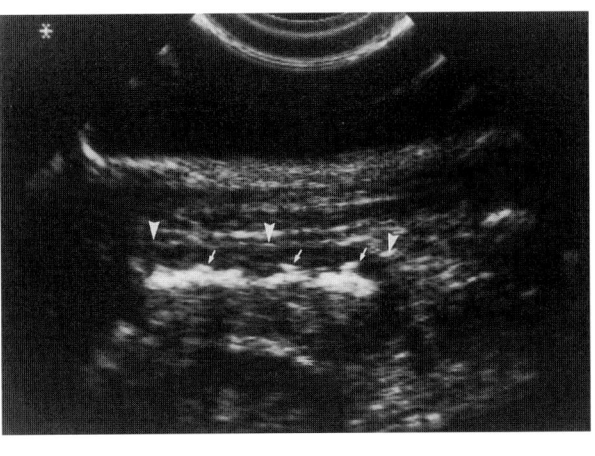

(a) (b)

Fig. 8-24. US features of a Crohn's ileitis with ulcerations.
(a) The thickened ileum (below arrowheads) presents with distinct wall layering. Bright, echogenic air in its lumen allows the visualization of deeper ulcerations (arrows). It should be noted that the hyperechoic fat of the submucosa near the ulcerations is decreased in thickness or completely absent. (By permission from Rioux.[3]) (b) Histologic correlation demonstrates a thickening of all the layers of the bowel wall. Near deeper mucosal (m) ulcerations (arrows), an inflammatory infiltrate in the submucosa (s) decreases its usual fatty hyperechogenicity at US. This is best shown in the area of the white dot. (mp = muscularis propria.)

(Fig. 8-27). The nodes are over 4 mm in diameter and up to 15 mm in thickness. Ileal peristalsis is normal or slightly decreased. No ulcerations are found. The pain disappears in a few days, but US findings may persist for a while.

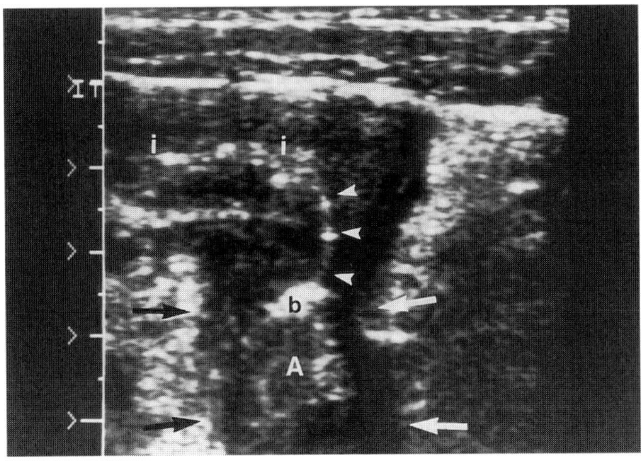

Acute Ileocolitis

Yersiniosis is an example of this condition. US findings are often impressive. Thickening of the ileal wall may reach 10 mm and the size of nodes a diameter of 20 mm. The ileum is usually aperistaltic. The cecum is often involved and shows an increase of the "mucosa-

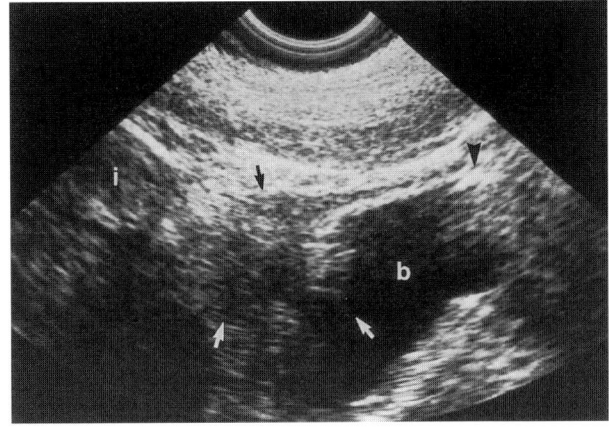

Fig. 8-25. US of Crohn's ileitis complicated by an abscess.
Underneath a longitudinal segment of ileitis (i) showing thickening of all the wall layers, there is an ill-defined oval collection (between arrows) of mixed echotexture. Interior bright echogenic areas suggested gas bubbles (b) in an abscess (A). The hyperechoic curved line (arrowheads) connecting the gut lumen to the abscess represents a minute transiently visible ulceration related to perforation of the ileal wall.

Fig. 8-26. Crohn's ileitis with an enterovesical fistula.
Below the level of the umbilicus, a longitudinal US scan of the abdomen demonstrates a thickened ileum in transverse view (i) adjacent to an intense hypoechoic inflammatory infiltration of the anterosuperior wall of the bladder (arrows). In the bladder (b), the presence of bright hyperechoic gas confirms the existence of an enterovesical fistula.

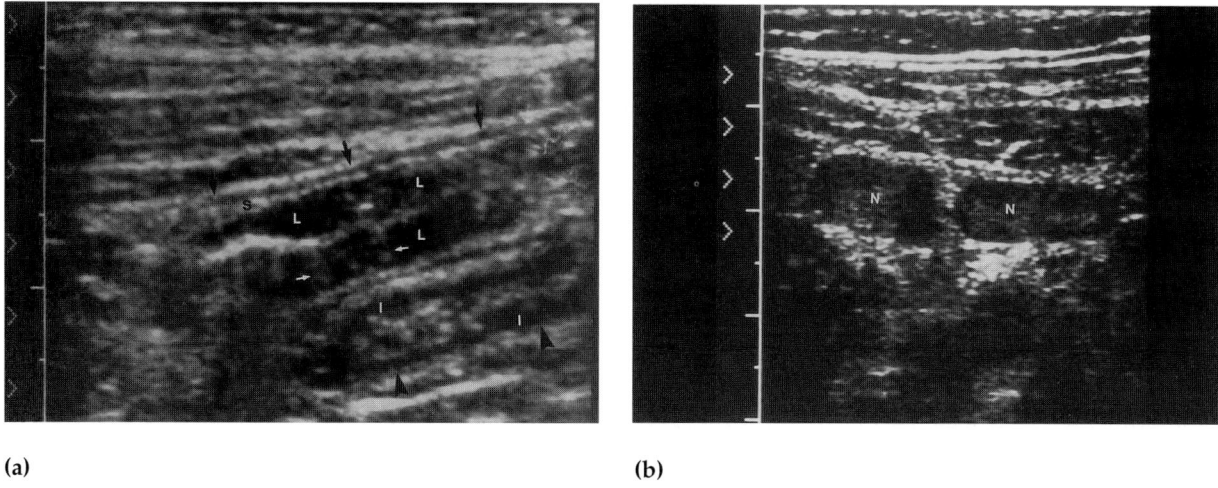

(a) (b)

Fig. 8-27. US of mesenteric adenitis in a 14-year-old patient. Right abdominal pain three days after influenza. Diarrhea was absent and stool cultures were negative. Complete clinical recovery after a week.
(a) US longitudinal view of ileum (below arrows) and appendix (above arrowheads) shows hypoechoic asymmetry in the layers of their walls (L = ileal wall; I = wall of appendix.) They represent benign lymphoid hyperplasia. This lymphoid tissue is sharply demarcated from the hyperechoic submucosal layer (s), which is reduced in thickness. Peristalsis was normal at real-time US. Small white arrows indicate subtle hyperechoic interfaces between folds thickened by the lymphoid tissue. (b) Enlarged hypoechoic lymphadenopathies are seen in the same area (N).

submucosa complex" (Fig. 8-28). This finding is highly suggestive of any bacterial ileocolitis. Superficial and even deeper ulcerations are observed, especially in Yersinia infections.[30] Unlike in Crohn's disease, neither fistulas, abscesses, or mesenteric fibrofatty hypertrophy are encountered. Return to normality occurs within 1 to 2 weeks. Stool cultures or serologic tests can be expected to be positive in only half the cases.[3] This emphasizes the usefulness of a noninvasive ultrasonic diagnostic tool like HRS in a patient with an indication of inflammatory change in the ileocecal area.

The major objective for the sonographer when examining patients with an acute inflammatory process in the right lower abdomen is to rule out appendicitis. Nonvisualization of the appendix is not sufficient evidence. A clearly demonstrated normal appendix should be the only clinically acceptable basis for the exclusion of appendicitis.[30]

Whipple's Disease

Infiltration of the small bowel by Whipple's bacilli is a rare event. Sonography may demonstrate a diffuse, nonspecific thickening of the small bowel with normal peristalsis. The bowel walls have been found homogeneously hyperechoic. Typical for a US diagnosis of Whipple's disease is the demonstration of fat-containing, hyperechoic mesenteric and retroperitoneal lymphadenopathies.[31]

Small Bowel Tumors

Benign Tumors

A *lipoma* is a hyperechoic, homogeneous mass of submucosal origin that projects into the gut lumen. It has

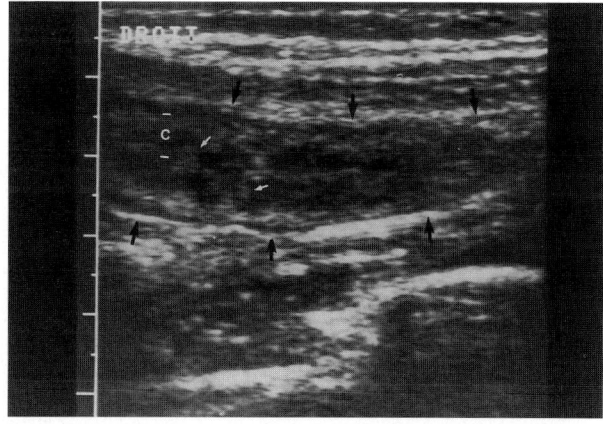

Fig. 8-28. US features of ileitis caused by *Yersinia enterocolitica.*
Longitudinal view of the ileum (between arrows) shows an enlarged mucosa-submucosa complex (c). The enlarged submucosa appears unsharp. White arrows indicate echogenic interfaces between thickened mucosal folds. Their mobility during real-time US distinguished them from mucosal ulcerations.

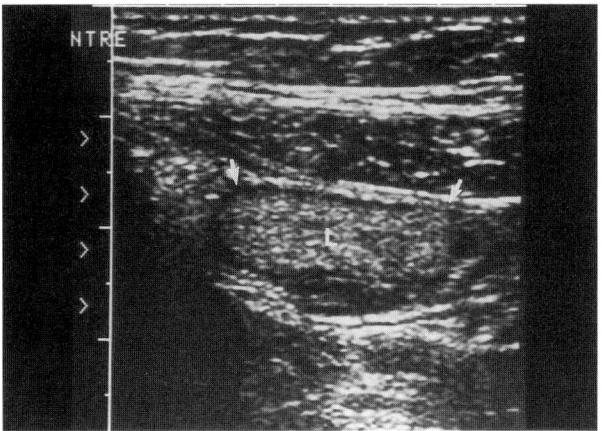

Fig. 8-29. Lipoma of the ileum.
During the US examination of a patient with appendicitis, a hyperechoic, homogeneous, well-delineated, and compressible endoluminal mass (arrow) was fortuitously demonstrated. During appendectomy the presence of a lipoma (L) was confirmed.

smooth, well-delineated contours and is compressible (Fig. 8-29). *Adenomatous polyps,* which originate from the mucosa, are multilobulated, hypoechoic masses projecting into the gut lumen, often at the end of a stalk of variable length. *Fibroid inflammatory polyps* and *hamartomatous polyps* may have similar US appearances (Fig. 8-30). *Neurofibroma* may present as a pedunculated endoluminal mass, usually with smooth contours. *Lymphangiomas* are rarely detected at US. They are pliable, multicystic, sonolucent masses containing fine septa and are located eccentrically in the gut wall (Fig. 8-31). Doppler flow is not detected in them.

Malignant Tumors

The diagnosis of a malignant tumor is often delayed and made only at an advanced stage of the disease.[32] Being able to recognize tumors of the small intestine by sonography is relevant for two main reasons: 1) Ultrasonography is one of the most frequent screening examinations in patients with vague abdominal symptoms; and 2) US departments that routinely carry out complete abdominal HRS have shown that it is possible to detect these tumors (clinically suspected or not) more often, sooner, and at a less advanced stage. Information obtained by ultrasound regarding location, shape, outline, mobility, compressibility, echogenicity, vascularity, and relation to bowel walls (and their layers) can be clinically important. Local or distant dissemination to liver, adrenals, spleen, lymph nodes, and others should also be assessed and reported.

Malignant or potentially malignant lesions are often large and ulcerated. Even when of different histologic origins, their macroscopic and sonographic findings often overlap.[33]

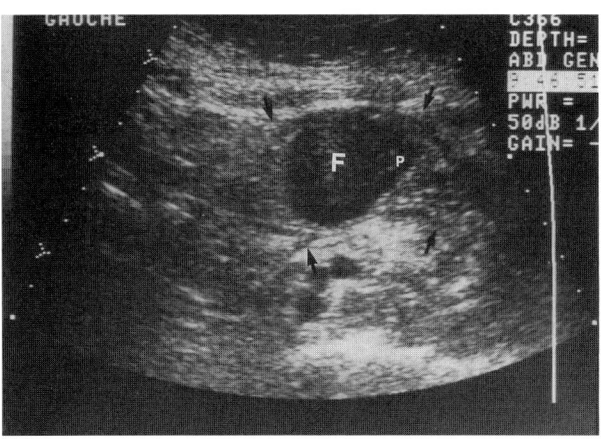

(a)

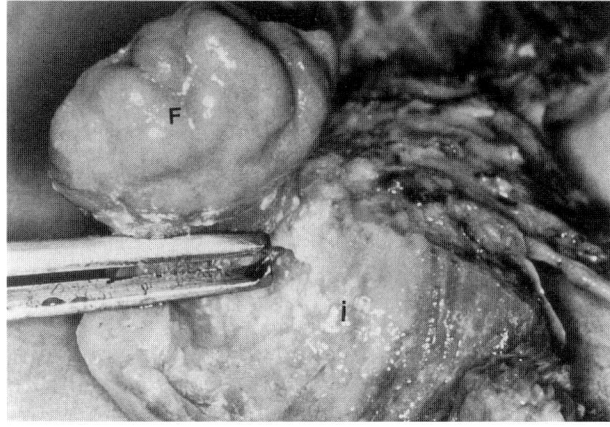

(b)

Fig. 8-30. Inflammatory fibroid polyp in the jejunum.
(a) In a segment of jejunum (arrows), US demonstrates a hypoechoic round mass (F) that seems to have an elongated pedicle (p). (b) Photograph of the opened surgical specimen shows a fibroid polyp (F) lifted from its attachment to the bowel wall. (i = intestinal lumen.)

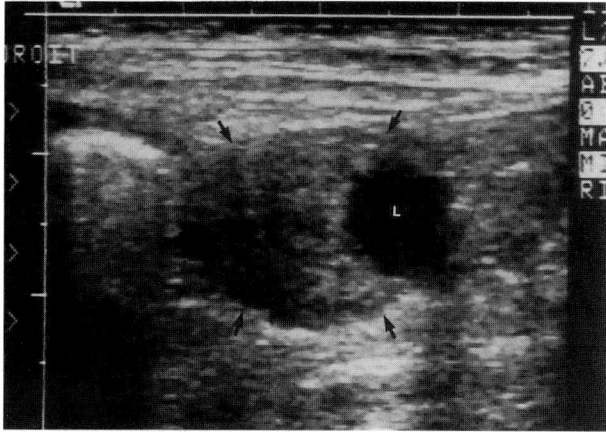

Fig. 8-31. Lymphangioma of the jejunum.
In a 74-year-old patient the US transverse view of a segment of jejunum (arrows) demonstrates a parietal, well-defined, compressible, sonolucent mass (L) with posterior acoustic enhancement. US could demonstrate eight other similar lesions in the jejunum. Doppler flow analysis of these lesions demonstrated absence of vascularity (corroborated by angiographic studies).

Metastases

These are the most frequent malignant lesions of the small bowel. They are mainly hypoechoic masses, eccentric to the gut wall, and may be associated with a hyperechoic lumenal ulceration (Fig. 8-32). A circumscribed hypoechoic mural nodule or a short segment of hypoechoic, annular wall thickening with lumen narrowing may be a further manifestation of metastases.

Adenocarcinoma

This classically presents as a single, annular, mostly proximal jejunal hypoechoic mass (Fig. 8-33). Wall layering is lost and ulceration occurs in about 40% of the tumors.[34] The associated lymphadenopathies are usually less impressive than in lymphoma.

Lymphoma

Most are non-Hodgkin's lymphomas and ultrasonically present as complex mesenteric/intestinal masses. The bowel component of the lymphoma is usually hypoechoic; it may be eccentric, is ulcerated, and substantially infiltrates the mesentery. Tumor-encircled hyperechoic perivascular mesenteric fat is characteristically preserved in lymphoma. Lymphoma may also present as an endoluminal mass, or as an annular, hypoechoic infiltration of the gut wall of atypical shape and with preservation of the submucosa (Fig. 8-34).

Stromal Tumors

These appear as hypoechoic masses difficult to differentiate from lymphoma, metastases, or adenocarcinoma. On the other hand, the finding of a predominantly exophytic or dumbbell-shaped mass, or one with little contact with the gut wall, suggests a possible stromal tumor. Although other small bowel tumors develop necrosis and/or ulceration, the presence of a hyper- or anechoic crescent-shaped necrosis extending to the periphery of the mass may indicate a stromal tumor (Fig. 8-35).[35] Associated lymphadenopathies are characteristically absent.

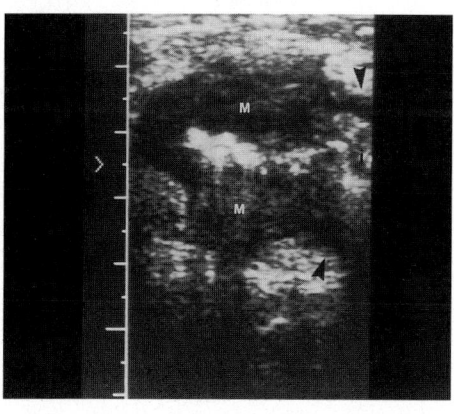
(a)

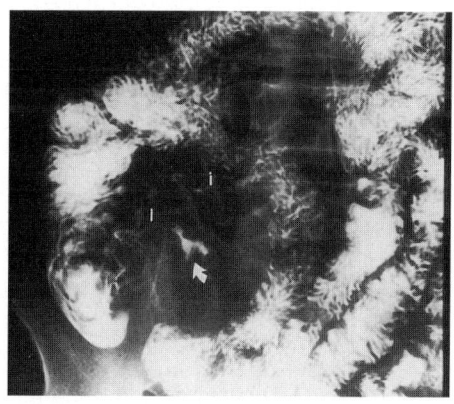
(b)

Fig. 8-32. US features of an ileal metastatic melanoma.
(a) Connected to a segment of ileum (i, arrowheads), a well-defined extraluminal hypoechoic mass (M) was demonstrated with a central hyperechoic ulceration. (b) Barium small bowel study shows an ulcerated (curved arrow) exophytic mass connected to the overlying ileum (i). There is a mass effect on adjacent bowel.

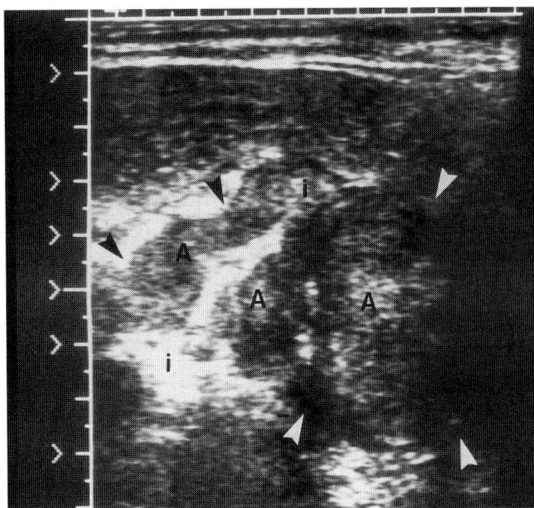

Fig. 8-33. Small bowel adenocarcinoma.
In the left abdomen, a longitudinal segment of the small intestine (i) presented a typical, hypoechoic, concentric narrowing (black arrowheads). Adenocarcinomatous tissue (A) interrupts the normal gut layers and produces an exophytic, exoenteric, hypoechoic rounded mass (between white arrowheads). The region of the tumor was fixed and adynamic.

spective of their echotexture. The interstitial pattern initially represents a woven appearance of the fat; at a later stage, the fat presents as a firm band of omentum with subtle irregular, nodular contours made visible when surrounded by ascites or when indenting the anterior peritoneum (Fig. 8-37). When presenting a pancake pattern, the omentum appears as a bulky mass, often hypoechoic with irregular and lobular contours.

Mesenteric involvement is suggested when the hyperechoic fat between the mesenteric vessels and small bowel walls appears heterogeneous, firm, or fixed, or presents distinct nodules. Nodules or diffuse hypoechogenicity affecting the serosa of the antimesenteric aspect of small bowel loops are considered to be serosal implants. A further US finding has recently been described,[2] namely an interruption of the anterior hyperechoic peritoneal line (Fig. 8-38), a result of involvement by tumor of the transperitoneal capillary network. In the same publication,[2] involvement of the omentum was the most frequently found diagnostic sign of PC (seen in 97% of cases).

Carcinoid Tumors

Although the most common small bowel neoplasms, these are extremely difficult to diagnose by ultrasound. Of nine carcinoid tumors found by sonography, the mean diameters of the lesions were 22 × 17 mm.[37] In all cases, the sonographic appearance was that of a hypoechoic, homogeneous, mostly intraluminal mass with a smooth contour, attached to the bowel wall by a broad base; it may cause interruption of the hyperechoic submucosal layer and thickening of the muscularis (Fig. 8-36).[36] A puckered indrawing of the bowel wall relates to desmoplasia and may be a sign of transserosal mesenteric invasion. The mesenteric metastases frequently show partial calcification. Carcinoids are hypervascular by Doppler study. They almost never become necrotic but infrequently ulcerate.

Peritoneal Carcinomatosis (PC)

US can be very useful in the detection of PC in patients with or without a known primary carcinoma.[2] A systematic US examination of the entire abdomen (using a 5- or 7.5-MHz transducer) should be carried out, as initially described. The omentum is considered abnormal if it presents a nodular, interstitial, or pancake pattern.[2] The pattern is termed nodular when one or many clearly delineated nodules are seen, irre-

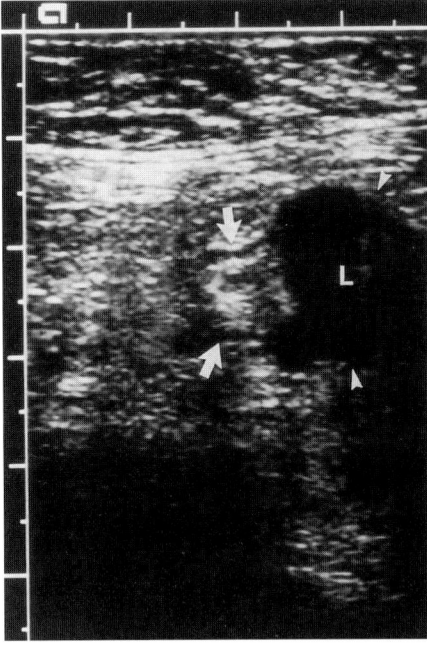

Fig. 8-34. US features of an ileal non-Hodgkin's lymphoma.
US transverse view of the ileum (between arrows) reveals a large hypoechoic mass (L), almost sonolucent, without posterior acoustic enhancement. Although the mass (between arrowheads) is fixed and originates from the gut wall, there is preservation of the contiguous hyperechoic submucosa with molding of the lymphomatous tissue on this layer. These findings are highly suggestive of lymphoma. (L = lymphoma.)

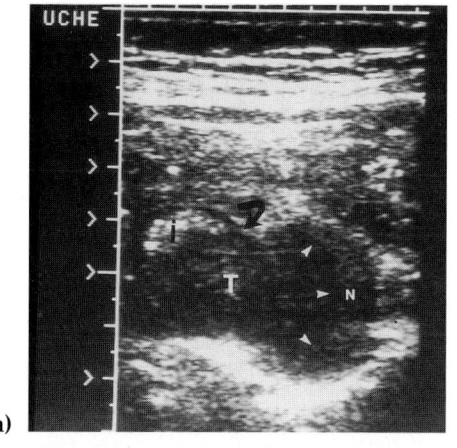
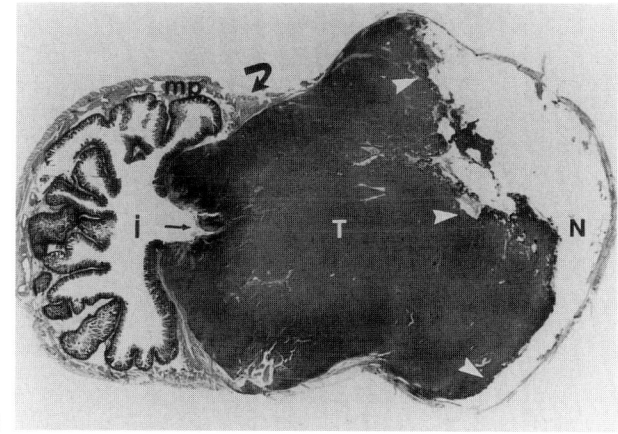

Fig. 8-35. US of crescent-shaped necrosis in a stromal tumor.
(a) Case of an intestinal (i) stromal tumor (T) in a 67-year-old man with unexplained repeated episodes of melena. US discloses a 3.5 × 4.5 cm hypoechoic solid mass. The dumbbell-shaped lesion has a large exoenteric and a small endoenteric component. At the periphery of the extraluminal component, there is a well-delineated echogenic crescent of necrosis (N, arrowheads). At the transition (curved arrow) between the gut wall and the tumor, the muscularis propria (MP) is of normal thickness. (b) Demonstrates the histology of the above-shown changes. (c) A peritoneal implant in a patient with disseminated leiomyosarcomatosis appears as a round, hypoechoic tumor mass (T), including at its periphery a sharply defined, transonic, crescent-shaped zone of necrosis (n) (arrowheads). (Arrow = ulceration in the tumor.) (By permission from Rioux and Mailloux.[35])

The sonographic differential diagnosis of PC should include tuberculous or lymphomatous peritoneal dissemination and primary abdominal mesothelioma.

Congenital Disorders

Small Bowel Duplication

The ileum is the most frequent site of small bowel duplication, which may be multiple in 20% of cases.[37] Sonography has found most duplications to be spherical and cystic, less than 10 cm in diameter, firm, and adherent to the bowel.[38] Duplications occupy the mesenteric border of a bowel segment and share its hyperechoic submucosal and hypoechoic muscularis propria layers as well as its arterial supply. A cystic duplication may be located endoenterically, exoenterically, or both. Intraluminal echoes represent mucosal secretions or hemorrhage. As 20% of the duplications contain gastric mucosa,[39] ulceration or perforation may occur. Observation of peristaltic contractions of the cyst wall during real-time scanning is strongly in support of the diagnosis.[39]

Meckel's Diverticulum (MD)

Most diverticula are asymptomatic and unexpected radiologic findings. However, nearly 20% of the MDs contain gastric mucosa, and acid-secretion-related complications may occur.

The patients are often referred for sonography to rule out appendicitis. The first step, therefore, is to identify the normal appendix. The ileum is then studied as far as is possible. The demonstration of inflamed mesenteric fat together with local tenderness demands close attention to such a focal area. The US aspect of a Meckel's diverticulum is that of a circular or oval, hypoechoic or sonolucent mass, 1 to 2 cm or more in diameter (Fig. 8-39). As with a duplication cyst, the wall of the MD is usually 2 to 5 mm thick and presents an inner hyperechoic SM and outer hypoechoic MP layer.

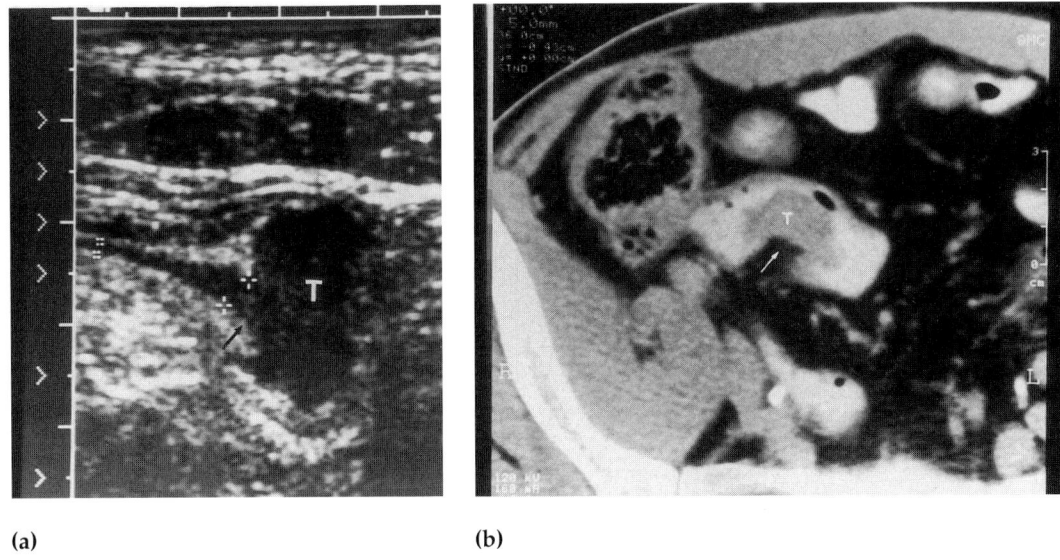

Fig. 8-36. Ileal carcinoid tumor with increased MP layer.
(a) A longitudinal US view of the terminal ileum exhibits an endoluminal hypoechoic tumor (T). The adjacent SM is interrupted and partly retracted toward the lumen. There is serosal transgression (arrow). The MP is thickened (3.5 mm) near the tumor (+) and normal (1.2 mm) away from it (h). (b) CT of the right inferior abdomen demonstrates the soft-tissue density of the tumor (T) in the lumen of the terminal ileum (arrow). (c) A macroscopic specimen (after longitudinal incision of the ileum) shows the endoluminal tumor (T). There is clear evidence of contiguous wall invasion and thickening of the muscularis propria layer (arrows) near the tumor base. At histology, beside the wall invasion by the tumor, there was hypertrophy of the adjacent uninfiltrated muscularis propria.

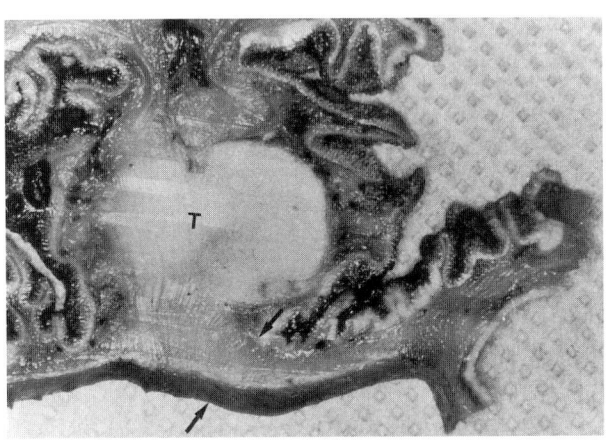

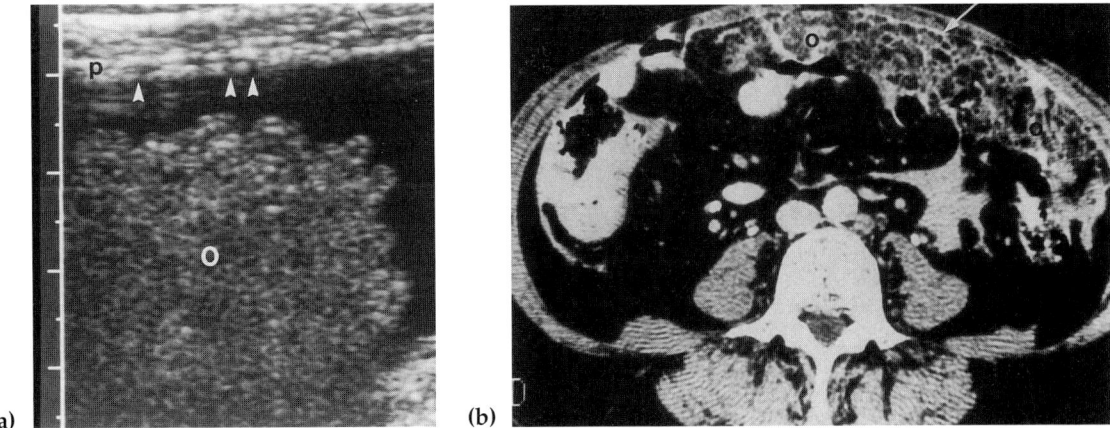

Fig. 8-37. Infiltration of the omentum in peritoneal carcinomatosis.
(a) Magnified view of a thickened, homogeneously hypoechoic, diffusely infiltrated omentum (O) in a patient with peritoneal carcinomatosis caused by an earlier resected endometrial carcinoma. The overlying parietal peritoneum (P) shows features of subtle hypoechoic linear infiltration by tumor (arrowheads). The anterior surface of the omentum is nodular. (b) CT of the same area shows a diffuse "honeycomb" pattern of omental infiltration (O). The nodular contour of the omentum observed at US is also seen. The peritoneum (arrow) is infiltrated and thickened.

Miscellaneous Disorders • 147

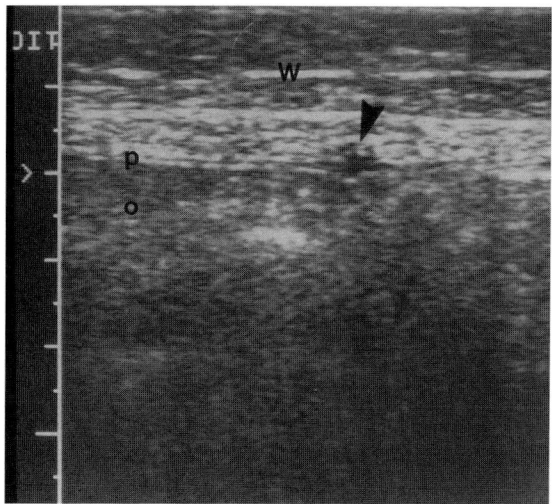

Fig. 8-38. Linear peritoneal implant of ovarian carcinoma. US shows a focal hypoechoic linear interruption (arrowhead) of the hyperechoic peritoneal lines (p). Both peritoneal layers are fixed at that level. Ascites is absent. (W = abdominal wall, O = omentum).

An MD can become inverted into the gut lumen, producing a single "target" sign in transverse view. A double target sign has also been reported in gut-gut intussusceptions headed by an inverted MD.[40] Rarely, an MD may be complicated by a tumor or an enterolith.[30]

Miscellaneous Disorders

Intussusception

Shown by US and in cross section an intussusception has a typical "doughnut" appearance. The hypoechoic outer rim (intussuscipiens) encircles an echogenic center (intussusceptum) composed of mesenteric fat containing the collapsed bowel, which is barely visible as a hypoechoic rim of muscularis propria (Fig. 8-40). If the intussusceptum is composed of more than one loop of bowel, the cross section will show multiple layers. Longitudinally imaged, an intussusception presents a pseudokidney appearance, with tubular hyperechoic invaginated mesenteric fat (the pseudosinus) adjacent to collapsed intestinal lumen, surrounded by hypoechoic layers (the pseudocortex). The amount of contiguous ascites and mesenteric edema varies with the duration and severity of the process.

Peristalsis may be observed in a larger, noninflamed Meckel's diverticulum. Unlike a cystic duplication, an MD should communicate with the bowel lumen and may, therefore, contain air.

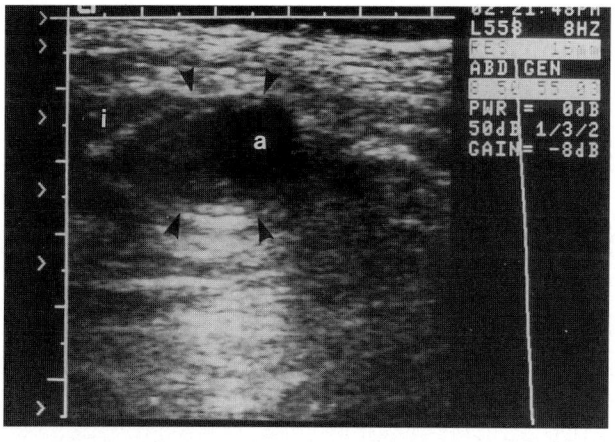

(a)

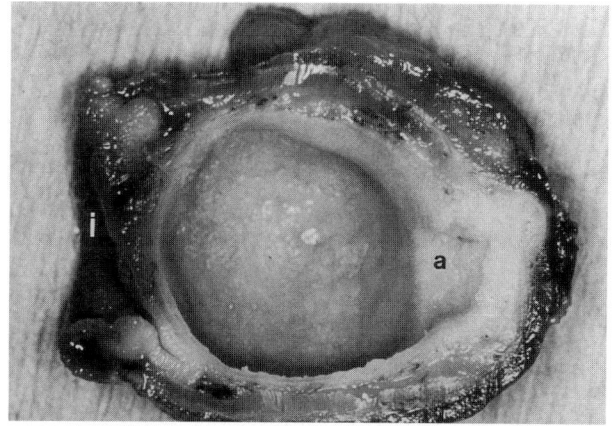

(b)

Fig. 8-39. US features of a cystic Meckel's diverticulitis in a 45-year-old woman clinically suspected of appendicitis. (a) Below a segment of ileum (i) (partially seen in transverse view) a fixed, constant and noncompressible mass (arrowhead) is demonstrated. Distinctive wall layers were observed and suggested a dilated Meckel's diverticulum. In addition to internal echogenic debris, the sonolucent area (a) was found to represent an abscess in the distal part of the diverticulum. Air was surprisingly absent from the diverticulum. (b) Photograph of the opened specimen revealed a Meckel's diverticulum that was sealed off from the ileal (i) lumen. The tip of the diverticulum contains a large erosion with contiguous white wall thickening. The abscess (a) had been in that location but was already evacuated when the picture was taken.

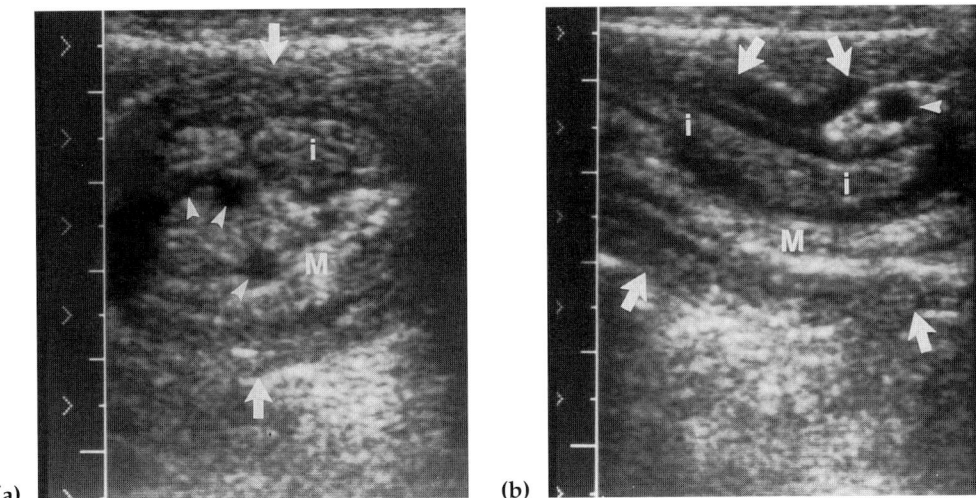

Fig. 8-40. US of ileocolic intussusception with mesenteric adenitis.
(a) A transverse view demonstrates the hypoechoic outer rim (between arrows) that represents the intussuscipiens, the walls of the colon. At its internal aspect is an echogenic center (the intussusceptum) composed of mesenteric fat (M), collapsed ileum (i), and small mesenteric nodes (arrowheads). (b) A longitudinal view of the same area again shows invaginated mesenteric fat (M) contained within the walls (arrows) of the colon. Mesenteric nodes (arrowhead) and the longitudinally seen ileum (i) are also outlined.

A sonographic objective is also the identification of the cause of the intussusception. A leading mass or a thickened segment of bowel wall is usually the cause of a fixed intussusception.

Intestinal Endometriosis

After the rectosigmoid and the appendix, the last 10 cm of the ileum are the third most frequent site for endometrial deposits affecting the gastrointestinal tract.[41] At US, endometrial masses firmly established on the wall of the gut create lumen constriction or wall retraction. These hypoechoic, cystic or echogenic, mural plaques create thickening of the hypoechoic MP, while preserving the inner submucosal and mucosal layers. The differential diagnosis includes mainly metastases and lymphoma.

Celiac Disease

Small bowel dilatation, hypersecretion, or increased separation of the jejunal folds would require enteroclysis to be radiographically specific. These changes are difficult to define by US. However, painless, transient intussusceptions may be found in clinically suspected or unsuspected celiac disease.

The cavitary mesenteric lymph node syndrome associated with severe hyposplenism is a rare and frequently fatal complication of long-standing celiac disease. Microsplenia is found in 30% to 50% of these patients.[42] At US, the normal mesentery is virtually replaced by sonolucent cystic lymphadenopathies with walls of variable thickness (Fig. 8-41). Posterior acoustic enhancement is present. Some cavities may contain echogenic deposits, which represent lipid-rich hyalin material, the fat component of the fat-fluid levels seen on CT.[43] In patients with known celiac disease, possible complications such as ulcerative jejunoileitis, small bowel lymphoma, and adenocarcinoma can be ruled out by sonography.

Gallstone Ileus

More often occurring in elderly female patients with other known medical disorders, gallstone ileus often has an unduly delayed diagnosis. In consequence, its reported mortality has ranged from 7% to 50%.[44] Sonography is the method of choice for making an early diagnosis in these patients. At US, the findings of a diseased gallbladder, pneumobilia, and ectopic gallstones with or without obvious signs of bowel obstruction suggest this diagnosis. Although the gallstones are found to be radiopaque in only 20% of plain abdominal X-ray films, they are all sonographically hyperechoic with frank posterior shadowing. They may be found in a fistula, the stomach, the duodenum (Bouveret's syndrome), the small bowel (the ileum in 60% of cases), and the colon (usually the sigmoid).

Roundworm Infestation

The sonographic appearance of small, endoluminal *Ascaris lumbricoides* has been described before.[45] An individual worm appears as a hypoechoic or echogenic

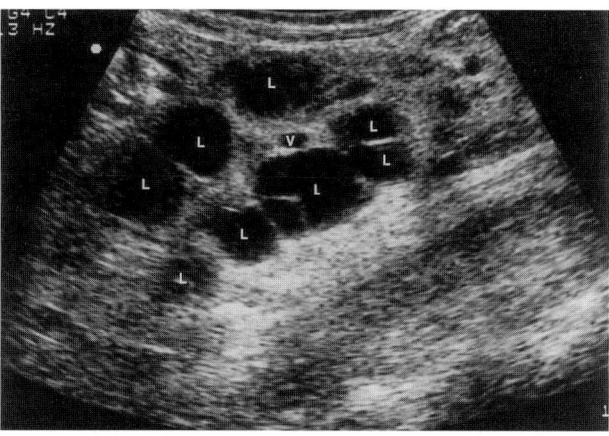
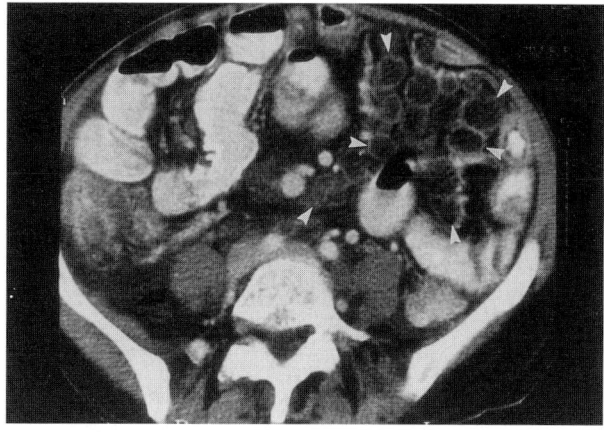

Fig. 8-41. Cavitary lymph node syndrome in celiac disease.
(a) A transverse view of the small bowel mesentery outlines numerous round, cystic, and sonolucent masses (L). Some masses show septa and thick walls. Posterior acoustic enhancement is also visible behind some of the cysts. All are cavitary lymph nodes (L). (V = mesenteric vessel.) (b) CT section at the same level shows thick-walled cystic mesenteric lymphadenopathies (arrowheads). This patient has proven celiac disease. The cavitary nodes gradually regressed over a period of weeks on a gluten-free diet and steroid treatment. (Courtesy of Professor Yves Menu, Clichy, France.)

tubular structure and ranges in width from 6 to 9 mm. Sometimes its alimentary canal is shown, either as an echogenic central line (when collapsed) or as two parallel well-defined hyperechoic bands with a hypoechoic center (when distended) (Fig. 8-42). In cross section, the alimentary canal appears as a small, single or double target. A bunch of worms usually presents an echogenic, complex mass. Curling movements of the worms can be identified on real-time US and confirm the diagnosis.

Bezoars

A bezoar may be the cause of small bowel obstruction. At sonography, it presents an endoluminal, arclike surface echo that casts a distinct posterior acoustic shadow. Compression of the bezoar by the transducer may induce fluid shift around it.[46] The differential diagnosis should include a trichobezoar, an enterolith, a gallstone, barium plug, lipoma, drug sachet, or, most unlikely, an endoluminal calcified tumor. If air is indicated within the mass, a bezoar or a drug sachet is the more likely diagnosis.

Toothpick Penetration

This nonopaque foreign body is a real challenge to the sonographer, who is often the first to suspect it. The most frequently found sonographic appearance of a toothpick is that of a hyperechoic, thin, straight line, with a variable degree of acoustic shadowing in the longitudinal view, and that of a hyperechoic dot with

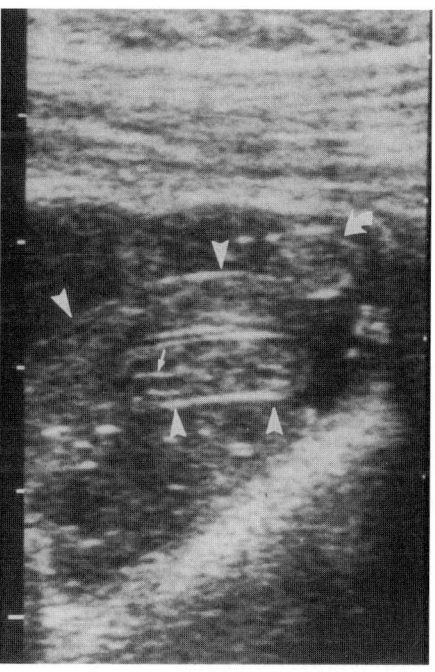

Fig. 8-42. US features of intestinal ascaris lumbricoides.
A transverse view of a fluid-filled segment of ileum demonstrates two echogenic tubular structures (arrowheads) delineated by hyperechoic walls. The lower ascaris contains a pair of subtle hyperechoic lines (arrow) representing the dilated alimentary canal. A curved arrow shows the transverse view of another worm. Both worms moved and curved as shown by real-time sonography. (Courtesy of Dr Laurent Garel, Montréal, Canada.)

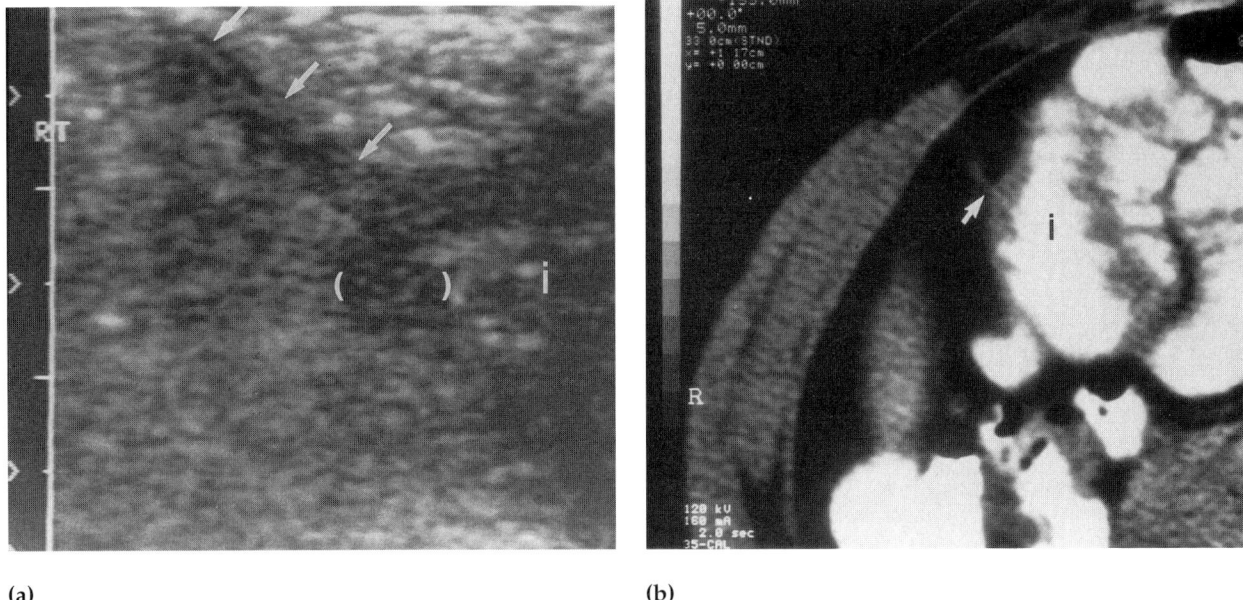

(a) (b)

Fig. 8-43. US features of a toothpick perforation of the jejunum in a patient clinically suspected of appendicitis.
(a) At the transition site from a small bowel dilatation, thickened intestine (i) is seen in transverse view. Emerging from the bowel wall into the omental fat (between parentheses) is an oblique hypoechoic thin line (arrows) associated with variable posterior shadowing. In transverse view (not shown here) there was a classic hyperechoic dot with clear posterior shadowing. (b) CT, in the area indicated by sonography, revealed a hyperdense line (arrow) perpendicular to the thickened intestinal (i) wall.

sharp posterior shadowing in the transverse view. An oblique position of the wooden object may decrease its hyperechogenicity and shorten its perceived length (Fig. 8-43).[47] In our experience of seven cases of US-detected, clinically unsuspected, swallowed toothpicks causing GI complications, all occurred in patients wearing dentures, and none of the patients could remember having swallowing the toothpicks.

Cystic Fibrosis

Distal intestinal obstruction syndrome is a frequent intestinal complication that occurs and recurs in about 15% of adult cystic fibrosis patients, particularly those with pancreatic insufficiency.[48] It is caused by the accumulation of thickened muco-fecal material in the terminal ileum and right colon.

By sonography, a thickened wall of the terminal ileal and cecum are the usual findings, without signs of adjacent inflammation.[49] In addition, the presence of small echogenic nodules fixed to the mucosa, which persist on serial ultrasound follow-ups, suggests dilated glands and crypts with inspissated mucus or muco-fecal material (Fig. 8-44).[50]

The editors express their appreciation of greatly valued advice given by Professors J.B.C.M. Pulyaert, MD, Beverly Coleman, MD, and Jill Langer, MD.

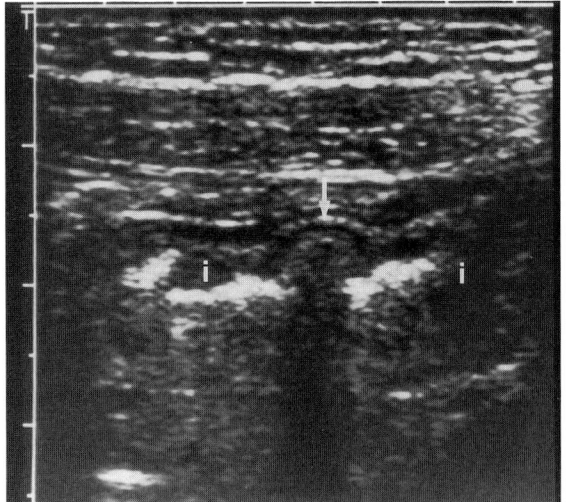

Fig. 8-44. US findings in an adult cystic fibrosis patient who complained of constipation and nausea.
Longitudinal US view of the ileum (i) shows hyperechoic foci that differed from other material in its lumen. Foci of moderate echotexture were also observed (arrow) and appeared to be embedded in the mucosa. Unlike the rest of the lumen contents, these nodules were fixed in position. Other similar nodules were seen on many US follow-ups. We believe they represent muco-feculent material classically encountered in adult cystic fibrosis patients.

The author wishes to thank Carole Johnston for secretarial assistance.

References

1. Ogata M, Imai S, Hosotani R, Aoyama H, Hayashi M, Ishikawa T. Abdominal ultrasonography for the diagnosis of strangulation in small bowel obstruction. *Br J Surg.* 1994;81:421–424.
2. Rioux M, Michaud C. Sonographic detection of peritoneal carcinomatosis: a prospective study of 37 cases. *Abdom Imaging.* 1995;20:47–51.
3. Rioux M. Echographie digestive: aspects échographiques des iléocolites. *Feuillets de Radiologie.* 1994;34(4):267–283.
4. Stoupis C, Ros PR, Abbitt PL, Burton SS, Gauger J. Bubbles in the belly: imaging of cystic mesenteric or omental masses. *Radiographics.* 1994;14:729–737.
5. Chou YH, Tiu CM, Lui WY, Chang T. Mesenteric and omental cysts: an ultrasonographic and clinical study in 15 patients. *Gastrointest Radiol.* 1991;16:311–314.
6. Fujita N, Noda Y, Kobayashi G, et al. Chylous cyst of the mesentery: US and CT diagnosis. *Abdom Imaging.* 1995;20:259–261.
7. Burke AP, Sobin LH, Shekitka KM, et al. Intra-abdominal fibromatosis: a pathologic analysis of 130 tumors with comparison of clinical subgroups. *Am J Surg Pathol.* 1990;144:335–341.
8. Chan YL, Cheng CSK, Ng PW. Mesenteric actinomycosis. *Abdom Imaging.* 1993;18:286–287.
9. Puylaert JBCM. Right-sided segmental infarction of the omentum: clinical, US, and CT findings. *Radiology.* 1992;185:169–172.
10. Rioux M, Langis P. Primary epiploic appendagitis: clinical, US and CT findings in 14 cases. *Radiology.* 1994;91:523–526.
11. La Bella A, Gimondo P, Camboni M. Eco-Doppler evaluation of intestinal peristalsis in normal and in some pathological conditions: preliminary data. *Ital J Gastroenterol.* 1993;25:13–18.
12. Lim JH, Ko YT, Lee DH, et al. Determining the site and causes of colonic obstruction with sonography. *AJR.* 1994;163:1113–1117.
13. Summers RW, Lu CC. Approach to the patient with ileus and obstruction. In: Yamada T, Alpers DH, Owyang C, et al, eds. *Textbook of Gastroenterology.* Philadelphia, Pa: JB Lippincott Co; 1991:715–731.
14. Balthazar EJ. CT of small bowel obstruction. *AJR.* 1994;62:255–261.
15. Ko YT, Lim JH, Lee DH, et al. Small bowel obstruction: sonographic evaluation. *Radiology.* 1993;188:649–653.
16. Taourel PG, Fabre JM, Pradel JA, et al. Value of CT in the diagnosis and management of patients with suspected acute small bowel obstruction. *AJR.* 1995;165:1187–1192.
17. Laufman H, Nora PF. Physiological problems underlying intestinal strangulation obstruction. *Surg Clin North Am.* 1962;42:219–229.
18. Smerud MJ, Johnson CD, Stephens DH. Diagnosis of bowel infarction: a comparison of plain films and CT scans in 23 cases. *AJR.* 1990;154:99–103.
19. Leonidas JC, Magid N, Soberman N, Glass TS. Midgut volvulus in infants: diagnosis with US. *Radiology.* 1991;179:491–493.
20. Smet MH, Marchal G, Ceulemans R, Eggermont E. The solitary hyperdynamic pulsating superior mesenteric artery: an additional dynamic sonographic feature of midgut volvulus. *Pediatr Radiol.* 1991;21(2):156–157.
21. Pracros JP, Sann L, Genin G, et al. Ultrasound diagnosis of midgut volvulus: the whirlpool sign. *Pediatr Radiol.* 1992;22:8–20.
22. Aizawa K, Tokuyama H, Yonezawa T, et al. A case of traumatic intramural hematoma of the duodenum effectively treated with ultrasonically guided aspiration drainage and endoscopic balloon catheter dilatation. *Gastroenterol Jpn.* 1991;26(2):18–22.
23. Couture A, Veyrac C, Baud C, et al. Evaluation of abdominal pain in Henoch-Schönlein syndrome by high frequency ultrasound. *Pediatr Radiol.* 1992;2:12–17.
24. Martinez-Frontanilla LA, Haase GM, Ernster JA, et al. Surgical complications in Henoch-Schönlein purpura. *J Pediatr Surg.* 1984;19:434–436.
25. Steinhard HJ, Loeschke K, Kasper H, et al. European Cooperative Crohn's disease study (ECCDS): clinical features and natural history. *Digestion.* 1985;1:97–108.
26. Glick SN. Crohn's disease of the small intestine. *Radiol Clin North Am.* 1987;25:25–45.
27. Frager DH, Goldman M, Beneventano TC. Computed tomography in Crohn's disease. *J Comput Assist Tomogr.* 1983;7:819–824.
28. Bronwyn J, Fishman EK, Hamilton SR, et al. Submucosal accumulation of fat in inflammatory bowel disease: CT/pathologic correlation. *J Comput Assist Tomogr.* 1986;10:759–763.
29. Wilson SR. US of the gastrointestinal tract: does it play a role? In: Rifkin MD, Charbonneau JW, Laing FC, eds. *Syllabus: A Special Course in Ultrasound 1991.* Chicago, Ill: Radiological Society of North America; 1991:307–318.
30. Rioux M. Sonographic detection of the normal and abnormal appendix. *AJR.* 1992;158:773–778.
31. Davis SJ, Patel A. Case report: distinctive echogenic lymphadenopathy in Whipple's disease. *Clin Radiol.* 1990;42:60–62.
32. Ashley SW, Wells SA Jr. Tumors of the small intestine. *Semin Oncol.* 1988;15(2):116–128.
33. Rioux M, Gariepy JL. Cystic lymphangioma of the colon: ultrasonographic and computed tomographic features. *Can Assoc Radiol J.* 1995;46:127–130.
34. Dudiak KM, Johnson CD, Stephens DH. Primary tumors of the small intestine: CT evaluation. *AJR.* 1989;152:995–998.
35. Rioux M, Mailloux C. Crescent shape necrosis: a new imaging sign suggestive of stromal tumor of the small bowel. *Abdom Imaging.* 1997;22:173–174.
36. Rioux M, Langis P, Naud F. Sonographic appearance of primary small bowel carcinoid tumor. *Abdom Imaging.* 1995;20:37–43.
37. Ducan BW, Adsick NS, Eraklis A. Retroperitoneal alimentary tract duplications detected in utero. *J Pediatr Surg.* 1992;27(9):1231–1233.

38. Balén EM, Hernàndez-Lisoàin JL, Pardo F, et al. Giant jejunoileal duplication: prenatal diagnosis and complete excision without intestinal resection. *J Pediatr Surg.* 1993; 28(12):1586–1588.
39. Spottswood SE. Peristalsis in duplication cyst: a new diagnostic sonographic finding. *Pediatr Radiol.* 1994;24: 344–345.
40. Itagaki A, Uchida M, Ueki K, Kajii T. Double target sign in ultrasonic diagnosis of intussuscepted Meckel diverticulum. *Pediatr Radiol.* 1991;21:148–149.
41. Gindoff PR, Jewelewicz R. Ileal resection in the operative treatment of endometriosis. *Obstet Gynecol.* 1987;69: 511–513.
42. Rubesin SE, Grumbach K, Herlinger H, et al. Adult celiac disease and its complications. *Radiographics.* 1989;9(6): 1045–1066.
43. Matuchansky C, Colin R, Hemet J. Cavitation of mesenteric lymph nodes, splenic atrophy and a flat small intestinal mucosa: report of 6 cases. *Gastroenterology.* 1984; 87:606–614.
44. Lasson A, Lorén I, Nilsson A, et al. Ultrasonography in gallstone ileus: a diagnostic challenge. *Eur J Surg.* 1995; 161:259–263.
45. Malde HM, Chadha D. Roundworm obstruction: sonographic diagnosis. *Abdom Imaging.* 1993;18:274–276.
46. Ko YT, Lim JH, Lee DH, Yoon Y. Small intestinal phytobezoars: sonographic detection. *Abdom Imaging.* 1993; 18:271–273.
47. Rioux M, Langis P. Sonographic detection of clinically unsuspected swallowed toothpicks: their gastrointestinal complications. *J Clin Ultrasound.* 1994;22:483–490.
48. Park RW, Grand RJ. Gastrointestinal manifestations of cystic fibrosis: a review. *Gastroenterology.* 1981;81:1143–1161.
49. Dik H, Nicolai JJ, Schipper J, et al. Erroneous diagnosis of distal intestinal obstruction syndrome in cystic fibrosis: clinical impact of abdominal ultrasonography. *Eur J Gastroenterol Hepatol.* 1995;7:279–281.
50. Keeling JW. Congenital abnormalities in the small and large intestine. In: McGee JOD, Isaacson PG, Wright NA, eds. *Oxford Textbook of Pathology.* Oxford, England: Oxford Medical Publications; 1992:1192–1193.

Computed Tomography of the Small Bowel
Technique and Principles of Interpretation

9

Bernard A. Birnbaum

Chapter Contents

Introduction
Technique
Principles of Interpretation

Introduction

Computed tomography (CT) is now established as one of the most important techniques for imaging the small intestine. Accumulated clinical experience using faster, high-resolution scanners and optimized scanning methodology has shown CT to be a highly accurate means of detecting and characterizing small bowel pathology. The value of CT lies in its cross-sectional imaging capability, which enables evaluation of both the inner and outer aspects of the alimentary tube. Though CT is capable of demonstrating the bowel lumen, it is generally agreed that barium examinations are superior to CT for evaluating intraluminal and mucosal disease. Barium studies display mucosal detail, but are only able to demonstrate indirect evidence of extramucosal disease. CT is complementary to barium examination of the gastrointestinal tract because of its ability to directly visualize the bowel wall, supporting mesentery, peritoneal cavity, retroperitoneum, and solid abdominal organs. Thus, CT provides a more accurate assessment of the extraluminal components of disease processes.[1]

Technological advances may soon enable CT to directly compete with barium examination of the bowel lumen. Investigators have recently demonstrated the feasibility of generating three-dimensional "endoscopic" views of the bowel using volumetric data sets obtained using helical CT scanners.[2,3] Though preliminary in nature, this research suggests a potential future role for CT to directly visualize the mucosal surface of the bowel and to provide a global assessment of both luminal and extraluminal abnormalities of the gastrointestinal tract.

The indications for CT evaluation of the small intestine continue to grow. CT may be used as an initial diagnostic screening examination in a patient with nonspecific abdominal complaints, or it may be performed as a specialized procedure where the study is prospectively tailored to provide important correlative information about a small bowel abnormality detected or suspected on the basis of another imaging examination. The focus of this chapter is to describe the imaging techniques necessary for optimized body CT and to review the principles of CT interpretation used to diagnose abnormalities of the small intestine.

Technique

The accurate detection of luminal, mural, and perienteric abnormalities of the small bowel on CT examination is critically dependent on the use of optimized scanning methodology.[1,4,5] An important goal of optimized body CT is to ensure acquisition of high-quality images without compromising patient throughput. This is primarily achieved on both helical and nonhelical CT scanners by the proper utilization of slice collimation, intravenous contrast material, and oral contrast agents. Although most survey studies of the abdomen are performed using 7- to 10-mm collimation, "high-resolution" imaging of the gastrointestinal tract is performed by judiciously using thin-section ($\leq$5 mm collimation) scanning technique over the region of interest at a time when both bowel and vascular opacification is maximal.

Thin-section imaging improves visualization of fine anatomic detail because image sharpness is improved by minimizing volume-averaging effects in the z-axis. The result is improved confidence in detecting subtle abnormalities. The disadvantage of using thinner collimation is that one begins to appreciate an increase in image noise due to a reduction in the photon flux as collimation reduction approaches 50%.[5] Image quality may be maintained by increasing patient dose (either milliamperes in helical mode or exposure time in conventional mode). Although this results in an increase in tube heating, the scanner's tube-heating capabilities will not be exceeded if acquisition of thin slices is restricted to the area of interest. With helical CT scanners, one may shorten the scan acquisition time while improving anatomic coverage by increasing the helical pitch (pitch is equal to the table increment per 360-degree rotation of the X-ray tube divided by slice collimation). Increasing the pitch to 1.5:1 using 5-mm collimation enables a 50% gain in high-resolution anatomic coverage while increasing the effective slice thickness (full width at half maximum) to only 5.5 mm.

Ideally, high-resolution images are prospectively acquired as intravenous contrast is administered to the patient. Although this requires prescan planning based on a priori knowledge of the location of a suspected bowel abnormality, it ensures accurate and optimized interrogation of the enhancement pattern of the bowel wall. If the location of a bowel abnormality is unknown, or a suspected finding is inadequately imaged prospectively, thin-section images may be obtained following completion of the initial examination. We believe that all patients with unexplained gastrointestinal pathology should undergo contrast-enhanced CT unless severe contrast allergy or medical contraindications exist. The bowel should be scanned during, or immediately following, the infusion of iodinated intravenous contrast material in order to improve conspicuity of subtle gastrointestinal lesions and to maximize visualization of the mural enhancement pattern. This is critical from a diagnostic standpoint, since the presence, degree, and pattern of mural enhancement are important imaging criteria used to differentiate benign from malignant etiologies of bowel wall thickening (see section on Principles of Interpretation).

Because mural wall thickening is the hallmark of intestinal disease, every effort must be made to first ensure a successful bowel prep. The lumen of the small bowel should be free of ingested material, well opacified, and well distended. The normal thickness of the intestinal wall is directly related to the degree of luminal distention. The normal intestinal wall is barely perceptible in a well-distended segment and should be no greater than 2 to 3 mm thick when measured from the luminal to the serosal surface (Fig. 9-1).[5] A wall thickness of 4 mm or greater in any segment of well-distended small bowel should always be considered abnormal.[6] Studies compromised by luminal underdistention should be cautiously evaluated. It may be impossible to determine the true thickness of the intestinal wall in cases of underdistention, and false-positive diagnoses may result when interpreting such studies. Inadequate contrast opacification of the intestinal lumen and incomplete luminal distention account for the vast majority of interpretative errors.[1,4] Poorly opacified, fluid-filled bowel loops and collapsed intestinal segments may present as soft-tissue density CT "pseudomasses." While pseudomasses may occur throughout the gastrointestinal tract, they most commonly involve the proximal jejunum, where they may be confused with a pancreatic tail neoplasm, mesenteric adenopathy, or primary bowel lesion (Fig. 9-2).

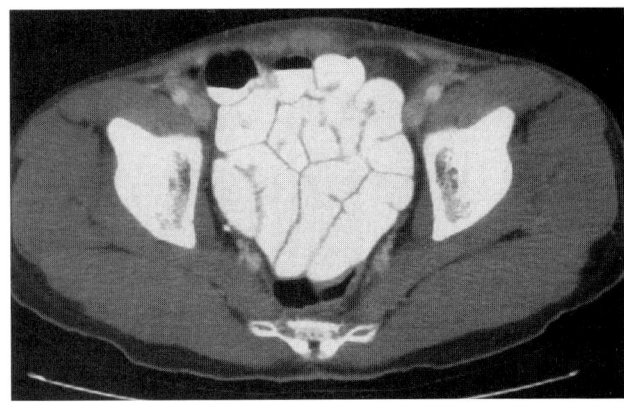

Fig. 9-1. Normal anatomy: ileum.
Pelvic ileal loops appear maximally distended with positive contrast material. The mucosal surface is featureless, and the intestinal wall is barely perceptible.

The small intestine is most commonly opacified with positive contrast agents. Luminal opacification is achieved by the oral administration of either a 1% to 2% barium sulfate suspension (Readi-CAT 2, E-Z-EM Co, Westbury, NY) or a 2% to 3% water-soluble iodinated solution (Gastrografin, diatrizoate meglumine, Bristol-Myers Squibb, Princeton, NJ). We prefer and routinely use barium suspensions because mucosal coating is often better, enabling improved evaluation of intestinal fold patterns.[5] Gastrografin is selectively used in patients presenting with abdominal trauma or suspected bowel perforation, for immediate preoperative patients, for intensive care unit patients, and for CT-guided interventional procedures.

Uniform opacification of the entire small bowel may be accomplished by the steady ingestion of 900 to 1000 ml of contrast over a 45-minute period immediately prior to the CT examination. At our institution, patients are asked to drink equal aliquots of contrast every 10 to 12 minutes and are specifically instructed not to ingest all the contrast at once. This helps prevent oral contrast "bolusing," which may result in nonuniform bowel opacification and poor luminal distention. In addition, a cup of contrast is always given

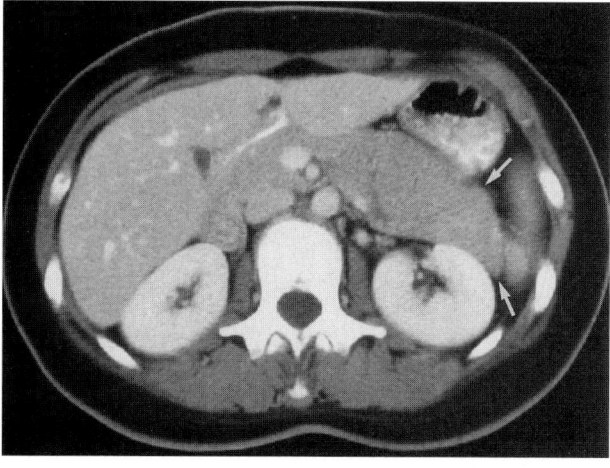 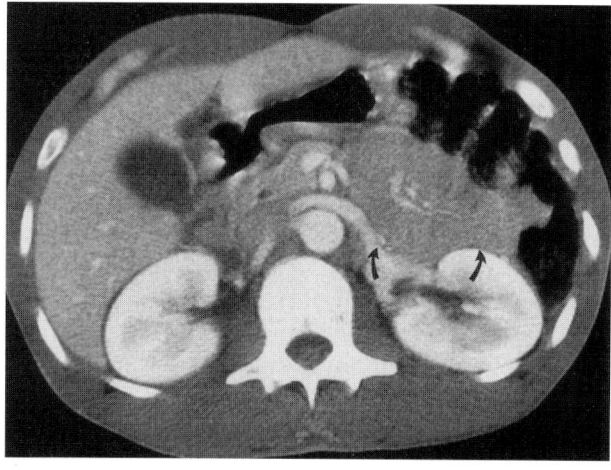

Fig. 9-2. Imaging pitfalls: left upper quadrant pseudomasses.
(a) Pancreatic tail pseudomass resulting from unopacified jejunum (arrows). (b) Pseudolymphoma appearance created by unopacified jejunal loops (arrows) that surround mesenteric vessels and mimic the "sandwich sign" of mesenteric adenopathy.

within 5 minutes of scanning to aid opacification of proximal jejunal loops. These bowel segments experience increased peristaltic activity relative to distal ileal loops and are more difficult to adequately distend. Our experience is similar to others in that we have not observed a significant difference between the intestinal transit times of barium and water-soluble agents.[5] We routinely administer 10 mg of oral metoclopramide with the first cup of contrast in order to improve ileal opacification.[7] Metaclopromide is contraindicated in patients with pheochromocytoma, mechanical bowel obstruction, and known allergies to this drug. This agent accelerates small bowel transit time, and the effects of its increased peristaltic activity usually subside by the time scanning is initiated 45 minutes later. Despite its use, some patients still require additional time for adequate opacification of the cecum and terminal ileum. In fact, when imaging patients with suspected right lower quadrant pathology, we routinely obtain an initial unenhanced scan at the level of the iliac crest prior to scan initiation. If the terminal ileum is not yet opacified, we wait and delay the study for another 15 to 20 minutes to ensure optimal evaluation of these bowel segments. Gastric distention is achieved using air as a negative contrast agent by administering effervescent granules with 25 ml of water prior to scan acquisition. Peristaltic artifacts are minimized by the routine administration of 0.1 mg of intravenous glucagon prior to scanning in all patients.

Negative contrast agents may also be used to opacify the mesenteric small bowel. Water and corn oil emulsions both provide reproducible luminal distention and negative contrast.[8-11] The fat content of concentrated corn oil emulsions provides greater negative contrast than water. Unfortunately, poor palatability, untoward gastrointestinal side effects, and high cost have limited its clinical acceptance. Water, on the other hand, is increasingly being used as a negative contrast agent for the upper gastrointestinal tract in the helical CT era.[11] Water's low attenuation enables it to serve as an acceptable bowel opacification agent without interfering with helical CT-angiography applications. The high attenuation of barium suspensions and water-soluble iodinated solutions leads to the depiction of undesired bowel anatomy when thresholding algorithms are used to generate three-dimensional shaded-surface display renderings. Despite use of editing techniques, the visualized bowel tends to obscure vascular detail and therefore complicate study interpretation. While this imaging pitfall may be avoided by withholding oral contrast altogether, a preferable solution is to use water as a negative opacification agent in these patients.

Water serves as an acceptable contrast agent for CT applications directed toward the upper gastrointestinal tract and abdomen because of its ability to provide excellent anatomic depiction of the gastric wall, duodenal wall, duodenal-pancreatic interface, and papilla.[11] In order to achieve reliable distention of the stomach, duodenum, and proximal jejunum, patients must ingest approximately 1050 to 1100 ml of water over a 30-minute time interval prior to scanning. Reliable opacification of the distal jejunum and ileum requires the ingestion of an additional 500 to 750 ml of water. Because most patients have difficulty drinking such volumes, water has not yet achieved acceptance as a routine oral contrast agent for imaging both the stomach and mesenteric small bowel. Moreover, water should be used with caution in patients with suspected abdominal inflammation, as fluid-containing abscesses may appear isodense with bowel (Fig. 9-3). Patients with suspected high-grade small bowel obstruction do not need additional oral contrast because of the retained intraluminal fluid. Moreover, these patients have already been vomiting. Scanning should be performed before implementing mechanical suction (see Chapter 21). Intravenous contrast is mandatory unless contraindicated.

Air is an excellent negative contrast agent that has been successfully employed in evaluating the stomach, duodenal sweep, and colon.[1,3-5,12,13] When viewed at routine CT window and level settings, air minimizes appreciation of the normal bowel wall thickness compared with water, enabling improved conspicuity of small lesions and subtle bowel pathology.[4,5] The use of air as a negative contrast medium for the jejunum and ileum remains investigational. Enteric-coated, time-released effervescent granules and tablets have been used to noninvasively introduce gas into the mesenteric small bowel.[14] The resulting air-contrast effect is often nonuniform, however, which has prevented these agents from achieving clinical acceptance.

We have recently begun to use rectal air insufflation as a retrograde means of achieving air contrast within the terminal ileum on CT. We do this as a problem-solving technique to clarify a finding detected during the initial scanning sequence. Patients are placed in the left lateral decubitus position prior to insufflation to take advantage of air's position-dependent properties. Air is then insufflated into the colon, and is usually well tolerated by patients when coupled with the intravenous administration of 0.5 to 1.0 mg of glucagon. Following acquisition of the scout view, targeted thin-section scans are obtained through the right lower quadrant. The resulting images are often dramatic, and facilitate demonstration of both luminal and mural ileal pathology (Fig. 9-4).

Principles of Interpretation

In order to achieve a correct CT diagnosis in a patient with small bowel disease, one must perform a methodical analysis of a gastrointestinal lesion's imaging features. A logical differential diagnosis may be constructed by first identifying the pertinent CT findings, and then categorizing the visualized abnormality as being benign or malignant in nature using established CT criteria. Though intestinal diseases often demonstrate overlapping CT features, the addition of relevant clinical history often narrows the differential to a

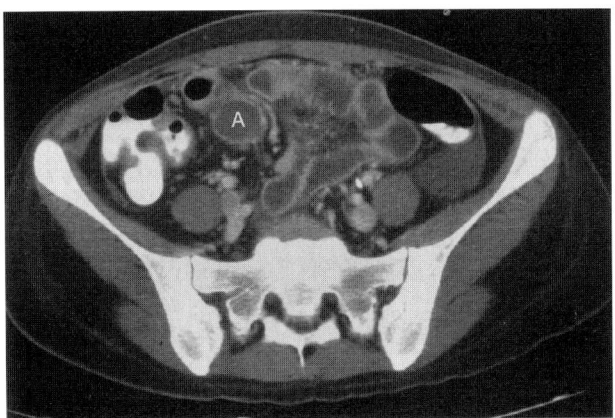

(a)

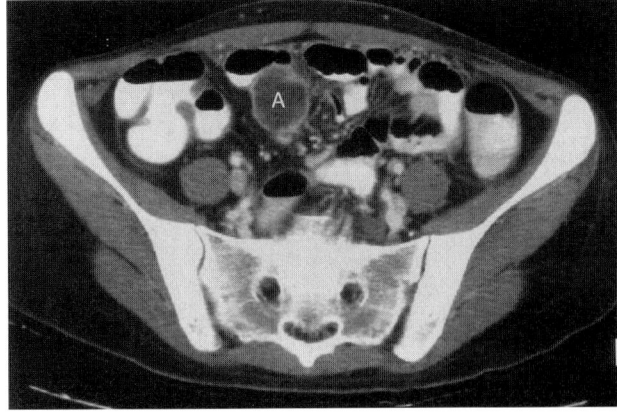

(b)

Fig. 9-3. Interloop abscess.
(a) Mesenteric abscess (A) appears similar to adjacent water-density ileal loops and was not prospectively identified. (b) Follow-up CT performed with positive contrast opacification of ileal loops clearly demonstrates peripherally enhanced abscess (A).

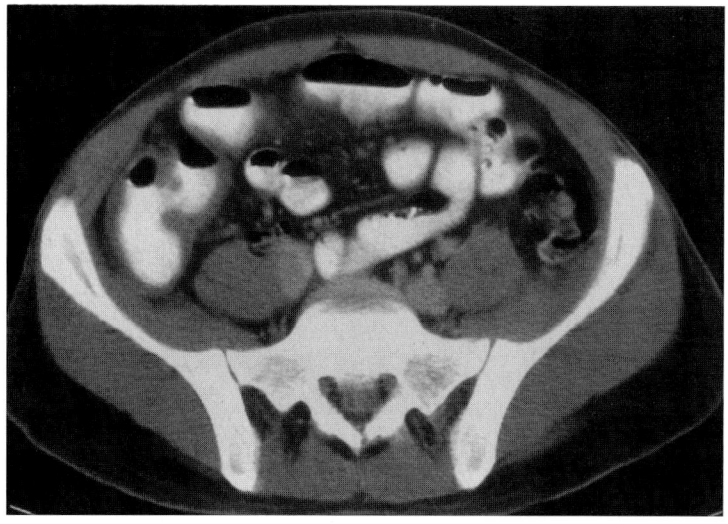 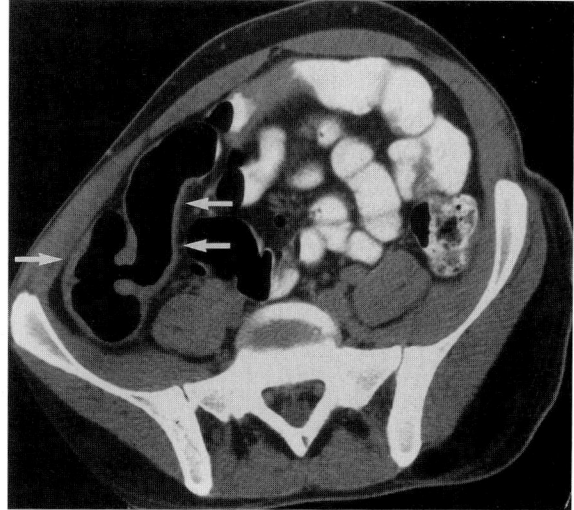

(a) (b)

Fig. 9-4. Air-contrast CT scan: evaluation of terminal ileum.
(a) Image with patient supine suggests pathologic thickening of the ileocecal region in a 25-year-old patient with suspected Crohn's disease. (b) After rectal air insufflation, repeat scanning in the left lateral decubitus position enables excellent bowel distention and confirms the presence of mural thickening in this location (arrows).

few diagnostic entities. In many primary gastrointestinal disorders, a constellation of CT findings may be noted that permits a precise diagnosis to be made.

A thorough analysis of a suspected pathologic lesion should include determination of lesion size, location, multiplicity, and length of involvement. Lesion localization is useful because certain diseases characteristically involve different segments of the small bowel. Familiar examples include preferential involvement of the proximal duodenum and jejunum by adenocarcinoma, and the known propensity for tuberculosis, cytomegalovirus (CMV), and Crohn's disease to affect the terminal ileum.[1,6,15,16] Lesion multiplicity suggests metastatic disease; however, one must exclude benign processes such as Crohn's disease or intestinal ischemia, which may also present with multiple sites of involvement. Extent of involvement is an especially important diagnostic parameter to consider. Benign intestinal disease is usually segmental in nature or tends to diffusely involve the entire small bowel. Malignant intestinal disease typically presents as a focal soft-tissue mass.[1] Though these rules often prove useful for disease categorization, important exceptions exist. For example, the mesenteric small bowel may be diffusely infiltrated by lymphoma, while CMV infection may result in focal wall thickening of the terminal ileum. Study interpretation is aided and the differential diagnosis further refined by carefully evaluating those features of gastrointestinal disease that are most efficaciously imaged by CT. These diagnostic parameters include the degree of intestinal wall thickening, the pattern of mural enhancement, and the presence or absence of perienteric, mesenteric, and peritoneal disease.

Bowel Wall Thickening

A CT diagnosis of intestinal wall thickening should be entertained only if the bowel segment in question appears adequately distended. Maximal distention is present if the suspicious segment and its afferent and efferent loops appear totally opacified with contrast. We have noted that the degree of distention of normal small bowel on CT closely parallels the degree of distention present on a well-performed small bowel follow-through barium examination. The maximum intraluminal diameter reported for the proximal jejunum on CT is 3.5 cm; however, this degree of dilatation is rarely seen unless the proximal bowel has been challenged by a large bolus of oral contrast, or CT enteroclysis has been performed.[17,18] More typically, the proximal mesenteric intestine measures 3.0 cm in diameter. As the bowel lumen narrows distally, this measurement decreases to approximately 2.5 cm at the level of the proximal ileum and 2.0 cm at the terminal ileum. These measurements may be used as a rough guide to help ascertain the degree of luminal distention. If wall thickening is suspected in an underdistended segment, this section of bowel should be flooded with contrast and rescanned with appropriate patient positioning using thin-section imaging to more accurately assess the mural anatomy. Though wall thickness varies with the degree of distention, the normal intestinal wall should measure no greater than 3 mm in thickness when measured in a true axial plane.[5,6]

Neoplastic, vascular, and inflammatory diseases can all result in abnormal thickening of the intestinal wall.[19] CT is extremely helpful in assigning patients with small bowel wall thickening to an appropriate disease category.[17] Benign intestinal lesions typically demonstrate circumferential and symmetric thickening of the bowel wall (Fig. 9-5).[1] The degree of thickening is variable depending on the etiology, but usually does not exceed 1.0 to 1.5 cm when measured from the luminal to the serosal surface.[1,17] The transition from normal to abnormal bowel is often gradual, and if luminal narrowing occurs, the inner mucosal surface retains its smooth contour. In contrast, neoplastic intestinal lesions characteristically demonstrate eccentric or asymmetric bowel wall thickening.[1] The degree of wall thickening is greater than that displayed by vascular and inflammatory conditions, and often exceeds 1.5 to 2.0 cm in thickness (Fig. 9-6).[1,17] Neoplasms typically show abrupt transition with adjacent normal bowel as well as lobulated and irregular contours. Luminal narrowing with obliteration of the normal fold pattern may be seen.

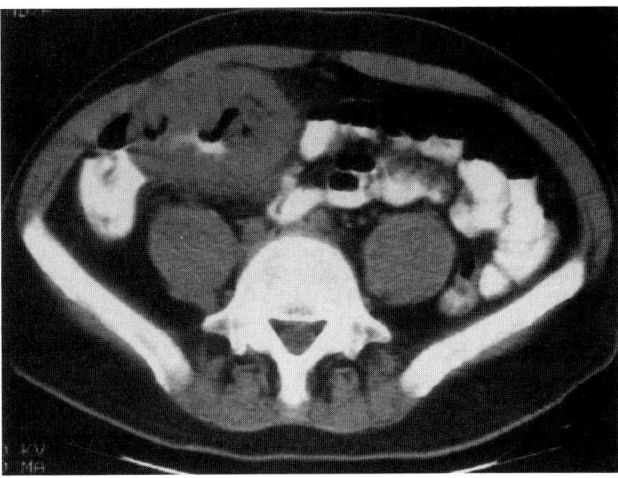

Fig. 9-6. Malignant bowel wall thickening in lymphoma. CT scan demonstrates an infiltrating circumferential, asymmetric soft-tissue mass of homogeneous attenuation involving the terminal ileum. A lobulated inner contour is seen within this nonobstructing neoplasm.

Subtle abnormalities of the intestinal fold pattern are best evaluated by barium studies. The intestinal folds may be demonstrated by CT when the small bowel is optimally opacified. The jejunal folds are more commonly demonstrated than their ileal counterparts, and typically measure less than 2 to 3 mm in thickness. The folds appear discrete and perpendicular to the bowel wall when the lumen is maximally distended, or show a feathery appearance when the bowel is partially opacified (Fig. 9-7). CT demonstration of fold thickening greater than 3 mm is a nonspecific finding that is often seen in benign diseases that cause abnormal bowel wall thickening. Examples include infectious enteritis, ischemic enteritis, hypoalbuminemic states, Whipple's disease, Crohn's disease, and reactive changes secondary to contiguous inflammation (eg, pancreatitis) (Fig. 9-8).

Bowel Enhancement Pattern

The appearance of the mural enhancement pattern is one of the most important CT diagnostic parameters used to differentiate neoplastic from non-neoplastic causes of intestinal wall thickening. The most significant observation is the presence of the "double halo" or "target" sign.[1,5,20] These signs refer to the cross-sectional imaging appearance of a thickened bowel loop that demonstrates concentric, alternating rings of high and low attenuation. In both cases, a variably

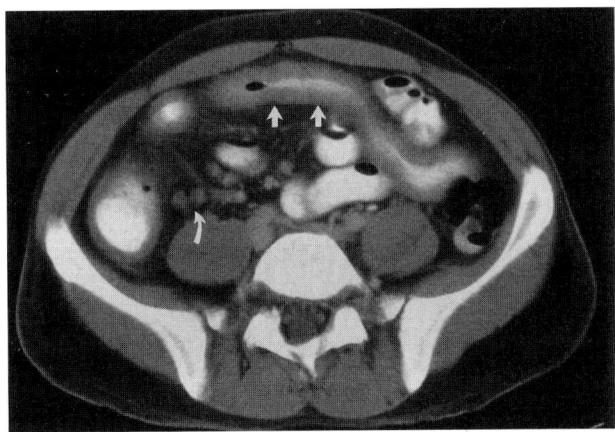

Fig. 9-5. Benign bowel wall thickening in Crohn's disease.
Segmental involvement of distal ileum with mild, circumferential, and symmetric mural thickening with a homogeneous appearance to the bowel wall (arrows). Reactive mesenteric nodes (curved arrow) are seen adjacent to thickened cecum.

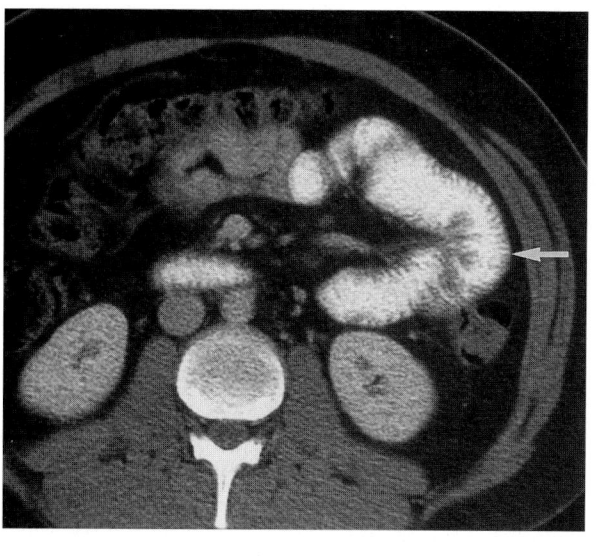
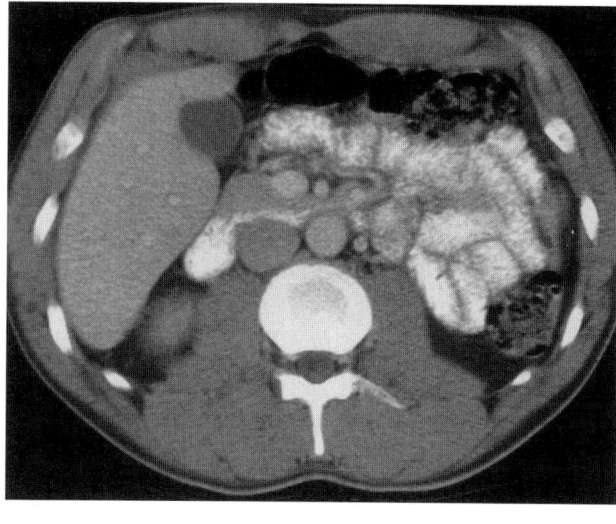

Fig. 9-7. Normal anatomy: jejunum.
(a) Small linear folds are identified within a maximally opacified jejunal loop (arrow). (b) A feathery fold pattern is present in a less distended bowel segment.

thickened, hypoattenuating layer of submucosa is seen to parallel the intestinal lumen. The double halo sign signifies the presence of an associated outer, high-attenuation ring; the target sign is used if both an inner and outer high-attenuation ring is present (Fig. 9-9). Both signs have the same clinical significance and differ only in the number of bowel layers appreciated.

The target sign was originally reported in Crohn's disease, but it is now known to be a nonspecific finding that reflects the underlying presence of submucosal edema, inflammation, or fat deposition.[1,20–22] Its

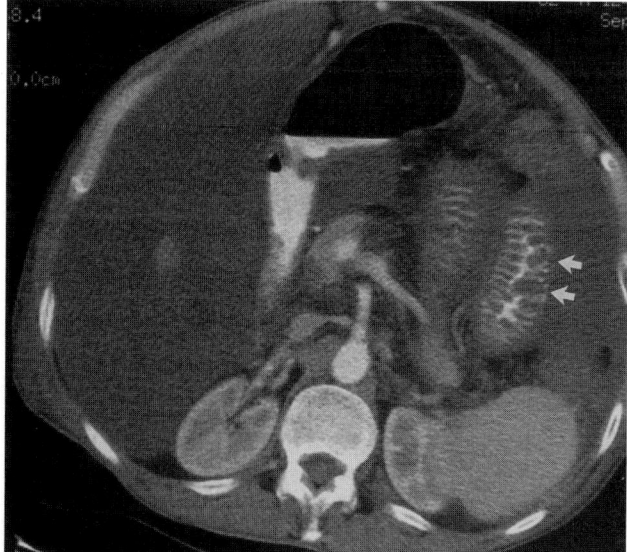

Fig. 9-8. Intestinal fold thickening.
CT scan of a 62-year-old male with cirrhosis, portal hypertension, ascites, and hypoalbuminemia reveals marked abnormal thickening of the jejunal folds (arrows).

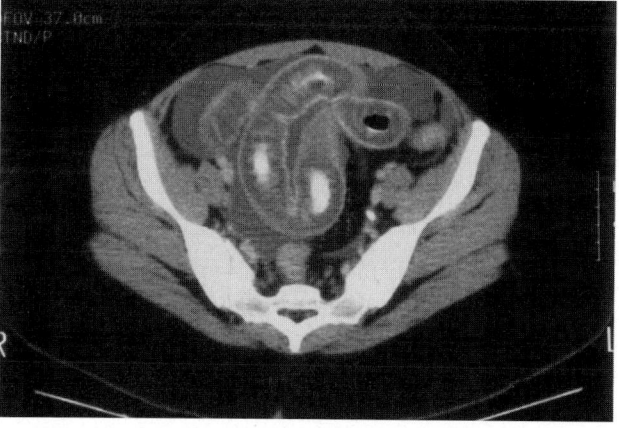

Fig. 9-9. Cross-sectional appearance of benign intestinal disease.
CT scan of a 27-year-old patient with systemic lupus erythematosis shows alternate rings of high, low, and high attenuation in a symmetrically and circumferentially thickened segment of bowel wall. Associated pelvic hemoperitoneum is present in this patient with vasculitis.

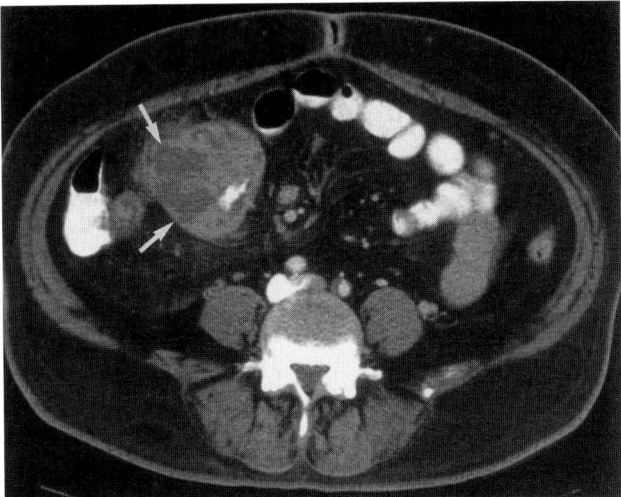

Fig. 9-10. Metastatic melanoma.
There is marked asymmetric wall thickening of the distal ileum, with luminal displacement and narrowing. Irregular regions of heterogeneous enhancement (arrows) are indicative of tumoral necrosis.

differential diagnosis in the mesenteric small bowel includes Crohn's disease, ischemia, infectious enteritis, radiation enteritis, vasculitis, graft-versus-host disease, bowel edema secondary to portal hypertension, bowel inflammation secondary to contiguous inflammatory processes, and strangulated small bowel obstruction. The importance of the target sign is that its presence nearly always signifies a benign etiology for intestinal wall thickening, making this sign one of the most useful in gastrointestinal radiology. Although scirrhous carcinomas of the stomach may demonstrate a laminated enhancement pattern, this author has never seen a malignant lesion of the small bowel display such features.[23] It must be stressed that the target sign is useful only when seen. Some benign diseases do not cause its appearance, and absence of this sign does not imply the presence of neoplastic bowel wall thickening.

Visualization of the target sign is usually dependent on performing a contrast-enhanced CT examination. It is best appreciated if the bowel is scanned during the arterial phase of enhancement when maximal contrast exists between the hyperemic mucosal and edematous submucosal bowel layers. In our experience, a 4- to 5-minute temporal window exists to image this enhancement pattern.[5] This requirement is easily met with the use of CT power injectors coupled with helical or dynamic incremental scanning techniques. The target sign can be detected on unenhanced images in patients with long-standing Crohn's disease, where mural thickening is caused by submucosal fat deposition. It is occasionally seen on unenhanced studies in the setting of severe bowel edema, but never to the same degree as on a contrast-enhanced exam.

When a region of abnormal bowel wall thickening demonstrates irregular areas of heterogeneous enhancement, one must exclude the presence of neoplastic intestinal disease (Fig. 9-10). Small primary adenocarcinomas present as focal masses that typically demonstrate uniform soft-tissue density. Larger lesions display patchy enhancement as a result of tumoral necrosis and ischemia.[24] Leiomyosarcomas (gastrointestinal stromal tumors) present as bulky, exophytic masses that arise from the muscularis or submucosal layers of the bowel wall. Tumor growth is frequently complicated by central ulceration, necrosis, and variable degrees of liquefaction. These pathologic features are manifested on CT as irregular hypoattenuating cavities, internal fluid-fluid levels, and cystic degeneration.[25] Intestinal lymphomas demonstrate a spectrum of CT appearances depending on their size, extent of mural involvement, and presence or absence of central ulceration. If extensive submucosal infiltration is present, these neoplasms demonstrate marked concentric thickening of a relatively long segment of small bowel. Interestingly, most lymphomas demonstrate homogeneous soft-tissue attenuation on contrast-enhanced CT. The malignant nature of this tumor is suggested by the degree of wall thickening (typically exceeding 1 cm), lobulated bowel contour, abrupt transition, and presence of associated adenopathy (Fig. 9-11).[26,27] A different appearance is noted

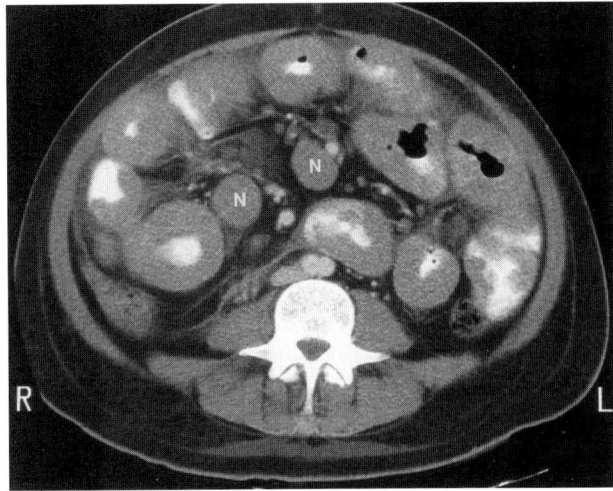

Fig. 9-11. Burkitt's lymphoma.
CT scan reveals diffuse, homogeneous, concentric thickening of the entire small bowel with associated mesenteric lymph nodes (N).

when intestinal lymphoma arises in a patient with Acquired Immune Deficiency Syndrome (AIDS). These patients have aggressive non-Hodgkin's lymphomas with highly malignant histologic subtypes.[28] Intestinal AIDS-related lymphomas present as large, heterogeneously enhancing complex masses that appear to engulf the involved bowel segment. Significant adenopathy is characteristically absent in this patient population.

Although use of intravenous contrast is strongly advocated when performing abdominal CT studies, the presence of intramural hemorrhage is best appreciated on an unenhanced examination. Mural hemorrhage presents as a segment of circumferentially thickened bowel wall that demonstrates homogeneous high attenuation (50 to 80 Hounsfield units).[29,30] The diagnosis is usually straightforward, as most patients have a known history of trauma, anticoagulation, or bleeding diathesis.

Perienteric Disease

The ability of CT to directly visualize the bowel wall, serosal surface, and perienteric fat has led to its successful application in the evaluation of extraluminal complications of intestinal disease. A confident diagnosis of extraluminal disease extension can be made by the identification of characteristic changes in the perienteric fat. These changes may be subtle in nature, and the use of thin-section scanning technique is advocated to enhance their recognition.

Perienteric inflammation increases the soft-tissue composition of the normal low-attenuation perienteric fat.[31,32] Minimal exudate appears as thin, wispy, soft-tissue density strands that approximate the bowel surface. As the severity of disease increases, the inflammation becomes more conspicuous, appearing as hazy or cloudlike regions of increased attenuation. The inflammatory process is termed a phlegmon if these cloudy regions coalesce into an ill-defined inflammatory mass. The most severe cases of inflammation are associated with fluid density collections. A spectrum of findings may be seen, ranging from poorly defined, interloop collections to encapsulated abscesses that contain gas bubbles or gas-fluid levels.

Fistulas and sinus tracts appear on CT as sharply defined, soft-tissue attenuation lines or stripes that extend from the bowel's serosal surface into the adjacent perienteric fat and mesentery.[5,32] These streaky bands can demonstrate a jagged or curvilinear course (Fig. 9-12). Identification of extraluminal air or extravasated oral contrast is confirmatory. On CT, fistulas may be hidden by the presence of matted bowel loops or significant perienteric inflammation. Barium studies re-

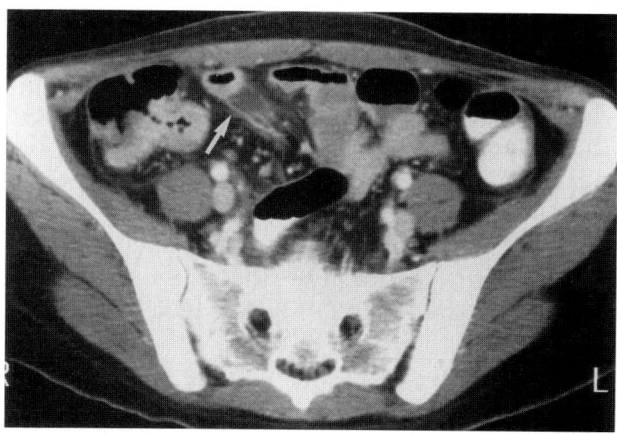

Fig. 9-12. Mesenteric sinus tract in a 23-year-old female with Crohn's disease.
A well-defined, curvilinear sinus tract (arrow) extends from the serosal surface of a circumferentially thickened ileal loop to a small mesenteric collection. Mild perienteric exudate results in increased attenuation to the bowel's subtended mesentery.

main the procedure of choice for documenting their presence and for delineating their origin and course. CT is complementary to barium examinations because of its ability to outline the full extent of fistulae and to demonstrate extension to other organs.

Changes in the perienteric fat may result from both neoplastic and inflammatory disease. Though overlap exists in the appearance of these findings, the changes due to transmural tumor extension typically appear thicker and more sharply defined compared with those seen with inflammation.[5,32] On occasion, it may be difficult to differentiate a perforated intestinal neoplasm from non-neoplastic causes of bowel wall thickening associated with perienteric inflammation. We have found the "fifty percent rule" to be helpful in such cases. This rule is based on our experience that perforated neoplasms typically demonstrate a prominent soft-tissue mass that outweighs the inflammatory component present. Inflammatory conditions, such as perforated diverticulitis, demonstrate the opposite findings. Although regions of eccentric bowel wall thickening may be seen, the degree of perienteric inflammation outweighs the degree of bowel wall thickening (soft-tissue component).

Mesenteric Disease

The small bowel mesentery functions as a suspensory ligament that connects the jejunum and ileum to the posterior abdominal wall. Derived from a reflection of the posterior parietal peritoneum, the mesentery consists of two peritoneal layers that pass forward to encase the mesenteric small bowel. Its leaves contain branches of the superior mesenteric vessels, lymphatic channels, lymph nodes, nerves, and a variable amount of fat. On CT, the mesentery appears as a fat-containing structure whose attenuation normally approximates the density of subcutaneous adipose tissue. If sufficient fat is present, the jejunal and ileal neurovascular bundles are readily appreciated and appear as round, oval, or short tubular structures (Fig. 9-13).[33]

Mesenteric lymph nodes are readily detected by CT. Normal mesenteric nodes can occasionally be seen and appear as discrete round or oval soft-tissue density masses that typically measure less than 5 mm in diameter. Mesenteric lymphadenopathy demonstrates a spectrum of CT appearances, ranging from clusters of small lymph nodes to large irregular, bulky masses.[34–36] Its presence is often a nonspecific finding. Adenopathy may exist in both benign and malignant disease, and significant overlap exists in the appearance of inflammatory and neoplastic nodes. Nevertheless, differentiation of neoplastic from nonneoplastic adenopathy may be possible in certain CT settings. Adenopathy is likely to be neoplastic in nature when a mesenteric mass exceeds 1.5 cm in size and is associated with abnormal thickening of the intestinal wall.[17] Extensive mesenteric adenopathy suggests a diagnosis of lymphoma. In particular, advanced cases of non-Hodgkin's lymphoma may demonstrate a characteristic "sandwich sign" in which large confluent soft-tissue masses encase the superior mesenteric vessels (Fig. 9-14).[35] Mesenteric carcinoid may also present with a pathognomonic appearance.

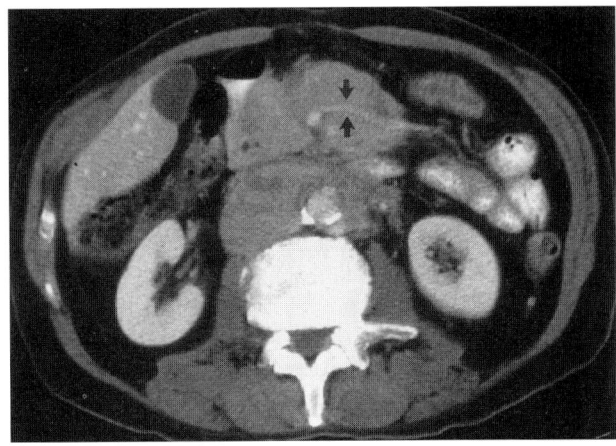

Fig. 9-14. Non-Hodgkin's lymphoma.
Extensive retroperitoneal adenopathy is present in addition to a confluent region of mesenteric adenopathy that has encased the mesenteric vasculature (arrows).

These tumors typically appear as a partially calcified, hypervascular mesenteric mass that induces an intense desmoplastic reaction.[37] This results in a retractile appearance to the mesentery with secondary angulation and tethering of adjacent small bowel loops (Fig. 9-15). The differential diagnosis for such desmoplastic changes includes desmoid tumors, metastases from scirrhous tumors (breast and pancreas carcinoma), and retractile mesenteritis.

The presence of reactive adenopathy is an important finding in the CT evaluation of patients with acute right lower quadrant pain. Enlarged mesenteric nodes may be associated with Crohn's disease, mesenteric adenitis, tuberculosis, and infectious enteritis (eg, salmonella), but are uncommonly seen in adult patients with acute appendicitis.[5] The attenuation and enhancement features of mesenteric lymph nodes can also assist in the differential diagnosis. Low-attenuation adenopathy may be seen in a variety of disorders. Mesenteric nodes in Whipple's disease may contain fat and fatty acids and demonstrate CT attenuation similar to that of adipose tissue.[38] This diagnosis is favored when low-attenuation adenopathy is seen in association with jejunal fold thickening. Characteristic lipid-fluid levels can be seen in enlarged mesenteric lymph nodes in cavitary mesenteric lymph node syndrome, a complication of hyposplenism and poorly controlled celiac disease.[39] Necrotic mesenteric adenopathy may be seen with neoplasms, particularly treated lymphomas, as well as with infection. Necrotic adenopathy in an AIDS patient suggests a diagnosis of *Mycobacterium tuberculosis* or *M avium-intracellulare* (MAI). If intestinal

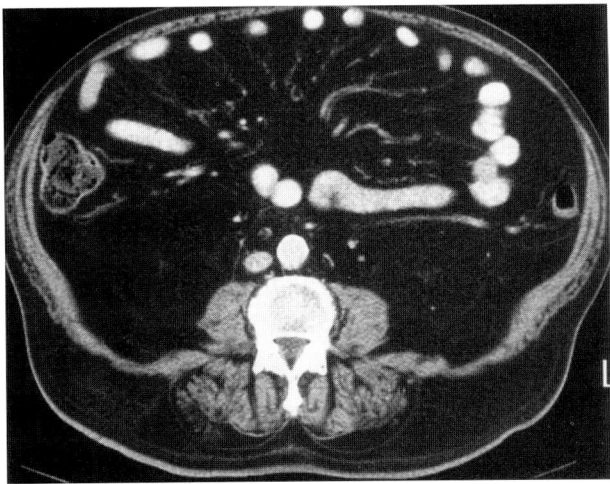

Fig. 9-13. Normal mesentery appears as a fat-containing structure traversed by vessels supplying the mesenteric intestine.

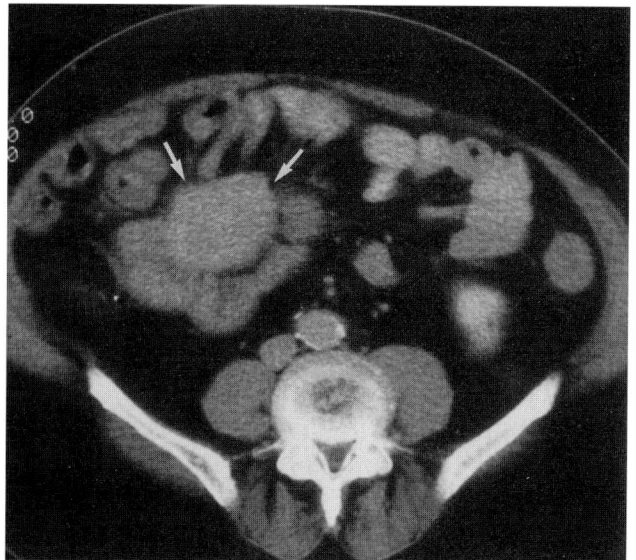 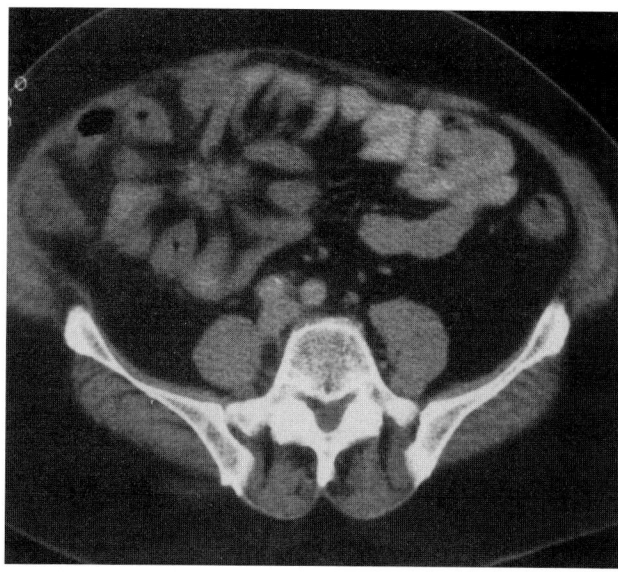

Fig. 9-15. Ileal carcinoid tumor with mesenteric spread and desmoplastic reaction.
(a) CT scan demonstrates a hypervascular mass within the ileal mesentery (arrows). (b) Tethered small bowel loops at the undersurface of the mass show a radiating, retractile appearance.

disease is present, these entities may be differentiated by the propensity of M tuberculosis to involve the ileocecal region and for MAI to produce a pseudo-Whipple's appearance that often involves the proximal mesenteric intestine.[40]

Inflammatory disease of the mesentery results in increased density to the mesenteric fat. This is commonly seen in Crohn's disease, where the mesentery can be secondarily involved by fistula, phlegmon, or abscess formation. Fibrofatty proliferation of the ileal mesentery is a characteristic finding of Crohn's disease.[6] On CT, one sees fat hypertrophy with secondary separation of right lower quadrant bowel loops (Fig. 9-16). The attenuation of the mesenteric fat may be increased due to the influx of inflammatory exudate, and hypervascularity of the vasa recta can be seen in cases of active inflammation.[41] Mesenteric lipodystrophies also result in fibrofatty proliferation; however, the jejunal mesentery is most frequently involved. A spectrum of CT findings may be seen depending on the degree of inflammation or fibrosis present. If inflammation dominates, an ill-defined region of hazy, increased density is seen within the mesentery. If significant fibrosis is present, well-defined soft-tissue masses can be seen with secondary desmoplastic retraction of bowel.[42] Mesenteric edema also presents with increased density to the mesenteric fat; however, the process is diffuse and is associated with thickening and indistinctness of the mesenteric vessels.[43] There is usually concomitant thickening of the intestinal folds and bowel wall. Though most commonly seen in systemic hypoalbuminemic states, mesenteric edema may be present with cirrhosis, nephrotic syndrome, and mesenteric venous thrombosis. If seen in the setting of closed-loop obstruction, one should exclude the complication of ischemic incarcerated bowel.[44]

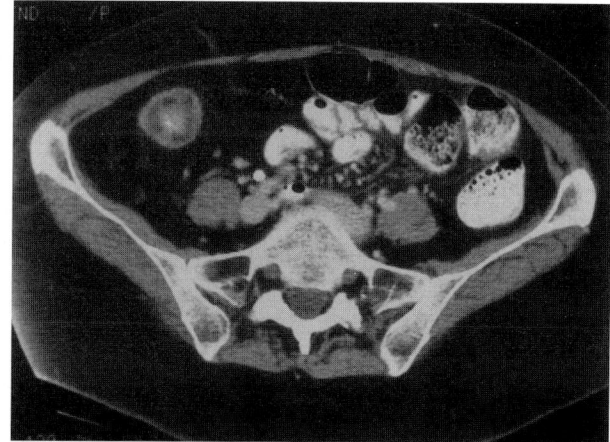

Fig. 9-16. Ileal Crohn's disease.
CT scan shows a circumferentially thickened ileal loop with a target appearance due to submucosal fat deposition. Fibrofatty proliferation has resulted in separation of this intestinal segment from adjacent bowel.

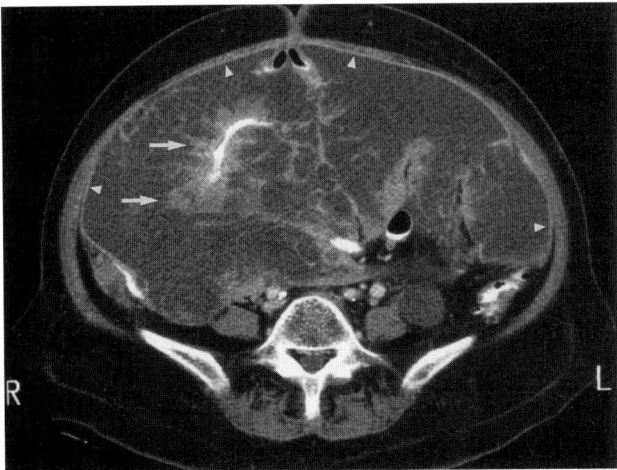

Fig. 9-17. Pseudomyxoma peritonei secondary to ovarian cystadenocarcinoma.
CT scan reveals complex ascites characterized by thickened septations within the ascites, thickened enhancing peritoneal surfaces (arrowheads), and soft-tissue implants along the serosal surface of an ileal bowel loop (arrows).

Peritoneal Disease

Peritoneal fluid collections are well demonstrated by CT. Simple ascites characteristically presents as low-attenuation fluid that measures between 0 and 20 Hounsfield units. Exudative and hemorrhagic collections usually demonstrate higher attenuation because the CT density of fluid rises with increasing protein content. Despite these general rules, the CT attenuation values of benign and malignant ascites overlap and it is therefore difficult to characterize the underlying cause of ascites on the basis of CT density alone.[45,46] Helpful findings include the distribution of bowel and peritoneal fluid. Patients with large amounts of free ascites present with free-floating, centrally located small bowel loops that approximate the anterior abdominal wall. Significant accumulation of fluid within the lesser sac is rarely seen with benign ascites unless a local etiologic factor exists (eg, pancreatitis). In contrast, the small bowel does not float freely and may appear tethered to the posterior abdominal wall in patients with malignant ascites. Malignant ascites may also present with significant accumulations of fluid in both the greater and lesser peritoneal sacs.[47]

Loculated ascites is a nonspecific finding that can result from both benign and malignant adhesions. If seen, one must exclude the presence of pseudomyxoma peritonei, which can present in similar fashion. Pseudomyxoma peritonei occurs secondary to rupture of a primary mucin-producing cystadenocarcinoma of the appendix or ovary or following rupture of a metastatic, cystic, mucin-producing peritoneal implant.[36] The CT manifestations of this uncommon condition reflect the amount of gelatinous material present within the peritoneal cavity. Advanced cases

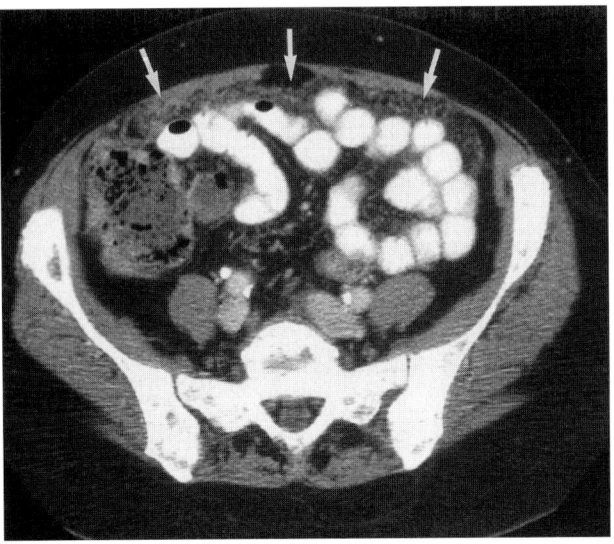

(a)

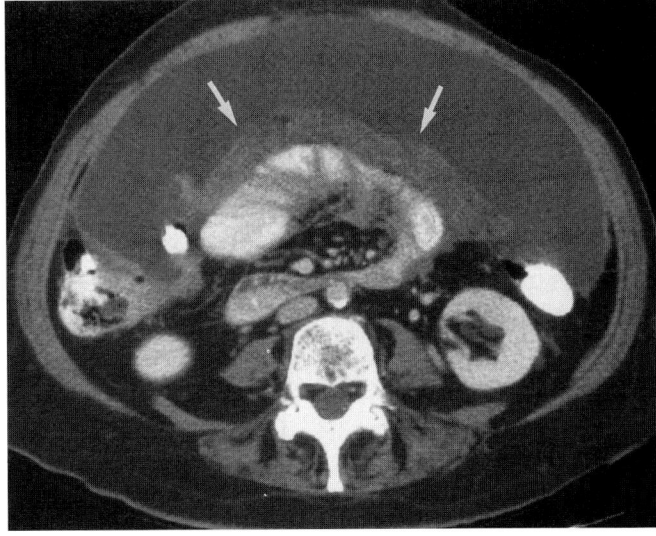

(b)

Fig. 9-18. Peritoneal seeding in ovarian carcinoma.
(a) Early peritoneal implants presenting as reticulonodular studding of the greater omentum (arrows). (b) CT scan in a patient with advanced disease shows omental caking (arrows) and posteriorly tethered small bowel loops.

manifest voluminous ascites, thickened septations within the ascites, and associated scalloping of the liver contour (Fig. 9-17).[48]

A diagnosis of malignant ascites is best made when ascitic fluid is seen in association with peritoneal implants and metastases to the solid abdominal organs. In cases of early peritoneal seeding, CT may demonstrate a fine reticular or reticulonodular appearance to the greater omentum and peritoneal surfaces. In advanced cases, these nodules coalesce into confluent soft-tissue masses that replace the omental fat and appear as "omental cakes" (Fig. 9-18). Though peritoneal implants are typically of soft-tissue density, these may calcify or appear cystic depending on the histology of the underlying neoplasm. Serosal implants may be predicted by identifying mural thickening adjacent to a solid or cystic peritoneal nodule.[32] The differential diagnosis of peritoneal carcinomatosis includes severe tuberculous peritonitis and peritoneal histoplasmosis.[49,50] Unlike bacterial and fungal peritonitis, which result in generalized thickening of the peritoneal surfaces, these infections may produce focal nodularity of the peritoneum as seen with metastatic disease.

References

1. Balthazar EJ. CT of the gastrointestinal tract: principles and interpretation. *AJR.* 1991;156:23–32.
2. Rubin GD, Beaulieu CF, Argiro V, et al. Perspective volume rendering of CT and MR images: applications for endoscopic imaging. *Radiology.* 1996;199:321–330.
3. Hara AK, Johnson CD, Reed JE, et al. Colorectal polyp detection with CT colography: two- versus three-dimensional techniques. *Radiology.* 1996;200:49–54.
4. Megibow AJ, Zerhouni EA. Techniques of gastrointestinal CT. In: Megibow AJ, Balthazar EJ, eds. *Computed Tomography of the Gastrointestinal Tract.* St. Louis, Mo: CV Mosby, Co; 1986:1–31.
5. Megibow AJ. Computed tomography of the gastrointestinal tract: techniques and principles of interpretation. In: Gore RM, Levine MS, Laufer I, eds. *Textbook of Gastrointestinal Radiology.* Philadelphia, Pa: WB Saunders Co, 1993:103–112.
6. Gore RM, Balthazar EJ, Gharemani GG, et al. CT features of ulcerative colitis and Crohn's disease. *AJR.* 1996;167:3–15.
7. Thoeni RF, Filson RG. Abdominal and pelvic CT: use of oral metoclopromide to enhance bowel opacification. *Radiology.* 1988;169:391–393.
8. Raptopoulos V, Davis MA, Smith EH. Imaging of the bowel wall. Computed tomography and fat density oral-contrast agent in an animal model. *Invest Radiol* 1986;21:847–850.
9. Raptopoulos V, Davis MA, Davidoff A, et al. Fat density oral contrast agent for abdominal CT. *Radiology.* 1987;164:653–656.
10. Raptopoulos V, Davidoff A, Karellas A, et al. CT of the pancreas with a fat-density oral contrast regimen. *AJR.* 1988;150:1303–1306.
11. Winter TC, Arger JD, Nghiem HV, et al. Upper gastrointestinal tract and abdomen: water as an oral administered contrast agent for helical CT. *Radiology.* 1996;201:365–370.
12. Megibow AJ, Zerhouni EA, Hulnick DA, et al. Air insufflation of the colon as an adjunct to computed tomography of the pelvis. *J Comput Assist Tomogr.* 1984;8:797–800.
13. Karantanas AH, Tsianos EB, Kontogiannis DS, et al. CT demonstration of normal gastric wall thickness: the value of administering gas-producing and paralytic agents. *Comput Med Imaging Graph.* 1988;12:333–337.
14. Klein HM, Gunther RW. Double contrast small bowel follow-through with an acid-resistant effervescent agent. *Invest Radiol.* 1993;28:581–585.
15. Balthazar EJ, Gordon R, Hulnick DH. Ileocecal tuberculosis: CT and radiologic evaluation. *AJR.* 1990;154:499–503.
16. Megibow AJ, Balthazar EJ, Hulnick DH. Radiology of nonneoplastic gastrointestinal disorders in acquired immune deficiency syndrome. *Semin Roentgenol.* 1987;22:31–41.
17. James S, Balfe DM, Lee JKT, et al. Small-bowel disease: categorization by CT examination. *AJR.* 1987;148:863–868.
18. Bender GN, Timmons JH, Williard WC, et al. Computed tomographic enteroclysis—one methodology. *Invest Radiol.* 1996;31:43–49.
19. Desai RK, Tagliabue JR, Wegryn SA, et al. CT evaluation of wall thickening in the alimentary track. *Radiographics.* 1991;11:771–783.
20. Megibow AJ. Imaging insights in gastrointestinal radiology. The target sign. *Radiol Soc North Am Today.* 1990;4:1.
21. Frager, DH, Goldman M, Beneventano TC. Computed tomography in Crohn's disease. *J Comput Assist Tomogr.* 1983;7:819–824.
22. Jones B, Fishman EK, Hamilton SR, et al. Submucosal accumulation of fat in inflammatory bowel disease: CT/pathologic correlation. *J Comput Assist Tomogr.* 1986;10:759–763.
23. Balthazar EJ, Siegel SE, Megibow AJ, et al. CT in patients with scirrhous carcinoma of the GI tract: imaging findings and value for tumor detection and staging. *AJR.* 1995;165:839–845.
24. Balthazar EJ, Megibow AJ, Hulnick DH, et al. Carcinoma of the colon: detection and preoperative staging by CT. *AJR.* 1988;150:301–306.
25. Megibow AJ, Balthazar EJ, Hulnick DH, et al. CT evaluation of gastrointestinal leiomyomas and leiomyosarcomas. *AJR.* 1985;144:727–731.
26. Megibow AJ, Balthazar EJ, Naidich DP, et al. Computed tomography of gastrointestinal lymphoma. *AJR.* 1983;141:541–547.
27. Dudiak KM, Johnson CD, Stephens DH. Primary tumors of the small intestine: CT evaluation. *AJR.* 1989;152:995–998.

28. Nyberg DA, Jeffrey RB, Federle MP, et al. AIDS related lymphomas: evaluation by abdominal CT. *Radiology.* 1986;159:59–63.
29. Plojoux O, Hauser H, Wettstein P. Computed tomography of intramural hematoma of the small intestine: a report of 3 cases. *Radiology.* 1982;144:559–561.
30. Balthazar EJ, Hulnick D, Megibow AJ, et al. Computed tomography of intramural hemorrhage and bowel ischemia. *J Comput Assist Tomogr.* 1987;11:67–72.
31. Hulnick DH. Small intestine. In: Megibow AJ, Balthazar EJ, eds. *Computed Tomography of the Gastrointestinal Tract.* St. Louis, Mo: CV Mosby Co;1986:217–278.
32. Megibow AJ. Imaging insights in gastrointestinal radiology. Perienteric changes—signs and significance in abdominal CT. *Radiol Soc North Am Today.* 1990;4:5.
33. Thoeni RF, Moss AA. The gastrointestinal tract. In: Moss AA, Gamsu G, Genant HK, eds. *Computed Tomography of the Body with Magnetic Resonance.* 2nd ed. Philadelphia, Pa: WB Saunders Co; 1993:643–734.
34. Bernardino ME, Jing BS, Wallace S. Computed tomography diagnosis of mesenteric masses. *AJR.* 1979;132:33–36.
35. Mueller PR, Ferrucci JT Jr, Harbin WP, et al. Appearance of lymphomatous involvement of the mesentery of ultrasonography and body computed tomography: the "sandwich sign." *Radiology.* 1980;134:467–473.
36. Jeffrey RB Jr. The peritoneal cavity and mesentery. In: Moss AA, Gamsu G, Genant HK, eds. *Computed Tomography of the Body with Magnetic Resonance Imaging.* 2nd ed. Philadelphia, Pa: WB Saunders Co; 1993:1139–1181.
37. Seigel RS, Kuhns LR, Borlaza GS, et al. Computed tomography and angiography in ileal carcinoid tumor and retractile mesenteritis. *Radiology.* 1980;134:437–440.
38. Li DKB, Rennie CS. Abdominal computed tomography in Whipple's disease. *J Comput Assist Tomogr.* 1981;5:249–252.
39. Holmes GKT. Mesenteric lymph node cavitation in coeliac disease. *Gut.* 1986;27:728–733.
40. Vincent ME, Robbins AH. Mycobacterium avium-intracellulare complex enteritis: pseudo-Whipple's disease in AIDS. *AJR.* 1985;144:921–922.
41. Meyers MA, McGuire PV. Spiral CT demonstration of hypervascularity in Crohn's disease: "vascular jejunization of the ileum" or the "comb sign." *Abdom Imaging.* 1995;20:327–332.
42. Katz ME, Heiken JP, Glazer HS, et al. Intraabdominal panniculitis: clinical, radiographic and CT features. *AJR.* 1985;145:293–296.
43. Silverman PM, Baker ME, Cooper C, et al. CT appearance of diffuse mesenteric edema. *J Comput Assist Tomogr.* 1986;10:67–70.
44. Balthazar EJ, Birnbaum BA, Megibow AJ, et al. Closed-loop and strangulating intestinal obstruction: CT signs. *Radiology.* 1992;185:769–775.
45. Bydder GM, Kreel L. Attenuation values of fluid collections within the abdomen. *J Comput Assist Tomogr.* 1980;4:145–150.
46. Haaga JR. The peritoneum and mesentery. In: Haaga JR, Alfidi RJ, eds. *Computed Tomography of the Whole Body.* 2nd ed. St. Louis, Mo: CV Mosby Co; 1988;1137–1199.
47. Gore RM, Callen PW, Filly RA. Lesser sac fluid in predicting the etiology of ascites. *AJR.* 1982;142:701–705.
48. Mayes GB, Chuang VP, Fisher RG. CT of pseudomyxoma peritonei. *AJR.* 1981;136:807–810.
49. Hanson RD, Hunter TB. Tuberculous peritonitis: CT appearance. *AJR.* 1985;144:931–932.
50. Alterman DD, Cho KC. Histoplasmosis involving the omentum in an AIDS patient: CT demonstration. *J Comput Assist Tomogr.* 1988;12:664–665.

Magnetic Resonance Imaging for Small-Bowel-Related Diagnosis
Contrast Agents and MR Angiographic Techniques

Evan S. Siegelman and Pablo R. Ros

Chapter Contents

Introduction
Technique
Contrast Agents
Clinical Applicants of Oral Contrast Agents for the Small Bowel
Conclusions

Introduction

The small bowel is the only portion of the gastrointestinal (GI) tract that is still primarily studied radiologically since, except for the duodenum, it is difficult to evaluate endoscopically. Traditionally, radiological examination of the small bowel has been performed by fluoroscopy (small bowel series and enteroclysis) using barium opacification. However, the use of cross-sectional abdominal imaging techniques (ultrasound [US], computed tomography [CT], and magnetic resonance [MR] imaging) is increasing, with a concomitant decrease in fluoroscopically guided barium examinations.[1]

MR imaging represents a powerful imaging tool, with its superb soft-tissue contrast and direct multiplanar imaging, as well as lack of ionizing radiation. MR can show the nonmucosal portions of the small bowel and detect extraluminal disease.[2] However, the application of MR imaging to the small bowel has lagged behind US and CT due to a number of technical limitations. These include limited signal to noise, motion artifacts resulting from a combination of long imaging times and physiologic motion due to respiration and peristalsis, and, finally, lack of suitable oral contrast agents. Finally, the current financial climate within health care delivery dictates that a new imaging tool should clearly demonstrate its superiority compared to existing methods regarding not only clinical efficacy, but also cost-effectiveness.

The development of fast imaging techniques has solved for the major part the problem of motion artifact. Breath-hold sequences for T1-[3–5] and T2-weighted[6–8] images are now widely available, minimizing motion artifacts. In addition, the development of phased-array coils for the abdomen[9–11] and pelvis[12] have markedly improved the signal-to-noise ratio, allowing for the use of smaller field-of-view, thinner slices, and thus higher-resolution images. The last obstacle, absence of oral contrast agents, has given rise to a particularly active area of clinical research, with a wide variety of oral MR imaging contrast agents being investigated, approved, or available for clinical use. Therefore, with the appropriate technique, MR imaging can be a useful technique for studying a number of disorders of the small bowel.

Technique

Although there are no definitive recommendations for the optimum MR imaging protocol to image the small bowel, due to variations of the different commercial units available and individual radiologists' preferences, there are some general principles that can be applied. A comprehensive MR examination of the small bowel usually requires both T1- and T2-weighted images. As stated, the choice of sequences depends upon equipment, available software, personal preferences, and experience, as well as the region being imaged (the duodenum, the pelvic small bowel, etc), and the clinical questions to be answered.

The use of an antiperistaltic agent such as glucagon, hyoscine butylbromide, or dicyclomine has also been advocated[13,14] and one of us (ESS) routinely uses intramuscular glucagon when performing abdominal and pelvic MR examinations (Fig. 10-1). Currently, we only occasionally use one of the intraluminal contrast agents described below, due to advances in fast imaging, half Fourier transformation, and cost of the approved oral contrast agents. However, in certain situations (see below), oral contrast agents may be of clinical value.

Contrast Agents

As in CT of the abdomen, there is a potential need with MR imaging to use an appropriate luminal contrast agent to allow differentiation of the normal GI tract from adjacent normal organs and extraluminal pathology. The mechanisms for achieving contrast with intraluminal GI contrast agents for MR imaging are quite different from the ones in CT, since instead of altering the absorption of X-ray photons there is a need with MR imaging to alter the proton environment within the bowel.

The ideal MR bowel contrast agent has to comply with certain requirements, such as palatability, safety, low cost, effectiveness with both T1- and T2-weighted pulse sequences, and homogeneous distribution throughout the GI tract with reliable bowel marking and preferably some degree of bowel distention.[15] An ideal bowel agent would not stimulate peristalsis, cause MR artifacts, or be absorbed from the gut.

A multitude of contrast agents have been investigated and found safe, palatable, and efficacious. Reviews of the different kinds of bowel contrast agents[16–18] have all suggested that an MR exam of the small bowel may be optimized with the use of intraluminal contrast (Fig. 10-2). However, to date an ideal and universally available agent has yet to find widespread clinical use.[19] Key areas to be outlined are the duodenum (which allows an improved visualization of the pancreatic head) and pelvic small bowel, where differentiation between normal bowel segments and adenopathy can be difficult without an intraluminal contrast agent, especially when using MR systems that cannot perform breath-hold imaging (Fig. 10-3).

GI contrast agents can be classified as positive or negative, depending upon the resultant increase or decrease of the signal intensity of the intraluminal bowel contents.[18] Some agents display biphasic characteristics, acting as both positive and negative contrast agents depending on concentration and imaging parameters.[18] At high concentration and long TE (echo delay time), the T2 effects of a biphasic agent may dominate to produce low-signal-intensity luminal con-

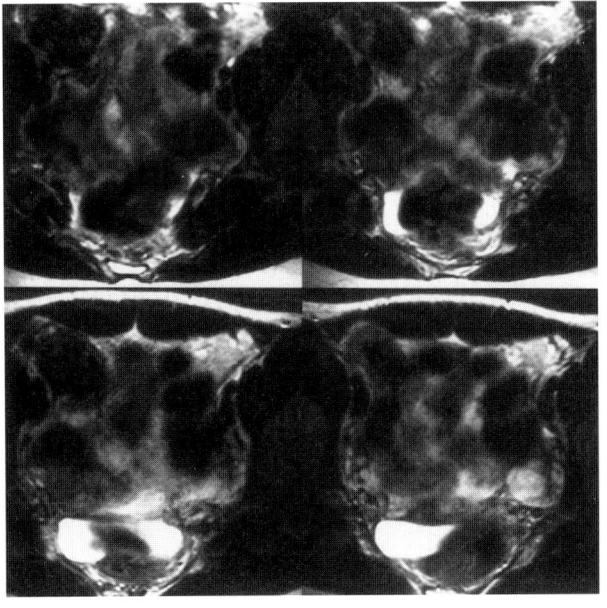

(a)

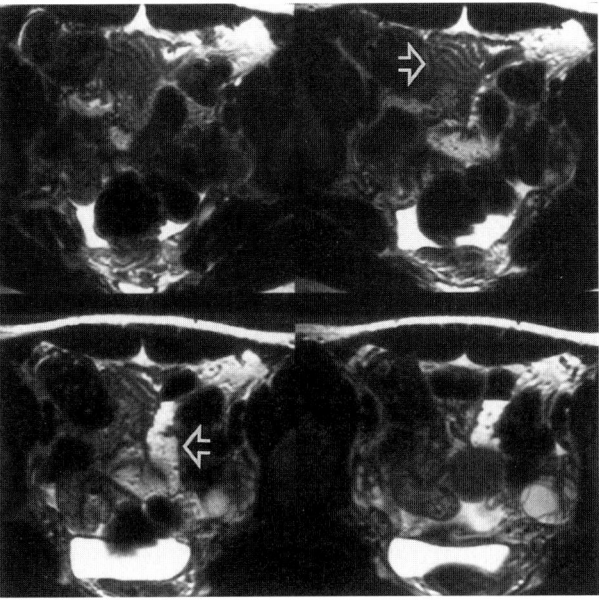

(b)

Fig. 10-1. The value of glucagon in a 16-year-old girl without bowel disease.
Four consecutive axial T2-weighted fast spin echo images obtained before (a) and after (b) the intramuscular administration of glucagon. No contrast agent was given orally. Once peristalsis is eliminated, the small bowel (arrows) becomes well delineated.

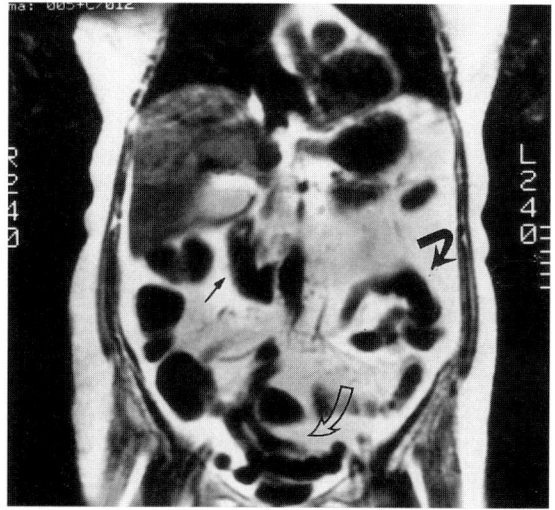 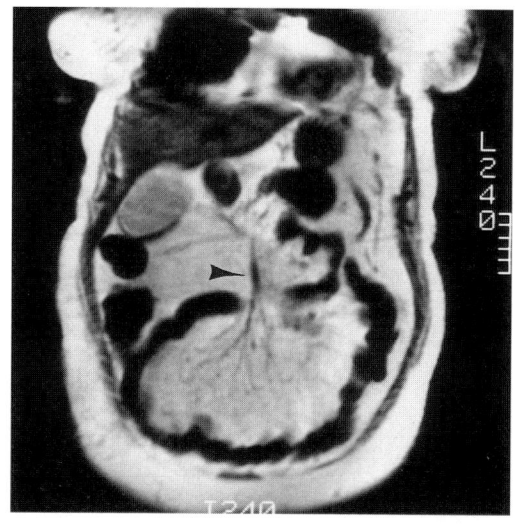

Fig. 10-2. Coronal demonstration of duodenum, jejunum, and ileum.
(a) After administration of a negative oral contrast material, coronal T1-weighted spin echo (SE) image allows clear depiction of the duodenum (small arrow), jejunum (curved arrow), and ileum (open arrow). (b) Section, slightly more anterior than A, demonstrates the superior mesenteric artery (SMA) branching into the mesentery (arrowhead) that appears bordered by jejunal loops. There is no resultant susceptibility artifact from the contrast material.

tents, with the converse occurring at low concentration and short TE. A classic example for this mixed behavior contrast agent is manganese chloride and substances containing significant quantities of manganese such as blueberry juice and green tea.[20,21]

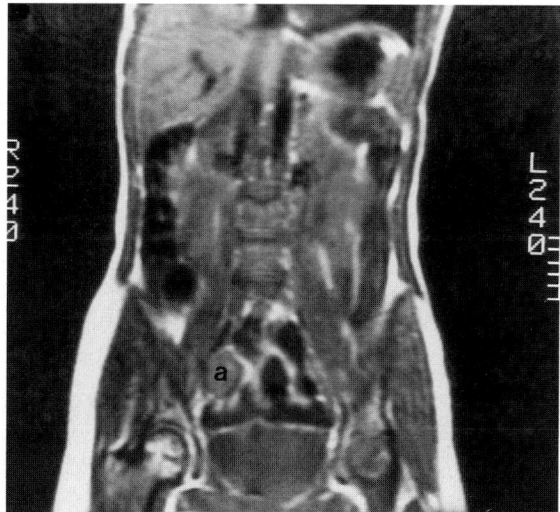

Fig. 10-3. Pelvic small bowel.
Coronal T1-weighted SE image of a woman with cervical cancer demonstrates after administration of a 60% wt/wt barium solution good marking of multiple pelvic bowel loops. This allows the visualization of right pelvic adenopathy (a) that cannot be confused with a loop of pelvic bowel.

Oral contrast agents can be further classified into miscible or immiscible with water. The former mix with bowel contents to alter the signal, while the latter act by displacing the bowel contents. Miscible agents are susceptible to concentration-dependent changes in signal intensity due to varying dilutions in different segments of the bowel. Immiscible agents usually need to be given in large volumes as they need to displace bowel contents in order to achieve their contrast effect.[22]

Positive contrast agents increase intraluminal signal by either a paramagnetic T1-shortening effect or by having intrinsically short T1-relaxation times. Paramagnetic agents are more common than short T1 agents. A variety of paramagnetic agents have been tested, such as ferric ammonium citrate (FAC) (Fig. 10-4), gadolinium solutions, manganese chloride (Fig. 10-5), and substances containing significant quantities of manganese (blueberry juice and green tea). FAC has been available as a dietary iron supplement since the early development of MR imaging in the 1980s as Geritol (Beechman; Bristol, Tenn). However, this formulation contains a large amount of ethanol, making it unsuitable for use as a contrast agent. Oral agents containing FAC (eg, Oral Magnetic Resonance—Onomembrane; Seattle, Wash) have been shown to be efficacious on T1-weighted images[23–25] but prone to motion-induced "ghost" artifacts due to peristalsis.[26] This is a frequent problem with all positive agents that can be minimized with the administration of an an-

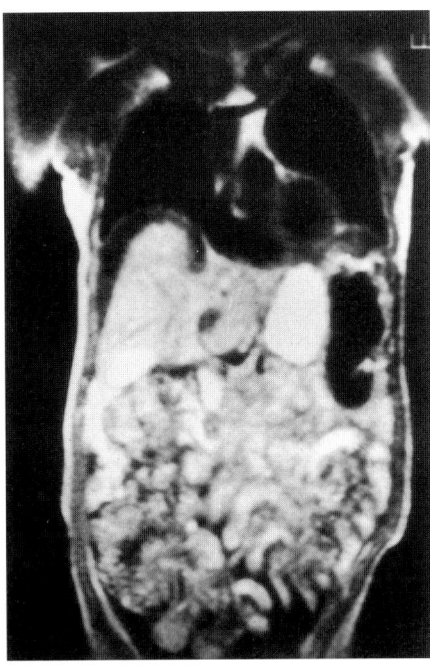

Fig. 10-4. Ferric ammonium citrate (FAC).
Coronal T1-weighted SE image after the oral administration of FAC demonstrates good distribution of this positive contrast agent with resultant high signal intensity of the stomach and small bowel.

tiperistaltic agent, such as glucagon and/or the use of breath-hold imaging sequences.[26–28]

Gadolinium chelate solutions (gadolinium-DTPA) have a biphasic action, but are predominantly positive contrast agents.[28,29] To counteract dilutional and concentrational effects, gadolinium chelate solutions are sometimes administered with Mannitol (Abbott Laboratories, Chicago, IL), which increases osmolality and reduces water absorption.[30–32] Oral gadolinium contrast agents have reported side effects that are primarily related to osmotic load of the Mannitol or to the antiperistaltic agent, which have to be given concomitantly to minimize motion artifact.[28] A recently published multicenter trial of a gadolinium-containing oral suspension that used neither Mannitol nor an antispasmodic agent showed good patient tolerance and increased diagnostic accuracy of the post-contrast scans.[33]

Manganese chloride is another biphasic agent that results in increased signal intensity on T1-weighted images and decreased signal on T2-weighted images (Fig. 10-5).[34] A manganese chloride formulation has been commercially available (Lumenhance, Bracco Pharmaceuticals; Princeton, NJ). Manganese is found also as an ingredient in natural products, such as blueberry juice and green tea.[21]

Short T1–relaxation time luminal contrast agents include mineral oil, oil emulsions, and sucrose polyester.[35,36] Of these, corn oil emulsions have been the

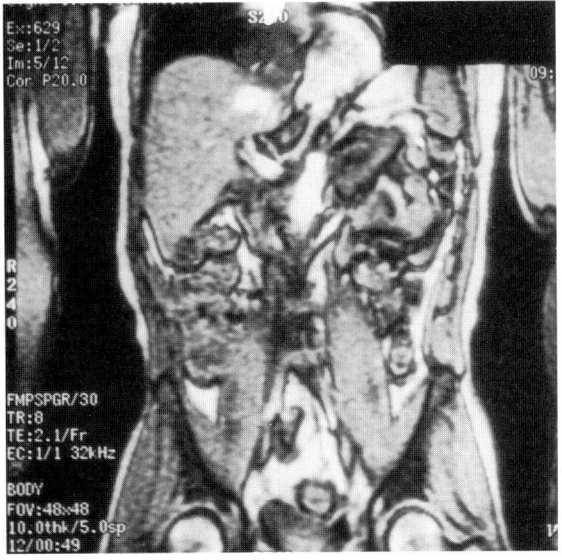
(a)

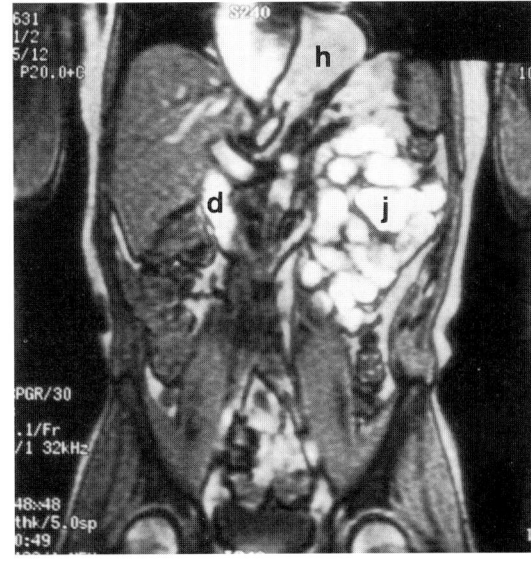
(b)

Fig. 10-5. Manganese chloride solution.
Coronal T1-weighted spoiled gradient echo images before (a) and after (b) the administration of a manganese chloride solution. After contrast administration, the duodenum (d) and the jejunum (j) appear clearly delineated with this biphasic contrast agent that is positive on T1-weighted images. A hiatal hernia (h) is present.

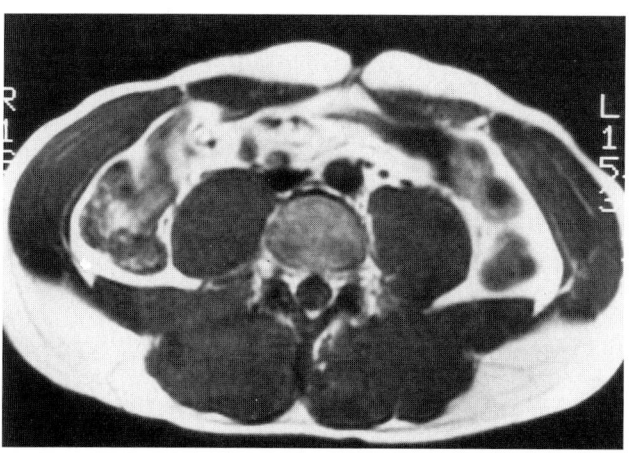 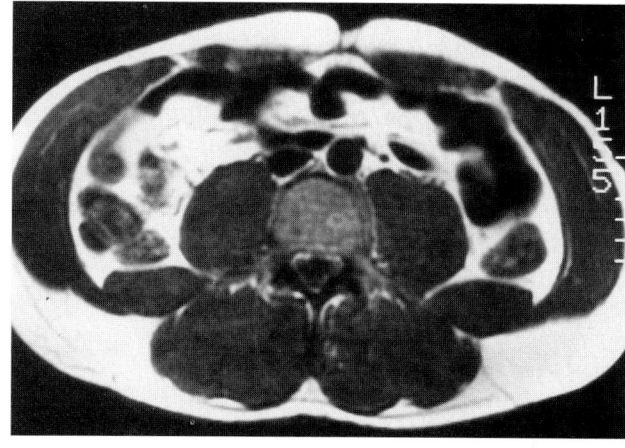

(a) (b)

Fig. 10-6. Superparamagnetic iron oxide solutions.
T1-weighted SE image at the level of the umbilicus, before (a) and after (b) administration of Gastromark. There is satisfactory distension and resultant low signal intensity of multiple small bowel segments after contrast administration.

most successfully tested (once blended with milk and ice cream), producing a positive contrast in both T1- and T2-weighted images.[18] In addition, a variety of nutritional support formulas and baby foods have been used as bowel markers, which have the advantages of low cost, excellent safety profile, and widespread availability.[37,38] In these cases, positive enhancement is present on both T1- and T2-weighted images due to a combination of lipids and paramagnetic trace elements in these solutions. A major disadvantage is partial intestinal absorption, resulting in heterogeneous distribution and irregular intestinal passage of the agent.[37]

Negative contrast agents have been, to date, the most successful intraluminal MR imaging agents. Negative GI contrast can be divided into three groups: 1) superparamagnetic iron oxide (SPIO) solutions, 2) diamagnetic agents, and 3) perfluorocarbons and gases. The first two are water-miscible, while the third group is immiscible. A clear advantage of this group of contrast is the reduction in severity of motion-induced artifacts from peristalsis secondary to the resultant decrease of intraluminal signal intensity.[39,40] To date, several SPIO solutions have been investigated, and some are available for clinical use—in Europe, Oral Magnetic Particles, or OMP (Abdoscan; Nycomed, Oslo, Norway) and in the US, Gastromark (Mallinckrodt; St. Louis, Mo). SPIO solutions act by creating local magnetic field inhomogeneities that lead to proton dephasing and resultant decrease in intraluminal signal intensity.[23,41–52] Both Gastromark and OMP particles have been proven to be clinically efficacious and generally well tolerated, with mild side effects of nausea and diarrhea in about 5% of patients (Figs. 10-2, 10-6).[18] Although SPIO solutions are effective in all pulse sequences, a significant amount of susceptibility artifacts on T2*-weighted gradient images has been reported primarily with OMP likely due to particle aggregation.[50] The current formulations (such as Gastromark) have a more viscous carrier matrix, resulting in minimal or no susceptibility artifacts. An alternative approach to minimize susceptibility artifacts has been to combine iron oxide solutions with barium sulfate or methylcellulose suspensions, resulting in a combination of superparamagnetic and diamagnetic contrast effects that lead to a cancellation of positive and negative susceptibility components.[53,54]

Diamagnetic contrast agents correspond to barium sulfate suspensions and clay compounds.[55–57] Clay compounds, such as kaolin and bentonite, are low-cost contrast agents, which may be found as food additives. Although they produce both T1 and T2 shortening, the T2-shortening effect predominates.[18] A problem associated with clay compounds is poor palatability and constipation.

Barium sulfate has been the most widely evaluated negative contrast agent.[58–63] It has several advantages, including a very well known safety and tolerance record based on over 50 year's experience of its use as a GI contrast agent, its wide availability, and low cost. A further advantage is that MR imaging can be performed following a small bowel series or enteroclysis, a situation where CT is often precluded.[60] The mechanism of action is a combination of T2 shortening due to diamagnetic susceptibility effects and replacement of intraluminal water by barium suspension, thus decreasing proton density.[18,60] The best results are achieved with high-density barium (larger than 60% wt/wt), with typical volumes of 600 to 900 ml given orally (Fig. 10-7).[64] Lower concentrations of barium have been shown to exhibit positive contrast effects, particularly in gradient-echo images. Also, a combination of a low barium concentration with either SPIO particles or a diamagnetic clay (eg, bentonite) results in a synergistic effect such that negative contrast is maintained on T1- and T2-weighted images.[54] The use of these less concentrated barium preparations increases patient tolerance.[18]

Perfluorocarbon and gases (such as air or carbon dioxide) reduce intraluminal signal by a third mechanism different from superparamagnetic and diamagnetic effects. Perfluorocarbons and gases decrease intraluminal signal by displacing normal bowel contents with contrast that lacks mobile protons and thus produce no MR signal.[65]

Perfluorocarbons are organic compounds in which protons have been replaced by fluorine, resulting in virtually absent signal in all pulsing sequences.[65] Perflubron ([imagent GI], Alliance Pharmaceuticals; San Diego, Calif) was approved by the Food and Drug Administration in October 1994. Due to its high cost, it was withdrawn from the market in 1996. Perflubron is an odorless, tasteless liquid with a very low surface tension that has therefore a rapid transit time through the bowel, reaching the colon in about 30 minutes.[66] Perflubron is an excellent intraluminal contrast agent that has the ability to insinuate itself through fistula tracts and partially obstructed bowel segments.[67] Perflubron constitutes an important example of how an excellent contrast material was removed from the market due to high cost and subsequent lack of use.[67–70]

Gas in the form of air or carbon dioxide can be introduced in the GI tract.[71] So far, its use has been described only in the stomach or rectum, distending the bowel and creating a negative contrast effect.[72,73] Antiperistaltic agents have to be used due to a tendency for gas to induce peristalsis. Due to limited anatomical coverage and difficulty in controlling the distribution of the contrast agent, gas has not been extensively used for the study of the small bowel. Using rectal insufflation or air with reflux into the small bowel, Chou and colleagues have used MR to establish the location and etiology of distal small bowel obstructions.[74]

In summary, there is a wide gamut of luminal contrast agents for MR imaging, each with varying properties and its own advantages and disadvantages. The choice of contrast agent may depend on the particular clinical situation, suspected pathology, region of the bowel to be imaged, and pulse sequences to be used. The major choices for the radiologists are between the two negative contrast agents that are commercially available—that is, barium compounds and iron oxide (Gastromark) solutions—or to simply attempt to image the patient with an antiperistaltic agent alone.

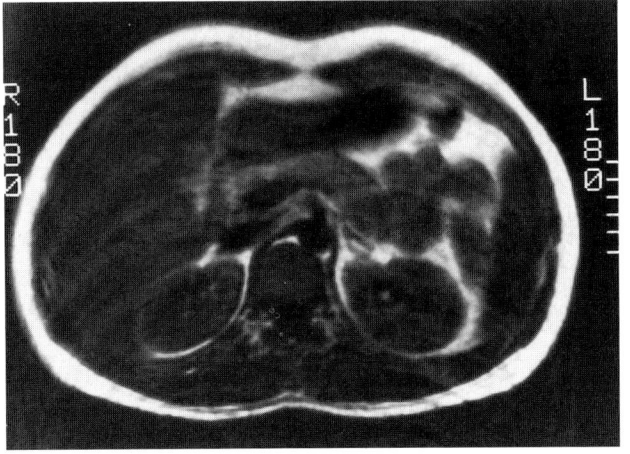
(a)

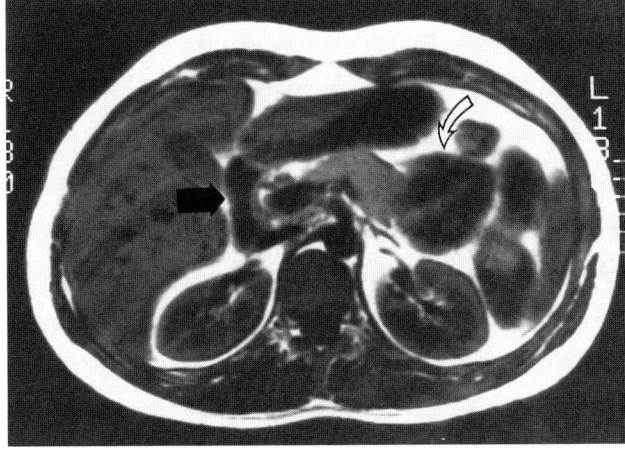
(b)

Fig. 10-7. Duodenum and jejunum before and after barium administration.
T1-weighted SE images before (a) and after (b) the administration of a high-density barium solution demonstrate how the duodenum (arrow) and proximal jejunum (curved arrow) can be visualized. Note how after barium administration the duodenal wall can be seen and the pancreas and kidneys are better identified.

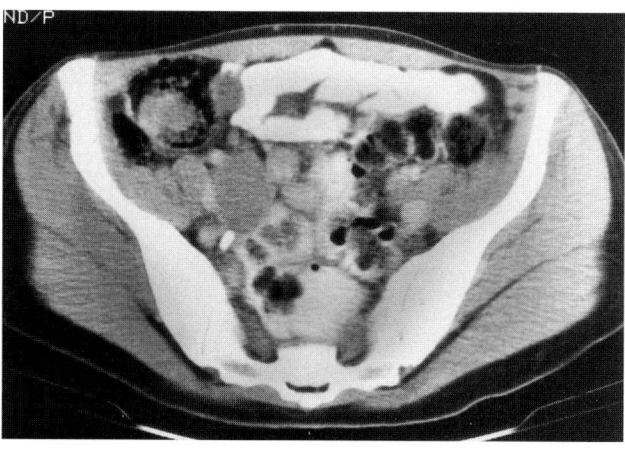 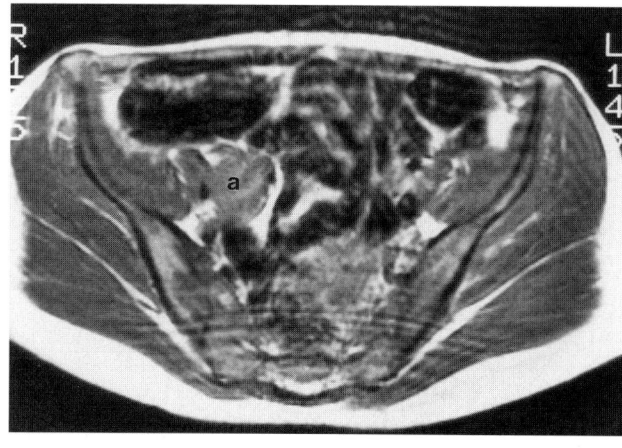

(a) (b)

Fig. 10-8. Pelvic adenopathy, CT versus MR imaging.
(a) In this standard CT section of the pelvis, it is difficult to differentiate what is adenopathy versus poorly opacified bowel. (b) T2-weighted SE image after administration of a negative contrast material (Gastromark) demonstrates only right iliac adenopathy (a). With the use of negative contrast agents the entire small bowel is well opacified, eliminating the common confusion in CT between pathology and poorly opacified loops of bowel.

Clinical Applications of Oral Contrast Agents for the Small Bowel

The applications of MR imaging of the small bowel with the optional use of oral contrast agents can be divided into three categories: 1) to differentiate normal small bowel from adenopathy (Fig. 10-8),[75] 2) to better appreciate parenteric masses (ie, pancreatic, mesenteric, and omental neoplasms and peritoneal carcinomatosis (Fig. 10-9),[58,59,76] and 3) to better define intrinsic small bowel pathology (Figs. 10-10, 10-11), including neoplasms,[77] inflammatory bowel disease (Figs. 10-12, 10-13),[66,78–87] and fistulous tracts (Fig. 10-14).[87–91] The pathophysiology and imaging findings of these entities are discussed elsewhere in this textbook.

Of the conditions mentioned above, two are worthy of additional discussion. Low and colleagues have shown that MR (contrast-enhanced, fat-suppressed, breath-hold gradient echo images obtained both with and without a negative bowel contrast agent) outperforms CT in the evaluation of malignant peritoneal implants (Fig. 10-9).[58,59,92] Thus MR could be considered the primary imaging test of choice in patients suspected of peritoneal malignancy or could evaluate ambiguous cases already imaged by other modalities.

While the mucosal changes of inflammatory bowel disease are best evaluated with conventional barium studies, the extraluminal manifestations of the disease (abscess and fistula) are better evaluated with cross-sectional imaging methods. The benefit of MR over CT is the fact that MR could be performed immediately after an upper GI or enteroclysis study. The retained barium and/or methylcellulose is actually beneficial as a bowel marker for MR as opposed to being a contraindication to CT.

With the continuing improvement of enhanced gradients, bowel contrast agents, and fast scan techniques, and the use of breath-hold T2-weighted images (Fig. 10-15), the field of MR fluoroscopy[93] may play an important role in the evaluation of small bowel disease in the future.

MR Angiographic Techniques

The pathology, pathophysiology, and imaging findings of vascular disorders of the small bowel are discussed in Chapter 20. This section provides an introduction to MR angiographic (MRA) techniques and their application to the evaluation of the mesenteric circulation.

The goal of any MR angiographic technique is to produce high contrast between the protons contained within flowing blood and the protons contained within stationary tissue.[94] The most common MR angiographic technique used in the abdomen is the two-dimensional (2D) time-of-flight (TOF) gradient echo sequence,[95] in part because of its wide availability without software modification, sensitivity to slow flow, and ability to be performed in a single breath-

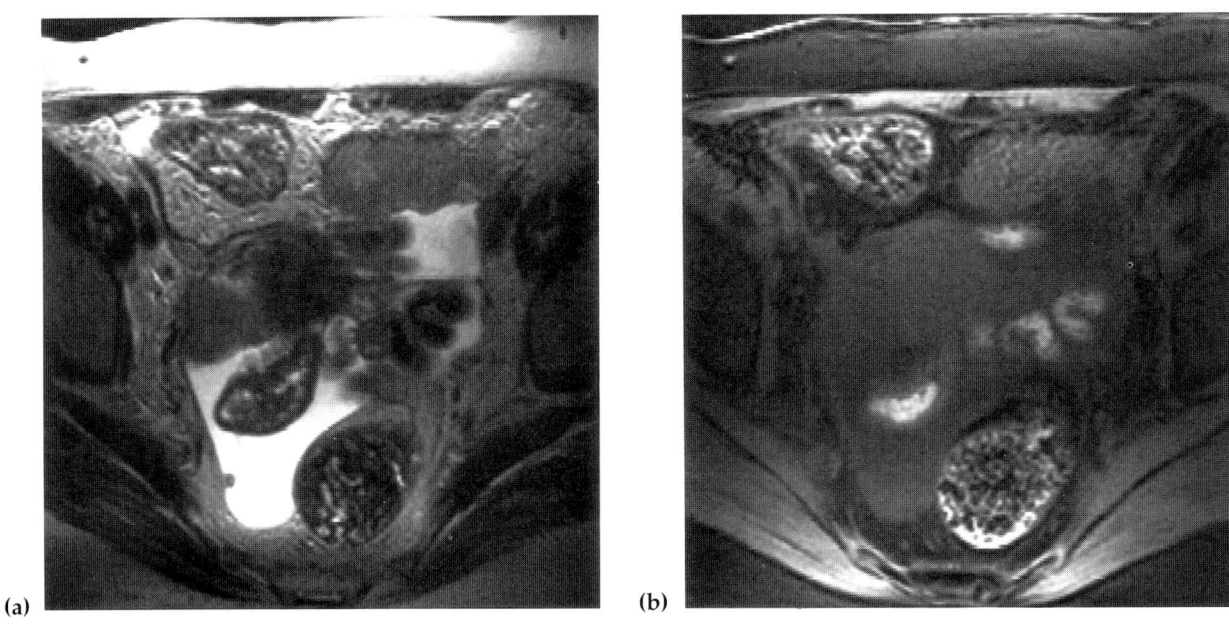

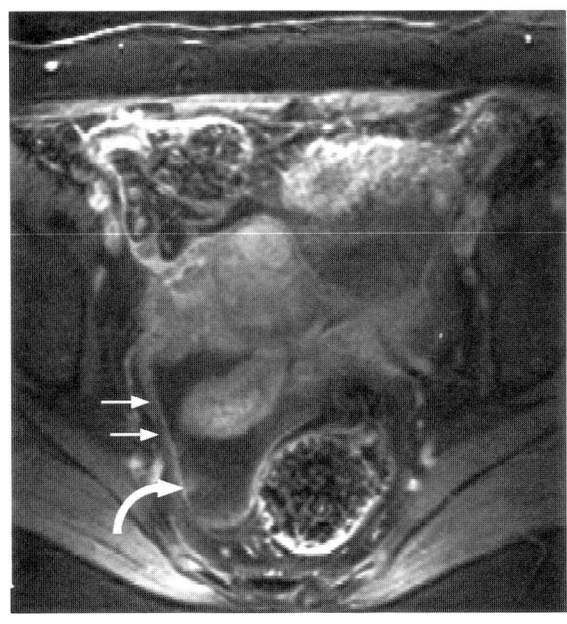

Fig. 10-9. Peritoneal enhancement in a patient with ovarian carcinoma metastatic to the peritoneum. (a) Axial T2-weighted fast spin echo image and axial, breath-hold, fat-saturated, T1-weighted gradient echo images obtained before (b) and after (c) gadolinium enhancement show cul-de-sac fluid. Peritoneal enhancement is present surrounding the fluid collection (straight arrows) as well as an enhancing nodular implant (curved arrow). Peritoneal spread of tumor was confirmed surgically. (Case courtesy of Eric Outwater, MD, Thomas Jefferson University Hospital.)

hold. In TOF techniques, unsaturated protons present within flowing blood that enter an imaging section have higher magnetization (ie, result in greater signal intensity) compared to saturated protons within stationary tissue in the imaging section.[96–102] One has to adjust the imaging parameters (TR [repetition time], TE, flip angle, slice thickness, flow compensation, saturation bands) of a 2D-TOF sequence in order to

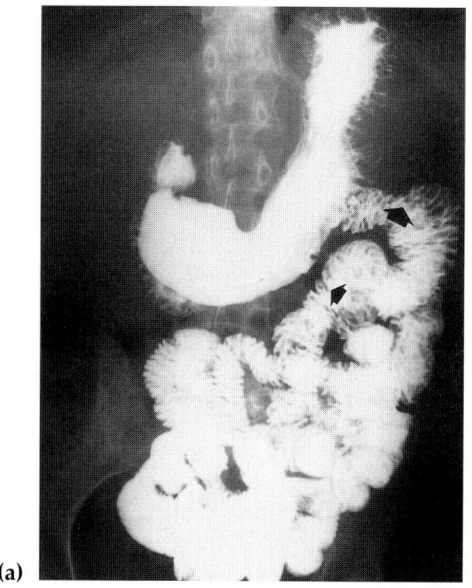 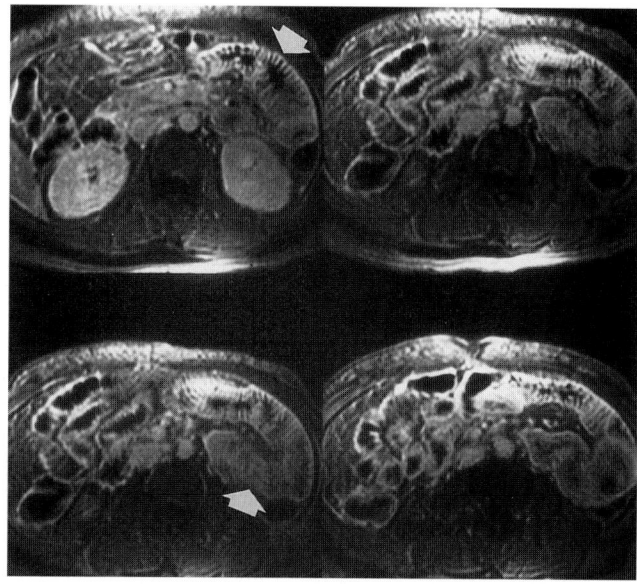

Fig. 10-10. Small bowel changes of lupus vasculitis in a 30-year-old woman with systemic lupus.
(a) Overhead film of an upper GI exam shows jejunal fold thickening (arrows). (b) Four fat-suppressed, breath-hold, T1-weighted gradient echo images obtained after gadolinium showed jejunal wall thickening and hyperemia. In this case, no oral contrast agent was administered.

achieve a balance between suppressing stationary tissue magnetization suppressing magnetization from flowing blood.[95,100,101,103]

The TR should be short enough to promote stationary proton saturation and to minimize imaging time. However, the TR should be long enough to allow a sufficient number of unsaturated flowing spins to enter the imaging slice. On 1.5 tesla systems, an optimized TR is usually between 25 and 45 msec. The flip angle should be large in order to increase stationary spin saturation and to increase the transverse magnetization of blood flowing into the slice. However, at very large flip angles there is a potential for saturating spins from slowly flowing blood that may be present in an imaging slice for more than one TR interval (for example, during diastole). As a compromise, we use a flip angle of 40 to 60 degrees.

Thicker slices result in images with greater signal-to-noise ratio and will decrease the time to image the volume of tissue to be evaluated. However, thick slices can result in decreased intravascular signal due to saturation of flowing spins that are present within the imaging plane for more than one TR interval. Thin slices will allow a greater relative number of unsaturated flowing spins to enter the slice for each repetition and will increase the resolution in the cranial-caudal plane (assuming one is acquiring axial images).

While slice thickness of 5 mm would be adequate to determine whether there is thrombosis of the superior mesenteric artery, a focal stenosis could be missed.

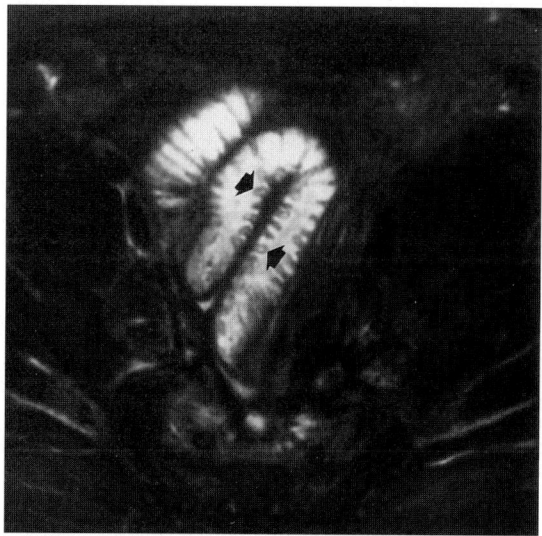

Fig. 10-11. Radiation enteritis in a 60-year-old man with rectal carcinoma.
Fat-suppressed, T2-weighted fast spin echo image shows prominent small bowel segments with minimally thickened walls and submucosal edema (arrows).

176 • 10. Magnetic Resonance Imaging for Small Bowel Related Diagnosis

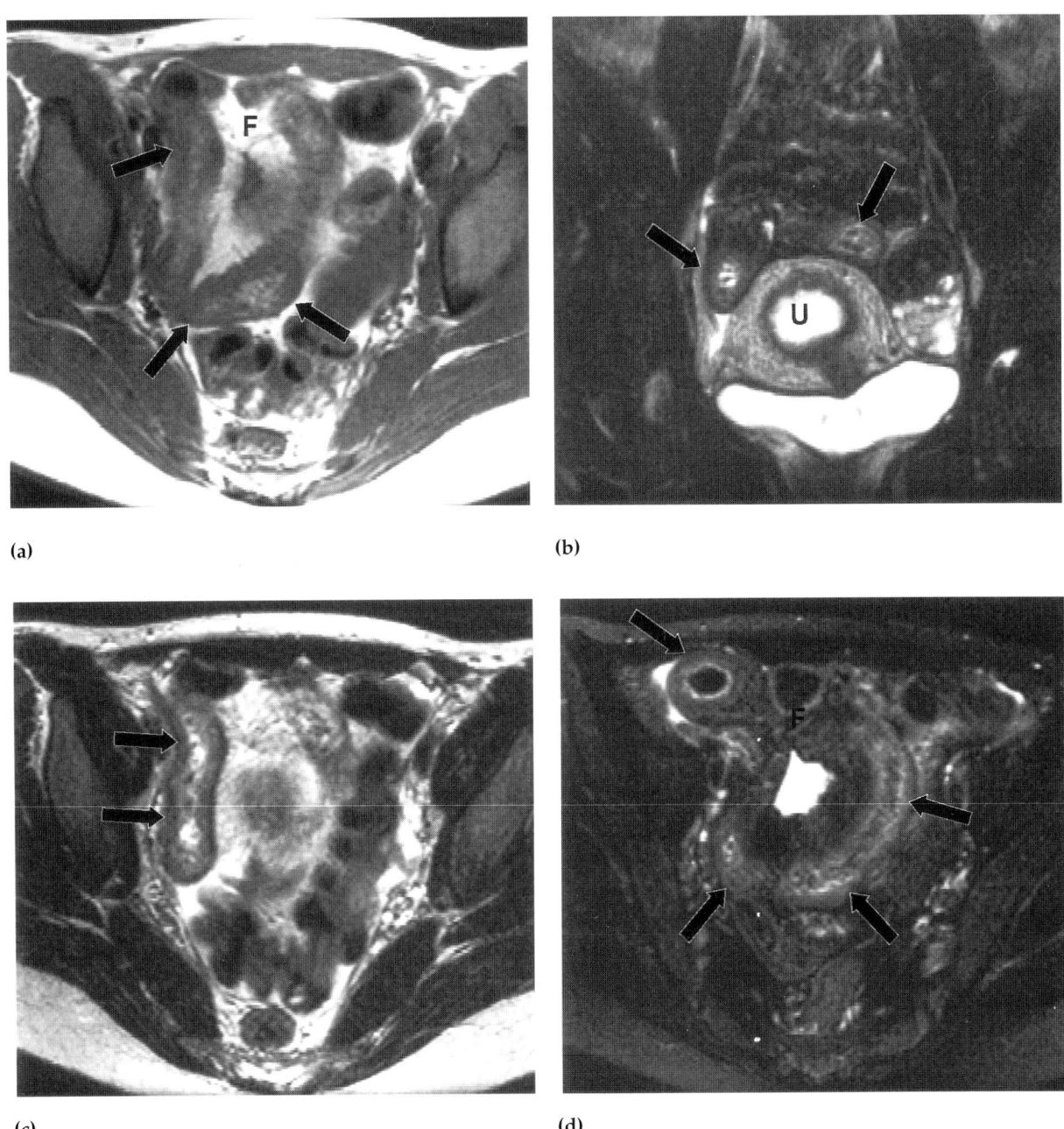

Fig. 10-12. Crohn's disease in a 26-year-old pregnant woman.
(a) Axial T1-weighted image shows bowel wall thickening in a segment of terminal ileum (arrows). There is stranding of the mesenteric fat. (b) Coronal T2-weighted fast spin echo image shows thick wall small bowel segments (arrows) adjacent to the uterus, which contains a gestational sac (U). Axial T2-weighted fast spin echo images without (c) and with (d) fat saturation show transmural thickening of the small bowel segment. (Case courtesy of Eric Outwater, MD, Thomas Jefferson University Hospital.)

Therefore, we recommend a slice thickness of 2 to 3 mm when performing 2D-TOF imaging of the abdomen.

Gradient moment nulling (motion artifact suppression technique [MAST] or "flow compensation") is an artifact reduction method[104] used with 2D-TOF technique. The gradient moment nulling technique alters the gradient waveforms to correct for motion-induced phase changes that occur during the application of gradients during image acquisition.[105] This results in decreased motion artifact and increased intravascular signal. The TE selected should always be minimized in order to maximize signal-to-noise ratio and to minimize any dephasing of the flowing spins that can oc-

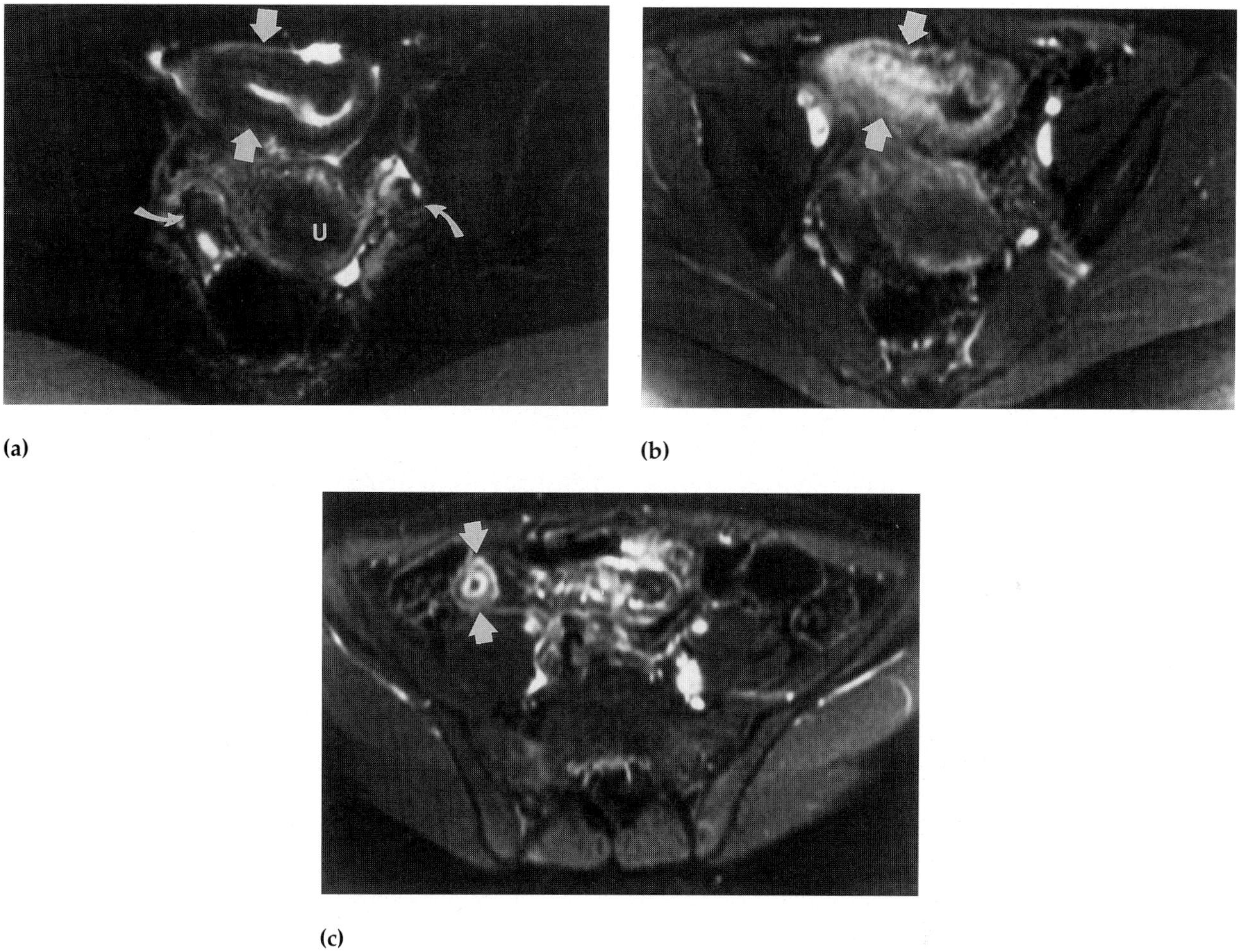

Fig. 10-13. Crohn's disease in a 25-year-old woman.
(a) Axial fat-suppressed T2-weighted fast spin echo image shows a distal small bowel segment with a moderate transmural thickening (arrows). Note the uterine fundus (U) and normal ovaries (curved arrows). (b) Fat-suppressed, breath-hold, T1-weighted gradient echo image obtained after gadolinium shows moderate enhancement of this bowel segment. Enhancing small bowel is more conspicuous if fat suppression is used as well as if a negative contrast agent is used orally (ie, one that results in low signal intensity), such as barium or iron oxide particles.[145] In this patient no contrast was given by mouth. The fluid present within this segment of bowel acted as a negative bowel agent on this enhanced T1-weighted image. (c) Additional enhanced T1-weighted image obtained at a higher level shows a thickened segment of enhancing distal ileum in cross section (arrows). This segment of bowel shows a target sign with enhancing mucosa and muscularis propria. Bowel wall thickening and the degree of bowel wall enhancement correlate well with disease severity. Although the morphological information obtained with MR imaging is comparable to that obtained with CT, the improved contrast resolution with MR imaging is helpful to identify active areas.[78]

cur. Both the use of thin slices and flow compensation utilize gradients that lengthen the minimal TE that can be achieved. On 1.5 tesla systems, the minimal TE is often in the range of 4 to 8 msec, depending on whether the system has enhanced gradients.

When performing axial 2D-TOF abdominal imaging, saturation bands can be placed either superiorly or inferiorly in order to eliminate signal from caudally or cranially directly blood flow, respectively. Such saturation techniques do not necessarily result in pure "MR venograms" and "MR arteriograms." For example, retrograde superiorly directed flow in the gastroduodenal artery (as may occur in a high-grade stenosis or occlusion of the celiac artery) would be saturated and not produce high signal intensity if an inferior saturation band was used.

2D-TOF techniques are often sufficient for detecting occlusions or high-grade stenoses involving the

178 • 10. Magnetic Resonance Imaging for Small Bowel Related Diagnosis

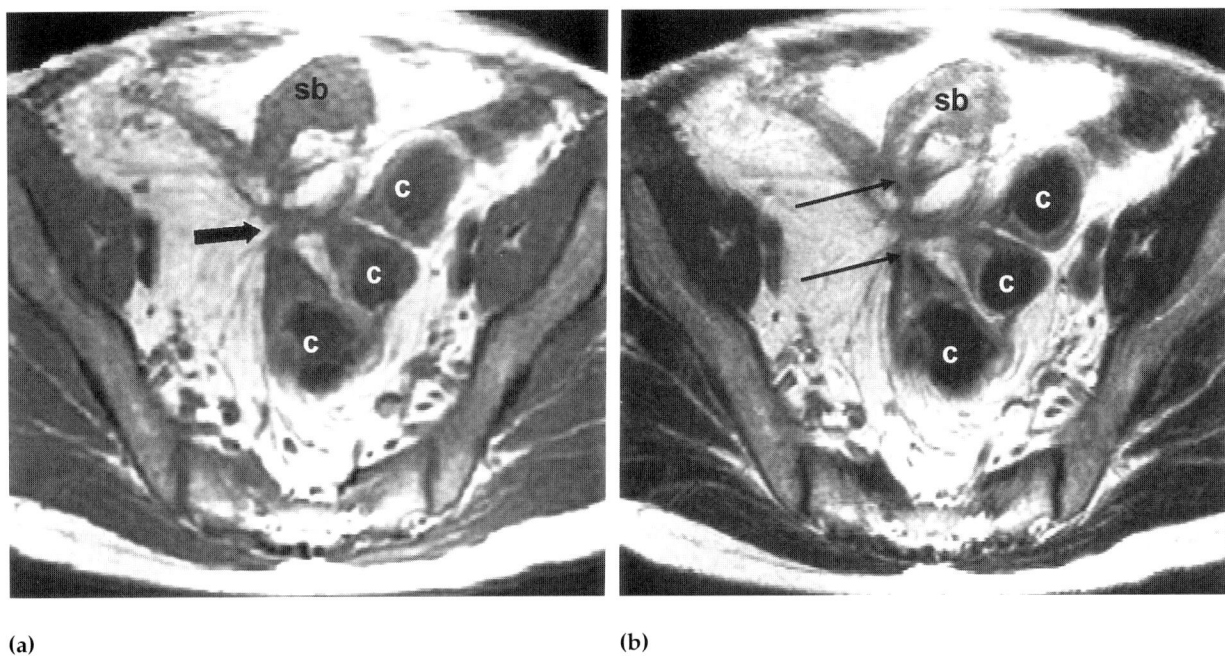

Fig. 10-14. Enterocolic fistulas in a 55-year-old man with Crohn's disease.
(a) Axial T1-weighted spin echo image shows a complex fistula tract (arrow) extending from the ileum (sb) to the sigmoid colon (c). (b) Axial T2-weighted fast spin echo image shows focal discontinuities in the bowel wall (thin arrows) at the entrance of fistula tracts. Note the asymmetric reactive wall thickening of the mesenteric side of the sigmoid colon (c). (Case courtesy of Eric Outwater, MD, Thomas Jefferson University Hospital.)

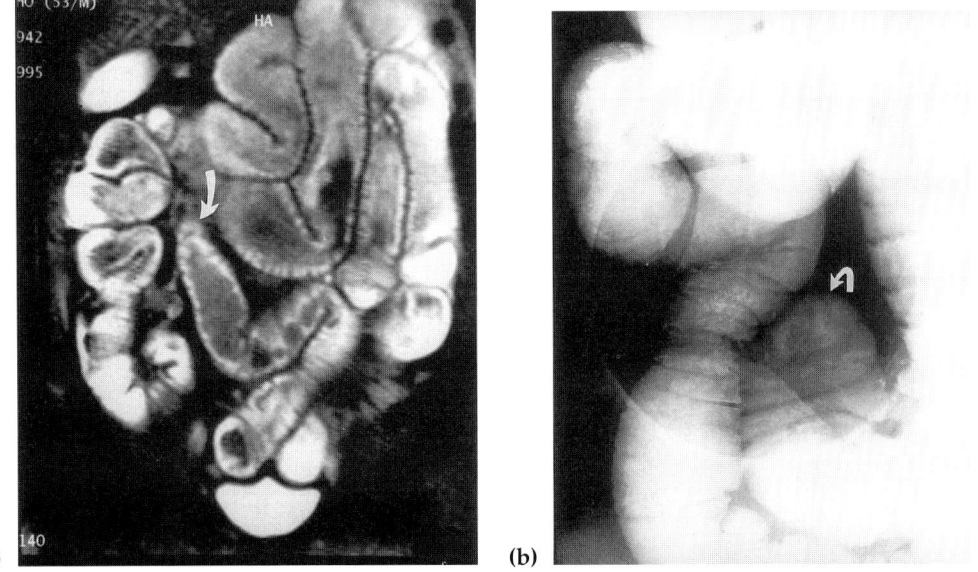

Fig. 10-15. Small intestinal obstruction secondary to an adhesive band.
(a) Coronal T2-weighted breath-hold image performed after the ingestion of water shows a beaklike focus of luminal narrowing (arrow) of a distal small bowel segment. (b) A spot radiograph of a small bowel follow-through shows a high-grade small bowel obstruction (arrow) at the same site. (Case and photos courtesy of Hyun Kwon Ha, MD, University of Ulsan College of Medicine, Seoul, Korea.)

aorta and its major branches (celiac, superior and inferior mesenteric arteries, and renal arteries) (Fig. 10-16). The most commonly used postprocessing algorithm used to view a set of 2D data is the maximum intensity projection (MIP) technique.[94,106,107] The postprocessed MIP images resemble conventional arteriograms and are often accepted by our referring vascular surgeons as a substitute for conventional arteriography.

Three-dimensional TOF imaging offers the advantages of greater spatial resolution in the section-select direction and higher signal-to-noise ratio compared to 2D methods[108] and would be desirable when one was trying to depict abnormalities of smaller vessels. The biggest disadvantage of 3D-TOF techniques is the presence of saturation of moving spins contained within the imaging volume. This is most pronounced within smaller, distal arterial segments and results in "pruning" of the arterial branches. 3D techniques are also more sensitive to patient motion. If a patient moves during a 3D-TOF acquisition, the entire study becomes blurred and an examination may be uninterpretable. However, when a patient moves during a 2D-TOF sequence, only one or two slices (ie, the slices being acquired at time of the patient's motion) are affected and the study is often still diagnostic.[103]

Beginning in the early 1990s, investigators started to use dynamic injection of gadolinium in order to improve the performance of the 3D-TOF sequence.[109–112] By imaging the volume of interest while the gadolinium is primarily in the arterial system, the contrast selectively shortens the T1 relaxation of blood. The majority of flow artifacts and unwanted saturation effects that can affect 2D-TOF techniques are minimized or eliminated when using a contrast-enhanced 3D acquisition. One should deemphasize the term "time-of-flight" when describing such enhanced MRA sequences. The resulting vessel conspicuity in contrast-enhanced MRA no longer depends on the inflow of unsaturated spins; it is almost entirely based on the selective T1-shortening of arterial blood.

With the development of enhanced gradients[113] contrast-enhanced 3D-TOF arteriograms can now be performed in a breath-hold and are being used with increasing frequency in the evaluation of diseases of the aorta and its branches (Fig. 10-17).[114–128] There have been two reported series that used a breath-hold contrast-enhanced 3D MRA technique to evaluate the mesenteric vessels.[129,130] In the study by Meaney and colleagues, the 3D MRA exam had a 100% sensitivity and 95% specificity for the evaluation of celiac, superior mesenteric artery, and inferior mesenteric artery

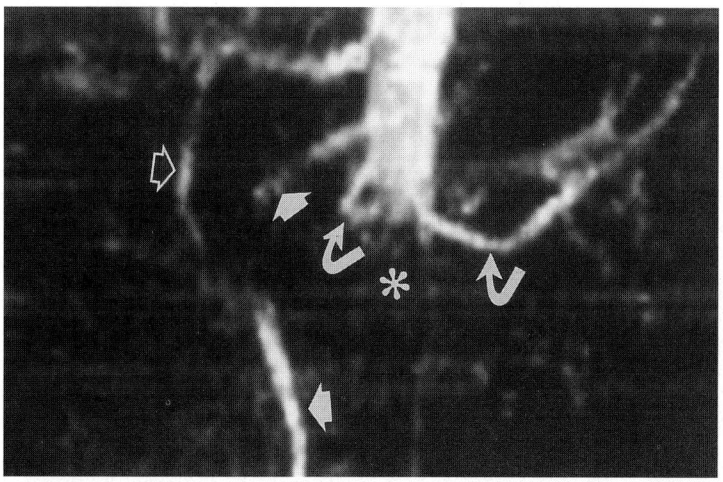

(a)

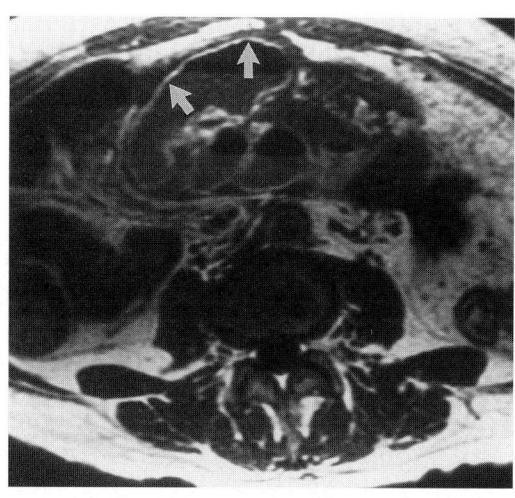

(b)

Fig. 10-16. Mesenteric ischemia in a 56-year-old woman.
(a) Steep left anterior oblique maximum intensity projection (MIP) MR arteriogram performed using a 2D-TOF sequence without contrast enhancement shows occlusion of the infrarenal abdominal aorta (*). The renal arteries were not thrombosed (curved arrows). There is occlusion of the proximal segment of the superior mesenteric artery (straight arrows) with reconstitution after a few centimeters by collateral vessels from the gastroduodenal artery (open arrow). (b) Axial T1-weighted spin echo sequence shows dilated small bowel segments with very high intramural signal intensity (arrows) suspicious for methemoglobin and subacute hemorrhage. Bilateral renal infarcts (not shown) were also present, suggesting embolic disease as the etiology. At subsequent surgery, small bowel segments with hemorrhagic infarction were removed.

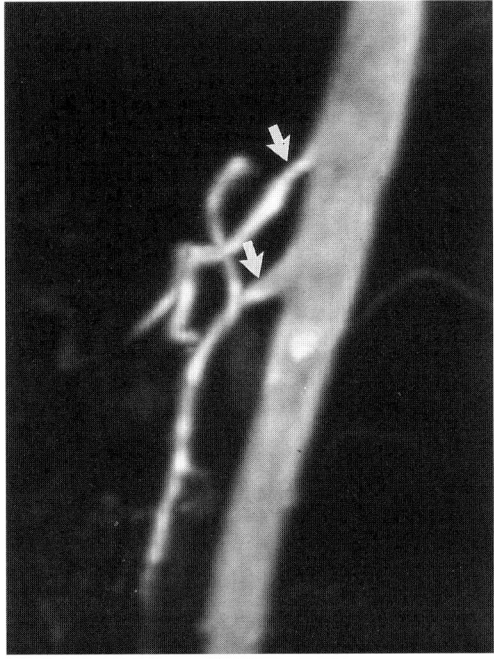 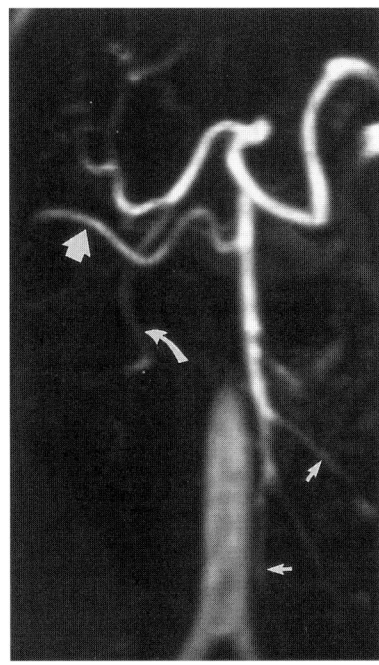

Fig. 10-17. Normal mesenteric arteries in a 39-year-old woman with suspected mesenteric ischemia.
(a) Sagittal MIP from a contrast-enhanced 3D MR arteriogram shows normal proximal segments of the celiac and superior mesenteric arteries (arrows). (b) Coronal MIP from the same sequence shows second-order branches of the SMA (small arrows), a replaced right hepatic artery (straight arrow), and a normal gastroduodenal artery (curved arrow).

stenosis [Fig. 10-18(a)].[130] Many centers are now using this technique as a first imaging test in patients with suspected mesenteric ischemia from stenosis/occlusion of the proximal mesenteric vessels. In the study by Shirkhoda, only 50% of third-order arterial branches were clearly delineated, thus limiting this technique in the evaluation of small vessel vasculitis, embolic disease of small vessels, and in some patients with distal vessel pruning in chronic mesenteric ischemia.[129] If one were concerned about disease in the mesenteric veins, a repeat breath-hold study performed 30 to 60 seconds after the arterial phase scan

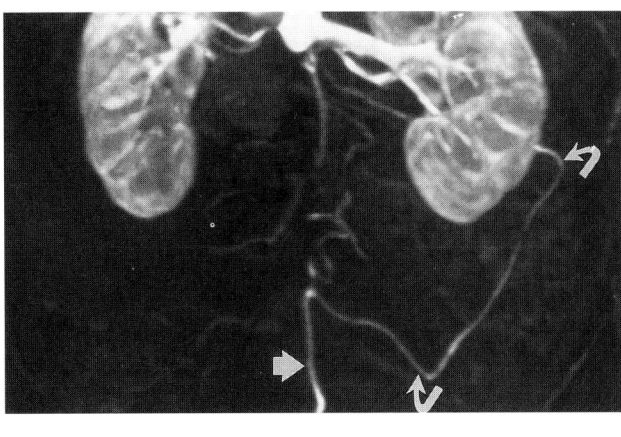 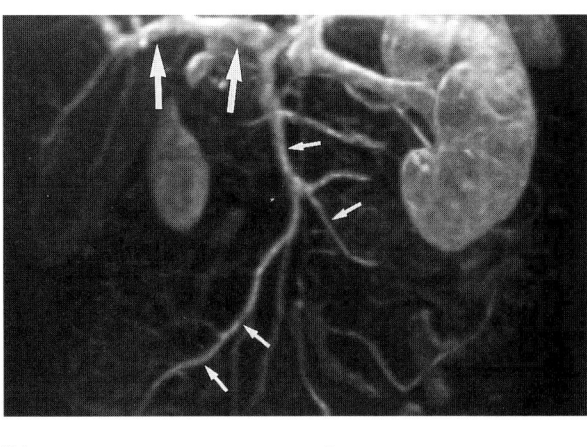

Fig. 10-18. Occluded origin of the inferior mesenteric artery with reconstitution by the arc of Riolan in a 59-year-old woman with occlusion of the infrarenal abdominal aorta.
(a) Coronal MIP from a contrast-enhanced MR arteriogram nicely demonstrates the collateral vessel (curved arrows) reconstituting the inferior mesenteric artery (straight arrow) after its origin. (b) Coronal MIP obtained during a second breath-hold acquisition shows branches of the superior mesenteric vein (small arrows), left renal vein, and portal vein (large arrows).

could delineate the inferior and superior mesenteric, splenic, and portal veins [Fig. 10-18(b)].

When performing a breath-hold contrast-enhanced 3D MRA, the injection of the contrast bolus should be performed such that the segment of aorta and its branches in question selectively contain gadolinium at the time of image acquisition. If one injects too late (or images too early), the arterial phase images may show no signal within the aorta. Conversely, if one injects too early (or images too late), then the resulting images could be degraded by enhanced venous structures (particularly the renal veins). The easiest method involves estimating the patient's circulation time and then prescribing the scan delay (typically 5 to 15 seconds after contrast injection). This method works with success approximately 70% of the time in my (ESS) experience. The majority of suboptimal first runs were scanned too early in patients with a prolonged circulation time. By simply repeating a second breath-hold scan immediately after the first one is completed, a reasonable arterial phase imaging can be obtained.

A second method involves the injection of a small "test dose" of contrast while the region of aorta to be evaluated is continuously scanned with a fast-gradient echo sequence (typically one scan every 1 to 2 seconds). This allows one to calculate a tailored circulation time for each patient.[120,131–133] The disadvantages of this technique are the increased scan time needed to perform the timing bolus and the resultant residual contrast that is often visible in the collecting system at the time of the second bolus injection. This technique also assumes that the patient's cardiac output remains stable between the test bolus and data acquisition, which may not always be the case.[134] The third technique uses specialized software that enables some MR systems to detect the arrival of contrast in a selected segment of aorta.[135–137] This technique offers the advantages of avoiding a test injection and having to calculate a patient-specific delayed time. One simply injects the contrast at any time and the system informs the user when to have the patient breath-hold and begin scanning. Such software is currently available on some systems (ie, "Smart Prep," General Electric, Milwaukee, Wi). A fourth technique of timing a bolus injection is similar to Smart-Prep, except the MR technologist or radiologist at the console visually monitors the contrast bolus by viewing consecutive fast sagittal images of the aortic segment in question. As the bolus is seen to arrive at the desired arterial segment, the patient is instructed to breath-hold and the 3D sequence is initiated.[134] The final method, which is not commercially available, involves a time-resolved scanning technique known as TRICKS[138] (Time Resolved Imaging of Contrast Kinetics). This method involves judicious sampling of k-space such that 3D images can be acquired once every 2 to 6 seconds. Such "MR fluoroscopic" methods would appear to guarantee that an optimal arterial phase scan be obtained.

Similar to conventional arteriography, contrast-enhanced MRA depicts true anatomic images of the arterial lumen. As discussed in Chapter 20, anatomic depiction of vessel stenosis or occlusion does not necessarily equate with a diagnosis of mesenteric ischemia that requires surgery. However, in patients with a high clinical suspicion of mesenteric ischemia, contrast-enhanced MRA techniques may be a "one-stop" imaging test that can be performed prior to a planned surgical procedure.

Phase-contrast MRA techniques can provide quantitative information concerning flow in mesenteric vessels (obtained while fasting and after a stress meal) that can suggest the clinical significance of any anatomically detected stenoses.[139–143] A second quantitative MR technique that has potential use in the evaluation of mesenteric ischemia is the use of MR to sample and measure the oxygen saturation in the superior mesenteric vein.[144]

Conclusions

The small bowel can be studied with MR imaging, particularly using fast imaging sequences, an antiperistalsis agent, and/or an oral contrast agent. When evaluating the small bowel and surrounding mesentery the use of an antiperistaltic agent and/or oral contrast agent should be considered, especially when using MR systems incapable of obtaining a breath-hold examination. In certain situations where barium examinations and CT do not provide all the clinical information needed, such as in bowel obstruction, inflammatory bowel disease, and extension of neoplasms; MRI, with its direct multiplanar capability, lack of ionizing radiation, and superb soft tissue contrast, may have clinical utility.

MR angiographic techniques can provide both qualitative and quantitative information concerning the presence and amount of flow to the small bowel. Contrast enhanced, breath-hold, 3D MR arteriography is a promising technique in the evaluation of patients with suspect mesenteric ischemia.

References

1. Gelfand DW, Ott DJ, Chen YM. Decreasing numbers of gastrointestinal studies: report of data from 69 radiologic practices. *AJR*. 1987;148:1133–1136.

2. Bagley AS, Semelka RC. Investigating bowel disease with ultrasound and MRI [comment]. *Abdom Imaging.* 1994;19:403–404.
3. Rofsky NM, Weinreb JC, Ambrosino MM, Safir J, Krinsky G. Comparison between in-phase and opposed-phase T1-weighted breath-hold FLASH sequences for hepatic imaging. *J Comput Assist Tomogr.* 1996;20:230–235.
4. Semelka RC, Willms AB, Brown MA, Brown ED, Finn JP. Comparison of breath-hold T1-weighted MR sequences for imaging of the liver. *J Magn Reson Imaging.* 1994;4:759–765.
5. Martin J, Sentis M, Puig J, et al. Comparison of in-phase and opposed-phase GRE and conventional SE MR pulse sequences in T1-weighted imaging of liver lesions. *J Comput Assist Tomogr.* 1996;20:890–897.
6. Gaa J, Hatabu H, Jenkins RL, Finn JP, Edelman RR. Liver masses: replacement of conventional T2-weighted spin-echo MR imaging with breath-hold MR imaging. *Radiology.* 1996;200:459–464.
7. Semelka RC, Kelekis NL, Thomasson D, Brown MA, Laub GA. HASTE MR imaging: description of technique and preliminary results in the abdomen. *J Magn Reson Imaging.* 1996;6:698–699.
8. Tang Y, Yamashita Y, Namimoto T, Abe Y, Takahashi M. Liver T2-weighted MR imaging: comparison of fast and conventional half-Fourier single-shot turbo spin-echo, breath-hold turbo spin-echo, and respiratory-triggered turbo spin-echo sequences. *Radiology.* 1997;203:766–772.
9. Campeau NG, Johnson CD, Felmlee JP, et al. MR imaging of the abdomen with a phased-array multicoil: prospective clinical evaluation. *Radiology.* 1995;195:769–776.
10. Gauger J, Holzknecht NG, Lackerbauer CA, et al. Breathhold imaging of the upper abdomen using a circular polarized-array coil: comparison with standard body coil imaging. *MAGMA.* 1996;4:93–104.
11. Yamashita Y, Yamamoto H, Namimoto T, Abe Y, Takahashi M. Phased array breath-hold versus non-breath-hold MR imaging of focal liver lesions: a prospective comparative study. *J Magn Reson Imaging.* 1997;7:292–297.
12. McCauley TR, McCarthy S, Lange R. Pelvic phased array coil: image quality assessment for spin-echo MR imaging. *Magn Reson Imaging.* 1992;10:513–522.
13. Marti-Bonmati L, Graells M, Ronchera-Oms CL. Reduction of peristaltic artifacts on magnetic resonance imaging of the abdomen: a comparative evaluation of three drugs. *Abdom Imaging.* 1996;21:309–313.
14. Laniado M, Gronewaller E, Kopp AF, et al. The value of hyocine butylbromide in abdominal MR imaging with and without oral magnetic particles. *Abdom Imaging.* 1997;22:381–388.
15. Kressel HY. Insights of an abdominal imager: what do we need for MRI enhancement? *Magn Reson Med.* 1991;22:314–318.
16. Balinger JR. Contrast agents. In: Ros PR, Bidgood WD, eds. *Abdominal Magnetic Resonance Imaging.* St. Louis, Mo: CV Mosby Co; 1993:116–120.
17. Brown JJ. Gastrointestinal contrast agents for MR Imaging. *Magn Reson Imaging Clin N Am.* 1996;4:25–35.
18. Pels Rijcken TH, Davis MA, Ros PR. Intraluminal contrast agents for MR imaging of the abdomen and pelvis. *J Magn Reson Imaging.* 1994;4:291–300.
19. Hahn PF. Advances in contrast-enhanced MR imaging. Gastrointestinal contrast agents. *AJR.* 1991;156:252–254.
20. Sato S. A study of green tea for a positive gastrointestinal MR imaging enhancing agent. *Nippon Igaku Hoshasen Gakkai Zasshi.* 1994;54:876–885.
21. Hiraishi K, Narabayashi I, Fujita O, et al. Blueberry juice: preliminary evaluation as an oral contrast agent in gastrointestinal MR imaging. *Radiology.* 1995;194:119–123.
22. Wan X, Wedeking P, Tweedle MF. Sources of heterogeneous contrast enhancement in the gastrointestinal tract. *Magn Reson Imaging.* 1994;12:1009–1012.
23. Jacobsen TF, Laniado M, Van Beers BE, et al. Oral magnetic particles (ferristene) as a contast medium in abdominal magnetic resonance imaging. *Acad Radiol.* 1996;3:571–580.
24. Van Beers BE, Grandin C, De Greef D, Lundby B, Pringot J. Ferristene as intestinal MR contrast agent. Distribution and safety of a fast ingestion procedure with oral metoclopramide. *Acta Radiol.* 1996;37:676–679.
25. Patten RM, Lo SK, Phillips JJ, et al. Positive bowel contrast agent for MR imaging of the abdomen: phase II and III clinical trials. *Radiology.* 1993;189:277–283.
26. Patten RM, Moss AA, Fenton TA, Elliott S. OMR: a positive bowel contrast agent for abdominal and pelvic MR imaging: safety and imaging characteristics. *J Magn Reson Imaging.* 1992;2:25–34.
27. Hirohashi S, Uchida H, Yoshikawa K, et al. Large scale clinical evaluation of bowel contrast agent containing ferric ammonium citrate in MRI. *Magn Reson Imaging.* 1994;12:837–846.
28. Kaminsky S, Laniado M, Gogoll M, et al. Gadopentetate dimeglumine as a bowel contrast agent: safety and efficacy. *Radiology.* 1991;178:503–508.
29. Young SW, Qing F, Rubin D, et al. Gadolinium zeolite as an oral contrast agent for magnetic resonance imaging. *J Magn Reson Imaging.* 1995;5:499–508.
30. Laniado M, Kornmesser W, Hamm B, Clauss W, Weinmann HJ, Felix R. MR imaging of the gastrointestinal tract: value of Gd-DTPA. *AJR.* 1988;150:817–821.
31. Tilcock C, Unger EC, Ahkong QF, Fritz T, Koenig SH, Brown RD III. Polymeric gastrointestinal MR contrast agents. *J Magn Reson Imaging.* 1991;1:463–467.
32. Squillaci E, Crecco M, Cecconi L, Lupoi D, Sergiacomi GL, Simonetti G. Gadolinium-DTPA dimeglumine administered orally for the study of the abdomen with magnetic resonance. Clinical evaluation and tolerance. *Radiol Med (Torino).* 1993;86:284–293.
33. Rubin DL, Falk KL, Sperling MJ, et al. A multicenter clinical trial of gadolite oral suspension as a contrast agent for MRI. *J Magn Reson Imaging.* 1997;7:865–872.
34. Bernardino ME, Weinreb JC, Mitchell DG, Small WC, Morris M. Safety and optimum concentration of a manganese chloride-based oral MR contrast agent. *J Magn Reson Imaging.* 1994;4:872–876.

35. Li KC, Ang PG, Tart RP, Storm BL, Rolfes R, Ho-Tai PC. Paramagnetic oil emulsions as oral magnetic resonance imaging contrast agents. *Magn Reson Imaging.* 1990;8:589–598.
36. Tart RP, Li KC, Storm BL, Rolfes RJ, Ang PG. Enteric MRI contrast agents: comparative study of five potential agents in humans. *Magn Reson Imaging.* 1991;9:559–568.
37. Balzarini L, Aime S, Barbero L, et al. Magnetic resonance imaging of the gastrointestinal tract: investigation of baby milk as a low cost contrast medium. *Eur J Radiol.* 1992;15:171–174.
38. Mirowitz SA, Susman N. Use of nutritional support formula as a gastrointestinal contrast agent for MRI. *J Comput Assist Tomogr.* 1992;16:908–915.
39. Hahn PF, Stark DD, Lewis JM, et al. First clinical trial of a new superparamagnetic iron oxide for use as an oral gastrointestinal contrast agent in MR imaging. *Radiology.* 1990;175:695–700.
40. Vlahos L, Gouliamos A, Athanasopoulou A, et al. A comparative study between Gd-DTPA and oral magnetic particles (OMP) as gastrointestinal (GI) contrast agents for MRI of the abdomen. *Magn Reson Imaging.* 1994;12:719–726.
41. Oksendal AN, Bach-Gansmo T, Jacobsen TF, Eide H, Andrew E. Oral magnetic particles. Results from clinical phase II trials in 216 patients. *Acta Radiol.* 1993;34:187–193.
42. Oksendal AN, Jacobsen TF, Gundersen HG, Rinck PA, Rummeny E. Superparamagnetic particles as an oral contrast agent in abdominal magnetic resonance imaging. *Invest Radiol.* 1991;26:S67–70; discussion S71.
43. Rinck PA, Myhr G, Smevik O, Borseth A. Oral magnetic particles as an MR contrast medium for the gastrointestinal tract. *Rofo Fortschr Geb Rontgenstr Neuen Bildgeb Verfahr.* 1992;157:533–538.
44. Lonnemark M. Superparamagnetic particles as an oral contrast medium in abdominal magnetic resonance imaging. *Acta Radiol Suppl (Stockh).* 1992;378:109–121.
45. Lonnemark M, Hemmingsson A, Bach-Gansmo T, et al. Effect of superparamagnetic particles as oral contrast medium at magnetic resonance imaging. A phase I clinical study. *Acta Radiol.* 1989;30:193–196.
46. Lonnemark M, Hemmingsson A, Carlsten J, Ericsson A, Holtz E, Klaveness J. Superparamagnetic particles as an MRI contrast agent for the gastrointestinal tract. *Acta Radiol.* 1988;29:599–602.
47. Rinck PA, Smevik O, Nilsen G, et al. Oral magnetic particles in MR imaging of the abdomen and pelvis. *Radiology.* 1991;178:775–779.
48. Bach-Gansmo T, Dupas B, Gayet-Delacroix M, Lambrechts M. Abdominal MRI using a negative contrast agent. *Br J Radiol.* 1993;66:420–425.
49. MacVicar D, Jacobsen TF, Guy R, Husband JE. Phase III trial of oral magnetic particles in MRI of abdomen and pelvis. *Clin Radiol.* 1993;47:183–188.
50. Niemi P, Katevuo K, Kormano M, Baksaas I, Bach-Gansmo T, Maenpaa J. Superparamagnetic particles as gastrointestinal contrast agent in magnetic resonance imaging of lower abdomen. *Acta Radiol.* 1990;31:409–411.
51. Johnson WK, Stoupis C, Torres GM, Rosenberg EB, Ros PR. Superparamagnetic iron oxide (SPIO) as an oral contrast agent in gastrointestinal (GI) magnetic resonance imaging (MRI): comparison with state-of-the-art computed tomography (CT). *Magn Reson Imaging.* 1996;14:43–49.
52. Haldemann Heusler RC, Wight E, Marincek B. Oral superparamagnetic contrast agent (ferumoxsil): tolerance and efficacy in MR imaging of gynecologic diseases. *J Magn Reson Imaging.* 1995;5:385–391.
53. Faber SC, Stehling MK, Holzknecht N, Gauger J, Helmberger T, Reiser M. Pathologic conditions in the small bowel: findings at fat-suppressed gadolinium-enhanced MR imaging with an optimized suspension of oral magnetic particles. *Radiology.* 1997;205:278–282.
54. Liebig T, Stoupis C, Ros PR, Ballinger JR, Briggs RW. A potentially artifact-free oral contrast agent for gastrointestinal MRI. *Magn Reson Med.* 1993;30:646–649.
55. Listinsky JJ, Bryant RG. Gastrointestinal contrast agents: a diamagnetic approach. *Magn Reson Med.* 1988;8:285–292.
56. Mitchell DG, Vinitski S, Mohamed FB, Mammone JF, Haidet K, Rifkin MD. Comparison of Kaopectate with barium for negative and positive enteric contrast at MR imaging. *Radiology.* 1991;181:475–480.
57. Li KC, Tart RP, Fitzsimmons JR, Storm BL, Mao J, Rolfes RJ. Barium sulfate suspension as a negative oral MRI contrast agent: *in vitro* and human optimization studies. *Magn Reson Imaging.* 1991;9:141–150.
58. Low RN, Francis IR. MR imaging of the gastrointestinal tract with IV gadolinium and diluted barium oral contrast media compared with unenhanced MR imaging and CT. *AJR.* 1997;169:1051–1059.
59. Low RN, Barone RM, Lacey C, Sigeti JS, Alzate GD, Sebrechts CP. Peritoneal tumor: MR imaging with dilute oral barium and intravenous gadolinium-containing contrast agents compared with unenhanced MR imaging and CT. *Radiology.* 1997;204:513–520.
60. Ros PR, Steinman RM, Torres GM, et al. The value of barium as a gastrointestinal contrast agent in MR imaging: a comparison study in normal volunteers. *AJR.* 1991;157:761–767.
61. Panaccione JL, Ros PR, Torres GM, Burton SS. Rectal barium in pelvic MR imaging: initial results. *J Magn Reson Imaging.* 1991;1:605–607.
62. Langmo L, Ros PR, Torres GM, Erquiaga E. Comparison of MR imaging after barium administration with CT in pelvic disease. *J Magn Reson Imaging.* 1992;2:89–91.
63. Ernst O, Sergent G, L'Hermine C. Oral administration of a low-cost negative contrast agent: a three-year experience in routine practice. *J Magn Reson Imaging.* 1997;7:495–498.
64. Kraus BB, Rappaport DC, Ros PR, Torres GM. Evaluation of oral contrast agents for abdominal magnetic resonance imaging. *Magn Reson Imaging.* 1994;12:847–858.
65. Mattrey RF, Hajek PC, Gylys-Morin VM, et al. Perfluorochemicals as gastrointestinal contrast agents for MR imaging: preliminary studies in rats and humans. *AJR.* 1987;148:1259–1263.

66. Anderson CM, Brown JJ, Balfe DM, et al. MR imaging of Crohn disese: use of perflubron as a gastrointestinal contrast agent. *J Magn Reson Imaging*. 1994;4:491–496.
67. Mergo PJ, Helmberger T, Cerda JJ, Urrutia M, Ros PR. Rectal perflubron: new application in MRI of perirectal fistulae. *J Comput Assist Tomogr*. 1997;21:259–264.
68. Brown JJ, Duncan JR, Heiken JP, et al. Perfluoroctylbromide as a gastrointestinal contrast agent for MR imaging: use with and without glucagon. *Radiology*. 1991;181:455–460.
69. Chou CK, Chen LT, Sheu RS, et al. MRI manifestations of gastrointestinal lymphoma. *Abdom Imaging*. 1994;19:495–500.
70. Mattrey RF, Trambert MA, Brown JJ, et al. Perflubron as an oral contrast agent for MR imaging: results of a phase III clinical trial. *Radiology*. 1994;191:841–848.
71. Chou CK, Chen LT, Sheu RS, Wang ML, Jaw TS, Liu GC. MRI manifestations of gastrointestinal wall thickening [see comments]. *Abdom Imaging*. 1994;19:389–394.
72. Chou CK, Liu GC, Chen LT, Jaw TS. Retrograde air insufflation in MRI: a technical note. *Abdom Imaging*. 1993;18:211–214.
73. Chou CK, Liu GC, Yang CW, Chen LT, Sheu RS, Jaw TS. Abdominal MR imaging following antegrade air introduction into the intestinal loops. *Abdom Imaging*. 1993;18:205–210.
74. Chou CK, Liu GC, Chen LT, Jaw TS. The use of MRI in bowel obstruction. *Abdom Imaging*. 1993;18:131–135.
75. Chou CK, Sheu RS, Yang CW, Wang ML, Chen LT. Abdominal pseudotumors and simulated lymphadenopathy in MRI: differential features with the use of retrograde air insufflation. *Abdom Imaging*. 1994;19:503–506.
76. Chou CK, Liu GC, Su JH, Chen LT, Sheu RS, Jaw TS. MRI demonstration of peritoneal implants. *Abdom Imaging*. 1994;19:95–101.
77. Semelka RC, John G, Kelekis NL, Burdeny DA, Ascher SM. Small bowel neoplastic disease: demonstration by MRI. *J Magn Reson Imaging*. 1996;6:855–860.
78. Semelka RC, Shoenut JP, Silverman R, Kroeker MA, Yaffe CS, Micflikier AB. Bowel disease: prospective comparison of CT and 1.5-T pre- and postcontrast MR imaging with T1-weighted fat-suppressed and breath-hold FLASH sequences. *J Magn Reson Imaging*. 1991;1:625–632.
79. Shoenut JP, Semelka RC, Silverman R, Yaffe CS, Micflikier AB. Magnetic resonance imaging in inflammatory bowel disease. *J Clin Gastroenterol*. 1993;17:73–78.
80. Shoenut JP, Semelka RC, Silverman R, Yaffe CS, Micflikier AB. MRI in the diagnosis of Crohn's disease in two pregnant women. *J Clin Gastroenterol*. 1993;17:244–247.
81. Shoenut JP, Semelka RC, Magro CM, Silverman R, Yaffe CS, Micflikier AB. Comparison of magnetic resonance imaging and endoscopy in distinguishing the type and severity of inflammatory bowel disease. *J Clin Gastroenterol*. 1994;19:31–35.
82. Kettritz U, Shoenut JP, Semelka RC. MR imaging of the gastrointestinal tract. *Magn Reson Imaging Clin N Am*. 1995;3:87–98.
83. Kettritz U, Isaacs K, Warshauer DM, Semelka RC. Crohn's disease. Pilot study comparing MRI of the abdomen with clinical evaluation. *J Clin Gastroenterol*. 1995;21:249–253.
84. Funt SA, Krinsky G, Horowitz L. Clinical image. MR demonstration of submucosal fat in a patient with Crohn's disease. *J Comput Assist Tomogr*. 1996;20:940–941.
85. Haggett PJ, Moore NR, Shearman JD, Travis SP, Jewell DP, Mortensen NJ. Pelvic and perineal complications of Crohn's disease: assessment using magnetic resonance imaging. *Gut*. 1995;36:407–410.
86. Rollandi GA, Martinoli C, Conzi R, et al. Magnetic resonance imaging of the small intestine and colon in Crohn's disease. *Radiol Med (Torino)*. 1996;91:81–85.
87. Madsen SM, Thomsen HS, Munkholm P, Schlichting P, Davidsen B. Magnetic resonance imaging of Crohn disease: early recognition of treatment response and relapse. *Abdom Imaging*. 1997;22:164–166.
88. Koelbel G, Schmiedl U, Majer MC, et al. Diagnosis of fistulae and sinus tracts in patients with Crohn disease: value of MR imaging. *AJR*. 1989;152:999–1003.
89. Outwater E, Schiebler ML. Pelvic fistulas: findings on MR images. *AJR*. 1993;160:327–330.
90. Semelka RC, Hricak H, Kim B, et al. Pelvic fistulas: appearances on MR images. *Abdom Imaging*. 1997;22:91–95.
91. Boudghene F, Aboun H, Grange JD, Wallays C, Bodin F, Bigot JM. Magnetic resonance imaging in the exploration of abdominal and anoperineal fistulas in Crohn's disease. *Gastroenterol Clin Biol*. 1993;17:168–174.
92. Low RN, Sigeti JS. MR imaging of peritoneal disease: comparison of contrast-enhanced fast multiplanar spoiled gradient-recalled and spin-echo imaging. *AJR*. 1994;163:1131–1140.
93. Li KC, Chan FP, Gold GE, Pauly JM, Ken AB, Macovski AE. Real time interactive MR imaging of the small bowel. *Radiology*. 1996;201:487.
94. Saloner D. MRA: principles and display. In: Higgins CB, Hricak H, Helms CA, eds. *Magnetic Resonance Imaging of the Body*. Philadelphia, Pa: Lippincott-Raven; 1997:1345–1368.
95. Mitchell DG. Abdominal MR angiography by two-dimensional time-of-flight techniques. *Appl Radiol*. 1995;24:34–44.
96. Laub GA. Time-of-flight method of MR angiography. *Magn Reson Imaging Clin N Am*. 1995;3:391–398.
97. Bradley WG Jr, Waluch V. Blood flow: magnetic resonance imaging. *Radiology*. 1985;154:443–450.
98. Bradley WG Jr. Carmen lecture. Flow phenomena in MR imaging. *AJR*. 1988;150:983–994.
99. Axel L. Blood flow effects in magnetic resonance imaging. *AJR*. 1984;143:1157–1166.
100. Mitchell DG. Vascular techniques. In: Mitchell DG, ed. *MRI Principles: A Guide for the Mathematically Illiterate*. Philadelphia, Pa: WB Saunders Co; 1998:187–191.
101. Mitchell DG, Nazarian LN. Hepatic vascular diseases: CT and MRI. *Semin Ultrasound CT MR*. 1995;16:49–68.
102. Rofsky NM. Vascular MR imaging. In: McCarthy SM, Ramsey RG, Weinreb JC, eds. *American Roentgen Ray*

Society. Reston, VA: American Roentgen Ray Society, 1997:89–98.
103. Anderson CM, Lee RE. Time-of-flight techniques. Pulse sequences and clinical protocols. *Magn Reson Imaging Clin N Am*. 1993;1:217–227.
104. Ehman RL, Felmlee JP. Flow artifact reduction in MRI: a review of the roles of gradient moment nulling and spatial presaturation. *Magn Reson Med*. 1990;14:293–307.
105. Mitchell DG, Stark DD. Motion artifact. In: Mitchell DG, Stark DD, eds. *Hepatobiliary MRI*. St. Louis, Mo: Mosby; 1992:11–14.
106. Laub G. Displays for MR angiography. *Magn Reson Med*. 1990;14:222–229.
107. Schreiner S, Paschal CB, Galloway RL. Comparison of projection algorithms used for the construction of maximum intensity projection images. *J Comput Assist Tomogr*. 1996;20:56–67.
108. Lewin JS, Laub G, Hausmann R. Three-dimensional time-of-flight MR angiography: applications in the abdomen and thorax. *Radiology*. 1991;179:261–264.
109. Prince MR. Gadolinium-enhanced MR aortography. *Radiology*. 1994;191:155–164.
110. Prince MR, Yucel EK, Kaufman JA, Harrison DC, Geller SC. Dynamic gadolinium-enhanced three-dimensional abdominal MR arteriography. *J Magn Reson Imaging*. 1993;3:877–881.
111. Kanal E, Talagala SL, Applegate GA, Rubin R. Fast three-dimensional time-of-flight MR angiography with timed injection of contrast material. *Radiology*. 1991; 181(P):119.
112. Krinsky GA, Rofsky NM, DeCorato DR, et al. Thoracic aorta: comparison of gadolinium-enhanced three-dimensional MR angiography with conventional MR imaging. *Radiology*. 1997;202:183–193.
113. Brown MA, Semelka RC. *MRI: Basic Principles and Applications*. New York, NY: Wiley-Liss, 1995:119–128.
114. Krinsky G, Rofsky N, Flyer M, et al. Gadolinium-enhanced three-dimensional MR angiography of acquired arch vessel disease. *AJR*. 1996;167:981–987.
115. Krinsky G, Rofsky N, Sandler M, DeCorato D, Weinreb J. Dynamic breath-hold 3D gadolinium-enhanced MRI of intraarterial masses: findings in two patients. *J Comput Assist Tomogr*. 1997;21:631–634.
116. Leung DA, McKinnon GC, Davis CP, Pfammatter T, Krestin GP, Debatin JF. Breath-hold, contrast-enhanced, three-dimensional MR angiography. *Radiology*. 1996; 201:569–571.
117. Snidow JJ, Johnson MS, Harris VJ, et al. Three-dimensional gadolinium-enhanced MR angiography for aortoiliac inflow assessment plus renal artery screening in a single breath hold. *Radiology*. 1996;198:725–732.
118. Holland GA, Dougherty L, Carpenter JP, et al. Breath-hold ultrafast three-dimensional gadolinium-enhanced MR angiography of the aorta and the renal and other visceral abdominal arteries [published erratum appears in *AJR*. 1996;167(2):541]. *AJR*. 1996;166:971–981.
119. Krinsky G, Weinreb J. Gadolinium-enhanced three-dimensional MR angiography of the thoracoabdominal aorta. *Semin Ultrasound CT MR*. 1996;17:280–303.
120. Steffens JC, Link J, Grassner J, et al. Contrast-enhanced, k-space-centered, breath-hold MR angiography of the renal arteries and the abdominal aorta. *J Magn Reson Imaging*. 1997;7:617–622.
121. Hany TF, Debatin JF, Leung DA, Pfammatter T. Evaluation of the aortoiliac and renal arteries: comparison of breath-hold, contrast-enhanced, three-dimensional MR angiography with conventional catheter angiography. *Radiology*. 1997;204:357–362.
122. Hany TF, Pfammatter T, Schmidt M, Leung DA, Debatin JF. Ultrafast contrast-enhanced 3D MR angiography of the aorta and renal arteries in apnea. *Rofo Fortschr Geb Rontgenstr Neuen Bildgeb Verfahr*. 1997; 166:397–405.
123. Prince MR, Narasimham DL, Stanley JC, et al. Breath-hold gadolinium-enhanced MR angiography of the abdominal aorta and its major branches. *Radiology*. 1995;197:785–792.
124. Prince MR, Narasimham DL, Stanley JC, et al. Gadolinium-enhanced magnetic resonance angiography of abdominal aortic aneurysms. *J Vasc Surg*. 1995;21:656–669.
125. Yamashita Y, Mitsuzaki K, Tang Y, Namimoto T. Gadolinium-enhanced breath-hold three-dimensional time-of-flight MR angiography of the abdominal and pelvic vessels: the value of ultrafast MP-RAGE sequences. *J Magn Reson Imaging*. 1997;7:623–628.
126. Gilfeather M, Holland GA, Siegelman ES, et al. Gadolinium-enhanced ultrafast three-dimensional spoiled gradient-echo MR imaging of the abdominal aorta and visceral and iliac vessels. *Radiographies*. 1997;17:423–432.
127. Siegelman ES, Gilfeather M, Holland GA, et al. Breath-hold ultrafast three-dimensional gadolinium-enhanced MR angiography of the renovascular system. *AJR*. 1997;168:1035–1040.
128. Shetty AN, Shirkhoda A, Bis KG, Alcantara A. Contrast-enhanced three-dimensional MR angiography in a single breath-hold: a novel technique. *AJR*. 1995;165:1290–1292.
129. Shirkhoda A, Konez O, Shetty AN, Bis KG, Ellwood RA, Kirsch MJ. Mesenteric circulation: three-dimensional MR angiography with a gadolinium-enhanced multiecho gradient-echo technique. *Radiology*. 1997; 202:257–261.
130. Meaney JFM, Prince MR, Nostrant TT, Stanley JC. Gadolinium-enhanced MR angiography of visceral arteries in patients with suspected chronic mesenteric ischemia. *J Magn Reson Imaging*. 1997;7:171–176.
131. Hany TF, McKinnon GC, Leung DA, Pfammatter T, Debatin JF. Optimization of contrast timing for breath-hold three-dimensional MR angiography. *J Magn Reson Imaging*. 1997;7:551–556.
132. Earls JP, Rofsky NM, DeCorato DR, Krinsky GA, Weinreb JC. Breath-hold single-dose gadolinium-enhanced three-dimensional MR aortography: usefulness of a timing examination and MR power injector. *Radiology*. 1996;201:705–710.
133. Earls JP, Rofsky NM, DeCorato DR, Krinsky GA, Weinreb JC. Hepatic arterial-phase dynamic gadolinium-enhanced MR imaging: optimization with a test examination and a power injector. *Radiology*. 1997;202: 268–273.

134. Wilman AH, Riederer SJ, King BF, Debbins JP, Rossman PJ, Ehman RL. Fluoroscopically triggered contrast-enhanced three-dimensional MR angiography with elliptical centric view order: application to the renal arteries. *Radiology.* 1997;205:137–146.
135. Prince MR, Chenevert TL, Foo TK, Londy FJ, Ward JS, Maki JH. Contrast-enhaned abdominal MR angiography: optimization of imaging delay time by automating the detection of contrast material arrival in the aorta. *Radiology.* 1997;203:109–114.
136. Foo TK, Saranathan M, Prince MR, Chenevert TL. Automated detection of bolus arrival and initiation of data acquisition in fast, three-dimensional, gadolinium-enhanced MR angiography. *Radiology.* 1997;203:275–280.
137. Foo TKF, Manojkumar S, Prince MR, Chenevert TL. MR smart prep: an automated method for detecting the bolus arrival time and initiating data acquisition in fast 3D gadolinium-enhanced MRA. Presented at the International Society for Magnetic Resonance in Medicine; 1966; Berkeley, Calif; 453.
138. Korosec FR, Frayne R, Grist TM, Mistretta CA. Time-resolved contrast-enhanced 3D MR angiography. *Magn Reson Med.* 1996;36:345–351.
139. Li KC, Whitney WS, McDonnell CH, et al. Chronic mesenteric ischemia: evaluation with phase-contrast cine MR imaging. *Radiology.* 1994;190:175–179.
140. Pelc NJ, Sommer FG, Li KC, Brosnan TJ, Herfkens RJ, Enzmann DR. Quantitative magnetic resonance flow imaging. *Magn Reson Q.* 1994;10:125–147.
141. Li KC, Hopkins KL, Dalman RL, Song CK. Simultaneous measurement of flow in the superior mesenteric vein and artery with cine phase-contrast MR imaging: value in diagnosis of chronic mesenteric ischemia. Work in progress. *Radiology.* 1995;194:327–330.
142. Li KC. MR angiography of abdominal ischemia. *Semin Ultrasound CT MR.* 1996;17:352–359.
143. Dalman RL, Li KC, Moon WK, Chen I, Zarins CK. Diminished postprandial hyperemia in patients with aortic and mesenteric arterial occlusive disease. Quantification by magnetic resonance flow imaging. *Circulation.* 1996;94:(II)206–210.
144. Li KC, Wright GA, Pelc LR, et al. Oxygen saturation of blood in the superior mesenteric vein: in vivo verification of MR imaging measurements in a canine model. Work in progress. *Radiology.* 1995;194:321–325.
145. Mirowitz SA. Contrast enhancement of the gastrointestinal tract on MR images using intravenous gadolinium-DTPA. *Abdom Imaging.* 1993;18:215–219.

Scintigraphy

Christopher F. Schultz, Abass Alavi, and Gary R. Lichtenstein

Chapter Contents

Acute Gastrointestinal Hemorrhage
Meckel's Diverticulum
Retained Gastric Antrum
Small Intestinal Transit
Postgastrectomy Transit Disorders
Crohn's Disease of the Small Intestine
Carcinoid Tumors of the Small Intestine

Scintigraphic imaging techniques play an increasingly important role in the evaluation of patients with small intestinal disease. These technologies are often used in combination with other diagnostic modalities and offer several advantages over contrast radiography, computed tomography, magnetic resonance imaging, ultrasound, endoscopy, and manometry. Scintigraphy is generally safe, noninvasive, simple to perform, moderate in cost, and superior in its ability to characterize tissue types and yield quantifiable physiologic and metabolic information. This chapter reviews the role of nuclear scintigraphy in the evaluation of intestinal hemorrhage, Meckel's diverticulum, retained gastric antrum, small bowel transit, postgastrectomy transit disorders, Crohn's disease of the small intestine, and small bowel carcinoid tumors. A detailed discussion of the basic principles of nuclear imaging and radiopharmaceutical chemistry is beyond the scope of this clinically oriented chapter. The reader is directed to texts within the field of nuclear medicine if a more comprehensive review of these topics is desired.

Acute Gastrointestinal Hemorrhage

Acute gastrointestinal (GI) hemorrhage is a common, potentially life-threatening condition. Accurate localization of the bleeding site is essential for the definitive management of these emergencies. Bleeding arising in the upper GI tract (defined as bleeding from a source proximal to the ligament of Treitz) often presents with melena or hematemesis and is probably best examined by endoscopic methods. Acute lower GI bleeding (ie, below the ligament of Treitz) is usually the result of colonic disease but may occasionally originate in the small intestine. The most common causes of massive small intestinal hemorrhage are angiodysplasia, Crohn's disease, lymphoma, vasculitis, Meckel's diverticulum, leiomyoma, juvenile polyps, carcinoma, and undetermined causes.[1] The diagnostic modalities utilized in the identification of the source of acute lower GI hemorrhage include colonoscopy, angiography, and nuclear scintigraphy. Colonoscopy permits identification of a variety of large bowel lesions and, occasionally, therapeutic intervention. Unfortunately, even in the absence of active hemorrhage, the endoscopic evaluation may be limited by the presence of retained blood throughout the entire length of colonic lumen, making localization of a specific source difficult. Alternatively, active hemorrhage may be so rapid that urgent colonoscopy after purge still will not allow for adequate visualization. Angiography is invasive, has significant morbidity in patients with renal or heart failure, and is less sensitive than the scintigraphic techniques but does afford the opportunity to intervene with selective intra-arterial infusion of vasopressin or embolization.

Nuclear scintigraphic methods are widely available, highly sensitive, can be performed quickly with relative ease, and are associated with minimal morbidity. When used in concert with arteriography or endoscopy (particularly in those patients where no bleeding site can be identified or in whom blood loss is intermittent), these studies have become a cornerstone of our diagnostic armamentarium.[2]

Technique

Two classes of scintigraphic tracers are currently available for the localization of GI hemorrhage. Agents that clear from the circulation include technetium-99m sulfur colloid (99mTcSC), the radiopharmaceutical commonly used for liver and spleen scanning, and technetium-99m albumin microcolloid.[3,4] Colloids are cleared rapidly from the blood and represent the most sensitive imaging tracer for GI hemorrhage.[5] The second class of radionuclide tracers are the blood-pool agents, which have a longer intravascular half-life that allows for delayed imaging in patients with intermittent bleeding. Several such radiotracers are now available for this purpose and include technetium-99m–labeled red blood cells (99mTc-RBC) and albumin.[4,6–10]

Because colloid is rapidly cleared by the reticuloendothelial system (RES), with a half-life of 2.5 to 3.5 minutes, and most being eliminated from the intravascular space by 15 minutes, the technique of 99mTcSC scintigraphy is probably best suited for the evaluation of patients who are believed to be actively hemorrhaging at the time of scanning.[3–5,11] The rapid RES clearance of circulating radionuclide results in very low vascular background activity, and the resultant high target-to-background ratio permits the identification of small amounts of extravasated tracer in the bowel lumen. In animal studies, 99mTcSC scintigraphy has detected bleeding rates of 0.05 to 0.1 ml/min.[5] A standard methodology for the 99mTcSC bleeding scan is outlined in Table 11-1. The addition of dynamic 5-second radionuclide angiography during the initial 60 seconds after injection may increase the sensitivity for nonbleeding hypervascular lesions such as leiomyomas, varices, and pseudoaneurysms.

Furthermore, because delayed images cannot reflect the rapid peristalsis (and retrograde movement) often observed in the presence of brisk hemorrhage, frequent imaging permits clearer definition of the exact or approximate location of active bleeding sites.[12]

Blood-pool labeling techniques include the in vitro, in vivo and the modified in vitro methods.[4,8–10] The in vitro RBC labeling technique (Ultra Tag, Mallinckrodt Medical Inc, St. Louis, Mo) results in the highest labeling efficiency available (greater than 95%) with minimal gastric mucosal and urinary tract secretion of free 99mTc pertechnetate and should be considered the method of choice for most GI bleeding studies.[13] Several medications may cause ineffective labeling of RBCs and the release of free 99mTc pertechnetate, which can be secreted by the gastric mucosa and may be misinterpreted as active upper GI hemorrhage. These medications include systemic heparin, methyldopa, hydralazine, quinidine, digoxin, propranolol, and doxorubicin.[4] As in the sulfur colloid technique, dynamic early imaging appears to increase the sensitivity and specificity of 99mTc-RBC bleeding scans. Maurer and colleagues performed "cinescintigraphy," obtaining continuous computerized dynamic images for 15 seconds per image in 15-minute sets (60 images per set). Image sets were then reviewed with a cinematic computer display screen while subsequent image sets were being obtained. This allows the physician to monitor the study and terminate imaging if a bleeding site is identified. More accurate localization or greater sensitivity over standard static images was

Table 11-1. Protocol for 99mTc sulfur colloid bleeding scan

Patient selection
   Nasogastric lavage negative for upper gastrointestinal hemorrhage
   Active bleeding believed to be on going

Radiopharmaceutical
   10 to 15 mCi of freshly prepared 99mTcSC injected intravenously

Data collection
   Large field-of-view gamma camera with low-energy all-purpose collimator
   Computer acquisition is preferable
   Intensity set to visualize bone marrow in every image
   Supine position, lower liver edge to pelvis
   Flow images immediately postinjection, 1 frame every 3 to 5 seconds for 60 seconds
   Static images for 750,000 to 1,000,000 counts every 1 to 2 minutes for 15 to 20 minutes.
   If negative, 1.5 million counts of the abdomen in anterior and left anterior oblique projections
   If negative, supplementary views of stool passed postinjection or glove postdigital rectal exam
   For repeat study minutes to hours later, increase all images by 200,000 to 500,000 counts

Source: Modified from Alavi and Ring.[3]

achieved in 8 of 21 patients (38%) with positive bleeding scans.[14] Because GI hemorrhage originating in the small intestine is perhaps the most difficult to localize correctly,[15,16] some investigators have used intravenous glucagon to inhibit peristalsis, aiding in the focal accumulation of extravasated radionuclide and improving localization of bleeding sites within the small bowel.[17]

Scan Interpretation

Normally a 99mTcSC bleeding scan demonstrates activity throughout the RES (liver, spleen, and bone marrow), conveniently providing easily recognizable anatomic landmarks for rapid study interpretation (Fig. 11-1). This normal level of upper abdominal signal intensity can, however, obscure intraluminal tracer in adjacent or superimposed bowel loops, resulting in a false-negative study or inaccurate site localization. The bladder and male genitalia may occasionally be seen. Renal transplants appear as discrete structures that remain unchanged over time. In patients with end-stage liver disease, the hepatic blood flow is impaired and relatively greater amounts of sulfur colloid are removed from circulation by the bone marrow and spleen. An ectopic spleen may demonstrate increasing levels of activity but should remain stationary with serial imaging. An abnormal or positive study is defined as a focal accumulation of radionuclide that increases in intensity over time and moves distally on sequential images, following a pattern typical for large or small bowel (Fig. 11-2). Normal vascular structures, vascular abnormalities (collateral vessels, aneurysms, pseudoaneurysms, or ectatic vessels) or hypervascular lesions may be detected on the sulfur colloid angiogram, even in the absence of active bleeding.

Blood-pool labeling with 99mTc-RBC results in high vascular background activity in the heart, aorta, vena cava, and other large vessels. Hepatic and splenic activity is present but appears less intense in comparison to 99mTcSC scintigraphy (Fig. 11-3). A focus of abnormal activity, not associated with the normal vascular landmarks, which appears to lie within the intestinal lumen and moves distally, is evidence of active GI hemorrhage. The accuracy of 99mTc-RBC bleeding scans in localizing the site of GI hemorrhage ranges in the medical literature from 41% to 94%.[18] Consequently, the utility of these technologies in the evaluation of the actively bleeding patient is controversial. Because of inaccuracies in localizing the bleeding sites, some have advocated abandoning labeled RBC scans for this purpose. A review of 16 positive-tagged RBC scans with corroborating studies (angiography, endoscopy, surgery, or a combination of these) found that 14 (88%) correctly localized the site of bleeding. Seventy-one percent of the accurately localized studies were abnormal during the early continuous phase of imaging (first 2 hours). Contrast angiography is reported to be diagnostic in only 65% of individuals who are actively bleeding at the time of study[16] (bleeding sensitivity of >0.5 ml/min). Suzman and others reported a retrospective analysis of 224 patients with active lower GI bleeding who underwent erythrocyte scintigraphy. Prognostically, patients with a positive/localizing scan were five times more likely to require surgical intervention than individuals with a negative study.[19] It was also reported that only 2% of

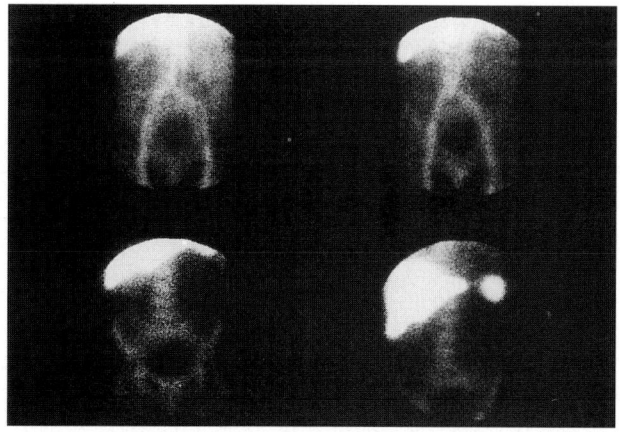

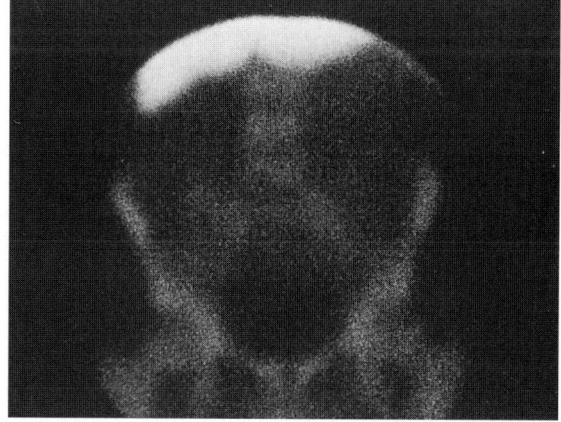

Fig. 11-1. Negative sulfur colloid scan.
(a) Images obtained immediately after the administration of the radiotracer reveal a vascular pattern that clears relatively fast. (b) Delayed images show uptake in the liver, spleen, and bone marrow without tracer activity in the GI tract.

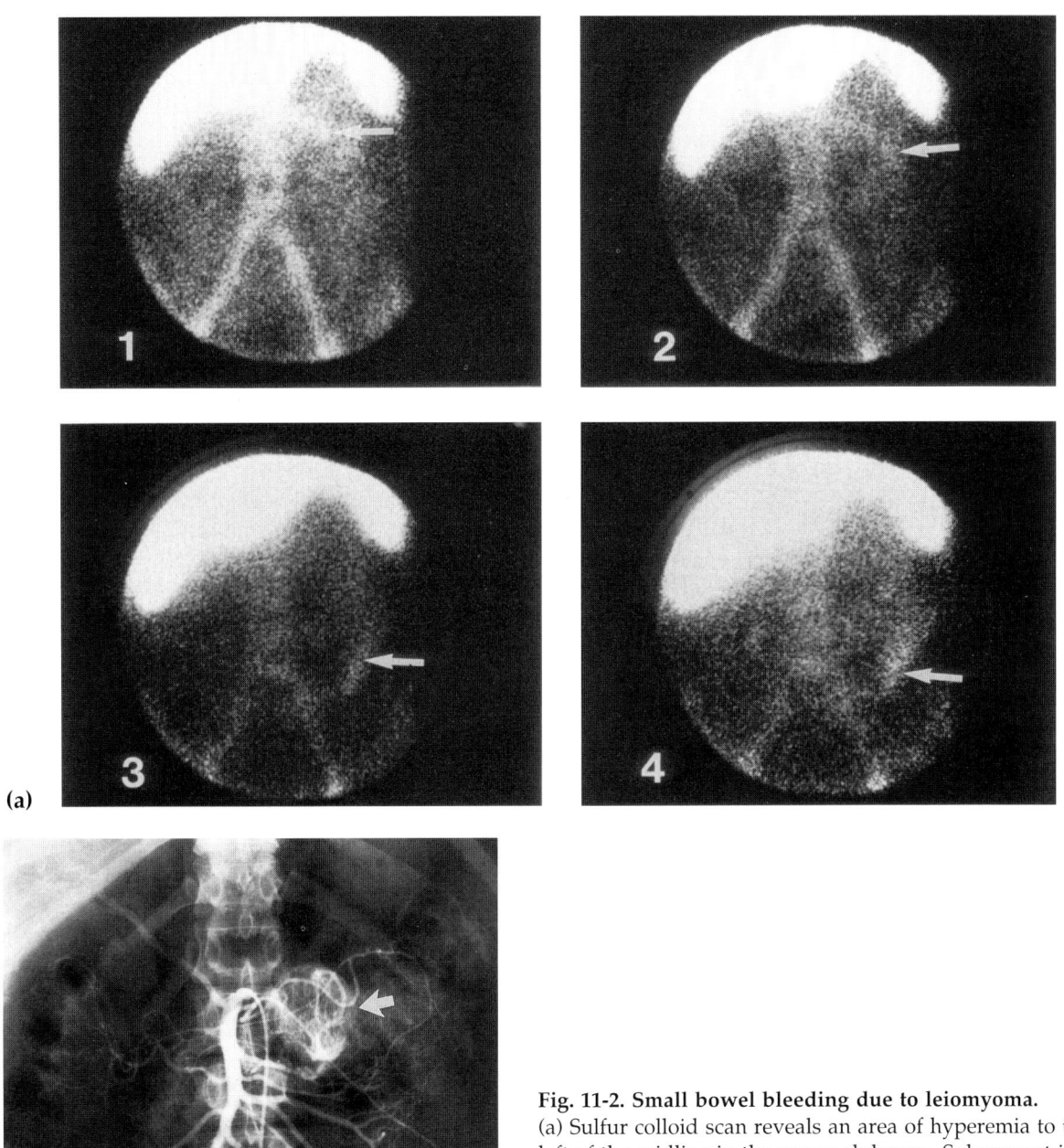

Fig. 11-2. Small bowel bleeding due to leiomyoma. (a) Sulfur colloid scan reveals an area of hyperemia to the left of the midline in the upper abdomen. Subsequent images reveal evidence of extravasation into an area most likely representing jejunum. Consecutive images (1 to 4) show the radioactive blood to move to the lower abdomen on the left (arrows). (b) A superior mesenteric arteriogram reveals a vascular lesion in the same location, most consistent with a leiomyoma (as confirmed by a histopathology after surgery).

patients with a negative bleeding scan ultimately required surgery.[20]

In summary, the 99mTc-labeled RBC scans are highly sensitive and compare favorably to the bleeding rates detected by sulfur colloid scanning.[21] Blood-pool labeling technologies are superior to colloid for the evaluation of intermittent lower GI bleeding because they permit repeated dynamic continuous imaging for up to 24 hours without reinjection. However, a positive result without continuous monitoring of the patient frequently misrepresents the true site of hemorrhage and should be interpreted with caution. Also,

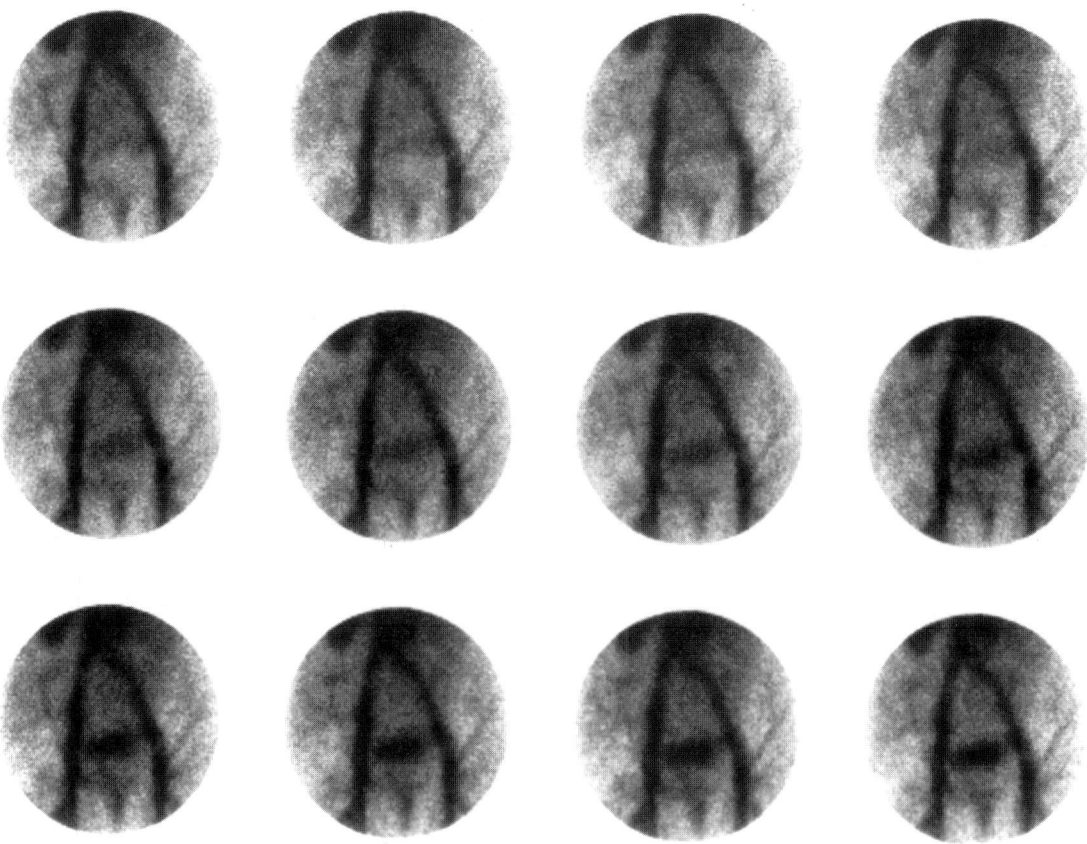

Fig. 11-3. Normal red blood cell scan.
Following the intravenous administration of labeled red blood cells, a normal vascular pattern is noted. There is also a significant level of background activity that remains the same throughout the examination. The latter represents blood pool in the small vessels and capillaries. Note gradual accumulation of radiotracer in the bladder, which is unavoidable in spite of significant improvement in labeling techniques.

false-positive tests can result from the gastric and small bowel secretion of free pertechnetate during the performance of 99mTc-RBC bleeding scans; however, careful assessment and exclusion of upper GI sources of bleeding by endoscopy should make it possible for this technology to accurately localize sites of small intestinal hemorrhage.[22] Ultimately, application of these technologies should assist those performing angiography by identifying patients who are not actively bleeding and by limiting angiographic studies to the most likely culprit vessels.

Meckel's Diverticulum

This represents the most common congenital anomaly of the GI tract, with a prevalence of approximately 1% to 2% in the general population. A true diverticula (ie, containing all layers of the bowel wall), Meckel's diverticulum usually occurs within 100 cm of the ileocecal valve and measures less than 2 in in length.[23] Heterotopic tissue is present in 50% of all diverticula and is most commonly composed of gastric mucosa, pancreatic tissue, or their combination.[24]

Acid secretion by heterotopic gastric mucosa may result in ulceration within or close to the diverticulum and consequent GI hemorrhage. Almost all bleeding diverticula contain gastric mucosa[25] and are thus theoretically detectable by 99mTc-pertechnetate imaging. Bleeding is the most common symptom in children but is a relatively rare complication of the anomaly in adults. A review of 402 cases found GI hemorrhage due to Meckel's to be age-specific, occurring in no one over 31 years of age.[23]

The risk of developing any complication due to a Meckel's diverticulum decreases with age. Of those individuals who become symptomatic, 50% of cases occur before the age of 2 years[26] and usually manifest as bleeding or obstruction. Only 2% of adults with Meckel's diverticulum appear to develop symptoms.[27] The most frequent complication in the adult is small bowel obstruction, often the result of intussusception or volvulus. Perforation, diverticulitis, carcinoma, and bleeding may also occur in the adult population.[24] When considering all patients with a complication of Meckel's diverticulum (including nonhemorrhagic presentations), the literature indicates a prevalence of only 34% to 57% of heterotopic tissue.[23,28] This may limit the sensitivity of 99mTc-pertechnetate scanning if nonbleeding patients are studied.

At the cellular level, defining the specific site of 99mTc-pertechnetate concentration and secretion has proved somewhat problematic and controversial. It now seems possible that the surface mucus-secreting cells in the stomach and the ectopic gastric mucosa of a Meckel's diverticulum are responsible for concentration and secretion of pertechnetate (although a dual mechanism with some concomitant parietal cell secretion cannot be excluded). This appears to be influenced by the surface area, blood flow, and viability of the gastric tissue. An additional hypothesis suggests that the movement of 99mTc-pertechnetate from cell to lumen may also be pH-dependent, with higher acid secretion promoting reflux of pertechnetate while inhibition of acid secretion could result in back diffusion and mucosal accumulation.[29]

Technique

A typical protocol is described in Table 11-2. Any patient suspected of having a Meckel's diverticulum is appropriate for 99mTc-pertechnetate scanning. Perhaps the best candidates for a Meckel's scan are those with suspected small intestinal hemorrhage or a previous history of GI bleeding, or persons under 40 years of age, because they are more likely to have functioning heterotopic gastric mucosa, which is necessary for a positive scan. Several pharmacologic modifications of this technique have been employed to improve the sensitivity and specificity. The administration of pentagastrin 6 μg/kg body weight subcutaneously 15 minutes before intravenous injection of 99mTc-pertechnetate to a 3-year-old patient with rectal bleeding rendered positive a previously negative Meckel's scan.[30] Pentagastrin increases gastric mucosal blood flow, gastric acid output, and intestinal motility. This results in conversion to a positive study, increased intensity of gastric mucosal uptake, and reduced background activity. A Meckel's diverticulum was subsequently confirmed at laparotomy.[30] Caution should be exercised when premedicating with pentagastrin because the augmentation of gastric mucosal acid secretion may worsen ileal ulceration and induce further bleeding. Cimetidine has also been used to reduce the rate of false-negative scanning. In a case report of a 33-year-old male patient with a previously negative Meckel's scan and recurrent lower GI hemorrhage,

Table 11-2. Protocol for Meckel's diverticulum scan

Patient preparation
  Nothing by mouth for 6 to 12 hours
  Frequent bladder emptying should be encouraged for visualization of a Meckel's diverticulum low in the pelvis
  Some patients positioned on left side to minimize emptying of pertechnetate into the duodenum; in others, nasogastric suction

Agent and dose
  99m technetium pertechnetate (TcO4)
  50 to 200 uCi/kg bodyweight or 10 to 15 mCi in adults as intravenous bolus

Data collection
  Large field-of-view gamma camera
  Angiogram during transient blood-pool phase (analogous to 99mTcSC and 99mTc-RBCs) obtaining 1 frame every 1 to 5 seconds, anterior abdominal images for 60 seconds
  Dynamic images for 500,000 to 750,000 counts per image for 60 minutes
  Delayed anterior, oblique, and lateral views as necessary
  Postvoid imaging should be obtained

Source: Adapted from Sfaidanakis and Conway[26] and Datz.[32]

treatment with intravenous cimetidine prior to a second study allowed for accumulation of tracer in the mid-lower abdomen. A Meckel's diverticulum containing gastric mucosa was identified at operation.[25] Cimetidine is believed to work by inhibition of mucosal secretion of pertechnetate, leading to an increase in the mucosal concentration of radionuclide. Glucagon has been used to delay the peristaltic movement of 99mTc-pertechnetate away from the lesion (improving sensitivity) and to slow the distal movement of secreted tracer by the stomach to the small bowel, theoretically reducing the likelihood of a false-positive result.[31]

Scan Interpretation

Following injection of 99mTc-pertechnetate, early flow images demonstrate blood-pool activity in the heart, liver, spleen, kidneys, and large vessels of the abdomen. Genitourinary activity is also seen early in the exam, and the renal pelvis is often quite prominent. Increasing gastric activity is noted during the first 5 to 20 minutes of the study, and radionuclide may subsequently be seen to leave the stomach and move distally into the small bowel. Rarely, a focal ureteral collection can be visualized at the level of the pelvic brim. Bladder activity is identified by its expected location and predictable increase in size and intensity as the study progresses.[32]

A positive scan is characterized by progressive accumulation of tracer as a discrete focus, usually of high signal intensity, appearing simultaneously with uptake of 99mTc-pertechnetate in the normal gastric mucosa[33] (Fig. 11-4). Although most commonly located in the anterior aspect of the right lower quadrant, a Meckel's diverticulum can appear anywhere

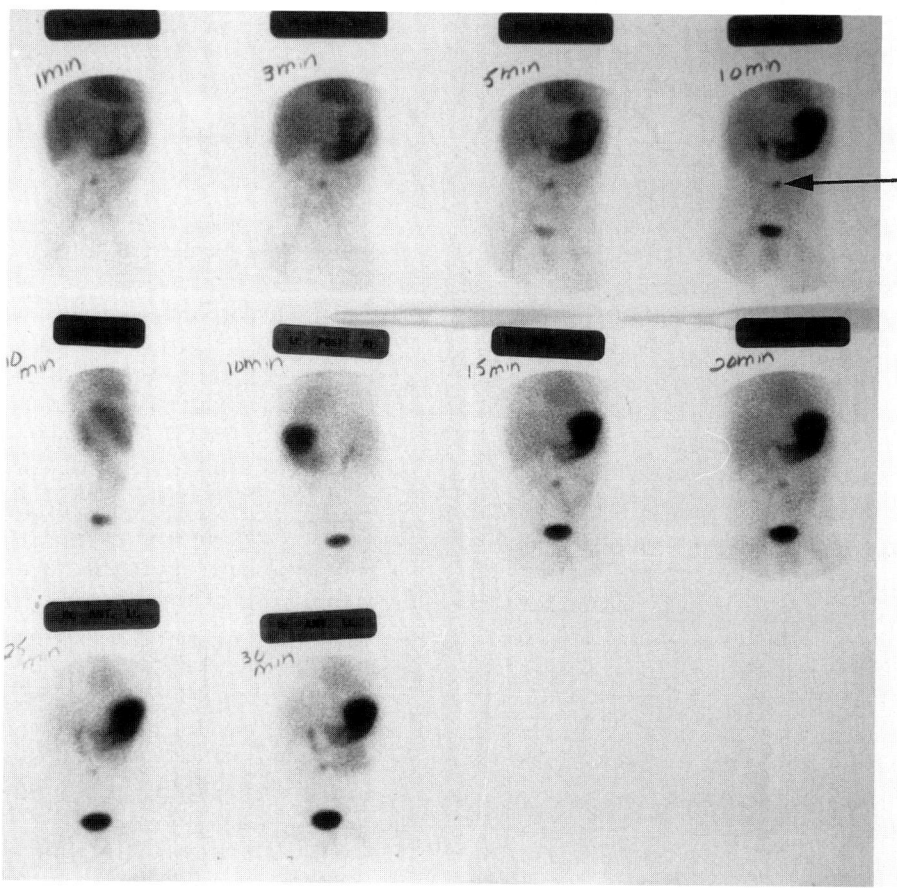

Fig. 11-4. Positive Meckel scan.
Following the intravenous administration of technetium-99m pertechnetate, there is rapid accumulation in the stomach, which remains intense throughout the examination. Simultaneous with stomach uptake a focus of mild concentration is noted in the midabdomen between the bladder and upper abdomen. The tracer activity becomes more intense over time, which is typical for ectopic gastric mucosa. This pattern is typical for Meckel's diverticulum. The first and second images in the middle row represent right lateral and posterior views, necessary for definitive diagnosis.

within the abdomen and may exhibit considerable movement, spontaneously or with changes in the patient's position. Abnormal but atypical results that do not meet "classic" criteria for a positive scan may still yield important diagnostic information. An actively bleeding Meckel's diverticulum was demonstrated during the radionuclide angiogram portion of a pertechnetate study as intraluminal tracer extravasated into the small bowel lumen.[34] Another atypical Meckel's scan was "transiently positive" then "faded," only to reappear in subsequent images. At surgery, a Meckel's diverticulum with gastric-type mucosa was found with an adjacent bleeding ileal ulcer.[35]

Since first described in 1970,[36] the use of pertechnetate scintigraphy to detect heterotopic gastric mucosa in a Meckel's diverticulum has gained widespread acceptance. As the technology advanced and with the introduction of the gamma camera, a surgically proven sensitivity of 85% to 91%, a specificity of 95% to 100%, and an accuracy of 90% to 94% was reported for 99mTc-pertechnetate scanning of ectopic gastric mucosa.[26,33] However, most of the patients in one of the reports[33] were children (greater than 90%) and considerable controversy arose over the applicability and usefulness of the Meckel's scan as a diagnostic tool in adults.[25] In a review of 49 patients[37] with surgically confirmed Meckel's diverticulum, 11 of the patients (mean age 26.1 years) had preoperative radiologic investigation of the small intestine. Only one of six patients had a positive radionuclide scan. The most common reason for a false-negative Meckel's scan was the absence of or insufficient amount of viable ectopic gastric mucosa within the diverticulum. As small as 1 square cm of ectopic gastric mucosa can be visualized by modern high-resolution techniques.[38] In a review of the literature including 184 adults with surgically proven Meckel's diverticulum a sensitivity of 62.5%, a specificity of 9%, and an accuracy of 46% were found.[39] It was postulated that the technology was more accurate in children because they were more likely to have larger areas of ectopic gastric mucosa within their diverticula.[40,41] Other causes of a false-negative Meckel's scan include 1) necrotic or ulcerated ectopic gastric mucosa, 2) impaired diverticular blood supply secondary to intussusception, volvulus, or ischemia, 3) "wash-out" of tracer by active bleeding, or 4) a variety of technical problems.[39] False positive Meckel scans have also been reported.[42]

Retained Gastric Antrum

The retained gastric antrum syndrome is a rare and unfortunate consequence of peptic ulcer disease surgery following antrectomy and Billroth II gastrojejunostomy.[43] It is characterized by inadequate gastric resection leaving a portion of gastric antrum within the duodenal stump. Because the antral remnant is not in contact with the acidic gastric stream, the remaining antral G cells are released from the normal negative feedback loop in which gastrin release is inhibited by low intraluminal pH. Hypergastrinemia and continuous stimulation of parietal cells results in increased acid output and recurrent marginal ulceration. Serum gastrin levels may rise to the range seen in the Zollinger-Ellison syndrome.

Technetium pertechnetate imaging can be used to identify the presence of a retained gastric antrum.[2] Following administration of 99mTc-pertechnetate, no activity should localize to the afferent loop. Dynamic imaging allows the physician to differentiate a confirmatory scan from retrograde filling of the afferent loop. Technetium pertechnetate imaging is reported to have a sensitivity of 73% and specificity of 100% for retained gastric antrum.[44]

Small Intestinal Transit

Patients frequently seek medical attention for a variety of nonspecific GI symptoms (abdominal pain, distension, bloating, nausea, vomiting, postprandial abdominal discomfort, diarrhea, constipation, etc). Individuals with chronic or recurrent symptoms referable to the alimentary tract, without an identifiable structural, infectious, or biochemical explanation, are often presumed to have a functional disorder. These symptoms can reflect the presence of a GI motility disorder. An understanding of the pathophysiology of a patient's symptom complex may facilitate a more directed therapeutic approach and alleviate patient anxiety. In disease states affecting small intestinal motility (ie, chronic idiopathic intestinal pseudo-obstruction [CIIP], diabetes mellitus, progressive systemic sclerosis [PSS], postvagotomy, amyloidosis, irritable bowel syndrome [IBS], etc). measurement of the small bowel transit time (SBTT), most commonly as a component of whole-gut transit time, can now be accomplished using scintigraphic methods.[45]

Historically, hydrogen breath testing with lactulose has been employed in the evaluation of patients with suspected abnormalities in SBTT. Breath testing, however, reflects only the leading-edge cecal arrival time of substrate and does not allow for measurement of the overall transit time for the bulk of the meal. Breath testing is also prone to errors in the assessment of small intestinal transit because correction for abnormalities or individual variations in gastric emptying is not feasible.[46,47] Furthermore, lactulose itself actually slows gastric emptying of solids and accelerates SBTT and the orocecal transit time (OCTT).[48] Lactulose breath tests are frequently difficult to interpret. Up to 25% of the population lack the necessary bacterial strains to metabolize this sugar,[49,50] and hydrogen production may be impaired due to low colonic pH.[51] Small intestinal bacterial overgrowth, systemic antibiotics, colonic enemas, oral flora, and smoking may result in artifactual data.[52,53]

Small bowel manometry (SBM) has also been performed in patients with functional disorders of the GI tract.[54] Assessment of motility patterns during the fasting and fed states can be achieved and differentiation between myopathic and neuropathic processes is frequently possible. Several disadvantages, however, limit the clinical application of SBM. First, the motility recording obtained represents only proximal small bowel motor function and provides no information regarding the distal two thirds of the small intestine. Second, SBM is invasive and fluoroscopy is often necessary to ensure proper catheter placement.[55] Third, the mere presence of a luminal gastroduodenal catheter has been implicated in altering SBTT.[56] Finally, manometry measures the "pressure profile" of small intestinal motor activity but does not actually assess its effect on the propagation of chyme over time and, hence, does not truly measure transit.[52]

Technique

In numerous studies designed to measure GI transit, various radionuclides (99mTc, 6-hour half-life),[47,57] indium-111 (111-In) (2.8-day half-life),[45] and iodine-131[58] have been used to label a heterogeneous group of materials—water,[59] mashed potatoes,[57] dietary fiber (the so-called "bran scan"),[58,60] scrambled eggs,[45] and polystyrene pellets,[61,62] which are then ingested by the study subject. Unless contraindicated, all medications known to affect GI motility should be discontinued 48 to 72 hours prior to the study and patients should be fasting for 8 to 12 hours. In premenopausal women, the examination should be performed in the first 2 weeks of the menstrual cycle because high serum progesterone levels in the latter half of the cycle are a likely cause of slow gastric emptying.

When performed as an adjunct to the gastric emptying scan, SBTT is measured by the use of dual isotopes and prolonged imaging. Because 99mTc and 111-In have different energies, both radiopharmaceuticals can be imaged separately, allowing for simultaneous assessment of the solid and liquid phases.[55,63] Maurer and Krevsky[45] recommend the use of two large scrambled eggs labeled with 500 uCi 99mTcSC served between two pieces of white bread. The sandwich is eaten within 5 minutes. The subject then drinks 300 ml of water containing 125 uCi 111-In-diethylenetriaminepentaacetic acid (DTPA). Gastric emptying is measured in standard fashion. Determination of SBTT generally requires an additional 4 hours of imaging over the usual 2 hours necessary for gastric emptying analysis.[55,59,64] After 120 minutes, sets of 60-second, anterior and posterior supine images (to better define the terminal ileum and cecum) are obtained every 20 to 30 minutes. Imaging is continued for up to 400 minutes or until at least 10% of total abdominal counts fill the cecum or ascending colon (cecal arrival time).[45] Alternatively, analysis of distal ileum filling can serve as an index of SBTT.[59] As described previously, all data are then analyzed using geometric mean-corrected counts.[65] A recently described similar technique used 250 uCi 111-In-polystyrene resin pellets in healthy subjects and patients with either gastroparesis or CIIP.[66] It demonstrated that a more limited number of scans taken at 2, 4, and 6 hours after ingestion of a radiolabeled solid meal could provide adequate sensitivity for identification of these disorders at considerable cost savings.

Scan Interpretation

In the absence of severe gastroparesis, 111-In-DTPA radiolabeled liquids empty quickly (and exponentially) from the stomach, while the passage of 99mTc-labeled solids into the duodenum is characterized by an initial lag phase followed by a slow, linear emptying phase. In the small intestine, however, solid and liquid components of chyme move at similar speeds, occasionally progressing in a "stop-and-go" fashion, with the bulk of liquid tracer maintaining the initial lead-time provided by its earlier gastric exit.[58] Chyme spreads out as it moves through the small intestine, passing distally, not as a bolus, but as a "spectrum of transit times".[58] The most rapid small intestinal transit is seen in the duodenum and jejunum. Ileal transit of chyme is somewhat slower,[67] and the terminal ileum appears to serve a reservoir function before filling of the right colon occurs.[68] Emptying of the distal ileum into the colon does not occur linearly but is associated with a series of bolus transfers[61] that may be impaired in myopathic disease processes such as PSS or delayed as in the visceral neuropathy seen in diabetes mellitus.[69] In the above protocol, the normal mean SBTT (measured as cecal arrival time) was 232 minutes, with a wide range (+/− 2SD) of 72 to 392 minutes.[45] Alternatively, if one uses colonic filling as the study endpoint, normal values are reported to range from 11% to 70% of scintigraphic tracer detectable in the ascending colon region of interest at 6 hours.[64]

The clinical utility of identifying an abnormal SBTT has been questioned.[46] Transit may or may not be abnormal in functional bowel disorders. Charles et al[64] reported on their experience with 65 patients with functional bowel disorders. In patients with functional constipation, SBTT was slow in only 12 of 35 patients (34%) and colonic transit was normal or fast in 32 (66%). Delayed ileal emptying has been shown by scintigraphic methods to affect at least a subset of patients with IBS irritable bowel syndrome.[60] Currently, however, there is little evidence that demonstration of these abnormalities in SBTT change patient management. Markedly prolonged SBTT in patients with CIIP is shortened following treatment with cisapride,[70] and scintigraphy could prove useful in the management of these patients. Talley has suggested that in the evaluation of patients with suspected isolated colonic inertia, confirmation of normal SBTT would help exclude patients with a more widespread motor disorder (ie, CIIP) that might preclude colectomy.[46] Further studies are clearly warranted to better define the clinical role of this promising technology in the evaluation and management of patients with functional disorders of the small intestine.

Postgastrectomy Transit Disorders

Afferent loop syndrome results from obstruction of the afferent segment of a gastrojejunostomy.[71] Acutely, patients complain of abdominal pain and nonbilious emesis with complete obstruction of the afferent limb. In its more common, chronic form (secondary to partial obstruction of the afferent loop), patients may present with right upper quadrant pain exacerbated by meals, with nausea, vomiting, and weight loss. Intestinal stasis may result in a "blind loop" syndrome characterized by bacterial overgrowth and malabsorption. The intestinal phase of cholescintigraphy has been reported to demonstrate (serendipitously) intermittent afferent loop obstruction[72] and may be considered in the diagnostic evaluation of these patients.

The Roux stasis syndrome may be seen in 10% to 50% of patients following Roux-en-Y gastroenterostomy.[71] Symptoms can include epigastric fullness, abdominal pain, nausea, and vomiting. Both the vagotomized gastric remnant and the Roux limb are believed to contribute to the development of the Roux stasis syndrome. Nuclear imaging appears to be useful in the diagnosis of this disorder. Scintigraphic evidence of Roux limb stasis has been reported in 18 of 28 symptomatic patients (64%) and in only 3 of 27 asymptomatic patients (11%) ($p < 0.01$).[73]

Crohn's Disease of the Small Intestine

Crohn's disease is an idiopathic, chronic disorder characterized by segmental and discontinuous transmural bowel inflammation involving the small bowel in 70% of patients. Patients usually present with symptoms of abdominal pain and diarrhea (see Chapter 15). Labeled leukocyte scintigraphy may be useful in the diagnosis and management of these patients by allowing for a rapid, noninvasive estimation of disease extent and severity with minimal associated morbidity. The use of 18F-fluorodeoxyglucose positron emission tomography (PET) may also prove to be of use in the evaluation of the patients.

Technique and Scan Interpretation

Leukocyte labeling is most commonly performed with 111-In-tropolonate or oxine[74] and 99mTc-hexamethyl propylene amine oxime (HMPAO).[75] Leukocytes are obtained from the study subject, separated, and labeled by incubation with the radiopharmaceutical in saline (111-In) or plasma (99mTc). After injection, labeled granulocytes marginate and then migrate to areas of inflammation before being shed into the bowel lumen.[76] Indium-111 leukocyte (111-In-WBC [white blood cell]) imaging is usually carried out at 2 to 4 hours after injection.[77] Technetium-99m-HMPAO images are routinely obtained soon after injection, often demonstrating activity at 15 to 30 minutes postinjection and becoming intense in areas of inflamed bowel over 1 hour.[78] Late imaging is rarely indicated unless assessment for intra-abdominal abscesses is the indication for the examination[79,80] or, perhaps, when differentiating between fibrotic and inflammatory strictures.[81] Both cell preparations distribute early to liver, spleen, and bone marrow.

While the precise role of leukocyte scintigraphy in the evaluation and management of patients with small intestinal Crohn's disease has yet to be fully defined, at the very least, this technology serves as a useful adjunct to more traditional diagnostic modalities. The sensitivity of 111-In-WBC scanning when compared to small bowel radiography is approximately 70%.[76,82,83] Technetium-99m-HMPAO-labeled WBC scans appear to have greater sensitivity in defining the extent of small bowel disease, particularly terminal ileal involvement. Of 18 patients with known small bowel Crohn's disease who underwent 99Tc-HMPAO-WBC scintigraphy and barium radiography (up to 9 months between studies), all those with terminal ileal disease by contrast radiography (12 patients) had positive scans with good correlation as to site and disease extent.[74] In another report, 99mTc-HMPAO-WBC scanning could reliably determine the location of disease and, to a lesser degree, the severity of disease activity. Scintigraphic activity weakly correlated with the Crohn's disease activity index (CDAI) and erythrocyte sedimentation rate (ESR).[84] Nuclear imaging has also demonstrated complications of Crohn's disease including abscesses,[79] fistulae, and sinus tracts.[85] Comparative studies have shown leukocyte scanning with 99mTc-HMPAO-WBC to be superior to 111-In-WBC scans[86,87] and radioimmunoscintigraphy[88,89] for imaging Crohn's disease of the small intestine. It was concluded that "except when fecal excretion studies are contemplated, 99mTc-HMPAO should be the preferred leukocyte label, on the grounds of availability, image quality, ease of use, and radiation dosimetry."[76]

Carcinoid Tumors of the Small Intestine

Carcinoid tumor is the second most common malignancy affecting the small bowel, accounting for 17% to 39% of all small intestinal tumors.[90] Seventy-eight percent of small bowel carcinoids occur in ileum, 18% in the duodenum, and 4% in the jejunum.[90] All small intestinal carcinoids have metastatic potential, but the majority of these lesions are clinically silent and are often discovered incidentally at endoscopy, computed tomography, or during small bowel contrast radiography (see Chapter 19). This discussion will be limited to the scintigraphic diagnostic approach to primary lesions of the small intestine and will not address the use of this technology in the evaluation and treatment of distant metastases.

Technique and Scan Interpretation

Since the introduction of somatostatin receptor (SSTR) scintigraphy for the localization of neuroendocrine tumors by Krenning et al in 1989,[91] octreotide scanning has become the preferred method for imaging solitary, resectable, small intestinal carcinoids. Octreotide is a long-acting synthetic octapeptide homologous with somatostatin at the four amino-acid sequence that confers its biologic activity.[92] Derived from neural crest cells, carcinoid tumors express somatostatin (analogue) receptors in over 80% of cases.[93] The most frequently expressed somatostatin receptor subtype is SSTR 2, which also has the highest binding affinity for octreotide.[94] Radioisotope bound to modified octreotide is used to target cell surface–expressed somatostatin receptors.[92] Indium-111-DTPA-D-Phe-octreotide has emerged as the radiopharmaceutical of choice for SSTR scintigraphy because of its long physical half-life, low vascular background activity, lack of significant biliary excretion, and ease of preparation

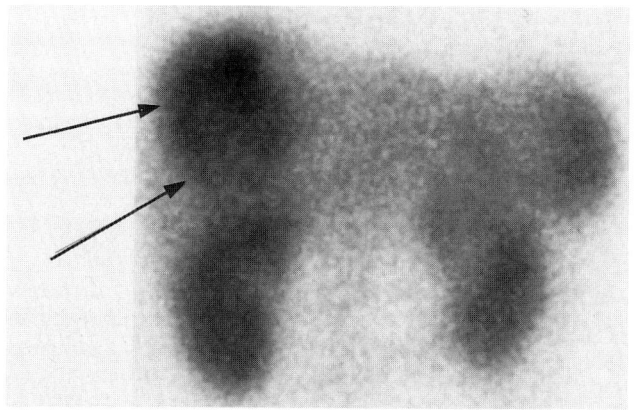 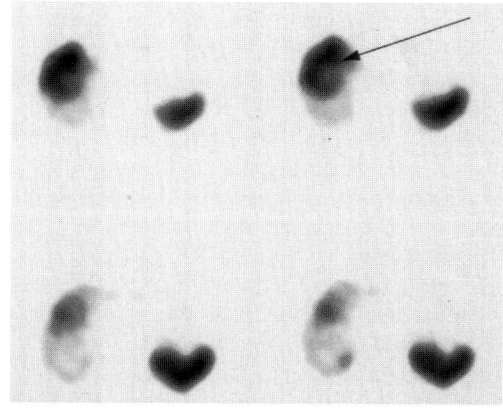

(a) (b)

Fig. 11-5. A 52-year-old white male presented with episodes of tachycardia and paroxysmal flushing. MRI revealed a 7 × 7 × 8 cm necrotic mass in the anterior aspect of the right lobe of the liver. No other lesions were identified. An upper GI series and detailed small bowel study demonstrated a 5-mm smooth polyp in the distal ileum.
(a) An anterior view of the abdomen after the administration of octreotide shows a large focus of increased uptake in the upper right lobe of the liver (arrows). (b) Transaxial single-photon emission-computed tomography images show large focal area of increased uptake in the anterior aspect of the right lobe of the liver (arrow). Follow-up selective hepatic angiography revealed a large hypervascular mass in the right lobe of the liver and a smaller similar mass in the left lobe. Pathologic diagnosis revealed metastatic carcinoid tumors to the liver and small carcinoid nodules in the ileum and 5 of 12 positive lymph nodes. A 4-month postoperative follow-up octreotide scan revealed no lesions.

relative to the earlier radiolabeled somatostatin analogue, 123I-Tyr-3-octreotide.[95]

It is difficult to determine the true sensitivity of 111-In-DTPA-D-Phe-octreotide scintigraphy in localization of isolated small bowel disease since most studies have examined a variety of neuroendocrine tumors, often at advanced stages. What can be concluded from a review of the literature is that the 111-In-DTPA-D-Phe-octreotide scan is highly sensitive, superior to 123-I-Tyr-3-octreotide scanning, and compares favorably to conventional imaging modalities (Figs. 11-5, 11-6). A sensitivity of 96% was reported in a study of

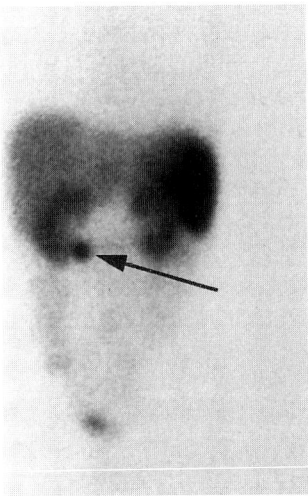

Fig. 11-6. **A 35-year-old white male was admitted complaining of recent onset of nausea, vomiting, and weakness.**
Five years ago he underwent a heart transplant. Lab tests revealed impaired liver and renal function and anemia. An MRI scan showed mildly dilated intra- and extrahepatic bile ducts down to the level of the ampulla. No pancreatic or ampullary mass was seen, and the patient was treated medically and discharged only to be readmitted 2 months later with the same complaints. Ultrasound study revealed moderately dilated biliary ducts and a mildly dilated pancreatic duct along with a 1.2 × 0.8 cm gallstone. Endoscopic retrograde cholangiopancreatography revealed abrupt irregular termination of the pancreatic duct. A biliary stent was inserted.

Shortly thereafter, an octreotide scan showed a small but prominent focus of increased uptake in the right upper quadrant area (arrow) medial to the lower pole of the right kidney. A hepatobiliary scan localized the focal site of uptake to the ampulla of Vater.

At surgery the only abnormality was an encapsulated 10 × 12 mm tumor at the distal common duct obliterating the opening of the pancreatic duct. A transduodenal submucosal resection was done and the biliary stent left in place. Pathology diagnosis was a low-grade ampullary neuroendocrine tumor extending deep into submucosa with clear surgical margins.

72 carcinoid tumors.[96] A further report demonstrated all 12 known extrahepatic carcinoid tumors with 111-In-DTPA-D-Phe-octreotide scintigraphy and found it to have greater sensitivity than 123-I-Tyr-3-octreotide scanning.[97] When compared with other diagnostic techniques, octreotide scintigraphy appears to be more sensitive in detecting extrahepatic disease than the traditional noninvasive imaging methods and comparable to invasive modalities such as intraoperative ultrasound, endoscopic ultrasound, arteriography, and transhepatic portal venous sampling.[92] Additionally, intraoperative scintigraphy has been reported to aid in the operative management of these patients, by the demonstration of additional (ie, occult) foci of disease.[98] A recent study addressing the cost-effectiveness of 111-In-DTPA-D-Phe-octreotide scintigraphy concluded that this technology was highly effective in confirming the diagnosis, demonstrating disease extent, and planning therapeutic intervention.[99] False-negative scans result from 1) low tumor cellularity combined with a low receptor density, 2) high tumor somatostatin content with occupancy of the available somatostatin receptors, 3) SSTR subtypes that are not recognized by the ligand, and 4) inadequate localization of tumor in an area of high background activity (ie, kidney, spleen, gut, liver).[93]

Scintigraphy with 111-In-DTPA-D-Phe-octreotide is a simple, safe, and cost-effective diagnostic modality to functionally localize somatostatin receptor–positive carcinoid tumors of the small intestine. When used in concert with other traditional imaging techniques, this technology has become an important adjunct in the evaluation and management of these patients.

References

1. Meeroff JC. Management of massive gastrointestinal bleeding. *Hosp Prac*. 1986;21:154A.
2. Mauer AH, Fischer RS. Current applicability of scintigraphic methods in gastroenterology. *Bailleres Clin Gastroenterol*. 1995;9:71–95.
3. Alavi A, Ring EJ. Localization of gastrointestinal bleeding: superiority of 99mTc sulfur colloid compared with angiography. *Radiology*. 1981;137:741–748.
4. Parekh JS, Teates CD. Emergency nuclear medicine. *Radiol Clin North Am*. 1992;30:455–474.
5. Alavi A, Dann RW, Baum S, et al. Scintigraphic detection of acute gastrointestinal bleeding. *Radiology*. 1977;124:753–756.
6. Miscowiak J, Nielsen SL, Munck O, et al. Abdominal scintiphotography with 99mTc labeled albumin in acute gastrointestinal bleeding. An experimental study and a case report. *Lancet*. 1977;2:852–854.
7. Miscowiak J, Nielsen SL, Munck O, et al. Acute gastrointestinal bleeding detected with abdominal scintig-

raphy using technetium-99m-labeled albumin. *Scand J Gastroenterol.* 1979;14:389–394.
8. Smith TD, Richards P. A simple kit for the preparation of 99mTc-labeled red blood cells. *J Nucl Med.* 1976;71:126–132.
9. Pavel DG, Zimmer AM, Patterson VN. In vivo labeling of red blood cells with 99mTc: a new approach to blood pool visualization. *J Nucl Med.* 1977;18:305–308.
10. Callahan RJ, Froelich JW, McKusick KA, et al. A modified method for the in vivo labeling of red blood cells with 99mTc: concise communication. *J Nucl Med.* 1982;23:315–318.
11. Winzelberg GG, Froelich JW, McKusick KA, et al. Radionuclide localization of lower gastrointestinal hemorrhage. *Radiology.* 1981;139:465–469.
12. Berger RB, Zeman RK, Gottschalk A. The technetium-99m-sulfur colloid angiogram in suspected gastrointestinal bleeding. *Radiology.* 1983;147:555–558.
13. Maurer AH. Gastrointestinal bleeding and cine-scintigraphy. *Semin Nucl Med.* 1996;26:43–50.
14. Maurer AH, Rodman MS, Vitti RA, et al. Gastrointestinal bleeding: improved localization with cine scintigraphy. *Radiology.* 1992;185:187–192.
15. Winzelberg GG, McKusick KA, Froelich JW, et al. Detection of gastrointestinal bleeding with 99mTc-labeled red blood cells. *Semin Nucl Med.* 1982;12:139–146.
16. McKusick KA, Froelich JW, Callahan RJ, et al. 99mTc red blood cells for detection of gastrointestinal bleeding: experience with 80 patients. *AJR.* 1981;137:1113–1118.
17. Froelich JW, Juni J. Glucagon in the scintigraphic diagnosis of small-bowel hemorrhage by Tc-99m-labeled red blood cells. *Radiology.* 1984;151:239–242.
18. Emslie JT, Zarnegar K, Siegel ME, et al. Technetium-99m-labeled red blood cell scans in the investigation of gastrointestinal bleeding. *Dis Colon Rectum.* 1996;39:750–754.
19. Suzman MS, Talmor M, Jennis R, et al. Accurate localization and surgical management of active lower gastrointestinal hemorrhage with technetium-labeled erythrocyte scintigraphy. *Ann Surg.* 1996;224:29–36.
20. Orecchia PM, Hensley EK, McDonald PT, et al. Localization of lower gastrointestinal hemorrhage. *Arch Surg.* 1985;120:621–624.
21. Thome DA, Datz FL, Remley K, et al. Bleeding rates necessary for detecting acute gastrointestinal bleeding with Tc-99m-labeled red blood cells in an experimental model. *J Nucl Med.* 1987;28:514–520.
22. Dusold R, Burke K, Carpentier W, et al. The accuracy of technetium-99m-labeled red cell scintigraphy in localizing gastrointestinal bleeding. *Am J Gastroenterol.* 1994;89:345–348.
23. Mackey WC, Dineen P. A fifty year experience with Meckel's diverticulum. *Surg Gynecol Obstet.* 1983;156:56–64.
24. Rubin DC. Small intestine: anatomy and structural anomalies. In: Yamada T, ed. *Textbook of Gastroenterology.* Philadelphia, Pa: JB Lippincott Co; 1995:1555–1576.
25. Diamond RH, Rothstein RD, Alavi A. The role of cimetidine-enhanced technetium99m-pertechnetate imaging for visualizing Meckel's diverticulum. *J Nucl Med.* 1991;32:1422–1424.
26. Sfakianakis GN, Conway JJ. Detection of ectopic gastric mucosa in Meckel's diverticulum and in other aberrations by scintigraphy: 11. Indications and methods—a 10 year experience. *J Nucl Med.* 1981;22:732–738.
27. Soltero MJ, Bill AH. The natural history of Meckel's diverticulum and its relation to incidental removal: a study of 202 cases of diseased Meckel's diverticulum found in King county, Washington, over a fifteen year period. *Am J Surg.* 1976;132:168–171.
28. Sfakianakis GN, Conway JJ. Detection of ectopic gastric mucosa in Meckel's diverticulum and in other aberrations by scintigraphy: 1. Pathophysiology and 10-year experience. *J Nucl Med.* 1981;22:647–654.
29. Williams JG. Pertechnetate and the stomach—a continuing controversy. *J Nucl Med.* 1983;24:633–636.
30. Treves S, Grand RJ, Eraklis AJ. Pentagastrin stimulation of technetium-99m uptake by ectopic gastric mucosa in a Meckel's diverticulum. *Radiology.* 1978;128:711–712.
31. Sfakianakis GN, Anderson GF, King DR, et al. The effect of gastrointestinal hormones on the pertechnetate imaging of ectopic gastric mucosa in experimental Meckel's diverticulum. *J Nucl Med.* 1981;22:678–683.
32. Datz FL. Gastrointestinal imaging. In: Taylor A and Datz FL, editors. *Clinical Practice of Nuclear Medicine.* New York, NY: Churchill Livingstone, 1991:317–360.
33. Sfakianakis GN, Haase GM. Abdominal scintigraphy for ectopic gastric mucosa: a retrospective analysis of 143 studies. *AJR.* 1982;138:7–12.
34. Lotfi K, Oates E. Bleeding Meckel's diverticulum presenting as focal extravasation on pertechnetate scintigraphy. *Clin Nucl Med.* 1996;21:1–3.
35. Delberke D, Frexes-Steed M. The "fading" Meckel's diverticulum: an unusual scintigraphic presentation. *Clin Nucl Med.* 1992;17:701–704.
36. Jewett TC, Duszynski DO, Allen JE. The visualization of Meckel's diverticulum with 99mTc pertechnetate. *Surgery.* 1970;68:567–570.
37. Dixon PM, Nolan DJ. The diagnosis of Meckel's diverticulum: a continuing challenge. *Clin Radiol.* 1987;38:615–619.
38. Heinzelman M, Schob O, Schlumpf R, et al. Preoperative diagnosis of Meckel's diverticulum by pertechnetate scan and laparoscopic resection. *Surg Laparosc Endosc.* 1994;4:378–381.
39. Schwartz MJ, Lewis JH. Meckel's diverticulum: pitfalls in scintigraphic detection in the adult. *Am J Gastroenterol.* 1984;79:611–618.
40. Ho JE, Konieczny KM. The sodium pertechnetate Tc 99m scan: an aid in the evaluation of gastrointestinal bleeding. *Pediatrics.* 1975;56:34–40.
41. Tauscher JW, Bryant DR, Gruenther RC. False positive scan for Meckel's diverticulum. *J Pediatr.* 1978;92:1022–1023.
42. Siddiqui A, Ryo UY, Pinsky SM. Arteriovenous malformation simulating Meckel's diverticulum on 99mTc-pertechnetate abdominal scintigraphy. *Radiology.* 1977;122:173–174.
43. DelValle J, Lucey MR, Yamada T. Gastric secretion. In: Yamada T, ed. *Textbook of Gastroenterology.* Philadelphia, Pa: JB Lippincott Co; 1995:295–326.
44. Lee C, P'eng FK, Yeh PH. Sodium pertechnetate Tc 99m

antral scan in the diagnosis of retained gastric antrum. *Arch Surg.* 1984;119:309–311.
45. Mauer AH, Krevsky B. Whole-gut transit scintigraphy in the evaluation of small bowel and colon transit disorders. *Semin Nucl Med.* 1995;25:326–338.
46. Talley NJ. Measurement of whole-gut transit: a new test comes of age? *Mayo Clin Proc.* 1995;79:193–194.
47. Caride VJ, Prokop EK, Troncale FJ, et al. Scintigraphic determination of small intestinal transit time: comparison with the hydrogen breath technique. *Gastroenterology.* 1984;86:714–720.
48. Miller MA, Parkman HP, Brown KL, et al. The lactulose breath test is not a physiologic standard for orocecal transit: lactulose delays gastric emptying and accelerates small bowel transit. *Gastroenterology.* 1995;108:A650 Abstract.
49. Gilat T, Ben Hur H, Gelman-Malachi E, et al. Alterations of colonic flora and their effect on the hydrogen breath test. *Gut.* 1978;19:602–605.
50. Ravich WJ, Bayless TM, Thomas M. Fructose: incomplete intestinal absorption in humans. *Gastroenterology.* 1983;84:26–29.
51. Perman JA, Modlers S, Olson AC. Role of pH in production of hydrogen from carbohydrates by colonic bacterial flora. Studies *in vivo* and *in vitro. J Clin Invest.* 1981;67:643–650.
52. von der Ohe MR, Camilleri M. Measurement of small bowel and colonic transit: indications and methods. *Mayo Clin Proc.* 1992;67:1169–1179.
53. Thompson DG, Binfield P, De Belder A, et al. Extra intestinal influences on exhaled breath hydrogen measurements during the investigation of gastrointestinal disease. *Gut.* 1985;26:1349–1352.
54. Parkman HP, Harris AD, Krevsky B, et al. Gastroduodenal motility and dismotility: update on techniques for evaluation. *Am J Gastroenterol.* 1995;90:869–892.
55. Parlcman HP, Miller MA, Fisher RS. Role of nuclear medicine in evaluating patients with suspected gastrointestinal motility disorders. *Semin Nucl Med.* 1995;25: 289–305.
56. Read NW, Aljanabi MN, Bates TE, et al. Effect of gastrointestinal intubation on the passage of a solid meal through the stomach and small intestines in humans. *Gastroenterology.* 1983;84:1568–1572.
57. Read NW, Miles CA, Fisher D, et al. Transit of a meal through the stomach, small intestine and colon in normal subjects and its role in the pathogenesis of diarrhea. *Gastroenterology.* 1980;79:1276–1282.
58. Malagelada J-R, Robertson JS, Brown ML, et al. Intestinal transit of solid and liquid components of a meal in health. *Gastroenterology.* 1984;87:1255–1263.
59. Krevsky B, Maurer AH, Niewiarowski T, et al. Effect of verapamil on human intestinal transit. *Dig Dis Sci.* 1992;37:919–924.
60. Trotman IF, Price CC. Bloated irritable bowel syndrome defined by dynamic 99mTc bran scan. *Lancet.* 1986;2: 364–366.
61. Camilleri M, Colemont LJ, Phillips SF, et al. Human gastric emptying and colonic filling of solids characterized by a new method. *Am J Physiol.* 1989;257:G284–G290.
62. Proano M, Camilleri M, Phillips SF, et al. Transit of solids through the human colon: regional quantification in the unprepared bowel. *Am J Physiol.* 1990;258:G856–G862.
63. Christian PE, Datz FL, Sorensorn JA, et al. Technical factors in gastric emptying studies. *J Nucl Med.* 1983;24:264–268.
64. Charles F, Camilleri M, Phillips SF, et al. Scintigraphy of the whole gut: clinical evaluation of transit disorders. *Mayo Clin Proc.* 1995;70:113–118.
65. Hardy JG, Perkins AC. Validity of the geometric mean correction in the quantification of whole bowel transit. *Nucl Med Commun.* 1985;6:217–224.
66. Camilleri M, Zinsmeister AR, Greydanus MP, et al. Towards a less costly but accurate test of gastric emptying and small bowel transit. *Dig Dis Sci.* 1991;36:609–615.
67. Camilleri M, Malagelada JR, Brown ML, et al. Relation between antral motility and gastric emptying of solids and liquids in humans. *Am J Physiol.* 1985;245: G580–G585.
68. Read NW, Aljanabi MN, Holgate AM, et al. Simultaneous measurement of gastric emptying, small bowel residence and colonic filling of a solid meal by the use of the gamma camera. *Gut.* 1986;27:300–308.
69. Greydanus MP, Camilleri M, Colemont LJ, et al. Ileocolonic transfer of solid chyme in small intestinal neuropadiies and myopathies. *Gastroenterology.* 1990;99: 158–164.
70. CaniiHeri M, Brown ML, Malagelada JR. Impaired transit of chyme in chronic intestinal pseudoobstruction: correction by cisapride. *Gastroenterology.* 1986;91: 619–626.
71. Eagon JC, Miedema BW, Kelly KA. Postgastrectomy syndromes. *Surg Clin North Am.* 1992;72:445–465.
72. Chandramouli B, Gupta SM. Scintigraphic detection of transient afferent loop obstruction. *Clin Nucl Med.* 1993;18:68–69.
73. van der Mijle HCJ, Beekhuis H, Bleichrodt RP, et al. Transit disorders of the gastric remnant and Roux limb after Roux-en-Y gastrojejunostomy: relation to symptomatology and vagotomy. *Br J Surg.* 1993;80:60–64.
74. Saverymuttu SH, Peters AM, Crofton ME, et al. Indium-111 autologous granulocytes in the detection of inflammatory bowel disease. *Gut.* 1985;26:955–960.
75. Kennan N, Hayward M. Tc HMPAO-labelled white cell scintigraphy in Crohn's disease of the small bowel. *Clin Radiol.* 1992;45:331–334.
76. Giaffer NM. Labeled leukocyte scintigraphy in inflammatory bowel disease: clinical applications. *Gut.* 1996;38: 1–5.
77. Saverymuttu SH, Peters AM, Hodgson HJ, et al. Indium-111 autologous leukocyte scanning: comparison with radiology for imaging the colon in inflammatory bowel disease. *Br Med J.* 1982;285:1255–1257.
78. Roddie ME, Peters AM, Danpure HJ, et al. Inflammation: imaging with Tc-99m HMPAO-labeled leukocytes. *Radiology.* 1988;166:767–772.
79. Rothstein RD, Alavi A. The role of scintigraphy in the management of inflammatory bowel disease. *J Nucl Med.* 1991;32:856–859.

80. Peters AM. Imaging inflammation: current role of labeled autologous leukocytes. *J Nucl Med.* 1992;33:65–67.
81. Slaton GD, Navab F, Boyd CM, et al. Role of delayed indium-111 labeled leukocyte scan in the management of Crohn's disease. *Am J Gastroenterol.* 1985;80:790–795.
82. Poitras P, Carrier L, Chartrand R, et al. Indium-111 leukocyte scanning of the abdomen. Analysis of its value for diagnosis and management of inflammatory bowel disease. *J Clin Gastroenterol.* 1987;9:418–423.
83. Crama-Bohbouth GE, Arndt JW, Pena AS, et al. Value of indium-111 granulocyte scintigraphy in the assessment of Crohn's disease of the small intestine: prospective investigations. *Digestion.* 1988;40:227–236.
84. Scholmerich J, Schmidt E, Schumichen C, et al. Scintigraphic assessment of bowel involvement and disease activity in Crohn's disease using technetium 99m-hexamethyl propylene amine oxine as leukocyte label. *Gastroenterology.* 1988;95:1287–1293.
85. Even-Sapir E, Bames DC, Martin RH, et al. Indium-111-white blood cell scintigraphy in Crohn's patients with fistulae and sinus tracts. *J Nucl Med.* 1994;35:245–250.
86. Allan RA, Sladen GE, Bassingham S, et al. Comparison of simultaneous 99mTc-HMPAO and 111-In oxine labelled white cell scans in the assessment of inflammatory bowel disease. *Euro J Nucl Med.* 1993;20:195–200.
87. Arndt JW, van der Sluys Veer A, Blok D, et al. Prospective comparative study of technetium-99m-WBCs and indium-111-granulocytes for the examination of patients with inflammatory bowel disease. *J Nucl Med.* 1993;34:1052–1057.
88. Papos M, Nagy F, Narai G, et al. Anti-granulocyte immunoscintigraphy and 99m Tc hexamethylpropyleneamine-oxime-labeled leukocyte scintigraphy in inflammatory bowel disease. *Dig Dis Sci.* 1996;41:412–420.
89. Mairal L, de Lima PA, Martin-Comin J, et al. Simultaneous administration of 111-In-human immunoglobulin and 99mTc-HMPAO labelled leukocytes in inflammatory bowel disease. *Euro J Nucl Med.* 1995;22:664–670.
90. Lance P. Tumors and other neoplastic diseases of the small bowel. In: Yamada T, ed. *Textbook of Gastroenterology.* Philadelphia, Pa: JB Lippincott Co; 1995:1696–1714.
91. Krenning EP, Bakker VM, Breeman WAP, et al. Localisation of endocrine-related tumours with radioiodinated analogue of somatostatin. *Lancet.* 1989;1:242–244.
92. Modlin IM, Cornelius E, Lawton GP. Use of an isotopic somatostatin receptor probe to image gut endocrine tumors. *Arch Surg.* 1995;130:367–373.
93. Reubi JC. Neuropeptide receptors in health and disease: the molecular basis for in vivo imaging. *J Nucl Med.* 1995;36:1825–1835.
94. John M, Meyerhof W, Richter D, et al. Positive somatostatin receptor scintigraphy correlates with the presence of somatostatin receptor subtype 2. *Gut.* 1996;38:33–39.
95. Krenning EP, Bakker VVH, Kooij PPM, et al. Somatostatin receptor scintigraphy with indium-111-DTPA-D-Phe-l-octreotideinman: metabolism, dosimetry and comparison with iodine-123-Tyr-3-octreotide. *J Nucl Med.* 1992;33:652–658.
96. Krenning EP, Kwekkeboom DJ, Reubi JC, et al. 111-In-octreotide scintigraphy with 111-In-DTPA-D-Phe- and 123I-Tyr-3-octreotide: the Rotterdam experience with more than 1000 patients. *Euro J Nucl Med.* 1993;20:716–731.
97. Lamberts SWJ, Reubi J-C, Krenning EP. Validation of somatostatin receptor scintigraphy in the localization of neuroendocrine tumors. *Acta Oncol.* 1993;32:167–170.
98. Ahlman B, Wangberg B, Tisell LE, et al. Clinical efficacy of octreotide scintigraphy in patients with midgut carcinoid tumors and evaluation of intraoperative scinfillation detection. *Br J Surg.* 1994;81:1144–1149.
99. Kwekkeboom DJ, Lamberts SWJ, Habbema JDF, et al. Cost-effectiveness analysis of somatostatin receptor scintigraphy. *J Nucl Med.* 1996;37:886–892.

Angiography and Interventional Radiology

12

James E. Jackson and David J. Allison

Chapter Contents

Introduction
Small Intestinal Hemorrhage
Management of Small Bowel Hemorrhage
Chronic GI Bleeding
Visceral Ischemia
Nonvascular Interventional Radiology
Conclusions

Introduction

The indications for conventional *diagnostic* angiography of the small intestine are relatively few. Most often carried out is the angiographic investigation of acute and chronic gastrointestinal bleeding. Intestinal ischemia, either of acute onset due to a superior mesenteric embolus or chronic due to stenotic disease, is an uncommon indication; the diagnosis is often suspected on the basis of the clinical history and then confirmed or refuted using noninvasive imaging, especially Doppler ultrasound; angiography may be necessary if the diagnosis remains in doubt. Other indications include diagnosis of classical polyarteritis nodosa and other arteritides that may rarely affect the small intestine (eg, Behçet's, Wegener's, Churg-Strauss).

While the use of conventional angiography may have diminished for diagnostic work because of the development of better noninvasive imaging methods, the indications for *therapeutic* angiographic techniques are increasing (Table 12-1). Embolization of sites of hemorrhage in the small bowel has become much safer since the introduction of small catheters that allow more distal catheterization, and there are now many reports of its successful use. Small bowel varices due to portal hypertension or a localized venous stenosis may be treated either by the insertion of a transjugular intrahepatic portosystemic stent shunt (TIPSS) or by venous angioplasty with or without stenting. Acute visceral ischemia can be effectively treated by recanalization and local thrombolysis if an early diagnosis is made; the development of angioplasty balloons and of a variety of metallic stents has also allowed the safe and effective treatment of visceral arterial stenoses causing chronic intestinal angina. Carcinoid tumors of the small bowel may metastasize to the liver and give rise to the carcinoid syndrome. Palliative treatment of this condition may be achieved by hepatic arterial embolization. This technique lies outside the scope of this chapter and will not be discussed further; interested readers are referred to other texts.[1]

Small Intestinal Hemorrhage

The choice of radiological investigation in a patient with lower gastrointestinal hemorrhage (ie, that which occurs beyond the ligament of Treitz or duodeno-jejunal flexure) depends upon whether the bleeding is acute and life-threatening or chronic; these different presentations will be discussed separately.

Diagnosis of Acute Small Bowel Hemorrhage

When bleeding is acute and life-threatening, and endoscopy has failed to detect the responsible site, the patient should be referred for immediate angiography. While it is the present authors' opinion (and that of others[2]) that scintigraphy is of limited value in the investigation of patients with acute lower gastrointestinal bleeding because of its inability accurately to define the source of hemorrhage in most individuals, in those centers where angiography is not available scintigraphy may provide some information of use to the surgeon prior to laparotomy.[3] The different scintigraphic agents used for the detection of gastrointestinal hemorrhage are described in Chapter 11 and will not be discussed further here.

Table 12-1. Indications for therapeutic angiographic techniques

Acute gastrointestinal hemorrhage
    Embolization
    Vasopressin infusion
    Per-operative localization
    TIPSS for small bowel varices
    Portal vein angioplasty with or without stent insertion for localized stenosis or occlusion

Acute visceral ischemia
    Recanalization with or without local thrombolysis

Chronic visceral ischemia
    Visceral artery angioplasty with or without stent insertion

Embolization of liver metastases from a small bowel primary tumor (eg, carcinoid)

Barium studies have no place in the investigation of *acute* gastrointestinal hemorrhage. Not only are they unlikely to detect the source of bleeding, but the barium within the bowel loops will seriously compromise the efficacy of any subsequent diagnostic or therapeutic procedure entailing angiography.

Massive hemorrhage from the lower gastrointestinal (GI) tract is most common in patients who are more than 50 years old.[4] Table 12-2 lists a variety of possible causes, many of which are more likely to present with chronic blood loss (eg, small and large bowel neoplasms, inflammatory bowel disease) but which may occasionally present with an acute, life-threatening bleed:

Angiographic Localization

The angiographic localization of GI bleeding relies on the detection of contrast extravasation into the bowel lumen. Owing to the typically intermittent nature of GI blood loss, however, this feature is only seen in approximately 50% to 70% of patients even when there is clinical evidence of recent active bleeding. One has to remember that during each arteriogram the injected contrast medium will only be present for a few seconds within the vessel from which the bleeding has occurred and if there is no active bleeding during that short period, contrast extravasation will not be seen. In many patients, therefore, the angiographer has to rely on other angiographic abnormalities, which may be subtle. The most useful secondary sign is that of abnormal venous return (Fig. 12-1), which is usually early but may sometimes be delayed; this finding should prompt the radiologist to study in greater detail the area from which it emanates, using superselective catheterization and magnified images. The introduction of a catheter into a more selective position (and the injections associated with this maneuver) may provoke GI bleeding, and contrast extravasation will then be evident (Fig. 12-5).

Digital Subtraction Angiography (DSA)

It is worth discussing the role of DSA at this point. The superior contrast resolution of DSA when compared with a conventional film will in most cases make the detection of contrast extravasation into the bowel lumen much easier using the former technique, although care has to be taken to ensure that movement is kept to a minimum so as to avoid the generation of confusing DSA artifacts. Bowel peristalsis is usually easily abolished by the use of antiperistaltic agents, but patient respiration may be more difficult to control, especially in this group of individuals who are often unwell. A useful technique in such patients is the acquisition of images during normal respiration, with

Table 12-2. Causes of massive gastrointestinal hemorrhage from the small intestine

Small bowel diverticular disease

Small bowel angiodysplasia

Postradiotherapy telangiectasia

Inflammatory bowel disease

Small bowel varices

Small bowel neoplasms

Meckel's diverticulum

Anastomotic ulcers

Recent surgery (anastomosis or biopsy)

Vasculitis (eg, polyarteritis nodosa)

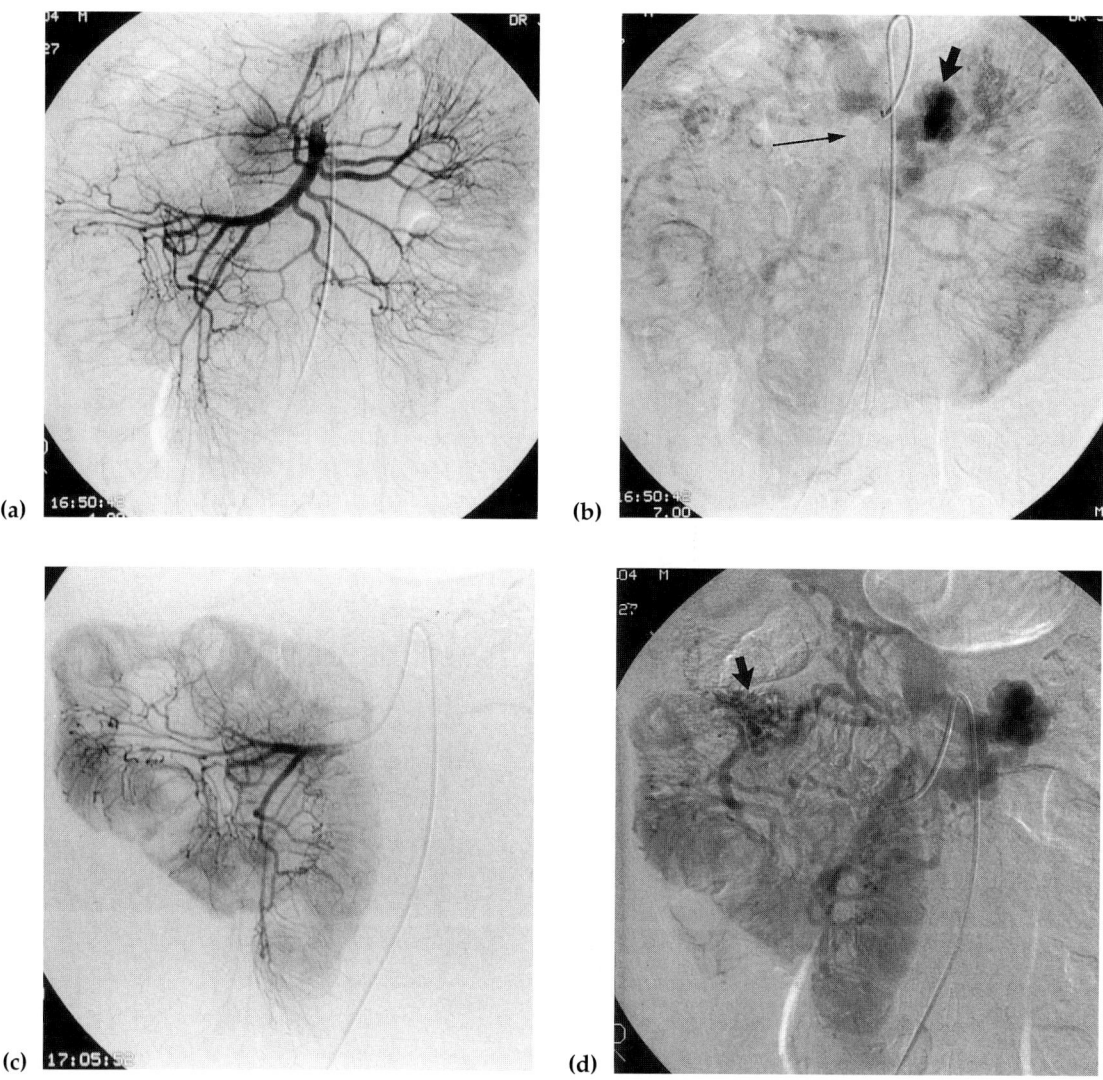

Fig. 12-1. A 34-year-old man with several episodes of acute gastrointestinal bleeding. Patient has undergone a previous right hemicolectomy.
(a) Main superior mesenteric arteriogram demonstrates marked attenuation and proximal occlusion of the ileocolic artery consistent with his previous surgery. No other significant abnormality is seen. (b) Venous phase of superior mesenteric artery (SMA) angiogram demonstrates a tight stenosis of the main superior mesenteric vein (thin arrow) with resultant jejunal varices (thick arrow). (c) Catheter has been introduced into the distal SMA to study the distal ileal vessels. The arterial phase appears normal. (d) Venous phase of the same angiographic run again demonstrates the main superior mesenteric venous stenosis and jejunal varices and also shows varices crossing the ileocolic anastomosis (arrow), which were poorly visualized on (b). This case serves to illustrate the importance of closely scrutinizing the venous drainage of the small bowel when studying patients with gastrointestinal bleeding and also shows the usefulness of selective studies.

multiple masks being obtained before the injection of contrast medium. A suitable mask will then be for DSA of most of the subsequent opacified images.

Subtle vascular irregularities may be missed because of the relatively poor spatial resolution of DSA, but this is rarely a significant problem so long as magnified selective images are obtained.

The use of DSA becomes even more important (almost mandatory) during embolization procedures, as it allows rapid angiography to be performed with immediate review. There is no doubt that DSA has made embolization considerably safer both for this reason and because it allows the use of smaller quantities of contrast agent in patients who are often very unwell.

The Source of Bleeding

As anyone who has managed patients with acute gastrointestinal hemorrhage will know, it is very difficult to determine the likely source of bleeding solely on the basis of clinical history and the endoscopic findings. The upper gastrointestinal tract is, for example, the source of hemorrhage in up to 10% of patients with severe rectal bleeding.[5] Blood may clear very rapidly from the stomach and duodenum into the more distal bowel, and an apparently normal upper GI endoscopy does not, therefore, exclude a bleeding point from this portion of the gut. Conversely, hematemesis may rarely occur from a bleeding point beyond the ligament of Treitz. Finally, blood from a bleeding source in the descending colon or the rectum can reflux into the more proximal bowel and may, therefore, be seen in the right side of the colon and even the terminal ileum on colonoscopy. The message, therefore, for the angiographer is that a full study of all of the vessels supplying the gastrointestinal tract (inferior mesenteric artery, superior mesenteric artery, celiac axis) is mandatory in the majority of cases regardless of the history and endoscopic findings.

It is also important that the finding of a bleeding site should not stop the angiographer from completing a full "three vessel" study. The reasons for this are threefold: Firstly, there may rarely be more than one source of hemorrhage; secondly, the site of origin of an intra-abdominal tumor might be incorrectly determined, or its full extent underestimated, if a "limited" study is performed because of the propensity for certain tumors to parasitize a blood supply from adjacent organs (Fig. 12-2); and thirdly, abnormalities in other vascular territories may provide clues as to the etiology of the gastrointestinal bleeding. For example, the finding of small intrahepatic aneurysms on a celiac axis arteriogram in a patient with contrast extravasation from a small bowel vessel would suggest the diagnosis of polyarteritis nodosa. Similarly, the finding of numerous vascular liver lesions would suggest the presence of malignant disease.

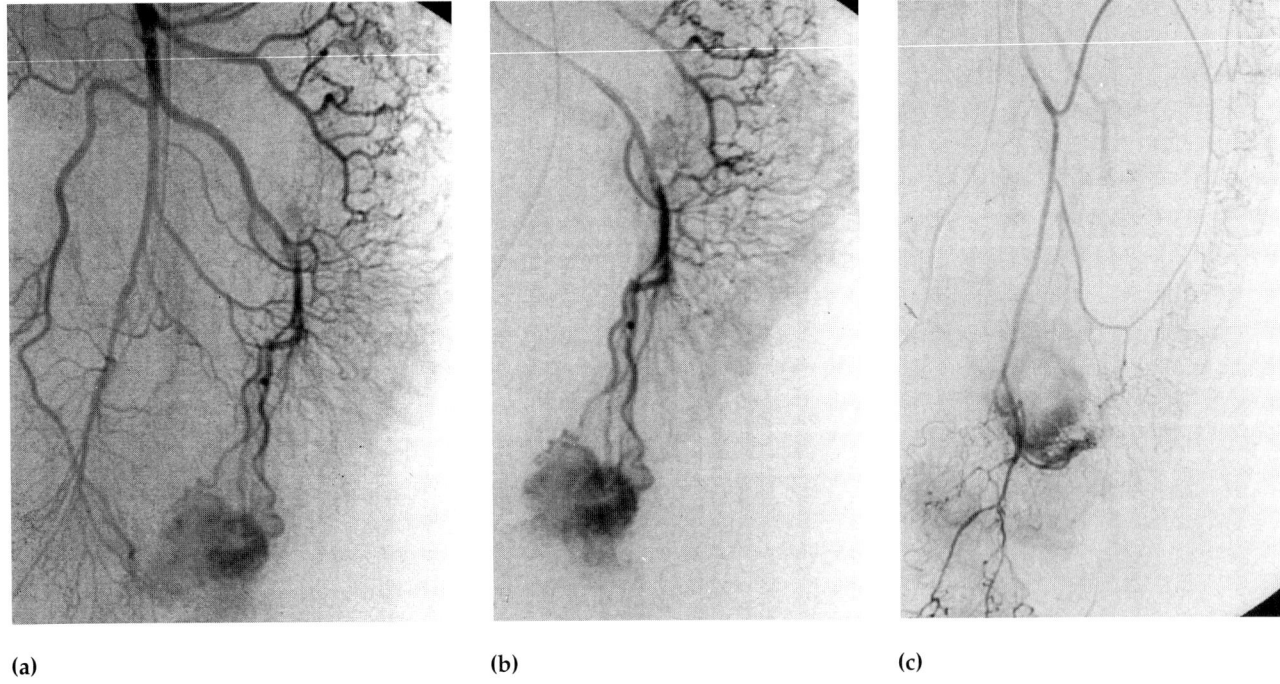

Fig. 12-2. A 45-year-old woman with several episodes of melena.
(a) Main superior mesenteric arteriogram demonstrates an approximately 4-cm-diameter hypervascular mass in the left lower abdomen being supplied by hypertrophied branches of the last jejunal artery. Appearances would be consistent with a distal jejunal leiomyoma (subsequently confirmed at surgery). (b) A selective distal jejunal arteriogram better demonstrates the arterial supply to the neoplasm. (c) An inferior mesenteric arteriogram shows that the tumor has parasitized an arterial supply from sigmoid branches.

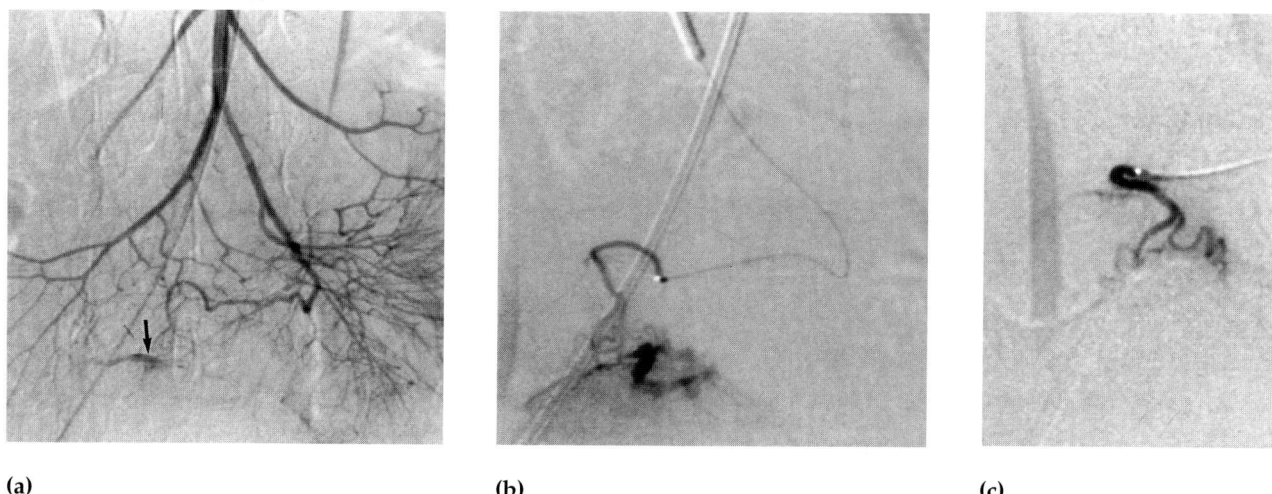

Fig. 12-3. A 42-year-old man with several severe episodes of severe gastrointestinal hemorrhage.
(a) Distal superior mesenteric arteriogram demonstrates active contrast medium extravasation from the second ileal artery (arrow). (b) A coaxial 3-French catheter has been introduced into the vessel, from which contrast medium extravasation is still apparent. The cause of the bleeding is not obvious. (c) Embolization was performed using a small amount of polyvinyl alcohol in order to stabilize the patient prior to surgery. No further contrast medium extravasation is seen on this image. At laparotomy the next day a necrotic leiomyoma of the proximal ileum was resected.

The Provocation Technique

As has been mentioned above, active contrast extravasation will not be seen in up to half the patients who have had a recent acute gastrointestinal hemorrhage; nor will many of these have any other angiographic signs suggesting the likely source of bleeding. It might be useful in some of these individuals to try and provoke rebleeding by the use of vasodilators, heparin, and/or thrombolytic agents injected directly into the vessel (usually the superior mesenteric artery) thought to be the most likely pathway to the source of hemorrhage. This "provocation" technique should not be undertaken lightly, as there is a risk of producing catastrophic bleeding, but it has proved useful in some patients with a history of several life-threatening bleeds in whom the source of hemorrhage has not been found at previous angiography or laparotomy.[6–8] Needless to say, it is imperative that appropriate resuscitation facilities are available if this technique is to be used.

Interest has been expressed in the use of carbon dioxide as the injected contrast medium in this group of patients with acute gastrointestinal bleeding.[9] It is suggested that the use of this agent improves the sensitivity of angiography for the detection of contrast medium extravasation owing to its reduced viscosity compared with liquid agents and the fact that if it enters the bowel lumen it rapidly expands and is thus easier to visualize. The initial results for the detection of the bleeding site using this method have been promising, and it will be interesting to see if they are confirmed by further experience with the technique.

Management of Small Bowel Hemorrhage

In most individuals with bleeding from the jejunum or ileum, angiography is used to localize the source of gastrointestinal hemorrhage and treatment is then surgical. One of the major reasons for this is that contrast extravasation into the small bowel is a very nonspecific angiographic finding and the underlying cause for the bleeding is often not apparent. Thus an acutely bleeding small bowel angiodysplastic lesion may have the same appearance as an actively bleeding avascular small bowel tumor or an area of ulceration due to a vasculitis or inflammatory bowel disease (Fig. 12-3). In some patients, however, the use of arterial embolization or the localized infusion of vasopressin may be useful as a definitive treatment in cases where there is a confident diagnosis, as a palliative treatment in a patient with inoperable disease, or as a means of stabilizing the patient prior to later surgery. Small bowel hemorrhage due to varices related to portal venous hypertension may be successfully treated by insertion of a TIPSS; a localized venous stenosis or occlusion causing segmental portal venous hypertension (see Fig. 12-1) may be treated by angioplasty with or without insertion of a stent (see below).

Embolization[4,10–16]

Embolization is undoubtedly the procedure of first choice for traumatic (accidental and iatrogenic) arterial bleeding from the liver[17–21] and should also, arguably, be the procedure of first choice for aneurysmal disease of the visceral arteries in the upper gastrointestinal tract.[11,22–28] The surgical treatment of many of these lesions is associated with considerable morbidity and mortality, while embolization can be successfully performed in the majority of patients under local anesthesia.

Severe bleeding from benign duodenal or gastric ulcers is usually managed successfully by a combination of endoscopic methods and medical therapy, but the occasional patient will continue to bleed. The choice between embolization or surgery in these individuals will often depend upon the expertise that is locally available. In most centers, however, surgical oversewing is usually performed, with embolization reserved for poor anesthetic risk patients and for those who continue to bleed postoperatively.

Persistent severe hemorrhage in patients with erosive or hemorrhagic gastritis is perhaps best managed by the selective infusion of vasopressin into the left gastric artery.[10] There are two main reasons why a trial of selectively administered vasopressin should be attempted in the first instance in these patients: Firstly, as mentioned above, diffuse bleeding may be difficult to control by embolization because of the very rich collateral supply to the stomach and duodenum; secondly, gastric infarction is a recognized risk of vasopressin therapy after failed embolization.[29]

Contraindications

There are few, if any, absolute contraindications to embolization in acute upper gastrointestinal hemorrhage, other than those related to angiography itself such as an uncorrectable, severe bleeding diathesis or a previous history of a severe reaction to contrast medium. Particular care should be exercised, however, in those patients who have severe visceral arterial atheromatous disease, those who have undergone (failed) vasopressin therapy, or those who have a history of previous upper gastrointestinal surgery that involved the ligation of normal branches supplying the stomach. These individuals are at an increased risk of gastric infarction following embolization.[29,30]

Duodenum

Causes of duodenal bleeding include peptic ulcers, pancreatico-duodenal arcade aneurysms (duodenum), neoplasms (duodenal or pancreatic in origin), and iatrogenic causes such as biopsy and surgery. While the extensive vascular supply to this portion of the bowel reduces the risk of ischemia following embolization, it also means that the successful control of hemorrhage is more difficult, as an occlusion created in one vessel supplying a bleeding point is rapidly bypassed through collateral channels that may be difficult or impossible to catheterize. The treatment of duodenal bleeding, therefore, often requires the use of small particulate embolic material to achieve a relatively distal block.

Peptic Ulceration

Persistent bleeding from duodenal peptic ulceration that does not respond to local transendoscopic therapy is often due to erosion of the ulcer into an adjacent large artery, usually the main trunk of the gastroduodenal artery or the retroduodenal (posterior superior pancreatico-duodenal) artery. Such patients can be successfully treated operatively and this may be usefully combined, in certain individuals, with a more definitive antiulcer surgical procedure (eg, highly selective vagotomy).

Alternatively, and particularly in those patients who are poor candidates for general anesthesia owing to old age, poor lung function, severe hypovolemia, etc, angiography and embolization can be performed.[10,31] The method of embolization performed will depend upon the angiographic findings. When a defect is demonstrated within the wall of a large artery with brisk contrast extravasation, occlusion is performed on either side of the abnormality, usually with metallic coils. The results of this form of treatment in terms of arresting bleeding are likely to be extremely good.

More difficulty will be experienced when the source of bleeding is seen to be a small peripheral branch of the pancreatico-duodenal arcade or when no angiographic abnormality is visualized. In such cases an attempt should be made to reduce the perfusion pressure to this vascular territory while avoiding the occlusion of normal visceral vessels; the superior mesenteric artery is at particular risk during occlusion of the pancreatico-duodenal arcade. Embolization of duodenal bleeding may, therefore, involve occlusion of the distal anterior superior pancreatico-duodenal artery, the distal retroduodenal artery, and the proximal right gastroepiploic artery with metallic coils (so as to protect normal vessels) prior to the injection of small particulate polyvinyl alcohol into the gastroduodenal artery.

Aneurysmal Disease of the Pancreatico-Duodenal Arcade

This may be associated with acute or chronic pancreatitis (which is discussed below) or may be secondary to atheromatous disease.[32] The latter combination of atheromatous disease and aneurysm formation is often associated with hypertrophy of the pancreaticoduodenal vessels resulting from either atheromatous stenosis of the celiac axis or, more commonly, compression of the celiac axis origin by the median arcuate ligament of the hemidiaphragm. Whatever the cause, embolization is the procedure of first choice, as the aneurysm can be successfully isolated from the circulation in the majority of cases. When there is associated arterial hypertrophy of the pancreaticoduodenal arcade, embolization is usually most easily performed via the inferior pancreatico-duodenal artery arising from the proximal superior mesenteric or first jejunal arteries.

Neoplastic Disease

The duodenum may be involved by primary tumors (eg, carcinoma, stromal cell tumor), by neoplasms in adjacent viscera (eg, pancreas, gallbladder), or by secondary deposits (eg, breast, melanoma). The treatment of first choice must be surgical resection, but this may be neither possible nor in the patient's best interests because of tumor size or the presence of extensive metastatic disease, in which case embolization may be attempted. Those tumors most commonly referred for embolization because of severe, unremitting bleeding are inoperable primary leiomyosarcomas and large, vascular, pancreatic neuroendocrine tumors. In the present authors' experience one is more likely to find a focal arterial abnormality on angiography in patients who give a history of intermittent severe bleeds, rather than in those who have a persistent slow or moderate "ooze." When a focal lesion is seen, particularly if contrast extravasation is also demonstrated, embolization can be directed toward this abnormality. In many patients, however, the only angiographic abnormality visualized is that of extensive neovascularity, often with evidence of venous occlusion and resultant variceal formation. In such cases one can only aim to try to reduce perfusion pressure to the site of bleeding by occlusion of the tumor vessels. Great care has to be taken to avoid the embolization of adjacent normal structures that may be infiltrated by the tumor.

The results in this group of patients are not good and although some improvement may be obtained this is usually short-lived.

Pancreas

Acute and chronic pancreatitis may both be associated with severe gastrointestinal bleeding owing to the involvement of adjacent vessels.[17,23–28,33–36] Arterial erosion, either by pancreatic enzymes during an episode of acute pancreatitis (Fig. 12-4) or by pressure from an adjacent pseudocyst in chronic pancreatitis (Fig. 12-5), may cause life-threatening hemorrhage. This may occur into the pancreatic duct—*hemosuccus pancreaticus* (see Fig. 12-5),[23,28]—in which case each episode of bleeding is usually associated with severe epigastric pain, directly into the duodenum or into the retroperitoneum. The surgical treatment of acutely bleeding peripancreatic pseudoaneurysms is associated with quoted mortality rates of 16% for lesions around the pancreatic tail and up to 50% for those around the pancreatic head.[34,37,38] There are no comparable series documenting the results of embolization in a similar group of patients, but several small series and case reports suggest that this method of treatment should be the procedure of first choice, with surgery reserved for those patients in whom embolization is not possible.[23–28]

Embolization should be aimed at isolating the involved portion of the vessel from the circulation, and this is usually possible by placing metallic coils on either side of neck of the aneurysm (see Figs. 12-4, 12-5). Filling the pseudoaneurysm with metallic coils should be avoided, if possible, as the cavity is likely to expand during embolization (owing to the presence of intraluminal thrombus and the lack of a true wall) with the potential risk of rupture, but, on occasion, this method of occlusion has to be employed if unfavorable anatomy precludes the use of a more satisfactory technique.

Jejunum and Ileum

While embolization in the upper gastrointestinal tract is generally very safe, beyond the ligament of Treitz there is a moderate risk of gut infarction owing to the presence of a poor collateral circulation. The aim of embolization should be to reduce the perfusion pressure to the area of contrast extravasation, thus allowing hemostasis while preserving the collateral circulation to the gut wall. Occlusion of the vasa recta should, therefore, be avoided, as these vessels do not anastomose with one another and gut infarction is likely to ensue. In the present authors' opinion embolization is best performed with metallic coils, as their deployment can be accurately controlled (Fig. 12-6), although particulate agents such as polyvinyl alcohol and absorbable gelatin sponge may also be used (Fig. 12-3).

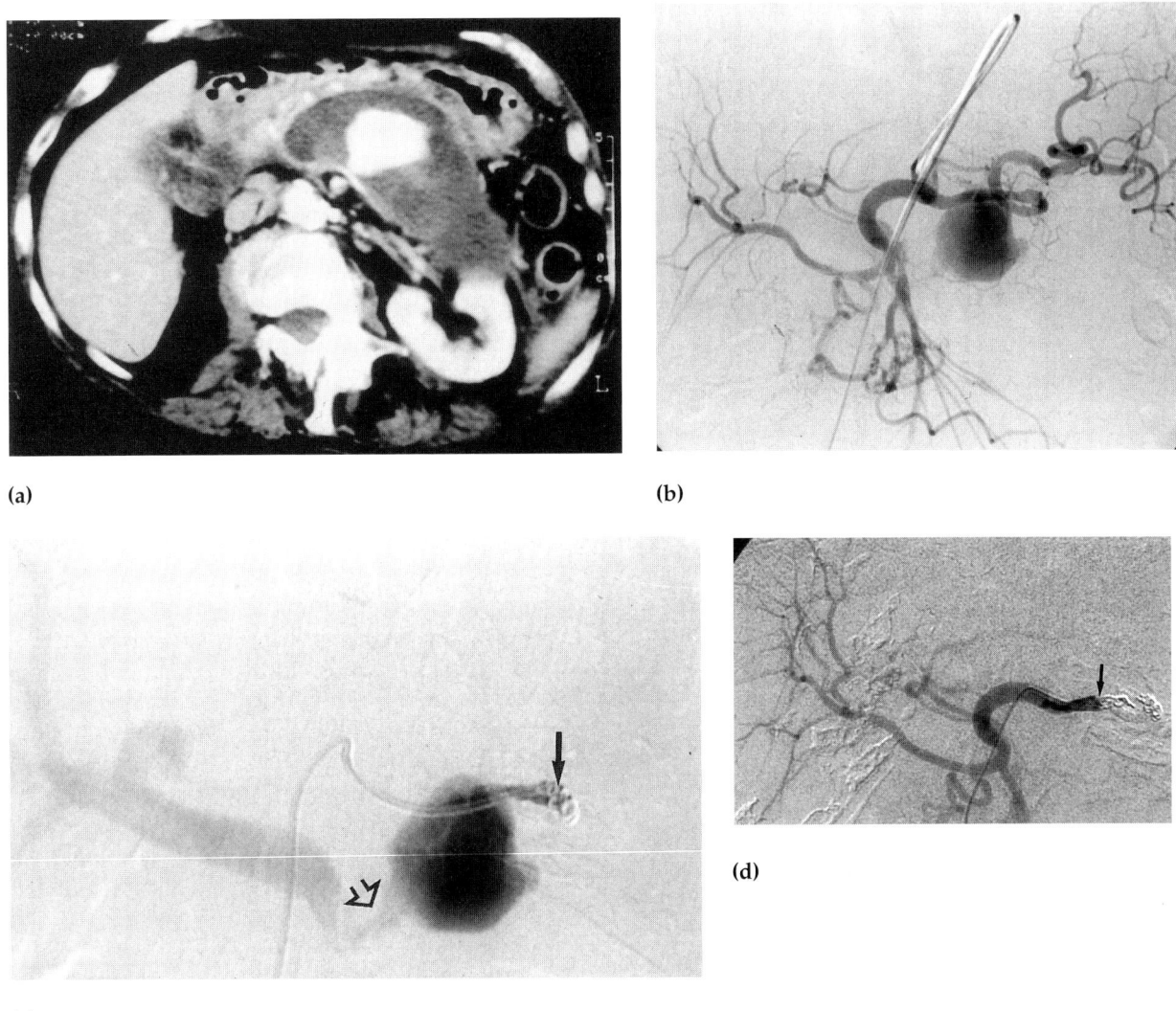

Fig. 12-4. A 66-year-old woman with an episode of acute pancreatitis complicated by massive upper gastrointestinal bleeding.
(a) A contrast-enhanced axial computed tomography (CT) scan demonstrates an enhancing cavity within a large peripancreatic fluid collection consistent with a pseudoaneurysm. (b) Celliac axis arteriogram demonstrates a pseudoaneurysm arising from the proximal splenic artery. Later images in the same run showed that this aneurysmal cavity also communicated directly with the splenic vein. (c) The splenic artery immediately beyond the pseudoaneurysm has been occluded with metallic coils (arrow). A check arteriogram to confirm occlusion of the "back door" shows the communication of the pseudoaneurysm with the portal venous system (open arrow). (d) Coils have now been placed immediately proximal to the pseudoaneurysm (arrow), thus isolating it from the circulation. Splenic supply was preserved via the left gastric artery. The patient made an uneventful recovery.

Complications

The possible complications of angiography and selective catheterization include general problems such as puncture site hematoma, contrast medium reaction, arterial dissection, etc, and there is a higher incidence of such problems in patients undergoing complex interventional procedures than in those undergoing simple diagnostic studies.[39] The reasons for this are obvious and include the fact that patients are usually unwell and are often not very cooperative; they may also be hypovolemic and have abnormal clotting mechanisms as a result of repeated tranfusions.

Complications specific to the embolization procedure are those of inadvertent occlusion of a normal vascular territory (which should be avoidable if one adheres to the general principles of embolization), bowel infarction, and persistent bleeding.

Arterial embolization above the ligament of Treitz is associated with a low risk of ischemic complications because of the extensive collateral vascular supply to this area. Small branches of the pancreatico-duodenal arcades may be safely occluded when treating duodenal hemorrhage.

Poor embolization technique whereby proximal arterial occlusion is performed without distal occlusion is a common cause of recurrent bleeding. This lapse in technique usually results in continued retrograde perfusion of the bleeding site via collaterals and makes subsequent treatment by further embolization extremely difficult or impossible because of a lack of direct vascular access to the lesion.

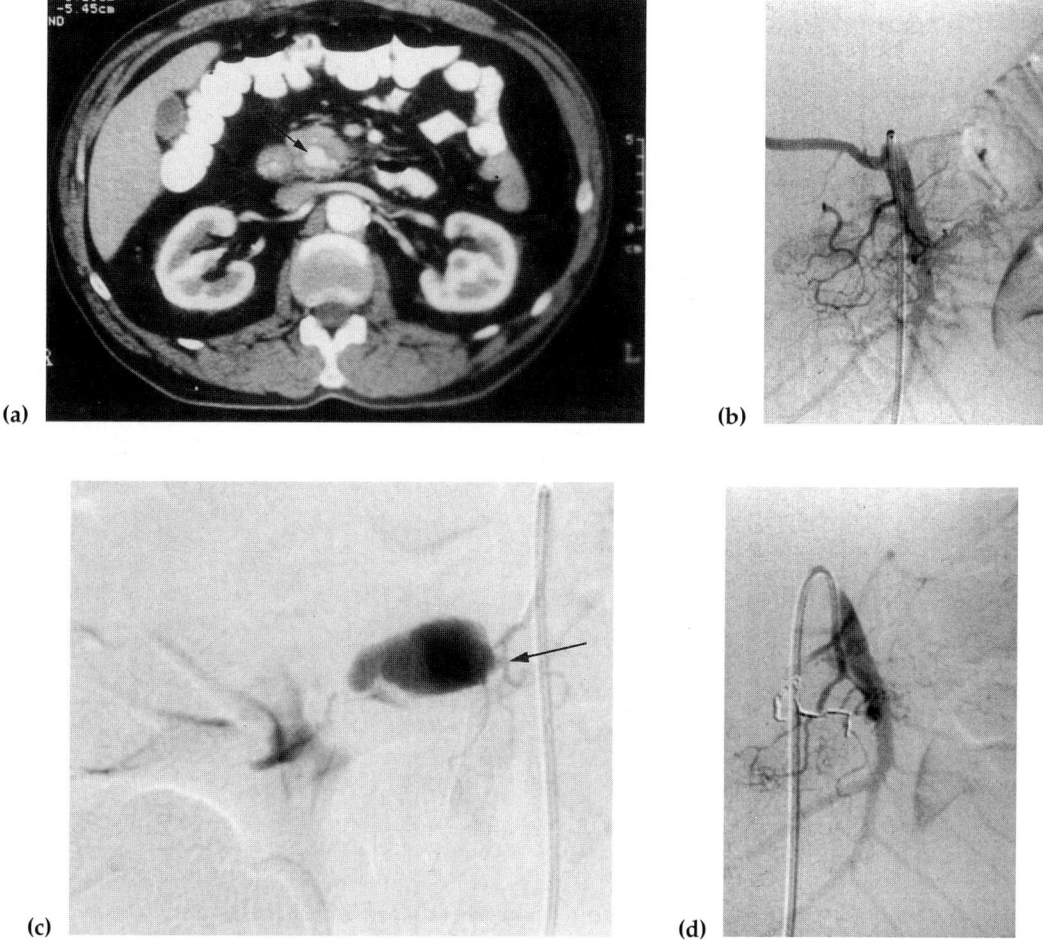

Fig. 12-5. A 53-year-old man with a history of chronic pancreatitis and several episodes of acute upper gastrointestinal bleeding associated with severe epigastric pain radiating through to his back.
(a) Contrast-enhanced axial CT scan through the abdomen demonstrates a brightly enhancing cavity within the uncinate process of the pancreas consistent with a pseudo-aneurysm (arrow). (b) Selective first jejunal arteriogram, from which the inferior pancreatico-duodenal (IPD) artery arises, shows no definite abnormality. (c) The catheter has been introduced selectively into the IPD artery and there is now contrast opacification of the pseudoaneurysm, which communicates with the pancreatic duct. Contrast medium is seen to spill through the ampulla into the duodenum. The origin of the pseudoaneurysm from a branch of the IPD artery has been arrowed. (d) No further contrast medium extravasation is seen after embolization across the neck of the pseudoaneurysm with platinum microcoils. The patient made an uneventful recovery.

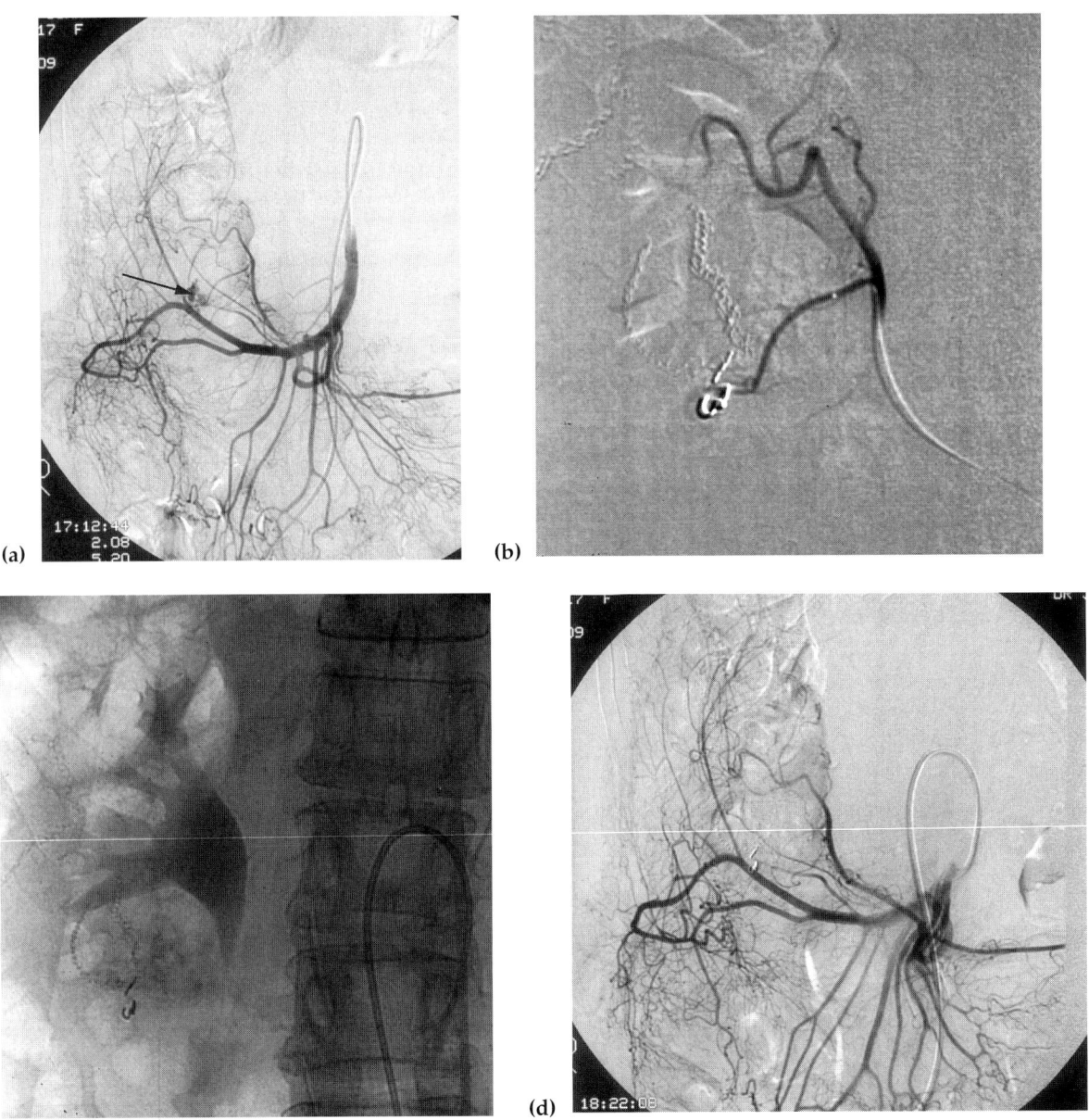

Fig. 12-6. A 66-year-old woman presenting with brisk per rectal bleeding ten days following a right hemicolectomy for an ischemic cecal volvulus.
(a) Main superior mesenteric arteriogram demonstrates brisk contrast medium extravasation (arrow) from the region of the ileocolic anastomosis. (b) A distal branch of the right colic artery supplying the anastomotic bleeding point has been selectively catheterized and embolized with platinum microcoils. (c) Control film following embolization demonstrates the microcoils adjacent to the surgical staples at the ileocolic anastomosis. (d) Postembolization superior mesenteric arteriogram shows no further bleeding and preservation of adjacent gut vessels. The patient had no further bleeding and was discharged home three days later.

Vasopressin

The use of intra-arterial vasopressin for acute upper or lower gastrointestinal hemorrhage gained widespread acceptance in the United States in the 1970s and 1980s[10] but was never as popular in the United Kingdom and other parts of Europe. While it will often successfully control hemorrhage during the infusion itself, rebleeding is common when the agent is discontinued, and there are a number of serious side effects associated with its use. Cardiovascular complications such as arrhythmia, bradycardia, hypertension, cardiac arrest, myocardial infarction, visceral infarction,[40,41] and vascular occlusion at the puncture site have all been reported and may occur in up to 43% of patients.[42] As well as these complications, there is the problem of maintaining the selective catheter position during the infusion. For these reasons the use of vasopressin has fallen out of favor in many centers. In the present authors' own institution, if the patient is not a surgical candidate, intra-arterial vasopressin is no longer used, and embolization is performed as the procedure of first choice.

Per-Operative Localization of Bleeding Site

When a source of hemorrhage is localized to the small bowel at arteriography, the angiographer can inform the surgeon from which jejunal or ileal artery the bleeding is arising. Even so, the site of bleeding may be extremely difficult to find at surgery despite the use of on-table enteroscopy and small bowel transillumination, and it is our own practice to localize the abnormality for the surgeon by introducing an angiographic catheter into the vessel supplying this area prior to transferring the patient to the operating room. The abnormal segment of bowel is then easily delineated at the time of surgery by injecting fluorescein or methylene blue via the catheter.[43]

Transjugular Intrahepatic Portosystemic Stent Shunt (TIPSS)

This procedure is most commonly performed for the treatment of upper gastrointestinal bleeding from esophageal or gastric varices that has not responded to treatment by endoscopic sclerotherapy or banding, and a full description of the technique, therefore, falls outside the scope of this chapter. Occasionally patients with portal hypertension may preferentially bleed from small intestinal varices, and in such cases insertion of a TIPSS may be lifesaving.[44–45] This procedure may be combined, if necessary, with embolization of the small bowel varices, although this is generally not required if a satisfactory reduction in the portosystemic pressure gradient is achieved.

Small intestinal varices may occasionally be due to "segmental" portal venous hypertension secondary to a localized venous stenosis or occlusion (Fig. 12-1). This is uncommon but if present may be treated by percutaneous transhepatic (or transjugular) venous angioplasty with or without stent insertion.[46]

Chronic GI Bleeding

The approach to chronic or occult lower gastrointestinal bleeding is different. If upper and lower gastrointestinal endoscopy have failed to detect a source of bleeding then barium studies should be performed. A barium enema will often be performed first, especially if there is a suspicion that the entire colon was not imaged at colonoscopy. The small bowel should then be investigated with an intubated study (small bowel enema). Isotope scans have little place in the investigation of this group of patients. The one exception to this is perhaps the young patient in whom a Meckel's diverticulum is a more likely cause of bleeding.

Cross-sectional imaging techniques such as ultrasound and computed tomography are rarely useful in the investigation of chronic gastrointestinal bleeding. It is perhaps worthwhile performing an abdominal ultrasound study, however, in those patients in whom the above investigations have failed to locate the source of hemorrhage before proceeding to the more invasive procedure of angiography. Occasionally unsuspected but relevant abnormalities will be detected (eg, liver metastases from an undetected primary bowel tumor; portal, splenic, or superior mesenteric venous occlusion with associated varices; hydronephrosis due to a desmoplastic reaction surrounding a carcinoid tumor extending down to the root of the mesentery and involving the ureter).

The cause of GI hemorrhage will be detected by endoscopy and the above "routine" radiological investigations in the majority of patients with chronic blood loss. Angiography will, therefore, be required only in a relatively small number of patients.

Investigations

As mentioned above, many of the causes of gastrointestinal bleeding will be detected using "routine" investigations including endoscopy, barium studies, and scintigraphy (eg, labeled white cell scans for inflammatory bowel disease and technetium-99m pertechnetate scans for a Meckel's diverticulum). These investigations are discussed in detail in Chapter 13 and will not be described further here.

When these investigations have failed to detect the source of chronic gastrointestinal blood loss, angiography should be performed. It must be remembered that contrast extravasation will not be seen in this group of patients because of the slow rate of blood loss. The radiologist has to rely, therefore, on other angiographic abnormalities, which may be very subtle. These include focal areas of early venous return, areas of increased or decreased vascularity, neovascularity, vascular irregularity, and aneurysm formation. It is not enough, in the majority of patients, to perform a conventional "three-vessel" visceral arteriogram in which only the inferior mesenteric artery, superior mesenteric artery, and celiac axis are selectively catheterized and studied. Superselective studies of some or all of the following vessels—jejunal, ileal, ileocolic, right colic, middle colic, splenic, common hepatic, left gastric, and gastroduodenal arteries—will be necessary in many individuals if subtle abnormalities are to be detected. Images will be of sufficiently good quality using a DSA technique (on a state-of-the-art machine) in most individuals.

Unlike acute gastrointestinal hemorrhage, where the finding of contrast extravasation can be caused by a number of different pathologies, a specific diagnosis can often be suggested from the angiographic findings when an abnormality is detected in a patient with chronic gastrointestinal bleeding:

Meckel's Diverticulum[47–50]

Most Meckel's diverticula are supplied by a persistent vitelline artery, which is visualized as a long, often nonbranching vessel arising from a distal ileal artery (Fig. 12-7). In some cases this vessel may be obvious on the selective superior mesenteric arteriogram, but superselective studies of the distal ileal vessels are often necessary with oblique views in order to "open up" overlapping bowel loops. An area of increased vascularity may occasionally be visualized within the Meckel's diverticulum itself or in the ileal loop at the base of the diverticulum that presumably represents ectopic gastric mucosa or ulceration.

Carcinoid Tumors[51]

These tumors have a very characteristic angiographic appearance (Fig. 12-8). The primary tumor itself is often hypervascular and the surrounding vessels are irregular with a "corkscrew" pattern owing to the surrounding desmoplastic reaction. Many of the arteries may be occluded and there is almost always occlusion of the draining veins, with some resultant variceal formation. There may be vascular liver metastases.

Leiomyomas[52]

These tumors are almost always hypervascular and exhibit early venous drainage (Fig. 12-2). Most are

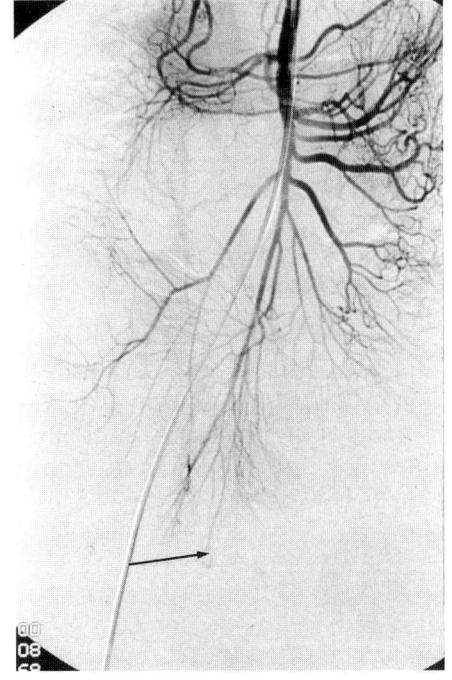
(a)

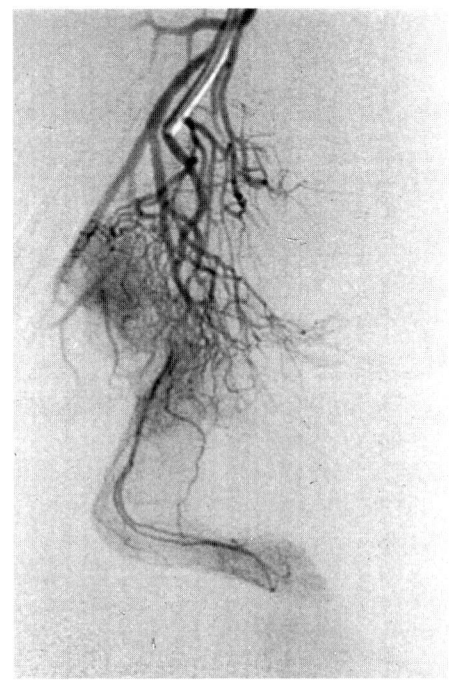
(b)

Fig. 12-7. A 23-year-old woman with several episodes of gastrointestinal bleeding.
(a) Main superior mesenteric arteriogram demonstrates long, apparently nonbranching, vessel arising from a distal ileal artery in the lower abdomen (arrow). (b) Selective fifth ileal arteriogram shows that this is a persistent vitelline artery supplying a Meckel's diverticulum.

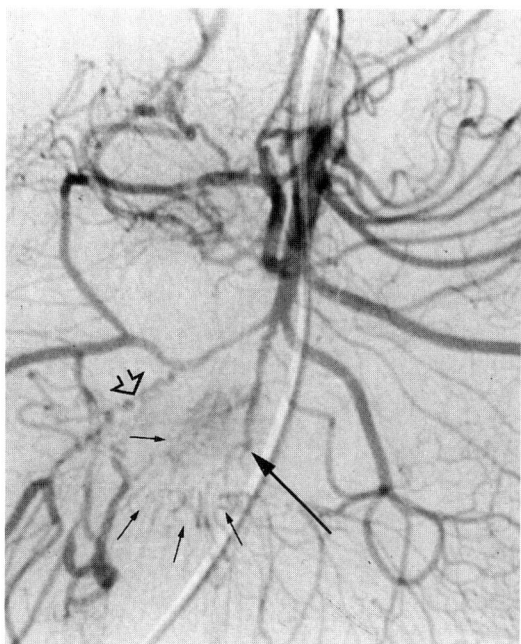

Fig. 12-8. A 57-year-old man with carcinoid syndrome. Main superior mesenteric arteriogram demonstrates the typical appearances of an extensive small bowel primary tumor with arterial irregularity ("corkscrewing") (open arrow), and arterial occlusions involving the ileocolic (arrow), distal ileal, and distal superior mesenteric arteries and distortion of small branches (fine arrows) due to the associated desmoplastic reaction.

well defined and rounded, although this is not invariable, and do not show the vascular irregularity and venous occlusions seen in carcinoid tumors.

Adenocarcinomas

These tumors are usually hypovascular with areas of patchy increased tumor staining, although occasionally marked generalized hypervascularity may be present. Areas of neovascularity are usually present with vascular irregularity, but these changes may be subtle.

Visceral Ischemia

Acute Mesenteric Ischemia

This is uncommon and presents with the sudden onset of cramping abdominal pain and vomiting. These are nonspecific signs and this means that diagnosis, and therefore therapy, are often delayed. As the cause is most commonly an embolus from a cardiac source, the diagnosis should always be considered in a patient with an acute abdomen who also has preexisting heart disease, especially atrial fibrillation, mitral valve disease, or a previous myocardial infarction. If an early diagnosis is made before irreversible ischemia has occurred, then revascularization of the mesenteric vessels may be possible angiographically using a combination of catheter and guide wire recanalization and thrombolysis (Fig. 12-9).[53–55]

Chronic Visceral Ischemia

This is most commonly due to atheromatous disease involving the origins of the mesenteric vessels. Once again the symptoms tend to be relatively nonspecific and the diagnosis is, therefore, often delayed. Once the diagnosis has been made, usually by angiography, treatment may be by angioplasty with or without stent insertion (Fig. 12-10).[56–58] Alternatively, following diagnosis by mesenteric angiography, treatment may occasionally be by surgical removal of a partially occluding embolus (Fig. 12-11) or by other surgical means. Good results may be obtained with either of these therapeutic options.

Nonvascular Interventional Radiology

In the abdomen the commonest nonvascular interventional procedures are biopsies and drainages of collections. In the small bowel itself, most interventional procedures are directed toward the relief or prevention of obstruction; these may involve the dilatation of strictures and tight anastomoses in benign obstruction, stent insertion in the palliation of malignant disease, assistance in the positioning of intraluminal feeding and decompression tubes, and the creation of percutaneous enterostomies.

Biopsy

The value of percutaneous biopsy in the evaluation of soft-tissue masses in the abdomen, retroperitoneal space, and pelvis is now firmly established. The technique may obviate the need for an exploratory laparotomy or laparoscopy, and the result frequently has a significant influence on the subsequent clinical management of the patient. Although biopsies of tumors arising from the small bowel are performed this is rarely necessary, as the vast majority of these lesions will require surgical removal, and preoperative knowledge of the tumor type will not affect the sub-

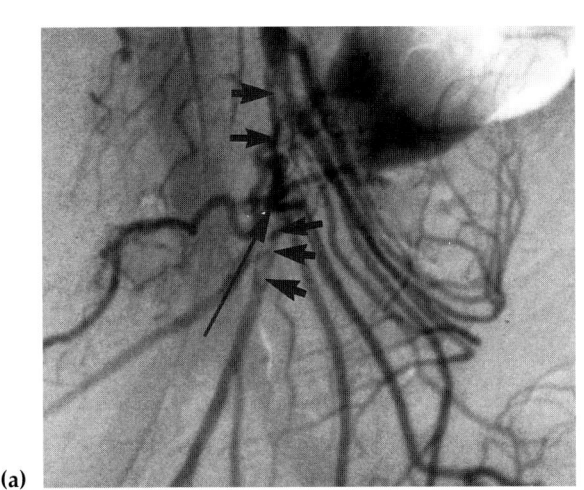 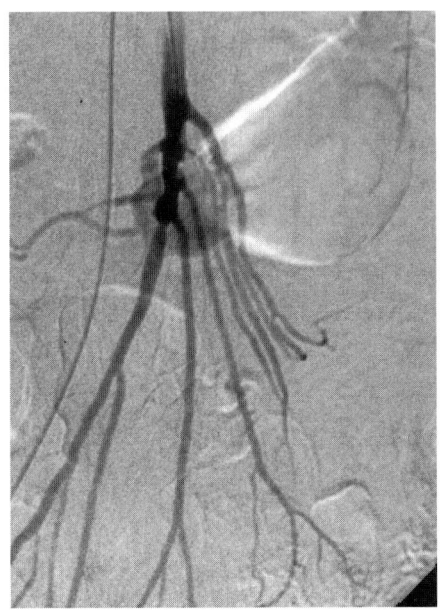

Fig. 12-9. A 85-year-old female patient with congestive heart failure presented with increasing lower abdominal pain. A CT scan showed small bowel edema and pelvic ascites.
(a) A superior mesenteric arteriogram demonstrated elongated emboli (arrows) partially occluding the mainstem (long arrow). Urokinase was infused. (b) A further arteriogram demonstrated restitution of flow through the SMA and its branches.

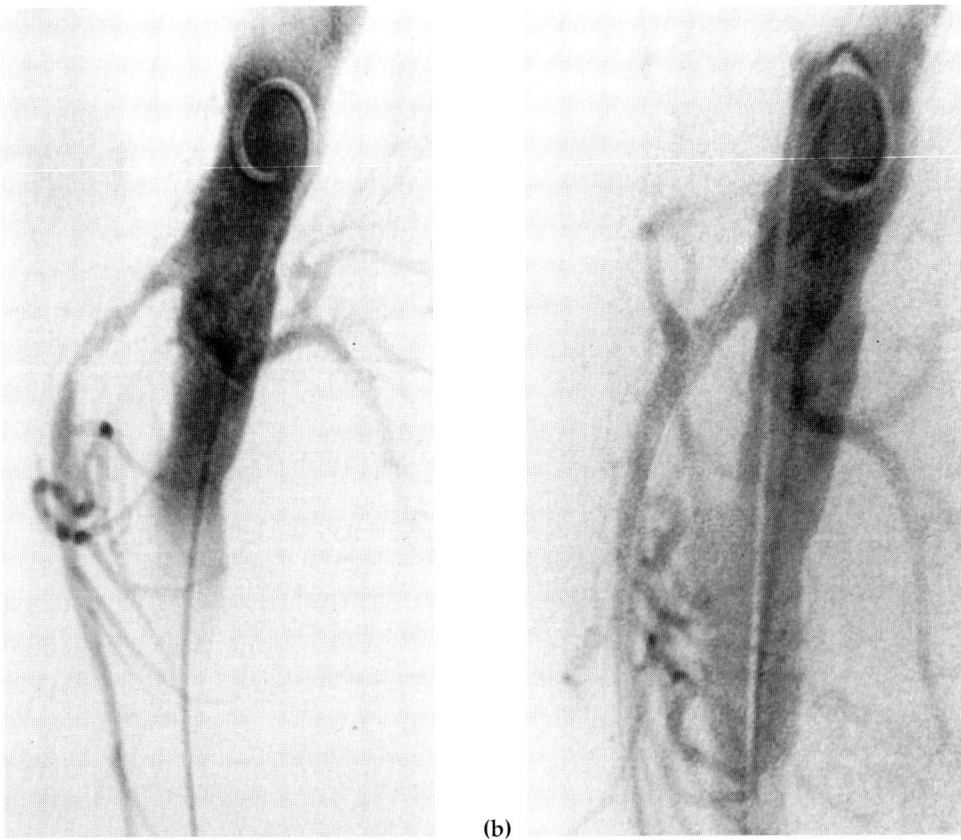

Fig. 12-10. A 62-year-old woman with severe visceral angina associated with loss of weight.
(a) Lateral abdominal aortogram demonstrates occlusion of the celiac axis and a tight irrregular stenosis of the proximal superior mesenteric artery. The inferior mesenteric artery was also occluded. (b) Lateral adominal aortogram after angioplasty and metallic stent placement across the superior mesenteric artery stenosis demonstrates wide patency of the SMA. The patient's symptoms were abolished.

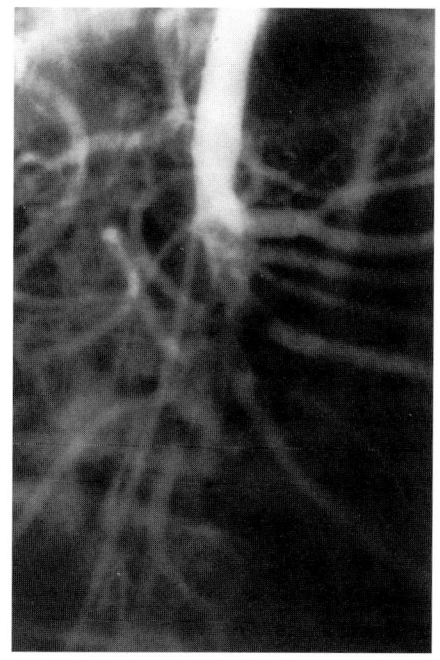 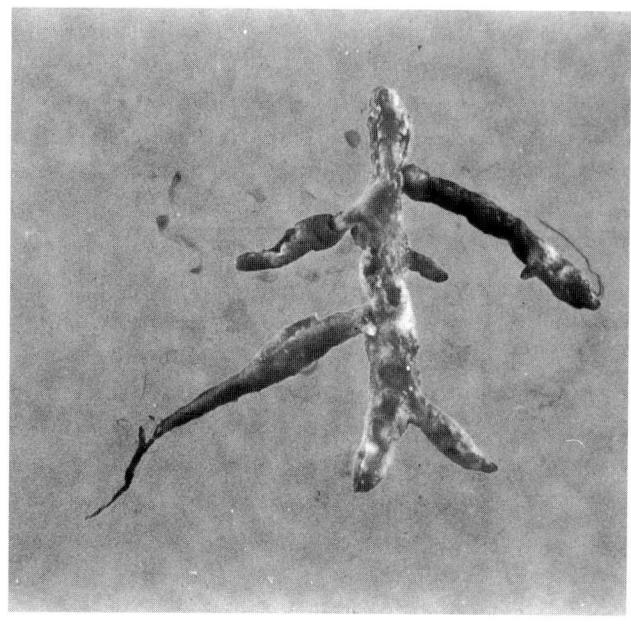

Fig. 12-11. A 60+-year-old man complaining of increasing abdominal pain of recent onset.
(a) A superior mesenteric arteriogram demonstrates embolus in the mid-superior mesenteric artery and extending into some of the branches. (b) Patient had surgery, the embolus was removed, and its shape closely resembles the focal distribution of the side branches of the SMA.

sequent management. A possible exception to this rule is when small bowel lymphoma is suspected and there is no suitable lesion amenable to endoscopic biopsy. In such cases a percutaneous transabdominal biopsy using ultrasound, computed tomography, and/or fluoroscopy with intraluminal contrast medium may be useful to confirm the diagnosis prior to chemotherapy. The most commonly biopsied lesions related to specific small bowel pathology include lymph node or hepatic metastases from a small intestinal tumor (eg, carcinoid).

The needle type used will depend to a large extent on the site of the lesion to be biopsied and the likely diagnosis. Fine needle aspiration biopsy (FNAB) permits diagnostic material to be obtained from deep-seated lesions without significant risk. The safety record of this technique is extraordinarily good despite the potential risks of hemorrhage, sepsis, and tumor seeding. Serious complications of the procedure are so rare that FNAB is now routinely performed on an outpatient basis in many centers.

Cutting needle biopsies are also safe, and there is some evidence to suggest that their use does not significantly increase the complication rate in solid organs such as the liver when compared with FNAB, providing that a good imaging guidance system is used to direct the needle to the target. Certain pathologies demand a core of tissue for a correct diagnosis, the most notable of which is lymphoma, and when this diagnosis is suspected a cutting needle biopsy is recommended.

The choice of imaging guidance during the biopsy will depend on a number of factors. Within the abdomen ultrasound is arguably the most important imaging modality for percutaneous biopsies. It is versatile, usually quick to perform, does not involve ionizing radiation, and is available as a portable technique. Computed tomography–guided biopsy is usually more time-consuming than ultrasound but is not adversely influenced by gas shadows (an important consideration in the abdomen), and it gives good resolution of different tissue components.

Drainage Procedures

Interventional techniques for the percutaneous drainage of abnormal fluid collections and abscesses have become established as routine management procedures in a large number of centers. Abscesses and collections may arise as a complication of intra-abdominal operations, small bowel perforation, or pancreatitis. Common sites include the lesser sac, the subphrenic space, and the pelvis, and these can usually be managed nonoperatively by the placement of a percutaneous drain. Computed tomography, ultrasound, and fluoroscopy can all be helpful for abscess drainage,[59] the most useful modality (or combination of modalities) depending upon the site or nature of the collection and the preference of the operator.

Enterocutaneous fistulae may be associated with abscesses or other fluid collections, and this connection may not be evident without radiologic intervention. There is a subset of high-output enterocutaneous fistulae, defined to have an output exceeding 200 mL per day. However, as much as 4 L of intestinal fluid has been known to drain per day in some of the patients. The associated massive loss of electrolytes and nutrients poses considerable problems of clinical management. The outpouring of the fluid containing gastric and pancreatic secretions also increases inflammation and necrosis in surrounding tissue. For healing to have a chance, outflow has to be controlled by placement of a T tube though the rent in the bowel wall and extending it craniad and caudad into the bowel lumen.[60] Drainage tubes have also to be placed into adjacent tissue spaces. Radiology has been an important factor in reducing the previous mortality rate of 45% to 67% to a more recent 6% to 20%.[61]

Dilatation Procedures

The esophagus is the part of the gastrointestinal tract most commonly treated by balloon dilatation and/or the insertion of a metallic endoprosthesis, and therapeutic techniques in this organ lie outside the scope of this chapter. Similar techniques may, however, be employed in the small bowel. The relief of obstruction at anastomotic sites is particularly useful and has been described for virtually all anastomoses that can be thought of, including gastroenterostomies, antralpyloric strictures, and entero-enterostomies.

Duodenal strictures due to involvement by pancreatic tumors or, less commonly, to primary duodenal malignancies can be successfully palliated by insertion of a metallic stent.[62,63] This procedure may be performed entirely under fluoroscopic control; it is often easier, however, to combine fluoroscopy with endoscopy (Fig. 12-12). Gastric dilatation, which is often present because of outlet obstruction, can make catheterization of the gastric pylorus and duodenum difficult due to looping of the catheter, and the use of an endoscope overcomes this problem, thereby shortening the procedure. The stent most commonly employed for duodenal stenoses is now the Wallstent owing to a combination of factors including its flexibility in comparison with other stents and the small size of its delivery device, which allows its passage through the working channel of an endoscope.

Percutaneous Jejunostomy

Percutaneous *gastrostomy* is established as an important procedure that allows the maintenance of adequate nutrition in patients with major swallowing difficulties or debilitating diseases while obviating the discomfort, infective complications, and management problems associated with long-term parenteral nutrition.

Percutaneous *jejunostomy* can be performed in patients in whom gastric surgery has rendered the stomach unsuitable as the organ of access. The gas-filled (or fluid-filled if ultrasound is used) jejunum is punctured directly through the anterior abdominal wall. Anchoring sutures are inserted to attach the jejunal loop to the abdominal wall to ensure positional stability during subsequent track dilatation; a catheter (usually 8- or 10-French) is then inserted through which feeding can immediately commence.

The complications of percutaneous jejunostomy include dislodgement of the catheter and leakage of intestinal contents, although these can be avoided by attention to details of technique. Catheter occlusion is usually easily managed by catheter exchange over a guide wire.

Percutaneous small bowel access may also be required for biliary interventional procedures in patients who have undergone a previous choledochojejunostomy. It is common practice in many centers in which these operations are routinely performed to form, at the time of the original surgery, a special access loop that is attached to the anterior abdominal wall, where it is marked with a metallic ring or surgical clips.[64,65] This allows easy percutaneous access to the biliary tree, without transgressing the liver, if the patient returns with a stricture at the choledochojejunal anastomosis.

Conclusions

While the indications for diagnostic visceral arteriography in small bowel disease have diminished over recent years owing to improvements in noninvasive vascular imaging, this investigation still plays an important role in the identification of the source of acute and chronic gastrointestinal bleeding. A variety of angiographic therapeutic options are now available for the control of hemorrhage that are of proven safety and efficacy.

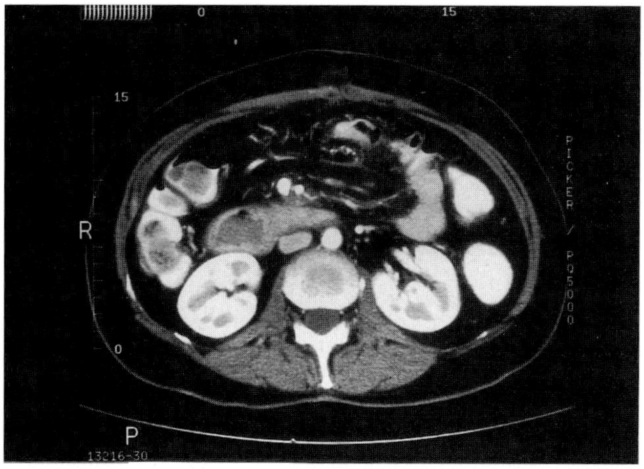

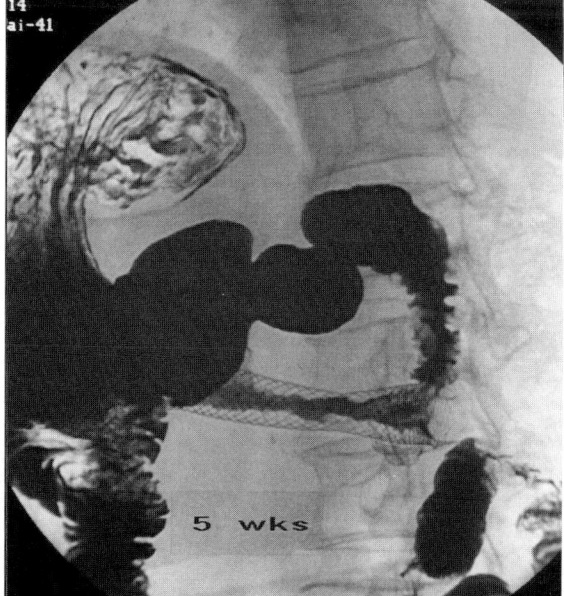

Fig. 12-12. **A 56-year-old woman with pancreatic carcinoma associated with obstruction of the third part of the duodenum. A previous surgical gastroenterostomy had failed.**
(a) Contrast-enhanced axial CT scan through the midabdomen demonstrates a markedly dilatated and fluid-filled second part of the duodenum proximal to a strictured third part. (b) A guide wire has been placed across the long stricture involving the third and fourth parts of the duodenum using a combination of endoscopy and fluoroscopy. (c) The loaded stent (Wallstent, 16 mm diameter, 5.6 cm long) has been introduced across the strictured segment. (d) The stent has been deployed. (e) A view from a barium meal performed 5 weeks later shows wide patency of the stent.

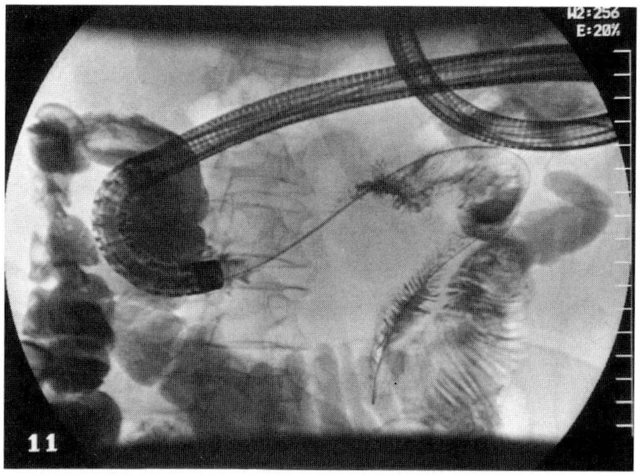

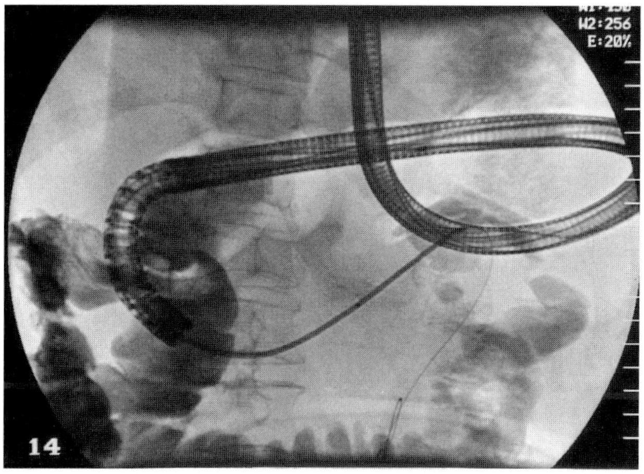

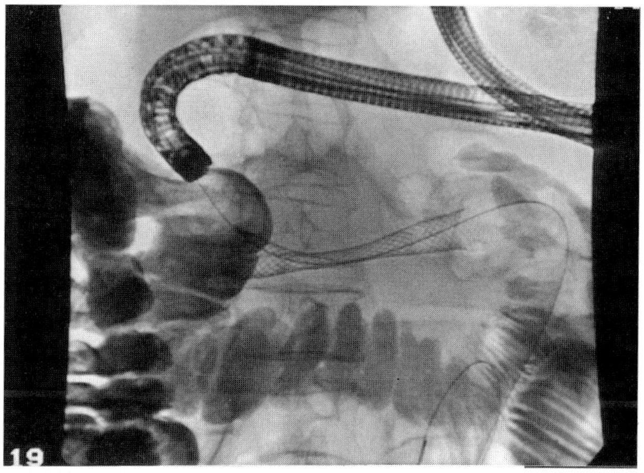

This patient was still feeding normally 9 months after stent placement. (Case courtesy of Professor C Zollikofer, Department of Radiology, Kantonsspital Winterthur, Brauerstrasse 15, Postfach 834, 8401 Winterthur, Switzerland.)

Nonvascular interventional radiological techniques in small bowel disease are becoming more common in most centers, and include biopsies, abscess drainages, stricture dilatation and stent insertion, and small bowel access for enteral nutrition.

References

1. Jackson JE, Allison DJ. Transcatheter embolization of hepatic neoplasms. In: Freeny PC, Stevenson GW, eds. *Margulis and Burhenne's Alimentary Tract Radiology.* 5th ed. St. Louis, Mo: CV Mosby Co; 1994:1722–1734.
2. Hunter JM, Pezim ME. Limited value of technetium 99m-labelled red cell scintigraphy in localization of lower gastrointestinal bleeding. *Am J Surg.* 1990;159:504–507.
3. Smith R, Copely DJ, Bolen FH. ^{99m}Tc RBC scintigraphy: correlation of gastrointestinal bleeding rates with scintigraphic findings. *AJR.* 1987;148:869–874.
4. Zuckerman DA, Bocchini TP, Birnbaum EH. Massive hemorrhage in the lower gastrointestinal tract in adults: diagnostic imaging and intervention. *AJR.* 1993;161: 703–711.
5. Boley SJ, Brandt LJ. Vascular ectasias of the colon. *Dig Dis Sci.* 1986;31:265–425.
6. Rösch J, Keller FS, Wawrukiewicz AS, Krippaehne WW, Dotter CT. Pharmacoangiography in the diagnosis of recurrent massive lower gastrointestinal bleeding. *Radiology.* 1982;145:615–619.
7. Koval G, Benner KG, Rösch J, Kozak BE. Aggressive angiographic diagnosis in acute lower gastrointestinal hemorrhage. *Dig Dis Sci.* 1987;32:248–253.
8. Glickerman DJ, Kowdley KV, Rösch J. Urokinase in gastrointestinal tract bleeding. *Radiology.* 1988;168:375–376.
9. Textor HJ, Wilhelm K, Strunk H, Schuller H, Schild HH. The diagnosis of intra-abdominal hemorrhage with CO_2 as the contrast medium. [in German] *Rofo.* 1997;166: 51–53.
10. Athanasoulis CA, Waltman AC, Novelline RA, Krudy AG, Sniderman KW. Angiography. Its contribution to the emergency management of gastrointestinal hemorrhage. *Radiol Clin North Am.* 1976;14:265–280.
11. Reuter SR. Embolization of gastrointestinal hemorrhage. *AJR.* 1979;133:557–558.
12. Chuang VP, Wallace S, Zornoza J, Davis LJ. Transcatheter arterial occlusion in the management of rectosigmoid bleeding. *Radiology.* 1979;133:605–609.
13. Walker WJ, Goldin AR, Shaff MI, Allibone GW. Percatheter control of hemorrhage from the superior and inferior mesenteric arteries. *Clin Radiol.* 1980;31:71–80.
14. Rosenkrantz H, Bookstein JJ, Rosen RJ, Goff WB, Healy JF. Postembolic colonic infarction. *Radiology.* 1982;142: 47–51.
15. Palmaz JC, Walter JF, Cho KJ. Therapeutic embolization of the small-bowel arteries. *Radiology.* 1984;152:377–382.
16. Gomes AS, Lois JF, McCoy RD. Angiographic treatment of gastrointestinal hemorrhage: comparison of vasopressin infusion and embolization. *AJR.* 1986;146: 1031–1037.
17. Fagan EA, Allison DJ, Chadwick VS, Hodgson HJF. Treatment of hemobilia by selective arterial embolization. *Gut* 1980;21:541–544.
18. Kadir S, Athanasoulis CA, Ring EJ, Greenfield A. Transcatheter embolization of intrahepatic arterial aneurysms. *Radiology.* 1980;134:335–339.
19. Kelley CJ, Hemingway AP, McPherson GAD, Allison DJ, Blumgart LH. Non-surgical management of postcholecystectomy haemobilia. *Br J Surg.* 1983;70:502–504.
20. Clouse ME. Hepatic artery embolization for bleeding and tumors. *Surg Clin North Am.* 1989;69:419–432.
21. Adam A, Jackson JE, Mueller PR, Dick R, Allison DJ. Interventional techniques in the hepatobiliary system. In: Grainger RG, Allison DJ, eds. *Diagnostic Radiology: A Textbook of Medical Imaging.* 3rd ed. Edinburgh, Scotland: Churchill Livingstone; 1997:1235–1258.
22. Blomley MJK, Jackson E. Case report: a gastroduodenal artery pseudoaneurysm presenting with obstructive jaundice and treated by arterial embolization. *Clin Radiol.* 1994;49:715–718.
23. Camilleri M, Hemingway AP, Chadwick VS, Blumgart LH, Hodgson HJF, Allison DJ. Embolization of an intrapancreatic aneurysm. *Br J Radiol.* 1982;55:685–687.
24. Mandel SR, Jaques PF, Mauro M, Sanofsky S. Nonoperative management of peripancreatic arterial aneurysms. A 10-year experience. *Ann Surg.* 1987;205:126–128.
25. Huizinga WKJ, Kalideen JM, Bryer JV, Bell PSH, Baker LW. Control of major haemorrhage associated with pancreatic pseudocysts by transcatheter arterial embolization. *Br J Surg.* 1984;71:133–136.
26. Baker KS, Tisnado J, Cho S-R, Beachley MC. Splanchnic artery aneurysms and pseudoaneurysms: transcatheter embolization. *Radiology.* 1987;163:135–139.
27. Walker TG, Waltman AC. Angiographic management of massive hemorrhage caused by pancreatic disease. *Semin Interven Radiol.* 1988;5:61–63.
28. Ryan CM, Benjamin IS, Allison DJ. The diagnosis and management of haemosuccus pancreaticus. *J Interven Radiol.* 1989;4:130–134.
29. Goldman ML, Land WC, Bradley EL, Anderson J. Transcatheter therapeutic embolization in the management of massive upper gastrointestinal bleeding. *Radiology.* 1976;120:513–521.
30. Prochaska JM, Flye MW, Johnsrude IS. Left gastric artery embolization for control of gastric bleeding; a complication. *Radiology.* 1973;107:521–522.
31. Keller FS, Barton RE, Rösch J. Angiographic diagnosis and therapy of gastrointestinal tract bleeding. In: Freeny PC, Stevenson GW, eds. *Margulis and Burhenne's Alimentary Tract Radiology.* 5th ed. St. Louis, Mo: CV Mosby Co; 1994:994–1016.
32. Granke K, Hollier LH, Bowen JC. Pancreaticoduodenal artery aneurysms: changing patterns. *South Med J.* 1990; 83:918–921.
33. Stanley JC, Frey CF, Miller TA, Lindenauer SM, Child CG. Major arterial hemorrhage. A complication of pancreatic pseudocysts and chronic pancreatitis. *Arch Surg.* 1976;111:435–440.
34. White AF, Baum S, Buranasiri S. Aneurysms secondary to pancreatitis. *AJR.* 1976;127:393–396.

35. Eckhauser FE, Stanley JC, Zelenock GB, Borlaza GS, Freier DT, Lindenauer SM. Gastroduodenal and pancreaticoduodenal artery aneurysms: a complication of pancreatitis causing spontaneous gastrointestinal hemorrhage. *Surgery*. 1980;88:335–344.
36. Bretagne J-F, Heresbach D, Darnault P, et al. Pseudoaneurysms and bleeding pseudocysts in chronic pancreatitis: radiological findings and contribution to diagnosis in 8 cases. *Gastrointest Radiol*. 1990;15:9–16.
37. Kiviluoto T, Kivisaari L, Kivilaakso E, Lempinen M. Pseudocysts in chronic pancreatitis. Surgical results in 102 consecutive patients. *Arch Surg*. 1989;124:240–243.
38. Stabile BE, Wilson SE, Debas H. Reduced mortality from bleeding pseudocysts and pseudoaneurysms caused by pancreatitis. *Arch Surg*. 1983;118:45–51.
39. Allison DJ, Jackson JE. Arteriography: In: Grainger RG, Allison DJ, eds. *Diagnostic Radiology: A Textbook of Medical Imaging*. 3rd ed. Edinburgh, Scotland: Churchill Livingstone; 1997:2345–2424.
40. Berardi RS. Vascular complications of superior mesenteric artery infusion with pitressin in treatment of bleeding esophageal varices. *Am J Surg*. 1974;127:757–761.
41. Roberts C, Maddison FE. Partial mesenteric arterial occlusion with subsequent ischemic bowel damage due to pitressin infusion. *AJR*. 1976;126:829–831.
42. Conn HO, Ramsby GR, Storer EH, et al. Intra-arterial vasopressin in the treatment of upper gastrointestinal hemorrhage: a prospective, controlled clinical trial. *Gastroenterology*. 1975;68:211–221.
43. Ohri SK, Jackson JE, Desa LA, Spencer J. The intraoperative localization of the obscure bleeding site using fluorescein. *J Clin Gastroenterol*. 1992;14:331–334.
44. Cohen GS, Ball DS, Flynn DE. Transjugular transhepatic placement of a superior mesenteric vein stent for small bowel varices. *J Vasc Interv Radiol*. 1995;6:707–710.
45. Scaletscky R, Wright JK Jr, Shaw J, Smith JA Jr. Ileal conduit venous varices from portal hypertension as a cause of recurrent, massive hemorrhage: case report and review of the literature. *J Urol*. 1994;151:417–419.
46. Mathias K, Bolder U, Lohlein D, Jager H. Percutaneous transhepatic angioplasty and stent implantation for prehepatic portal vein obstruction. *Cardiovasc Interven Radiol*. 1993;16:313–315.
47. Oglevie SB, Smith DC, Gardiner GA. Angiographic demonstration of bleeding in an unusually located Meckel's diverticulum simulating colonic bleeding. *Cardiovasc Intervent Radiol*. 1989;12:210–212.
48. Routh WD, Lawdahl RB, Lund E, Garcia JH, Keller FS. Meckel's diverticula: angiographic diagnosis in patients with non-acute hemorrhage and negative scintigraphy. *Pediatr Radiol*. 1990;20:152–156.
49. Okazaki M, Higashihara H, Saida Y, et al. Angiographic findings of Meckel's diverticulum: the characteristic appearance of the vitelline artery. *Abdom Imaging*. 1993;18:15–19.
50. Mitchell A, Spencer J, Allison DJ, Jackson JE. Meckel's diverticulum; angiographic findings in 16 patients. *AJR*. In press.
51. Jeffree MA, Barter SJ, Hemingway AP, Nolan DJ. Primary carcinoid tumours of the ileum: the radiological appearances. *Clin Radiol*. 1984;35:451–455.
52. Valls C, Sancho C, Bechini J, Dominguez J, Montana X. Intestinal leiomyomas: angiographic imaging. *Gastrointest Radiol*. 1992;17:220–222.
53. Schoenbaum SW, Pena C, Koenisberg P, Katzen BT. Superior mesenteric artery embolism: treatment with intraarterial urokinase. *J Vasc Interv Radiol*. 1992;3:485–490.
54. Turégano F, Simó G, Echenagusia AJ, Fiuza C, De Tomás J, Pérez D. Successful intraarterial fragmentation and urokinase therapy in superior mesenteric artery embolism. *Surgery*. 1995;117:712–714.
55. Simó G, Echenagusia AJ, Camúñez F, Turégano F, Cabrera A, Urbano J. Superior mesenteric arterial embolism: local fibrinolytic treatment with urokinase. *Radiology*. 1997;204:775–779.
56. Allen RC, Martin GH, Rees CR, et al. Mesenteric angioplasty in the treatment of chronic intestinal ischemia. *J Vasc Surg*. 1996;24:415–421.
57. Hallisey MJ, Deschaine J, Illescas FF, et al. Angioplasty for the treatment of visceral ischemia. *J Vasc Interv Radiol*. 1995;6:785–791.
58. Lindblad B, Lindh M, Chuter T, Ivancev K. Superior mesenteric artery occlusion treated with PTA and stent placement. *Eur J Vasc Endovasc Surg*. 1996;11:493–495.
59. Bernini A, Spencer MP, Wong WD, Rothenberger DA, Madoff RD. Computed tomography-guided percutaneous abscess drainage in intestinal disease: factors associated with outcome. *Dis Colon Rectum*. 1997;40:1009–1013.
60. McLean GK, Mackie JA, Freiman DB, Ring EJ. Enterocutaneous fistulae interventional radiologic management. *AJR*. 1982;138:615–619.
61. McLean GK. Interventional radiology of the gastrointestinal tract. *Curr Probl Diagn Radiol*. 1990;19:85–132.
62. Strecker EP, Boos I, Husfeldt KJ. Malignant duodenal stenosis: palliation with peroral implantation of a self-expanding nitinol stent. *Radiology*. 1995;196:349–351.
63. Binkert CA, Jost R, Steiner A, Zollikofer CL. Benign and malignant stenoses of the stomach and duodenum: treatment with self-expanding metallic endoprostheses. *Radiology*. 1996;199:335–338.
64. Cameron DC, Frazer CK. The Hutson loop and prosthesis: clinical uses in hepato-biliary intervention. *Australas Radiol*. 1995;39:159–165.
65. Perry LJ, Stokes KR, Lewis WD, Jenkins RL, Clouse ME. Biliary intervention by means of percutaneous puncture of the antecolic jejunal loop. *Radiology*. 1995;195:163–167.

Enteroscopy

13

Lewis R. Felder and J. S. Barkin

Chapter Contents

Introduction
Push Enteroscopy
Sonde Enteroscopy
Intraoperative Enteroscopy
Ileoscopy
Indications for Enteroscopy
Enteroclysis and Enteroscopy
Risks
Conclusion

Introduction

The second half of the twentieth century has ushered in the era of modern endoscopy in which flexible endoscopes are used to examine the upper and lower gastrointestinal tracts. Standard upper endoscopes can routinely be advanced to the second portion of the duodenum and may allow careful inspection of the duodenal mucosa past the ampulla of Vater. Conversely, standard colonoscopes may successfully examine the entire large bowel and achieve ileal intubation, with inspection of the distal portion of the ileum in greater than 90% of examinations done by experienced endoscopists.[1] Therefore, the entire mucosal surface between the mid-duodenum and the distal ileum was beyond the reach of standard endoscopes. Before the advent of longer endoscopes (enteroscopes), small bowel radiography remained the gold standard of diagnostic testing for disorders of the small intestine; biopsy sampling was performed by using small peroral capsules. These options clearly have limitations, as radiography cannot visualize mucosal lesions that do not protrude above or extend below the surface, and capsule biopsies cannot be guided and may, therefore, miss patchy or isolated lesions. However, this combination of methodologies continued until the early 1980s, when the introduction of longer endoscopes with improved techniques made it possible to advance the operating end of the scope deep into the small bowel. Enteroscopy can be divided into push and sonde types.

Push Enteroscopy

A push enteroscope is longer than the standard, upper endoscope and is constructed to permit rapid advancement into the proximal jejunum. It has four-way tip deflection that allows visualization of the small bowel mucosa of the entire lumen as well as a biopsy channel through which biopsy instruments can be passed. Standard pediatric or adult colonoscopes can only be advanced to approximately 50 cm past the ligament of Treitz,[2] as looping within the stomach inhibits greater penetration of the small bowel. Enteroscopy overcomes this limitation by the use of an overtube, which is back-loaded onto the enteroscope before insertion through the mouth. It is then advanced over the scope to the pylorus after the tip of the enteroscope has passed beyond the ligament of Treitz. The overtube straightens the scope within the stomach, prevents the forming of loops, and allows passage further into the small bowel. Fluoroscopic guidance is used during the advance and placement of the overtube and for the documentation of the distance the endoscopic tip has reached into the small bowel. Barkin et al described the passage of a newer-generation enteroscope, the SIF 10L, that has a working length of 271 cm and can be inserted an average of 94 cm past the ligament of Treitz.[2]. The only complications noted in this study were a Mallory-Weiss tear, likely caused by placement of the overtube, and an unexplained episode of pancreatitis, possibly from temporary occlusion of the ampulla of Vater by the overtube. Overall, complications resulting from push enteroscopy are rare and usually related to overtube placement.

Sonde Enteroscopy

While push enteroscopy allows almost total mucosal visualization of the proximal small bowel, it cannot visualize the entire bowel. A sonde enteroscope may allow endoscopic evaluation of the entire small bowel. This long, slender, flexible endoscope may be passed nasally and transits the small bowel by peristaltic movement, stimulated by a balloon at its tip. There are several differences between sonde and push enteroscopy, such as: 1) Visualization of the small bowel mucosa occurs upon withdrawal of the sonde endoscope, with only limited mucosal cover. A Mayo clinic study estimated that only 50% of the lumen could be viewed during controlled withdrawal[3]; 2) Active tip deflection is not possible with most sonde enteroscopes and lateral movement can be varied only by inflation of the distal balloon or by palpation over the anterior abdominal wall; 3) Duration varies from 4 to 6 hours but can take more than 24 hours for complete transit of the enteroscope; this period can be shortened by actively placing the tip of the sonde enteroscope into the duodenum with the aid of a standard upper endoscope, a technique described by Lewis and Waye[4]; and 4) biopsy capabilities are non-existent or limited. Sonde enteroscopy and intraoperative endoscopy were found to be comparable for depth of penetration and ability to detect small arteriovenous malformations (AVMs).[5]

Intraoperative Endoscopy

This technique requires peroral intraoperative passage of an endoscope into the duodenum by the endoscopist. The endoscopic advance through the small bowel is aided by the surgeon, who telescopes the small bowel over the endoscope. This technique may be thought to represent the most complete form of endoscopic evaluation of the small intestine. This approach allows for the examination of the small bowel by endoluminal visual inspection as well as visualization of the bowel wall by transillumination to the serosal surface, using the endoluminal light of the endoscope for this purpose. When lesions are visualized, the surgeon places a surgical loop at that site as a guide for later resection. This technique has a role in patients who have ongoing occult bleeding that requires transfusions. Another method of intraoperative endoscopy requires the passage of endoscopes through multiple enterotomies. Unfortunately, this technique is associated with significant morbidity, as there may be leakage at enterotomy sites with subsequent infection.

Ileoscopy

Routine colonoscopy can reach the cecum and provides an opportunity to intubate the terminal ileum and inspect its mucosa. Endoscopists can traverse the ileocecal vale in approximately three of four patients. In a unique combination of radiographic and endoscopic approaches, a guide wire is inserted through the biopsy channel of the colonoscope and is inserted into the ileum. A catheter is then threaded over the wire and advanced into the terminal ileum, and the colonoscope is then removed, leaving the catheter in place. Contrast material introduced via the catheter can provide excellent visualization of the distal small bowel.[6]

Indications for Enteroscopy

Enteroscopy is most frequently used in patients with occult gastrointestinal bleeding, which is defined as ongoing or intermittent, that was not diagnosed by routine upper and lower endoscopy, nor by small bowel radiographic studies.[7] Push enteroscopy has been useful in discovering sources of occult bleeding in 13% to 38% of patients.[8–10] Angiodysplasia is the most common finding and accounts for 80% of lesions.[9] The use of combined push and sonde enteroscopy has been described in a group of patients with bleeding of obscure origin.[5] They reported 40% abnormal endoscopic examinations beyond the reach of routine upper endoscopy,[9] similar to rates in the experience of the authors. These reports emphasize the need to visualize the small bowel in patients with occult bleeding. In addition to AVMs, small bowel tumors accounted for 10% of lesions, several of which had not been visualized by enteroclysis. Using push enteroscopy, a possible bleeding site was found in 21 of 28 patients (75%) with occult intestinal bleeding.[11] The sources of bleeding were almost equally divided between sites proximal and distal to the ligament of Treitz. Eight of 10 lesions distal to the ligament of Treitz were AVMs (Fig. 13-1), and two were small bowel tumors, none of which had been detected by radiological imaging. Malabsorption may also be assessed by enteroscopic evaluation (Fig. 13-2). The biopsy specimens obtained by push enteroscopy have been shown to be adequate in 76% to 100% of patients.[12,13] It is recommended that only one specimen be obtained with each passage of the biopsy forceps to minimize crush artifacts and that six biopsy specimens be obtained to ensure that multiple areas are sampled. The pathological processes that have been diagnosed include Whipple's disease, eosinophilic enteritis, and lymphoma.

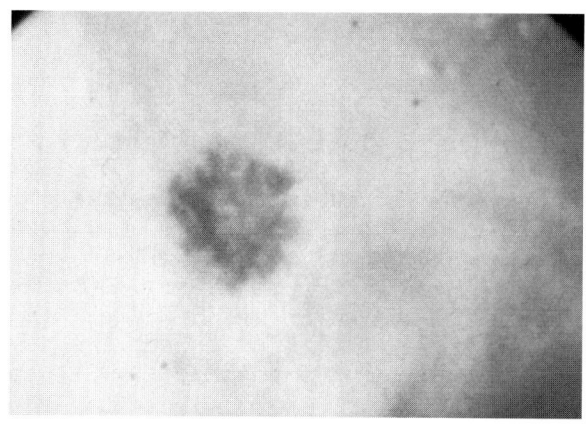

Fig. 13-1. Magnified enteroscopic image of an AVM.

Enteroscopy has become the method of choice for obtaining small bowel biopsies.

Enteroclysis and Enteroscopy

Enteroscopy can visualize lesions overlooked by small bowel follow-through examinations, but enteroclysis can visualize the entire small bowel; thus it should be regarded as complementary study to enteroscopy. Enteroclysis can be combined with push enteroscopy to permit total small bowel visualization. In this technique, enteroscopy allows placement of a catheter for the performance of the enteroclysis. It involves placing a guide wire into the biopsy channel of the enteroscope, advancing it once the tip of the enteroscope is in the jejunum. The enteroscope is then withdrawn, leaving the wire in place; the enteroclysis tube with a distal balloon is advanced over the wire. Once the appropriate jejunal site is reached, the balloon is inflated, fixing the tube in place, and the wire is withdrawn.

Contrast and air are then infused to perform the enteroclysis.[14] Similarly, as colonoscopy detects lesions in patients who have undergone a negative air contrast barium enema, enteroscopy may detect mucosal lesions not seen by enteroclysis. These include AVMs and small bowel tumors. Enteroclysis was performed in 128 patients with obscure intestinal bleeding and lesions were found in 21%. Interestingly, 63% of the lesions were small bowel tumors and 11% were AVMs.[15] The findings are in contrast to the approximately 40% yield reported with enteroscopy, with the majority of lesions comprising vascular malformations. This is not unexpected as enteroclysis will find mucosal abnormalities caused by tumors and will overlook most AVMs in which the mucosa appears normal. Enteroclysis as complementary test to enteroscopy is most useful in identifying more distal small bowel tumors; however, it is not a sensitive modality for identifying AVMs, which comprise the most common etiology of occult gastrointestinal blood loss. Enteroscopy can also obtain tissue for histological identification of small bowel lesions that have been visualized by radiographic techniques (see also Chapter 7).

Risks

The same risks reported with upper gastrointestinal endoscopy and with small bowel suction biopsy may be assumed with standard enteroscopy. Morbidity associated with push-type enteroscopy is related to overtube passage.

Conclusion

Enteroscopy has gained wide acceptance over the past 20 years and is now an accepted diagnostic and ther-

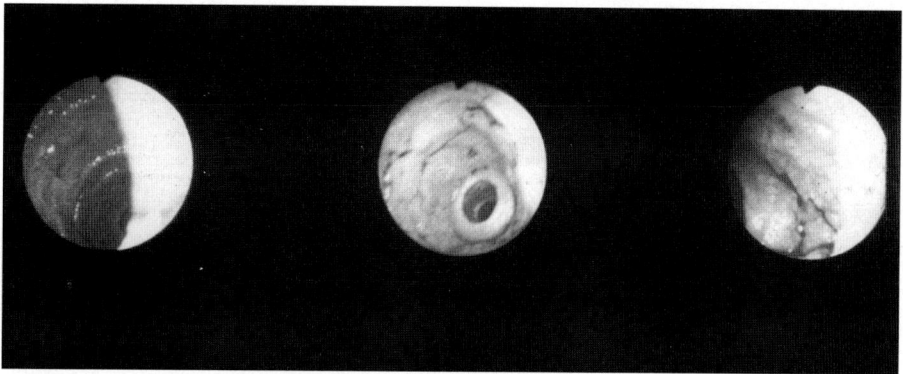

Fig. 13-2. Findings of villous atrophy in duodenum and jejunum of a patient with celiac disease.

apeutic procedure. This technique is most useful for evaluating patients with occult gastrointestinal bleeding, suspected malabsorption, or occult causes of diarrhea and for the histological identification of radiographically shown lesions. Two methods, push and sonde enteroscopies, are most commonly employed, and each has its own distinct advantages. Push enteroscopy allows for more thorough viewing of the mucosa and has biopsy and therapeutic capabilities, but cannot access the entire small bowel. Sonde enteroscopy allows passage through the entire small bowel, but with limited viewing and without therapeutic or biopsy diagnostic capabilities. Given the limitations of each type of enteroscopy, no single method exists for directly evaluating the small bowel in its entirety with the necessary diagnostic capability. At present, push endoscopy is the best method in most scenarios and, when combined with radiographic evaluation via enteroclysis, provides the most complete evaluation of the small bowel. Intraoperative enteroscopy remains the gold standard for diagnosis and therapy of patients who continue to have occult bleeding and require therapy.

References

1. Foutch P, Sawyer P, Sanowski R. Push enteroscopy for the diagnosis of patients with gastrointestinal bleeding of obscure origin. *Gut.* 1987;28:869–877.
2. Barkin JS, Chong J, Reiner DK. First generation video enteroscope: fourth generation push-type small bowel enteroscopy utilizing an overtube. *Gastrointest Endosc.* 1994;40(6):743–747.
3. Gostout CJ, Schroeder KW, Burton DD. Small bowel enteroscopy. An early experience in gastrointestinal bleeding of unknown origin. *Gastrointest Endosc.* 1991;37:5–8.
4. Lewis BS, Waye JD. Total small bowel enteroscopy. *Gastrointest Endosc.* 1987;33:435–438.
5. Lewis BS, Wenger J, Waye JD. Small bowel enteroscopy and intraoperative endoscopy for obscure gastrointestinal bleeding. *Am J Gastroenterol.* 1991;86:171–174.
6. Rokkas T, Psara C, Stefanopoulous T, et al. Endoscopic retrograde ileography. *Gastrointestinal Endoscopy.* 1991;37:A274.
7. Waye JD. Small bowel endoscopy. *Endoscopy.* 1992;24:68–72.
8. Foutch PG, Sawyer R, Sanowski R. Push enteroscopy for diagnosis of patients with gastrointestinal bleeding of obscure origin. *Gastrointestinal Endoscopy.* 1990;36:337–341.
9. Lewis BS, Waye JD. Small bowel enteroscopy: a comparison of findings with push and sonde enteroscopy in 81 patients with gastrointestinal bleeding of obscure origin. *Gastrointest Endosc.* (abstract) 1988;34:207.
10. Messer J, Romeu J, Waye JD, et al. The value of proximal jejunoscopy in unexplained gastrointestinal bleeding. *Gastrointest Endosc.* (abstract) 1984;30:151.
11. Barkin JS, Lewis BS, Waye JD, et al. Diagnostic and therapeutic jejunoscopy with a new longer enteroscope. *Gastrointest Endosc.* 1992;38(1):55–58.
12. Koren E, Foroozan P. Endoscopic biopsies of normal duodenal mucosa. *Gastrointest Endosc.* 1997;21:51–54.
13. Scott BB, Jenkins D. Endoscopic intestinal biopsy. *Gastrointest Endosc.* 1981;27:162–167.
14. McGovern R, Barkin JS. Enteroscopy and enteroclysis: an improved method for combined procedures. *Gastrointest Radiol.* 1990;15:327–328.
15. Moch A, Herlinger H, Kochman ML, et al. Enteroclysis in the evaluation of obscure gastrointestinal bleeding. *AJR.* 1994;163:1381–1384.

Congenital and Developmental Anomalies of the Small Bowel in Adolescents and Adults

14

Dean D.T. Maglinte and George S. Bisset III

Chapter Contents

Introduction
Early Development of Midgut
Midgut Rotation
Midgut Duplications
Omphalomesenteric Duct Anomalies
Anomalies of Intestinal Rotation
Anomalies of Intestinal Fixation
Idiopathic Localized Dilatation of the Ileum (Ileal Dysgenesis)

Introduction

Congenital anomalies of the small intestine can evade detection into adulthood because they cause only moderate and nonspecific clinical symptoms. The mesenteric small intestine (jejunum and ileum) in common with the duodenum distal to the entry of the common bile duct, the liver, pancreas, appendix, and the colon proximal to its midtransverse segment are derivatives of the fetal midgut. Congenital anomalies of the midgut, often encountered in infants and children, are uncommon in adolescents and adults.[1] Anomalies of the foregut predominate in adults.[2] Adults are also less likely than infants and young children to have multiple anomalies. Most midgut malformations are related to the following three events in the development of the fetus[3]:

1. Separation of the notochord from the endoderm beginning the 3rd week of development. A variety of intestinal duplications result from failure of separation.
2. Regression of the vitelline stalk starting the 5th week of development. Failure of regression results in Meckel's diverticulum or other rare omphalomesenteric duct vestiges.
3. Return of the intestines to the abdomen in the 10th week. Anomalies of intestinal rotation and fixation of the mesenteries arise from improper return of the midgut from its extracoelomic position to the abdominal cavity.

An adequate awareness of the embryology of the fetal midgut is necessary for the understanding of the pathophysiologic consequences of its aberrations, the symptoms of which may manifest in later life.

Early Development of Midgut

The primitive gut of the human embryo is already demarcated into three segments at the beginning of the 3rd week of development.[3,4] Ventrally the primitive midgut communicates with the yolk sac, the primary source of nutrition for the fetus at this stage of development (Fig. 14-1). During the 3rd and 4th weeks, the embryo grows rapidly while the yolk sac and open midgut lag behind. This results in elongation and constriction of the connecting segment, the vitellointestinal duct (yolk stalk or omphalomesenteric duct). This structure is obliterated by the 7th to 8th week of gestation, when the placenta replaces the yolk sac as the source of nutrition for the fetus.[5] At the 4th week of gestation, the primitive midgut is a straight tube supported by a dorsal mesentery attached to the midline in front of the aorta. It is supplied by the superior mesenteric artery (SMA), which lies in the dorsal mesentery.

The further elongation of the midgut is accompanied by a series of intestinal movements that culminate in the final position of the small and large bowel within the abdomen. This series of movements can be divided into three stages.[3,6,7]

Midgut Rotation

Rotation within the Hernia

The first stage of rotation occurs from the 6th to 10th weeks. The midgut elongates, forming a hairpin-

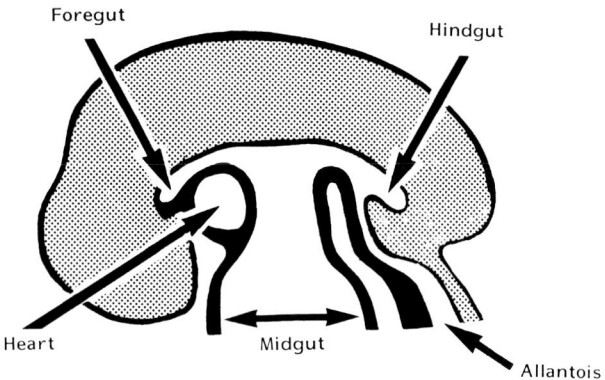

Fig. 14-1. Diagrammatic longitudinal section of a 3-week-old human embryo.
The midgut develops from the roof of the secondary yolk sac between the anterior and posterior intestinal portals and opens ventrally into the yolk sac between them. The transverse septum forms the anterior boundary of the embryonic midgut. Into its substance will grow the primordium of the liver. The pancreas will grow dorsally within the mesentery.

shaped loop in the sagittal plane, extending ventrally into the umbilical cord. The SMA forms the axis of this loop and extends to its apex, which is marked by the attachment of the vitellointestinal duct. The SMA divides the umbilical loop into a *prearterial* (cephalic or proximal) segment that will develop into the distal half of the duodenum, the jejunum, and part of the ileum and a *postarterial* (caudal or distal) segment that will develop into the distal ileum, cecum, appendix, ascending colon, and most of the transverse colon. While the umbilical loop is being extruded, it rotates 90 degrees counterclockwise around its axis, bringing the prearterial segment to the right and the postarterial segment to the left of the SMA. A further 90-degree counterclockwise rotation occurs while the midgut is still in the umbilical cord. Completion of the first stage brings the prearterial segment caudal and the postarterial segment cephalad to the SMA (Fig. 14-2).

Stage of Reentry

The second stage starts in the 10th week when the midgut loop starts returning to the abdomen. The prearterial segment returns first and enters the abdomen to the left of the SMA, displacing the hindgut and its mesentery to the left (Fig. 14-3). The ascending colon and the cecum, which have become larger than the small bowel, are the last to enter the abdomen. As the midgut enters the abdomen, it undergoes a further 90-degree counterclockwise rotation. This simultaneous two-phase "rotation" during its return to the abdominal cavity results in the intestines assuming normal anatomic relationships. In the first phase, the duodenojejunal junction passes behind the SMA and becomes fixed to the upper left retroperitoneum. In the second phase, the cecum passes from the left of the abdomen, anterior to the SMA, and assumes its normal position right of midline (Fig. 14-4).

Stage of Fixation

The third stage starts by the 11th week when the cecum starts to descend to reach the right iliac fossa between the 12th and 20th weeks (Fig. 14-5). The mesenteries of most of the duodenum and the ascending and descending colon fuse with the parietal peritoneum of the posterior abdominal wall, and thus these segments become secondarily retroperitoneal. The base of the small bowel mesentery fuses with the posterior peritoneum in a diagonal line from the ligament of Treitz to the cecum. Fixation continues until shortly before birth.

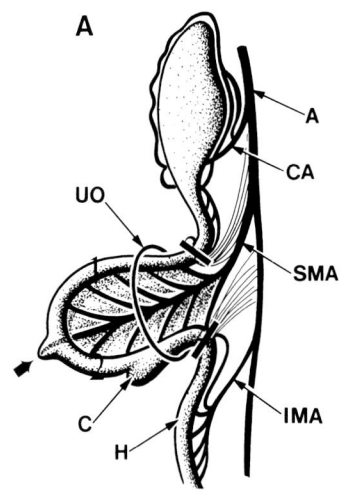

Fig. 14-2. Schematic drawing during the 6th week of fetal life.
The blood supply of the primitive gut is shown (A = aorta; CA = celiac artery; SMA = superior mesenteric artery; IMA = inferior mesenteric artery). The umbilical loop is divided by the attached vitellointestinal duct (arrow) into prearterial and postarterial limbs. A superior condensation band or ligament of Treitz fixes the midgut a short distance below its commencement. Most of the midgut is extended into the base of the umbilical cord (uo = umbilical orifice), where it will normally remain until approximately the tenth week (C = cecum; H = hindgut).

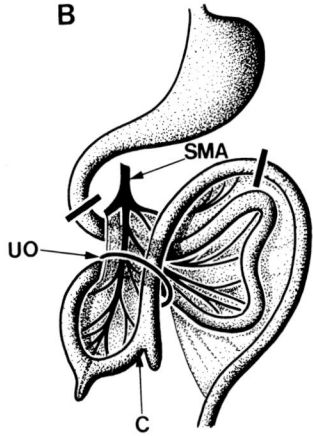

Fig. 14-3. The physiologic umbilical hernia is partly reduced.
In this frontal schematic drawing, the midgut has reentered the abdomen on the right side of the superior mesenteric vessels and has passed to the left side of the abdomen behind the vessels. The intestine is elongating, and the hindgut is displaced to the left side of the abdomen. A portion of the midgut still protrudes into the base of the cord (uo = umbilical orifice; c = cecum; SMA = superior mesenteric artery).

Midgut Duplications

Embryogenesis

Alimentary tract duplications are uncommon congenital anomalies that are usually identified in the first decade of life. Sixty percent to 85% are diagnosed by age 2 years.[8, 9] Only a few patients older than 15 years with isolated duplications have been described in the literature.[10–20] The duplications occur along the mesenteric aspect of the alimentary tract and are most commonly discovered in the ileum, followed by the esophagus, stomach, and duodenum, although they can occur throughout the gastrointestinal tract (Fig. 14-6).

Duplications result from disturbances in embryonic development of the gut. Intracellular vacuoles are formed during the "solid" stage of alimentary tract development in the 6th embryonic week. These vacuoles may develop into cysts or coalesce into chains, forming tubular duplications. The duplication wall contains all layers except where it is fused with the bowel, where a common muscular wall is shared (Fig. 14-7). No plane of cleavage can be established between duplication and adjacent bowel, and blood supply to the normal alimentary tract may be disrupted by local excision of the duplication.

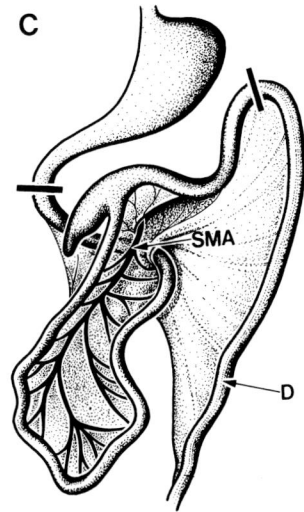

Fig. 14-4. In the early 11th week of fetal life the physiologic umbilical hernia is completely reduced.
The cecum is initially located in the epigastrium beneath the stomach and as the colon continues to rotate lies in the right upper quadrant (D = descending colon; SMA = superior mesenteric artery).

Types of Duplications

Three types of duplications are described[21]: 1) *"double-barrel"* duplication with two communications, 2) *"tubular"* duplication with either proximal or distal com-

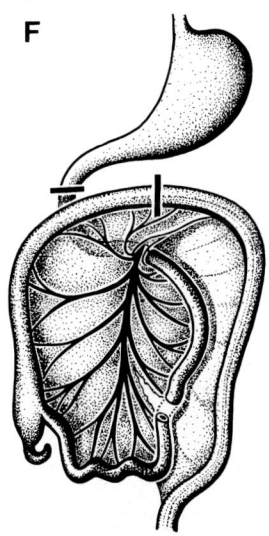

Fig. 14-5. The midgut loop has rotated 270 degrees counterclockwise.
Rotation of the colon is complete, and the cecum is in its final position. The dotted segment of the small bowel denotes the transition zone between jejunum and ileum.

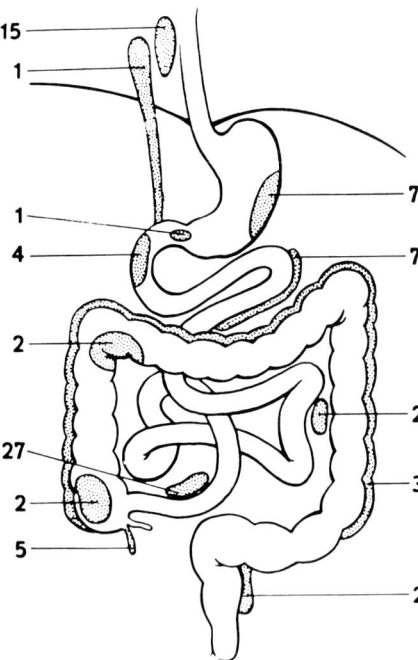

Fig. 14-6. Sites of duplications. This diagram records the number of sites in a series of 78 duplications. (With permission from Bower, Sieber, and Kiesewether.[23])

munication, and 3) the *spherical* type with no communication. Overall only 20% communicate with the lumen.[22] They may vary in size from several centimeters to large cystic masses. Multiple lesions have been reported in 15% of all gastrointestinal duplications and in 3% to 6% of all small bowel duplications.[23,24] It is worth noting that Meckel's diverticulum may coexist with duplications in different segments of bowel.[25]

Clinical Considerations

The clinical presentation of ileal duplications is most commonly related to complications such as intestinal obstruction or hemorrhage. Pain is a common symptom in adolescents and adults. An asymptomatic mass can be palpated in approximately one half of patients.[9] Cystic duplications in the inner layers of the bowel wall produce obstruction by intussusception.[26] Duplications can also cause obstruction of the gut lumen by direct compression or volvulus if the duplication assumes the form of a pendulous mass. Perforated peptic ulcer (due to acid-secreting mucosa in the duplication) and volvulus were the most common complications in one series.[26] Of the small number of ileal duplications presenting in adults, malignancy occurred in three (23%) of 13 patients.[27] The diverse potential of embryonic endoderm at the time these duplications arise may offer an explanation for the heterotopic mucosa.

Diagnosis

The diagnosis is not usually a clinical consideration in the adult.[2] The discovery may be incidental at laparotomy for other conditions. Barium examinations and ultrasonography have greatly facilitated recognition.

Plain film radiography may show evidence of a mass displacing gas-filled adjacent bowel or evidence of intestinal obstruction. An echogenic inner rim that indicates mucosa and mucus is surrounded by a sonolucent band of smooth muscle (Fig. 14-8). This has been termed the muscular rim sign and is diagnostic of duplication cyst. The diagnosis is most commonly made when an ultrasound examination, performed to investigate an abdominal mass, demonstrated an anechoic mass adjacent to bone. Diagnosis of duplication can be made directly by barium study when the communication is wide enough to permit entry of barium into the duplicated segment (Fig. 14-9).[27] Otherwise barium studies will often demonstrate an extrinsic mass deforming the mesenteric border of the small bowel occasionally causing obstruction by its mass effect or by intussusception (Fig. 14-10). These findings have been shown by computed tomography (CT),[28] which will demonstrate the absence of calcification, a differential diagnostic feature against a teratoma.[29]

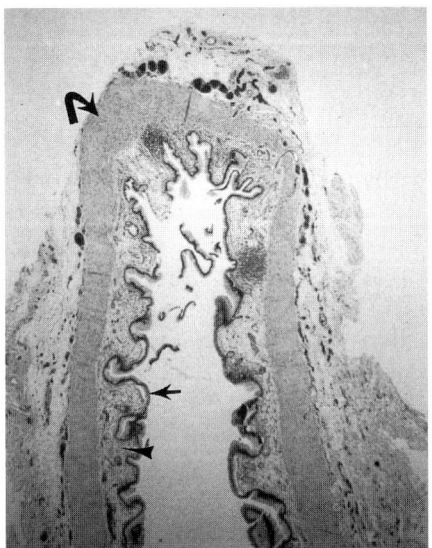

Fig. 14-7. Photomicrograph of duplication cyst. All three layers of a bowel wall are identified in this cyst (mucosa [arrow], submucosa [arrowhead], and the muscularis [curved arrow]).

Midgut Duplications • 231

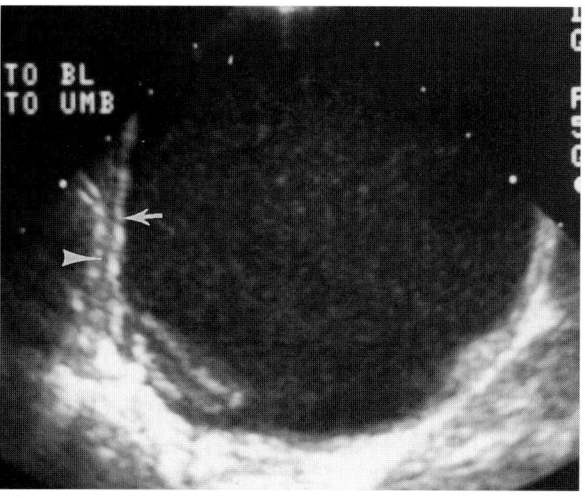 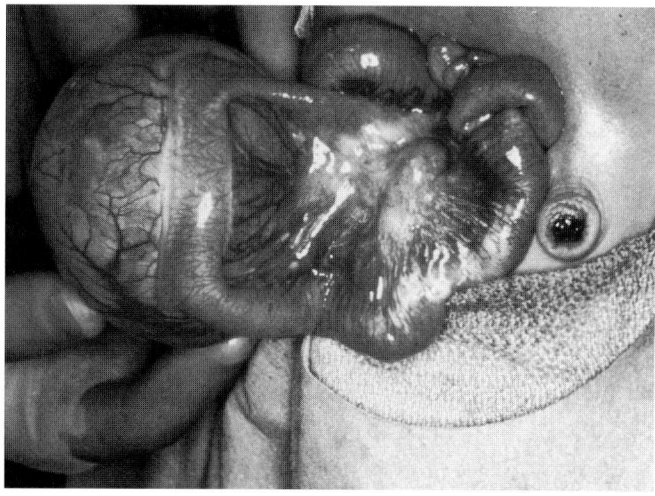

(a) (b)

Fig. 14-8. Cystic ileal duplication.
(a) Ultrasound examination of a patient with a palpable mass in the right lower quadrant demonstrates a large hypoechoic mass that contains multiple internal echoes. The mucosa (arrow) and a band of smooth muscle (arrowhead) are well demonstrated. The echogenic debris centrally is most likely mucus. The increased through transmission is typical of these cystic masses. (b) At surgery, this large duplication cyst was found at the mesenteric aspect of the bowel. There was no significant obstruction.

Technetium-99m scintigraphy is used for the detection of ectopic gastric mucosa, with an 86% sensitivity and a low false-positive rate.[30] The value of radionuclide scintigraphy in the detection of gastric mucosa within duplication has been reported.[31,32] They resemble a Meckel's diverticulum with ectopic gastric mu-

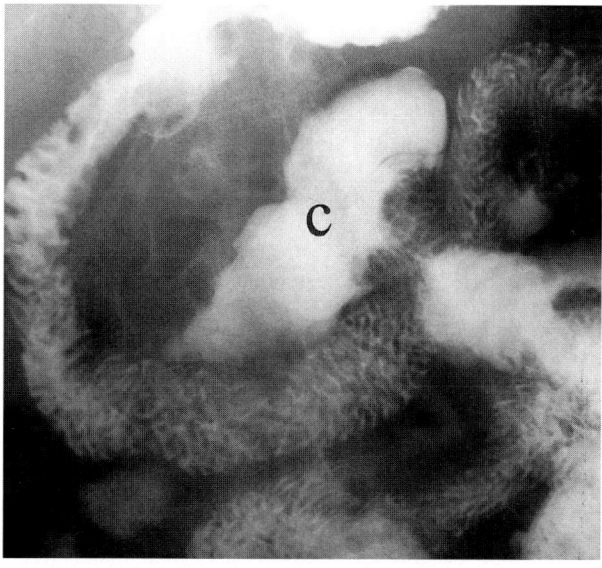

Fig. 14-9. Communicating midgut duplication.
Barium has entered a tubular structure (c) at duodenojejunal segment.

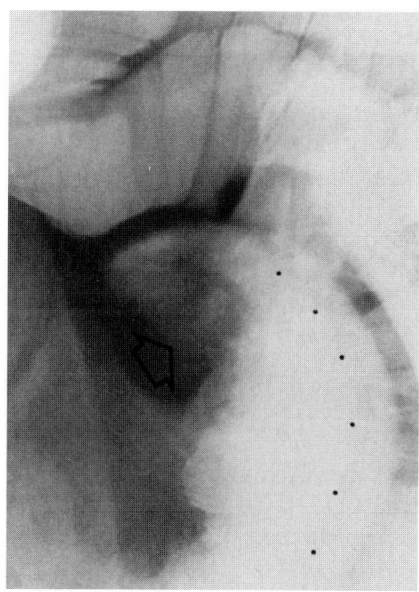

Fig. 14-10. Enteroclysis radiograph of a noncommunicating intestinal duplication in a young man presenting as a mass.
A fixed filling defect involving two superimposed limbs of ileum (dots) with thickened folds in apposition to the mass (open arrow). At surgery, the mass was an inflamed cyst.

cosa. Ectopic gastric mucosa within the duplication may secrete acid and pepsin, causing ulceration or perforation of the duplication or the adjacent normal mucosa.

Omphalomesenteric Duct Anomalies

Types and Development

Failure of obliteration of the omphalomesenteric duct may result in an omphalomesenteric fistula, an enterocyst, a fibrous band connecting the small intestines to the umbilicus, or a Meckel's diverticulum.[33,34] All reported omphalomesenteric duct anomalies can be summarized as follows:

1. Meckel's diverticulum.
2. Persistent fibrous cord.
3. Mesodiverticular vascular band.
4. Umbilical fecal fistula.
5. Umbilical sinus.
6. Umbilical polyp.
7. Omphalomesenteric duct cyst.

In approximately 95% of individuals, the omphalomesenteric duct becomes obliterated in its entire extent by the 7th or 8th week of fetal life. A local portion of the duct remains open at its junction with the ileum in 1% to 3% of the population. This remnant is referred to as a Meckel's diverticulum.[33] It is the most common congenital anomaly of the gastrointestinal tract. The rest of the vitelline duct may disappear completely or transform into a fibrous cord, attaching the blind end of Meckel's diverticulum to the umbilicus. The vestige of the vitelline duct may persist as a solid cord between an ileal loop and the umbilical region of the anterior abdominal wall. On rare instances, there might be a complete failure in the closure of vitelline ducts, resulting in an umbilico-intestinal fistula (Fig. 14-11). This congenital fistula provides a pathway for discharge of intestinal contents and may even be wide enough to permit prolapse of an ileal loop to be visible as a sausagelike umbilical mass.[33,35] The omphalomesenteric duct may occasionally remain patent in its distal segment and produce an umbilical sinus. In such instances, the more proximal portion of the duct often persists as a fibrous cord attached to the ileum. Another related anomaly is the vitelline cyst. This occurs when the omphalomesenteric duct is obliterated at both ends, while the intermediate or central portion of it has retained a patent lumen. This segment may gradually enlarge to form an intraabdominal lesion known as enterocystocele. It can be located within the anterior abdominal wall and present as an umbilical cyst.

Meckel's Diverticulum

This accounts for 90% of all omphalomesenteric duct anomalies. Meckel's diverticulum is a true diverticulum and contains all layers of the intestinal wall. There are different types of Meckels, which account for their variable appearance on contrast examination (Fig. 14-12). The diverticulum receives its blood supply through a remnant of the vitelline artery originating directly from the SMA or from an ileal branch close to its origin from the SMA (Fig. 14-13). The position of the diverticulum is highly variable. Although it has been reported as far proximal as the ligament of Treitz,[36] it is usually found within 100 cm of the ileocecal valve on the antimesenteric aspect of the ileum.[35,37] Because of lengthening of the intestines during growth, diverticula are located at a greater distance from the ileocecal valve in adults than in children. The mean distance from the diverticulum to the ileocecal valve in a large study group was 34 cm in children <2 years old, and 67 cm in adults.[37] The average diverticulum is about 3 cm long,[35,38] nearly 90% are 1 to 10 cm long, but record lengths of up to 100 cm have been reported.[35,39] Approximately 50% contain heterotopic mucosa, 16% pancreatic acinar tissue, and the remainder Brunner's glands, pancreatic islets, colonic mucosa, hepatobiliary tissue, or a combination of tissues.[37] An increased incidence of Meckel's diverticulum is seen in cases with other congenital anomalies such as cleft palate, bicornuate uterus, and annular pancreas.[40,41] An association between Meckel's diver-

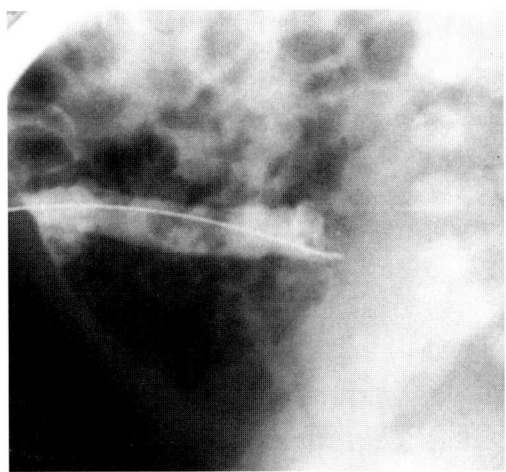

Fig. 14-11. Everted mucocele of the umbilicus (omphalomesenteric duct remnant).
The lateral radiograph obtained following injection of water-soluble contrast through an umbilical catheter demonstrates filling of a loop of bowel. The catheter was inserted through the cord attachment into the ileum.

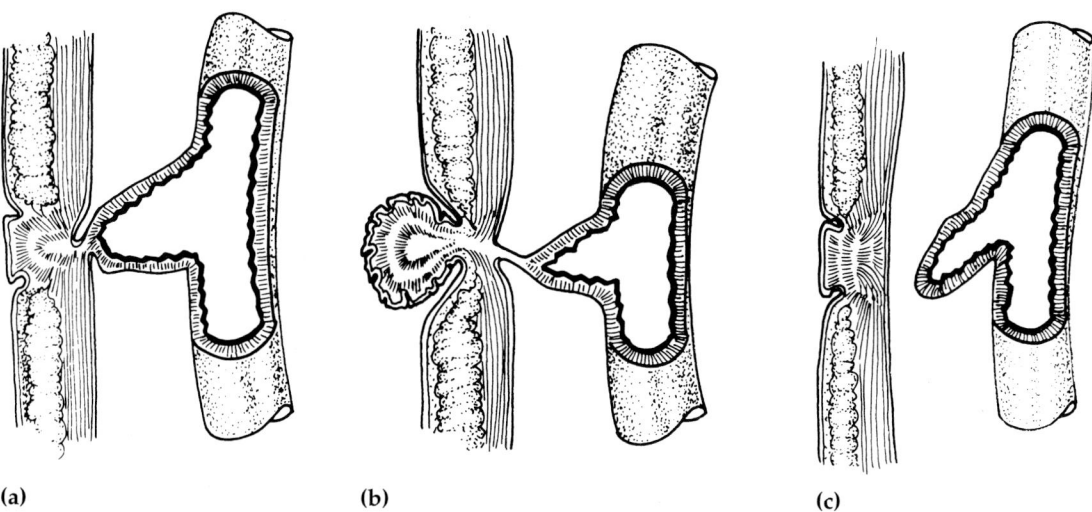

Fig. 14-12. Types of Meckel's diverticulum.
(a, b) In approximately 25% of cases, the diverticulum is attached to the umbilicus or to another portion of the abdominal wall by a fibrous cord of varying length. (c) In the remainder of the cases, the diverticulum is free.

ticulum and inflammatory bowel disease has been raised. Two operative series found 6% to 18% prevalence of Meckel's diverticulum in patients with Crohn's disease, compared with autopsy prevalence rates of 1% to 3%.[42,43] A recent review indicates that Meckel's diverticulum is incidental in most such cases.[44] Separation of distal ileal loops by the inflammatory process of Crohn's disease renders the diverticulum more readily identified by radiology (Fig. 14-14). The importance to the radiologist who may be confronted with this possible association is to study more carefully the state of the Crohn's disease, which is the likely cause of the patient's symptomatology.[44]

Clinical Considerations

The incidental finding of a Meckel's diverticulum at laparotomy and the 1% to 3% of incidence in the general population are evidence for the usual asympto-

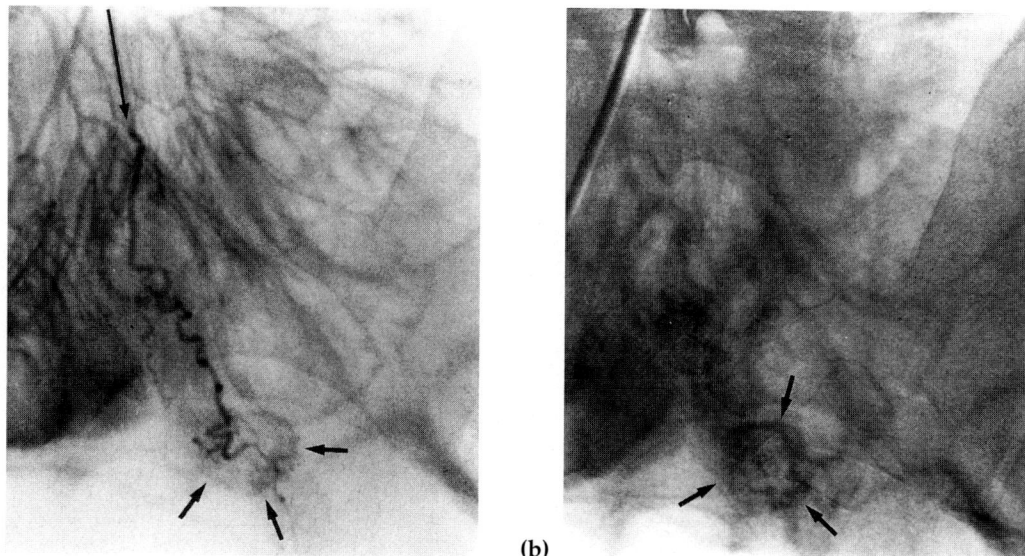

Fig. 14-13. Superior mesenteric angiogram of a Meckel's diverticulum.
(a) Vitelline artery (arrow) branches out over the diverticulum (arrows). (b) Later phase shows mural opacification (arrows) and start of returning veins.

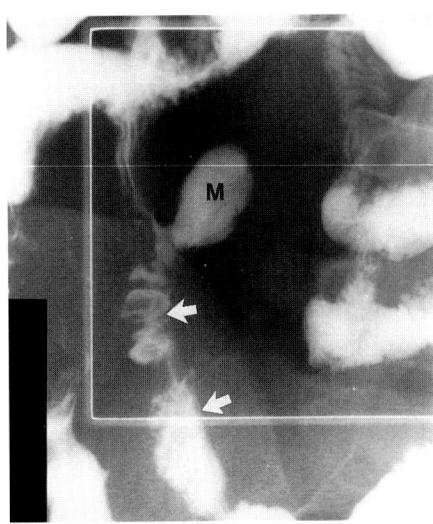

Fig. 14-14. Simple visualization of a Meckel's diverticulum (M) arising within the increased space around a segment of ileal Crohn's disease (arrows).

matic nature of a Meckel's diverticulum. Meckel originally quoted a 25% complication rate,[5] but a survey by Soltero and Bill has identified a total lifetime complication rate of 4%, which decreases to near zero with old age.[45] However, in view of the pattern of this survey, the result is likely to be an underestimate. Over 40% of those experiencing complications are under 10 years old.[37] Although this anomaly occurs with equal frequency in both sexes, males have a 3:1 incidence of complications.[35] When a symptomatic lesion does occur, it is difficult to diagnose because its signs and symptoms resemble those of more common disorders. The high mortality rate of 6% to 7% for Meckel's diverticulum–related complications is probably due to delay in diagnosis.[34] The symptomatic complications of Meckel's diverticulum fall into three major categories: bleeding, obstruction, and inflammation.

Although *bleeding* is the most common presentation in children,[45] there are numerous reports of adults presenting with bleeding from Meckel's diverticula.[46–52] Ninety percent of bleeding diverticula contain heterotopic mucosa.[53] Significant acid peptic secretion may be responsible for the bleeding by causing ulceration of the unprotected adjacent mucosa. More commonly, bleeding is due to peptic ulceration within the ectopic gastric mucosa and was the most frequent clinical manifestation of a Meckel's diverticulum in one adult series.[46,51] Adults are more likely to present with melena and children with hematochezia.[38] Slower colonic transit in the adult population or alternatively a less severe hemorrhage may account for this difference. Abdominal pain of varying severity often accompanies the bleeding.

Several reports have shown *obstruction* to be the most common presentation in the adult[35,37,45,54] and to have exceeded bleeding by more than three to one.[37] Obstruction may be caused by entanglement of the small bowel around a fibrous cord, by entrapment of an ileal loop within a mesodiverticular band, by intussusception, volvulus, incarceration within a hernia sac, or chronic diverticulitis. Symptomatic intussusception may develop when an invaginated diverticulum serves as the lead point (Fig. 14-15). However, inversion of the diverticulum may occur without symptoms.[55] Only anatomically free diverticula can invaginate. Volvulus can occur when a persistent fibrous band relates to the shape and degree of fixation of the diverticular tip.[45] Fixation of the tip may also allow torsion of the diverticulum around its own axis.[34] Occasionally, Meckel's diverticula prolapse into an inguinal, or less commonly, femoral or umbilical hernia and may become strangulated.[56] This has been called a hernia of Littré after the author who reported three cases nearly 300 years ago.[57] Chronic Meckel's diverticulitis can cause obstruction when the inflammation extends to the adjacent small intestine, producing adhesive narrowing. The various mechanisms of obstruction secondary to omphalomesenteric duct anomalies can be summarized as follows:[58]

1. Volvulus around a vitelline duct remnant.
2. Fibrous band remnant with closed-loop obstruction.
3. Intussusception.
4. Cicatricial narrowing of the small bowel secondary to ulceration.
5. Inflammation of the diverticulum with resulting obstruction.
6. Prolapse of intestine through an umbilical fistula.
7. Incarceration of the diverticulum in hernia (Littré).

The third most common clinical presentation relates to an *inflammatory process* such as diverticulitis, peptic ulceration of ileal mucosa, or rarely a foreign body with the diverticular lumen.[34] Obstruction of the diverticular opening with subsequent bacterial infection can occur in a fashion analogous to appendicitis, the most common preoperative diagnosis in patients presenting with Meckel's diverticulitis.[38] Peptic ulceration may cause tissue necrosis with diverticulitis or even perforation with peritonitis. In about 15% of cases, the inflammation and perforation may relate to the presence of a foreign body in the diverticulum. Fish bones, gallstones, marbles, bullets, and pennies have been shown to have lodged in a Meckel's diverticulum.[39,59]

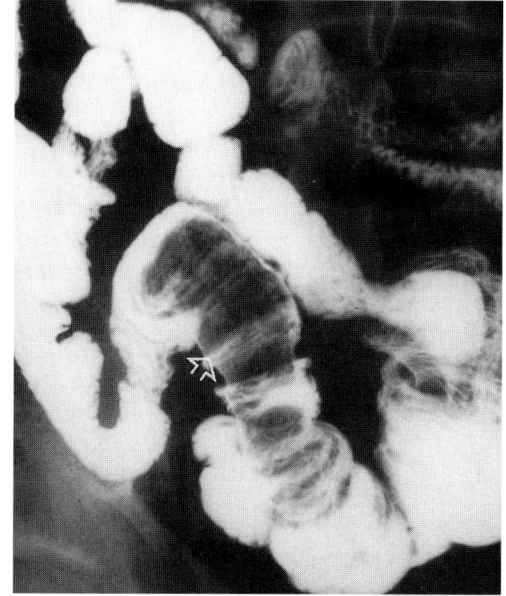
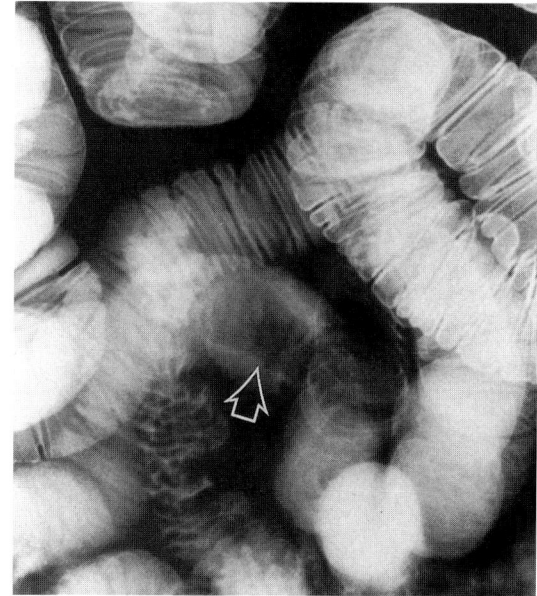
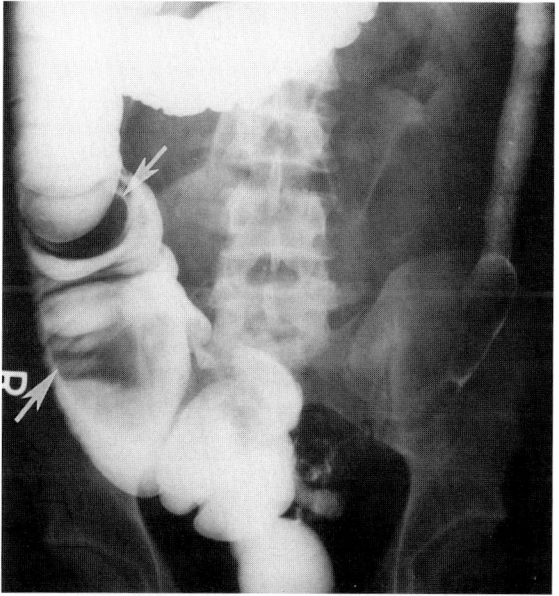

Fig. 14-15. Intussusception of a Meckel's diverticulum. (a) Diagnosis by small bowel follow-through. A long intraluminal filling defect (arrow) in distal ileum of a patient who presented with gastrointestinal bleeding and abdominal pain, probably caused by recurring intussusception. At laparotomy, the inverted diverticulum was found to contain ulcerated ectopic gastric mucosa. (Courtesy of L. De Gaeta, MD.) (b) Diagnosis by enteroclysis. Invaginated Meckel's diverticulum (arrow) in a male patient 66 years of age with lower gastrointestinal bleeding. At laparotomy, ulceration and ectopic gastric mucosa were revealed. (c) A barium enema performed in a young man with obstructive symptoms demonstrates an intussusception into the cecum and proximal ascending colon (arrows). At surgery, this was found to be an intussuscepted ileal Meckel's diverticulum.

Tumors occasionally develop in Meckel's diverticula. A recent review of neoplasms in Meckel's diverticulum found that of a total of 209 cases reported through 1985, 33% were carcinoid tumors, 27% sarcomas, 23% benign mesenchymal tumors, 12% adenocarcinomas, and the remainder miscellaneous lesions.[60] Although carcinoid is the most common neoplasm found in a Meckel's diverticulum, these lesions represent only 2% of all small intestinal carcinoids.[61]

The clinical diagnosis of a symptomatic Meckel's diverticulum may be difficult, especially in the adult, because symptoms resemble those of more common abdominal disorders. Even when the clinical index of suspicion is high, the preoperative diagnosis can be difficult.

Radiology

The spectrum of radiologic findings of Meckel's diverticulum has been reviewed by Ghahremani.[62] Plain abdominal radiographs are generally of no value, although occasionally a large diverticulum may contain sufficient gas to indicate its lumen.[63] This diverticulum is visualized as a well-demarcated round- or oval-shaped lucency in the subumbilical region or the right lower abdomen or pelvis. There is usually very little

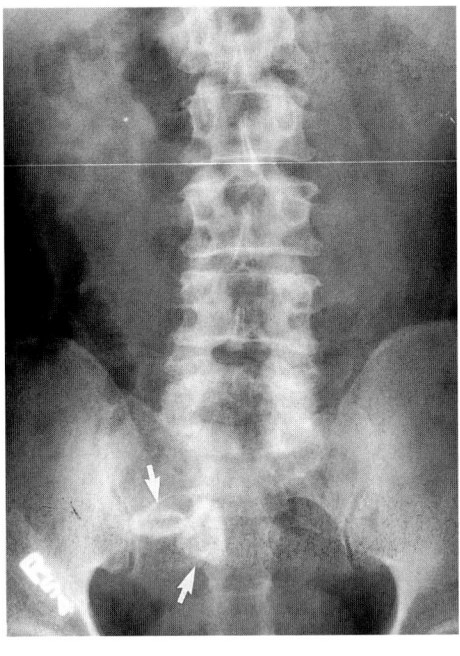
(a)

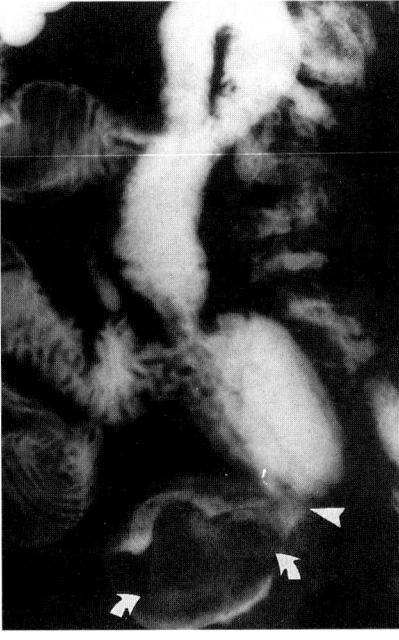
(b)

Fig. 14-16. Enteroliths shown to be situated in a Meckel's diverticulum.
(a) Faceted calculi (arrows) in the right lower abdomen of a patient with recurrent abdominal pain. (b) Barium study (oblique compression radiograph) differentiates stones in the Meckel's diverticulum (arrows) from colonic enteroliths, appendicoliths, gallstones, or stones in a bladder diverticulum. Arrowhead points to neck of diverticulum; barium has entered into the diverticulum.

change in the configuration and location between serial radiographs. This has been observed in Meckel's diverticulitis, where the retention of gas reflects the loss of contractility of the diverticulum due to edema and thickening of its walls [See Fig. 14-19(a)]. Evidence for coexistent small bowel obstruction is often present. The intradiverticular gas collection has permitted visualization of rugal folds covering the inner surface of a Meckel's diverticulum in some reports.[62] The most useful, although uncommon, plain film finding is demonstration of a single or multiple radiopaque enteroliths in a Meckel's diverticulum. A limited degree of mobility of the calculi with change in the position of the patient suggests their confinement within a well-defined structure (Fig. 14-16). Approximately one third of enteroliths are sufficiently opaque to be visible on plain radiography (see Chapter 5). Their formation relates to stasis and alkalinity of the intestinal contents. Of interest may be the observation that Meckel's diverticula containing stones are without ectopic mucosa, suggesting that enteroliths do not form in the presence of secreting tissue.[64] Calculi are faceted, single or multiple, composed primarily of calcium carbonate and calcium oxalate with an admixture of nonopaque elements. Some patients have presented with radiographic features of small bowel obstruction associated with a cluster of enteroliths.[63,65–67]

An extremely rare complication of enteroliths forming in a Meckel's diverticulum is a Meckel's stone ileus. This complication results from the extrusion of the enterolith with secondary mechanical small bowel obstruction.[68,69] There is a strong male predominance. The diagnosis should be entertained in an elderly male with obstruction from an opaque stone in the absence of a history of gallstones or of air in the biliary tract (Fig. 14-17).

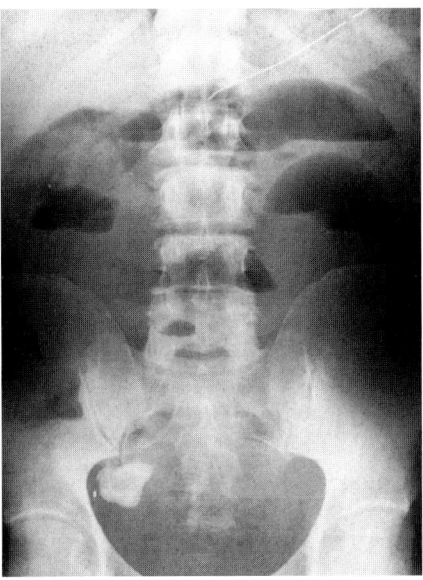

Fig. 14-17. Meckel's stone ileus.
An upright abdominal radiograph demonstrates a pattern typical of mechanical small bowel obstruction in an elderly patient without a history of gallstones. Note configuration of large dense calcification in right hemipelvis at site of distal small bowel obstruction. (Courtesy of Ed Stewart, MD.)

The "conventional" overhead-film-based barium follow-through study may demonstrate a Meckel's diverticulum when excessive mesenteric fat separates loops of small bowel (Fig. 14-18). More often the diverticulum is not demonstrated by this technique. The diverticulum may fail to fill with barium, either due to stenosis of its neck, presence of intestinal material, or contraction of its muscularis with expulsion of contents. Even if filled with barium, the diverticulum is more often obscured by overlying opacified bowel loops.[63,70,71] The "fluoroscopic" small bowel follow-through may improve the demonstration of a Meckel's diverticulum mainly because of fluoroscopic compression to separate bowel loops.[71] The yield of barium examinations for the diagnosis of Meckel's diverticulum has been significantly improved by the enteroclysis technique.[46,47,49,72] Maglinte et al[46] performed enteroclysis in 415 patients and preoperatively diagnosed Meckel's diverticula in 11 symptomatic patients. All but 1 presented with unexplained chronic blood loss (Fig. 14-19). Salomonowitz et al[47] found 7 Meckel's diverticula among 400 patients examined by enteroclysis. The detection rate of 1.75% in this study and 2.65% in the series by Maglinte et al approximates the autopsy incidence of this congenital anomaly. Intermittent, short-interval fluoroscopy during enteroclysis allows careful evaluation of individual segments at time of optimal filling and distention of the diverticulum (Fig. 14-20). The variable position of the diverticulum due to its mobile tip is minimized by the distention at enteroclysis. Although a Meckel's diverticulum is frequently asymptomatic, once identified, its walls should be carefully scrutinized. An abnormal outline of the diverticulum, an irregularity, distortion, or edema of a segment are good indicators of the presence of ectopic tissue, usually gastric mucosa (Fig. 14-21).[46]

The radiologic features by barium examination reflect the morphology of the anomaly, ie, a blind sac attached to the antimesenteric border of the distal small bowel. The identification of the sac as a Meckel's diverticulum rests on the demonstration of the *junctional fold pattern* at its base, the site of exit of the omphalomesenteric duct.[46] With the ileum and diverticulum distended, the junctional fold pattern appears as a mucosal triangular plateau [Fig. 14-20(d)]. When loops are partially collapsed, the mucosal fold junction takes on a triradiate pattern [Fig. 14-21(c)]. Either appearance of the junctional fold pattern mandates a diagnosis of Meckel's diverticulum, as this feature has not been seen in any other small bowel abnormality. A herniated Meckel (Littré's hernia) should also be identified by the demonstration of the junctional fold pattern.

Demonstration of a saccular outpouching or of an abnormal collection of barium in this area of the small

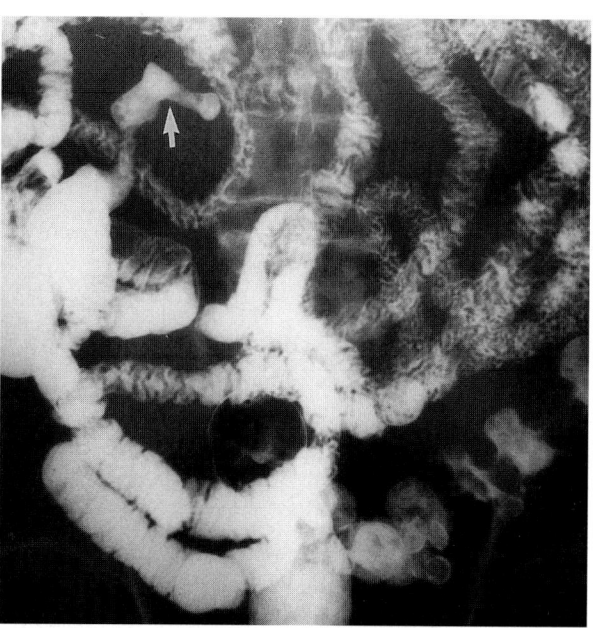

Fig. 14-18. Small bowel follow-through demonstration of Meckel's diverticulum.
Prone overhead radiograph of conventional examination in an obese male patient demonstrates a Meckel's diverticulum (arrow) in distal small bowel. Separation of bowel loops by increased amount of fat in the mesentery allowed follow-through diagnosis. (Courtesy of Richard Stephens, MD.)

bowel should lead to a search for the junctional fold pattern. In some instances, however, this may be difficult to display. Too much barium in the diverticulum or too dense a barium mixture may obscure the fold pattern. Adequate compression during infusion or the double-contrast phase of enteroclysis will avert this problem. A common pitfall in the diagnosis of a Meckel's diverticulum by contrast examination is shown in Fig. 14-22.

There have been few recent reports on the use of CT and ultrasound in the diagnosis of a Meckel's diverticulum and of some of its complications—especially invagination.[73-76] On CT, the diverticulum appears as a well-demarcated cyst or sausagelike structure attached to the distal small bowel. The fibrous remnant of the vitelline duct may be visible as a soft-tissue density between the diverticulum and the umbilicus. CT has had problems with inverted diverticula that were mistaken for a lipoma until ultrasound could demonstrate peristalsis.[74] It is possible to identify the soft-tissue wall of the diverticulum to distinguish the lesion from a purely fatty structure.[75] Of interest is the CT report of a strictly vegetarian patient with a Meckel containing a phytobezoar that was expelled into the ileal lumen to cause bowel obstruction.[76]

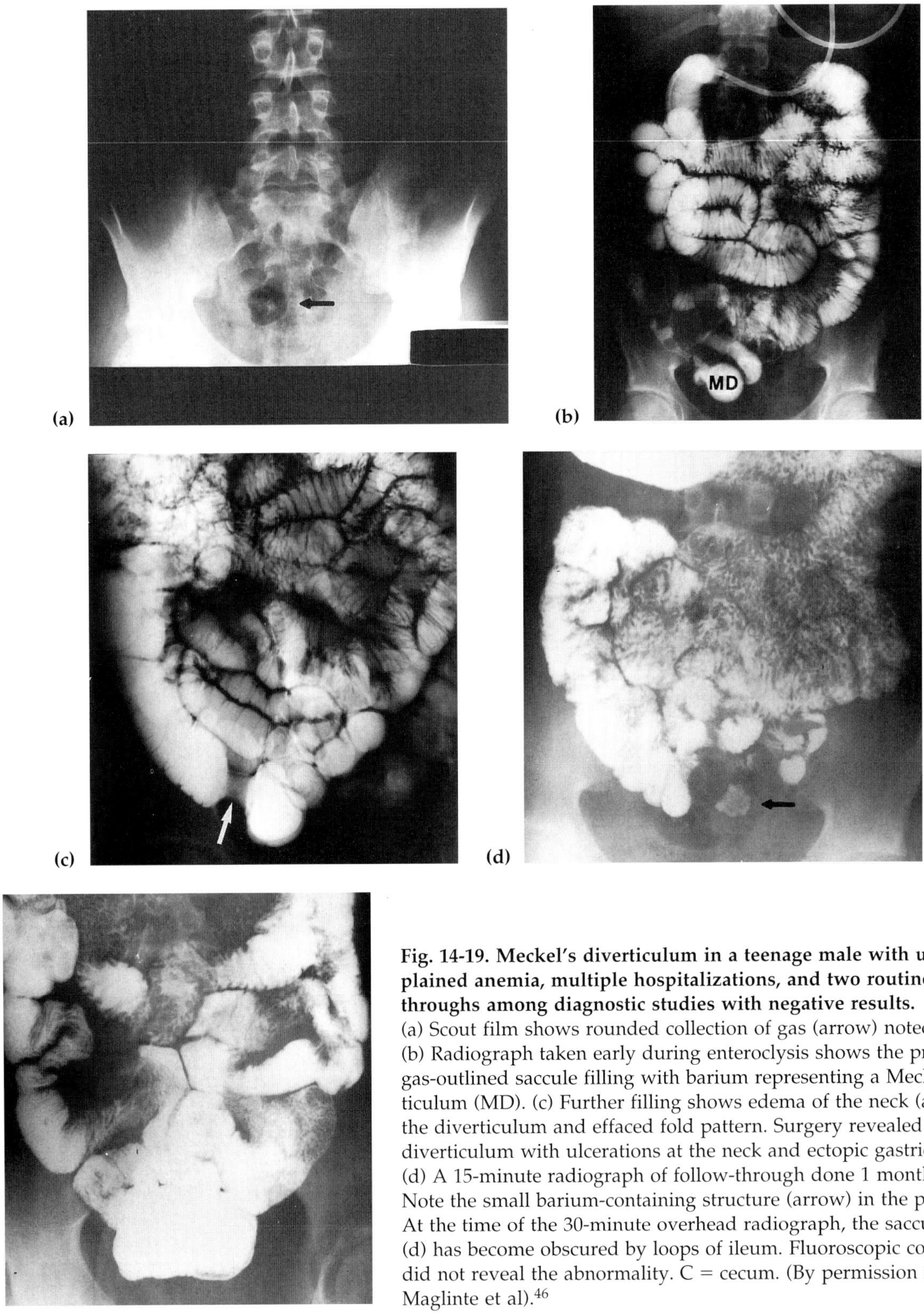

238 • 14. Congenital and Developmental Anomalies of the Small Bowel in Adolescents and Adults

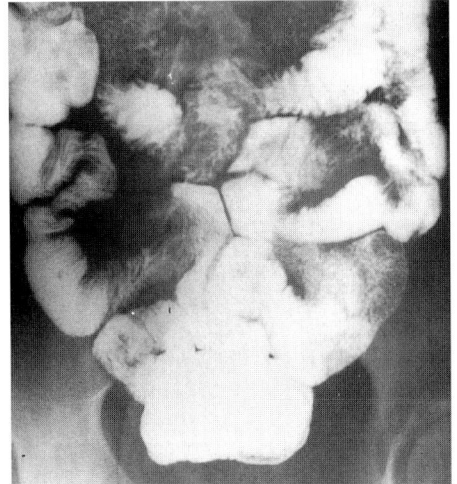

Fig. 14-19. Meckel's diverticulum in a teenage male with unexplained anemia, multiple hospitalizations, and two routine follow-throughs among diagnostic studies with negative results.
(a) Scout film shows rounded collection of gas (arrow) noted in pelvis. (b) Radiograph taken early during enteroclysis shows the previous gas-outlined saccule filling with barium representing a Meckel's diverticulum (MD). (c) Further filling shows edema of the neck (arrow) of the diverticulum and effaced fold pattern. Surgery revealed Meckel's diverticulum with ulcerations at the neck and ectopic gastric mucosa. (d) A 15-minute radiograph of follow-through done 1 month earlier. Note the small barium-containing structure (arrow) in the pelvis. (e) At the time of the 30-minute overhead radiograph, the saccule seen in (d) has become obscured by loops of ileum. Fluoroscopic compression did not reveal the abnormality. C = cecum. (By permission from Maglinte et al).[46]

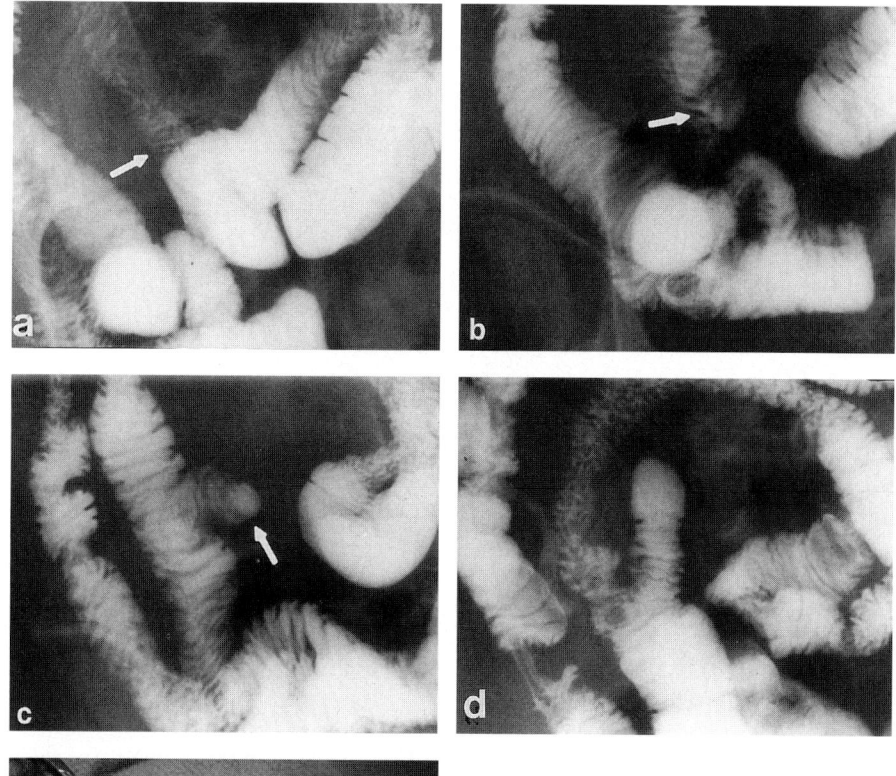
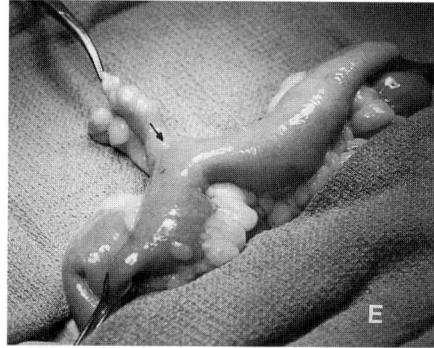

Fig. 14-20. Technique considerations for identification of a Meckel's diverticulum.
(a) Initial compression spot film during enteroclysis shows no abnormality. The site of the Meckel's diverticulum (arrow) is not apparent. (b, c) Further compression during barium infusion shows a small sac (arrow) starting to fill and distend. (d) With further filling, the Meckel's diverticulum becomes obvious. Arrowhead points to the "mucosal triangular plateau" (the junctional fold pattern). (e) Surgical specimen. Junction (arrow) of diverticulum with ileum. (By permission from Maglinte et al.[46])

CT may be able to differentiate an intussuscepting Meckel's diverticulum from an intussuscepting lipoma.[76,77] A Meckel's diverticulum will show the diverticulum surrounded by a thick collar of soft tissue, corresponding to the wall of the inverted diverticulum. Sonography has shown the Meckel as a saccular structure containing fluid and some echogenic material.[62,78]

The clinical and radiologic diagnosis of a symptomatic Meckel's diverticulum continues to be a challenge. It is possible that magnetic resonance imaging may, in time, make a significant contribution to the diagnosis of Meckel's diverticulum and its complications. In children, radionuclide scanning has been shown to be practical and reliable. In adolescents and adults, a detailed barium examination, particularly enteroclysis, appears to be the most reliable technique at the present time.[72]

Treatment and Management of Incidental Meckel's Diverticulum

The standard treatment of symptomatic diverticula remains surgical resection.[78] A laparoscopic approach to Meckel's diverticulectomy has been reported.[79] Many diverticula, however, are found incidentally at laparotomy or during radiographic studies performed for unrelated indications. Most current recommendations are that the removal of incidentally discovered Meckel's diverticula in adults is probably not justifiable unless there are risk factors present, such as 1) a past history of unexplained abdominal pain or lower gastrointestinal bleeding, 2) a narrow diverticular neck, which would predispose to diverticulitis and obstruction, 3) a palpable mass within the diverticulum, which suggests ectopic tissue or tumor, or 4) a fibrous band tethering the diverticulum to the umbili-

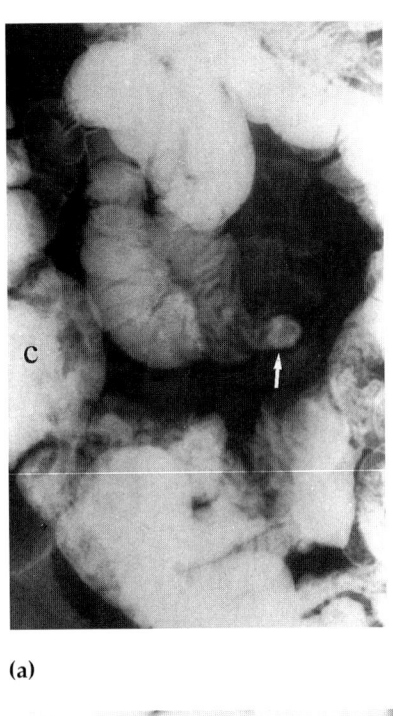
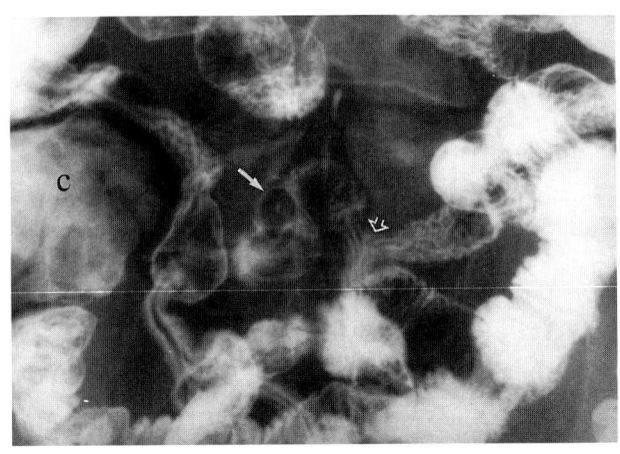
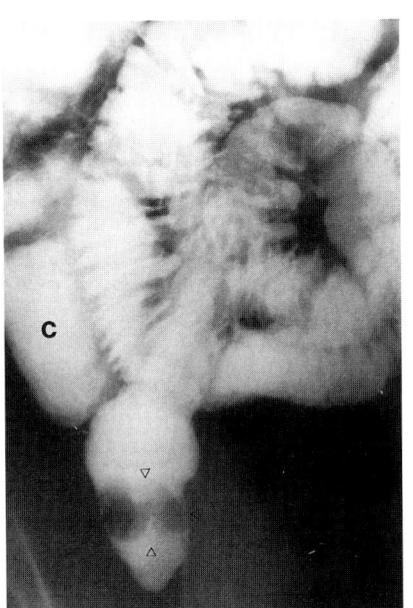
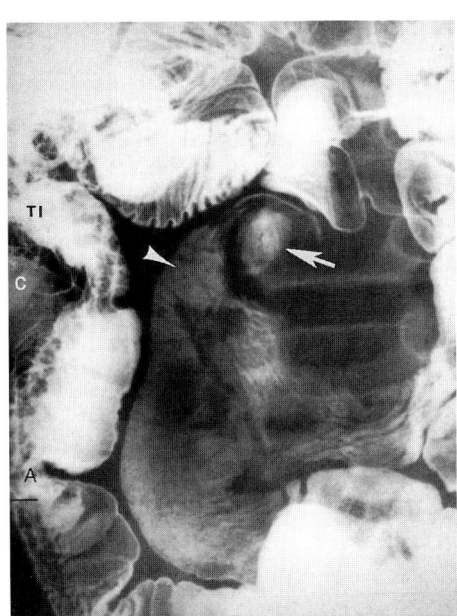
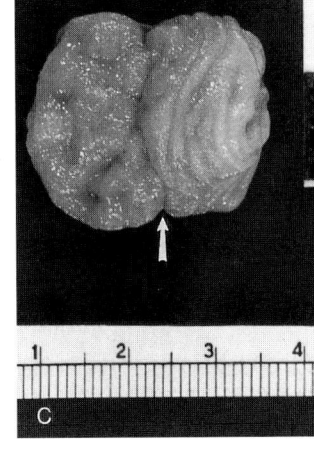

Fig. 14-21. Findings on barium examination that suggest ectopic mucosa in a Meckel's diverticulum.
(a) Small distorted antimesenteric diverticulum (arrow) without appreciable fold pattern in mid ileum in an elderly male with unexplained bleeding. (C = cecum.) At surgery ulcerated ectopic mucosa was found in the diverticulum. (b, c) A small umbilicated defect (arrow) and a large lobulated polypoid defect (between open arrowheads) in two different patients with surgically confirmed Meckel's diverticula containing ectopic tissue. Note triradiate junctional fold pattern (open arrow). (C = cecum.) (d) Barium collection (arrow) inside incompletely filled Meckel's diverticulum in an 8-year-old boy with anemia. Arrowhead points to junction of diverticulum with ileum. (C = cecum; TI = terminal ileum.) (e) Surgical specimen shows distorted diverticulum (arrows) and defect (arrowhead) in fundus representing ectopic gastric mucosa. (f) Diverticulum opened longitudinally with gastric mucosa on left and small bowel mucosa on right.

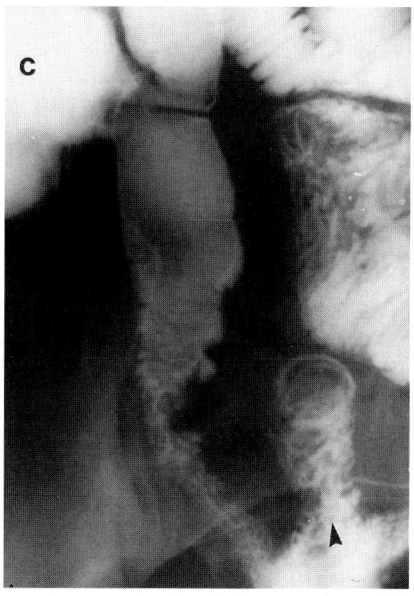
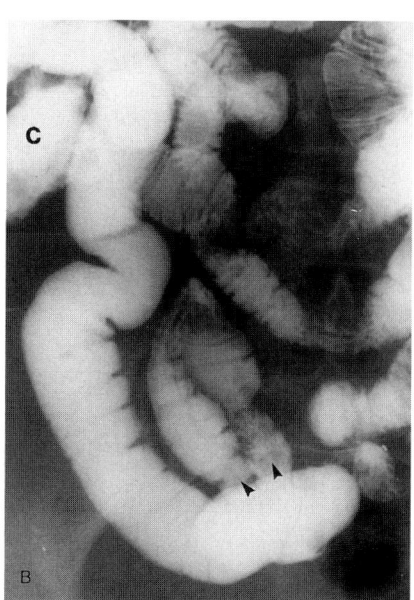

Fig. 14-22. Pitfall in the diagnosis of Meckel's diverticulum by barium examination.
(a) Pseudojunctional segment (arrowhead) produced by superimposition of two intestinal loops. (b) With the patient in oblique position, compression radiograph shows two superimposed loops (arrowheads). Their conjoined course inferiorly has produced a pseudotriangular plateau. A pseudosaccule can be produced by the axial projection of a loop of bowel especially when fixed by adhesions. Proper positioning will clarify this finding.

(a) (b)

cus, thus predisposing to volvulus and obstruction.[80] However, in the case of children, because of their higher incidence of complications some pediatric surgeons continue to advocate removal of incidental Meckel's diverticula.[34]

Anomalies of Intestinal Rotation

"Malrotation," actually a misnomer, encompasses nonrotation, incomplete rotation, hyperrotation and anomalies of fixation. Anomalies of midgut rotation account for 1% of all intestinal obstructions seen in neonates and children; its incidence in adults is much less.[81] Most symptomatic midgut malrotations are found in the neonatal period and present with high intestinal obstruction due either to adhesive bands extending from the duodenum to the cecum (Ladd's bands) or to midgut volvulus.[82] Many individuals remain asymptomatic and the condition is discovered incidentally during imaging studies or at autopsy. Others have recurrent, chronic vague or acute abdominal pain frequently mistaken clinically for more common clinical conditions (functional illness, adhesions, chronic pancreatitis, appendicitis, or Crohn's disease). Occasionally older children may present with a spruelike malabsorption syndrome related to chronic, intermittent volvulus. Resultant lymphatic and venous obstruction leads to protein loss. Most symptomatic adult patients have many features in common.[1] The most frequent presentation of intestinal obstruction is midgut volvulus. Less frequently, duodenal obstruction due to peritoneal bands or to internal hernias is seen. Symptoms in the adult usually goes back to childhood. In a few adult patients, however, acute episodes may occur without the history of intestine related problems.

Specific anomalies occur with each stage of rotation:

Stage 1

During the first stage, failure of the abdominal contents to return to the coelomic cavity leads to an *omphalocele*, a herniation into the umbilical cord. This can be diagnosed prenatally by ultrasound. It differs from an umbilical hernia in that the intestines are not covered by skin but by a thin peritoneal sac (Fig. 14-23).

Stage 2

It is during the second stage of rotation that most of the anomalies of development occur.[83] Stage 2 errors include nonrotation, incomplete rotation, hyperrotation, and reversed rotation. Gastroschisis, or herniation of the abdominal contents lateral to the umbilicus, occurs during stage 2.

If rotation stops at 90 degrees, this will result in *nonrotation* (Fig. 14-24). The small bowel is located on the right side of the abdomen; the colon on the left side. The ligament of Treitz (duodenojejunal flexure)

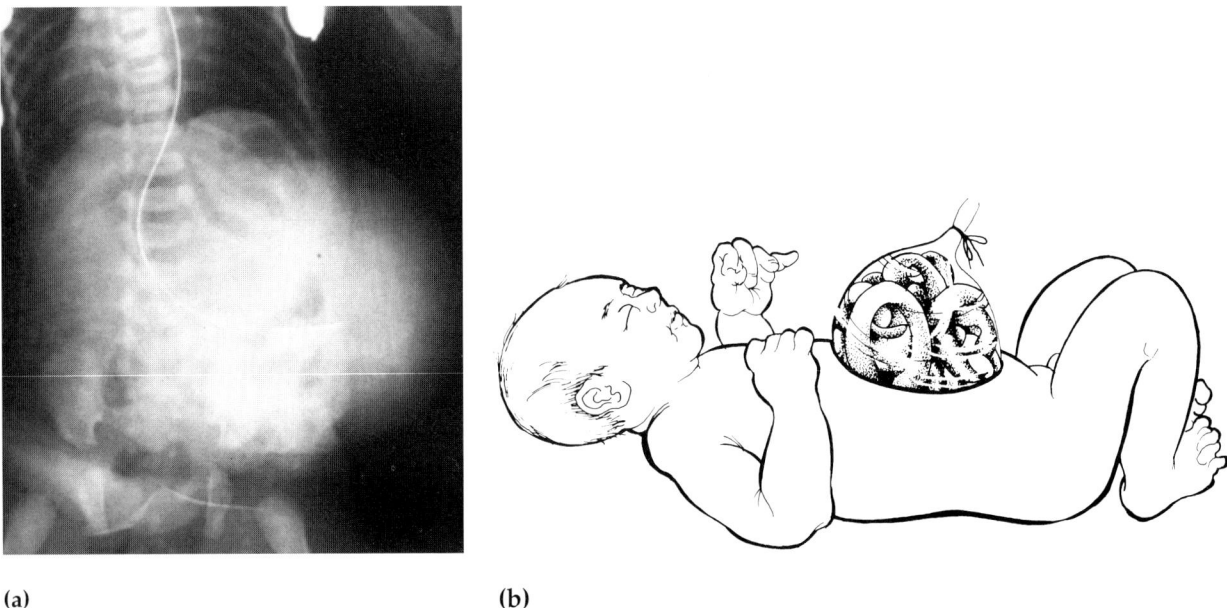

Fig. 14-23. Omphalocele.
(a) Anteroposterior view of abdomen in a newborn demonstrates a large omphacocele, which deviates toward the left. The nasogastric tube position denotes the position of the stomach within the central herniation. Incidentally noted is dextrocardia. (b) Diagram in lateral position to show that most or all of the intestine and, frequently, other abdominal organs are outside the body covered by a thin sac. Omphalocele differs from an umbilical hernia in that the intestines are not covered by skin.

is absent.[84] The terminal ileum joins the cecum by crossing the midline from the right. Although the gut may become fixed in these positions by abnormal peritoneal bands (Ladd's bands), fixation usually does not occur; hence a common mesentery exists with a narrow pedicle, prone to volvulus. If the rotation of the prearterial segment stops between 90 degrees and 180 degrees, the postarterial part may complete its full 270-degree rotation to result in *mixed rotation or malrotation*, the most common type of anomaly. The duo-

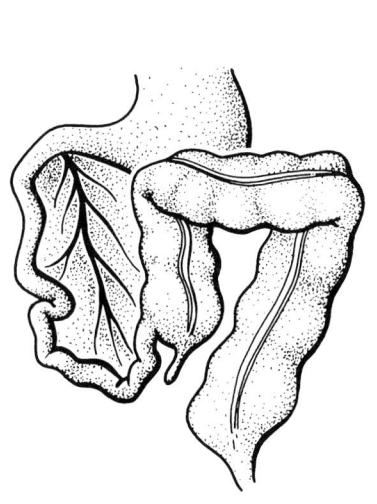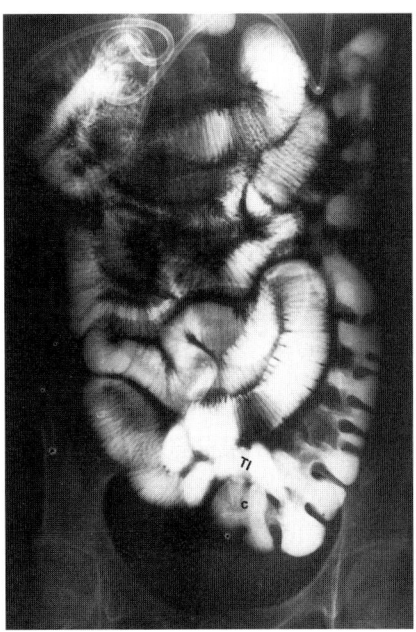

Fig. 14-24. Nonrotation.
(a) The postarterial segment has reentered the abdomen first instead of last. The ascending portion of the duodenum and the duodenojejunal flexure are absent. The jejunum appears as the direct continuation of the second portion of the duodenum and lies with the ileum in the right hemiabdomen. The terminal ileum terminates at the right side of the cecum which, with the entire colon, lies in the left hemiabdomen. (b) Enteroclysis radiograph shows the terminal ileum (TI) crossing midline to reach left-sided cecum (c).

denojejunal flexure is not in its normal position to the left of L2. The small bowel has a right, median, or partial left-sided position. Peritoneal bands may hold the cecum in an abnormal position and compress the duodenum, usually in its third segment (Fig. 14-25). In *reversed rotation*, the rarest abnormality, the postarterial segment returns to the abdomen first and a 180-degree clockwise rotation occurs (Fig. 14-26). The duodenum is on the right side of the abdomen and the transverse colon retroduodenal.[85] *Hyperrotation* is a continuation of rotation beyond the normal 270 degrees (Fig. 14-27). The colon is longer than normal and the cecum can reach the splenic flexure instead of remaining in the right lower quadrant.

Stage 3

Stage 3 anomalies consist of a mobile cecum, unattached duodenum, and/or unattached small bowel mesentery that can lead to cecal volvulus and internal hernias.[86] Cecal inversion results when there is premature fixation of the cecum in a subhepatic position (Fig. 14-28). Developmental anomalies are more frequent in males than females. A mobile cecum, however, occurs more often in females but males are more susceptible to the volvulus that may complicate it.

Radiology

In symptomatic adolescents or adults radiologic evaluation begins with plain abdominal radiography. The plain film findings of midgut volvulus include: 1) normal or abnormal intestinal pattern, 2) duodenal obstruction, 3) gastric distention with paucity of intraluminal gas distally, and 4) small bowel distention with air fluid levels. In the adult, additional imaging is frequently needed.

When an upper gastrointestinal barium study is performed for abdominal pain, the position of the duodenojejunal flexure should be ascertained. If this is not projected to the left of the left spinal pedicles and at least as cephalad as the duodenal bulb, the study

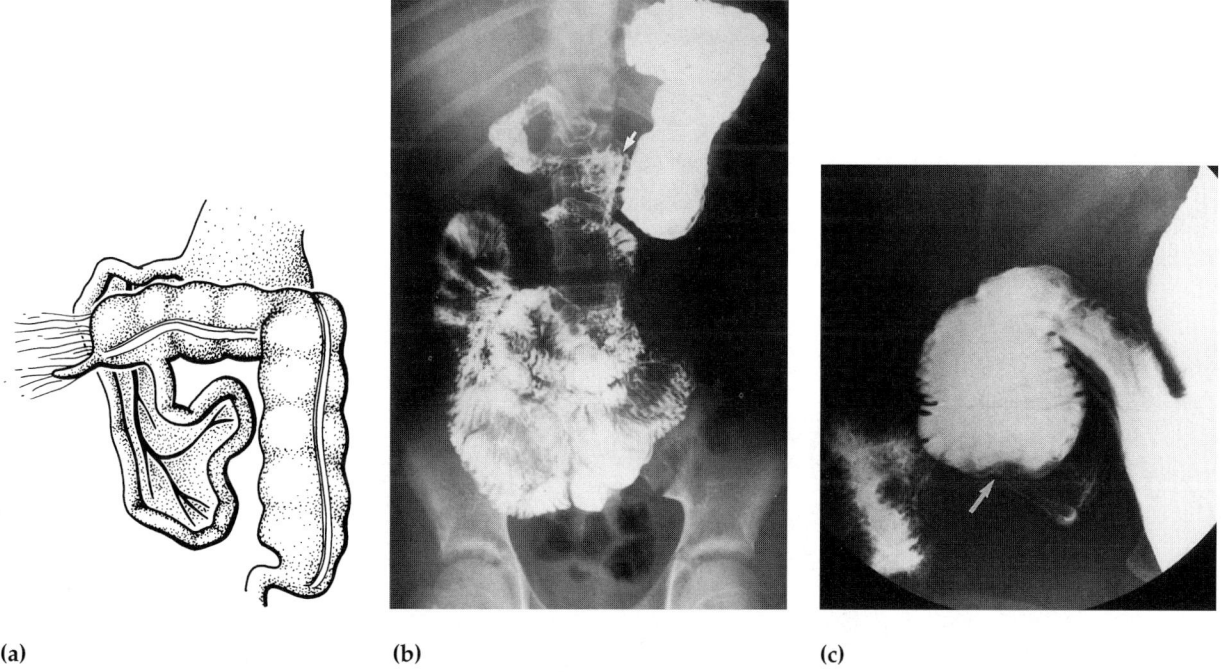

(a)   (b)   (c)

Fig. 14-25. Mixed rotation or malrotation, the most common anomaly during the second stage.
(a) During reentry, the midgut has failed to complete the entire arc of 180 degrees of counterclockwise rotation. The terminal ileum enters the abdomen first. The prearterial segment has failed to rotate. The cecum becomes fixed to the abdominal wall and usually lies anterior to the second portion of the duodenum. Mesenteric bands from the liver and posterolateral abdominal wall pass to the cecum (Ladd's bands) and compress the duodenum. Volvulus may be a complication. (b) The upper gastrointestinal follow-up film demonstrates multiple jejunal loops in the right midabdomen. The duodenojejunal junction (arrow) is below the level of the duodenal bulb and passes just to the left of the left L2 pedicle. The duodenum has a shortened appearance. (c) Cecal transduodenal bands (Ladd's bands). A transverse defect (arrow) is caused by the bands, obstructing the descending duodenum.

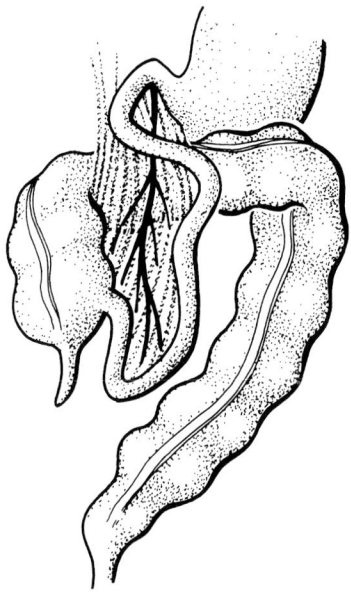

Fig. 14-26. Reversed rotation.
Usually the postarterial segment reenters the abdomen first, and the colon comes to lie behind the superior mesenteric artery. The small bowel is ventral to the artery and the colon. Periduodenal bands may be present and cause obstruction. (Adapted from Gray SW, Skandalakis JE. *Embryology for Surgeons.* Philadelphia, Pa: WB Saunders Co, 1972.)

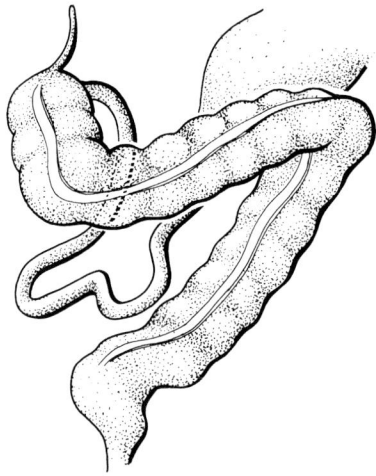

Fig. 14-28. Cecal inversion.
Early fixation before elongation of the colon has ceased forces the cecum to remain in the right upper abdomen. The appendix points cephalad but in a case with the more common undescended cecum, the appendix points downward. (Adapted from Gray SW, Skandalakis JE. *Embryology for Surgeons.* Philadelphia, Pa: WB Saunders Co, 1972.)

should be extended to determine the position of the cecum [see Fig. 14-25(b)]. Alternatively, a barium enema should be performed for the same purpose. Duodenojejunal obstruction secondary to malrotation and volvulus may occasionally occur in the presence of a normally positioned cecum.[87] However, as the cecum is mobile in 16% of people, the barium enema alone may not be able to differentiate between a patient with malrotation who is symptomatic for reasons other than volvulus and a patient with volvulus not due to malrotation.[88] Finding the jejunum in the right upper quadrant does not in itself mean malrotation, provided the duodenojejunal junction is in its normal position. In children, the conventional barium findings include a midline or high cecum and a partially obstructed duodenum leading to a "corkscrew" duodenojejunal junction.[89] These findings usually make a diagnosis possible (Fig. 14-29). However, in the adolescent or adult, when a barium study is done in a symptom-free period or with mild symptoms, the finding of an abnormal duodenojejunal position may be incidental.[90] An abnormal duodenojejunal junction in a symptomatic patient may have to become a reason for surgery, and must not to be dismissed as a normal variant.[91] In some patients, a "Z" pattern at the duodenojejunal junction is seen on barium studies. The "Z" may be related to extrinsic pressure by congenital bands and may look identical to the corkscrew of a volvulus, in which case the pattern is produced by bowel winding round the SMA.[92] The twisting is always clockwise.[93] A 180-degree twist is tolerable, but 270-degree to 720-degree twisting leads to significant obstruction that can cause lymphatic blockage (with chylous ascites and protein-losing enteropathy) or

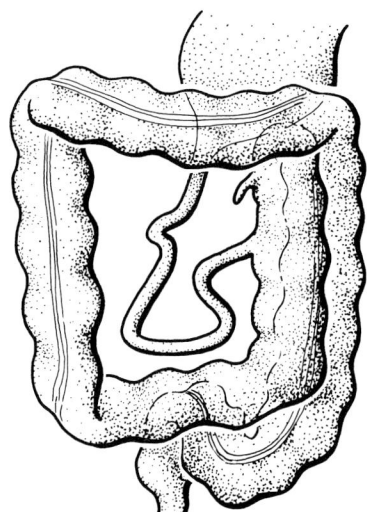

Fig. 14-27. Hyperrotation.
The general intestinal pattern is normal but the excessive length of the colon allows cecum to reach the left upper quadrant.

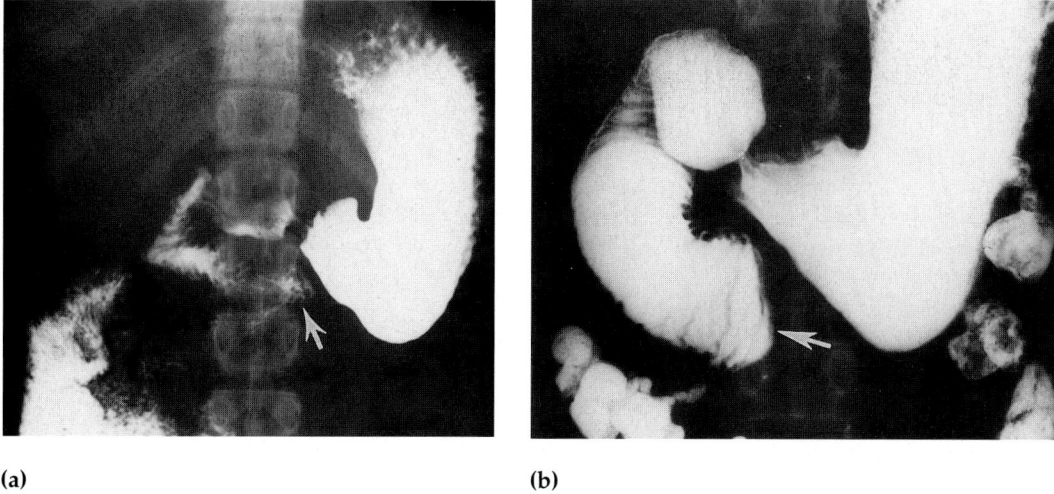

Fig. 14-29. Malrotation.
(a) In this 13-year-old, the upper gastrointestinal series demonstrates the duodenojejunal junction (arrow) to be located below the duodenal bulb and it does not extend to the left of the left L2 pedicle. Jejunal loops are noted in the right midabdomen. The "Z" pattern of the duodenojejunal junction is typical. (b) The upper gastrointestinal series performed 8 months later during an acute bout of abdominal pain and vomiting demonstrates a markedly dilated duodenum, typical of malrotation with midgut volvulus. Note the blind ending duodenum (arrow). (The patient had a prior barium enema, explaining the appearance of barium in the colon.)

cause venous engorgement. Finally, arterial occlusion can lead to ischemic pain and ultimately infarction (Fig. 14-30).

Ultrasound or CT may give useful additional information. On ultrasound, the malrotation manifests as a change of position of the superior mesenteric vein (SMV) from the normal—to the right of the SMA—to being anterior or to the left of it. Studies of volvulus by ultrasound in a newborn may have shown a "whirl" image [Fig. 14-31(a)] of thickened bowel twisted on itself; at times there may be vascular signals at the periphery.[89,91] On CT, the diagnosis has been suggested

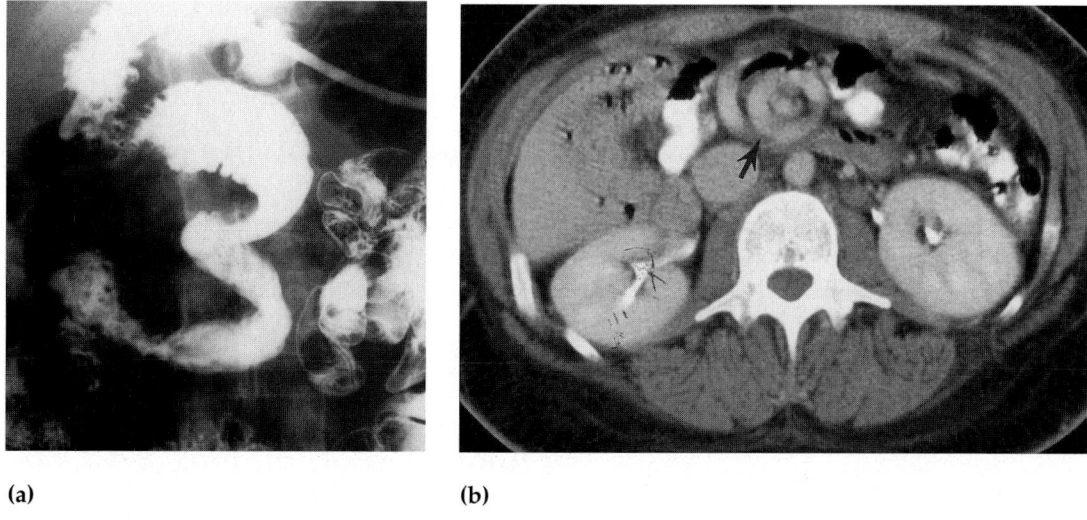

Fig. 14-30. Enteroclysis in a young patient with nonrotation and partial volvulus.
(a) Without normal peritoneal anchoring, the abnormally mobile midgut has twisted around the (SMA), producing the "corkscrew" of a volvulus. Note the clockwise twist. The twisting occurs at the only attachment and fulcrum, the SMA. (b) CT study of patient (a) shows encircling loops of bowel around SMA (arrow) creating a distinctive "whirl-like" pattern. (Courtesy of F.M. Kelvin, MD.)

14. Congenital and Developmental Anomalies of the Small Bowel in Adolescents and Adults

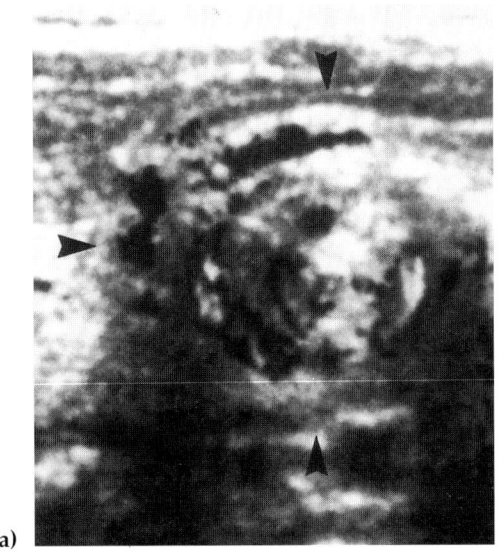
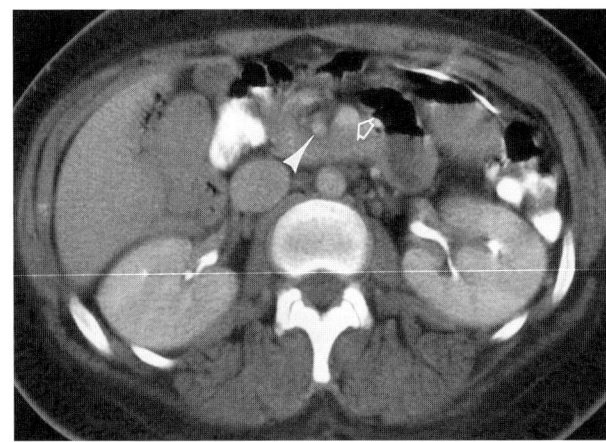
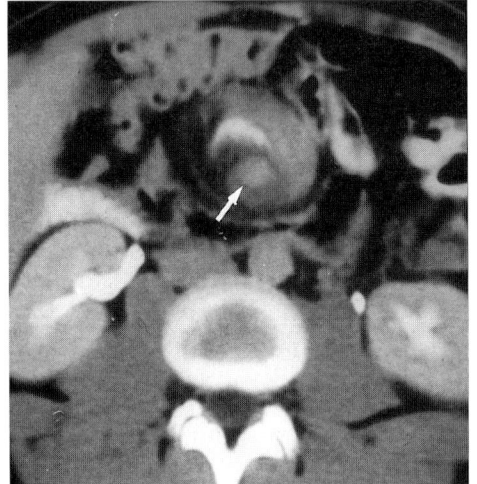

Fig. 14-31. Diagnosis of malrotation and midgut volvulus by ultrasound and CT.
(a) Midgut volvulus in a neonate. Transverse ultrasound scan through the midabdomen shows a characteristic "whirl" sign (arrowheads) due to clockwise rotation of small bowel around the mesenteric root. (Courtesy of M. Rioux, MD, Québec.) (b) In an 18-year-old female with intermittent abdominal pain, the CT examination demonstrates reversal of the relative positions of the superior mesenteric artery (arrowhead) and superior mesenteric vein (open arrow). (c) At a slightly lower level, the "whirl-like" arrangement of the mesenteric vessels and proximal jejunum (arrow) diagnostic of a volvulus is demonstrated.

by the abnormal course of the mesenteric vessels and of the proximal jejunum to form a "whirl-like" arrangement, distorted by the malrotation [Fig. 14-31(b), (c)]. As with ultrasound, reversal of the normal relative position of the SMV and SMA suggests intestinal malrotation[94–96] and is not a sign of volvulus.[97] The "whirlpool" or "whirl-like" patterns seen both on ultrasound and CT are the features to suggest volvulus.

Treatment and Management of the Asymptomatic Adult

The management of midgut rotational anomalies encountered in the asymptomatic adult population is complicated by anecdotal reports and small patient series.[98] In light of the rarity of complications in patients more than 2 years of age, a nonoperative approach has been emphasized.[98,99] Should the patient develop unexplained abdominal symptoms, urgent laparotomy has been advised to exclude small bowel volvulus.[98] In contrast, others recommend prophylactic surgery, citing cases of bowel infarction occurring without preliminary symptoms and the catastrophic outcome of a misdiagnosed small bowel volvulus.[90,100] Surgical intervention is indicated in the setting of chronic symptoms.[101]

Anomalies of Intestinal Fixation

Congenital Internal Hernias

Although postsurgical or traumatic defects of the mesentery and omentum are more common causes of internal hernias in adults, anomalies of intestinal rotation and peritoneal fixation are important factors that predispose to internal herniation.[102] The reason why some congenital internal hernias do not produce symptoms in the early years of life is unclear.

Congenital internal hernias are rare and account for only 0.5% to 3% of all cases of intestinal obstruction.[103,104] The autopsy incidence of internal hernias has been stated to be between 0.2% and 0.9%[105] Many of these hernias are easily reducible and may remain asymptomatic or only intermittently symptomatic throughout life. Some patients may present with acute small bowel obstructions that may recur. In these instances, the radiologic diagnosis is best made if the contrast examination is performed during the period of symptoms, before spontaneous reduction has occurred. The preoperative radiologic diagnosis of an internal hernia is important since, at laparotomy, the hernia may be reduced, either spontaneous or caused by inadvertent traction. A full evaluation of all significant peritoneal fossae and mesenteric recesses may not be possible during the usual exploratory laparotomy.[106] Contrast small bowel examination can provide the most useful diagnostic demonstration of an internal abdominal hernia.[107] These radiologic findings include the following:[107] 1) crowding together of several small intestinal loops due to encapsulation within a hernial sac, from which position they can usually not be displaced, 2) dilatation and prolonged stasis of barium in dilated herniated loops, and 3) disturbed arrangement and abnormal location of small intestinal loops.

The following classification is based upon the anatomic regions in which internal hernias occur: A) paraduodenal, B) foramen of Winslow, C) paracecal, D) intersigmoid, E) transmesenteric, F) transomental. Paraduodenal hernias are the most common and make up 53% of all reported internal hernias.[104] In another review 13% of internal hernias were related to the cecum and terminal ileum, 8% passed through the foramen of Winslow, 8% were transmesenteric, and 6% occurred in the sigmoid region.[95] A review of a smaller series of cases found the transomental hernia to be the most frequent (38% of congenital internal hernias).[108]

Paraduodenal Hernias

Paraduodenal hernias are subdivided into left and right depending upon their direction and passage through defined openings leading into a retroperitoneal position.[81] They are more frequent on the left than right in a ratio of 3:1[109] and three times more common in men than women.[81,108]

A *left paraduodenal hernia* results when, during return of the small intestine into the abdominal cavity, an intestinal loop passes through the fossa of Landzert into the as yet unfused descending mesocolon. This fossa is situated to the left of the ascending duodenum and is demarcated anterolaterally by a fold that is elevated by containing the inferior mesenteric vein and the ascending branch of the left colic artery. Bowel loops extend into the hernia in a left and inferior direction (Fig. 14-32).[107] Subsequent fusion of the descending mesocolon forms a pocket to accommodate the hernia, which may contain a single intestinal loop, or sometimes the whole of the small intestine (Fig. 14-33). The afferent limb enters the hernia posteriorly directly from the retroperitoneal position of the duodenum and is usually not identified at barium studies. Only the efferent limb will be seen to pass through the hernial orifice.[107] The cecum is completely rotated and lies in the right iliac fossa.[81,103]

In *right paraduodenal hernia*, the hernial orifice is to the right of the midline and the peritoneal sac is directed posteriorly and to the right. The mesentericoparietal fossa of Waldeyer is the usual entry site for a right paraduodenal hernia. This fossa is situated below the duodenum and behind the superior mesenteric artery. The hernia extends into a space behind the ascending colon and the right portion of the transverse colon.[107] The two limbs of the hernia should be

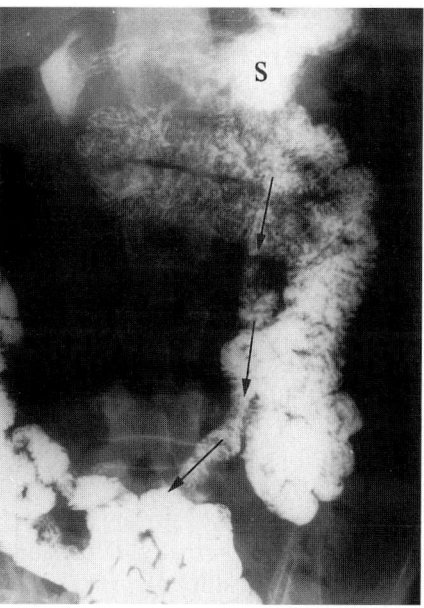

Fig. 14-32. Left paraduodenal hernia.
Moderate-size left paraduodenal hernia with inferior convexity shows mild dilatation of crowded loops of jejunum posterior and below the stomach. The exiting segment is seen to emerge from the direction of the fossa of Landzert (arrows). (S = stomach.)

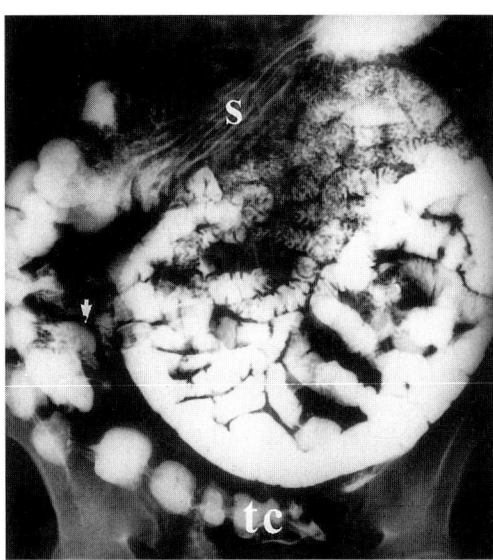

Fig. 14-33. Large left paraduodenal hernia.
Except for a few inches of distal ileum (arrow), the mesenteric small bowel is contained in a well-circumscribed configuration, with its inferior border being convex downward. The ovoid mass has displaced the transverse colon (TC) inferiorly and indented the posterior gastric wall (S = stomach). Note minimal dilatation of herniated loops inside the hernial sac. (Courtesy of F.M. Kelvin, MD.)

seen in close apposition and are usually somewhat narrowed at their passage through the fossa. In a review of the reported cases of right paraduodenal hernia most patients were adults, with a mean age of 36.6 years.[110] No patients were younger than 8 years of age.[111]

Small paraduodenal hernias may remain asymptomatic through life. Left paraduodenal hernias may reduce spontaneously; right paraduodenal hernias usually do not. Clinical manifestations result from partial or complete obstruction of the small intestine, usually in adulthood and more often affecting the right sided hernia.

Radiology

Plain film radiography during acute presentation and higher grades of obstruction may demonstrate dilated loops of small bowel confined to one area. When fluid-filled, a pseudotumor is produced. The plain film findings, however, are not pathognomic.

The findings of barium contrast examination of paraduodenal hernias are diagnostic. Displaced bunched loops of small bowel when outlined by barium are seen to be confined to a space lateral to the midline with a convex inferior border. Fluoroscopic palpation leaves the bowel loops in virtually unchanged relative position, suggesting encapsulation.[105,107] A large left paraduodenal hernia, a circumscribed ovoid crowded loop of jejunum, occupies the left upper quadrant immediately lateral to the ascending duodenum, indents the posterior wall of the stomach, and may depress the distal transverse colon (Fig. 14-33). More distal bowel loops can be displaced from the encapsulated loops by compression during fluoroscopy. Dilatation of the involved segments and stasis of contrast material may be evident. Smaller hernias may not appear well encapsulated. In order to differentiate a small left paraduodenal hernia from crowded loops of bowel secondary to adhesions, the efferent loop should be visualized emerging from the area of the fossa of Landzert (Fig. 14-32).

Right paraduodenal hernias show a similar crowding of loops that extend to the right at the level of the inferior duodenal flexure. A small hernia shown by follow-through is diagnosed on the basis of the displacement, the constancy of the bunching, and the demonstration of entering and exiting limbs at the likely orifice position (Fig. 14-34). In another patient plain films showed dilated fluid levels containing bowel loops in the right upper abdomen [Fig. 14-35(a)]. An enteroclysis was done. The small bowel catheter was seen to deviate from its expected course, turning abruptly down and to the right long before reaching the ligament of Treitz area. Bunched right-sided jeju-

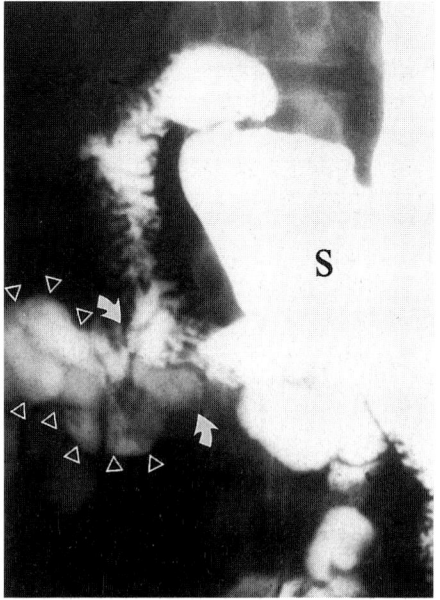

Fig. 14-34. Right paraduodenal hernia.
Both afferent and efferent loops of a small right paraduodenal hernia can be identified at the hernial orifice (white arrows). Open arrowheads outline hernial sac. (S = stomach). (Courtesy of A. Friedman, MD.)

nal loops were then opacified, and a diagnosis of right paraduodenal hernia was very likely (Fig. 14-35). It is a requirement for a positive diagnosis, however, to image the efferent loop close to and parallel with the entering segment [Fig. 14-35(c)]. This should be im-

aged at an early still single-contrast stage of the enteroclysis. If not identified then, later filming, when bowel distention has reached more distal loops, may find it difficult or impossible to make this positive diagnosis. Mostly overhead-film-based follow-through

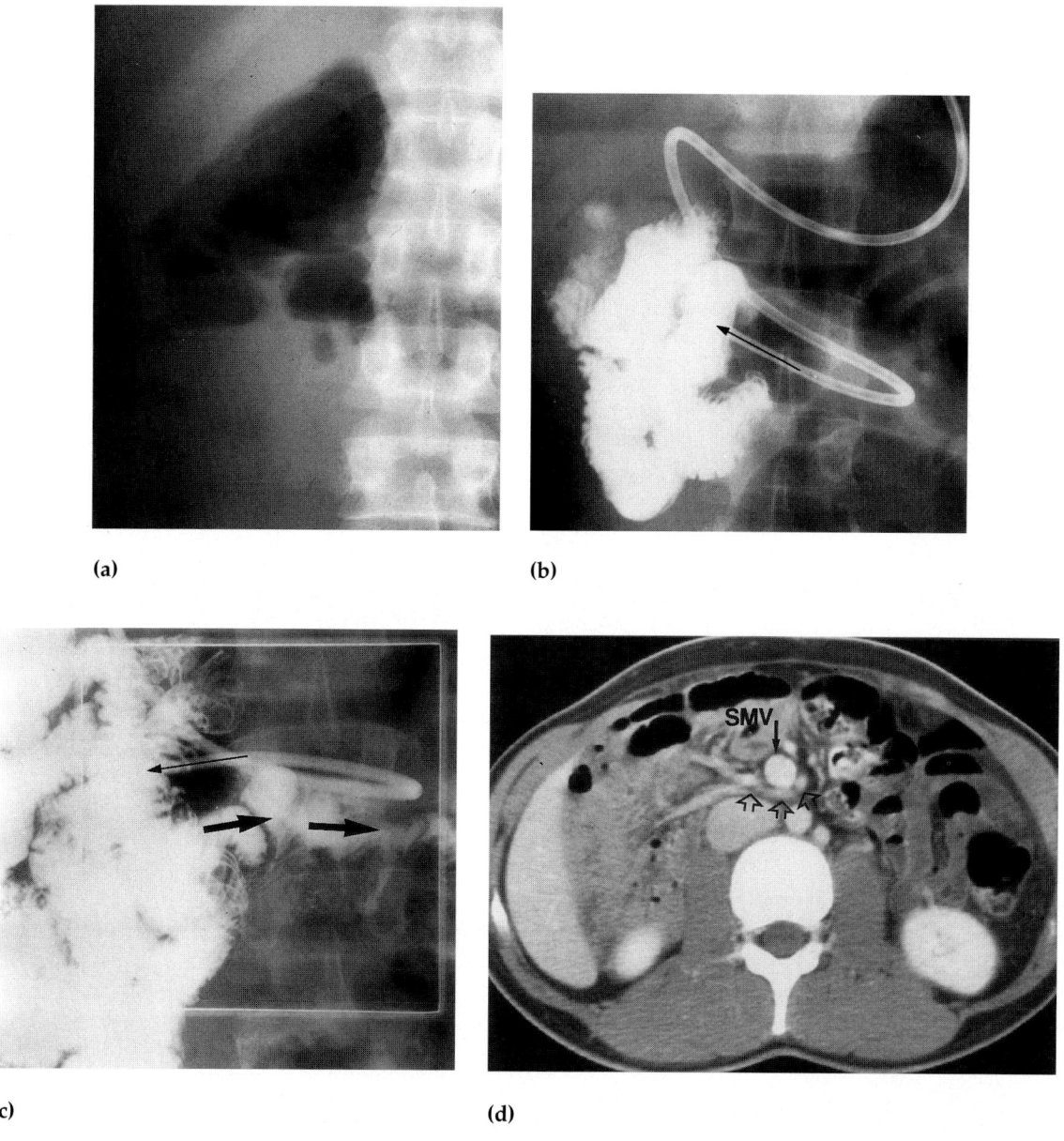

Fig. 14-35. Right paraduodenal hernia presenting with intermittent low-grade small bowel obstruction. Diagnosis by plain films, enteroclysis, and CT.
(a) Moderately dilated loops of duodenum and proximal small bowel containing fluid levels are seen in the right upper abdomen. (b) Early enteroclysis film shows the catheter to have entered into a segment of jejunum coursing towards the right (arrow). No ascending duodenum was present. (c) Further opacification could demonstrate the exiting limb of jejunum in close and parallel relation (arrows) to the entering segment (both have passed through the fossa of Waldeyer). (d) Subsequent CT scans could demonstrate a jejunal mesenteric vein (open arrows) returning to the SMV by passing through the fossa of Waldeyer behind the SMV, then joining it from its normal left. Findings in (c) and (d) are proof positive of right paraduodenal herniation.

examinations may entirely miss a diagnosis of right paraduodenal hernia, being unable to identify the exiting limb after it has become obscured by overlying bowel loops distal to the hernia. A CT scan adds important further confirmation of the diagnosis of right paraduodenal hernia [Fig. 14-35(d)]. A right paraduodenal hernia must be differentiated from isolated malrotation of the proximal limb of the fetal umbilical loop. In that condition there will not be adjacency and parallelism lying in front of the ascending colon (Fig. 14-36).

The CT features of paraduodenal hernias have been described in several reports.[112–115] In left paraduodenal hernias the findings involve: 1) confined bowel loops at the level of the ligament of Treitz or interposed between the stomach and pancreas, behind the pancreas, or in front of the left psoas muscle; and 2) dilatation and air-fluid levels in the herniated loops. In right paraduodenal hernias, the primary CT findings are 1) looping of SMA and superior mesenteric vein (SMV) jejunal branches posteriorly and to the right, and 2) clustering or apparent encapsulation of small bowel loops in the right midabdomen. The hernial sac may not be discerned. CT findings of right paraduodenal hernia–associated malrotation are: 1) SMV rotated more toward the left and ventral aspect of the SMA than normal, and 2) absence of the normal ascending duodenum. The anterior and lateral posi-

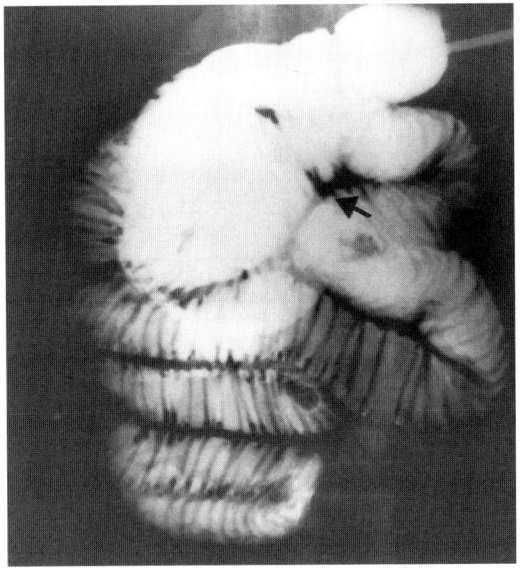

(a)

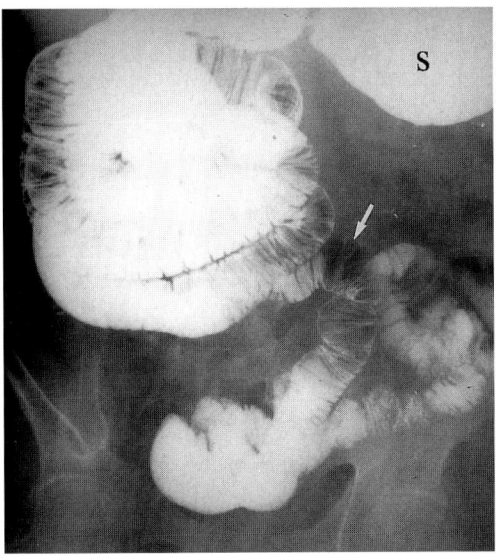

(b)

Fig. 14-36. Isolated malrotation of cephalic loop of midgut.
(a) The duodenojejunal junction (arrow) at tip of enteroclysis catheter is not in its normal position to the left of L2. (b) During enteroclysis, a loop of bowel (arrow) is seen coursing toward the left lower abdomen. Excessive infusion flow rates have artificially distended malrotated loops in the right upper abdomen and produced a pseudoencapsulation. (S = refluxed contrast in stomach.) (c) Radiograph obtained following cessation of infusion shows the right colon posterior to the malrotated segment in the right hemiabdomen. The loops could be separated by compression, and no sac or hernial orifice could be identified. (C = cecum).

(c)

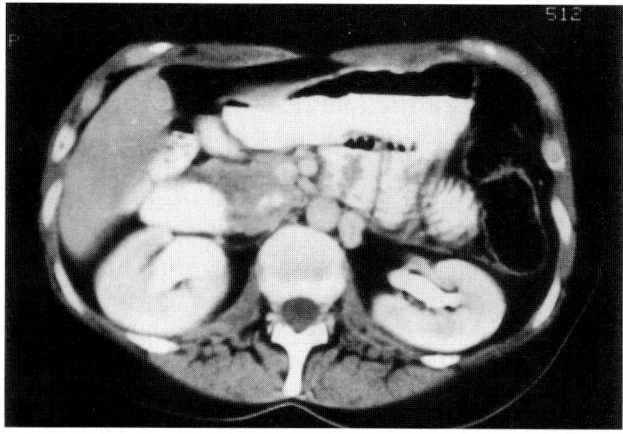
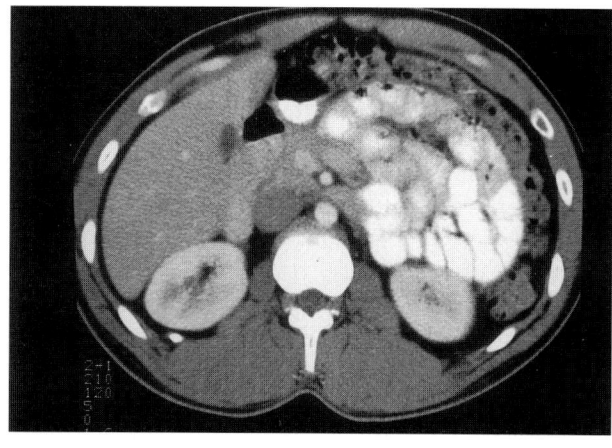
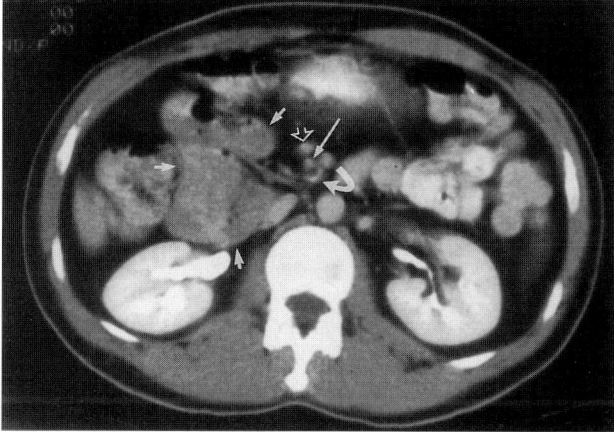

Fig. 14-37. CT of paraduodenal hernias.
(a) CT section shows a cluster of mildly dilated small bowel loops with air-fluid levels behind the stomach at the level of the ligament of Treitz in a case of left paraduodenal hernia. (From Warshauer[114] with permission.) (b) CT section shows clustering of nondilated small bowel loops in left upper abdomen adjacent to ligament of Treitz with well-defined outer convex margins suggestive of encapsulation in another case of left paraduodenal hernia. (Courtesy of David M. Warshauer, MD.) (c) CT section demonstrates encapsulated nonrotated small bowel loops in the right midabdomen (arrows). The normally rotated ascending colon lies lateral to these small bowel loops. The SMA (open arrow) is rotated anterior and to the left of its normal position, and there is looping of arterial and venous jejunal branches (curved arrow) behind the SMV (long arrow). Surgery disclosed a right paraduodenal hernia. (From Warshauer[114] with permission.)

tion of the ascending colon will also be apparent. The CT features of paraduodenal hernias are illustrated in Figs. 14-35(d) and 14-37.

The arteriographic appearance of paraduodenal hernias reflects the CT findings and is equally characteristic but is now rarely required.[106]

Treatment

Even small and asymptomatic hernias are potentially dangerous and should be considered an operable condition. Operative management consists of reduction of the hernia and obliteration of the defect.[116]

Other Internal Hernias

Foramen of Winslow herniations account for approximately 8% of congenital internal hernias.[104] The cecum is the most common organ herniated (68%), followed by the small intestine.[117] Other organs such as the ascending colon, appendix, transverse colon, omentum, or gallbladder are found in it occasionally. The majority of the patients present with intestinal obstructions, and there may be a history of previous intermittent episodes of abdominal pain. The only suggestive physical sign is a palpable tender mass in the perigastrium. The correct preoperative diagnosis is made in less than 10% of cases reported.[118]

Any of five factors is believed to contribute to the development of herniation through the foramen of Winslow:[118] 1) a common mesentery for the entire intestine, 2) a failure of fusion of the ascending colon to the posterior abdominal wall (conducive to increased mobility), 3) an abnormal length of the mesentery, 4) an abnormally large foramen, and 5) a possible pressure gradient between the greater and lesser peritoneal sacs produced by a heavy meal or by straining.

If the cecum is the lead point, the diagnosis can be made if there is: 1) failure to visualize the cecum in its usual position, 2) collection of gas or gas and fluid in the lesser sac displacing the stomach anteriorly and to the left, and 3) displacement of the first and second parts of the duodenum to the left.[108] There is possible confusion with a cecal volvulus.[119,120] Both conditions will demonstrate a gas-filled, kidney-shaped loop of bowel in the upper abdomen and absence of cecum in its usual position. In cecal volvulus, the "hilum" of the distended kidney-shaped loop of bowel may point toward the right iliac fossa. In cecal herniation through the foramen of Winslow, the "hilum" points toward the foramen of Winslow.[121] This may be observed on plain film or contrast radiography. If the stomach is filled with gas, it can be seen to be displaced to the left and anteriorly by the mass of herniated loops. The proximal duodenum may also be displaced to the left (Fig. 14-38). If the stomach or duodenum is obstructed by the intestines passing into the lesser sac, then air will not pass distally and the typical signs of obstruction will not be evident.[122] If the small bowel is the lead point, plain radiographs of the abdomen show evidence of mechanical small bowel obstruction, with gas-containing loops behind the stomach. Small bowel contrast examination shows dilatation and increased peristalsis with a focal point of obstruction at or near the location of the foramen of Winslow, between the duodenal bulb and the hilus of the liver.

Paracecal hernias comprise a very small percentage of congenital intestinal hernias (6% to 13%).[104,108] A minor error of rotation of the midgut with incarcera-

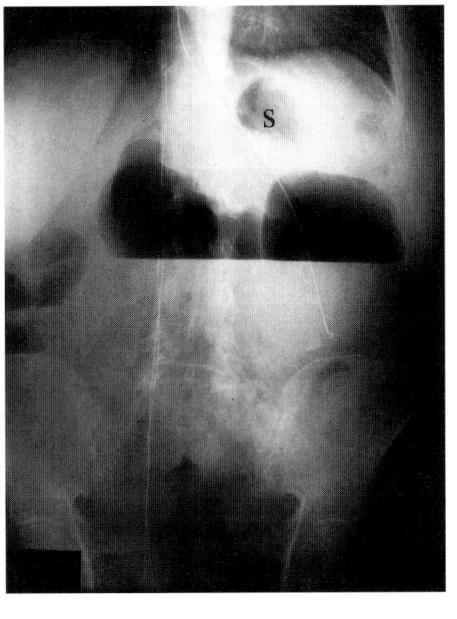

(a)

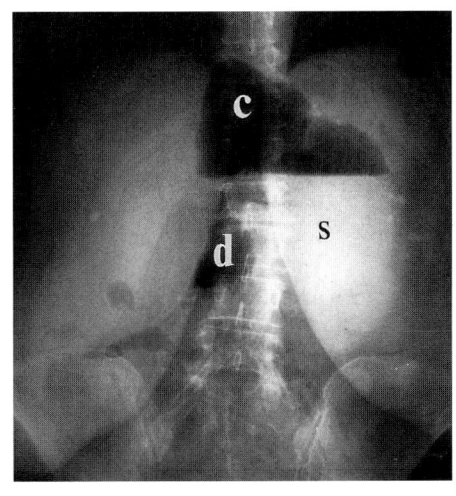

(b)

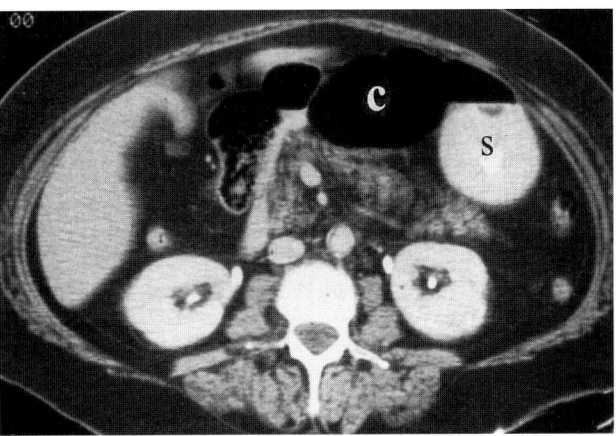

(c)

Fig. 14-38. Imaging of foramen of Winslow herniation. (a) Upright abdominal radiograph of an elderly patient with severe upper abdominal pain and vomiting shows two confluent air-fluid levels in the upper midabdomen and absence of the cecum in the right lower abdomen. (S = stomach). (b) CT shows contrast-filled stomach (S) displaced to the left and anteriorly by a distended gas-filled cecum (c). Mild medial displacement of contrast-filled descending duodenum by a segment of right colon is also noted (d = duodenum).

Transomental hernias are very rare with the exception of a single report, as already mentioned earlier. Focal dilatation of a loop of small bowel is observed, and contrast radiography suggests encapsulation of the dilated loop (Fig. 14-41). Bowel protruding through the often indurated margin of the omental defect may become strangulated. A case has been reported of a hernia that entered the lesser sac through the gastrocolic ligament, to pass behind the stomach and reenter the peritoneal cavity through an incarcerating secondary defect in the lesser omentum.[123]

Idiopathic Localized Dilatation of the Ileum (Ileal Dysgenesis)

During the last two decades this uncommon entity of congenital or idiopathic nature has been described in a group of children and adults.[124–130] This rare entity is characterized by a sharply demarcated dilatation of a focal segment of ileum.

Pathogenesis

It is believed that a congenital neuromuscular dysfunction accounts for the isolated atonic segment of

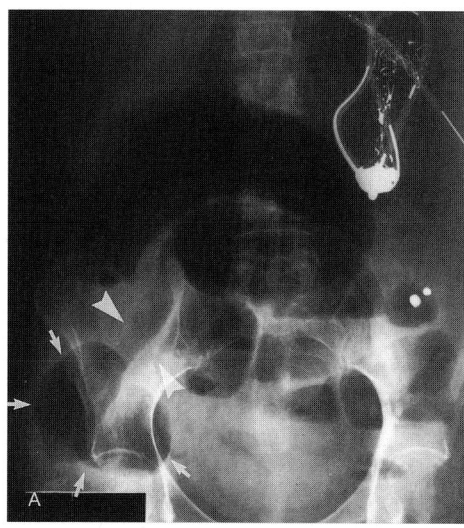

Fig. 14-39. Paracecal hernia.
Plain abdominal radiograph shows mechanical distal small bowel obstruction. Two narrowed loops of bowel are seen in close approximation (arrowheads) suggesting passage to a space with dilated and fixed loops (arrows) beyond the expected position of the cecum. Small bowel loops proximally are markedly distended. (By permission from Ghahremani GG, Meyers MA. *Radiology*. 1975;5:1-30.)

tion of a loop of ileum behind the cecum during the final stages of descent and fixation of the right colon can result in the formation of a paracecal hernia. Herniation may also take place into one of four fossae in the cecal area or through congenital or acquired defects in the cecal or appendiceal mesentery. The correct diagnosis may be suggested on plain abdominal radiographs. The distal ileum may be seen to pass through the area of the cecum to protrude into the periphery of the right lower abdomen. Gaseous distention of the proximal small bowel is noted. Contrast examinations, however, are more informative. Demonstration of the fixed position of the herniated loops posterolateral to the cecum suggests a diagnosis of paracecal hernia (Fig. 14-39).[98]

Intersigmoid hernia. An intersigmoid recess, forming an inverted "V" directed upward behind the attachment of the sigmoid mesocolon, has been reported to occur in 65% of adults. Of internal hernias, 6% are found in the sigmoid region[104] and they are usually reducible. A contrast examination will show the small bowel trapped and encapsulated between two loops of the sigmoid. Occasionally, the sigmoid colon is elevated and displaced to the right. This finding occurs when a large defect of the sigmoid mesentery allows herniation of the small bowel loops toward the left abdomen posterolateral to the sigmoid colon (Fig. 14-40).

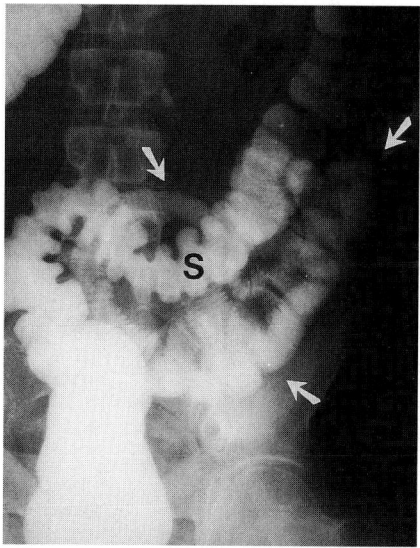

Fig. 14-40. Intersigmoid hernia.
During a barium enema there is retrograde filling of small bowel loops (arrows) that are crowded toward the left and below the sigmoid (S), suggesting the diagnosis of an intersigmoid hernia. The sigmoid is elevated and displaced toward the midline. (Courtesy of G. Ghahremani, MD.)

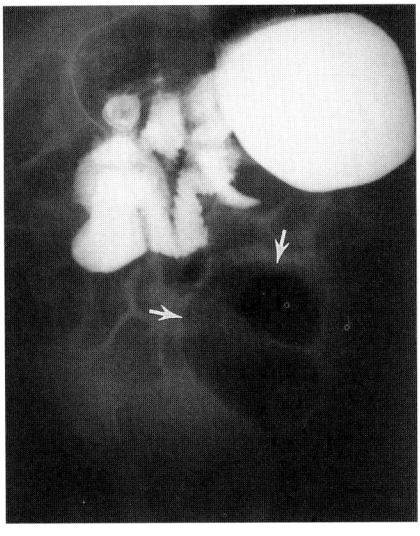
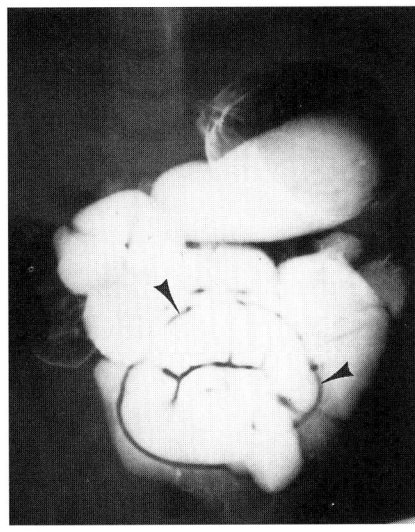

Fig. 14-41. Transomental hernia. (a) Upper gastrointestinal series of pediatric patient who presented with vomiting. A gas-filled loop of bowel in the left lower abdomen (arrows) appears to be focally dilated. (b) Delayed radiograph shows the dilated loop of bowel encapsulated within a hernial sac (arrowheads). At surgical exploration, this was a transomental hernia.

ileum or that a temporary obstruction of a loop early in its development may have been caused by vitelline vessels that later involuted. Stasis of contents subsequently led to the dilatation. Microscopy demonstrates normal ganglion cells and nerve plexuses in the wall of the localized dilatation. However, ectopic gastric mucosa and other aberrant tissues are occasionally found in the mucosal lining, supporting its congenital origin.[130] The mucosa may be ulcerated, but otherwise the bowel wall appears to be normal.

Clinical Considerations

Despite a widely patent lumen, the atonic segment functions as a peristaltic barrier. The majority of patients hitherto reported have presented with recurrent obstructive symptoms. Bleeding may also be present. Some 15% of childhood cases have been associated with omphaloceles[130] and others with Meckel's diverticula.[125] Segmental resection of the dilated segment and end-to-end anastomosis are curative.

Radiology

During contrast radiography, idiopathic localized dilatation of the ileum has been mistaken for a Meckel's diverticulum.[128] Careful fluoroscopy will show absence of peristalsis in the dilated segment, whereas the caliber and motility of adjacent segments are normal. It is further differentiated from a Meckel's diverticulum by the direct continuity of the dilated lumen with the normal ileum. The dilated segment is sharply demarcated and is lobulated (Fig. 14-41). It may be spherical or tubular. An ulcer can occasionally be demonstrated within the lesion (Fig. 14-41b).[128]

References

1. Wang C, Welch CE. Anomalies of intestinal rotation in adolescents and adults. *Surgery.* 1963;54:839–855.
2. Samaniego AG, Wilson WH, Chandler JG. Symptomatic congenital lesions of the alimentary tract in adults. *Am J Surg.* 1991;162:545–552.
3. Gray SW, Skandalakis JE. The small intestine. Embryology for surgeons. In: Gray SW, Skandalakis JE, eds. *The Embryological Basis for Treatment of Congenital Defects.* Philadelphia, Pa: WB Saunders Co; 1972:130–141.
4. Hamilton WJ, Mossman HW. *Human Embryology. Prenatal Development of Form and Function.* Baltimore, Md: Williams and Wilkins Co; 1972:339–359.
5. Meckel JF. Ueber die divertikel am darmkanal. *Arch die Physiol.* 1809;9:421–453.
6. Dott NM. Anomalies of intestinal rotation, their embryology and surgical aspects: with report of five cases. *Br J Surg.* 1923;11:251–286.
7. Snyder WH Jr, Chaffin L. Embryology and pathology of the intestinal tract: presentation of 40 cases of malrotation. *Ann Surg.* 1954;140:368–380.
8. Bissler JJ, Klein RL. Alimentary tract duplication in children: case and literature review. *Clin Pediatr (Phila).* 1988;27:152–157.
9. Grosfeld JL, O'Neal JA Jr, Clatworthy HW Jr. Enteric duplications in infancy and childhood: an 18-year review. *Ann Surg.* 1970;172:83–90.
10. Moore TC, Battersby JS. Congenital duplications of the small intestine: report of 11 cases. *Surg Gynecol Obstet.* 1952;95:557–567.
11. Nolan JJ, Lee JG. Duplications of the alimentary tract in

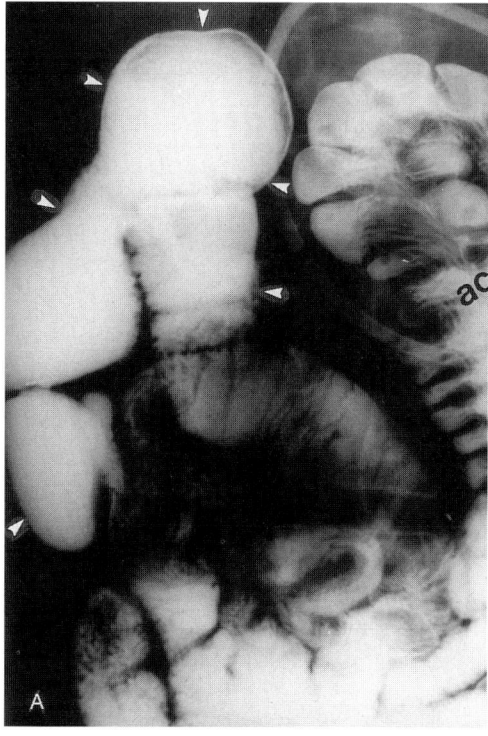
(a)

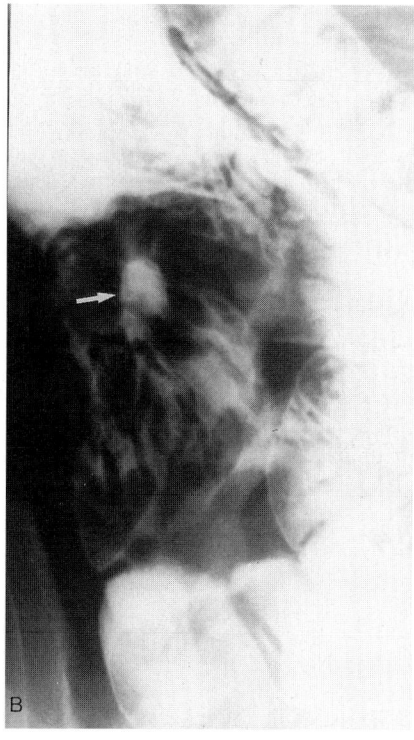
(b)

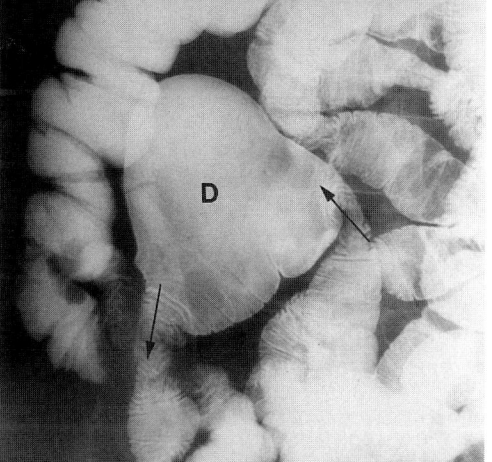
(c)

Fig. 14-42. Idiopathic localized dilatation of ileum in a patient presenting with unexplained gastrointestinal bleeding.
(a) Focal dilatation of a segment of distal ileum (arrowheads). The small bowel mesentery is long, and ileal segments extended lateral to the ascending colon (ac). The lumen of the dilated segment is continuous with the rest of the ileum. The dilated segment was aperistaltic fluoroscopically. (b) Compression radiograph of the midportion of the dilated segment shows a chronic ulcer (arrow). Findings were confirmed at surgery. (c) Enteroclysis of a further case of a short segment of ileal dysgenesis (D). Entering and exiting limbs (arrows) are unobstructed.

adults with a report of three cases. *Ann Surg*. 1953;137: 342–348.
12. Anderson MC, Silberman WW, Shields TW. Duplications of the alimentary tract in the adult. *Arch Surg*. 1962;85:94–108.
13. Thomson TJ, Wilson JH, Cunningham GLW. Gastrointestinal tract duplication: massive hemorrhage from ulcer. *Gastroenterology*. 1954;26:774–777.
14. Hartl H. Duplication of the small intestine. *Wien Klin Wschr*. 1951;63:795–806.
15. Mazingarbe A. Un cas de peritonite par rupture d'un kyste enteroide. *Arch Mal Appar Dig*. 1956;45:83–89.
16. Aalameh RN, Hausner RJ, Thomas SJ, Johnson CD. Massive hemorrhage in an ileal duplication cyst. *South Med J*. 1984;77:1606–1607.
17. Staunton DA, Jacobson AF, Thorning D, Lynch MK. Coumadin-induced gastrointestinal hemorrhage associated with an ileal duplication. *J Clin Gastroenterol*. 1990;12:685–689.
18. Micolonghi T, Meissner GF. Gastric-type carcinoma

arising in duplication of the small intestine. *Ann Surg.* 1958;147:124–127.
19. Orr MM, Edwards AJ. Neoplastic change in duplications of the alimentary tract. *Br J Surg.* 1975;62:269–274.
20. Adair HM, Trowell JE. Squamous cell carcinoma arising in a duplication of the small bowel. *J Pathol.* 1981;133:25–31.
21. Van Twisk R. A congenital diverticulum of the small intestine: Meckel's diverticulum or duplication. *Neth J Surg.* 1984;36:107–111.
22. Scully RE, Galdabini JJ, McNeely BV. Case records of the Massachusetts General Hospital. *N Engl J Med.* 1980;17:958–962.
23. Bower RJ, Sieber WK, Kiesewether WB. Alimentary duplications in children. *Ann Surg.* 1978;188:669–674.
24. Buras RR, Guzetta PC, Majd M. Multiple duplications of the small intestine. *J Pediatr Surg.* 1986;21:957–959.
25. Anderson MC, Silberman WW, Shields TW. Duplications of the alimentary tract in the adult. *Arch Surg.* 1962;85:94–108.
26. Forshall I. Duplications of the intestinal tract. *Postgrad Med J.* 1961;37:570–589.
27. Johnson JA III, Poole GV. Ileal duplications in adults. Presentation and treatment. *Arch Surg.* 1994;129: 659–661. Also, Gilchrist AM, Sloan JM, Logan CJH, Mils JOM. Case report: gastrointestinal bleeding due to multiple ileal duplications diagnosed by scintigraphy and barium studies. *Clin Radiol.* 1990;41:134–136.
28. Kelly RB, Mahoney PD, Johnson JF. CT demonstration of an unusual enteric duplication cyst. *J Comput Asst Tomogr.* 1986;10:506–507.
29. Ros PR, Olmsted WW, Moser RP Jr, et al. Mesenteric and omental cysts: histologic classification with imaging correlation. *Radiology.* 1987;164:327–332.
30. Sfakianakis GN, Conway JJ. Detection of ectopic gastric mucosa in Meckel's diverticulum and in other aberrations by scintigraphy Indications and methods—a 10 year experience. *J Nucl Med.* 1981;22 (part I): 647–654; 22 (part II):732–738.
31. Schwesinger WH, Croom RD, Habibian MR. Diagnosis of an enteric duplication with pertechnetate 99m TC scanning. *Ann Surg.* 1975;181:428–438.
32. Newmark H, Ching G, Halls J, Levy IJ. Bleeding peptic ulcer caused by ectopic gastric mucosa in a duplicated segment of jejunum. *Am J Gastroenterol.* 1981;75:158–162.
33. Souderlund S. Meckel's diverticulum. A clinical and histologic study. *Acta Chir Scand.* 1959;248:13–23.
34. Turgeon DK, Barnett JL. Clinical review: Meckel's diverticulum. *Am J Gastroenterol.* 1990;85:777–781.
35. Mackey WC, Dineen P. A fifty-year experience with Meckel's diverticulum. *Surg Gynecol Obstet.* 1983;156:56–64.
36. McSwain GR, Anderson MC. Meckel's diverticulum of the proximal jejunum. *Arch Surg.* 1979;114:212–213.
37. Yamaguchi M, Takeuchi S, Awazu S. Meckel's diverticulum: investigation of 600 patients in the Japanese literature. *Am J Surg.* 1978;136:247–249.
38. Weinstein EC, Cain JC, ReMine WH. Meckel's diverticulum: 55 years of clinical and surgical experience. *JAMA.* 1962;182:131–133.
39. Moses WR. Meckel's diverticulum. Report of two unusual cases. *N Engl J Med.* 1947;237:118–122.
40. Caylor HD. Meckel's diverticulum. *Gastroenterology.* 1949;33:31–46.
41. Kiernan PD, ReMine SG, Kiernan PC, et al. Annular pancreas. *Arch Surg.* 1980;115:46–50.
42. Bondeson L, Starck-Bondeson AG. Crohn's disease in heterotropic gastric mucosa in a Meckel's diverticulum. *Acta Pathol Microbiol Scand.* 1974;82:427–430.
43. Ekman CN. Regional enteritis associated with Meckel's diverticulum: a report of five cases. *Gastroenterology.* 1958;34:130–134.
44. Glick SN, Maglinte DDT, Herlinger H. Association of Meckel's diverticulum and Crohn's disease. *Gastrointest Radiol.* 1988;13:67–71.
45. Soltero MJ, Bill AH. The natural history of Meckel's diverticulum and its relation to incidental removal. *Am J Surg.* 1976;132:168–173.
45. Rutherford RB, Akers DR. Meckels diverticulum: a review of 148 pediatric patients, with special reference to the pattern of bleeding and to mesodiverticular vascular bands. *Surgery.* 1966;59:618–626.
46. Maglinte DDT, Elmore MF, Isenberg M, Dolan PA. Meckel diverticulum: radiologic demonstration by enteroclysis. *AJR.* 1980;134:925–932.
47. Salomonowitz E, Wittich G, Hajek P, et al. Detection of intestinal diverticula by double contrast small bowel enema: differentiation from other intestinal diverticula. *Gastrointest Radiol.* 1983;8:271–278.
48. Veith FJ, Botsford TW. Disease of Meckel's diverticulum in adults. *Am Surg.* 1962;28:674–677.
49. Ho CS, Shewchun J, Greenberg GR. Diagnosis of Meckel's diverticulum in adults. *Mt Sinai J Med.* 1984;51:378–381.
50. Weinstein EC, Cain JC, Remine N. Meckel's diverticulum: 55 years of clinical and surgical experience. *JAMA.* 1962;182:251–253.
51. Maglinte DDT, Jordan LG, et al. Chronic gastrointestinal bleeding from Meckel's diverticulum: radiological considerations. *Clin Gastroenterol.* 1981;3:47–52.
52. Hirschy JC, Thorpe JJ, Cortese AF. Meckel stones. *Radiology.* 1976;119:19–20.
53. Berman EJ, Schnieder A, Potts WJ. Importance of gastric mucosa in Meckel's diverticulum. *JAMA.* 1954;156:6–7.
54. Leijonmarck CE, Bonman-Sandelin K, Frisell J, et al. Meckel's diverticulum in the adult. *Br J Surg.* 1986;73:146–149.
55. Ponka JL. Intussusception due to invaginated Meckel's diverticulum: presentation of two cases and an analysis of 52 cases collected from the literature. *Am J Surg.* 1956;92:545–557.
56. Castleden WM. Meckel's diverticulum in an umbilical hernia. *Br J Surg.* 1970;57:932–934.
57. Perlman JA, Hoover HC, Safer PK. Femoral hernia with strangulated Meckel's diverticulum (Littre's hernia). *Am J Surg.* 1980;139:286–289.
58. Goldsmith EA, Gotfried EA. Meckel's diverticulum: re-

59. Velanovich V, Ledbetter D, McGahren E, et al. Foreign bodies within a Meckel's diverticulum. *Arch Surg.* 1992;127:864.
60. Dixon AY, McAnaw M, McGregor DH, et al. Dual carcinoid tumors of Meckel's diverticulum presenting as metastasis in an inguinal hernia sac: case report with literature review. *Am J Gastroenterol.* 1988;83:1283–1288.
61. Warner RRP. Carcinoid tumor. In: Berk EJ, ed. *Bockus, Gastroenterology*. Philadelphia, Pa: WB Saunders Co; 1985:1874–1886.
62. Ghahremani GG. Radiology of Meckel's diverticulum. *Crit Rev Diagn Imaging.* 1986;26:1–43.
63. Dalinka MK, Wunder JF. Meckel's diverticulum and its complications, with emphasis on roentgen demonstration. *Radiology.* 1973;106:295–298.
64. Bergland RM, Gump F, Price JB. An unusual complication of Meckel's diverticulum seen in older patients. *Ann Surg.* 1963;154:6–8.
65. Benhamou G. Small intestinal obstruction by an enterolith from a Meckel's diverticulum. *Int Surg.* 1979;64:43–45.
66. Christiansen KH, Cancelmo RP. Meckel's stone ileus. *AJR.* 1967;99:139–141.
67. Newmark H, Halls J, Silberman EL, et al. Two cases showing the radiographic appearance of Meckel's stones. *Am J Gastroenterol.* 1979;72:193–196.
68. Donaldson WG. Calculi in a Meckel's diverticulum: a case report and a review. *Aust N Z J Surg.* 1978;48:644–646.
69. Rudge FW. Meckel's stone ileus. *Mil Med.* 1992;157:98–100.
70. Meguid MM, Wilkinson RH, Canty T, et al. Futility of barium sulfate in diagnosis of bleeding Meckel's diverticulum. *Arch Surg.* 1974;108:361–362.
71. Maglinte DDT, Burney BT, Miller RE. Lesions missed on small bowel follow-through: analysis and recommendations. *Radiology.* 1982;144:737–739.
72. Dixon PM, Nolan DJ. The diagnosis of Meckel's diverticulum: a continuing challenge. *Clin Radiol.* 1987;38:615–619.
73. Ikard RW. Diagnosis of Meckel's diverticulum by computerized tomography. *Tenn Med.* 1996;89:164–165.
74. Daneman A, Myers M, Shuckett B, Alton DJ. Sonographic appearance of inverted Meckel diverticulum with intussusception. *Pediatr Radiol.* 1997;27:295–298.
75. Blakeborough A, McWilliams RG, Raja U, et al. Pseudolipoma of inverted Meckel diverticulum: clinical, radiological and pathological correlation. *Eur Radiol.* 1997;7:900–904.
76. Frazzini VI Jr, English WJ, Bashist B, Moore E. Case report. Small bowel obstruction due to phytobezoar formation within Meckel diverticulum. CT findings. *J Comput Assist Tomogr.* 1996;20:390–392.
77. Hamada T, Ishida O, Yasutomi M. Inverted Meckel diverticulum with intussusception: demonstration by CT. *J Comput Assist Tomogr.* 1995;19:808–810.
78. Halstead AE. Intestinal obstruction from Meckel's diverticulum. *Ann Surg.* 1902;35:471–494.
79. Crosthwaite GL, Leather AJ. Laparoscopy: the ultimate diagnostic tool for a bleeding Meckel's diverticulum. *Aust N Z J Surg.* 1997;67:223–224.
80. Petrokubi RJ, Braum S, Rohrer GV. Cimetidine administration resulting in improved pertechnetate imaging of Meckel's diverticulum. *Clin Nuc Med.* 1978;3:385–388.
81. Berardi RS. Anomalies of midgut rotation in the adult. *Surg Gynecol Obstet.* 1980;151:113–124.
82. Snyder WH, Chaffin L. Embryology and pathology of the intestinal tract: presentation of 40 cases of malrotation. *Ann Surg.* 1954;140:368–379.
83. Rees JR, Redo SF. Anomalies of intestinal rotation and fixation. *Am J Surg.* 1968;116:834–841.
84. Balthazar EJ. Intestinal malrotation in adults: roentgenologic assessment with emphasis on isolated complete and partial nonrotation. *AJR.* 1976;126:358–367.
85. DePrima SJ, Hardy DC, Brant WE. Reversed intestinal rotation. *Radiology.* 1985;157:603–604.
86. Deitch EA, Engel JM. Anomalies of gut rotation mimicking appendicitis in the adult. *Am Surg.* 1988;46:226–229.
87. Berdon WE, Baker DH, Bull S, et al. Midgut malrotation and volvulus. *Radiology.* 1970;96:367–383.
88. Andrassy RJ, Mahour GH. Malrotation of the midgut in infants and children. *Arch Surg.* 1981;116:158–160.
89. Pracros JP, Sann L, Genin G, et al. Ultrasound diagnosis of midgut volvulus: the whirlpool sign. *Pediatr Radiol.* 1992;22:18.
90. Fukuya T, Brown BP, Lu CC. Midgut volvulus as a complication of intestinal rotation in adults. *Dig Dis Sci.* 1993;38:438–444.
91. Loyer E, Eggli KD. Sonographic evidence of superior mesenteric vascular relationship in malrotation. *Pediatr Radiol.* 1989;19:173–175.
92. Ablow RC, Hotter FA, Seashore JH, et al. Z-shaped duodenojejunal loop: sign of mesenteric fixation and congenital bands. *AJR.* 1983;141:461.
93. Berdon WE. The diagnosis of malrotation and volvulus in the older child and adult: a trap for radiologists. *Pediatr Radiol.* 1995;25:101–103.
94. Paul AB, Dean DM. Computed tomography in volvulus of the midgut. *Br J Radiol.* 1990;63:893–894.
95. Nichols DM, Li DK. Superior mesenteric vein rotation. A CT sign of midgut malrotation. *AJR.* 1983;141:707–708.
96. Shatzes D, Gordon PH, Haller JD, et al. Malrotation of the bowel: malalignment of the superior mesenteric artery-vein complex shown by CT and MR. *J Comput Assist Tomogr.* 1990;14:93–95.
97. Zerin JM, DiPietro MA. Mesenteric vascular anatomy at CT: normal and abnormal appearance. *Radiology.* 1991;199:739–742.
98. Sing RF, Blasko EC, Kefalides PT, Wolferth CC. Management of anomalous rotation in adults. *Am Surg.* 1994;60:938–941.
99. Gilbert HW, Armstrong CP, Thompson MH. The presentation of malrotation of the intestine in adults. *Ann R Coll Surg Engl.* 1990;72:239–242.
100. Cathgart RS, Williamson B, Gregorie HB, Glasgow PF.

Surgical treatment of midgut nonrotation in the adult patients. *Surg Gynecol Obstet.* 1981;152:207–210.
101. Kern IB, Curie BG. The presentation of malrotation of the intestine in adults. *Ann R Coll Surg Engl.* 1990;72:239–242.
102. Zimmerman LM, Laufman HL. Intraabdominal hernias due to developmental and rotational anomalies. *Ann Surg.* 1953;138:82–91.
103. Bertelsen S, Christiansen J. Internal hernia through mesenteric and mesocolic defects: a review of the literature and a report of two cases. *Acta Chir Scand.* 1967;133:426–428.
104. Hansmann GH, Morton SA. Intraabdominal hernia. Report of a case and review of the literature. *Arch Surg.* 1939;39:973–986.
105. Ghahremani GG. Internal abdominal hernias. *Surg Clin North Am.* 1984;64:393–406.
106. Meyers MA. Paraduodenal hernias. Radiologic and arteriographic diagnosis. *Radiology.* 1970;95:29–37.
107. Meyers MA. *Dynamic radiology of the abdomen: Normal and Pathologic Anatomy.* 3rd ed. Chapter 10, Internal Abdominal Hernias. New York, NY: Springer Verlag; 1988:424–435.
108. Newsom BD, Kukora JS. Congenital and acquired internal hernias: unusual causes of small bowel obstruction. *Am J Surg.* 1986;152:279–285.
109. Bartlett MK, Wang C, Williams WH. The surgical management of paraduodenal hernia. *Ann Surg.* 1968;108:249–254.
110. Turley K. Right paraduodenal hernia. A source of chronic abdominal pain in the adult. *Arch Surg.* 1979;114:1072–1074.
111. Murphy DA. Internal hernias in infancy and childhood. *Surgery.* 1964;55:311–316.
112. Day DL, Drake DG, Leonard AS, Letourneau JG. CT findings in left paraduodenal hernia. *Gastrointest Radiol.* 1988;13:27–29.
113. Passas V, Karavias D, Grilias D, Birbas A. Computed tomography of left paraduodenal hernia. *J Comput Asst Tomogr.* 1986;10:542–543.
114. Warshauer DM, Mauro MA. CT diagnosis of paraduodenal hernia. *Gastrointest Radiol.* 1992;17:13–15.
115. Dole SD. Left paraduodenal hernia: report of a case, with radiographic findings, including abdominal computed tomography. *J Am Osteopathic Assoc.* 1987;87:556–559.
116. Ohkuma R, Miyazaki K. Hernia through the foramen of Winslow. *Jpn J Surg.* 1977;7:151–157.
117. Richardson JB, Anastopoulos HA. Hernia through the foramen of Winslow. *Md Med J.* 1981;30:56–59.
118. Henisz A, Matesanz J, Westcott JL. Cecal herniation through the foramen of Winslow. *Radiology.* 1974;112:575–578.
119. Harned RK, Farley GE. Herniation of cecum and terminal ileum through the foramen of Winslow. *Am J Gastroenterol.* 1974;61:304–307.
120. Stankey R. Intestinal herniation through the foramen of Winslow. *Radiology.* 1967;89:929–930.
121. Lemish W, Cameron D. Cecal herniation through the foramen of Winslow. *Australas Radiol.* 1989;33:109–110.
122. Dainko EA. Incarcerated foramen of Winslow hernia. *Surg Clin North Am.* 1970;50:1015–1020.
123. Yasuda S, Inatsugi N, Sakurai T, et al. A case of intestinal obstruction due to a hernia traversing the lesser sac. *Jpn J Surg.* 1989;19:70–73.
124. Ratcliffe J, Tait J, Lisle D, Leditschke JF, Bell J. Segmental dilatation of the small bowel: report of three cases and literature review. *Radiology.* 1989;171:827–830.
125. Morewood DJW, Cunningham ME. Case report: segmental dilatation of the ileum presenting with anaemia. *Clin Radiol.* 1985;36:267–268.
126. Usselman JA, Ghahremani GG, Bordin GM, et al. Idiopathic localized dilatation of the ileum in adults. *Gastrointest Radiol.* 1981;6:313–317.
127. Maglinte DDT. The small bowel: miscellaneous considerations. In: Taveras JM, Ferrucci JT, eds. *Radiology.* Philadelphia, Pa: JB Lippincott Co; 1986:1–8.
128. Javors BR, Gold RP, Ghahremani GG, et al. Idiopathic localized dilatation of the ileum in adults: findings on barium studies. *AJR.* 1995;164:87–90.
129. Herlinger H. Miscellaneous disorders. In: Gore RM, Levine MS, Laufer I, eds. *Textbook of Gastrointestinal Radiology.* Philadelphia, Pa: WB Saunders Co; 1994:997–1016.
130. Bell MJ, Ternberg JL, Bower RJ. Ileal dysgenesis in infants and children. *J Pediatr Surg.* 1982;17:395–399.

Crohn's Disease

15

Frederick M. Kelvin and Hans Herlinger

Chapter Contents

Etiology
Clinical Considerations
Pathology
Imaging Techniques
Radiology of Barium Examinations
Evolution of Disease
Diffuse Jejunoileitis
Complications
Assessment of Disease Activity
Differential Diagnosis

Excluding malignant neoplasms, Crohn's disease is the most devastating disease commonly involving the gastrointestinal tract. Initially, this disease was not recognized as a separate identity but was regarded as a nonspecific granuloma usually related to chronic appendicitis or ileal tuberculosis.[1] It was not until 1932 that Crohn, Ginzburg, and Oppenheimer described the clinical and pathologic findings as a distinct disease entity.[2]

Crohn's disease has a worldwide distribution with different levels of prevalence. The disease is most common in Northern Europe and in North America and is infrequent in Asia (except for Japan), Central America, and South America. Its incidence has increased in recent years and now seems to have reached a plateau.[3] The disease most commonly affects young adults, with a peak between 15 and 25 years.[3] A previously suggested second peak in the elderly is probably due to unrecognized ischemic colitis. However, patients who develop Crohn's disease when over 50 years old have a significantly greater likelihood of left colonic involvement.[4] Both sexes are equally affected. The disease appears to be more common in Jews, particularly those born in Europe or America as opposed to Israeli-born Jews.[3] There is a tendency for the disease to cluster in families.

Etiology

One of the earliest lesions in Crohn's disease is an ulceration that overlies lymph follicles, a lesion that is associated with active inflammation and contiguous granulomatous change. This association suggests that an infectious agent may have gained access through the overlying epithelium. Possible causal agents include the mycobacterium *M paratuberculosis*,[5] which has been isolated from some patients with Crohn's disease, and the measles virus, as this has been found at sites of vascular damage in Crohn's disease.[6] It has also been suggested that the disease may be caused by immune-mediated injury rather than a specific infection.[7] Furthermore, as Crohn's disease often occurs in several members of a family, there appears to be a genetic predisposition. Clearly, the precise etiology of Crohn's disease remains elusive.

Clinical Considerations

Most patients present with recurrent episodes of diarrhea, abdominal pain, and sustained weight loss. This chapter will deal almost exclusively with small intestinal Crohn's disease; however, differences in presentation from colonic Crohn's disease need to be recognized. For example, Crohn's colitis is more likely to be associated with rectal bleeding, perianal fistulae, and extraintestinal complications.[8] Disease confined to the ileum has a better prognosis, though complications such as abscess formation and obstruction may develop. Diarrhea is usually moderate in severity. Abdominal pain is frequently localized to the right lower quadrant, is usually steady, and reflects involvement of the terminal ileum. Cramping pain may indicate partial small bowel obstruction. Fever is present in about half the patients, is usually low grade, and is possibly caused by absorption of bacterial toxins or products of tissue breakdown. Weight loss is common and is related to anorexia and to protein-losing enteropathy. A secondary dissaccharidase deficiency may increase diarrhea by its osmotic effect and cause further weight loss. Anemia is a frequent finding and is due to a combination of malabsorption of folate, vitamin B_{12}, and iron, and to low-level blood loss. Clinical evidence of malabsorption suggests extensive small bowel involvement. A mass in the right lower quadrant is a fairly common finding. Usually, the mass is small and represents thickened and inflamed distal ileum. More severe inflammation may cause matting of adjacent loops of ileum and may lead to the formation of a larger palpable mass.[8]

Gastrointestinal symptoms may be minimal in children, in whom the disease may be present with predominantly extraintestinal manifestations. It is important to recognize that a child with Crohn's disease may present with growth retardation.

Extraintestinal manifestations may occur at any age. Hepatobiliary complications are the most frequent. About 30% of patients develop gallstones as a result of bile salt malabsorption caused by ileal disease or resection. Sclerosing cholangitis, and occasionally bile duct carcinoma, may occur. Hydronephrosis, generally on the right side, may result from ureteric compression by an adjacent inflammatory mass. Oxalate or urate stones in the urinary tract are a recognized complication. Sacroiliitis or a peripheral arthritis occurs in about 20% of patients. Other systemic complications include erythema nodosum, uveitis, and amyloidosis. Many of the skin, joint, and ocular manifestations appear to be related to the activity of the Crohn's disease itself, and in particular to the severity of colitis.

The disease is characterized by a prolonged and unpredictable course, with periods of exacerbation separated by remissions. In addition to episodes of small bowel obstruction, its course is often complicated by the development of abscesses or fistulae, as well as a high incidence of recurrence after surgical resection. An initial surgical procedure increases the likelihood of subsequent surgery.

Medical therapy is the mainstay of management in Crohn's disease. The specific therapeutic agents employed depend on the severity, location, and extent of the disease.[9] Corticosteroid therapy is used in moderate or severe disease in order to induce a remission, whereas sulfasalazine and mesalamine are preferred for maintenance therapy when the disease is mild. Assessment of disease activity is difficult because the clinical patterns of disease are relatively heterogeneous. The Crohn's Disease Activity Index has been developed as an indicator of activity but has been criticized because of its subjective elements.[9] Other methods of evaluating disease severity, including radiologic techniques, have therefore been proposed.[10]

Surgery is reserved for the treatment of complications or failure of medical therapy. Common indications for surgery include stricture causing persistent obstruction, symptomatic fistulae, and abscess formation. Less frequent indications include uncontrollable hemorrhage, free perforation, and inability to control extraintestinal manifestations.[11] For terminal ileal disease, the cecum and appendix are resected as well as the diseased small bowel. Appendicitis is thereby eliminated as a possible future cause of recurrent right lower quadrant pain.[11] Surgery should preserve as much small bowel as possible in order to prevent the short-bowel syndrome. To facilitate this goal, the technique of strictureplasty has been developed as an alternative to bowel resection.

Pathology

Noncaseating granulomas are considered a hallmark of the disease, but are only found in up to two thirds of biopsy specimens.[12] They are not essential for diagnosis, and other histopathologic features are often available. These include lymphocytic aggregates of transmural distribution, plasma cell infiltrates, and crypt abscesses.[12]

As mentioned previously, the main macroscopic findings at the earliest stage of disease are small erosions (aphthous ulcers) often located over enlarged lymph follicles. Histologic examination of biopsy specimens taken from areas of mucosa that appear normal by endoscopy or radiology may show active inflammation and even granulomas.[13]

The inflammatory process in more established disease extends discontinuously through the lamina propria, is most intense in the submucosa, but tends to involve all layers of the bowel wall. The aphthous ulcers may heal or may enlarge and coalesce to form deeper, usually linear ulcerations or fissures, which frequently assume a longitudinal or transverse orientation. Progression of the disease results in bowel wall thickening due to a combination of edema and fibrosis, and the fibrosis eventually leads to stricture formation. Adjacent loops of bowel often become matted together because the transmural inflammation has involved the serosa and mesentery. As a result, ulcers that have extended through the bowel wall may give rise to fistulae between contiguous loops. Alternatively, sinus tracts may end blindly within abscess cavities in the mesentery, the peritoneal cavity, or the extraperitoneal space. Free perforations are unusual.

"Fat Wrapping"

A thickened layer of subserosal fat is a frequent finding in advanced Crohn's disease. This finding has been referred to as "creeping fat" and "fibrofatty proliferation." Both terms are inappropriate; fat is incapable of self-propulsion and lipocytes do not proliferate. However, lipocytes can hypertrophy by an increased intracellular accumulation of fat globules. Two events have been suggested to explain the increase of subserosal fat in the bowel wall.[14] Transmural perivascular inflammation fans out into the mesentery; fibrosis and contraction develop and tether hypertrophied fat into the bowel wall. In addition, the muscularis propria contracts longitudinally to accentuate the subserosal accumulation of the fat.[14]

Granulomas do not occur in Crohn's disease only. Aphthous ulcers, and even fissures, can be observed in other inflammatory conditions. Diagnosis based on macroscopic or microscopic pathology is often inconclusive and usually requires correlation with clinical findings and radiologic and/or endoscopic interpretation, as well as the response to treatment. Diagnosis is optimally based on a team approach.

Distribution

Crohn's disease may involve any portion of the digestive tract from mouth to anus. Combined involvement of colon and terminal ileum is the most frequent pattern and is seen in approximately 55% of patients. Disease confined to the small bowel occurs in about 30% of patients. Of this group; 14% have involvement of the terminal ileum alone, 13% have disease extending from the terminal ileum into the more proximal intestine, and 3% have disease of proximal small bowel with sparing of the terminal ileum.[13] In children, sparing of the terminal ileum occurs more frequently (approximately 20%); there is a significantly higher frequency of duodenal/jejunal disease in this age group.[15] In about 15% of cases, only the colon is diseased. Characteristically, diseased segments are separated by intervening lengths of apparently normal bowel. This discontinuous involvement is another hallmark of Crohn's disease.

Imaging Techniques

Radiologic investigation has a diverse role in Crohn's disease. It may be used to confirm or exclude the diagnosis, to show the extent of disease prior to surgery, to help assess disease activity, to diagnose its complications, and to detect postoperative recurrence.

Plain Abdominal Radiography

Plain abdominal radiographs should be obtained in a patient who presents with an acute abdomen. The most common abnormality is small bowel obstruction. In a patient with chronic disease, the presence of gas-filled loops in the right lower quadrant suggests complicated disease. Gallstones or urinary tract calculi may be identified. Pneumoperitoneum is highly unusual.

Barium Studies

An accurate, well-performed barium examination is pivotal for detecting and showing the extent of Crohn's disease. Even though an experienced endoscopist can enter the terminal ileum in approximately 80% of patients during colonoscopy, enteroscopy is currently not available in routine clinical practice. The traditional small bowel follow-through study is associated with a significant number of false-negative results.[16] This contributes to the considerable delay between onset of symptoms and diagnosis, which is as much as 2 to 4 years when the disease is limited to the small bowel.[17] In addition, a number of patients in whom the diagnosis of Crohn's disease is based on follow-through studies are shown not to have the disease when examined by more sensitive methods. The National Cooperative Crohn's Disease Study published in 1979 was based mostly on follow-through examinations, many done with inadequate amounts of barium.[18] In many cases, one or more segments of bowel were inadequately defined and could not be evaluated. The panel of radiologists reviewing this cooperative study concluded that the nature and extent of Crohn's disease in these patients should be interpreted with caution.[18] The problem of incomplete radiographic demonstration of the small bowel persists to this day. Because the majority of the small bowel is not generally evaluated by endoscopy, barium radiology retains a major responsibility in Crohn's disease, and it is the duty of the radiologist to select that method of barium examination that is most appropriate to the clinical situation.[19]

Although diagnostic problems related to Crohn's disease are often best demonstrated by enteroclysis, a small bowel follow-through that tests the entire intestinal tract by intermittent fluoroscopy and combines it with adequate palpation can approach the accuracy of enteroclysis.[20] The radiologic literature provides the following range of detection rates for small bowel Crohn's disease: 89% to 97% for peroral methods[21] and 83% to 100% for enteroclysis.[22-25] The addition of a peroral pneumocolon[26] to the "dedicated" barium follow-through has been strongly recommended by Glick[27]; this approach is valuable whenever distal ileal Crohn's disease is suspected (Fig. 15-1). By this technique, the distal 20 to 50 cm of ileum can be shown in double contrast in 80% of patients. It is particularly effective in the presence of ileal resection. In such patients, the usually unimpeded retrograde flow of barium and air during a double-contrast barium enema may produce even more reliable images of the neoterminal and distal ileum than the peroral pneumocolon. Obviously, both the peroral pneumocolon and the barium enema suffer from the disadvantage of not providing any demonstration of the more proximal small bowel.

At one of the authors' institutions, enteroclysis is used routinely for evaluating patients with known or suspected small bowel Crohn's disease. However, there are certain circumstances in which the use of enteroclysis has particular merit. These include: 1) to rule out or confirm Crohn's disease in patients already treated, but in whom there is doubt concerning the validity of the original diagnosis; 2) when there is an exacerbation of obstructive features and it may be useful to distinguish a fibrous stricture from an actively ulcerated stenotic segment; 3) preoperatively, to assess the extent of disease and rule out the presence of skip lesions; and 4) to demonstrate the early mucosal changes of Crohn's disease.

The radiologic findings of small bowel Crohn's disease are described in detail in a subsequent part of this chapter.

Computed Tomography (CT)

The early mucosal changes of Crohn's disease cannot be shown by CT. The strength of CT lies in its ability to demonstrate the transmural extent of inflammation, associated mesenteric inflammatory changes, abscess and fistula formation, and the extraintestinal complications of Crohn's disease.[28-30] The CT features of Crohn's disease have been elegantly described and illustrated in a review by Gore et al.[31]

Bowel wall thickening (greater than 3 mm when fully distended and imaged transaxially) is clearly depicted by CT (Fig. 15-2). When acute inflammation is present, the thickened wall often shows a "target" or "double-halo" appearance (Fig. 15-3) in which the intermediate low-density ring represents submucosal edema or fat infiltration. The inner ring of mucosa and the outer ring of muscle layer and serosa may demonstrate intense enhancement if the inflammation is severe.

A palpable mass or separation of small bowel loops on barium examination may be due to a variety of

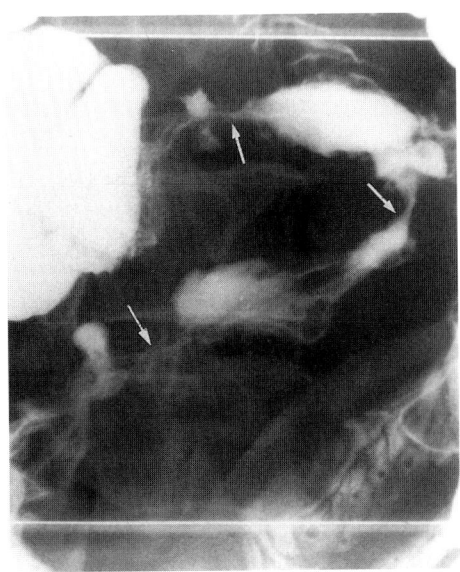 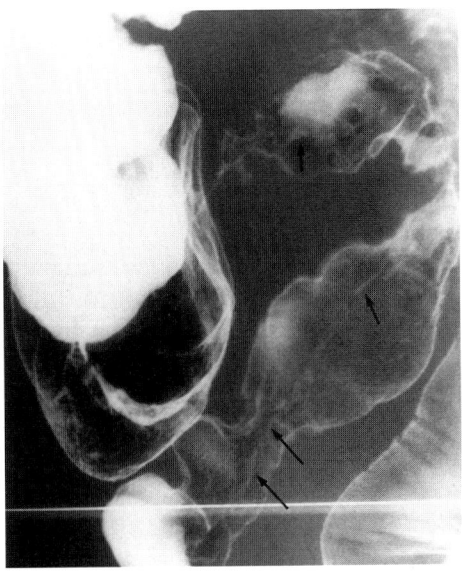

(a) (b)

Fig. 15-1. Benefit of performing peroral pneumocolon in Crohn's disease.
(a) Small bowel follow-through shows severe involvement of the terminal ileum. The appearances suggest multiple tight strictures (arrows) but there is no mucosal detail. (b) Peroral pneumocolon at end of follow-through examination shows much better luminal distention. The strictures are less severe than suggested by the follow-through, and there are numerous linear ulcerations (arrows) indicating the presence of active inflammation.

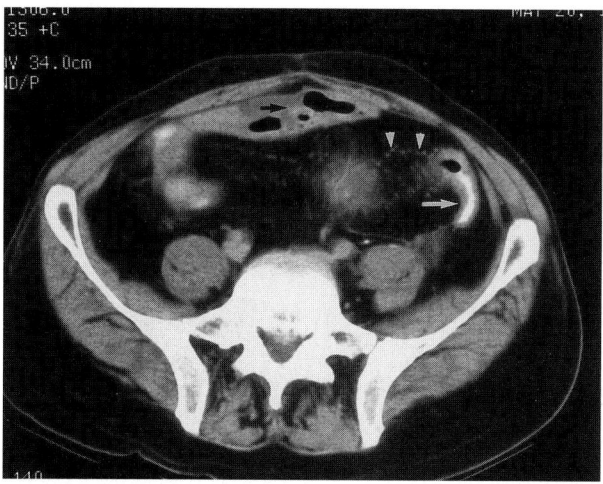

Fig. 15-2. Bowel wall thickening and mesenteric vascular dilatation shown by CT.
A segment of small bowel exhibits mural thickening and luminal narrowing (white arrow). Minimally dilated vessels (arrowheads) are present in the adjacent mesentery. There are matted loops of small bowel (black arrow) located underneath the anterior abdominal wall.

causes: abscess, phlegmon, fibrofatty proliferation, bowel wall thickening, and enlarged mesenteric nodes.[31] CT distinguishes between these causes, which helps direct patient management. This is particularly relevant during an acute flare-up of the disease, as CT is the procedure of choice for detection of an intra-abdominal or pelvic abscess and, if appropriate, for percutaneous drainage of the abscess. So-called fibrofatty proliferation of the mesentery is manifested by blurring of the interface between bowel and mesentery and increased attenuation of mesenteric fat (Fig. 15-3).

Extraintestinal manifestations that may be identified on CT scans include gallstones, sclerosing cholangitis (Fig. 15-4), urinary tract calculi, hydronephrosis, sacroileitis, and osteomyelitis (usually secondary to an adjacent pelvic abscess or fistula).[31] When performing abdominopelvic CT in Crohn's disease, it is important to include the entire perineum, as CT may demonstrate perianal or perirectal abscesses or fistulae.

Spiral CT has the added capability of demonstrating alterations of the vascular pattern near or within the bowel wall. These changes consist of vascular dilatation (see Fig. 15-3), tortuosity, and prominence of the vasa recta; the last appearance has been referred to as the "comb sign".[32]

CT enteroclysis, which involves the performance of CT following an infusion of a large volume of methylcellulose solution or water-soluble contrast, is a recently developed alternative to standard enteroclysis examination.[33,34] This technique combines some of the intraluminal findings seen on biphasic enteroclysis with the ability of CT to show extraluminal changes (Fig. 15-5).

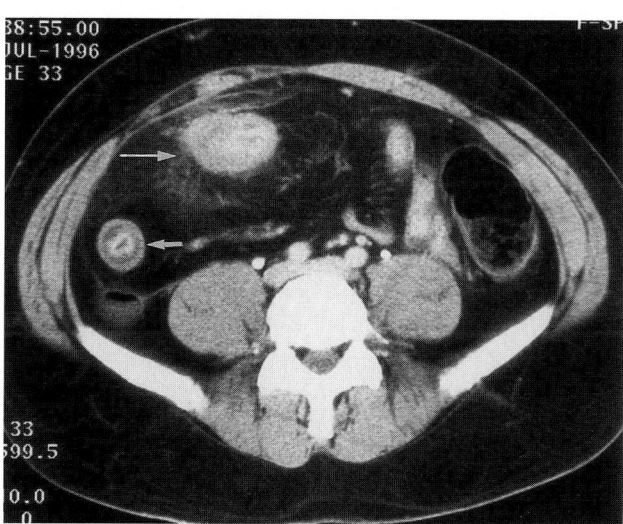

Fig. 15-3. "Target" appearance of acutely inflamed small bowel.
A section of small bowel imaged transaxially shows marked stratification (short arrow) with an enhancing inner ring of mucosa and an outer enhanced ring of muscularis and serosa, separated by edematous submucosa; this constitutes the "target" sign. An adjacent loop of small bowel (longer arrow) demonstrates mild perienteric inflammatory change.

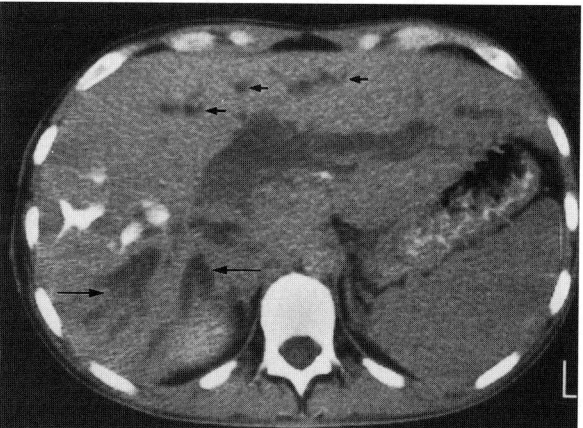

Fig. 15-4. Changes of sclerosing cholangitis complicating Crohn's disease demonstrated by CT.
The presence of a focal cluster of dilated intrahepatic ducts (long arrows) and discontinuous areas of minimal intrahepatic bile duct dilatation (short arrows) is suggestive of sclerosing cholangitis. Note residual contrast in dilated branches of right hepatic duct from preceding endoscopic retrograde cholangiopancreatography. (Courtesy of Dr Richard Gore, Evanston, IL.)

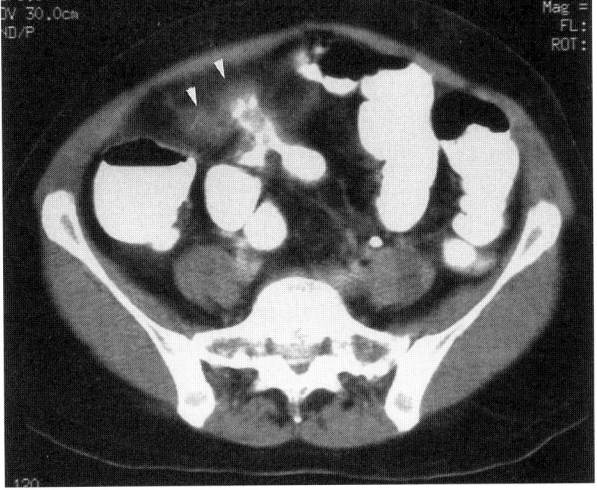

(a)

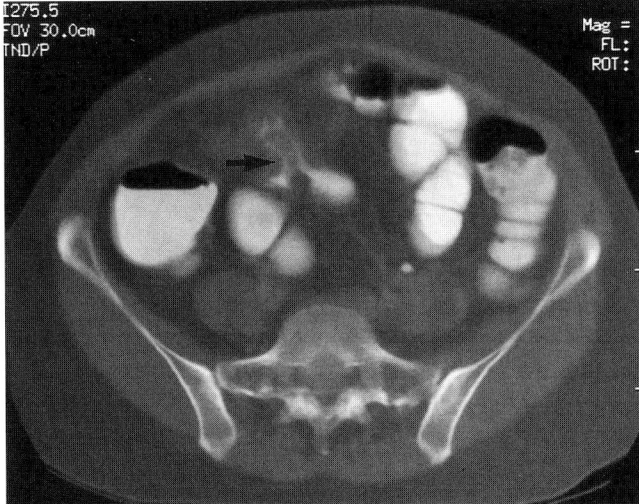

(b)

(c)

Fig. 15-5. CT enteroclysis of small bowel Crohn's disease. (a) Section through upper abdomen shows normal, well-distended loops of proximal small bowel. "Small bowel window" setting (W = 3665, L = 808). (b) Section at lower level demonstrates a segment of irregular narrowing in the distal ileum (arrow). Same setting as in (a). (c) Same section as (b) but at soft-tissue window setting shows soft-tissue mesenteric inflammatory changes (arrowheads) contiguous with involved segment (W = 400, L = 40). (Courtesy of Col Greg Bender, MD, Washington, DC.)

Ultrasonography (US)

US has a variety of applications in Crohn's disease.[35] Because many patients are young and undergo repeated evaluations of their disease process, there is considerable interest in utilizing US. On transabdominal US, thickened small bowel produces the "target" or "pseudokidney" sign when imaged transversely and the rigid loop sign when shown in longitudinal section (Fig. 15-6).[36] These US changes are nonspecific, as they may be seen in a wide variety of inflammatory disorders. A sensitivity of 87% to 95% for the detection of Crohn's disease has been shown, and it has therefore been suggested that US can be used to select patients for barium examination.[36,37] A more recent study emphasized that, while US is a sensitive method of detection, it clearly underestimates the extent of involvement because of its inability to identify mildly diseased segments.[38] In some institutions, high-resolution US is the modality of choice for screening patients with suspected inflammatory bowel disease and is performed if standard abdominal US is negative.[39] (See also Chapter 8.)

Nuclear Medicine Studies

Mucosal infiltration with leukocytes is a characteristic histological feature in inflammatory bowel disease. This forms the basis for the use of labeled leukocyte imaging in Crohn's disease. The most widely used radioisotopes for labeling leukocytes are indium-111 tropolonate (^{111}In) and technetium-99m hexamethyl propylene amine oxime (^{99m}Tc HMPAO).[40] Scanning with ^{111}In has been shown to have a sensitivity of 70% compared with barium examination[41]; results with [99mTc] HMPAO are somewhat better.[40] (For further information see Chapter 11.)

Magnetic Resonance Imaging (MRI)

MRI of the abdomen was initially hampered by motion artifact and poor contrast resolution. These limitations have been overcome by the use of breath-hold techniques. Gadolinium-enhanced fat-suppressed MRI is a sensitive method for detecting Crohn's disease. The typical appearance in Crohn's disease is a segment of bowel wall showing high signal intensity and a thickness exceeding 4 mm.[42] MR findings of bowel wall thickness, length of involved bowel, and degree of contrast enhancement all showed a significant correlation with the endoscopic and histologic findings.[43] A further application of MRI is the assessment of perianal fistulae and sinus tracts, for which it has already emerged as the procedure of choice.[44] It is almost certain that MRI will be increasingly used in the future for the evaluation of small bowel disease. As with US, it has the benefit of avoiding radiation exposure in a frequently young patient population. (See Chapter 10.)

Radiology of Barium Examinations

The barium findings in Crohn's disease are numerous and depend upon the stage of the disease and its location. Alterations can be functional or organic.

Functional Disturbances

Motor disturbances, either hypermotility or hypomotility, are a result of the inflammatory process. The "string sign" is an expression of marked irritability and spasm; the area of narrowing often widens as the peristaltic wave reaches the affected segment. Hyperperistalsis may occur proximal to an area of narrowing. An early recurrence may be associated with motility disturbances, the small bowel being dilated and hypotonic.

In the acute phase or when an extensive jejunoileitis is present, excessive luminal fluid and exudate can produce flocculation and dilution of peroral barium. Radiographically, the interface between the intraluminal barium and the mucosa then appears blurred instead of sharply demarcated.[45] This may be a factor in favor of the use of enteroclysis, which can achieve a more detailed fold pattern in these circumstances.[46,47]

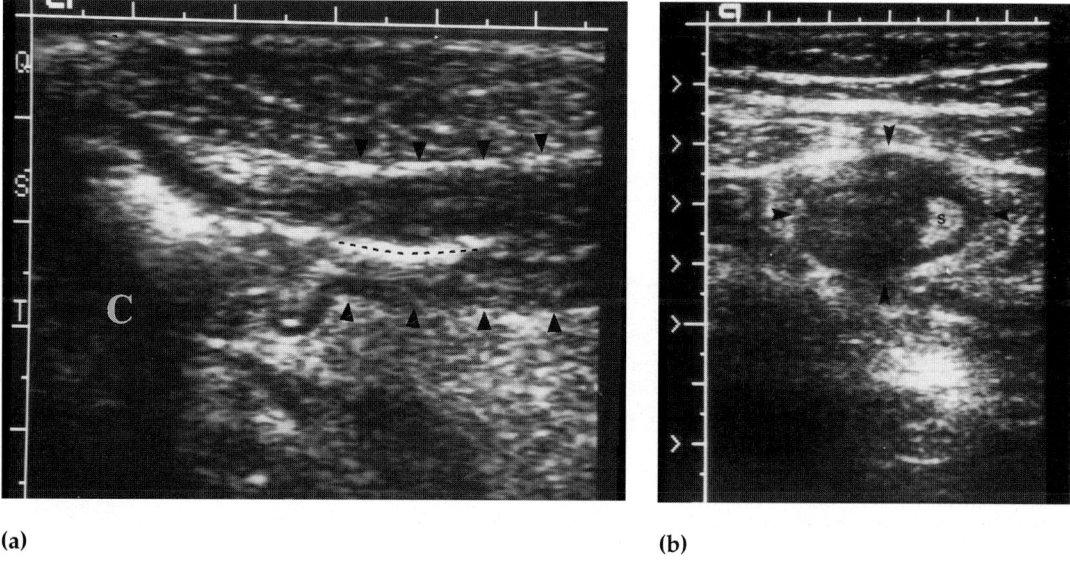

(a) (b)

Fig. 15-6. Appearances by ultrasonography.
(a) Longitudinal section shows markedly thickened bowel wall between bowel lumen (dotted black line) and serosal margin (arrowheads) due to severe changes of Crohn's disease in terminal ileum. (C = cecum). (Courtesy of Dr Bill Charboneau, Rochester, MN.) (b) Crohn's ileitis with fibrosis. Transverse section shows an almost completely hypoechoic wall without differentiation of its layers (arrowheads). Only a small amount of hyperechoic submucosa (s) is preserved. Such asymmetry is characteristic of Crohn's disease. Surrounding fat is slightly edematous. (Courtesy of M. Rioux, MD, Quebec, Canada.)

Organic Abnormalities

Organic abnormalities may be classified as alterations of the villous pattern, fold abnormalities, polypoid lesions, ulcerations, signs of fibrosis, and mesenteric abnormalities.

Abnormalities of the Villous Pattern

Normally, three to seven intestinal villi occupy an area of 1 mm^2; they are infrequently demonstrated during enteroclysis. A granular pattern coarser than that due to normal villi has been reported in 39 of 46 consecutive cases of Crohn's disease[48]; in some of these cases it was the only evidence of small bowel involvement. A later publication confirmed this finding in Crohn's disease, as well as in other inflammatory conditions, ischemia, and radiation damage.[49] We have also seen this coarse villous pattern in *Yersinia ileitis* and in the proximal jejunum after Billroth II gastric surgery. In our experience, supported by the study of surgical specimens, a diffuse reticular network of round or occasionally angular radiolucent foci, 0.5 to 1.0 mm in diameter, is a frequent finding on the mucosal surface of the small intestine in Crohn's disease [Fig. 15-7(a–c)]. At times these foci are slightly larger (1 to

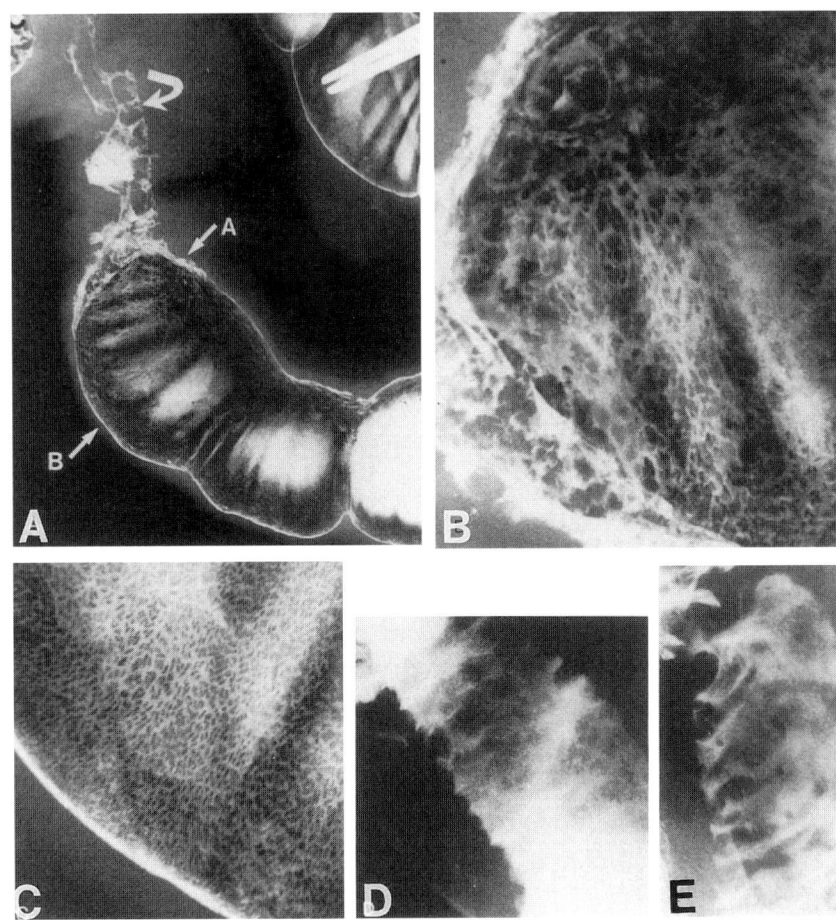

Fig. 15-7. Villous pattern in Crohn's disease.
(a) Resected specimen of terminal ileum outlined in double contrast. The distal terminal ileum (curved arrow) shows advanced Crohn's disease. Next to it (arrow, zone A), there is an intermediary zone of coarse granularity. Proximal to it (arrow, zone B), the degree of granularity seems to be fading. (b) Photographic enlargement of zone A. The foci of this pattern are large and irregular, imparting a very coarse granularity. The intervillous grooves are pronounced. Histology showed marked villous atrophy. (c) Photographic enlargement of zone B. The foci are small and of similar size. The intervillous grooves produce a regular pattern. This appearance of coarse granularity resembles but exceeds the normal villous pattern; the latter can occasionally be demonstrated on high-definition radiographic systems, using high-density barium suspensions. (d) In another patient, diffuse coarse granularity is shown in single contrast with compression and in association with fold thickening, nodularity, and a few aphthous ulcers. The margin of the mucosal surface shows a shaggy outline. (e) Coarse granularity, aphthous ulcers, and fold thickening can be features of early recurrent Crohn's disease in the neoterminal ileum.

2 mm) and have a patchy distribution. The granularity increases in coarseness adjacent to erosions or near a superficial abscess and may then be appreciated also on single-contrast barium studies [Fig. 15-7(d, e)]. It may also be seen in an otherwise normal-appearing segment between two areas of advanced disease, suggesting that what seem to be skip lesions are actually part of a continuous process.

Even when associated with other superficial mucosal changes, the granular pattern tends to occupy the more proximal bowel segments.[49] It has been observed proximal to an enterocolic anastomosis as well as proximal to more obvious radiologic changes (Fig. 15-8).[49] Histologic sections of areas of coarse granularity demonstrate a chronic inflammatory cell infiltrate, with blunted, clubbed villi or villi fused by exudate.

Fold Abnormalities

Mucosal and submucosal edema secondary to lymphatic obstruction and the inflammatory process may cause thickening and distortion of valvulae conniventes [Fig. 15-9(a)]. These fold changes are frequently seen in Crohn's disease[50,51] and may be the only evidence of an early, more proximal skip lesion [Fig. 15-9(b)]. The thickened folds may appear straightened, fused, or nodular [Fig. 15-9(c, d)]. Asymmetric thickening is not uncommon. These fold changes may be an early manifestation of recurrent disease in the neoterminal ileum [Fig. 15-9(e)] but are more frequently seen adjacent to more advanced lesions. Detailed radiography with compression often reveals associated aphthous ulcers and a coarse villous pattern. The thickened folds may then appear finely nodular and granular. At other times, folds of normal thickness may appear distorted, fused, or interrupted, with interspersed areas without folds. Many investigators[52–55] have considered fold abnormalities to be among the earliest features of enteric Crohn's disease. Similar changes can also be seen in radiation ileitis, ischemia, and occasionally lymphoma.[56]

Absence of folds is an uncommon finding (Fig. 15-10) and may be associated with focal widening of the lumen and loss of peristalsis. This is probably a reflection of mucosal atrophy associated with quiescent long-standing inflammation.[57]

Polypoid Lesions

A polyp is a mass that protrudes into the lumen, arising more often from the mucosa than the submucosa. The term has no histologic connotation and can be applied to neoplastic or focal inflammatory elevations ("inflammatory polyp").[58]

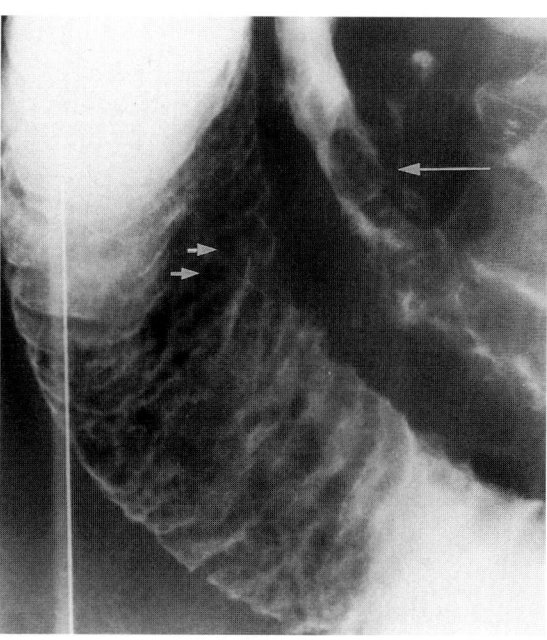

Fig. 15-8. Coarse villous pattern of Crohn's disease proximal to more severe disease.
An area of stricture formation with associated sinus tracts is present in the distal ileum (long arrow). A dilated loop of more proximal small bowel shows the superficial changes of a coarse granular pattern, fold thickening, and a few aphthous ulcers (short arrows).

The term "pseudopolyps" refers to islands of relatively normal mucosa surrounded by areas of mucosal denudation, giving the false impression of being elevated above mucosal level.[58] "Postinflammatory polyps" are focal excrescences of regenerated mucosa surrounded by healed epithelial surfaces. They are a frequent finding in colonic Crohn's disease but are rare in the small bowel. When seen in the small bowel they form well-defined, round- or oval-filling defects, usually in an area of absent folds (Fig. 15-11).[45,50,53,59]

Multiple polypoid elevations can produce a radiographic appearance to which the descriptive term "cobblestoning" has been applied. However, this pattern can be caused by two different pathologic entities that represent different stages of the disease process. It is therefore important to distinguish between these similar radiographic patterns. The infrequently seen "nodular pattern" is characterized by the juxtaposition of numerous polyps separated by grooves. The nodular defects are the main radiographic feature and are of fairly uniform size, usually less than 1 cm in diameter. The grooves may produce curved lines of barium trapped between the nodules. The presence of nodules causes notching of the bowel margin. Importantly, there is little or no luminal narrowing (Fig. 15-12). Ulcerations, if present, are shallow.

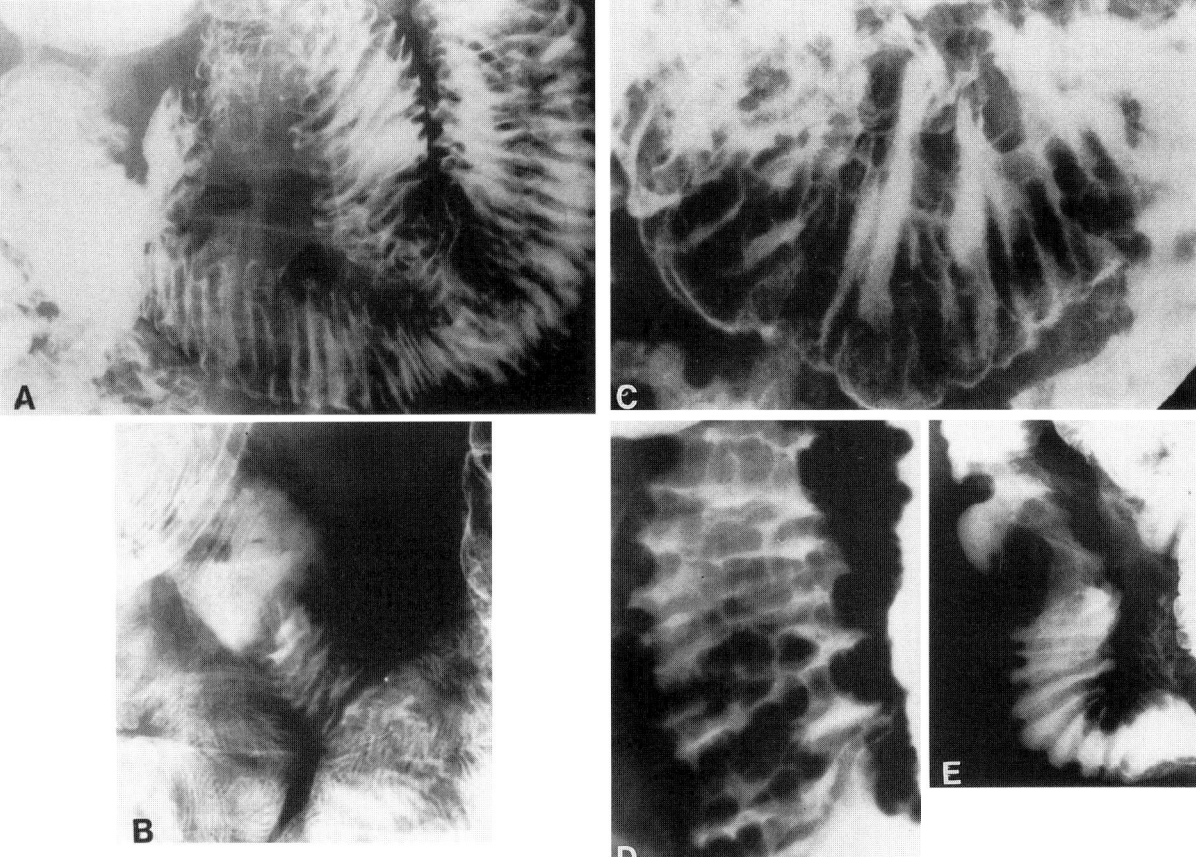

Fig. 15-9. Fold changes in Crohn's disease.
(a) Diffuse Crohn's disease of the jejunum appears as thick, straight folds indicating mucosal and submucosal inflammatory change. Some areas show mild lumen narrowing due to spasm. (b) Segment of proximal jejunum with fold thickening and restricted distensibility. This finding represents an early skip lesion with more advanced disease in the distal ileum. (By permission from Herlinger.[51]) (c) In a slightly more advanced stage of the disease, nodules are superimposed on fold thickening. A coarse villous pattern is also seen. (d) A more severely diseased segment of the ileum shows pronounced nodularity superimposed on thickened folds. (e) Crohn's disease recurrence in the neoterminal ileum shown as fold thickening with a few aphthous ulcers close to the anastomosis.

The "ulceronodular pattern" results from a combination of intersecting longitudinal, transverse, and oblique linear ulcers that surround residual islands of mucosa, which may be slightly elevated by underlying inflammatory edema ("pseudopolyps"). The main radiologic findings are barium-filled ulcerations that are larger, more irregular, and straighter than the curving lines seen with the "nodular pattern" [Fig. 15-13(a)]. The shallow elevations are of varying size and shape and do not cause the same degree of notching of the bowel margin that is seen with the "nodular pattern." This "ulceronodular pattern" represents a more advanced stage of the disease, with more pronounced fibrosis, reduced pliability, and luminal narrowing [Figs. 15-13(b–d)]. The term "cobblestone pattern" should be applied only to this more advanced form of Crohn's disease.

Ulcerations

The radiologic appearance of the ulcers depends upon their shape, size, and depth; upon the changes in the surrounding mucosa; and also upon the technique employed.

"*Aphthous ulcers*" appear radiologically as shallow depressions, 1 to 2 mm in diameter, often surrounded by elevations ("halos") [Fig. 15-14 and 15-15].[60,61] The same pattern of aphthous lesions has also been identified in Crohn's disease of the esophagus, stomach, duodenum, and colon. Aphthous ulcerations are usually multiple and sometimes diffuse. They may be the only radiographic abnormality or may be associated with larger ulcers and more extensive pathology. In their early stages, aphthous ulcers may be difficult to differentiate from nodular lymphoid hyperplasia.

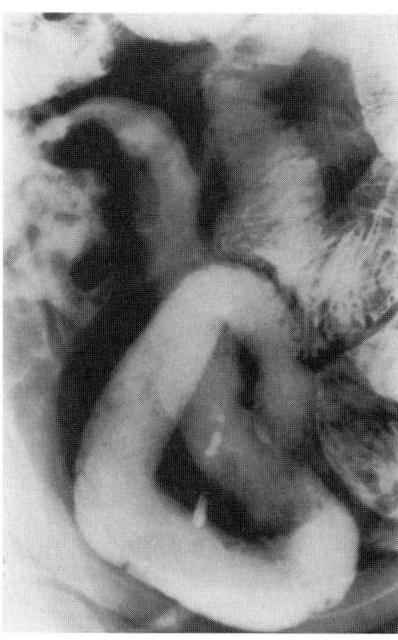

Fig. 15-10. Loss of fold pattern in patient with long history of Crohn's disease.
There is virtually complete loss of folds throughout a long segment of distal and terminal ileum.

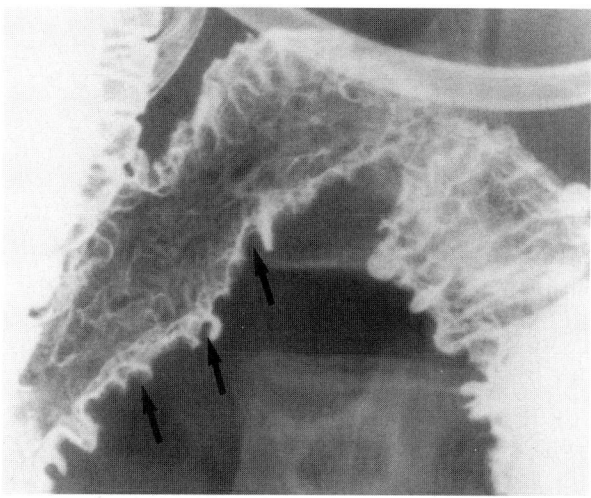

Fig. 15-12. "Nodular pattern" consists of a large number of inflammatory nodules of fairly uniform size.
Curving lines of barium represent depressions between nodules, not linear ulcers. The bowel margin is notched by the nodules (arrows).

However, nodules of lymphoid tissue are usually of similar size and may have central rounded umbilications, whereas aphthous ulcers vary in size and shape.

Aphthous ulcers are usually seen in less affected parts of the small intestine, often considerably proximal to more advanced disease (Fig. 15-14). When associated with fold thickening and a coarse villous pattern, they provide firm evidence of early disease. This combination of findings is usually seen in the terminal or neoterminal ileum [Fig. 15-7(e)]. The double-contrast small bowel enema or the peroral pneumocolon may demonstrate aphthous ulcers with greater precision, particularly if hypotonic agents are used.

The reported radiologic prevalence of aphthous ulcers in small bowel Crohn's disease varies from 25% to 52.5%.[50,55,62,63] Their frequency is underestimated by radiology, since histologic studies have identified them in 70% of surgical specimens.[64] Although aphthous ulcers are usually considered to be the earliest sign of Crohn's disease or of its recurrence,[60] follow-up has frequently failed to show progression to more established disease.[65] In the very early stages of Crohn's disease, small erythematous plaques with intact mucosa have been seen endoscopically, but were not demonstrable by radiography.[66]

Aphthous ulcerations are not pathognomonic of Crohn's disease as they may be observed in other diseases such as yersiniosis, tuberculosis, salmonellosis, Behçet's syndrome, ischemic colitis, amebiasis, and cytomegalovirus enteritis.

Larger, Nonstenosing Ulcers

These may be isolated or associated with aphthous ulcers and more extensive lesions (Fig. 15-15). Like aphthous ulcers, they are not specific for Crohn's disease.

Linear Ulcers Along the Mesenteric Border

These constitute one of the most important signs of small bowel Crohn's disease. The ulcers can exceed 15

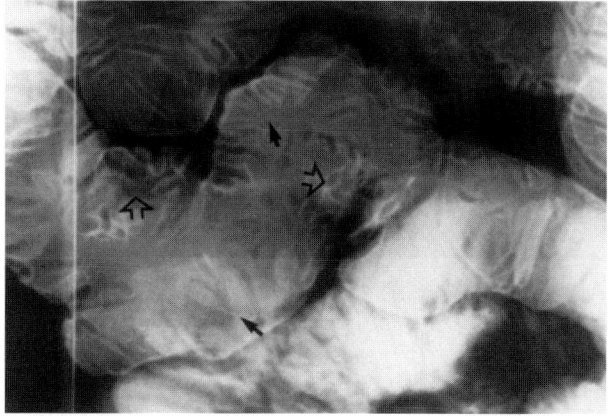

Fig. 15-11. Postinflammatory polyps and distorted folds.
No normal folds are present. Folds are interrupted and distorted (short arrows). Postinflammatory polyps are seen in groups with their tips close together (open arrows).

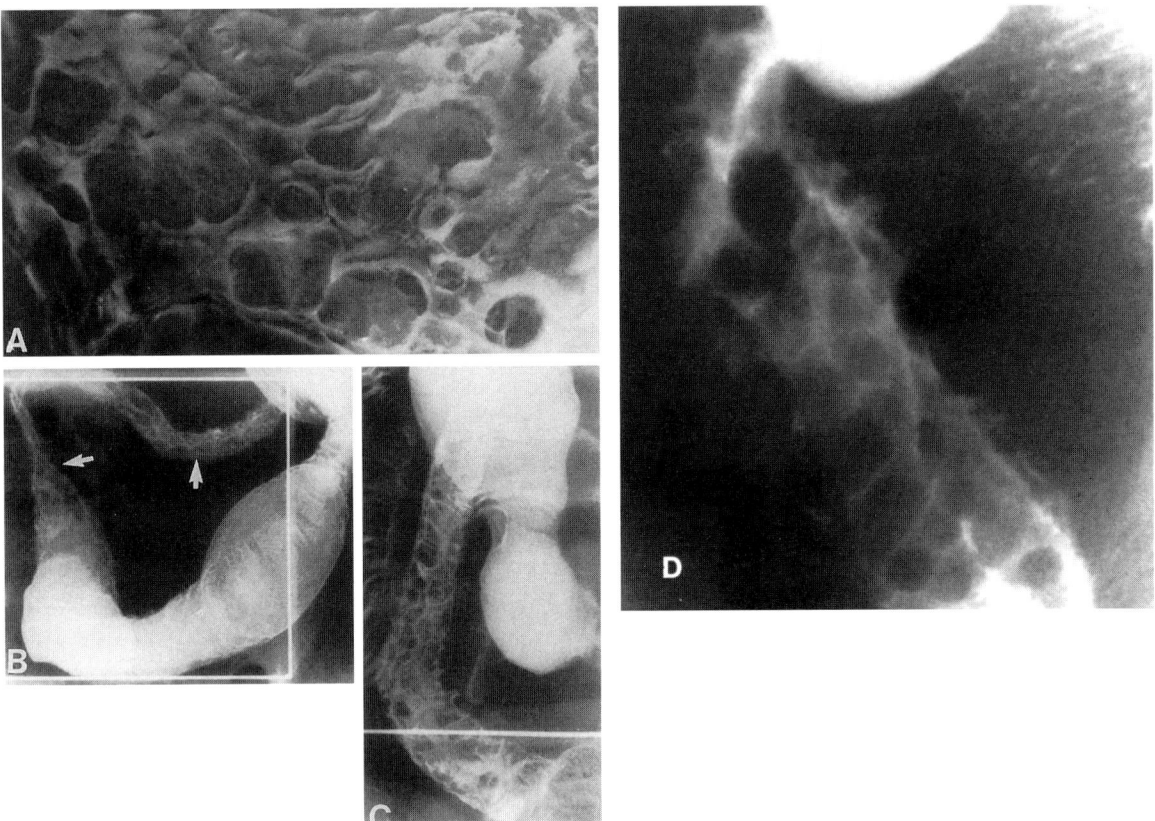

Fig. 15-13. The "ulceronodular" pattern.
(a) Barium-coated specimen. Longitudinal, transverse, and oblique linear ulcerations surround residual islands of elevated mucosa. This is the real "cobblestone" pattern. (b) In another patient, a dilated, featureless segment of ileum with only a few folds is seen proximal to more advanced disease, which shows linear ulcerations in an apparently stenotic segment (arrows). (c) Same patient as in (b). The lumen is outlined in double contrast and demonstrates a typical "cobblestone" pattern of linear ulcerations separating islands of protruding mucosa. Note the persistence of luminal narrowing.

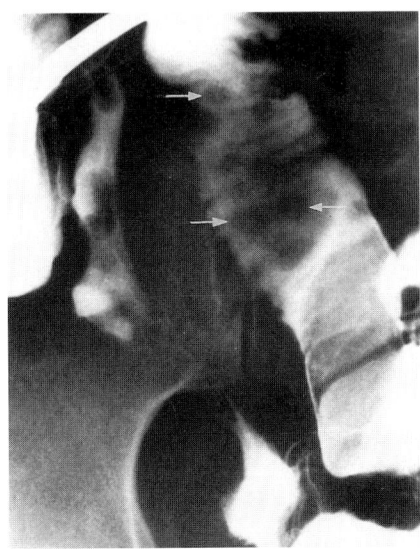

Fig. 15-14. Aphthous ulcers proximal to more severe disease.
Long segment of stenotic Crohn's disease represents the terminal ileum. A section of more proximal ileum contains several aphthous ulcers (arrows) as the only evidence of more proximal disease.

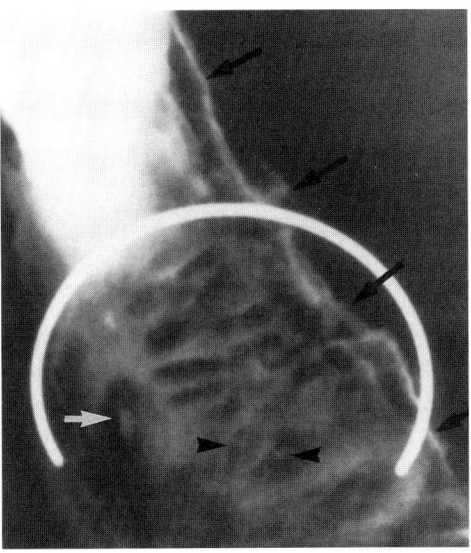

Fig. 15-15. Linear ulcerations along the mesenteric border.
The rigid-appearing mesenteric border shows extensive linear ulceration (black arrows). Note thickened, interrupted folds in middle of involved lumen, and scattered aphthous ulcers (arrowheads). A particularly large ulcer with a well-defined halo is present on the antimesenteric border (white arrow).

cm in length,[67] and run parallel to the shortened, concave, or straightened and somewhat rigid mesenteric border (Fig. 15-16). The adjacent mesentery is thickened and retracted, especially at its junction with the diseased bowel segment. While often readily identified, these linear ulcers can be shallow and only 1 to 2 mm wide; they are then best shown by double-contrast enteroclysis or by careful follow-through study using the proper degree of compression. Their recognition is aided by identifying a relatively radiolucent rim that separates the ulceration from thickened folds that approach it from the antimesenteric side. The radiolucent elevation is formed by fusion of these slightly thickened folds [Fig. 15-17(a, b)]. The rigidity of the mesenteric border is due to transmural inflammation that extends from the linear ulcer into the mesentery [Fig. 15-17(c)].[68] A further highly characteristic feature is the usual noninvolvement of the relatively redundant antimesenteric border, which retains pliability and forms folds or sacculations [Fig. 15-17(d, e)].[69] The combination of mesenteric border shortening and ulceration together with antimesenteric redundancy is virtually pathognomonic of small bowel Crohn's disease. The antimesenteric sparing does not last because, with time, the disease will progress transaxially [Fig. 15-18(a, b)]. However, there may, in some cases, remain sufficient difference between antimesenteric and mesenteric outlines to recognize the underlying Crohn's disease pattern, this even on barium studies of suboptimal quality [Fig. 15-18(c)].

Deeper Stenosing Ulcerations

These produce luminal narrowing that may appear as concentric or asymmetric strictures. These lesions are often multiple and commonly involve a relatively short segment of proximal ileum (Fig. 15-19). Short, dilated segments between the stenoses may show fold thickening and a coarse villous pattern. Deeper ulcerations in very active disease can reach the serosa through the thickened bowel wall and are best shown in the single-contrast phase of enteroclysis [Fig. 15-20(a)]. Deep ulcers can also show flask-shaped terminations that extend deep into the submucosa [Fig. 15-20(b)].

Signs of Fibrosis

Stenosis of the small intestinal lumen occurs frequently in Crohn's disease and results from a combination of fibrosis, inflammatory thickening, and spasm. Collagen, mostly of type I, is found in the wall of normal small bowel and nonstrictured Crohn's disease. When stricture formation occurs, collagen type V is present in large amounts throughout the submucosa and is associated with proliferation of smooth muscle cells, both muscularis mucosae and propria. This leads to fusion of the two muscle layers through the deepened submucosa to form a noncompliant thickened wall, ie, a fibrous stricture.[70]

During barium studies, a true fibrous stricture must not be confused with narrowing caused by ulceration and spasm. Luminal narrowing can be manifested by the "string sign," usually found in the terminal ileum. It is classically described as a thin line of barium, resembling a frayed cotton string [Fig. 15-21(a)]. The string sign represents intense irritability and spasm that is usually associated with extensive ulceration. The organic reality of the string sign is best revealed during the lumen distending phase of enteroclysis [Fig. 15-21(b)] or by a follow-through study done with metoclopramide. The "string sign" should now be an obsolete diagnosis, to be replaced either by the demonstration of spasm associated with an actively ulcerated stenotic segment (Fig. 15-22) or by a segment surrounded by intramural abscesses.[56] On the other hand, the ability of enteroclysis to challenge the distensibility of the intestinal wall may make it possible to confidently demonstrate the unchanging narrowed pattern of a true fibrous stricture (Fig. 15-23). In some patients, however, the distinction between active ulceration and true fibrosis may be difficult to make.

On barium examination, wall thickening can only be inferred by indirect signs. These include luminal narrowing, increased separation of adjacent loops, and relative rigidity of involved loops.

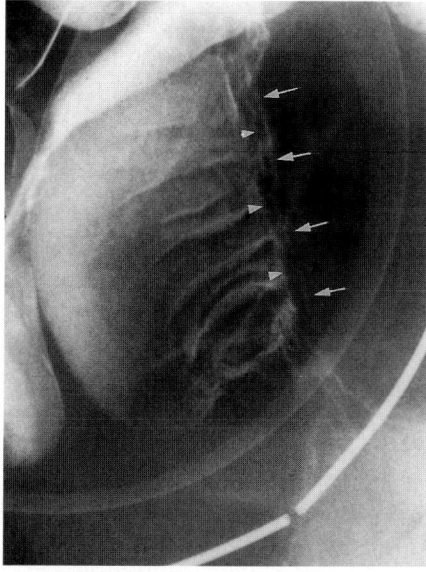

Fig. 15-16. Mesenteric border ulceration.
Extensive linear ulceration along mesenteric margin (arrows) is separated from thickened folds by a radiolucent rim (arrowheads). Note uninvolved and sacculated antimesenteric border.

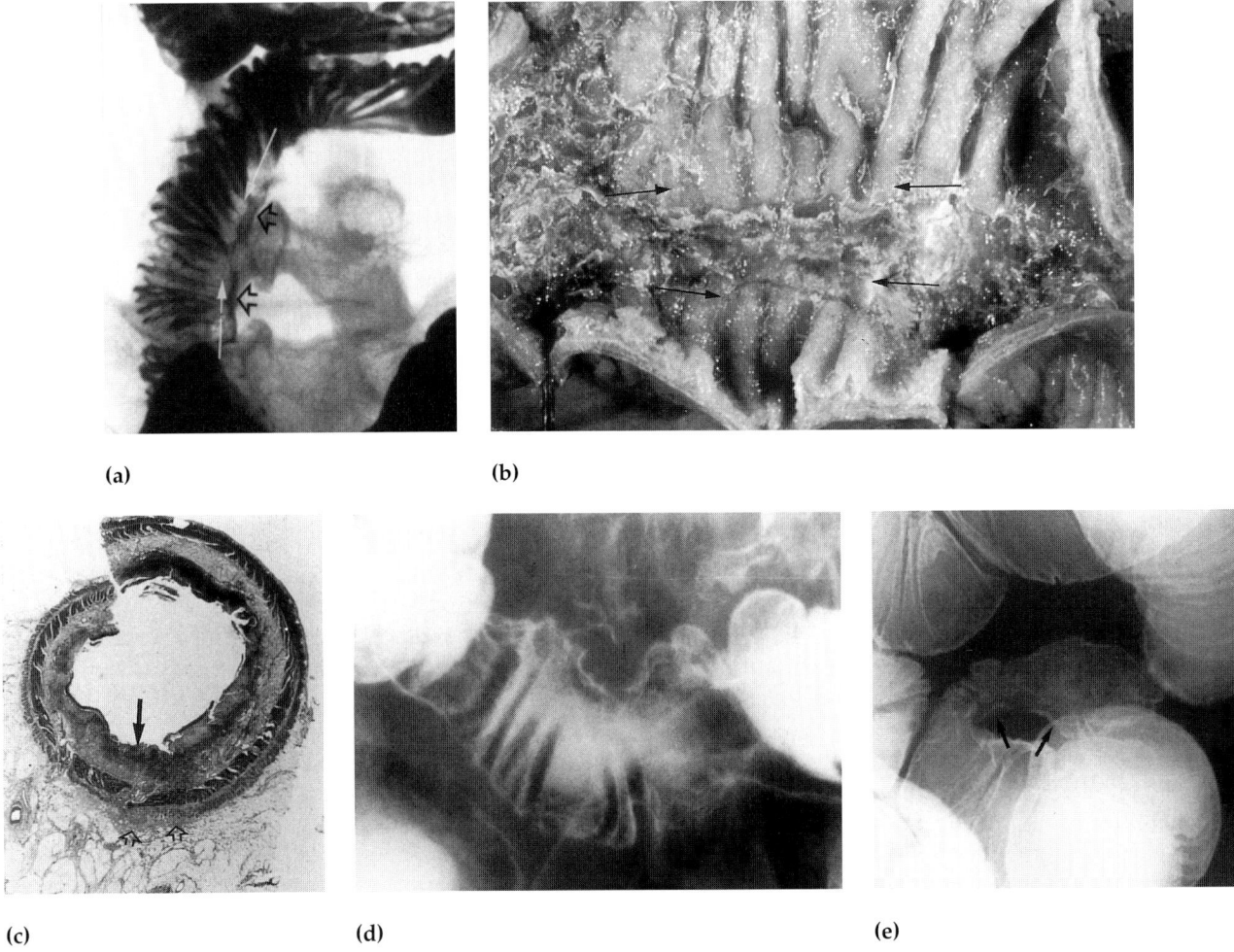

Fig. 15-17. **The mesenteric border linear ulcer.**
(a) Mesenteric border linear ulcer (open arrows) typically is demarcated by a linear elevation (long arrows). (Courtesy of M. Maruyama, MD.) (b) En face view of a specimen with mesenteric border ulcer demarcated on both sides by the fusion of thickened transverse folds (arrows). (c) Low magnification of cross-sectioned ileum showing mesenteric border ulcer (arrow) from which transmural disease extends into the mesentery (open arrow). (d) Skip lesion with mesenteric border linear ulcer demarcated by a radiolucent band; antimesenteric border redundancy expressed as infolding and sacculation. (e) Minimal length of mesenteric border linear ulcer (arrows) and antimesentric folding suffices for a confident diagnosis of a skip lesion in Crohn's disease.

Mesenteric Abnormalities

As with wall thickening, barium studies can only suggest mesenteric involvement. The demonstration of abnormal separation between loops implies mesenteric involvement and requires CT, ultrasonography, or MRI for its confirmation. Significant mesenteric involvement is usually associated with more advanced disease, including the presence of fibrosis.

Retraction of the mesentery may produce kinking and fixation of small bowel segments. These features are not specific and may be observed in other forms of mesenteric infiltration, eg, peritoneal carcinomatosis and fibrolipomatosis of the mesentery.[70]

Stages of Mesenteric Involvement

A classification system is presented that is based upon the degree of involvement as demonstrated radiographically. This system provides a useful framework for understanding the evolution of the radiographic changes. It should be recognized, however, that lesions representing different stages of the disease often coexist. This classification does not correlate with indices of disease activity. The stages of radiographic classification are represented diagrammatically in Fig. 15-24.

Stage 1: Early lesions. Fold thickening, aphthous ulcerations, and coarse granularity of the villi. The intestinal wall retains normal contractility.

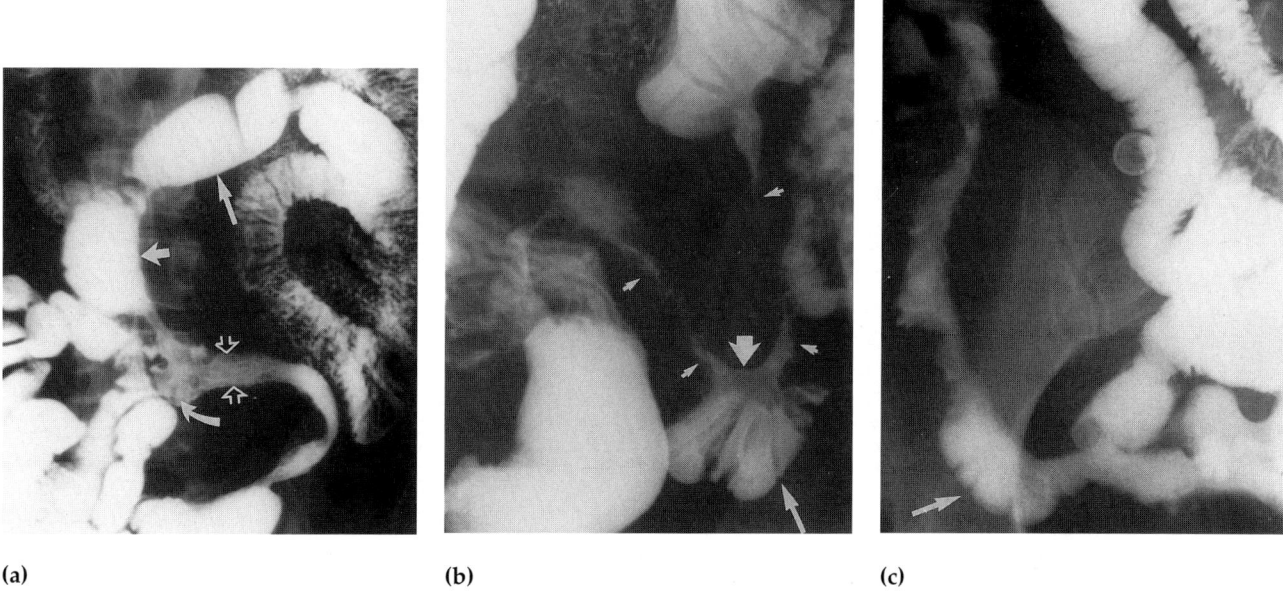

(a) (b) (c)

Fig. 15-18. Antimesenteric sacculations in Crohn's disease.
(a) Crohn's disease intensifies in caudad direction. The shortened, straight mesenteric border (straight arrows) expresses the likely presence of a linear ulcer. A more distal antimesenteric sacculation is being invaded by transaxial Crohn's ulcerations (curved arrow). More distally the previous pattern has become replaced by ulceronodular disease with lumen narrowing (between open arrows). (b) In the destruction of the mesenteric border ulcer/antimesenteric sacculation pattern an occasional saccule (large arrow) may survive, still retaining its demarcation against its mesenteric border ulcer (thick arrow). On either side of it, ileum is contracted and ulcerated (small arrows). (c) Distal and terminal ileum show extensive abnormality. Although mucosal detail is lacking in this follow-through study, antimesenteric sacculation (arrow) is sufficiently shown in the diseased segment to indicate ulceration or retraction of the straightened mesenteric margin and render Crohn's disease a firm diagnosis.

Stage 2: Intermediate lesions. This stage is characterized by the presence of nodular fold thickening and by mesenteric border ulceration, shortening, and rigidity together with scalloping of the still uninvolved antimesenteric border. The bowel wall is moderately thickened.

Stage 3: Advanced lesions. The ulceronodular ("cobblestone") pattern in a stiffened and narrowed seg-

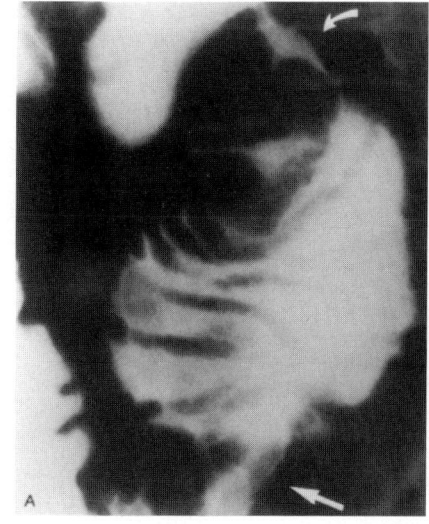
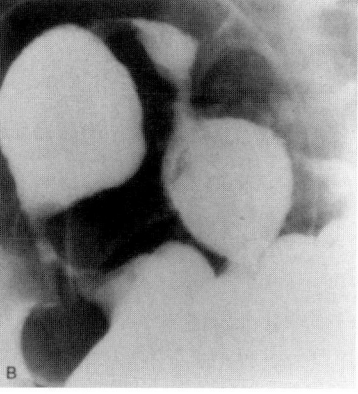

Fig. 15-19. Stenosing ulcerations in Crohn's disease.
(a) Two large ulcers in the proximal ileum. One of the ulcers produces a concentric stenosis (curved arrow). The other ulcer causes asymmetric narrowing (straight arrow). (b) Four short ulcerated segments involve a limited length of ileum with relatively unaffected, dilated segments between them. This not infrequent form of Crohn's disease is associated with partial small bowel obstruction and bacterial overgrowth.

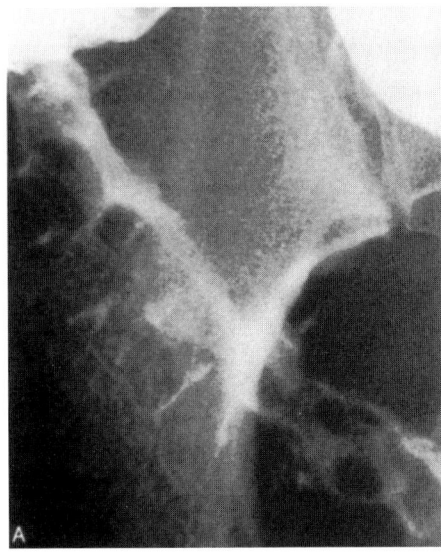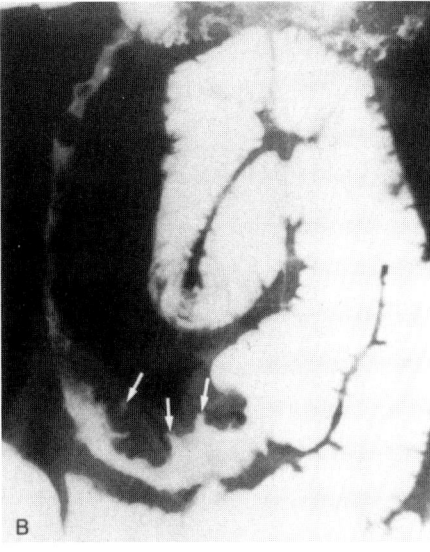

Fig. 15-20. Deep ulcerations and fissures.
(a) Deep transmural fissures in the terminal ileum shown in the single-contrast phase of enteroclysis. Note pronounced wall thickening and luminal narrowing. (b) Long stricture proximal to an ileocolic anastomosis. Several deep, flask-shaped ulcers (arrows) are seen at the proximal end of this stricture. Wall thickening is indicated by the increased distance of the diseased segment from an adjacent loop.

ment with more pronounced wall thickening and the possible development of a stricture indicates an advanced stage of transmural disease. Subserosal fat accumulation maps the extent of this transmural process.

Generally, the intensity of Crohn's disease progresses in a caudad direction. It is not unusual for the three radiographic stages of the disease to reflect this caudad progression in their sequential arrangement. The *anatomic extent* of Crohn's disease involvement, including the presence or absence of more proximally situated skip lesions, forms another aspect of radiographic classification. Enteroclysis is highly successful in delineating the proximal extent of the diseased bowel segment, sometimes shown as a fairly abrupt change from the apparently normal bowel (Fig. 15-25). Enteroclysis is also the ideal method for the demonstration of any skip lesions, which are always at a less advanced stage of the disease and may be some distance above the major lesion [see Figs. 15-8, 15-14, 15-17(e)].

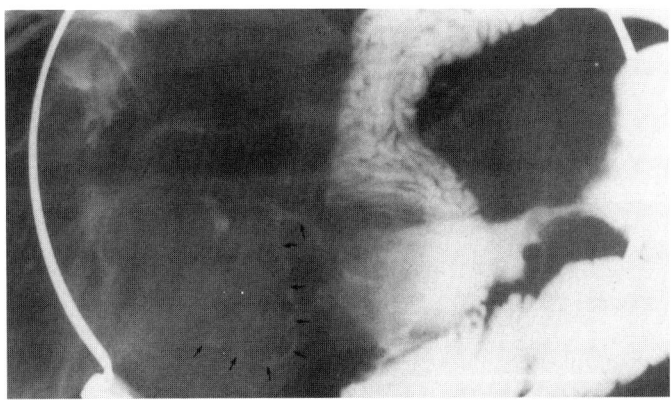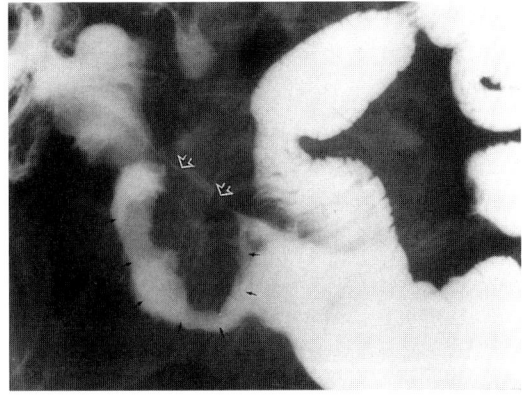

(a)   (b)

Fig. 15-21. The "string sign" is usually found in the terminal ileum and represents intense spasm associated with ulceration.
(a) Early stage of single-contrast enteroclysis. A thin line of barium is demonstrated, resembling a frayed cotton string (arrows). (b) Further luminal distention overcomes the spasm and outlines a distorted, ulcerated segment (small arrows), bypassing a narrow ileoileal fistula (open arrows).

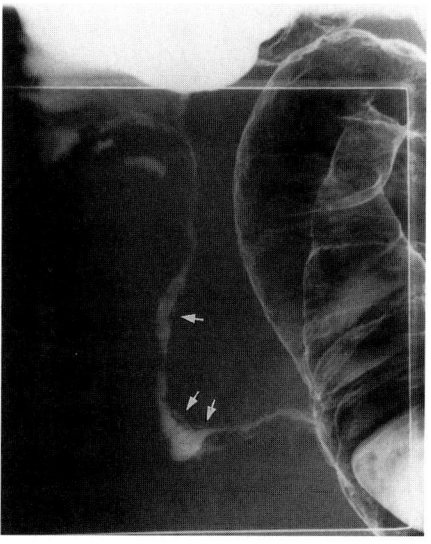
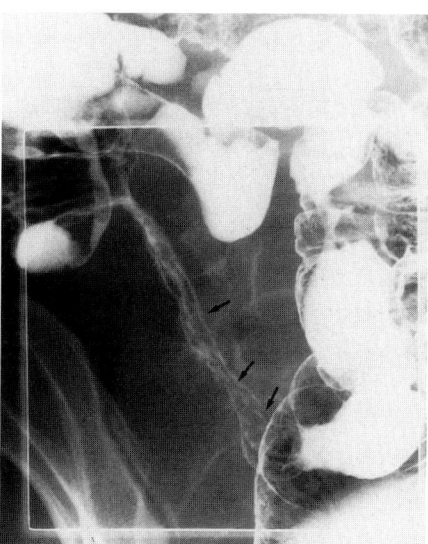

Fig. 15-22. Enteroclysis demonstration of spasm due to active ulceration.
(a) A long segment with marked luminal narrowing is shown in the distal and terminal ileum. Mesenteric border ulceration (arrows) is seen. (b) Following further infusion, the lumen is shown to be mildly distensible, and extensive linear ulceration (arrows) is evident. The presence of spasm and active inflammation excludes a fibrous stricture and suggests that medical therapy may be beneficial.

Evolution of Disease

Progression and Remission

As previously mentioned, Crohn's disease is clinically characterized by periods of exacerbation separated by remissions. The majority of cases show progression of the disease, with complications making an early appearance. In others, noncomplicated inflammatory disease may continue for many years with periods of even prolonged remission.[59] Lesions may even revert to apparent normality following intense and prolonged medical treatment, especially with corticosteroids.[71,72]

Longitudinal progression of small bowel disease in the absence of surgery is controversial. It is generally agreed that the disease remains confined to that length of bowel shown to have been involved at the time of the initial radiologic examination.[59,73] However, the National Cooperative Crohn's Disease Study documented that a minority of patients receiving only medical treatment showed disease extension in excess of 20 cm.[18] Extension into the proximal small bowel or spread into the colon has also been reported.[74] However, it is now believed that this apparent extension of disease merely reflects our inability to demonstrate the full extent of the early changes of Crohn's disease at the time of the first barium examination.

Recurrence

Surgical intervention in Crohn's disease carries the likelihood of recurrence with extension into previously uninvolved areas.[75,76] In one group of patients who had undergone ileal resection, 73% showed endoscopic evidence of recurrent disease within 1 year.[77] The severity of the ileoscopic changes had prognostic value; 80% of the patients with mild or no endoscopic lesions during the first year remained clinically stable

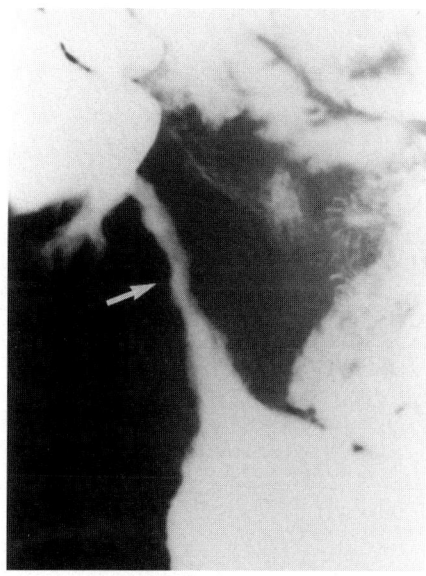

Fig. 15-23. Fibrous stricture due to advanced Crohn's disease.
(a) Relatively featureless stricture (arrow) in the terminal ileum is present. This persisted unchanged throughout the enteroclysis infusion. Obstructing fibrotic strictures such as this require surgical intervention.

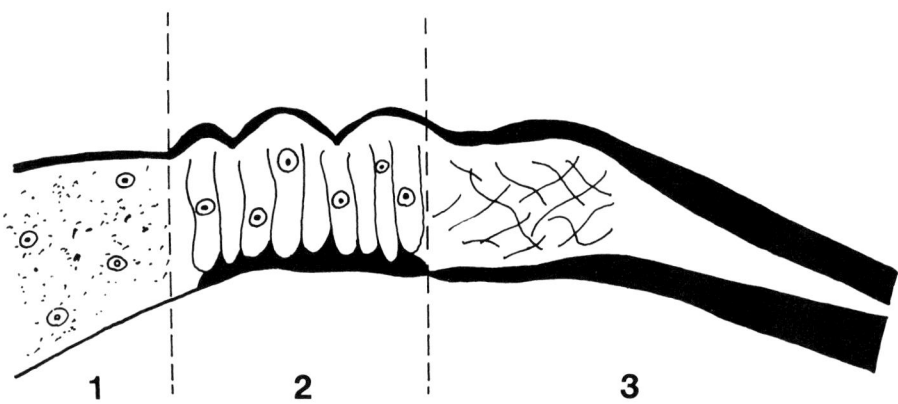

Fig. 15-24. Diagrammatic representation of the early (1), intermediate (2), and advanced (3) stages of the radiographic findings in Crohn's disease of the small bowel (see text).

during the next 3 years, whereas 92% of patients with more severe endoscopic changes developed progressive symptoms or more severe disease over the same period.[77] Ileoscopically shown recurrences may approach 100% over time.[78] Historically, resection with wide margins of normal bowel has been advocated to prevent anastomotic recurrence. Careful study, however, has shown that the rate of recurrence is not related to microscopic disease so that the margins of resection need only be in grossly normal appearing bowel.[11,79]

Similar to ileoscopic findings, radiographically

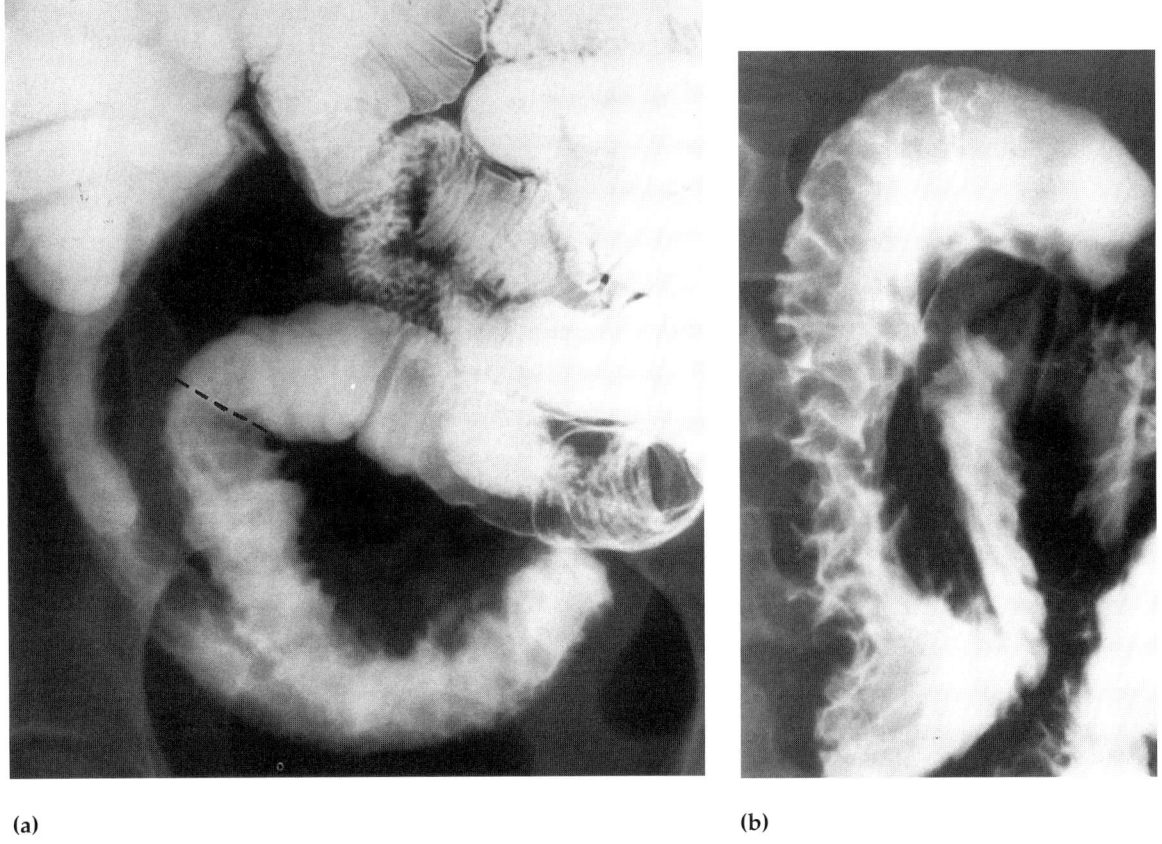

Fig. 15-25. Demonstration of proximal limit of small bowel involvement.
(a) Recurrent disease in neoterminal ileum is manifested by a long segment with ulceronodular changes ("cobblestoning"). Its demarcation from seemingly normal, more proximal ileum is clearly shown (dotted line). (b) Upper gastrointestinal series in same patient shows florid fold thickening in descending duodenum due to concomitant duodenal Crohn's disease.

shown changes mostly precede symptoms and can almost always be demonstrated within 2 years of surgery.[80] The early radiographic findings in recurrent disease of the neoterminal ileum are diffuse fold thickening and aphthous ulcerations [Fig. 15-7(e)]. Preanastomotic narrowing up to 4 cm in length without associated aphthous ulcers may be due to the surgical procedure itself.[80] Recurrences mostly involve the small bowel immediately proximal to the anastomosis with the colon [see Figs. 15-7(e), 15-9(e), 15-25(a)].[53] However, there are reports of recurrent disease both proximal and distal to the ileocolic anastomosis,[77,81] and also the formation of skip lesions, in one case in the duodenum [Fig. 15-25(b)].

Diffuse Jejunoileitis

Diffuse jejunoileitis is a subset of Crohn's disease in which the granulomatous process involves the proximal ileum and distal jejunum, not infrequently sparing the terminal ileum.[51] Jejunal involvement alone is the least common distribution of Crohn's disease in the small bowel.[51,82,83] Crohn and Yarnis encountered 40 patients with diffuse jejunoileal disease among a total of 676 patients with granulomatous enteritis.[84]

This condition differs from the more usual form of small bowel involvement in its progression and response to treatment. Diffuse jejunoileitis is less likely to respond to treatment and may, over the course of

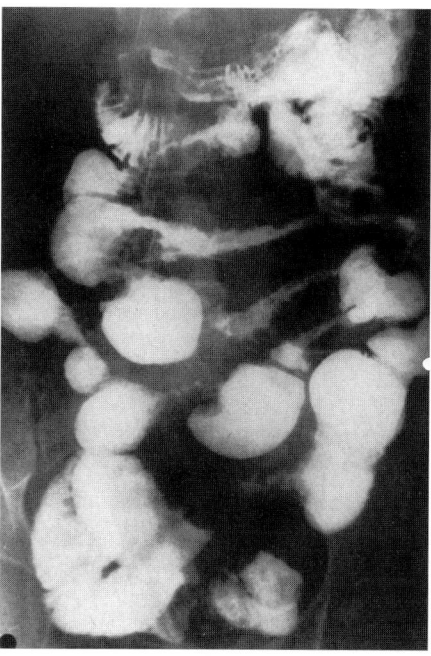

Fig. 15-27. Advanced jejunoileitis.
Long segments of severe stricturing and ulceration are present throughout the jejunum and proximal ileum. Marked separation of the involved loops implies considerable associated mesenteric inflammatory change.

years, develop significant proximal extension to involve even the duodenum. Of particular significance, cicatrized stenotic segments may develop simultaneously in separated areas and cause significant obstruction (Fig. 15-26).[45] In many centers, the use of strictureplasty has largely replaced resection for the surgical management of such strictures if short in length. This surgical approach, together with aggressive use of corticosteroids, has resulted in a much improved prognosis.[85]

Barium studies show the usual early changes that gradually evolve into more advanced disease with ulceration, cobblestone pattern, focal dilatations, and a stenotic phase. Eventually long segments are involved in stricture formation with chronically obstructed, dilated segments in between; alternatively, long narrowed loops separated from one another by wall thickening and mesenteric involvement may develop (Fig. 15-27).[86]

Complications

Obstruction

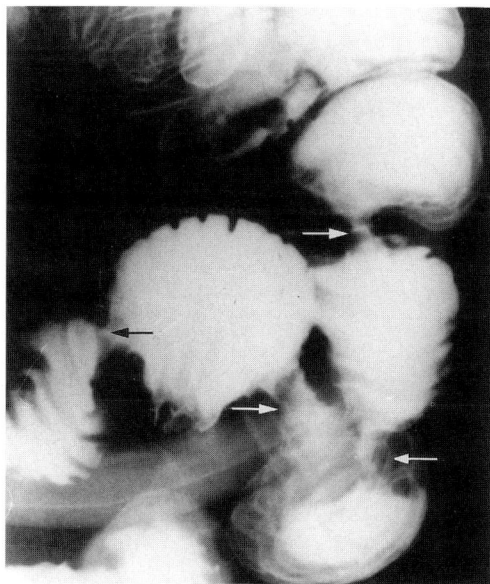

Fig. 15-26. Diffuse jejunoileitis with multiple strictures.
The jejunum contains multiple short strictures (arrows) with intervening segments of normal-appearing bowel.

Small bowel obstruction is a frequent problem once the disease advances into the stenotic stage. High-

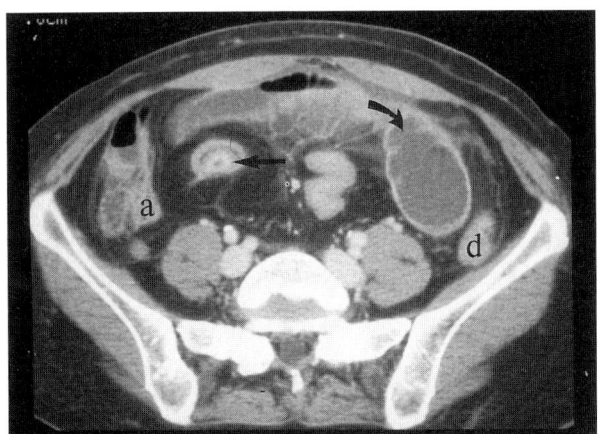

Fig. 15-28. Small bowel obstruction due to Crohn's disease of distal ileum.
Contrast-enhanced CT scan shows lumen narrowing and mural thickening (straight arrow) of distal ileum. Dilatation of fluid-filled small bowel proximally (curved arrow) and collapsed ascending colon (a) and descending colon (d) indicate the presence of small bowel obstruction caused by the distal ileal disease. Mural stratification ("target" sign) of the narrowed segment may imply active inflammation and suggests that the stenosis may be reversible with medical therapy. (Courtesy of Dr Richard Gore, Evanston, IL, from Gore et al,[31] with permission.)

grade obstruction is unusual, even in the presence of multiple strictures.[59] If surgery is needed because of recurrent obstructive episodes and inability to discontinue steroid therapy, it is usually performed on an elective basis.[11] In the National Cooperative Crohn's Disease Study, 13% of the patients had small bowel obstruction that eventually required surgical intervention.[87] Preoperative radiologic assessment of the extent of disease, particularly delineation of the proximal limit of involvement, can serve as a useful road map for the surgeon. Equally relevant is the demonstration or exclusion of more proximal skip lesions. Both purposes are optimally served by enteroclysis.[88] CT enteroclysis may also serve this function.

Intestinal obstruction caused by an actively inflamed stenotic segment (Fig. 15-28) will generally improve with conservative treatment, which includes corticosteroids and tube decompression. However, episodes of partial obstruction are likely to recur. Patients with fibrous strictures as defined by enteroclysis (see earlier) cannot improve, and should have surgical relief, preferably by strictureplasty.[89] Radiologists ought to be familiar with the postoperative appearance of a strictureplasty as shown by barium examination. A strictureplasty is characterized by a short annular narrowing with parallel margins and shouldering at both ends [Fig. 15-29(a)].[90] Adenocarcinoma is typically more irregular, and, in Crohn's disease, characteristically involves a longer segment of bowel. Follow-up of a strictureplasty may show virtual or complete return to a normal appearance [Fig. 15-29(b)]. Interestingly, the incidence of recurrence after strictureplasty does not appear to be greater than when bowel resection was performed.[91]

Postoperative obstruction may be due to recurrent stricture formation from continuing Crohn's disease

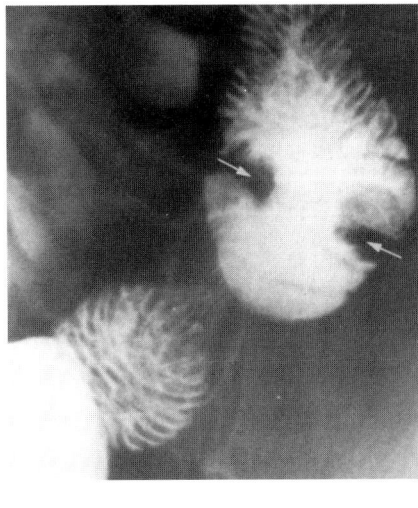
(a)

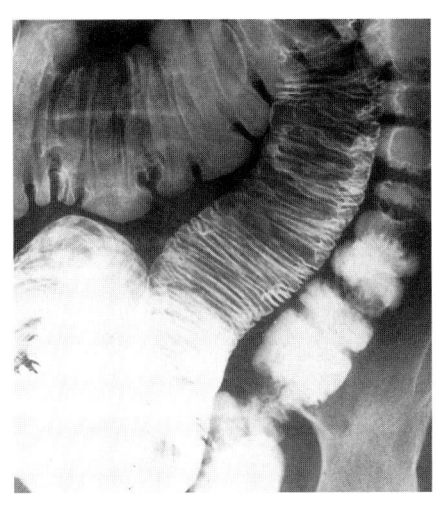
(b)

Fig. 15-29. Appearance of strictureplasty.
(a) Recent strictureplasty is manifested by short symmetric area of narrowing (arrows) with relatively smooth margins. (b) Enteroclysis 2 ½ years later shows complete resolution at the site of strictureplasty.

or to postsurgical adhesions.[51,83] Enteroclysis is capable of distinguishing one from the other, a contribution of radiology relevant to management.

Fistulae

Transmural extension of fissures or ulcers is responsible for the formation of fistulae and sinus tracts. The term fistula implies a communication between two epithelial lined organs (internal fistula) or a communication with the skin surface (external fistula). Sinus tracts are linear extensions into an exoenteric inflammatory process. Fistulae and sinus tracts are highly characteristic of advanced Crohn's disease and are often multiple. They typically originate in an area of active disease that is frequently proximal to a site of partial obstruction.[11] Internal fistulae are more common than the external type. Enteroenteric fistulae are often asymptomatic and may be discovered incidentally during a radiologic examination.[11] External fistulae most commonly extend to the anterior abdominal wall or the perianal area. Except for those in the perianal region, external fistulae occur mostly after surgery and tend to pass through the scar or incision. Unless due to an anastomotic leak, such fistulae are unlikely to close spontaneously. Surgical intervention with interruption of the fistula and resection of the actively diseased bowel is usually necessary.

It is unclear as to which radiologic technique is the most sensitive for the detection of fistulae complicating Crohn's disease. Fistulae and sinus tracts may be shown by fistulography, barium study,[51] ultrasound [Fig 15-30(a)], CT [Fig. 15-30(b)],[31] or MRI (Fig. 15-31).[92] Fistulae have been shown by enteroclysis in 19% of patients with small bowel involvement.[51] This percentage is likely to be an underestimate, since short, fistulous communications between matted bowel loops are missed by radiology, surgery, and even specimen study.[93] Barium entering narrow channels during the single contrast phase of enteroclysis is unlikely to be flushed away during the double-contrast phase and may remain very visible through the overlying transradiant bowel loops.[51] Direct injection of contrast material into the opening of an enterocutaneous fistula may establish its origin and relationships accurately (see Chapter 7). The most commonly shown internal fistulae are ileocecal, ileoileal (Fig. 15-32), and ileosigmoid. The ileocecal fistulae are often multiple[94] and extend through the inflammatory process, often bypassing an obstructed ileocecal valve area. An ileosigmoid fistula (Fig. 15-33) may short-circuit an obstructed distal ileum and serve a useful purpose, at least temporarily. However, ileosigmoid fistulae, if wide enough, may be associated with severe diarrhea, caused by bile salts bypassing the enterohepatic circulation and entering directly into the sigmoid colon.[11] It is important to recognize that the site of entry of a

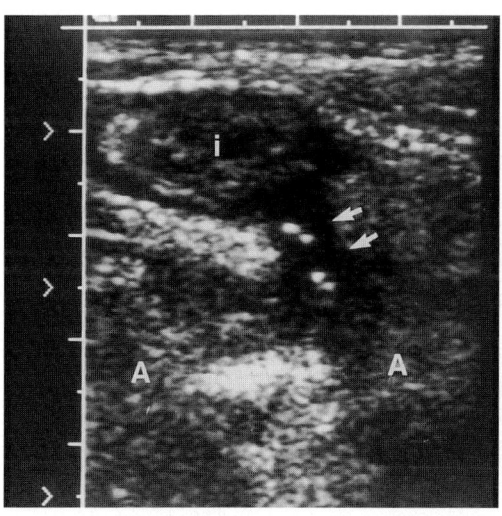
(a)

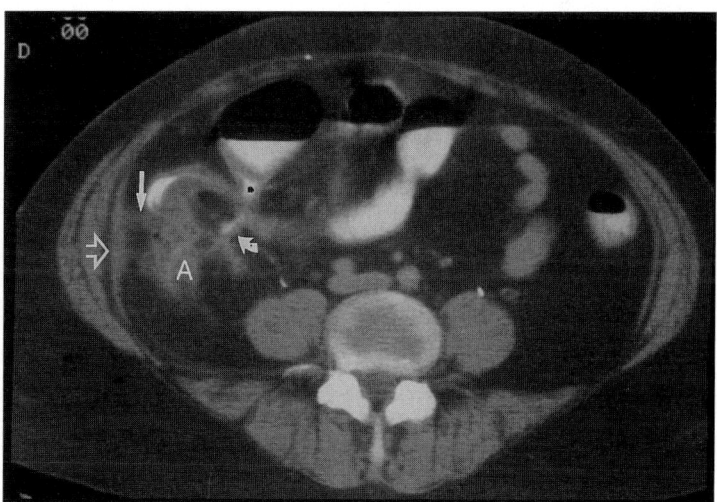
(b)

Fig. 15-30. Imaging demonstration of fistulae and sinus tracts due to ileocolic Crohn's disease.
(a) Ultrasound demonstrates a hypoechoic tract (arrows) that leads from a thickened Crohn's ileitis (i) into a large abscess (A). Gas bubbles are seen in the tract at the level of the arrows. (Courtesy of Michel Rioux, MD, Québec.) (b) A sinus tract (curved arrow) extends laterally from a loop of ileum into a pericolic abscess collection (A). Converging loops of bowel (black dot) indicate fistula formation. A further sinus tract (straight arrow) extends to the thickened transversus abdominis muscle (straight arrow) (Courtesy of Dr Richard Gore, Evanston, IL, from Gore et al,[31] with permission.)

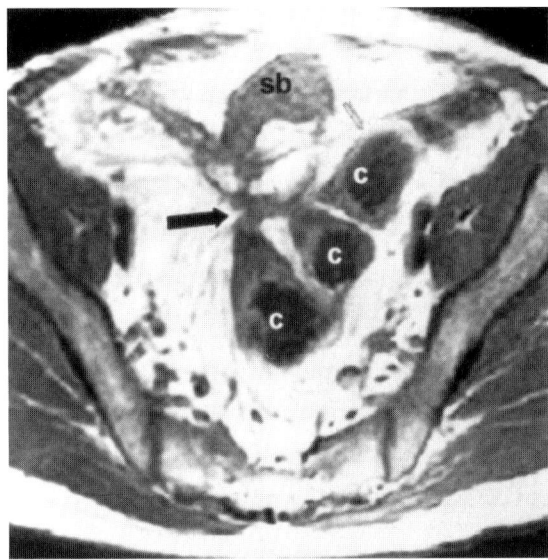

Fig. 15-31. Ileosigmoid fistulae shown by MRI.
T1-weighted image demonstrates multiple fistulous tracts of low signal intensity (arrow) between pelvic small bowel (sb) and sigmoid colon (c).

try into the duodenum.[95,97]

Enterovesical fistulae are infrequent and occur more often in men than women, in whom the uterus serves as a barrier to the spread of inflammation.[97,98] Enterovesical fistulae typically present with pneumaturia. Demonstration of the fistulous tract between the bowel and bladder is notoriously difficult. The presence of gas in the bladder in the absence of a Foley catheter or previous instrumentation is virtually diagnostic of an enterovesical fistula.[31] The traditional belief that enterovesical fistulae require surgical correction to prevent urinary sepsis is being reevaluated; such fistulae have been followed for up to 21 years without evidence of renal damage.[99] Enterovaginal fistulae are more likely to be found after hysterectomies.[100]

Most fistulae are of small diameter, and flow rates through them are insignificant. They may persist during disease inactivity. Occasional fistulae with wider lumens may have to be repaired because of malabsorption, diarrhea, and weight loss. Other than this, the presence of the fistula itself is not an indication for resection but rather of the severity of the underlying obstruction and extraintestinal inflammatory process.

Enteric fistulae are not exclusive to Crohn's disease and may develop in ileocolic tuberculosis, sigmoid diverticulitis, postradiation, or after chronic enteric infections. We have also encountered an adenocarcinoma of the ileum with fistulization to the sigmoid colon.

Perianal and perirectal fistulae are a frequent complication of Crohn's disease. They are more common

fistula into the sigmoid colon is unlikely to become the cause of colonic Crohn's disease; only the fistulous opening needs to be excised.[95,96] Similarly, small bowel fistulae to the duodenum, which are rare, have never been associated with Crohn's disease at the site of en-

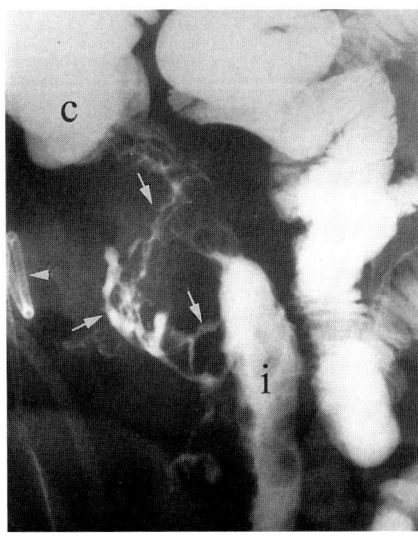

Fig. 15-32. Extensive ileoileal fistulae.
Numerous sinus tracts and ileoileal fistulae (arrows) arise from a long segment of Crohn's disease of the neoterminal ileum. An adjacent gas-containing abscess is present, which is drained by a percutaneously placed catheter (arrowhead). (c = right colon, i = neoterminal ileum.)

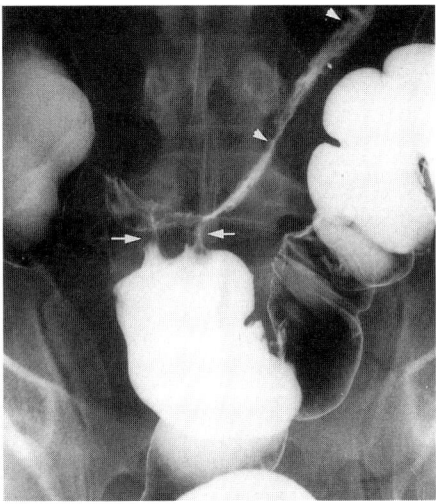

Fig. 15-33. Ileosigmoid fistula.
Two fistulous tracts (arrows) connect a markedly narrowed segment of ileum (arrowheads) with the sigmoid colon.

Complications • 281

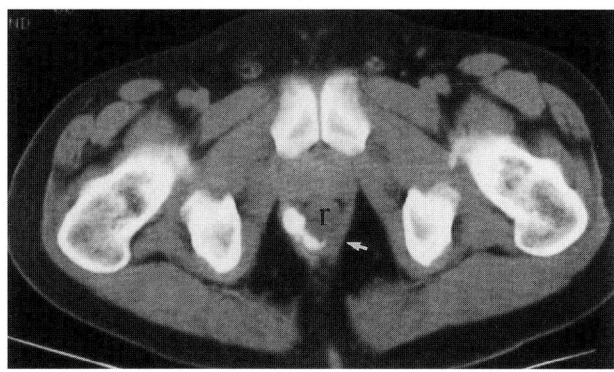

Fig. 15-34. Perirectal fistula.
A sinogram obtained preoperatively shows the relationship of a rectocutaneous fistula to the levator ani muscles (arrow). (r = rectum.) (Courtesy of Dr Richard Gore, Evanston, IL, from Gore et al,[31] with permission.)

in patients with ileocolic or colonic disease than with isolated small bowel involvement. Such fistulae are often poorly shown by barium studies, either because the enema tip has been inserted too deeply or because severe local pain limits adequate visualization effort.[31] MR imaging is the procedure of choice for showing these fistulae and their relationships to the anal sphinc-ters, the latter being essential for planning successful surgery.[44,101,102] CT can also be used to delineate perineal and perirectal fistulae (Fig. 15-34)[31] but lacks the multiplanar capabilities of MRI.

Abscesses

Abscess formation occurs in approximately 15% to 20% of patients with Crohn's disease.[103,104] Abscesses are often a consequence of transmural disease and subsequent sinus tracts, but may also occur as a postsurgical complication. An apparent subcutaneous or abdominal wall abscess may be the initial presentation of an incipient fistula.[11] The commonest site of origin is the terminal ileum. Abscesses may be found in a variety of locations, including the adjacent mesentery, the peritoneal cavity, in extraperitoneal location (Fig. 15-35), and at a retroperitoneal site including the ileopsoas, the ischiorectal fossa, and the presacral space (Fig. 15-36). Very occasionally an abscess turns out to be the lesser evil, as in the case shown in Fig. 15-36 where the abscess was next to abnormal ileal loops tethered to a thickened presacral area in which, at surgery and histology, adenocarcinoma was identified. Further abscess sites include the liver and the anterior abdominal wall (Fig. 15-37). Abscesses some-

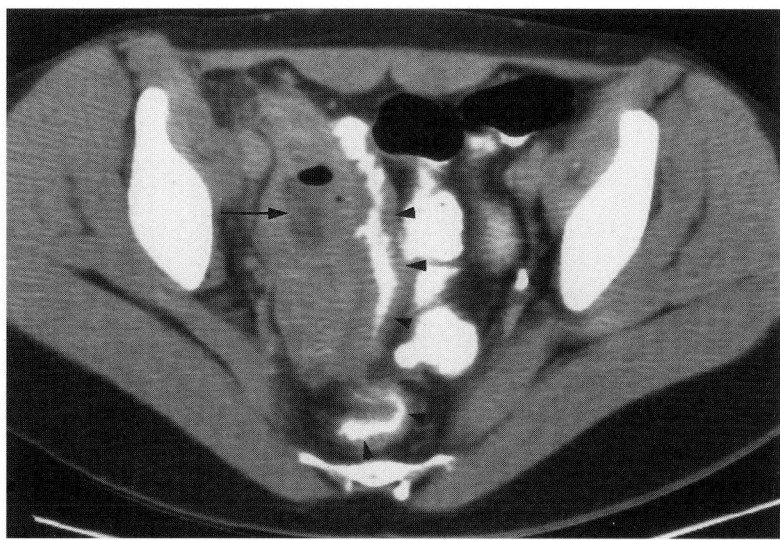

(a)

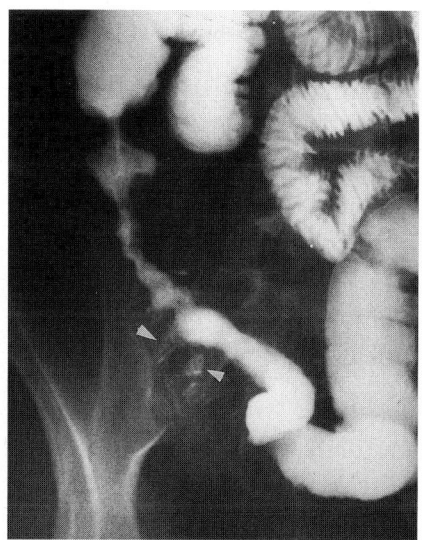

(b)

Fig. 15-35. Extraperitoneal abscess secondary to recurrent ileal Crohn's disease.
(a) A large mass containing a central collection of fluid and gas (long arrow) represents an abscess, which has arisen from a long area of Crohn's disease involving the distal ileum. The involved bowel segment shows irregular luminal narrowing and mural thickening (arrowheads). (b) Enteroclysis examination in same patient demonstrates the long segment of recurrent disease in the neoterminal ileum, from which several deep sinus tracts (arrowheads) originate. Although enteroclysis shows the sinus tracts, contrast material does not fill the abscess cavity itself.

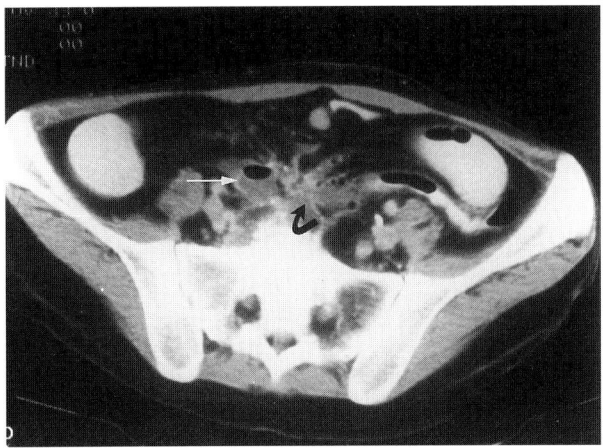

Fig. 15-36. Presacral abscess (arrow) in long-standing Crohn's disease.
Next to it abnormal bowel loops tethered to a thickened presacral area (curved arrow). Resection and subsequent histology identified an adenocarcinoma. (Courtesy of Dina Caroline, MD.)

times resolve spontaneously by discharging their contents into a bowel lumen.

Clinical findings include fever, chills, elevated leukocyte count, and a palpable, tender abdominal mass. Clinical diagnosis may be difficult because symptoms may be minimal, masked by corticosteroids, or mistaken for an exacerbation of the disease.[31,103] Barium studies are usually nondiagnostic as they show only a mass effect which, if close to the involved bowel, demonstrates the "proximity effect" of spiculated, edematous mucosal folds facing the lesion [Fig. 15-38(a)].[95] Occasionally an extraluminal gas collection is present [Fig. 15-38(a)], or barium may actually enter the communicating abscess [Fig. 15-38(b)].

CT is clearly the method of choice for diagnosis as well as percutaneous management. Abscesses are depicted as rounded or oval fluid-density masses, the wall of which may show contrast enhancement. Extraluminal gas within the mass is found in up to 50% of abscesses.[105] The gas is most often secondary to a sinus tract communicating with the skin surface or bowel. Complete opacification of bowel loops is desirable for a definitive CT diagnosis of an abscess. In contrast to an abscess, a phlegmon is seen on CT as an ill-defined mass of soft-tissue density. It may resolve completely with antibiotics or progress into an abscess.

Ultrasonography is often used as a primary imaging technique and can show the presence of an abscess. However, interference by air-filled bowel loops often limits the clinical utility of ultrasonography in this situation.[105] Ultrasonography would be a more cost-effective method for the follow-up of abscesses than CT.

Abscesses in Crohn's disease are often difficult to manage. Enthusiasm for percutaneous drainage was initially tempered by the knowledge that these abscesses are often associated with fistulae and may be multilocular.[31] In the past decade or so, percutaneous drainage has become well established either as a temporizing measure or as definitive therapy.[106–108] In cases without any evidence of fistulous communication, percutaneous drainage may prevent the need for any surgical intervention.[106] When there is a communication between diseased bowel and the abscess, percutaneous drainage may cause a two-stage surgical procedure to be replaced by a single-stage resection.[107] A very recent report analyzes the success and failure rates of percutaneous drainage of Crohn's abscesses.[108] Success was more likely when there were fewer fistulae and the abscesses were either primary or spontaneous (vs recurrent or postoperative).[108] Hospital stay was significantly shorter after successful drainage.[108]

Perforation

Deep fissures usually reach the serosal surface slowly enough to permit walling off by adhesions to a neighboring viscus, or by the parietal peritoneum or omen-

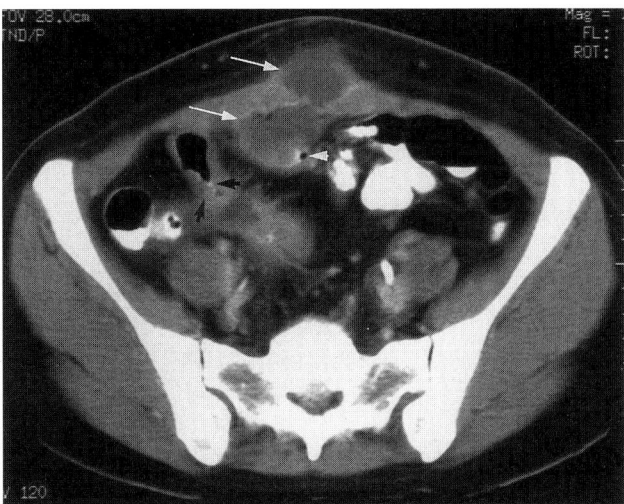

Fig. 15-37. Anterior abdominal wall abscess.
There is a dumbbell-shaped fluid collection (white arrows) both deep and superficial to the rectus abdominis muscle. A small adjacent area of contrast (arrowhead) suggests there may be a fistula leading to the abscess. Note the marked mural thickening in the distal ileum (short black arrow) with adjacent streaky mesenteric change. (Courtesy of Col Greg Bender, MD, Washington, DC.)

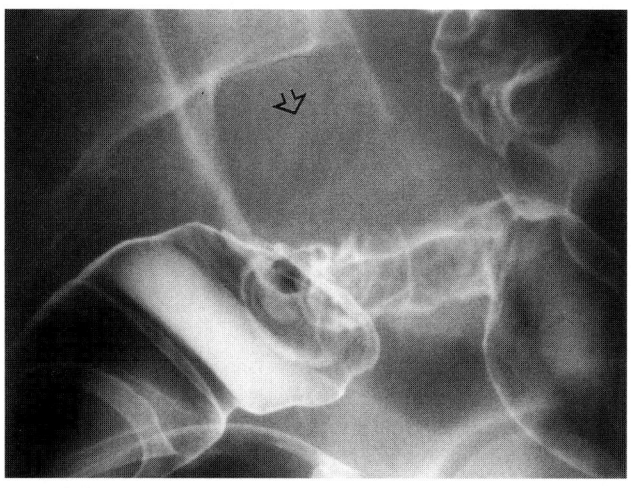 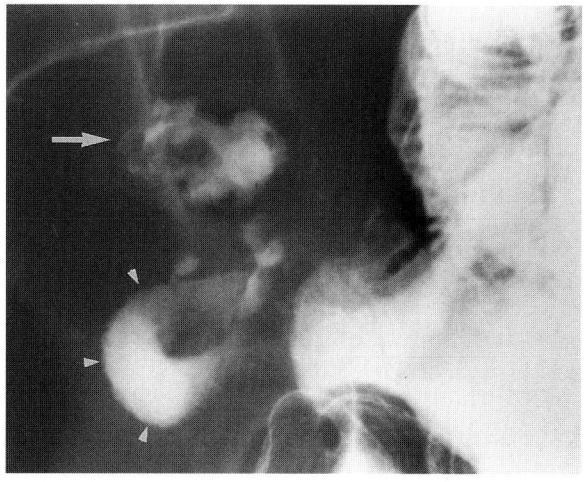

(a) (b)

Fig. 15-38. Demonstration of abscess cavity by enteroclysis.
(a) The presacral space is widened and contains an ovoid extraluminal gas collection (open arrow) suggestive of an abscess. The adjacent rectosigmoid colon is displaced with segmental narrowing and spiculated mucosal folds, indicating the proximity effect caused by the nearby abscess. (b) Enteroclysis film in same lateral position demonstrates a stenotic segment of involved ileum (arrowheads) from which contrast material has extravasated into the abscess cavity (arrow). The diseased ileum and abscess were resected and easily separated from the rectosigmoid. A later barium enema showed a normal rectum and distal sigmoid. (By permission from Herlinger et al.[95])

tum, thus preventing a free perforation.[2] The usual outcome of this transmural penetration is an abscess or fistula. Nevertheless, perforation with free intraperitoneal air is seen in 2% to 3% of cases. Perforation may be secondary to a more acute penetration of the bowel wall by ulceration, fissuring, necrosis, or the rupture of an intra-abdominal abscess.

Carcinoma and Lymphoma

The rarity of small bowel adenocarcinoma complicating small bowel Crohn's disease makes it impossible to assess the exact magnitude of the risk.[109] Although no exact numbers are available, it is evident that, when compared with the general population, an increased risk of small bowel cancer exists in Crohn's disease of many years' duration, especially situated in bypassed bowel loops. It must be important to keep the possibility of carcinoma in mind whenever there is prolonged Crohn's disease and an excessive amount of local fibrosis is shown (see Fig. 15-36!). (This problem has been more fully discussed in Chapter 19.) We only wish to add a single but alarming case report that describes the first case of carcinoma developed at a stricturoplasty site 7 years after the surgery.[110]

An increased number of lymphomas in patients with Crohn's disease has also been reported.[111] Lymphoma complicating Crohn's disease tends to develop in small bowel segments with preexisting inflammatory changes. Two other reports refer to lymphoma developing during immune suppressive therapy with azothiaprine.[112,113]

Assessment of Disease Activity

Attempts to assess and monitor the activity of Crohn's disease by either barium examination or endoscopy have been relatively unsuccessful. In recent years, a variety of imaging-related options have been advocated for the assessment of disease activity.[10] However, it is still unclear which of these options are to be preferred or whether even any of them may become incorporated into routine clinical practice.

As described previously, enteroclysis can often distinguish between the unyielding narrowing of a fibrous stricture and the actively inflamed luminal narrowing that can be distended by the continued infusion of contrast material. This should aid the selection of patients for surgical intervention.

On contrast-enhanced CT, acute inflammation may result in mural stratification that gives rise to the "target" or "double-halo" appearance. The intensity of contrast enhancement of the inflamed mucosa and serosa is believed to reflect the clinical activity of the disease.[31,114] This mural stratification is lost in long-standing disease if transmural fibrosis has supervened. In active disease, diminution of mural thickening and contrast enhancement may indicate success after a course of medical therapy (Fig. 15-39).

Similarly, contrast-enhanced MRI has been used to evaluate disease activity in inflammatory bowel disease (Fig. 15-40). MRI appears to be an ideal technology to depict both the small bowel abnormalities and their causes [Fig. 15-41(a, b)]. In one study that used histopathology as the gold standard, MRI correctly graded the severity of disease in 13 of 20 patients, whereas endoscopy did so in only 11 of these patients.[115] These authors found that the bowel wall thickness as measured by MRI showed good correlation with the degree of contrast enhancement. MRI has also successfully monitored treatment response and relapse.[116]

As with CT, the sonographic demonstration of mural stratification has been shown to indicate that transmural fibrosis has not taken place, and that medical treatment may still be successful (see Chapter 8) [Fig. 15-6(b)]. Another ultrasonographic approach for assessing disease activity has utilized Doppler flow measurements of the superior mesenteric artery.[117] Doppler blood flow values were found to be significantly higher in patients with active Crohn's disease than in those without evidence of activity.

Differential Diagnosis

In the majority of patients, the distinction between small bowel Crohn's disease and other disorders is not difficult. The following characteristic features of Crohn's disease can be of positive help in differential diagnosis: deep ulcerations, cobblestone pattern, predominant involvement of the mesenteric border, juxtaposition of lesions in different stages of evolution, and presence of an intermediary segment with superficial lesions interposed between stenotic disease below and normality above.[65] Occasionally, however, some of these appearances may be mimicked by other disorders. In children, care should be taken not to confuse Crohn's disease with the small (2 to 3 mm) nodules and prominent folds caused by lymphoid hyperplasia.

Infectious Ileitis

Infectious ileitis can radiologically resemble nonstenotic Crohn's disease. The radiologic features are mucosal fold thickening; nodular defects; mucosal ulcerations varying from aphthous ulcers to larger, oval, or longitudinal shapes; and the terminal ileum as the favored

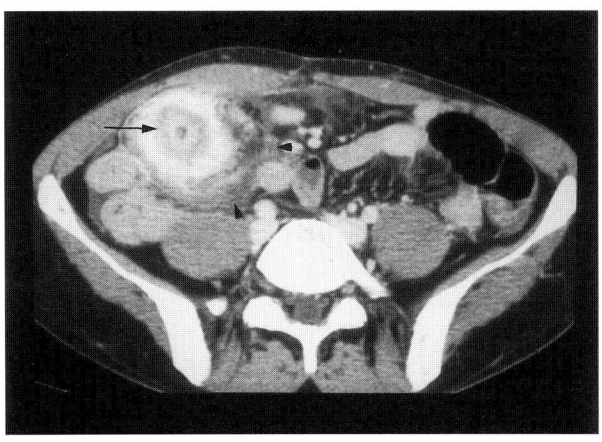

(a)

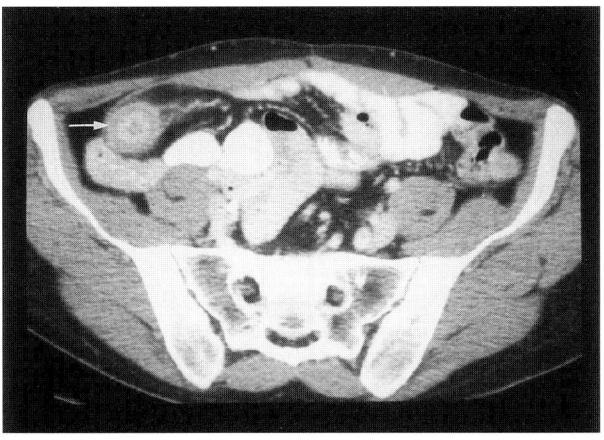

(b)

Fig. 15-39. Decreased inflammatory changes on CT following medical treatment.
(a) Contrast-enhanced CT scan of terminal ileum shows intense enhancement of mucosa and muscularis propria-serosa. The edematous, thickened submucosa shows low attenuation (straight arrow) in relation to the other layers of the bowel wall, producing target sign. Peri-intestinal fat also shows marked inflammatory change (arrowheads). Patient had low-grade small bowel obstruction and fever. (b) CT scan obtained for same patient as in (a) after 9-week course of antibiotic and steroid therapy shows diminution of mural thickening and of contrast enhancement of involved ileum (arrow) as well as marked reduction of inflammatory change in adjacent mesentery. Symptoms of obstruction have improved also. (Courtesy of Dr Richard Gore, Evanston, IL, from Gore et al,[31] with permission.)

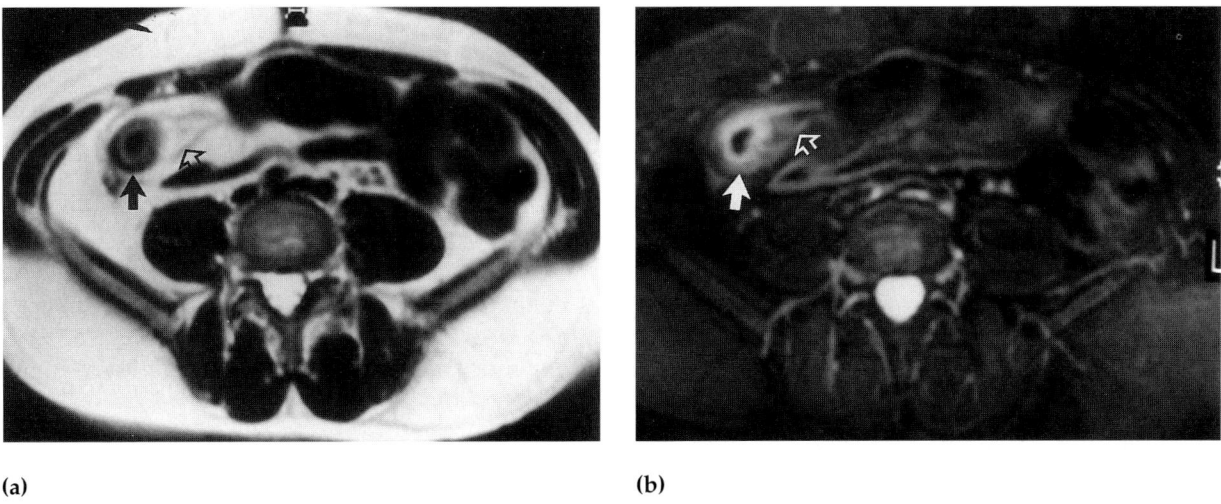

Fig. 15-40. MRI demonstration of active inflammatory change.
(a) MR examination performed 1 hour after oral administration of a negative superparamagnetic contrast agent (Lumirem, Guerbet). Axial T2-weighted turbo spin echo (TSE) image shows active mural inflammation manifested by hyperintense thickened wall of involved ileal loop (arrow) with inhomogeneous perivisceral fat. (b) In the fat-suppressed T2-weighted TSE image obtained at the same level, the visibility of wall hyperintensity (arrow) appears greatly increased, as is the hyperintensity of the perivisceral fat. (Courtesy of Francesca Maccioni, MD, Rome, Italy.)

site of involvement. The organisms responsible may be *Yersinia, Campylobacter, Shigella,* or *Salmonella.* The major differences between infectious ileitis and Crohn's disease are the usually self-limited nature of the former conditions and the absence of a stenotic phase. The isolation of microorganisms by stool culture and the search for a positive serologic diagnosis should be suggested by the radiologist at an early stage.

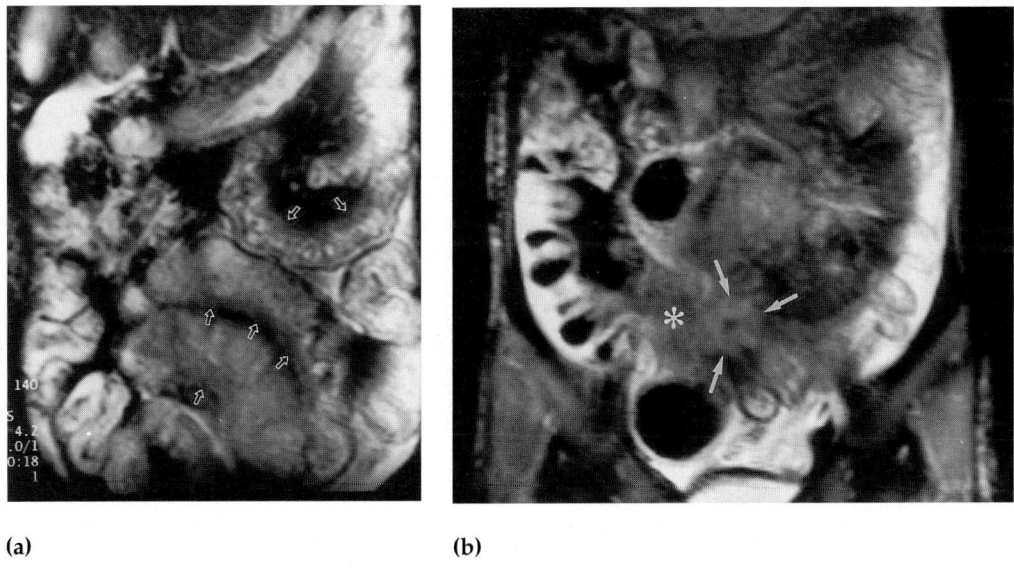

Fig. 15-41. MRI features of Crohn's disease activity with partial obstruction.
(a) Coronal T2-weighted Half-Fourier Acquisition Single-shot Turbo Spin-Echo sequence (HASTE) image shows diffuse wall thickening affecting three bowel loops with mesenteric border ulcerations (arrows) and increasing lumen dilatation. (b) T2-weighted coronal HASTE image clearly demonstrates a thick walled stricture (arrows) with fairly extensive perienteric inflammatory infiltrate (asterisk). (Courtesy of H.K. Ha, MD, Seoul, Korea.)

Tuberculosis

Isolated involvement of the terminal ileum is rare. Cecal involvement is more intense than that of the terminal ileum, with retraction and fibrosis involving the cecal wall opposite the ileocecal valve. Mucosal alterations are coarser than in Crohn's disease, and ulcerations are more irregular and sometimes annular. Despite these differences, differentiation on radiological grounds can be difficult. Some patients show evidence of active pulmonary tuberculosis on chest radiographs, but this is often absent.

Lymphoma

The infiltrative form of lymphoma can occasionally mimic nonstenotic Crohn's disease. Deep ulceration, excavation into the mesentery, skip lesions, and frequent involvement of the terminal ileum are shared by the two conditions. If CT is performed, lymphoma shows considerably more wall thickening. Lymphoma lacks the hyperperistalsis and segmental spasm of Crohn's disease and rarely causes stenosis. The coarse granular pattern of Crohn's disease and of other inflammatory conditions does not occur in lymphoma.

Ischemia

Ischemia of the small intestine, if shown by barium study, can closely resemble Crohn's disease. However, rapid change in appearance is the hallmark of ischemia, either with return to normality, deterioration to stricture formation, or breakdown. In the elderly, distinction between the two conditions can be more difficult.

Miscellaneous Conditions

Metastatic disease, usually distributed by seeding, predominantly affects mesenteric borders and the ileocecal area. It can be associated with mesenteric retraction and lumen distortions to resemble sacculation. The scattered distribution of the lesions, the absence of an intermediary segment, and the clinical background should point away from Crohn's disease.

Radiation enteropathy can resemble the radiologic findings of Crohn's disease. Awareness of a history of prior radiation therapy and a knowledge of the radiation portal employed are helpful in support of the correct diagnosis.

Adenocarcinoma of the ileum (not the usual site) has been an occasional differential diagnostic problem.[118]

Appendiceal abscesses or pelvic inflammatory disease can cause displacement and concave border mucosal edema of bowel loops in close proximity to the lesions. Crohn's disease would not present with features indicating an extrinsic origin.

It should be reassuring to know that, in the great majority of patients, the differential diagnosis of Crohn's disease is not difficult. There are rare occasions when a radiologic diagnosis may be impossible at the initial examination. Repeat enteroclysis, examination of the colon, CT, MRI, endoscopy, and/or a therapeutic trial may all have to be employed to reach a definitive diagnosis in an unusual situation.

References

1. Moschowitz E, Wilensky AO. Nonspecific granulomas of the intestines. *Am J Med Sci.* 1923;166:48–66.
2. Crohn DB, Ginzburg L, Oppenheimer GD. Regional ileitis: a pathologic and clinical entity. *JAMA.* 1932;99: 1323–1329.
3. Sandler RS, Golden AL. Epidemiology of Crohn's disease. *J Clin Gastroenterol.* 1986;8:160–165.
4. Feczko PJ, Barbour H, Halpert RD, et al. Crohn's disease in the elderly. *Radiology.* 1985;157:303–304.
5. Yoshimura HH, Merkel RS, Grahm DY. Association of *Mycobacterium* related to *Mycobacterium paratuberculosis* with Crohn's disease by culture and DNA hybridization. *Gastroenterology.* 1984;86:1306.
6. Pounder RE. The pathogenesis of Crohn's disease. *J Gastroenterol.* 1994;29(suppl 7):11–15.
7. MacDermott RP. Alterations in the mucosal immune system in ulcerative colitis and Crohn's disease. *Med Clin North Am.* 1994;78:1207–1231.
8. Meyers S, Janowitz HD. Crohn's disease, clinical features. In: Berk JE, ed. *Bockus Gastroenterology.* 4th ed. Philadelphia, Pa: WB Saunders Co; 1985:2240–2258.
9. Hanauer SB. Inflammatory bowel disease. *N Engl J Med.* 1996;334:841–847.
10. Wills JS, Lobis IF, Denstman FJ. Crohn's disease: state of the art. *Radiology.* 1997;202:597–610.
11. Kahng KU, Roslyn JJ. Surgical treatment of inflammatory bowel disease. *Med Clin North Am.* 1994;78: 1427–1441.
12. Hamilton SR, Morson BC. Crohn's disease, pathology. In: Berk JE, ed. *Bockus Gastroenterology.* 4th ed. Philadelphia, Pa: WB Saunders Co; 1985.
13. Mekhjian HS, Switz DM, et al. Clinical features and natural history of Crohn's disease. *Gastroenterology.* 1979;77:898–906.
14. Herlinger H, Furth EE, Rubesin SE. Fibrofatty proliferation of the mesentery in Crohn's disease. The query corner. *Abdom Imaging.* In press.
15. Halligan S, Nicholls S, Bartram CI, et al. The distribution of small bowel Crohn's disease in children compared to adults. *Clin Radiol.* 1994;49:314–316.

16. Maglinte DDT, Burney BT, Miller RE. Lesions missed on small-bowel follow-through: analysis and recommendations. *Radiology.* 1982;144:737–739.
17. Steinhardt JH, Loeschke K, Kasper H, et al. European Cooperative Crohn's Disease Study (ECCDS): clinical features and natural history. *Digestion.* 1985;31:97–108.
18. Goldberg HI, Caruthers SB, Nelson JA, et al. Radiographic findings of the National Cooperative Crohn's Disease Study. *Gastroenterology.* 1979;77:925–937.
19. Dyer NH, Rutherford C, Visick JH, et al. The incidence and reliability of the individual radiographic signs in the small intestine in Crohn's disease. *Br J Radiol.* 1980;43:401–408.
20. Carlson HC. Perspective: the small bowel examination in the diagnosis of Crohn's disease. *AJR.* 1986;147:63–65.
21. Hildell J, Lindstrom C, Wenckert A. Radiographic appearance in Crohn's disease. I. Accuracy of radiographic methods. *Acta Radiol: Diagn.* 1979;20:609–625.
22. Sanders DE, Ho CS. The small bowel enema. Experience with 150 examinations. *AJR.* 1976;127:743–751.
23. Vallance R. An evaluation of the small bowel enema based on an analysis of 350 consecutive examinations. *Clin Radiol.* 1981;31:227–232.
24. Gurian L, Jendrzejewski J, Katon R, et al. Small bowel enema. An underutilized method of small bowel examination. *Dig Dis Sci.* 1982;27:1101–1108.
25. Maglinte DDT, Chernish SM, Kelvin FM, et al. Crohn's disease of the small intestine: accuracy and relevance of enteroclysis. *Radiology.* 1992;184:541–545.
26. Kelvin FM, Gedgaudas RK, Thompson WM, et al. The peroral pneumocolon: its role in evaluating the terminal ileum. *AJR.* 1982;139:115–121.
27. Glick SN. Crohn's disease of the small intestine. *Radiol Clin North Am.* 1987;25:25–45.
28. Goldberg HI, Gore RM, Margulis AR, et al. Computed tomography in the evaluation of Crohn's disease. *AJR.* 1983;140:277–282.
29. Kerber GW, Greenberg M, Rubin JM. Computed tomographic evaluation of local and extraintestinal complications of Crohn's disease. *Gastrointest Radiol.* 1984;9:143–148.
30. Goldman SM, Fishman EK, Gatewood OMB, et al. CT in the diagnosis of enterovesical fistulae. *AJR.* 1985;144:1229–1233.
31. Gore RM, Balthazar EJ, Ghahremani GG, et al. CT features of ulcerative colitis and Crohn's disease. *AJR.* 1996;167:3–15.
32. Meyers MA, MacGuire PV. Spiral CT demonstration of hypervascularity in Crohn's disease: "vascular jejunization of the ileum" or the "comb sign." *Abdom Imaging.* 1995;20:327–332.
33. Bender GN, Timmons HJ, Williard WC. Computed tomographic enteroclysis. One methodology. *Invest Radiol.* 1996;31:43–49.
34. Schober E, Turetschek K, Schima W. Methylcellulose enteroclysis spiral-CT: technique, examination quality and side effects—experience in 160 patients. Presented at the Eighth annual meeting of the European Society of Gastrointestinal Radiology; June 1997; Amsterdam, The Netherlands.
35. Sarrazin BJ, Wilson SR. Manifestations of Crohn's disease at US. *Radiographics.* 1996;16:499–520.
36. Sheridan MB, Nicholson DA, Martin DF. Transabdominal ultrasonography as the primary investigation in patients with suspected Crohn's disease or recurrence: a prospective study. *Clin Radiol.* 1993;48:402–404.
37. Solvig J, Ekberg O, Floren C-H, et al. Ultrasound examination of the small bowel: comparison with enteroclysis in patients with Crohn's disease. *Abdom Imaging.* 1995;20:323–326.
38. Pradel JA, David XR, Taourel P, et al. Sonographic assessment of the normal and abnormal bowel wall in nondiverticular ileitis and colitis. *Abdom Imaging.* 1997;22:167–172.
39. Rioux M, Gagnon J. Imaging modalities in the puzzling world of inflammatory bowel disease. *Abdom Imaging.* 1997;22:173–174.
40. Giaffer MH. Labeled leukocyte scintigraphy in inflammatory bowel disease: clinical applications. *Gut.* 1996;38:1–5.
41. Poitras P, Carrier L, Chartrand R, et al. Indium-111 leukocyte scanning of the abdomen. Analysis of its value for diagnosis and management of inflammatory bowel disease. *J Clin Gastroenterol.* 1987;9:418–423.
42. Kettritz U, Shoenut JP, Semelka RC. MR imaging of the gastrointestinal tract. *Magn Reson Imaging Clinics N Am.* 1995;3:87–98.
43. Shoenut JP, Semelka RC, Silverman R, et al. Magnetic resonance imaging in inflammatory bowel disease. *J Clin Gastroenterol.* 1993;17:73–78.
44. Barker PG, Lunniss PJ, Armstrong P. Magnetic resonance imaging of fistula-in-ano: technique, interpretation and accuracy. *Clin Radiol.* 1994;49:7–13.
45. Marshak RH, Lindner AE. *Radiology of the Small Intestine.* 2nd ed. Philadelphia, Pa: WB Saunders Co; 1976:158–273.
46. Nolan DJ, Piris J. Crohn's disease of the small intestine: a comparative study of the radiological and pathological appearances. *Clin Radiol.* 1980;31:591–596.
47. Ekberg O. Crohn's disease of the small intestine examined by double contrast technique. A comparison with oral technique. *Gastrointest Radiol.* 1977;1:355–359.
48. Glick SN, Teplick SK. Crohn's disease of the small intestine: diffuse mucosal granularity. *Radiology.* 1985;154:313–317.
49. Jones B, Hamilton SR, et al. Granular small bowel mucosa: a reflection of villous abnormality. *Gastrointest Radiol.* 1987;12:219–225.
50. Nolan DJ, Gourtsoyiannis NC. Crohn's disease of the small intestine: a review of the radiological appearances in 100 consecutive patients examined by a barium infusion technique. *Clin Radiol.* 1980;31:597–603.
51. Herlinger H. The small bowel enema and the diagnosis of Crohn's disease. *Radiol Clin North Am.* 1982;20:721–742.
52. Sellink JL. *Radiological Atlas of Common Disease of the Small Bowel.* Leiden, The Netherlands: HE Stenfert Kroese BV; 1976.
53. Ekberg O. Barium/air double contrast examination of

54. Nolan DJ. Radiology of Crohn's disease of the small intestine: a review. *J Roy Soc Med.* 1981;74:294–300.
55. Ekberg O, Lindstrom C. Superficial lesions in Crohn's disease of the small bowel. *Gastrointest Radiol.* 1979;4:389–393.
56. Goldberg HI, Sheft DJ. Abnormalities in small intestinal contour and caliber. *Radiol Clin North Am.* 1976;14:461–475.
57. Kelvin FM, Maglinte DDT. Small bowel: Crohn's disease. In: Taveras JM, Ferrucci JT, eds. *Radiology. Diagnosis—Imaging—Intervention.* Philadelphia, Pa: Lippincott-Raven. In press.
58. Buck JL, Dachman AH, Sobin LH. Polyps and pseudopolypoid manifestations of inflammatory bowel disease. *Radiographics* 1991;11:293–304.
59. Marshak RH, Wolf BS. Roentgen findings in regional enteritis. *AJR.* 1955;74:1000–1014.
60. Engelholm L, Mainguet P, Potvliege P. Radiology in early Crohn's disease of the small intestine. In: Wetterman IT, Pena AS, Booth CC, eds. *The Management of Crohn's Disease.* New York, NY: Excerpta Medica; 1976.
61. Laufer I, Costopoulos L. Early lesions in Crohn's disease. *AJR.* 1978;130:307–311.
62. Pringot J, Goncette L, Ponette E, et al. Nonstenotic ulcers of the small bowel. *Radiographics.* 1984;2:357–375.
63. Schmutz G, Kempf F, Schutz JF, et al. Le transit du grele en double contraste dans la maladie de Crohn. *J Radiol.* 1980;61:235–241.
64. Rickert RR, Carter HW. The "early" ulcerative lesion of Crohn's disease: correlating light and scanning electron microscopic studies. *J Clin Gastroenterol.* 1980;2:11–19.
65. Ekberg O, Bath L, Sostrom B, et al. Are superficial lesions of the distal part of the ileum early indicators of Crohn's disease in adult patients with abdominal pain? A clinical and radiologic long-term investigation. *Gut.* 1984;25:341–346.
66. Watier A, Devroede G, et al. Small erythematous mucosal plaques: an endoscopic sign of Crohn's disease. *Gut.* 1980;21:835–839.
67. Yamagata S, Baba S, Hosoda S, et al. Crohn's disease in Japan. *Gastroenterol Jpn.* 1979;14:366–373.
68. Herlinger H, Rubesin SE, Furth EE. Mesenteric border linear ulcer in Crohn's disease: historical, radiologic and pathologic perspectives. *Abdom Radiol.* In press.
69. Meyers MA. Clinical involvement of mesenteric and antimesenteric borders of small bowel loops. *Gastrointest Radiol.* 1976;1:49–58.
70. Graham MF, Diegelmann RF, Elson CO, et al. Collagen content and types in the intestinal strictures of Crohn's disease. *Gastroenterology.* 1988;84:257–265.
71. Marshak RH. Granulomatous disease of the intestinal tract (Crohn's disease). *Radiology.* 1975;114:3–22.
72. Goldstein F, Murdock MG. Clinical and radiologic improvement of regional enteritis and enterocolitis after treatment with salicylazosulfapyridine. *Am J Dig Dis.* 1971;16:421–431.
73. Hildell J. Radiographic patterns of Crohn's disease. Malmo, Sweden: University of Lund; 1978. Thesis.
74. Truelove SC, Pena AS. Course and prognosis of Crohn's disease. *Gut.* 1976;17:192–201.
75. Softly A, Myren J, Clamp SE, et al. Factors affecting recurrence after surgery for Crohn's disease. *Scand J Gastroenterol.* 1988;(suppl 144)23:31–34.
76. Greenstein AJ, Sachar DB, Pasternack BS, et al. Reoperation and recurrence in Crohn's colitis and ileocolitis, crude and cumulative rates. *N Engl J Med.* 1975;193:656–690.
77. Rutgeerts P, Geboes K, Vantrappen G. Predictability of the postoperative course of Crohn's disease. *Gastroenterology.* 1990;99:956–963.
78. Olaison G, Smedh K, Sjodahl R. Natural course of Crohn's disease after ileocolic resection: endoscopically visualized ileal ulcers preceding symptoms. *Gut.* 1992;33:331–335.
79. Pennington L, Hamilton SR, Bayless TM, et al. Surgical management of Crohn's disease: influence of disease at margin of resection. *Ann Surg.* 1980;192:311–318.
80. Hildell J, Lindstrom C, Wenckert A. Radiographic appearance in Crohn's disease. IV. The new distal ileum after surgery. *Acta Radiol: Diagn.* 1980;21:221–229.
81. Koch TR, Dave DR, Ford H, et al. Crohn's ileitis and ileocolitis. A study of the anatomical distribution of recurrence. *Dig Dis Sci.* 1981;26:528–531.
82. Bartram CI. *Radiology in Inflammatory Bowel Disease.* New York, NY: Marcel Dekker; 1983. pp 121–125.
83. Bartram CI. The radiological demonstration of adhesions following surgery for inflammatory bowel disease. *Br J Radiol.* 1980;53:650–653.
84. Crohn BB, Yarnis H. *Regional Ileitis.* 2nd ed. New York, NY: Grune & Stratton; 1958.
85. Tan WC, Allan RN. Diffuse jejunoileitis of Crohn's disease. *Gut.* 1993;34:1374–1378.
86. Cooke WT, Swan CJ. Diffuse jejunoileitis of Crohn's disease. *Q J Med.* 1974;43:583–601.
87. Mekhjian HS, Switz DM, Watts HD, et al. National Cooperative Crohn's Disease Study: factors determining recurrence of Crohn's disease after surgery. *Gastrointest Radiol.* 1979;77:907–913.
88. Fanucci A, Letto F, Cerro P, et al. X-ray assessment of the extent of lesions in small intestinal Crohn's disease. *Ital J Gastroenterol.* 1985;17:23–24.
89. Deli TCB, Kettlewell MGW, Mortensen NJM, et al. Ten years experience of strictureplasty for obstructive Crohn's disease. *Br J Surg.* 1989;76:339–341.
90. Kelly IMG, Bartram CI. Pseudotumoral appearance of small bowel strictureplasty for Crohn's disease. *Abdom Imaging.* 1993;18:366–368.
91. Sayfan J, Wilson DAL, Allan A, et al. Recurrence after strictureplasty for Crohn's disease: it is no more likely than after resection. *Br J Surg.* 1989;767:335–338.
92. Koelbel G, Schmiedl U, Majer MC, et al. Diagnosis of fistulae and sinus tracts in patients with Crohn's disease: value of MR imaging. *AJR.* 1989;152:999–1003.
93. Steinberg DM, Cooke WT, Alexander-Williams J. Abscess and fistulae in Crohn's disease. *Gut.* 1973;14:865–869.

94. Givel JC, Hawker P, et al. Entero-enteric fistula complicating Crohn's disease. *J Clin Gastroenterol.* 1983;5: 321–323.
95. Herlinger H, O'Riordan D, Saul S, et al. Nonspecific involvement of bowel adjoining Crohn's disease. *Radiology.* 1986;159:47–51.
96. Korelitz BI. The ileosigmoidal fistula in Crohn's disease: a clinical radiological correlation. *Mt Sinai J Med.* 1984;51:341–346.
97. Greenstein AJ, Sachar DB, Tzakis A, et al. Course of enterovesical fistulae in Crohn's disease. *Am J Surg.* 1984;147:788–792.
98. Schraut WH, Block GE. Enterovesical fistula complicating Crohn's ileocolitis. *Am J Gastroenterol.* 1984;79: 186–190.
99. Gorcey S, Katzka I. Is operation always necessary for enterovesical fistulas in Crohn's disease? *J Clin Gastroenterol.* 1989;11:396–398.
100. Givel JC, Hawker P, Allan RN, et al. Enterovaginal fistulae associated with Crohn's disease. *Surg Gynecol Obstet.* 1982;155:494–496.
101. Myhr GE, Myrvold HE, Nilsen G, et al. Perianal fistulas: use of MR imaging for diagnosis. *Radiology.* 1994;191:545–549.
102. O'Donovan AN, Somers S, Farrow R. MR imaging of anorectal Crohn's disease: a pictorial essay. *Radiographics.* 1997;17:101–107.
103. Keighley MR, Eastwood D, et al. Incidence and microbiology of abdominal and pelvic abscess in Crohn's disease. *Gastroenterology.* 1982;83:1271–1275.
104. Ribeiro MB, Greenstein AJ, Yamazaki Y, et al. Intraabdominal abscess in regional enteritis. *Ann Surg.* 1991;213:32–36.
105. Alexander ES, Weinberg S, Clark RA, et al. Fistulae and sinus tracts: radiographic evaluation, management and outcome. *Gastrointest Radiol.* 1982;7:135–140.
106. Lambiase RE, Cronan JJ, Dorfman GS, et al. Percutaneous drainage of abscesses in patients with Crohn disease. *AJR.* 1988;150:1043–1045.
107. Casola G, vanSonnenberg E, Neff CC, et al. Abscesses in Crohn disease: percutaneous drainage. *Radiology.* 1987;163:19–22.
108. Sahai A, Belair M, Gianfelice D, et al. Percutaneous drainage of intra-abdominal abscesses in Crohn's disease: short- and long-term outcome. *Am J Gastroenterol.* 1997;92:275–278.
109. Lasher BA. Risk factors for small bowel cancer in Crohn's disease. *Dig Dis Sci.* 1992;37:1179–1184.
110. Marchetta F, Fazio VW, Ozuner G. Adenocarcinoma arising from a stricturoplasty site in Crohn's disease: report of a case. *Dis Colon Rectum.* 1996;39:1315–1321.
111. Greenstein AJ, Mullin GE, Strauchen JA, et al. Lymphoma in inflammatory bowel disease. *Cancer.* 1992;69: 1119–1123.
112. Kelly MD, Stuart M, Tschuchnigg M. Primary intestinal Hodgkin's disease complicating ileal Crohn's disease. *Austr N Z J Surg.* 1997;67:485–489.
113. Larvol L, Soule JC, Le Tourneau A. Reversible lymphoma in the setting of azothiaprine therapy for Crohn's disease. *N Engl J Med.* 1994;331:883–884.
114. Tomei E, Diacinti D, Marini M, et al. Computed tomography of bowel wall in patients with Crohn's disease: relationship of inflammatory activity to biological indices. *Ital J Gastroenterol.* 1996;28:487–492.
115. Shoenut JP, Semelka RC, Magro CM, et al. Comparison of magnetic resonance imaging and endoscopy in distinguishing the type and severity of inflammatory bowel disease. *J Clin Gastroenterol.* 1994;19:31–35.
116. Madsen SM, Thomsen HS, Munkholm P, et al. Magnetic resonance imaging of Crohn disease: early recognition of treatment response and relapse. *Abdom Imaging.* 1997;22:164–166.
117. van Oostayen JA, Wasser MNJM, van Hogezand RA. Doppler sonography evaluation of superior mesenteric artery flow to assess Crohn's disease activity; correlation with clinical evaluation, Crohn's disease activity index and α1-antitrypsin clearance in feces. *AJR.* 1997;168:429–433.

Parasitic and Bacterial Inflammatory Diseases

16

Hans Herlinger

Chapter Contents

Introduction
Enteritis Caused by Parasites
Bacterial Enteritis
Infections by Fungi
Extrinsic Inflammations Affecting the Small Intestine

Introduction

The parasitic and inflammatory diseases of the small bowel can produce a wide spectrum of radiographic abnormalities. The appearance of involved segments will depend upon what layers of the wall are involved, what the natural history of the particular disease is, and at what point in the course of the disease the patient is examined. Although no one finding is disease-specific, a particular feature or combination of features may suggest one diagnosis rather than another. Colonic involvement is present in many. The radiologic appearances of specific enteritides can be mimicked by idiopathic inflammatory diseases. For precise diagnosis of a parasitic or specific inflammatory disease of the intestine, one must rely on laboratory findings, yet even these are not always straightforward. Therefore, other factors must be taken into consideration, and radiology is one of them. Diagnosis becomes particularly important, as this group of diseases is usually treatable and can often be cured.

The geographic location must affect the probability of a particular small bowel lesion being present. For example, where Crohn's disease would be diagnosed in Western countries, a parasitic infestation or tuberculosis would be a more likely diagnosis in the Philippines, India, or countries in Southern Africa. Parasitic infestations are uncommon outside endemic areas, but widespread emigration and travel have resulted in their importation into other countries. A knowledge of the mode of transmission and of the natural course of infection or infestation of the small bowel can aid the radiologist in the differential diagnosis.

Enteritis Caused by Parasites

Because of extensive American civilian and military travel throughout the world, parasitic infestations are now more frequently encountered in North America. The same applies to other countries in the Western world. In addition to the immigrant population, patients in psychiatric institutions are the segments of the population who have a significant parasitic burden in the United States and other countries in the West.[1]

In the diagnosis of parasitic infestation, the examination of the stool for parasites and ova must be the first step. Since the clinical symptoms are usually nonspecific, however, a radiologic examination is not infrequently obtained at the beginning. The radiologist, therefore, may be in a position to contribute to the diagnosis of the disease.

The parasites, having entered the host in their different ways, ultimately select their final location for continued existence.[2] While most protozoan parasites settle in the colon, helminths show a preference for the small intestine. Of the parasites that infest the small intestine, *Giardia lamblia*, *Ancylostoma*, and *Strongyloides* primarily cause inflammatory changes in the duodenum and proximal jejunum. *Ascaris lumbricoides* (roundworm) and the taeniae can cause localized, functional, and structural disorders throughout the small intestine. Ascariasis and ancylostomiasis are the most frequently encountered parasitic infestations involving the small bowel in the tropics.

Ascariasis

Ascaris lumbricoides is the largest intestinal nematode parasitic in humans. The roundworms are found in tropical and semitropical countries throughout the world and thrive with poor sanitation. As an example of the parasitic burden, it has been estimated that a total of 18,000 tons of *Ascaris* ova are produced annually in the intestinal tract of the population of China.[3]

Roundworms are transmitted without the need for an intermediate host. Embryonated eggs are swallowed and hatch in the duodenum. The larvae penetrate the bowel wall, enter venous channels, and pass through the liver and heart into the lungs; they then ascend the trachea, are swallowed, and again reach the small intestine to mature in the bowel wall. They then commence their tireless egg production.

Small bowel symptoms attributable to ascariasis are difficult to assess, mainly because of the usually associated presence of other parasites. Children are generally more severely affected. The smaller calibers of their intestinal lumens favor the development of obstructions by boluses of worms.[4] The use of 15 to 30 ml of water-soluble meglumine diatrizoate (MD gastroview, Mallinckrodt, St. Louis, Mo.) by nasogastric tube has been suggested to induce bowel movements in children who present with obstruction due to massive ascariasis; however, this should be done only after rehydration and in the absence of signs of peritonitis.[5] A single worm has also been reported to become the lead point of an intussusception.[6] Severe infestation may lead to malabsorption and malnutrition. Dyspeptic symptoms suggesting peptic ulcer disease are not infrequent. Extraintestinal migration of ascarides, for example into bile ducts, can be associated with a variety of complications.

Radiology

The worms can be identified on plain abdominal films in 70% of cases.[6] Mature worms within the small bowel are visible because of their soft-tissue density against surrounding intraluminal air (Fig. 16-1).[7] A larger bolus of parasites may create a so-called whirlpool effect and can be associated with ileuslike bowel distention or with obstruction. Edema of the intestinal mucosa may also be evident on plain films. On contrast examination, ascarides cause elongated tubular defects in the barium-filled bowel lumen (Fig. 16-2). Female worms are up to 35 cm in length; the male is somewhat shorter. Their linear intestinal tracts may take up barium, to appear as a thin, linear opacity within the soft-tissue density of the worm. This linear shadow may persist for some time after barium has been eliminated from the gut. Worms can also be recognized in the colon. A computed tomography (CT) identification of an ascaris has been reported.[8]

Diagnosis is confirmed by the finding of *Ascaris* ova on microscopic examination of the stool. Often, the

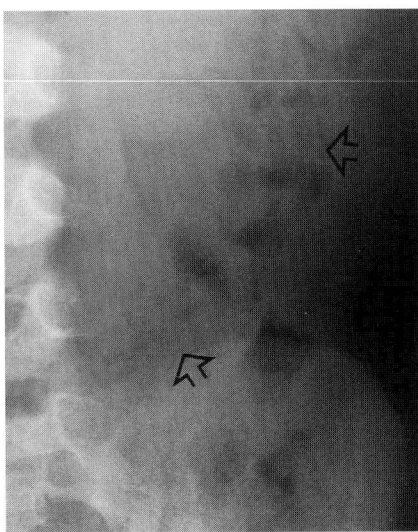

Fig. 16-1. Plain film in ascariasis.
A bolus of worms is outlined by intraluminal gas in the left abdomen (arrows). Ascarides can be identified on plain films in 70% of infested children.

patient will also describe a typical roundworm passed on defecation.

Ancylostomiasis

Hookworm infestation is endemic in the tropical areas of the world but can also occur in more temperate zones. The disease is produced by two varieties of ne-

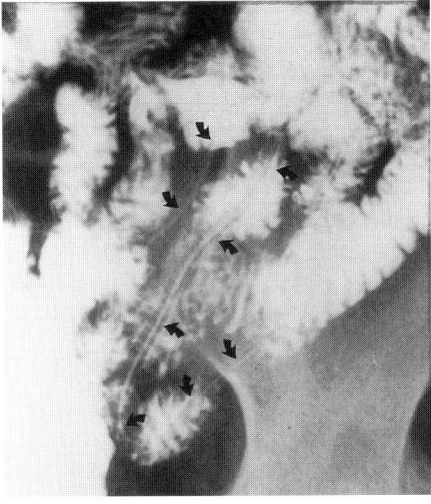

Fig. 16-2. Barium examination in ascariasis.
Small bowel meal shows ascarides as elongated tubular filling defects (arrows) in distal jejunum. Barium ingested by the worms opacifies their straight intestinal tracts. (Courtesy of G. Eidenschwank, MD, and C. Slywotzky, MD.)

matodes, *Ancylostoma duodenale* and *Necator americanus*. The Old World hookworm, *A duodenale*, is found in Southern Europe, the Mediterranean region, and the west coast of South America. *N americanus*, brought to America during the slave trade era, predominates in the southern United States, much of South America, and the Caribbean, and, together with *A duodenale*, is found in India, Southeast Asia, and the southwestern Pacific area.[9]

The adult worm lives attached to the small intestinal mucosa, mainly of the jejunum. Under suitable soil conditions, the many eggs discharged each day by the female worm rapidly develop into infective filariform larvae, ready to penetrate human skin. They find their way through the liver and heart to the lungs and then to the pharynx, to be swallowed and enter the intestine.

Adult hookworms anchor themselves to the jejunal mucosa, secreting an anticoagulant to ensure their intake of blood. They may change the site of attachment from time to time. Each adult *N americanus* causes a daily blood loss of approximately 0.03 to 0.15 ml.[10] The intestinal blood loss is proportional to the fecal egg count.[10] Persons with a light parasite load are usually asymptomatic. Severe infestation frequently leads to the insidious development of microcytic, hypochromic anemia (hookworm disease). Heavy infestation, especially in children, can cause severe anemia and retardation of growth and intellectual development. Hypoalbuminemia and eosinophilia are other features of hookworm disease.

Radiology

The 8- to 13-mm worms cannot be visualized in barium studies. However, the finding of fold thickening and motility disturbances with pronounced focal irritability usually limited to the duodenum and proximal jejunum should suggest the diagnosis. It can be confirmed by finding typical ova in the patient's stool. Endoscopic appearances take the form of gross duodenitis with areas of hemorrhage. Worms have been demonstrated on biopsy specimens.

Anisakiasis

The larvae of the anisakiad genera *Anisakis* and *Contracaecum* can invade the gastrointestinal tract of humans and cause herring worm disease or anisakiasis. Marine mammals and piscivorous birds pass the eggs with their feces. The eggs hatch in the sea, and are taken up by plankton and then by fish, such as herring. *Anisakis* larvae reside in the intestinal tract of fish but migrate into muscle when the fish dies and is not filleted shortly after being caught. Fish that are refrigerated at sea and are not filleted until later are the likely source of infection in humans, provided they prefer to eat the fish raw or pickled. Ingested *Anisakis* larvae develop to their fourth larval stage only and cannot develop further in humans.[11]

The invasive 50- to 100-mm-long *Anisakis* larvae burrow into the walls of the stomach and intestine where they cause eosinophilic granuloma formation and at times ulceration, perforation, or a mesenteric abscess. Larvae may be identified within these lesions. Although the majority of cases have been reported from Japan and Scandinavia, sporadic reports have come from most maritime areas, including the coastal parts of California and Alaska.[12]

Radiology

Radiology[13] and endoscopy[14] can be of value in the diagnosis of gastroduodenal anisakiasis. Yet, the diagnosis of intestinal anisakiasis has rarely been made radiologically.[15,16] Findings by barium study include irregular thickening of the wall of the small bowel or colon, mucosal edema, and luminal narrowing [Fig. 16-3(a)]. Ulceration with mass effect appears to be an unusual feature in anisakiasis [Fig. 16-3(b)]. The most common sites of involvement are the jejunum, ileum, and colon. Sonography has been used in the diagnosis of 18 cases of intestinal anisakiasis; all cases showed wall thickening, mostly with ascitic fluid close to the involved segment.[17]

The condition should be suspected when symptoms of abdominal pain and pyrexia are associated with both a history of raw fish ingestion and abnormal appearances during barium examination.

Strongyloidiasis

Strongyloides stercoralis is a nematode parasite. *S stercoralis* has worldwide distribution but is much more common in the tropics, where the soil provides a suitable environment for development. Penetration through the skin and subsequent migration through the lung to the small bowel resemble that described in hookworms. No male parasites are found in the gut. The females, only 2 to 3 mm in length, burrow into the superficial mucosa of the duodenum and jejunum and release ova into the bowel lumen. The ova produce rhabditiform larvae that normally reach the warm soil and there develop into infective filariform larvae, ready to restart the cycle of infestation.

In the majority of patients, clinical manifestations are few or none, infestation being light. Abdominal discomfort may be intensified by the intake of alcohol or greasy food. With more severe infestations there may

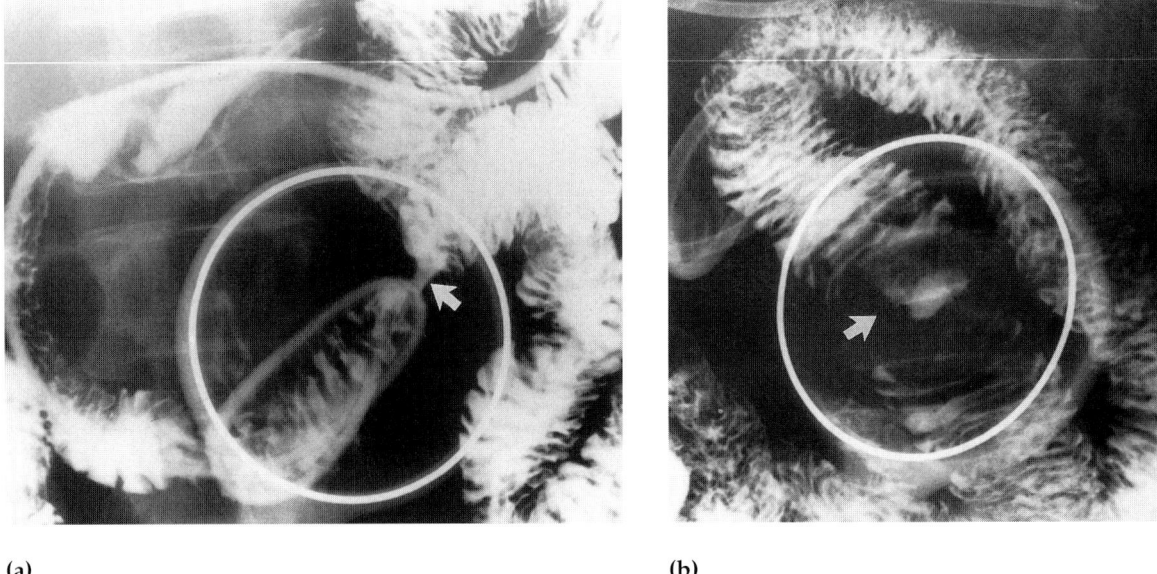

Fig. 16-3. Duodenojejunal anisakiasis in a Swedish male patient who had lived in Japan for several years. (a) Small bowel follow-through shows a short stricture (arrow) in the distal duodenum obstructing the further passage of the tube. Note mild thickening of folds proximal to stricture. (b) A short annular ulcerated lesion (arrow) with shouldering but without obvious mucosal destruction is seen in the proximal jejunum. In view of the patient's residence history and the compatible appearance, a radiologic diagnosis of anisakiasis was made. Both lesions were resected. Histology showed granulomata with an excess of eosinophils. Although no larvae could be identified, histology was considered consistent with the diagnosis of anisakiasis. (Courtesy of Anders Lunderquist, MD, Lund, Sweden.)

be nausea and vomiting, diarrhea, weight loss, and urticaria. Massive strongyloidiasis can develop in many conditions that depress the host's immune system—immunosuppressive drugs, corticosteroids, radiation therapy, advanced age, and infrequently, Acquired Immunodeficiency Syndrome (AIDS). Rhabditiform larvae may then transform into the infective filariform stage within the gut, to penetrate the wall again and start a cycle of repeated and progressively increasing internal autoinfection. External autoinfection can also occur and is usually associated with poor hygiene, allowing filariform larvae to penetrate the perianal skin and start on their passage to the small intestine.[18] It is possible for hyperinfestation to be associated with life-threatening dissemination, presenting with pulmonary infiltrates, meningitis, and intravascular coagulation.

Radiology

With light infestation, mucosal invasion produces only focal edema and spasm. A patient with a more significant parasite load may present with fold thickening in the duodenum and jejunum [Fig. 16-4(a, b)]. Radiologic findings in more prolonged infestation may include effacement of folds and a pipestem appearance of the jejunum [Fig. 16-4(c)] or a diffusely ulcerated, shortened, and narrowed jejunum [Fig. 16-4(d)] that will not return to a normal fold pattern after successful treatment. When the infestation is associated with immune deficiency, the duodenal folds are severely thickened and folds throughout the jejunum show thickening with indication of thickening of the bowel wall itself. Such changes may be partially reversible.[19] In overwhelming infestation, there may be toxic dilatation with paresis, usually permanent. The pronounced mucosal swelling in the duodenum has been considered the cause of papillary stenosis, which responded to treatment with thiabendazole.[20]

The abnormal radiologic pattern in the more severe forms of strongyloidiasis should suggest the diagnosis, especially if supported by a history of tropical origin or prolonged residence there. The demonstration of rhabditiform larvae in a wet saline stool preparation is not always successful. The diagnostic yield of duodenal aspiration or endoscopic biopsy is reported to exceed 90%.[21]

Tapeworm

Taenia saginata, the beef tapeworm, is the most common *Taenia* affecting humans and is found throughout the world, except where meat is not eaten for religious reasons. Humans are its only definitive hosts. The infestation is acquired by eating insufficiently cooked

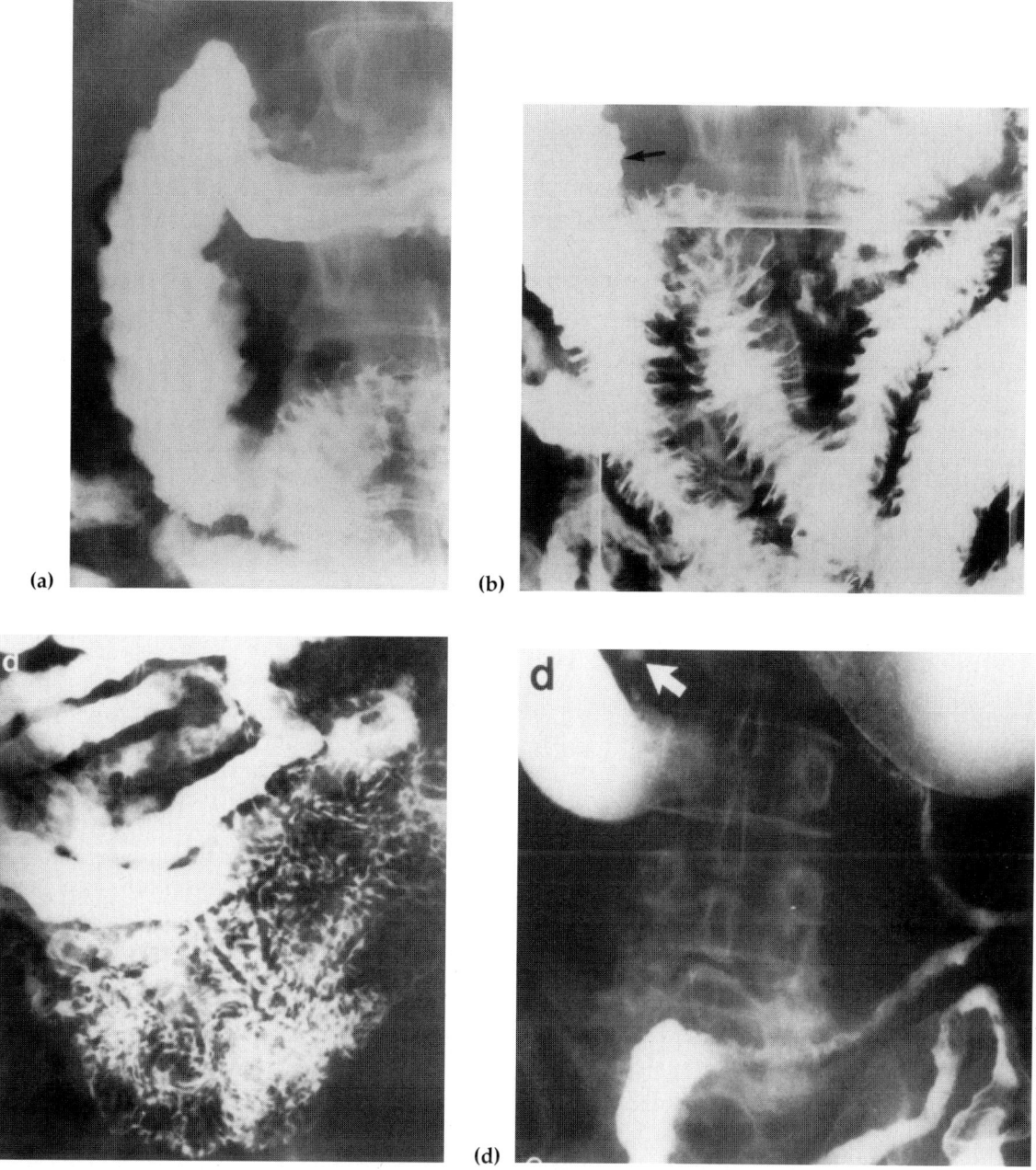

Fig. 16-4. Strongyloidiasis in a female human immunodeficiency virus–positive patient who presented with abdominal pain, pronounced weight loss, and diarrhea.
(a) Marked thickening of duodenal mucosal folds. (b) The small bowel follow-through shows gross fold thickening in the jejunum (arrow again indicates changes in the duodenum). (c) In a further patient positive for strongyloidiasis a barium study outlined a different but still typical small bowel pattern. Thickened folds are barely identified in the diffusely tubular jejunum and duodenum (d = duodenum). (Courtesy of J.C. Lappas, MD.) (d) In a third patient with prolonged infestation the jejunum is ulcerated, shortened, and narrowed (d = duodenum, arrow indicates reflux of barium into ampulla). Treatment achieved widening of the bowel lumen but without return of a normal fold pattern. (Courtesy of J. Farman, MD.)

meat that contains the encysted larvae. The considerable length of the adult worm (average 4.5 mm consisting of some 1500 proglottides) may occasionally give rise to obstructive symptoms. Some patients complain of abdominal discomfort, nausea, vomiting, and malaise. Eggs that are identical to those of *T. solium* can be found in the feces. A more specific diagnosis is possible when gravid proglottides are recovered from the feces. Occasionally the adult tapeworm has been demonstrated by barium study.[22]

T. solium, the pork tapeworm, is rare in the United States. It averages 4.5 mm in length and can live up to 25 years in the intestinal tract. *Cysticerci* are bladders of less than 1 cm that contain scoleces and are the infective larval stage. If consumed with insufficiently cooked pork, the larvae are released by digestion and then mature. Abdominal symptoms are vague, and there may be a moderate eosinophilia. The relevant complication is cysticercosis, an invasion of the skeletal muscle, brain, and other structures by the infective larvae that eventually die and calcify.

Diphyllobothrium latum, the fish tapeworm, is distributed worldwide. Infection is common in areas where improperly cooked freshwater fish forms a prominent part of the diet; Scandinavia, Alaska, Canada, and the lake areas of Minnesota and Michigan are examples. Similar to other tapeworms, it may be several meters in length and inhabits the small intestine, with its scolex attached high in the jejunum. There are usually no symptoms. However, *D latum* competes with the host's supply of vitamin B_{12} and has been found to absorb 80% to 100% of a single dose of radioactive B_{12}.[11] In patients who present with a macrocytic anemia in a country with a high prevalence of the parasite, infection with *D latum* should be suspected and the stool tested for the presence of typical ova or proglottides. Eradication of the worm cures the anemia.

Giardiasis

Giardia lamblia, a protozoan intestinal flagellate, is of global distribution, often occurring as a harmless commensal. However, it frequently presents with diarrhea and malabsorption and may be associated with immunologic abnormalities. It is the most widespread intestinal parasite in the United States, and the one most often identified in water-related outbreaks.[23]

Giardia is well adapted to its eventual location in the small bowel. In human volunteers only 10 cysts were capable of causing infection.[24] When mature infective cysts are swallowed, the low pH of the stomach induces excystment to liberate two trophozoites that later continue to multiply by binary fission.[11] The pear-shaped trophozoites of *G lamblia* inhabit the unstirred water layer over the intervillous spaces of the duodenum and proximal mesenteric small bowel, often attached to microvilli.[25] Cysts are formed in large numbers and mature during their passage through the alimentary tract. Trophozoites are passed also, especially at times of diarrhea.

Diarrhea and, in some cases, malabsorption are associated with giardiasis and are due to several likely mechanisms. *Giardia* avidly consumes bile salts and seems to be a factor in bile salt deconjugation.[24] Trophozoites were found to actively inhibit trypsin. *G lamblia* does not invade the epithelium. Lectin activity by *Giardia* may contribute to microvillous damage or may facilitate the action of toxins.[24] It is no longer suggested that a large jejunal population of *G lamblia* cause malabsorption by their mechanical barrier formation. Villous abnormalities from flattening to more diffuse atrophy have repeatedly been demonstrated. Giardiasis can be associated with several of the immunodeficiency syndromes, usually accompanied by low or absent IgA levels (see Chapter 17).

Radiology

The radiographic findings usually mentioned in the literature are an often considerable increase in the thickness of folds in the duodenum and proximal jejunum and a state of irritability (Fig. 16-5).[26] Radiology can be important toward the diagnosis of *Giardiasis*. The above-mentioned findings in a patient with prolonged diarrhea and a history of having been in an endemic area should induce the prominent mention of giardiasis in the differential diagnosis.

CT has demonstrated wall thickening in the jejunum as well as mesenteric adenopathy, both reverting to normal after treatment.[27] Radiology can also play a most useful role in further demonstrating pattern alterations, which would indicate associated immunodeficiencies (see Chapter 17).

A clinical diagnosis is of particular importance, since specific treatment for giardiasis is readily available. Stool examinations can be unrewarding, as cysts and trophozoites are passed intermittently and may have been suppressed by medication. Small intestinal biopsies, preferably at multiple sites, or the study of duodenal aspirates is more rewarding. Tests for anti-*Giardia* antibodies are becoming available; those testing IgM are preferred as they can distinguish current from previous infection.[28]

Schistosomiasis

Infection with flukes of the genus *Schistosoma* is one of the major health problems of the world. *S. japonicum*, which is endemic in Eastern Asia, especially China, has a predilection for mesenteric venous location. After penetrating the skin, the larvae pass through systemic veins to reach submucosal mesenteric venules where they produce up to 3500 eggs per day.[29] Some of the eggs reach the bowel lumen but the majority are retained in the bowel wall and cause further tissue damage. A granulomatous reaction leads to mucosal thickening, formation of polyps, eventually fibrosis, and possible calcification. However, involvement of

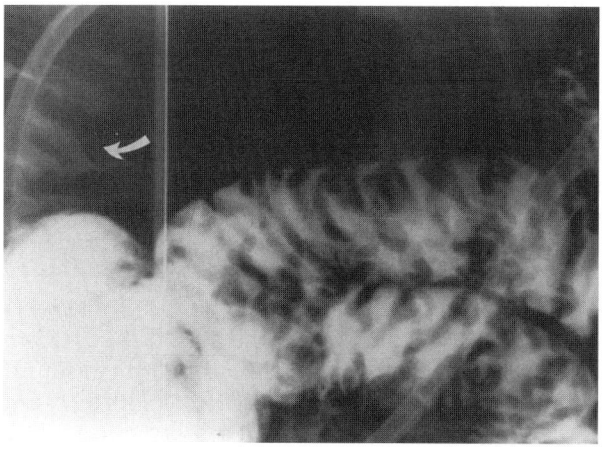 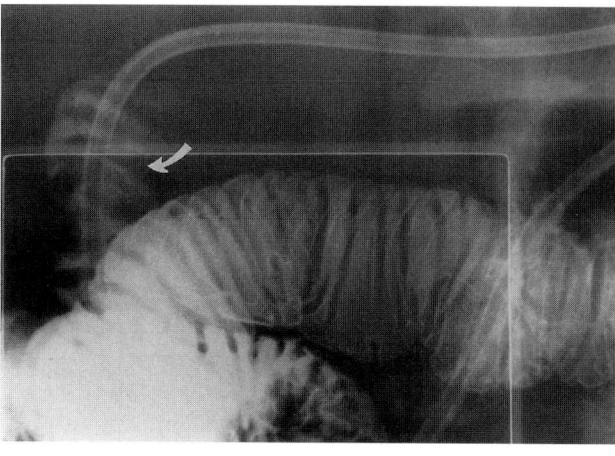

(a) (b)

Fig. 16-5. Giardiasis confirmed in an immunocompetent patient who presented with prolonged diarrhea. He had never traveled abroad but liked skiing in Colorado.
(a) Enteroclysis demonstrates fold thickening in an irritable proximal jejunum. (b) With rapid inflow of methylcellulose solution it was possible to distend the jejunum briefly and demonstrate fold thickening. Limited reflux of barium in (a) and (b) demonstrates severe thickening of duodenal folds (arrows). The radiologic report could suggest the likelihood of giardiasis.

the small intestine is overshadowed by that of the colon, and mural calcifications are usually seen there, best shown by CT. Some of the ova are swept back into the portal vein where they cause hepatic fibrosis of insidious onset, usually starting in childhood.[30]

Bacterial Enteritis

Mycobacterium tuberculosis

Until some 30 years ago, improved treatment of pulmonary tuberculosis, BCG immunization, pasteurization of milk, and awareness of the entity of Crohn's disease had rendered the diagnosis of abdominal tuberculosis uncommon in the Western world although it continued to be a significant health problem in developing countries, especially Asia.[31] Only 31 cases of intestinal tuberculosis but 503 of Crohn's disease were found in a New York hospital during a 44-year period to 1975.[32] In a report from India, on the other hand, 300 cases of intestinal tuberculosis and 13 of Crohn's disease were diagnosed during 14 years to 1978.[33] In recent years, however, there has been a resurgence of tuberculosis in the West. A number of factors are responsible, among them increased immigration, drug abuse, homelessness, and crowding in shelters.[34] The failure of many patients to complete the prolonged course of treatment has resulted not only in continued disease infectivity but also in the emergence of drug-resistant stains.[34] The epidemic of AIDS has added significantly to the clinical and public health problems of this "new tuberculosis." Extrapulmonary disease is encountered more frequently, its diagnosis more difficult and its progress more rapid. In the East and West there has been a relative ascendance of abdominal over pulmonary tuberculosis. Only a minority of patients with abdominal tuberculosis now show evidence of pulmonary disease.[35]

Pathology

Transaxial, often multiple ulcerations are typical features of tuberculous enteritis, increasing in frequency toward the distal ileum. Active, caseating granulomas are present there and in the involved regional nodes. Fibrous tissue is laid down, at times in excessive amounts, to merit the descriptive term ulcerohypertrophic tuberculosis. Later, often after treatment, these bowel segments may produce fibrous constriction, the ulcer-constrictive form.[31] Long segments of constrictive disease may be observed. The hypertrophic pattern predominates in the ileocecal area, giving rise to a palpable mass and to matting of involved and adjacent bowel with the diseased lymph nodes. Distinction from Crohn's disease can be difficult. Findings favoring tuberculous enteritis are the presence of miliary tubercles on the serosal surface of affected bowel segments, absence of deep fissures, the confluent nature of caseous granulomas, and their location in regional nodes.[36]

Clinical Aspects

It is important to keep the possible diagnosis of abdominal tuberculosis very much in mind, especially in the case of immigrants from Eastern countries. Weight loss, fever, diarrhea, an elevated sedimentation rate, a palpable mass, and ascites are clinical presentations that ought to suggest this diagnostic possibility. Patients with tuberculous enteritis predominantly affecting the ilocecal area are likely to present with right lower quadrant pain, which may be become generalized, severe, or insidious and may be associated with obstruction.[35] Unlike with Crohn's disease, diarrhea is a lesser feature and anal lesions are rare. But Crohn's disease remains the major differential diagnostic consideration (others are appendicitis, lymphoma, carcinoma, ameboma, and actinomycosis).

A definitive diagnosis ought to precede treatment, possibly with the exception of endemic regions where medical management may commence without a proven diagnosis. A radiograph of the chest without abnormal findings is not helpful in the differential diagnosis. Traditionally, a specific diagnosis rests either on the demonstration of *Myobacterium tuberculosis* in smear, culture, or guinea pig inoculation or on histologic evidence of tubercles with caseation. Cultures of ascitic fluid require up to 6 weeks and may be negative. Moreover, mycobacterium, once isolated, ought nowadays to be tested for sensitivity to the drugs available for its treatment, thus involving further delay. There are two procedures that can reach a definite diagnosis in shorter time. Laparoscopic biopsy may provide a sufficiently rapid and reliable diagnosis.[37] The serologic marker adenosine deaminase is reported to yield 95% sensitivity in the rapid diagnosis of tuberculous ascites.[37] A few reasons support the principle of diagnosis before treatment. Corticosteroids that may be beneficial in Crohn's disease are likely to be harmful in tuberculosis; however, an exception would be the beneficial effect of the additional use of prednisolone in patients with malabsorption of antituberculous drugs.[38] Antituberculous drugs, given in combination, need to be administered in adequate dosage and for 18 to 24 months to avoid the formation of resistant strains and achieve a cure. Moreover, once treatment has started, a bacteriologic diagnosis of tuberculosis may no longer be feasible.[39] Any surgical intervention intended for diagnosis or treatment should be based on sufficient clinical indications, and this becomes one of the purposes of diagnostic radiology in this disease.

Radiology

Barium studies. Earliest changes in tuberculous enteritis are altered motility with thickening and nodularity of folds [Fig. 16-6(a)]. Focal disappearance of folds, the demonstration of polyps, and ulcerations that are usually transaxial are other early findings [Fig. 16-6(b)]. These girdle ulcers and the subsequent development of short strictures [Fig. 16-6(c)] have been carefully documented by Yao and colleagues.[40] Radiological findings of ileocecal disease can be highly suggestive of *M tuberculosis*. In ileocecal disease cecal involvement in the tuberculous process can significantly exceed that of the terminal ileum.[41] A cephalad retraction of the cecum may be associated with straightening of the ileocecal junction angle.[41] Eventually, the cecum may become unrecognizable, with the terminal ileum continuing straight into the colon and the valve incompetent or no longer identifiable [Fig. 16-6(d–f)]. Predominant mass formation with ulceration involving the terminal ileum and usually more advanced ulcerative changes affecting the cecum or the ileocecal valve area are usually well demonstrated by CT (Fig. 16-7 and 16-8) or by a combination of barium and CT scans. Magnetic resonance imaging is at its best in the demonstration of changes in the mesentery and omentum (Fig. 16-9).

Complications are infrequent.[42] Strictures, typically short and of hourglass configuration, may become severe enough to cause obstruction (Fig. 16-8). More common are narrowed segments that are longer and tubular, involving small bowel and colon [Fig. 16-6(f)]. It would be unusual to find colonic disease alone. Fistulae may occur, mostly to the sigmoid colon. Perforation is rare.

Fig. 16-6. Enteroclyses or barium follow-through examinations in the demonstration of typical changes in ileocecal or more extensive tuberculosis.
(a) Korean immigrant presented with abdominal pain, diarrhea, and weight loss. Single-contrast enteroclysis shows localized fold thickening with nodularity (arrowheads) in the terminal ileum (TI). A similar lesion is seen in an adjacent segment of ileum (arrow). (Courtesy of Dan Nolan, MD, Oxford, England.) (b) Ileocecal tuberculosis with a star-shaped ulcer in the terminal ileum (curved arrow); the ileocecal valve area is more extensively ulcerated and narrowed (arrows). (c) Annular strictures (marked A, B, C) are a result of prior transaxial ulceration (illustration provided by the late Prof H. Shirakabe). (d) Patient from India with low-grade obstruction and weight loss. Enteroclysis outlines narrowing at the ileocolic junction (arrow) through which barium enters an irregularly narrowed colon. The cecum cannot be identified. (e) Linear and saccular ulcerations at the ileocecal junction; the ulcerated cecum is greatly reduced in size (arrows); the TI is in direct continuity with the ascending colon (long arrow). (f) Ileocolic tuberculosis in an Iranian immigrant living in Sweden with a long history of diarrhea and right abdominal pain. The TI (arrows) is minimally diseased (nodules, abnormal folds). The cecum and the ileocecal valve cannot be identified, and the ileocecal angle is lost; the extensively diseased colon is in continuity with the TI. (Courtesy of Anders Lunderquist, MD, Lund, Sweden.)

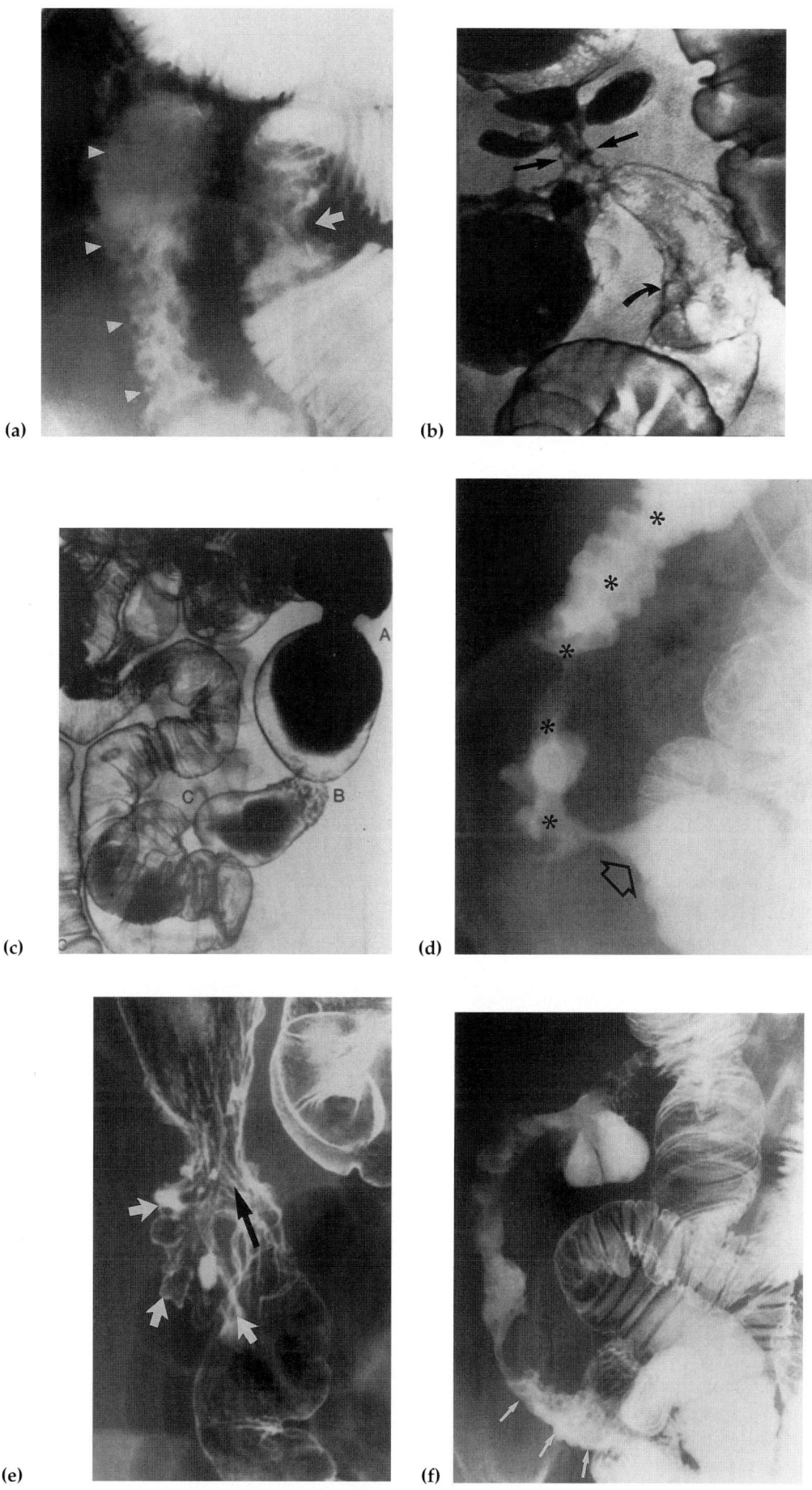

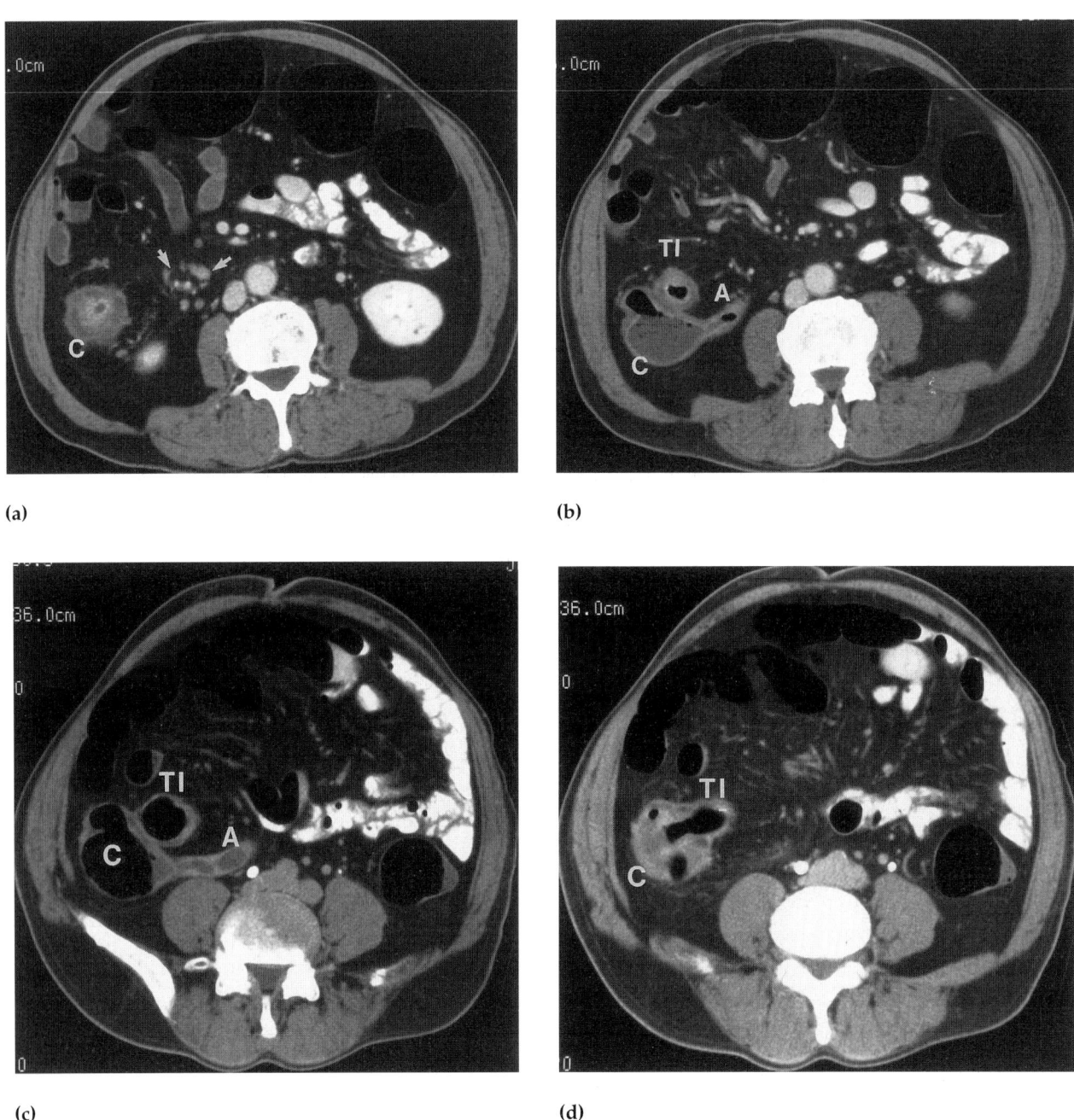

Fig. 16-7. Contrast-enhanced CT scans in ileocecal tuberculosis.
(a) The wall of the cecum (C) is greatly thickened. Irregular densities extend from the contrast enhanced mucosa into the thickened submucosa, indicating ulceration. Enlarged nodes are seen in the ileal mesentery (arrows). (b) A further image demonstrates contrast-enhanced wall thickening in the TI, appendix (A), and distal cecum (C). (c, d) Air contrast CT scans in left and right decubitus positions confirm the presence of cecal (C), ileal (TI), and appendiceal (A) wall thickening.

The differentiation of Crohn's disease from ileocecal tuberculosis can be difficult. Ulcers in tuberculosis tend to be oval in shape, transaxial, and large. The linear mesenteric border ulcers typical for Crohn's disease do not occur in tuberculous enteritis.[43] The contraction of the cecum with folds radiating to the site of old ulcerations and the predominance of cecal over terminal ileal pathology favor a diagnosis of tuberculosis over Crohn's disease. A short hourglass stricture is not seen in Crohn's disease. The change from normality to disease in the small bowel seems to be more abrupt in tuberculosis enterocolitis. A typical cobblestone pattern of Crohn's disease is not seen in tuberculosis.

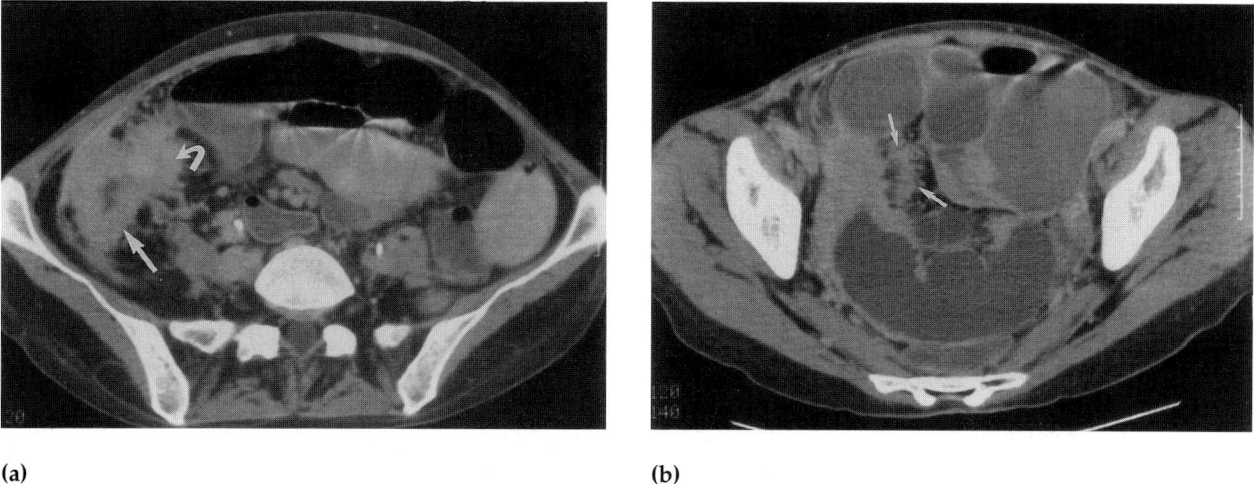

Fig. 16-8. Middle-aged male patient who complained of abdominal pain, diarrhea, and pyrexia.
The initial diagnosis was Crohn's disease, and he was treated with steroids, which caused significant worsening of his illness. Further investigations were done. (a) CT scan shows gross thickening of the wall of the cecum (arrow) with pericecal inflammation (curved arrow). (b) A more distal scan reveals small bowel obstruction caused by severe mural disease of the terminal ileum and disease extension into the mesentery (arrow). Prolonged antituberculous treatment was successful.

In cases of tuberculous peritonitis, an adynamic ileus may be present with or without ascites.[42] Calcifications may be seen in the lymph nodes or in the liver or spleen. Small bowel loops may show fixation outside the pelvis.

Sonography. A report from India describes the sonographic findings in 56 patients with abdominal tuberculosis. In all patients, the thickness of the mesentery was increased beyond 15 mm and was associated with lymphadenopathy. Ascites was found in 30% of patients. The diagnosis was confirmed by sonographically guided core biopsy of enlarged lymph nodes, by analysis of ascitic fluid, and (not recommended for nonendemic areas) by response to specific treatment.[44]

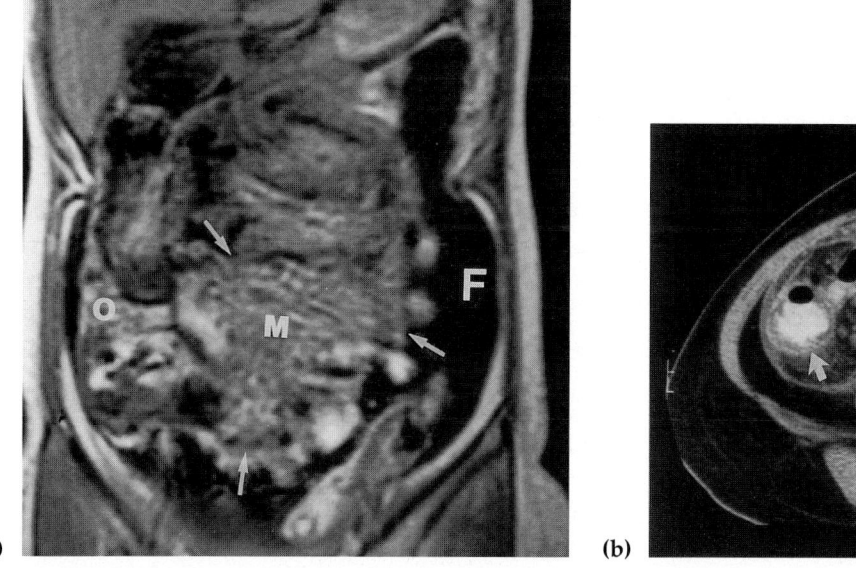
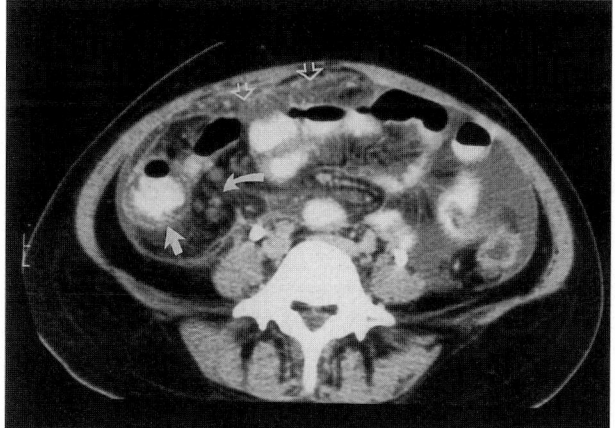

Fig. 16-9. Abdominal tuberculosis in young patient in Korea.
Turbo spin echo (TSE) breath-hold magnetic resonance images show (a) a coronal image demonstrating diffuse miliary implants in the mesentery (arrows) with involvement of the omentum (O) and a fluid collection (F). (b) Axial TSE image shows miliary implants in the omentum (open arrows) and a thickened cecal wall (arrow) with focal node enlargement (curved arrow). (Courtesy of H.K. Ha, MD, Seoul, Korea.)

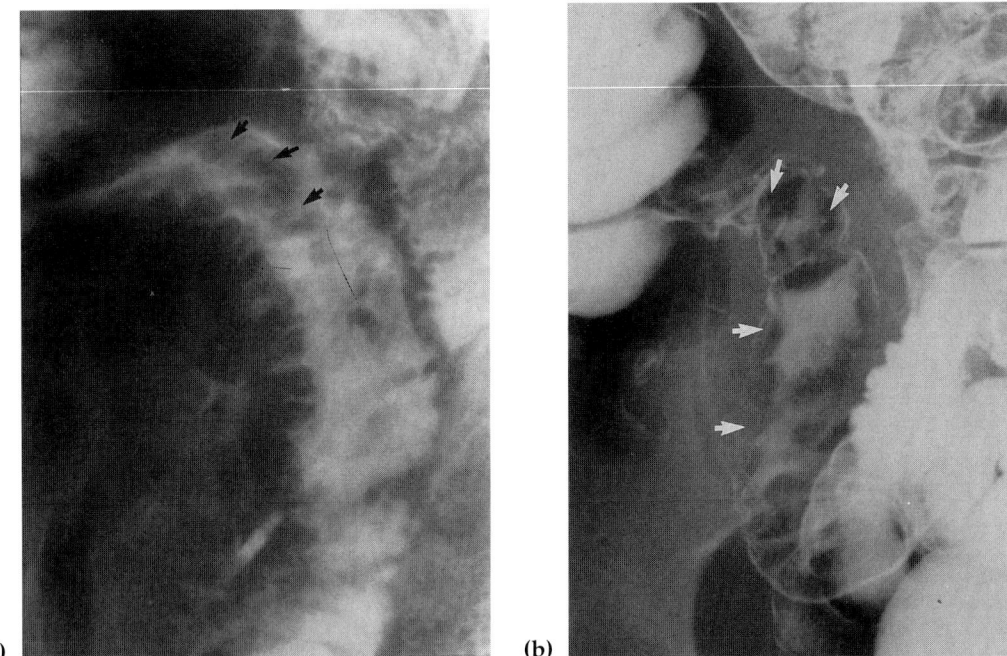

Fig. 16-10. *Yersinia* ileitis.
(a) Barium follow-through in a patient with a self-limited diarrheal illness and right lower quadrant pain shows edematous folds with few erosions (arrows) in a terminal ileum of normal lumen diameter. Diagnosis was confirmed by stool culture and serology. (b) In another patient, enteroclysis shows changes in TI yersiniosis. Numerous erosions (arrows) and fold thickening with normal lumen diameter would clearly distinguish this self-limited condition from Crohn's disease.

Yersiniosis

The infection is caused by gram-negative bacilli of two varieties, *Yersinia enterocolitica* and *Y pseudotuberculosis*.[45] Animal reservoirs include birds, dogs, and freshwater fish. Person-to-person spread occurs. *Yersinia* enters epithelial cells and produces an enterotoxin. It can multiply in Peyer's patches and from there spread into the lamina propria.[46] Human infection is more common in children or young adults, who usually present with fever and right-sided abdominal pain mimicking appendicitis. *Y enterocolitica* is the more likely organism in the United States and affects both sexes equally. *Y pseudotuberculosis* is more often encountered in Europe and has a male preponderance.[47]

The course of the illness tends to be self-limited. At times, a more protracted enterocolitis occurs with diarrhea mixed with blood and mucus accompanied by vomiting and fever. Ileal disease is characterized by shallow ulcerations of the mucosa at the site of lymphoid tissue, together with transmural edema and inflammation. Mesenteric lymph nodes show marked follicular and interfollicular hyperplasia without granulomas.[48] A bacteremia can lead to extraintestinal complications, in skin, liver, kidney, lung. Postinfection complications can be significant.[49] A 4- to 14-year-long follow-up of 458 patients who had been hospitalized in Norway with *Y enterocolitica* reported, among others, 53 cases with persistent joint pains, including 18 with ankylosing spondylitis; 17 patients with iridocyclitis; and 22 patients with chronic hepatitis.[50]

The diagnosis can be confirmed by combining bacteriologic or serologic techniques. It is important to warn the laboratory of a suspicion of *Yersinia* infection because standard processing of stool specimens may miss the diagnosis. Antibiotics are usually neither required nor helpful. They may have to be used in cases with complications or in immune deficiency states.

Radiology

Barium studies can demonstrate changes in the distal 20 cm of the ileum (Fig. 16-10) and these may be seen to extend into the cecum and ascending colon.[51] Thickened, nodular folds may be demonstrated, often with ulcers that may be aphthoid or larger, single or multiple. Aphthoid ulcers have also been demonstrated in the colon. The bowel mostly retains its normal lumen diameter. Thickened folds may later be replaced by fold effacement. Resolution of these changes is expected within 4 to 5 weeks.

The fact that changes in the terminal ileum eventually resolve aids the differential diagnosis from Crohn's disease, and so does the absence of fistulae or of linear ulcerations at the mesenteric border. The findings, however, appear similar to *Campylobacter* ileitis (see below). An inflammatory mass secondary to a *Yersinia* abscess has been shown by CT.[52]

Salmonellosis

In the United States, infection with nontyphoidal strains of *Salmonella* is responsible for 25% to 33% of cases of acute infectious diarrhea.[53] *Salmonella* invades the deeper layer of the small bowel mucosa, where it causes hyperemia and edema. It is usually contained there but can enter the portal system.[54] Enterotoxins contribute to the small bowel inflammation. Occasionally, a toxic megacolon develops.[55] Cases of acute *Salmonella* infection can occur person to person or through food or water. Salmonellosis is not as frequent a cause of traveler's diarrhea as are enteropathogenic strains of *Escherichia coli*. Diagnosis of this mostly self-limited disease depends upon stool culture, which should be done in all cases of acute diarrhea with a positive fecal leukocyte test.

Radiology

Plain film radiographs may show ileus of the small and large intestine. Barium studies are infrequently indicated. The radiologic appearance of the distal ileum is not unlike that of other inflammatory diseases. Aphthoid ulcers identified in the early stage of any acute inflammatory disease may also be seen in salmonellosis. CT scans of three patients with *Salmonella* enteritis have shown mild circumferential thickening of the terminal ileum; a corresponding barium study showed thickened folds.[56]

Campylobacter

Though *Campylobacter* infections are well documented among several species of animals, other infected persons are the more usual sources of human disease.[57] Infection mostly occurs through contaminated food or water. *Campylobacter fetus* and *C jejuni* are considered responsible for approximately 14% of cases of infectious diarrhea.[58] A diffuse, exudative enteritis with edema, ulceration, and bleeding results.[59] The disease is usually self-limited but relapses occur in about 20% of cases. Complications are rare and include toxic megacolon[60] and massive bleeds.[61]

Radiology

Small bowel changes revealed by barium examination are similar to those previously described. The distal ileum can be narrowed with irregular nodularity and thickening of the wall.[59] Shallow ulcers may be seen in more severely affected cases (Fig. 16-11). Findings

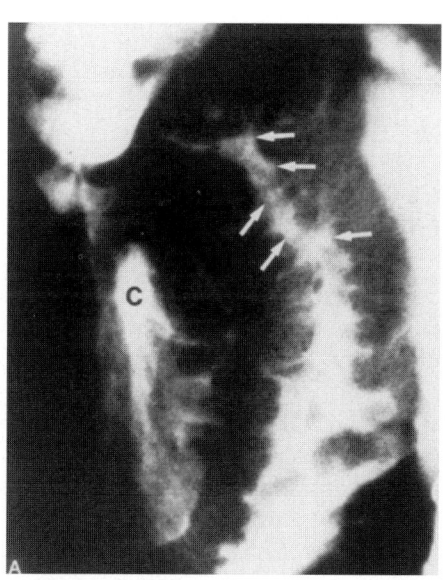 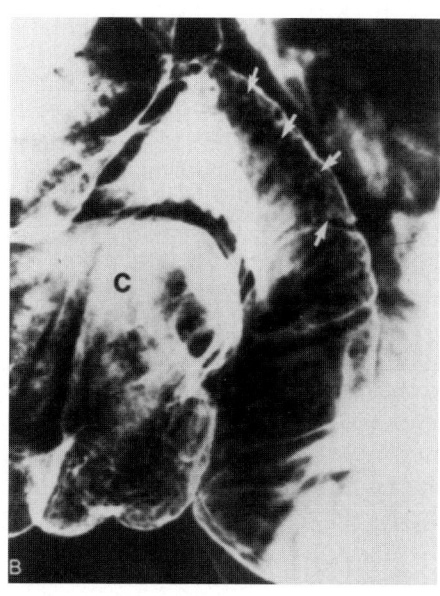

Fig. 16-11. *Campylobacter* **ileitis.**
(a) Compression spot radiograph of a small bowel examination in a 20-year-old medical student who presented with acute diarrhea. The terminal ileum shows fold thickening associated, in its distal portion, with lumen narrowing and shallow ulceration (arrows). The cecum (C) is in spasm. Appearances are compatible with *Yersinia* ileitis and Crohn's disease. *Campylobacter* was isolated from the stool. (b) A peroral pneumocolon 6 months later when symptoms had already resolved. However, lymphoid hyperplasis, minimal edema, and erosions (arrows), much smaller than before, are still seen. This appearance also resembles the resolution phase of *Yersinia* ileitis. (Courtesy of Frederick Kelvin, MD.)

in the colon are similar, usually indistinguishable from idiopathic colitis.

Diagnosis is made by isolation of *Campylobacter* by stool culture, which seldom remains positive for longer than two weeks.

Clostridium difficile

Antibiotic-associated pseudomembranous enteritis due to *Clostridium difficile* has been occasionally described in recent years. In one patient characteristic pseudomembranous lesions occurred together with colonic disease.[62] In another case a fulminant clostridial enteritis was diagnosed after colectomy.[63]

Shigellosis

The *Shigella* species is divided into four major groups, each with subgroups. Two mechanisms operate in causing bowel damage: the production of an enterotoxin and epithelial invasion. Virulent species are able to invade and multiply within epithelial cells.[64] Unlike *Salmonella*, which mainly affects the small intestine, *Shigella* causes a descending infection, which may damage the small intestine mostly by enterotoxic action on its way to the target organ, the colon. The most extensive and severe involvement is seen in the distal colon. The entire colon is affected in about 15% of cases, and it is then that the terminal ileum has been reported to be mildly inflamed.[65] However, exceptions occur. The report of a single case of shigellosis of the terminal ileum has demonstrated pronounced wall thickening (with target configuration shown by CT) and a severely ulcerated mucosa as shown with barium[56]; the colon in this case was unaffected.

Infections by Fungi

Two fungi are chiefly involved in producing inflammatory bowel disease: *Paracoccidioides brasiliensis*, mostly in South America, and *Histoplasma capsulatum*, in the United States.[66] Gastrointestinal involvement is almost always secondary and more common in immunosuppressed patients.

South American Blastomycosis

Paracoccidioidomycosis is common in Brazil. The organism locates in submucosal lymphoid tissue of the gut and then erodes the mucosa. Radiologic changes in the small bowel are nonspecific narrowing with mucosal irregularities.[67] Mesenteric nodes are region-

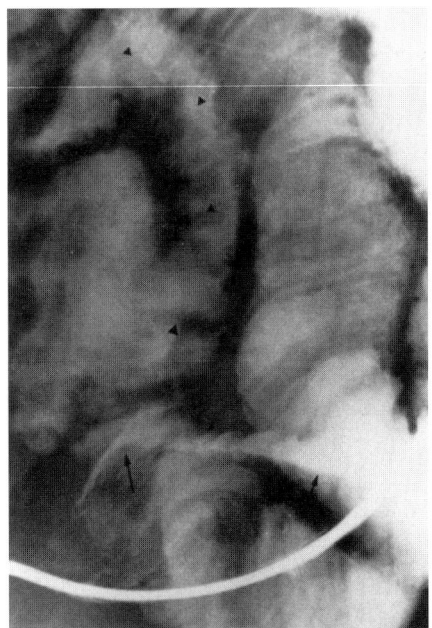

Fig. 16-12. **Young female patient was admitted with acute abdominal pain, pyrexia, and abdominal tenderness.** Enteroclysis demonstrates an extrinsic mass effect (arrows) elevating a proximal segment of terminal ileum out of the pelvis. The more distal terminal ileum was within normal limits. Fold thickening in the segment compressed by the mass suggests an inflammatory cause, probably a tuboovarian abscess. Surgery revealed an appendix abscess situated at the pelvis inlet.

ally enlarged. Diagnosis is based on identifying the organism in biopsy material, usually taken at laparotomy.

Histoplasmosis

Infection primarily involves the respiratory tract and affects small bowel or colon by dissemination. A granulomatous reaction similar to tuberculosis takes place, particularly in the localized form of the disease. In the small bowel it usually takes the form of discrete raised plaques that may undergo secondary ulceration and produce tissue destruction, sometimes with perforation.[68] The diagnosis is confirmed by demonstrating *Histoplasma* in tissue biopsy specimens, using methenamine silver stains. Radiology may demonstrate polypoid changes or ulcerations in the small bowel or in the ilocecal area, as well as strictures. Findings are nonspecific. A patient with AIDS and disseminated histoplasmosis with gastrointestinal involvement developed ileal perforations during antifungal therapy.[69] Small, rounded, and discrete calcifications in the liver and the spleen, especially if associated with pulmonary calcifications, would support a diagnosis of histoplasmosis.[70] (Cytomegalovirus and protozoan infections are discussed in Chapter 17.)

Extrinsic Inflammations Affecting the Small Intestine

Any inflammatory process arising within or extending into the inframesocolic space can secondarily affect the small intestine. The most common examples are abscesses of appendiceal or tubo-ovarian origin mostly involving the terminal ileum and inflammatory extensions of pancreatitis that can spread to bowel in the left upper quadrant of the abdomen or extend further via the small bowel mesentery.

Impressions on Bowel by Normal Extrinsic Structures, eg, fat

Obesity is often associated with hypertrophy of mesenteric fat. Bowel loops can be widely separated from one another, and this especially in the right abdomen. Loops are freely movable and are pliable when tested by manual compression. During the distended phase of enteroclysis the separation between loops becomes less obvious or may disappear.

Bowel loops may deform others, and impressions by the sigmoid or transverse colon are a frequent finding. In patients with a fairly narrow pelvis a linear impression on the ileum caused by the iliac artery is an occasional finding.[71] A pulsating impression by a dilated or tortuous aorta is readily identified during fluoroscopy.

Impression by an Extrinsic Mass

A general principle can be used to differentiate masses of mucosal or mural origin from those arising extrinsically. In the profile view of such a mass the angle at the junction of the mucosal plane and the base of the lesion indicates this distinction. A sharp angle, less than 90 degrees, indicates a mucosal origin; a 90-degree angle is in favor of mural origin; and a wide angle—90-degrees plus—an extrinsic origin. In the case of an extrinsic mass, palpation during fluoroscopy can distinguish simple displacement from infiltration.

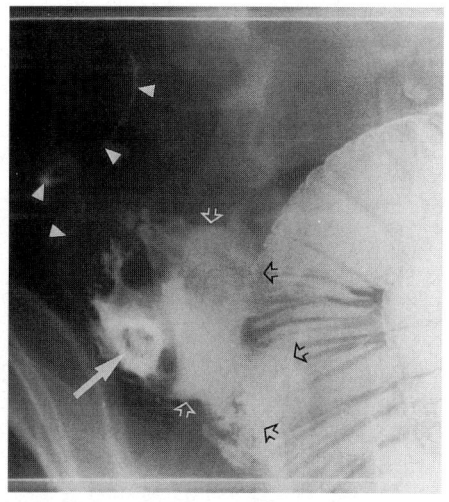
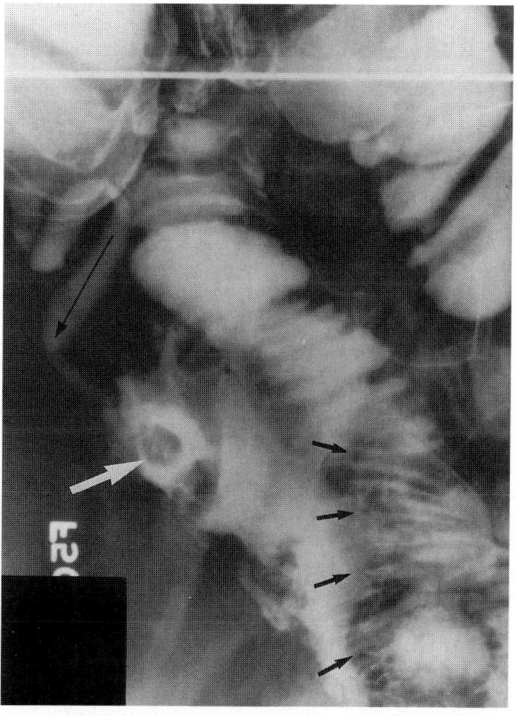

Fig. 16-13. An unusual enteroclysis demonstration of an appendiceal abscess that had ruptured into distal ileum. (a) Extravasation of barium into an exoenteric cavity (open arrows). An appendicolith is contained in part of this cavity (arrow). Faint opacification of what appears to be part of the appendix (arrowheads). (b) Later in the examination the appendix was opacified via the cecum (long arrow) and its continuity with the abscess cavity and the appendicolith was revealed. Note the diverging, slightly thickened mucosal folds now shown close to the cavity (arrows), a typical proximity effect of the inflammatory process.

16. Parasitic and Bacterial Inflammatory Diseases

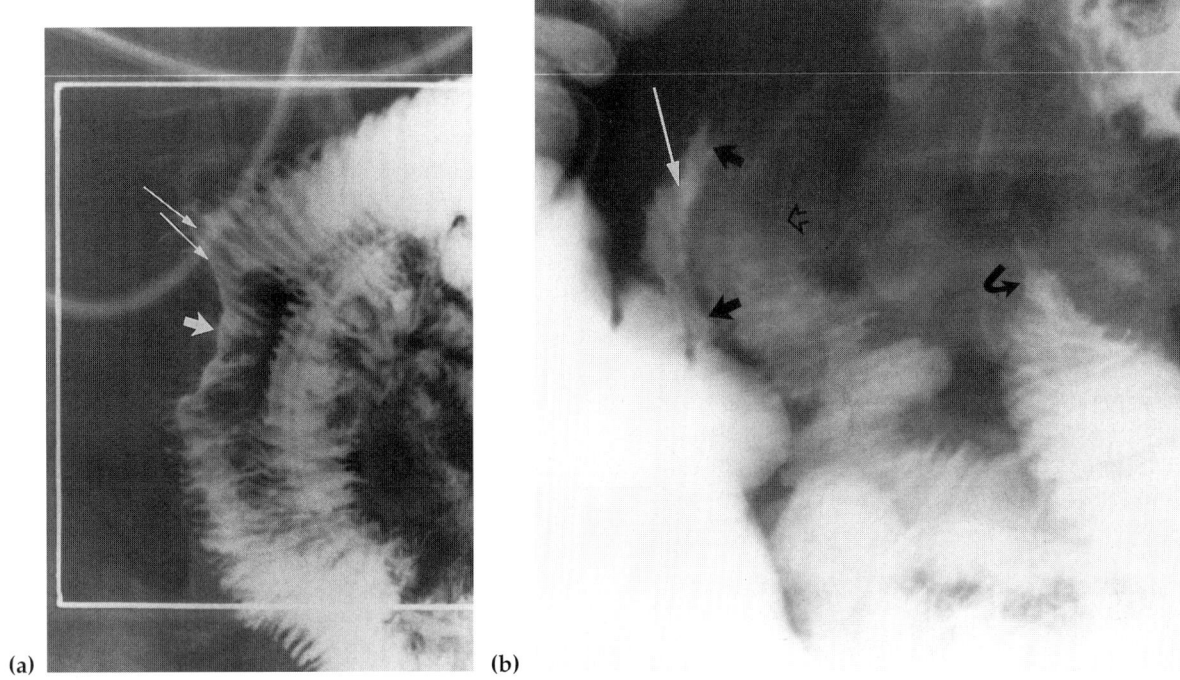

Fig. 16-14. An appendix abscess medial to the ascending colon.
(a) Extrinsic mass effect deforming proximal ileum (arrow). Thickened folds are displaced (long arrows) by the extrinsic mass. (b) Later during the enteroclysis, more distal ileum is demonstrated. The mass effect shown in (a) is indicated by a curved arrow. Another extrinsic mass effect (arrows) with the same displacement of thickened folds (long arrows) and the en face view of part of the same loop showing thickened, flattened, and stretched appearing folds (open arrow) all indicate that the extrinsic mass must be of an inflammatory nature, in this case an appendix abscess.

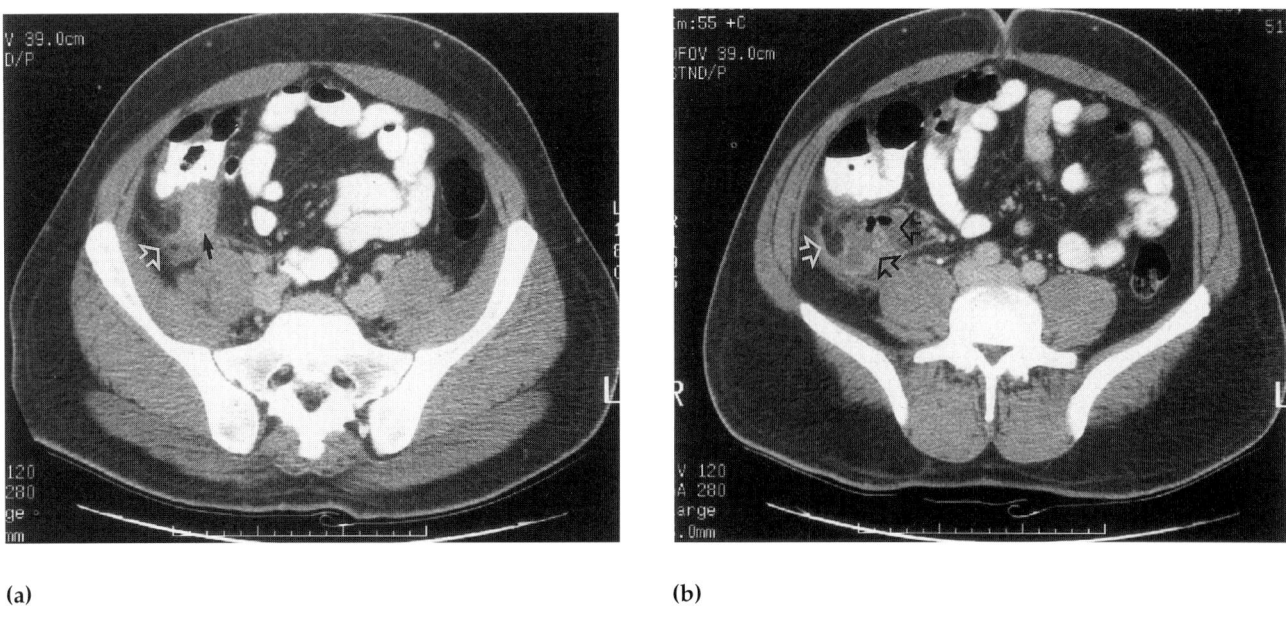

Fig. 16-15. CT can demonstrate the abscess and its appendiceal origin.
(a) Obstructed appendix (arrow) with related extrinsic inflammatory changes (open arrow). (b) More distal scan outlines the gas containing appendix abscess (open arrows).

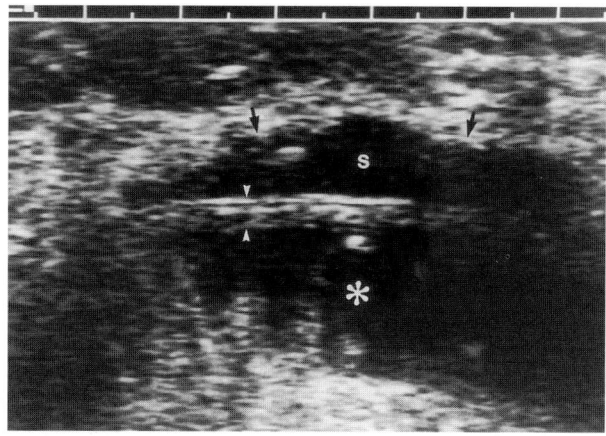

Fig. 16-16. A seroma, a not infrequent postoperative finding especially after gynecologic surgery, is demonstrated by ultrasound (S) in front of a fluid-distended small bowel* with normal wall layers (between arrowheads). Follow-up confirmed its gradual disappearance. (Courtesy of M. Rioux, MD, Quebec.)

Impression by an Extrinsic Inflammatory Process

An adjacent inflammatory mass, in addition to producing an extrinsic-type impression, may cause folds close to the inflammation to thicken without affecting folds away from the lesion.[72] These unilaterally thickened folds then diverge or are displaced sideways as they approach the inflammatory process close to them. Folds seen en face may merely show some thickening, flattening, and apparent stretching. Such changes are typically seen in the terminal or distal ileum in relation to an appendiceal or tubo-ovarian abscess and are well shown by enteroclysis (Figs. 16-12, 16-13, 16-14). CT, on the other hand, demonstrates the abscess itself and provides information as to its origin (Fig. 16-15).

Impression by a Postoperative Seroma

This is a not unusual finding after surgery. Lesions tend to disappear gradually. It is here shown by ultrasound (Fig. 16-16).

References

1. Weissberg DL, Berk RN. Ascariasis of the gastrointestinal tract. *Gastrointest Radiol.* 1978;3:415–418.
2. Archampong EQ. Tropical diseases of the small bowel. *World J Surg.* 1985;9:887–896.
3. Stoll NR. This wormy world. *J Parasitol.* 1947;33:1–18.
4. Wynne JM, Ellman BAH. Bolus obstruction by *Ascaris lumbricoides*. *S Afr Med J.* 1983;63:644–646.
5. Bar-Maor JA, deCarvalho JLAF, Chappell J. Gastrografin treatment of intestinal obstruction due to *Ascaris lumbricoides*. *J Pediatr Surg.* 1984;19:174–176.
6. Blumenthal DS, Schultz MG. Incidence of intestinal obstruction in children infected with *Ascaris lumbricoides*. *Am J Trop Med Hyg.* 1975;24:801–805.
7. Bean WJ. Recognition of Ascaris by routine chest or abdominal roentgenograms. *AJR.* 1965;94:379–384.
8. Hommeyer SC, Hamill GS, Johnson JA. CT diagnosis of intestinal ascariasis. *Abdom Imaging.* 1995;20:315–316.
9. Markell EK, Voge M. *Medical Parasitology.* 4th ed. Philadelphia, Pa: WB Saunders Co; 1976.
10. Martinez T, Ojeda A, Roche M, Layrisse M. Hookworm infection and intestinal blood loss. *Trans R Soc Trop Med Hyg.* 1967;61:373–378.
11. Monroe LS. Gastrointestinal parasites. In: Berk JE, ed. *Bockus Gastroenterology.* 4th ed. Philadelphia, Pa: WB Saunders Company; 1985:4250–4348.
12. Kliks MM. Anisakiasis in the western United States: four new case reports from California. *Am J Trop Med Hyg.* 1983;32:526–532.
13. Nakata H, Takeda K, Nakayama T. Radiological diagnosis of acute gastric anisakiasis. *Radiology.* 1980;35:49–53.
14. Namiki T, Morooha T, Kawanchi H. Diagnosis of acute gastric anisakiasis. *Stom Intest.* 1970;5:1437–1440.
15. Matsui T, Iida M, Murakami M, et al. Intestinal anisakiasis. Clinical and radiologic features. *Radiology.* 1985;157:299–302.
16. Richman RH, Lewicki AM. Right ileocolitis secondary to anisakiasis. *AJR.* 1973;119:325–331.
17. Shirahama M, Koga T, Ishibashi H, et al. Intestinal anisakiasis: US in diagnosis. *Radiology.* 1992;185:789–793.
18. Grove DI. Strongyloidiasis: a conundrum for gastroenterologists. *Gut.* 1994;35:437–440.
19. Medina LS, Heiken JP, Gold RP. Pipe stem appearance of small bowel in strongyloidiasis is not pathognomonic of fibrosis and irreversibility. *AJR.* 1992;159:543–544.
20. Astagneau ED, Hadengue A, Degott C, et al. Biliary obstruction resulting from *Strongyloides stercoralis* infection. Report of a case. *Gut.* 1994;35:705–706.
21. Hizawa K, Iida M, Aoyagi K, et al. Early detection of strongloidiasis using endoscopic duodenal biopsy: Report of a case. *J Clin Gastroenterol.* 1996;22:157–159.
22. Gold BM, Meyers MA. Radiologic manifestations of *Taenia saginata* infestation. *AJR.* 1977;128:493–494.
23. Lopez CE, Dykes AC, Juranek DD, et al: Waterborne giardiasis: a community wide outbreak of disease and a high rate of asymptomatic infection. *Amer J Epidemiology.* 1980;112:495–507.
24. Katelaris PH, Farthing MJG. Diarrhea and malabsorption in giardiasis: a multifactorial process? *Gut.* 1992;33:295–297.
25. Brandborg LL, Tankersley CB, Gottlieb S, et al. Histological demonstration of mucosal invasion by *Giardia lamblia* in man. *Gastroenterology.* 1979;75:757–769.
26. Brandon J, Glick SN, Teplick SK. Intestinal giardiasis: importance of serial filming. *AJR.* 1985;144:581.
27. Orchard JL, Petorak V. Abnormal abdominal CT findings in a patient with giardiasis: resolution after treatment. *Dig Dis Sci.* 1995;40:346–348.
28. Goka AKJ, Rolston DDK, Mathan VI, et al. Diagnosis of

giardiasis by specific IgM antibody enzyme-linked immunosorbent assay. *Lancet.* 1986;2:184.
29. Lee R-C, Chiang J-H, Chou Y-H, et al. Intestinal schistosomiasis japonica: CT-pathologic correlation. *Radiology.* 1994;193:539–542.
30. Strickland GT. Gastrointestinal manifestations of schistisomiasis. *Gut.* 1994;35:1334–1337.
31. Morson BC, Dawson IMP. *Gastrointestonal Pathology.* 2nd ed. Oxford, England: Blackwell Scientific; 1979:272–336.
32. Homan WP, Grafe WR, Dineen P. A 44-year experience with tuberculous enterocolitis. *World J Surg.* 1977;1:245–250.
33. Prakash A. Ulceroconstrictive tuberculosis of the bowel. *Int Surg.* 1978;63:23–29.
34. Snyder DE, Roper WI. The new tuberculosis. Editorial. *N Engl J Med.* 1992;326:703–705.
35. Palmer KR, Patil DH, Basran GS, et al. Abdominal tuberculosis in urban Britain—a common disease. *Gut.* 1985;26:1296–1305.
36. Mathan MM. The small intestine. In: Whitehead R, ed. *Gastrointestinal and Oesophageal Pathology.* New York, NY: Churchill Livingstone; 1989:446–447.
37. Grand Rounds, Hammersmith Hospital. Tuberculous enteritis. A serious problem in some patients. *Brit Med J.* 1996;313:215–217.
38. Grand Rounds, Hammersmith Hospital. Persistent fever in pulmonary tuberculosis. Drug malabsorption should be considered. *Brit Med J.* 1996;313:1543–1545.
39. Faustian FF, Marshall JB. Intestinal tuberculosis. In: Berk JE, ed. *Bockus Gastroenterology.* 4th ed. Philadelphia, Pa: WB Saunders Co; 1985:2019–2036.
40. Yao T et al. Roentgenographic analysis of tuberculosis of the small intestine. *Stom Intest.* 1977;12:1467–1480.
41. Brombart M, Massion J, et al. Radiologic differences between ileocecal tuberculosis and Crohn's disease. *Am J Dig Dis.* 1961;6:589–612.
42. Thoeni RF, Margulis AR. Gastrointestinal tuberculosis. *Semin Roentgenol.* 1979;14:283–294.
43. Meyers MA. Clinical involvement of mesenteric and antimesenteric borders of small bowel loops. II. Radiologic interpretation of pathological alterations. *Gastrointest Radiol.* 1976;1:49–58.
44. Jain R, Sawhney S, Bhargava DK, Berry M. Diagnosis of abdominal tuberculosis: sonographic findings in patients with early disease. *AJR.* 1995;165:1391–1395.
45. Vantrappen G, Janssens J, Hellemans J, Ghous Y: Yersinia enteritis and enterocolitis: gastroenterological aspects. *Gastroenterology.* 1977;72:220–227.
46. Hanski C, Autschka U, Schmoranzer HP, et al. Immunohistochemical and electron microscopic study of interaction of *Yersinia enterocolitica* serotype 08 with intestinal mucosa during experimental enteritis. *Infect Immun.* 1989;57:673–678.
47. Morain CO. Acute ileitis (editorial). *Br Med J.* 1981;283:1075.
48. Compton CC. Case records of the Massachusetts General Hospital, Scully E, ed, *N Engl J Med.* 1990;323:121–123. Case 28-1990.
49. Spiro HM. *Clinical Gastroenterology.* 4th ed. Chapter 30. New York, NY: McGraw-Hill; 1993:534–535.
50. Saebo A, Lasser J. *Yersinia enterocolitica,* an inducer of chronic inflammations. *Int J Tissue React.* 1994;16:51–57.
51. Ekberg O, Sjostrom B, Brahme F. Radiological findings in *Yersinia ileitis. Radiology.* 1977;123:15–19.
52. Coleman BG, Metzger RA, Kressel HY, Arger PH. Case report: computed tomography in the diagnosis of *Yersinia* infection in a patient with thalassemia major. *J Comput Assist Tomogr.* 1984;8:153–156.
53. Gertler S, Pressman J, Cartwright C, Dharmsathaphorn K. Management of acute diarrhea. *J Clin Gastroenterol.* 1983;5:523–534.
54. DuPont HL. Acute nonparasitic diarrhea. In: Berk JE, ed. *Bockus Gastroenterology.* 4th ed. Philadelphia, Pa: WB Saunders Co; 1985:1983–1995.
55. Bellary SV, Isaacs P. Toxic megacolon due to *Salmonella. J Clin Gastroenterol.* 1990;12:605.
56. Balthazar EJ, Charles HW, Megibow AJ. *Salmonella* and *Shigella*-induced ileitis: CT findings in four patients. *J Comp Assist Tomogr.* 1996;20:375–378.
57. Holt PE. Role of *Campylobacter spp.* in human and animal disease: a review. *J Roy Soc Med.* 1981;74:437–440.
58. Mee AS, Shield M, Burke M. Campylobacter colitis: differentiation from acute inflammatory bowel disease. *J Roy Soc Med.* 1985;78:217–223.
59. Brodey PA, Fertig S, Aron JM. Campylobacter enterocolitis: radiographic features. *AJR.* 1982;139:1199–1201.
60. McKinley MJ, Taylor M, Sangree MH. Toxic megacolon with Campylobacter colitis. *Conn Med.* 1980;44:496–497.
61. Michalak DM, Perrault J, Gilchrist MJ et al. *Campylobacter fetus jejuni*: a cause of massive lower gastrointestinal hemorrhage. *Gastroenterology.* 1980;79:742–745.
62. Tsutaoka B, Hansen J, Johnson D, Holodniy M. Antibiotic-associated pseudomembranous enteritis due to *Clostridium difficile. Clin Infect Dis.* 1994;18:982–984.
63. Yee HF Jr, Brown SR Jr, Ostroff W. Fatal *Clostridium difficile* enteritis after total abdominal colectomy. *J Clin Gastroenterol.* 1995;22:45–47.
64. Hale TI, Keren DF. Pathogenesis and immunology in shigellosis: application for vaccine development. *Curr Top Microbiol Immunol.* 1992;180:117.
65. Speelman P, Kabir I, Islam M. Distribution and spread of colonic lesions in shigellosis: a colonoscopic study. *J Infect Dis.* 1984;150:899.
66. Haggitt RC. The differential diagnosis of idiopathic inflammatory bowel disease. In: Norris HT, ed. *Pathology of the Colon, Small Intestine and Anus.* New York, NY: Churchill Livingstone, 1983:21–59.
67. Avritchir Y, Perroni AA. Radiological manifestations of small intestinal South American blastomycosis. *Radiology.* 1978;127:607–609.
68. Smith JMB. Mycoses of the alimentary tract. *Gut.* 1969;10:1035.
69. Heneghan SJ, Li J, Petrossian E, Bizer LS. Intestinal perfration from gastrointestinal histoplasmosis in acquired immunodeficiency syndrome. *Arch Surg.* 1993;128:464–466.
70. Eisenberg RL. *Gastrointestinal Radiology: A Pattern Approach.* Philadelphia, Pa: JB Lippincott Co; 1983:955
71. Sellink JL, Miller RE. *Radiology of the Small Bowel: Modern Enteroclysis Technique and Atlas.* The Hague, Netherlands: Martinus Nijhoff; 1982:18–20.
72. O'Riordan D, Herlinger H. Diagnosis of extrinsic abscesses affecting the small intestine. *Mt Sinai J Med.* 1984;51:347–350.

Immune Deficiency Diseases

17

Hans Herlinger

Chapter Contents

X-Linked Hypogammaglobulinema
Selective IgA Deficiency
Common Variable Immunodeficiency Syndrome (CVI)
Immunoproliferative Small Intestinal Disease (IPSID)
Graft-Versus-Host Disease
Acquired Immunodeficiency Syndrome (AIDS)
Secondary Immune Deficiencies
Solid Organ Transplantation (Immunosuppression)

General aspects of immunology and the special role of the gut in the immunologic defense of the body are described in Chapter 3. In purely general terms, the intestinal mucosal immune system has three functions: immune exclusion, immune elimination, and autoimmune regulation. Diseases affecting the immune system can be divided into two categories. Primary immune deficiencies result from intrinsic defects in the cellular components or in their secretory products and can be congenital or acquired. Secondary immune deficiencies occur more frequently and include the effects of malnutrition and aging, immune suppression, protein losing enteropathies, graft-versus-host disease, and the acquired immunodeficiency syndrome (AIDS).[1]

X-Linked Hypogammaglobulinemia

Only males are affected by this intrinsic B-cell disorder, a maturation block in pre–B-cell to B-cell differentiation. This results in an inability to produce functioning antibody. The thymus and T cells function normally. The disorder manifests itself with recurrent pyogenic infections during infancy or early childhood, once maternal IgG has disappeared. Gastrointestinal infections occur in 30% of patients.[2] *Campylobacter* is a common cause of diarrhea; giardiasis occurs infrequently but can cause severe mucosal changes. Patients may be exposed to viral infections, hepatitis, and enteroviral diseases. An increased risk is reported for lymphomas and leukemias.[1]

Radiologic findings are nonspecific. Parenteral immunoglobulin replacement is the best treatment option.[3]

Selective IgA Deficiency

This is the most common primary immune defect, variably reported to range from 1 in 500 to 1 in 3000 of the population.[1] Affected individuals are usually asymptomatic, since an increased output of secretory IgM can mask this defect. There is a strong association with celiac disease and pernicious anemia (intrinsic factor deficiency). Infections, if any, generally spare the gastrointestinal tract and are mainly sinopulmonary. *Giardia* infection is barely increased over the general population. An association with Crohn's disease is reported, with a prevalence of 1:73.[1] There is a risk of anaphylaxis if patients are given IgA-containing blood.

Nodular lymphoid hyperplasia (Fig. 17-1) with or without giardiasis may be the radiologic presentation.

Common Variable Immunodeficiency Syndrome (CVI)

CVI is the second most common primary immunodeficiency in adults. It is a heterogeneous disorder characterized by different combinations of B-cell and T-cell abnormalities. A decreased production of immunoglobulins, mostly IgG but also IgA and IgM, is a major feature of the disease. The number of B cells may be normal or decreased, but many fail to differentiate into Ig-secreting plasma cells. Ten percent to 20% of patients lack identifiable circulating B cells.[4] One third of the patients have an inverted $CD4^+$ to $CD8^+$ ratio, but T-cell deficiencies are much milder

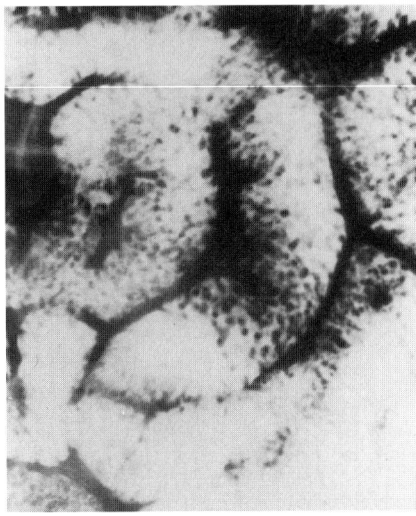

Fig. 17-1. Small bowel in IgA deficiency.
Nodular lymphoid hyperplasia, with nodules of 2- to 3-mm diameter evenly distributed through several loops of proximal small bowel against a normal fold pattern. Asymptomatic patient.

than in patients with AIDS.[4] Splenomegaly is seen in 70% A possible presentation is that of "hypogammaglobulinemic sprue," which shows subtotal villous atrophy but lacks increase of plasma cells in the lamina propria and is unresponsive to gluten withdrawal. Autoimmune diseases are a major component of CVI. One third of patients have atrophic gastritis and pernicious anemia with a distinct gastric cancer risk. Thrombocytopenia, autoimmune hepatitis, sclerosing cholangitis, thyroiditis, and aseptic arthritis are examples of associated autoimmune diseases.

There is an impaired response to many antigens and an increased susceptibility to infections. Patients usually present in the second or third decade with respiratory tract infections or diarrhea and steatorrhea. Giardiasis may cause extensive mucosal damage. Herpes virus infection, acquired in late childhood and continuing in a latent state, has caused severe reactivated disease in a minority of patients.[5] Development of viral hepatitis can be a problem, probably acquired with infusions of plasma or immunoglobulin preparations. Cytomegalovirus (CMV) infection, active or subclinical, can be detected in the majority of patients with CVI and may be linked to the development of an immune-mediated hemolytic anemia.[4] An increased incidence of malignant and nonmalignant lymphoproliferative disease exists. Long-term follow-up of CVI patients found the incidence of malignant tumors to be 5 to 10 times that of the general population, the majority of these tumors being gastric carcinomas.[6] Occasionally a more massive form of nonmalignant lymphoid hyperplasia develops in some of the CVI patients. This presentation is likely to be mistaken for lymphoma both by clinicians and radiologists.[7]

Radiology

Nodular lymphoid hyperplasia (NLH) is a frequent radiologic finding in CVI. It can extend through much of the small bowel [Fig. 17-2(a,b)] and may involve the colon. Individual nodules are slightly larger than in the self-limited lymphoid nodular hyperplasia of childhood and adolescence and may be more widely distributed.[8] Microscopically, the nodules reveal a polyclonal follicular reactive hyperplasia. Chronic antigenic stimulation together with deficient immune surveillance are considered to predispose to the formation of lymphoid hyperplastic nodules in the lamina propria or of larger aggregations of lymphoid tissue in the submucosa (Fig. 17-3). In only a minority of patients does NLH progress into malignancy. A recent CVI case report of documented progression to malignant lymphoma[9] could not demonstrate a histologic transition zone from adjacent NLH. However, another case report includes a literature review[10] and questions the benignity of NLH for three reasons: 1) NLH occurred in all small bowel lymphomas that complicated CVI; 2) NLH extended into the vicinity of the lymphomas; 3) Similarity was found in the monoclonal pattern of the lymphomas and that of the adjacent NLH.[10] Furthermore, a gradual morphologic transition from hyperplastic to monoclonal neoplastic tissue has been noted in lymphoid nodules close to lymphomas.[11] Attention has again been drawn to the likely sequential association of NLH and small bowel lymphoma even in the absence of immune deficiency.[11]

Immunoproliferative Small Intestinal Disease (IPSID)

In 1962 a new type of intestinal lymphoma was reported from Lebanon and the Near East.[12] It predominantly affected young people of Arab or Mediterranean Jewish origin but has also been discovered among South African blacks, Mexicans, and, recently, in an American who never left the country.[13] The term IPSID has been proposed for the overall disease process by the World Health Organization.[14]

Rudimentary hygiene by the mainly affected population leads to microbial colonization of the small bowel and an endemic parasite load. These factors are likely to be causally related to the development of the immunoproliferative intestinal infiltrate. An ill-

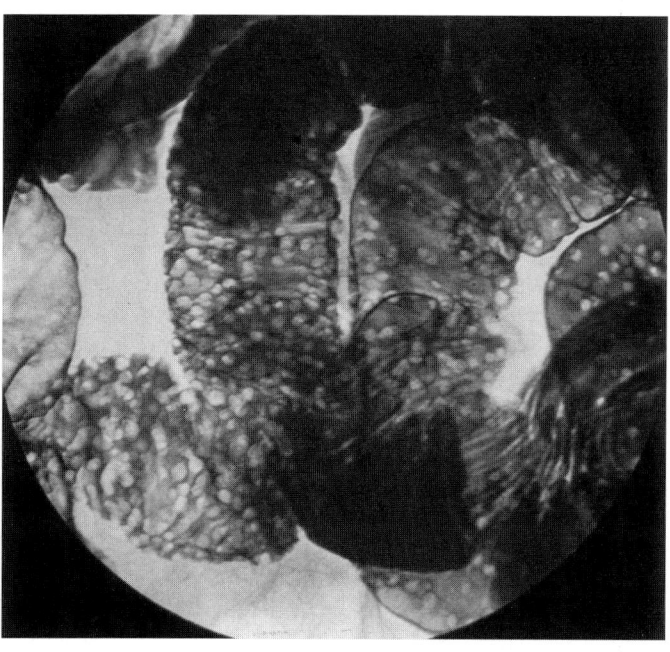 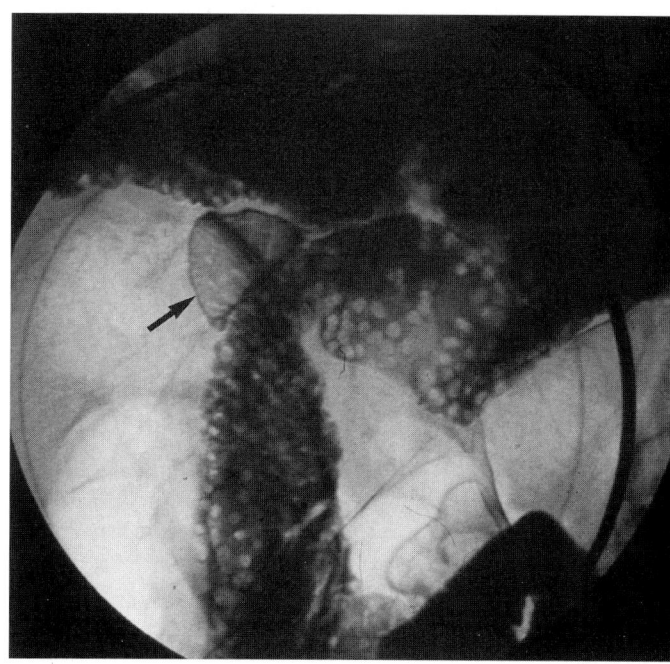

Fig. 17-2. Common variable immunodeficiency.
(a) Enteroclysis demonstration of crowded nodular lymphoid hyperplasia. Nodules vary between 2 and 4 mm in diameter with fusion of some of the nodules. (b) Incidentally shown Meckel's diverticulum (arrow) without nodules. Young patient, mild symptomatology.

defined immunological disturbance results in the frequent finding of a paraprotein consisting of incomplete alpha chains devoid of light chains. In over half the cases of IPSID the abnormal protein may be isolated from jejunal secretions or may be found in nonsecretory form as part of the mural infiltrate.

IPSID initially presents with diarrhea and weight loss and is characterized by a diffuse lymphoplasmacytic infiltrate of the lamina propria mainly of the proximal bowel, causing expansion of villi. The infiltrate soon spreads into the submucosa and produces nodular thickening of mucosal folds and may also involve lymph nodes. At this stage of the disease it may still be possible to prevent further progression by antibiotic therapy. If untreated or undiagnosed the disease advances from a polyclonal infiltrate to B-cell monoclonality with the formation of multiple lymphomatous tumors without a dominant mass, the Mediterranean lymphoma. Prognosis is now dismal.

Radiology

Virtually all barium studies in IPSID were done in the countries of their occurrence and only by the follow-through technique. These examinations merely show

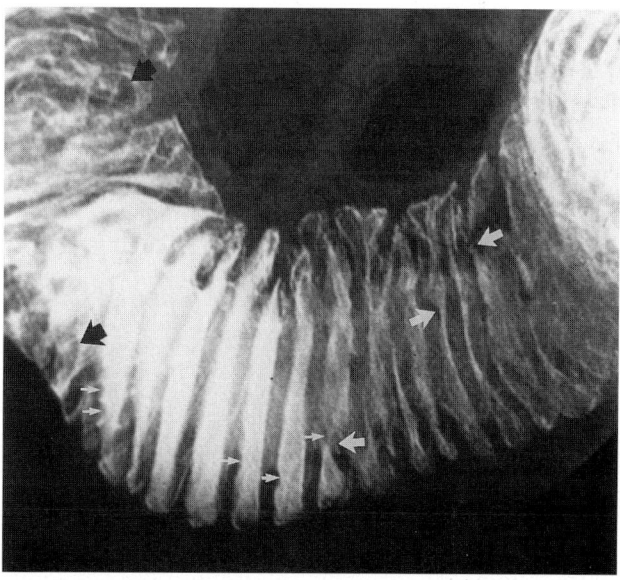

Fig. 17-3. Common variable immunodeficiency.
Female patient, 36 years, recurrent respiratory tract and enteric infections, continued professional life made possible by gamma globulin administration. Enteroclysis reveals fold thickening in the jejunum with evidence of fold-related nodules of various sizes (white arrows). Larger nodules are present, some indicated by arrows.

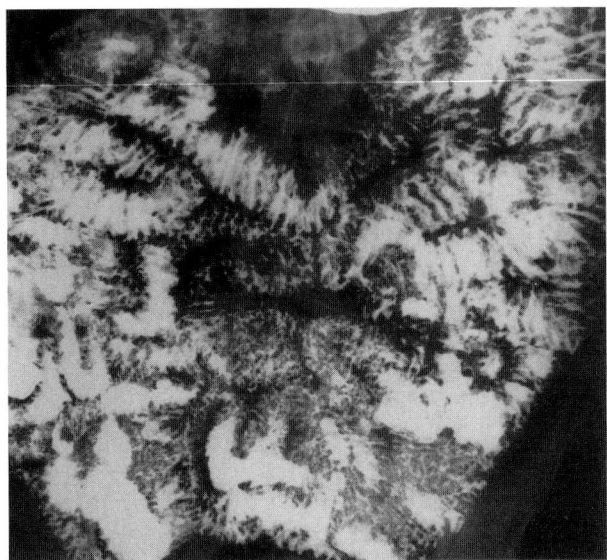

Fig. 17-4. Mediterranean lymphoma.
Young male patient, resident of Israel. Prone view of a follow-through barium examination shows fold thickening and irregular nodularity throughout the small bowel. (Courtesy of Dr E. Libson, MD, Israel.)

irregular nodularity, becoming increasingly coarse in the stage of Mediterranean lymphoma when lymph nodal enlargement produces separation of bowel loops (Fig. 17-4).[15] A notable exception is a report from Japan where enteroclysis was used in two patients with IPSID.[16] One patient was examined during the premalignant stage and showed diffuse and pronounced micronodularity, indicating infiltration of the lamina propria with dilatation of villi. Biopsy in the second patient showed IPSID in its malignant phase; enteroclysis demonstrated small nodules with thickened mucosal folds.[16]

Graft-Versus-Host Disease[17]

Bone marrow transplantation consists of the intravenous infusion of hematopoietic progenitor cells to renew bone marrow function in the recipient patient. The following are the more important indications for bone marrow transplantation: aplastic anemia, acute myeloid or lymphoblastic leukemia, multiple myeloma, non-Hodgkin's lymphoma, and some cancers. There are two major forms of transplantation: 1) using allogeneic bone marrow; and 2) using autologous marrow.

Allogeneic transplantation implies the use of marrow from another person. The donor's human leukocyte antigen (HLA) type should match that of the recipient as far as possible. Removal of T cells from the graft improves the success rate when adequate HLA matching could not be found. In autologous transplantation the recipient's own marrow is used; it has to be "purged" of any viable tumor cells. This form of transplantation is mostly used in older patients and is not suitable for nonmalignant conditions.

An *induction protocol* of high-dose chemotherapy or radiochemotherapy is used to achieve, in the allogeneic graft recipient, sufficient ablation of the residual marrow and the destruction of cancer cells, if present. Intestinal cell necrosis occurs immediately and takes some 3 weeks to heal. Abdominal pain and watery diarrhea occur. Eventually, the surface epithelium reverts to normal. Radiology is unhelpful. Ablation is followed by profound depression of leukocytes and platelets for a period of weeks before the donor marrow gets established within the host. During this highly susceptible time, bacterial, viral, and fungal infections are likely to occur. One of the major complications of allogeneic marrow transplantation is graft-versus-host disease.

Graft-versus-host disease (GVHD) is manifested and clinically graded on the basis of three parameters: A) skin lesions, B) liver damage, and C) intestinal tract involvement. Three factors make possible the occurrence of a GVHD reaction: 1) immunologically competent T lymphocytes within the graft; 2) the host differing genetically from the graft and perceived as antigenically foreign; or 3) the host's inability to reject the graft.[17] An acute and highly lethal form of GVHD is reported with increasing frequency following blood transfusions.[18] GVHD can present in acute, subacute, and chronic forms. It is usually preceded by features of intestinal damage caused by the induction protocol.

Acute graft-versus-host-disease[1] affects the lymphoid system, skin, liver, and gastrointestinal tract and starts 3 to 4 weeks after transplantation. There may be denudation of intestinal mucosa and profuse diarrhea with an output of 5 to 8 L/day with loss of electrolytes, protein, and blood. A maculopapular rash over palms, soles, and trunk appears. Hyperbilirubinemia indicates liver involvement. Cytomegalovirus infection is an important feature and is indicated by deeper gastrointestinal ulceration. Colorectal abnormalities are also present and rectal biopsy may demonstrate early changes, like apoptosis of crypt cells. Rectal biopsy can also indicate the severity of the graft-versus-host reaction, but the procedure can be dangerous and should be used sparingly. Barium radiology is a safer indication of the severity of the disease.

Subacute graft-versus-host disease develops 1 to 4 months after transplantation. Intestinal lesions predominate and are a continuation of the acute phase. Skin lesions may recur as liver disease intensifies.

Chronic graft-versus-host disease may occur 3 to 12

months after marrow grafting and involves the skin and liver as well as the gastrointestinal tract. In one fourth of the patients it can be the very first graft-versus-host reaction. Esophageal involvement with dysphagia may predominate in some patients. In the small bowel there can be patchy fibrosis of the lamina propria and submucosa.[1] Bacterial overgrowth, a result of dysmotility, may cause malabsorption. It is usually associated with profound immunodeficiency and recurrent infections, especially with cytomegalovirus.

GVHD rarely develops in patients younger than 5 years, and its incidence increases with age. Prior removal of mature T cells from the graft and initial chemotherapy have significantly reduced GVHD. Treatment or preventive treatment of cytomegalovirus infection has rendered GVHD a lesser problem. Prednisone alone or with azathioprine has been effective in the chronic phase of the disease.

Radiology

In acute graft-versus-host disease the barium studies can confirm the diagnosis and demonstrate the intensity of the inflammatory response. Mucosal folds are thickened or effaced; ulceration may be seen or areas of mucosal denudation indicated. Transit is accelerated, and luminal fluid is increased.[19] The ileum tends to be most severely affected [Fig. 17-5(a, b, c)]. The exclusion of acute radiation damage in the differential diagnosis of these findings presents no difficulty in view of the rapidly progressive and widespread changes of acute graft-versus-host disease. There may be evidence of incipient healing or of progression into lumen narrowing, wall thickening, and a ribbonlike appearance. An interesting observation in patients with pronounced mucosal sloughing was the persistence, over few days, of the barium coating of mucosal surfaces [Fig. 17-6(a, b)]. The mechanism of it was then not clear.[20] A further re-

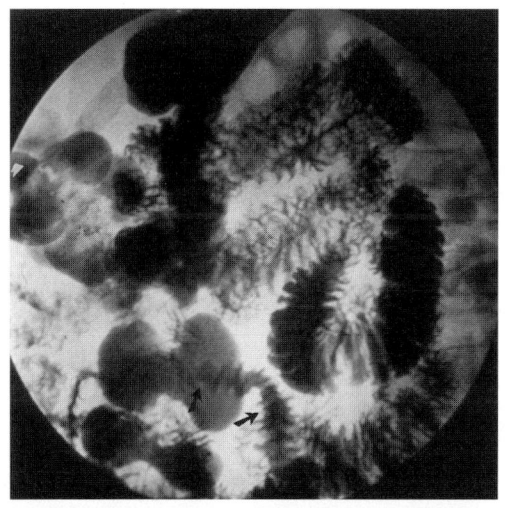
(a)

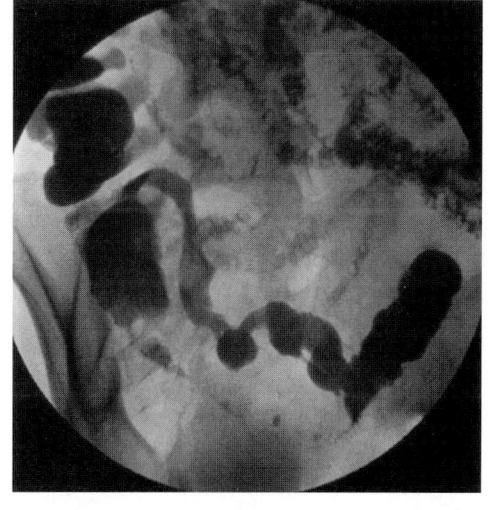
(b)

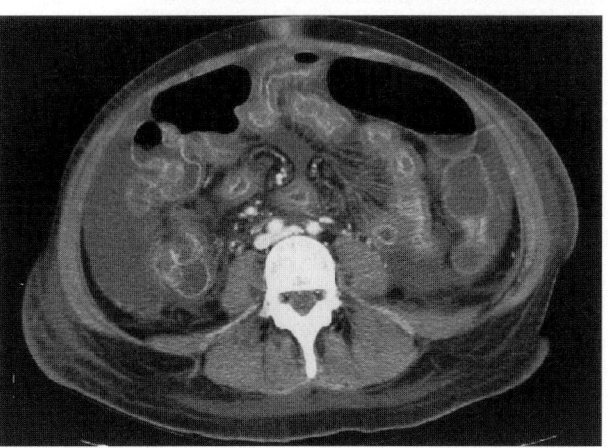
(c)

Fig. 17-5. Chronic graft-versus-host disease. Follow-through barium study (a,b) and CT examination (c) of the small bowel after bone marrow transplantation for myelodysplasia in a 29-year-old female patient.
(a) Thickened folds in proximal jejunum. Indication of wall thickening (arrows) commencing in distal jejunum. (b) Views of distal ileum show fold effacement, lumen narrowing, and wide separation of loops; transit was accelerated. (c) Contrast-enhanced CT demonstrates moderate circumferential wall thickening with a mural stratification pattern.

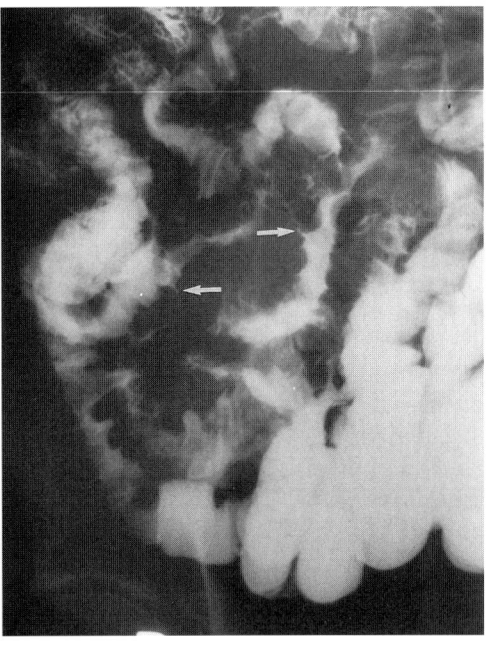
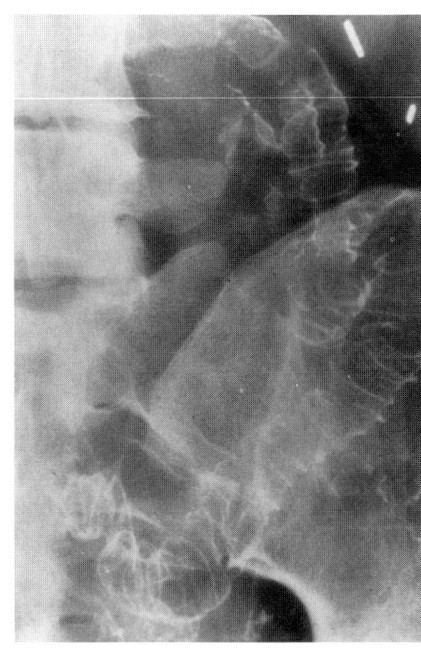

Fig. 17-6. Acute graft-versus-host disease.
Follow-through barium study (a) demonstrates ileal segments with thickened folds, loop separation, and several penetrating ulcers (arrows) suggesting associated CMV infection. (b) Plain film of the abdomen 48 hours later shows residual thin coating of barium of several bowel loops, likely to be a consequence of sloughing of the mucosa. (Courtesy of Bronwyn Jones, MD).

(a)   (b)

port dealing with cytomegalovirus-associated enterocolitis in a neutropenic patient could document that barium crystals initially overlying denuded lamina propria became trapped by the regenerating epithelium; they were slowly cleared over a period of 4 months.[21]

The subacute phase of graft-versus-host disease shows similar changes, but with more pronounced nodularity increase and lumen restriction. The distribution of the changes becomes more segmental, with wall thickening and, occasionally, areas of stenosis. Transit is rapid.[22]

In the chronic stage of graft-versus-host disease, residual small bowel abnormalities are complicated by supervening infections related to the patient's often profound immunodeficiency. Cytomegalovirus may cause an overwhelming infection with widespread ulceration. Other viral infections may cause similar changes.

Computed tomography (CT) can demonstrate thickening of the mesentery and of the wall of the small bowel and colon. A "target" sign can be demonstrated with intravenous contrast; there may also be ascites [Fig. 17-7(a, b)]. Interesting CT findings in two cases were the prolonged adherence of the peroral barium coating of the mucosal surface and the demonstration of a subepithelial halo of decreased attenuation.[23]

Treatment

Barium radiology can demonstrate typical changes of GVHD at an early stage and is highly relevant to management. The acute stage requires maintenance of fluid and electrolyte balances, and octreotide by injection. Treatment of the potentially lethal super-added infectious complications is important. High-dose corticosteroids in combination with cyclosporine or antithymocyte globulin may arrest the disease in about a third of patients.

Acquired Immunodeficiency Syndrome (AIDS)

Introduction

The pandemic spread of AIDS continues and may have affected 40 million people by the end of the century. Newer retroviral therapeutic agents are making an impact but are beyond the financial means of the majority of the patients, especially those in African countries. AIDS is a disorder of mainly cell-mediated immunity that predisposes the patient to multiple infections and to characteristic malignancies. The gastrointestinal tract is an important entry site for the AIDS virus as well as a major site for opportunistic infections that characterize the disease. The human immunodeficiency virus (HIV) is the third human retrovirus to be identified and differs from the human T-cell lymphotropic virus types I and II in its specific destructive effect on T-helper lymphocytes.

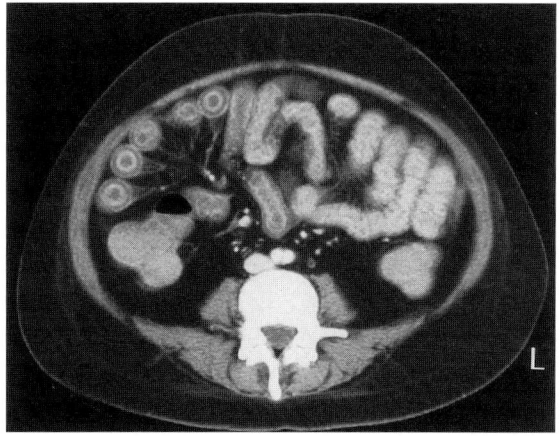 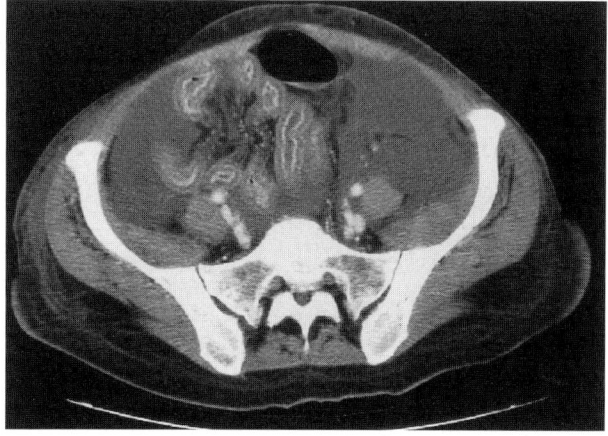

Fig. 17-7. Acute graft-versus-host disease with profuse watery diarrhea after allogeneic bone marrow transplantation for myelogenous leukemia.
CT scans (a) and (b) show circumferential mural thickening with a "target" enhancement pattern. Significant ascites is seen on image (b).

Whatever the route of entry into the body, and before seroconversion, primary infection leads to the appearance of HIV-specific cytotoxic T lymphocytes, mediated by $CD8^+$ cells.[24] Memory cytotoxic T lymphocytes are found but gradually decline over about 6 months to reach a stable level. High or low levels of stabilyzed memory T lymphocytes seem to affect the eventual intensity of the disease process.[24] Viral invasion relates to the binding of glycoprotein 120 of the AIDS virus to the CD4 molecule on the surface of helper T lymphocytes and, to a lesser extent, of macrophages and microglial cells.[25] The virus is then internalized into the cell, multiplies within the lymphocyte, and causes the release of a large number of new virions about 1½ days later and the death of the host cell.[26] It is estimated that during active disease some 10 billion virions are produced daily, killing about 2 billion $CD4^+$ lymphocytes, which are replaced as long as the body finds it possible.[27] Eventually, $CD4^+$ cell depletion and clinical immunodeficiency become evident.

Days or weeks after inoculation and coincident with a high plasma titer for HIV-RNA, 30% to 60% of infected persons develop an acute seroconversion syndrome that resembles infectious mononucleosis. Diarrhea may be part of this syndrome and will be discussed further below. Other features can be oral or esophageal ulcers, lymphadenopathy, and a maculopapular rash. This early stage is followed by a period of latency during which the plasma values for HIV-RNA decrease and the virus itself multiplies within the lymphoid system. There is progressive decline in the number of $CD4^+$ T cells, while the number of $CD8^+$ T cells remains fairly constant, resulting in a reduction in the ratio of $CD4^+$ to $CD8^+$ T cells. There is, furthermore, impairment of function of the still surviving $CD4^+$ T cells and, among its adverse effects, the inadequate terminal differentiation of IgA-bearing to IgA-secreting B cells.[28] In addition to impaired secretory antibody responses there is colonization of the small intestine by an increased bacterial load, aided by reduced gastric acid secretion and abnormal migrating motor complexes. Thus, bacterial overgrowth can contribute to diarrhea even before opportunistic infections take over.

When HIV infection has advanced to a degree when normally nonpathogenic organisms produce clinical infection, the late stage of AIDS is considered to have been reached. At this stage of the disease the $CD4^+$ T-cell count has been reduced to below 200 per microliter (normally 800 to 1200 cells per microliter). AIDS-defining illnesses involving the gastrointestinal tract are listed in Table 17-1.

HIV Enteritis

Increased frequency and altered consistency of stools are frequent symptoms in patients prior to opportunistic AIDS-defining infections. The identification of the HIV-associated antigen p24 in biopsy material taken from different sites in the small intestine and colon implies diffuse infiltration of the gastrointestinal tract HIV.[29] The same conclusions were reached by other investigators.[30,31] It can be difficult to rule out the presence of another unidentified pathogen. However, opportunistic enteric pathogens

Table 17-1. The more common AIDS-defining gastrointestinal illnesses[25]

Cause	CD4 T-cell count
Infectious agent:	
Cytomegalovirus	<100
Herpes simplex virus	<100
Candida albicans	<200
Histoplasma capsulatum	<200
Pneumocystis carinii	<200
Mycobacterium avium complex	<100
Neoplasms:	
Kaposi's sarcoma	<400
Non-Hodgkin's lymphoma	<200

could be found in 30 of 33 patients with AIDS and were found in only 1 of 23 non-AIDS, HIV-infected patients.[28] Furthermore, tissue p24 contents in intestinal mucosa were at their highest level in the pre-AIDS stages of the disease and then declined.[28] It has been shown that the presence of HIV genome in the intestinal mucosa is associated with histological and biochemical evidence of enteritis. So far, radiology has not contributed to a diagnosis in this stage of the disease.

Epidemiology

AIDS patients listed by the Centers for Disease Control (CDC) to 1986 were assigned to one of five high-risk groups.[32] Homosexual/bisexual males constituted 74% and intravenous drug abusers 17%, with an 11% overlap between the two groups. Hemophiliac disorders accounted for 1%, other recipients of blood and blood product transfusions for 2%. Heterosexual partners of any of the other subjects at risk constituted the fifth group. The remainder of the patients included the most unfortunate but small group of congenital AIDS, infants born to infected mothers. More recently, intravenous drug abusers present an ever-growing number of AIDS infections, partly held in check by the free distribution of hypodermic needles. Late figures show that women infected by heterosexual encounters make up 43% of AIDS cases in the United States.[33] There is also an increase in the number of congenital AIDS cases.

Definition of AIDS

Since a depressed level of T lymphocytes and reversal of the CD4/CD8 ratio can also occur in other immune deficiency states and since a positive test result for HIV antibodies can occur without overt disease, the CDC has established criteria for a diagnosis of AIDS, gradually widening the range over the years. Kaposi's sarcoma, multiple opportunistic infections, and primary central nervous system (CNS) lymphoma were the criteria mentioned in 1982. By 1985, lymphoreticular malignancies were included.[34]

Infections of the Small Intestine

The term *opportunistic infections* refers to agents that either are harmless to immunocompetent persons or cause only relatively mild and self-limited disease. In addition, there are infections by organism that can cause significant disease in persons with normal immune systems but occur with greater prevalence, in more severe form, and with certain differences of involvement in immunodeficient patients. Examples of such diseases are tuberculosis and histoplasmosis. Opportunistic infections eventually occur in most HIV-infected patients, and most of them affect the gastrointestinal tract, including the small bowel. Patients present with debilitating, often intractable diarrhea and weight loss, and often with malabsorption. When investigating such patients it should be remembered that the general homosexual population tends to be infected with a number of organisms, eg, *Giardia*, *Strongyloides*, and *Campylobacter*, which may cause diarrheal illnesses in the absence of HIV disease.[35]

Only the more common infective agents are described in greater detail. These are the protozoans *Cryptosporidium* and *Isospora belli*; the virus cytomegalovirus (CMV); and the bacterium *Mycobacterium avium intracellulare*. In addition, other less frequently diagnosed opportunistic infections will be mentioned only briefly.

Cryptosporidiosis

Cryptosporidiosis has been known as an infection in young calves and other animals and as a cause of time-limited diarrhea in immunocompetent persons who were in contact with them. The first human case was not described until 1976.[36] The tiny protozoan *Cryptosporidium parvum* completes its life cycle in a superficial parasitophorous vacuole among the microvilli of the small intestine, without penetrating the cytoplasm of the epithelial cells. Oocysts are passed into the stool and may release sporozoites for further maturation outside the body. Oocysts are thick-walled, can resist chlorination, or can survive in water for many months. Hence, the occasional water-borne outbreaks even in well-regulated Western countries. An acute diarrhea of self-limited 1 to 2 weeks' duration characterizes cryptosporidial infection of the immunocompetent patient. Patients with AIDS can develop a life-threatening prolonged diarrheal state or, less often, a cholera-like illness with the passage of up to 20 L of fluid per day. The exact mechanism for the diarrhea has not yet been determined. A parasite-produced enterotoxin could not be convincingly demonstrated.[37] Symptoms seem to parallel the intensity of infection, also expressed as percentage of surface epithelium occupied by the parasites.[38] Also found was an association with villous atrophy, nutrient malabsorption, and altered permeability.[37] Cryptosporidiosis has shown inconsistent response to treatment with numerous antibiotics. More recently, azithromycin therapy has been found effective in arresting severe diarrhea due to C parvum in children.[39]

Radiology. The usual findings by barium study are nonspecific fold thickening and intraluminal fluid increase [Fig. 17-8(a)]. These changes are most pronounced in the jejunum but may extend throughout the small bowel. A CT scan in a case of acute cryptosporidial enteritis clearly depicts the intense inflammatory change, with edema and increased mural and mesenteric vascularity [Fig. 17-8(b)]. Extension of the disease into biliary tracts is not unusual.

Isosporiasis

Isosporiasis, normally a zoonotic infection with an occasional mild and self-limited diarrhea in immunocompetent persons, can cause severe secretory diarrhea in AIDS patients. Diagnosis is by stool examination in which the oocysts of *Isospora belli* are readily distinguished from those of other coccidia.[40] Unlike cryptosporidium, oocysts of *I. belli* excyst within the small bowel and its sporozoites invade the epithelial cells. The incidence of isosporiasis in AIDS varies in different geographic areas, and is rather low in the United States. Clinical improvement has been reported after short administration of trimethoprim–sulfa-methoxazole.

Radiology. Barium follow-through examination gives a similar appearance to that described for cryptosporidiosis.

Cytomegalovirus

Cytomegalovirus (CMV) is a member of the herpesvirus group. Infection with CMV usually occurs during childhood, unaccompanied by characteristic clinical features. The virus then disseminates to multiple cellular reservoirs and continues in a latent phase throughout immunocompetent life.[41] CMV reactivation occurs in circumstances of immunosuppression (see later) or in immune deficiencies of any cause, including AIDS. With decreasing T-cell function reactivation can become persistent and can cause tissue in-

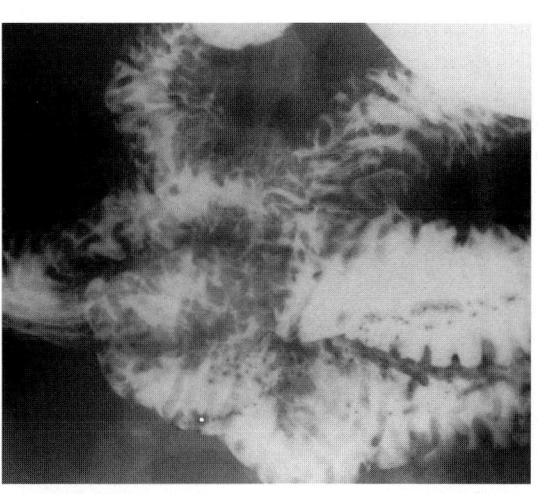

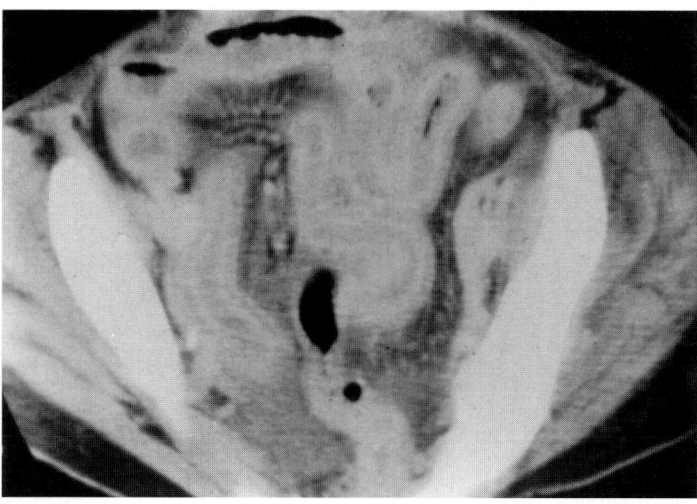

(a) (b)

Fig. 17-8. Cryptosporidial enteritis in AIDS.
(a) Barium study shows thickened folds in duodenum and jejunum, a nonspecific finding. Should radiology be required in more acute disease, CT would be preferred to barium. (b) CT in another patient with more acute cryptosporidiosis shows the bowel lumen to be filled with fluid, the bowel walls thickened and edematous with a faint stratification pattern. Mesenteric vessels are engorged.

jury. Typical CMV inclusion bodies are found in the endothelium of mucosal and submucosal capillaries. CMV vasculitis with vessel occlusion and associated necrosis and hemorrhage have been identified in terminal ileitis and as isolated lesions throughout the small intestine.[42] However, the cecum and terminal ileal area are the most commonly affected parts.[43] Massive bleeding from vasculitis-related CMV ulcers in the terminal ileum/cecum area have complicated immunodeficiency states in numerous cases.[44,45] Diagnosis is by immunohistological staining or by the demonstration of viral inclusion bodies. Effective treatment is presently achieved with ganciclovir or foscarnet.

Radiology. CMV-related deep ulcers affecting the terminal ileum have been demonstrated by barium examination and CT scans [Fig. 17-9(a, b)]; changes often extend into the cecum and may involve larger portions of the colon. More extensive CMV enteritis is characterized by segmental wall thickening with penetrating ulceration [Fig. 17-10(a, b)]. CT scans have demonstrated symmetrical wall thickening in the affected areas, usually the terminal ileum and cecum[46] [Fig. 17-11(a, b)].

Mycobacterium Avium–Intracellulare Complex

Mycobacterium avium–intracellulare complex (MAI) comprises mainly *M avium* together with a number of clinically less important strains. It is a virtually ubiquitous acid-fast bacillus found in soil and carried by animals, with little virulence to immunocompetent humans. As a cause of systemic disease, MAI was virtually unknown until the advent of AIDS, when it was found to occur in about 20% of patients.[35] Unlike tuberculosis (see below), MAI usually appears as a late complication of AIDS, when CD4 counts are below 100. The respiratory and gastrointestinal tracts are the usual portals of entry.

Dissemination of MAI can involve the lung, liver, spleen, bone marrow, lymph nodes, and the gastrointestinal tract. Blood samples in disseminated disease can be analyzed by culture or by the polymerase chain reaction method. Both are equally effective but the blood culture requires more time.[47] Duodenoscopy may demonstrate a granular mucosal pattern caused by the expansion of villi, reflecting the distended state of the lamina propria that forms the core of each villus.[48] Distention of the lamina propria results from a massive infiltration by macrophages, which contain large numbers of undigested bacilli. Biopsy of the altered or even normal-appearing duodenal mucosa can provide the diagnosis of MAI. (For comparison with Whipple's disease see Chapter 18.) Mesenteric and retroperitoneal lymph node enlargement can be characteristic. Treatment success has been claimed for rifabutin as a single agent or as part of a combination regimen.[49] Rifabutin given prophylactically to AIDS patients with a CD4 count at or below 75×10^9 cells/L has reduced the incidence of MAI infection by 55%.[49]

Radiology. With MAI involvement of the small bowel, enteroclysis can demonstrate a pattern of mucosal surface micronodularity that expresses the en-

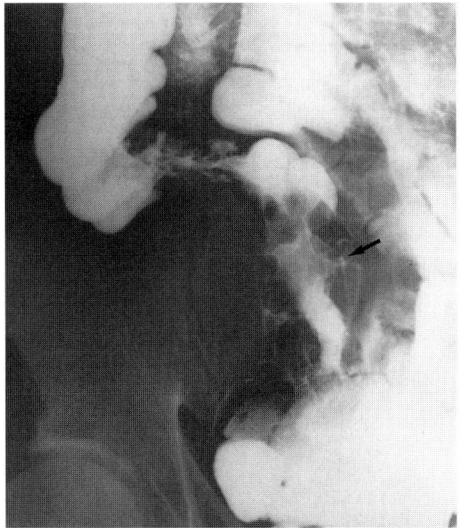
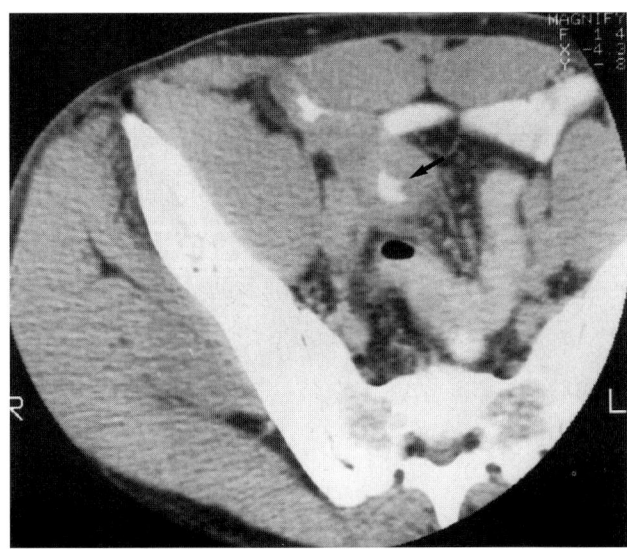

Fig. 17-9. Cytomegalovirus enteritis in AIDS.
(a) Barium follow-through into the terminal ileum demonstrates deep ulcers (arrow) and barium outlined tracks. (b) CT scan in the same area shows barium within a deep ulcer that has extended through the thickened bowel wall (arrow).

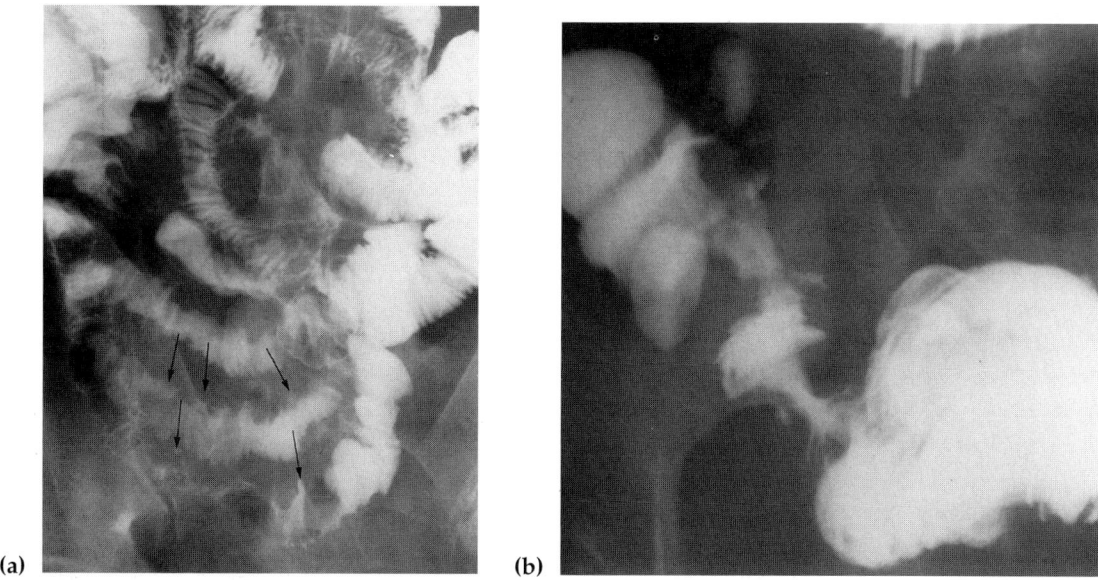

Fig. 17-10. Cytomegalovirus enteritis in AIDS.
(a) Barium follow-through study shows wide separation of loops of ileum, indicating mural thickening. Several ulcers are seen extending through the mucosa (arrows). (b) Terminal ileum, same examination. Lumen with limited distensibility and presence of several deeply penetrating ulcers.

largement of villi as described above [Fig. 17-12(a)]. In the setting of an AIDS-infected patient, a diffuse granular pattern of the mucosal surfaces shown by a follow-through examination is virtually diagnostic of MAI [Fig. 17-12(a)]; this diagnosis can be further sup-

ported by the CT demonstration of necrotic changes in enlarged and usually confluent mesenteric and retroperitoneal lymph nodes [Fig 17-13(b)]. Both radiological findings—micronodularity and a low attenuation nodal mass—can also be demonstrated in

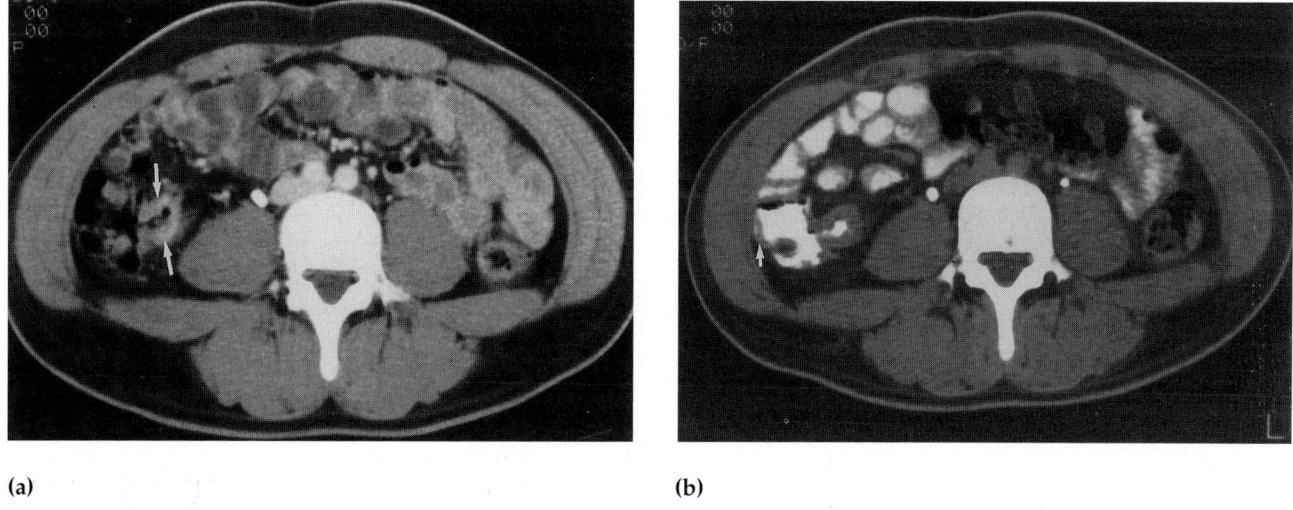

Fig. 17-11. Cytomegalovirus enterocolitis in AIDS. CT scans in 35-year-old male patient.
(a) Terminal ileum after IV contrast shows enhancement of its thickened wall (arrows). (b) Ingestion of barium demonstrates the narrowed lumen of terminal ileum with circumferential thickening of its wall (arrows). Biopsy was positive for CMV. The thickened lateral wall of cecum is indicated by an arrow.

320 • 17. Immune Deficiency Diseases

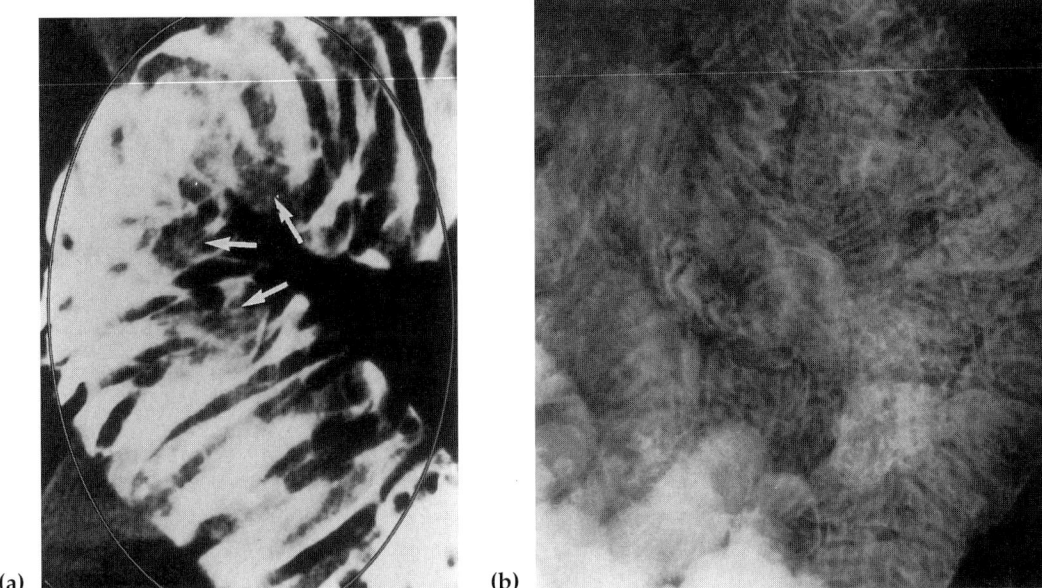

Fig. 17-12. *Mycobacterium avium-intracellulare* **infection in AIDS.**
(a) Enteroclysis (magnified view) shows jejunum with groups of micronodules of 1- to 2-mm diameter (arrows). (b) A follow-through barium study in another patient demonstrates thickened folds with a sandlike mucosal surface pattern.

Whipple's disease. The clinical background, disease history, and CD4 T-cell count (below 100 for MAI) will determine the differential diagnosis. Liver and spleen may be massively enlarged without focal lesions. MAI can also produce focal inflammatory changes, for example abscess formation related to bowel or located in the mesentery or the omentum and the abdominal wall [Fig. 17-14(a–c)].

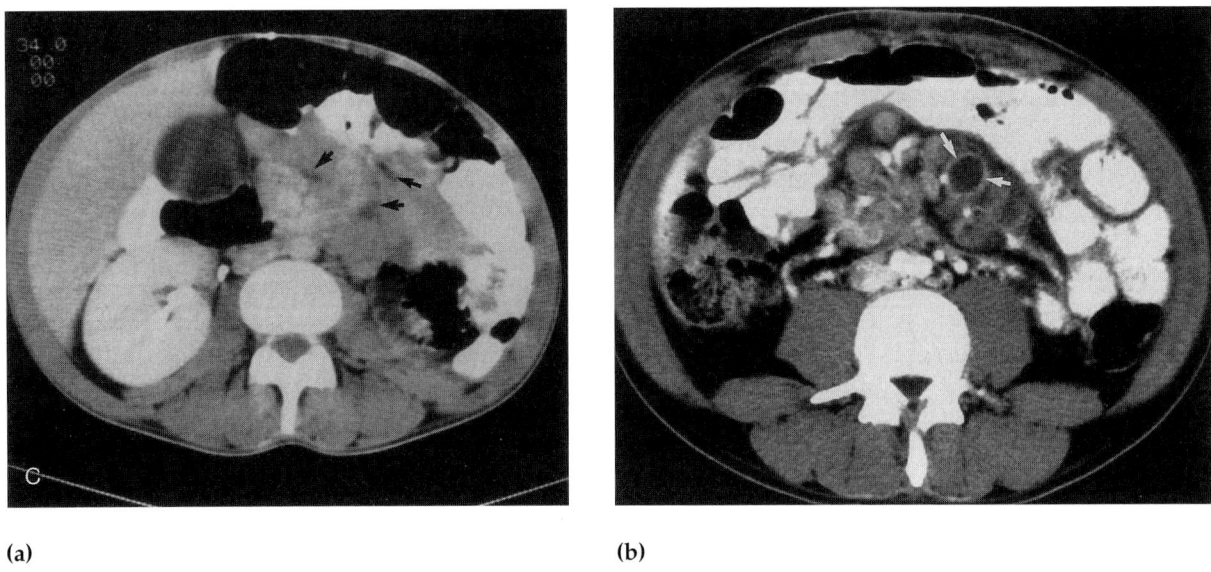

Fig. 17-13. *Mycobacterium avium-intracellulare* **infection in AIDS. CT demonstration of enlargement of mesenteric and retroperitoneal lymph nodes.**
(a) Matted nodal mass with areas of low attenuation indicating fat deposition or necrosis (arrows). (b) In a further patient there is evidence of necrosis of several enlarged lymph nodes (arrows to one of these).

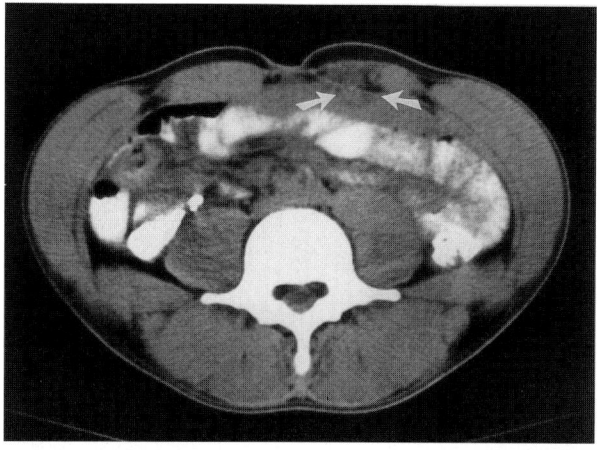
(a)

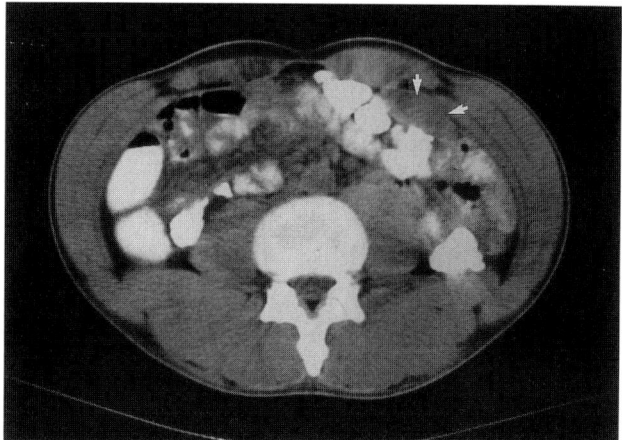
(b)

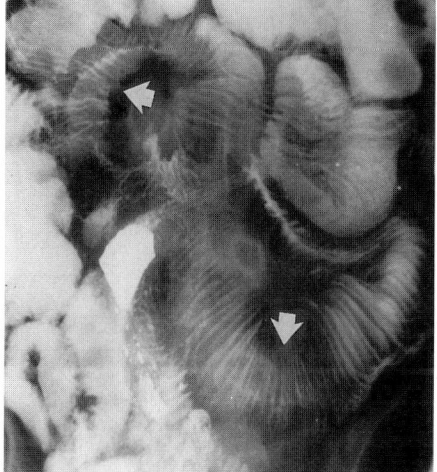
(c)

Fig. 17-14. *Mycobacterium avium-intracellulare* **infection in AIDS.**
(a) CT scan outlines an omental abscess (arrows) that extends into the left rectus muscle. (b) A further CT scan demonstrates extension of the omental abscess. (c) Enteroclysis demonstrates extrinsic inflammatory mass effect (arrows to displacement of thickened folds). Focal and disseminated MAI infection was confirmed by surgery.

Mycobacterium Tuberculosis

Small bowel localization of *mycobacterium tuberculosis* has been described in Chapter 16. Up to the early 1980s there had been an annual decrease of cases of tuberculosis reported in the United States. With the advent of AIDS this has changed into an annual increase of 16%.[50] Increased drug abuse, homelessness, crowding in shelters, and greater immigration have contributed to this increase. The major factor, however, has been the advent of the pandemic of AIDS. HIV infected persons with drug-susceptible M tuberculosis can respond favorably to treatment but fail to complete the full course of therapy in some 20% of cases.[50] About 90% of drug-resistant cases of tuberculosis have occurred in AIDS patients, in whom there has been a mortality rate between 70% and 90%.[49] Globally, tuberculosis is the most common opportunistic infection and the leading cause of death in AIDS.[51] The disease appears mostly before other opportunistic infections, when CD4 counts are still between 500 and 300.

Radiology. The ileocecal area, especially the valve and medial border of the cecum, are affected in some 90% of the cases. Compared to non-AIDS ileocecal tuberculosis, barium studies and CT scans have shown greater wall thickening and more pronounced regional nodal masses[52,53] (Figs. 17-15, 17-16). Enlarged nodes

322 • 17. Immune Deficiency Diseases

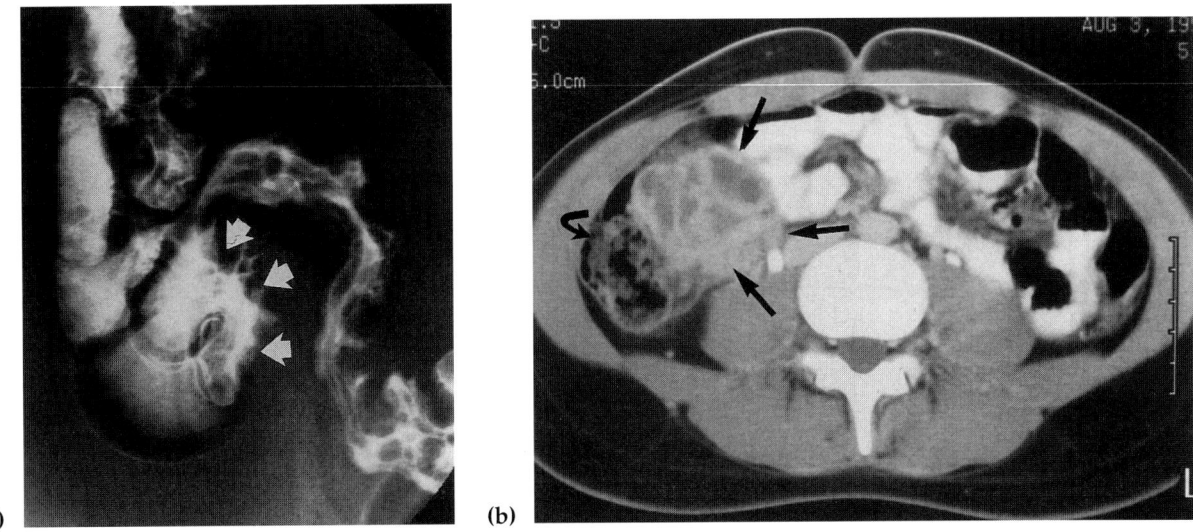

Fig. 17-15. Ileocecal tuberculosis in AIDS.
(a) Barium follow-through depicts ulceration of the medial border of the cecum (arrows) with displacement of the terminal ileum. (b) Large nodal mass (arrows) with areas of caseation necrosis close to the medial border of the cecum (curved arrow). (Courtesy of Emil J. Balthazar, MD.)

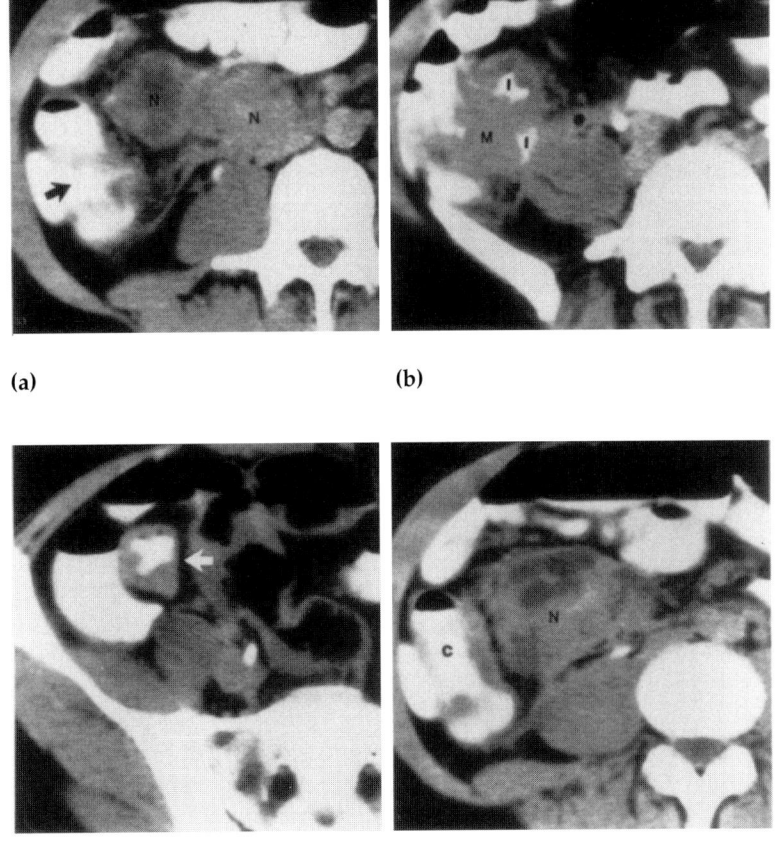

Fig. 17-16. Ileocecal tuberculosis in AIDS. CT scans after peroral contrast.
(a) Ileocecal valve thickening (arrow) and large mesenteric nodal masses (N) with caseation necrosis. (b) Medial border of cecum related soft tissue mass (M) engulfing terminal ileum (I). (c) More proximal scan of ileum with circumferential wall thickening (arrow). (d) Wall thickening of colon (C) of heterogeneous density and a large mesenteric nodal mass (N) with areas of caseation necrosis. (Courtesy of Emil J. Balthazar, MD.)

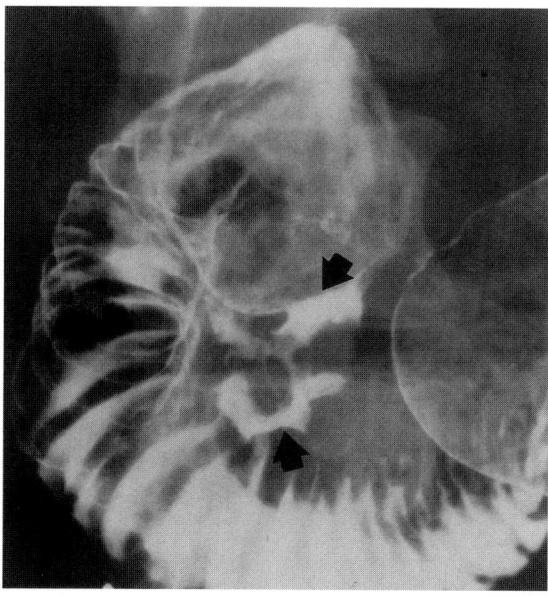

Fig. 17-17. Duodenal tuberculosis with cavity in AIDS. Barium study outlines descending duodenum in communication with a cavity in a regional nodal mass (arrow). (Courtesy of Kyunghee C. Cho, MD.)

may contain areas of necrosis. Focal disease may also affect proximal areas of the small bowel, at times with cavitation (Fig. 17-17).

Bacillary Angiomatosis

Bacillary angiomatosis refers to recently described vascular proliferative lesions in persons with AIDS. The infective agents belong to the *Bartonella* group of bacilli.[54] Highly vascular lesions resembling Kaposi's sarcoma can affect internal organs and produce enhancing mesenteric and retroperitoneal adenopathies when shown by CT. Raised, nodular, ulcerated mucosal lesions have been described in the GI tract, including the small intestine.[55] Antibiotics are usually effective therapy.

Microsporidia

Microsporidia are protozoan parasites and a cause of chronic diarrhea in AIDS patients whose CD4 count is less than 100. The parasites can be found in biopsies from the distal duodenum. Light microscopy shows them as clusters of microsporidial spores in the cytoplasm of absorptive enterocytes. Treatment with albendazole is curative.

Multiplicity and Multifocality

The aforementioned infective agents frequently occur in combination and at multiple sites in the gastrointestinal tract.[56] Cryptosporidiosis, for example, is frequently associated with other opportunistic infection. AIDS-related neoplasms may also be found in association with infections (see below).

AIDS-Related Neoplasms

Kaposi's Sarcoma (KS)

Classic Kaposi's sarcoma was a rare disease of elderly Europeans of Eastern or Mediterranean ancestry and involved the gastrointestinal tract in its late stage.[57] A much more aggressive endemic form of Kaposi's sarcoma affects young populations in equatorial Africa, has been known for a long time, and is unrelated to AIDS.[58] Kaposi's sarcoma has resurfaced in AIDS patients and is usually disseminated and progressive. KS has been detected in 44% of homosexual and bisexual men with AIDS but in only 4% of AIDS-infected intravenous drug abusers.[59] This pattern of prevalence points to a cofactor in the genesis of the sarcoma. It could very recently be determined by means of sequence-based detection techniques that a new herpesvirus related to virtually all KS lesions in AIDS patients.[60] The new virus has been designated Kaposi's sarcoma–associated herpesvirus (KSHV). A further study has detected KSHV sequences in 100% of AIDS-KS and 72% of classical KS.[61] The same new herpesvirus has also been detected in endemic KS and in posttransplantation KS.[62]

KS lesions contain thin-walled neovascular formations, extravasated red cells, inflammatory lymphocytes, and proliferating endothelium-derived spindle cells. Multicentric lesions, cutaneous and visceral, are usual and can appear synchronously. A recent paper concluded that multiple KS lesions in the same patient arise from a single clone of cells, and may be regarded a disseminated monoclonal cancer.[63] Almost all patients have skin lesions; about half have involvement of the gastrointestinal tract. Barium studies frequently show multiple lesions mostly in the stomach, duodenum, and colon.[64] They take the form of submucosal polypoid elevations, often centrally umbilicated. Earlier lesions are observed as nodules or focal fold thickening. They are infrequently found in the jejunum or ileum (Fig. 17-18(a, b)]. The presence of violaceous papules on the patient's back, on the lower extremities, or over the hard palate supports the diagnosis of Kaposi's sarcoma.

Radiology. CT demonstrates the KS-related lymphadenopathy. Retroperitoneal, mesenteric, and pelvic nodes can appear as abnormal clusters of nonenlarged nodes (0.5 to 1.0 cm) or as fewer enlarged or matted nodes (Fig. 17-19). Dynamic sequential CT scans in AIDS patients with disseminated KS have

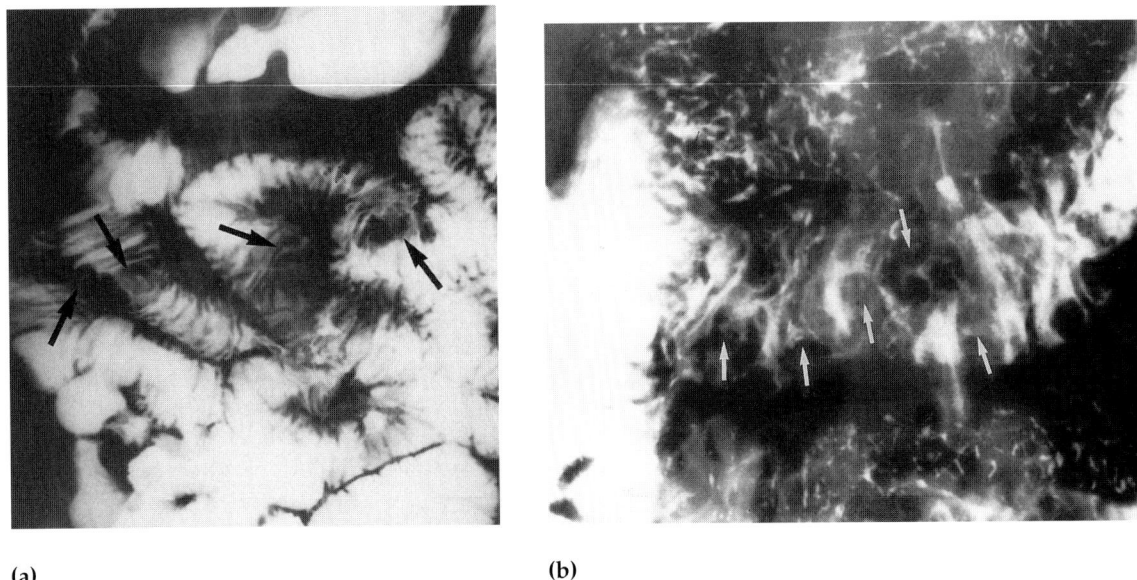

Fig. 17-18. Kaposi's sarcoma (KS) in AIDS.
(a) Barium studies demonstrate several small umbilicated, round, polypoid masses in the jejunum (arrows). (Courtesy of Emil J. Balthazar, MD.) (b) Young male homosexual AIDS patient who presented with severe diarrhea that was of cryptosporidial origin (see thickened folds and flocculation of barium). In addition, there were numerous ulcerated or umbilicated polypoid masses 1 to 3 cm in diameter representing Kaposi's sarcomas (arrows to some).

identified hyperattenuating adenopathy in 26 of 38 patients, with a positive predictive value of 79%.[65] Clustered nodes, usually of normal size, can also be seen during the latency stage of HIV disease and then in the absence of Kaposi's sarcoma. Lymph nodes in MAI (see earlier) tend to be larger and contain areas of lower density. An associated hepatospleno-megaly favors Kaposi's sarcoma.

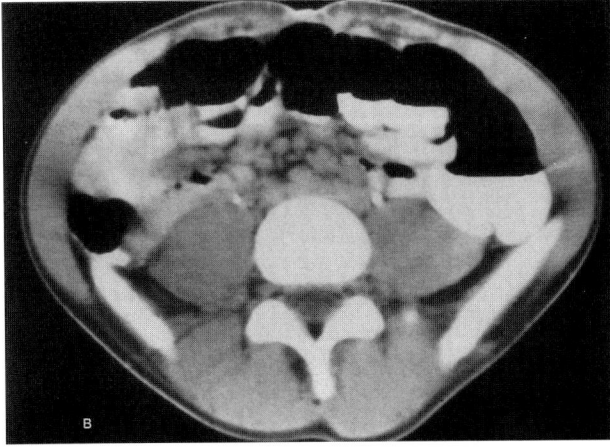

Fig. 17-19. Kaposi's sarcoma (KS) in AIDS.
CT demonstration of numerous 1 to 3 cm mesenteric and retroperitoneal nodes in a patient with KS of the stomach and skin.

AIDS-Related Lymphoma

The gastrointestinal tract and the central nervous system are the most frequent sites for AIDS-related lymphomas. The great majority are of B-cell origin and usually of aggressive large-cell type; some are Burkitt's lymphomas, possibly related to the Epstein-Barr virus. In one study of 869 AIDS patients, 108 (12%) developed malignant neoplasms; lymphoma accounted for 35%, Kaposi's sarcoma for 60%, and miscellaneous tumors for 5%.[66]

Radiology. CT has been the primary and follow-up radiological technique in the majority of cases. There is considerable similarity in the CT appearances of AIDS-related and non-AIDS abdominal lymphoma. Among the few features that may suggest AIDS-related lymphoma are 1) a mean age at diagnosis of 40 years (against 63 for non-AIDS) and 2) a higher incidence of mesenteric lymphadenopathy.[66] In AIDS patients with intra-abdominal lymphoma, the disease was extranodal in 86%, with lymph node enlargement found in 56%.[66] CT scans showed involvement of the gastrointestinal tract more often than of the liver; enlarged nodes were mostly homogeneous and usually more dense than muscle.[67] Hepatomegaly was rarely seen except in association with focal liver lesions. Splenomegaly was reported to be of minor degree and uncommon.[67] In the gastrointestinal tract the stomach was only slightly more often affected than the small bowel.

Lymphomatous changes demonstrated in the small

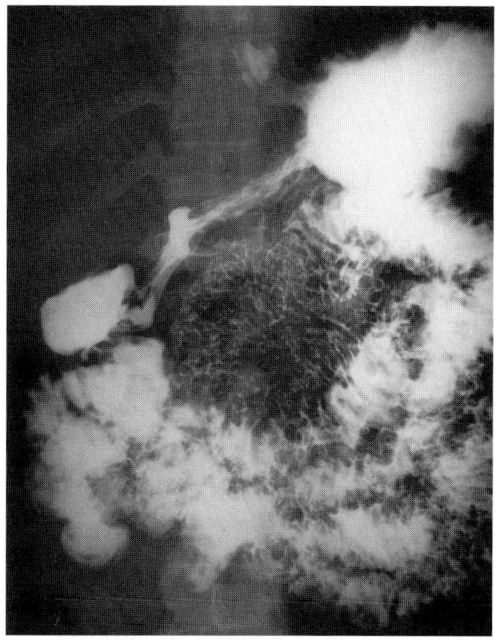

Fig. 17-20. Non-Hodgkin's small bowel lymphoma in AIDS Patient of 35 years.
(a) Barium follow-through with diffuse nodular fold thickening. (b) CT scan shows a segment of jejunum with multiple nodular masses (arrows) causing distortion of the barium outlined lumen. (c) In addition to multiple nodular masses affecting further segment of bowel outlined with barium (arrows), there is now extensive retroperitoneal adenopathy (open arrows). (With permission from Balthazar EJ et al, *AJR* 1997;168:675–680.)

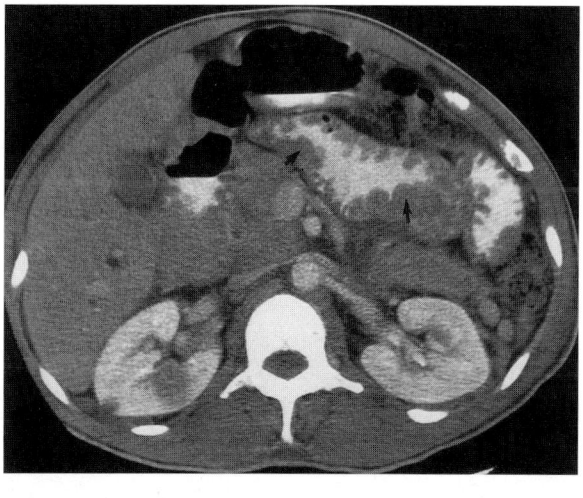

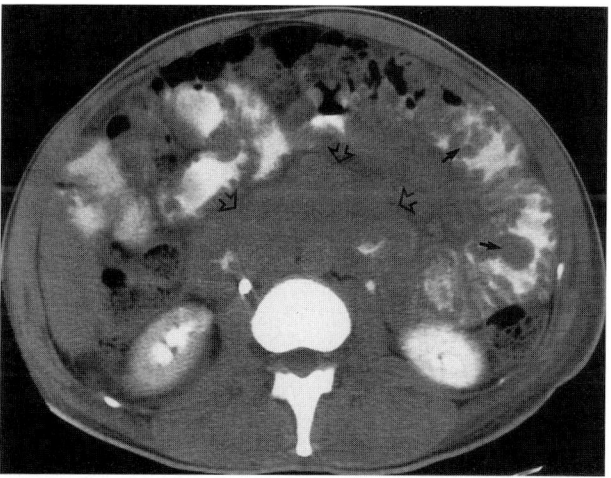

bowel were mostly circumferential wall thickening affecting single segments but more often multiple segments (Fig. 17-20). Focal cavitary lesions could be part of the presentation (Figs. 17-21, 17-22, 17-23). Extensive lymphadenopathy characterized a case of Burkitt's lymphoma (Fig. 17-24). The few CT-based differences already mentioned between AIDS-related and unrelated lymphoma are more of statistical than practical value. However, two clear points of difference have emerged: 1) Perianal lymphoma appears to be unique to AIDS; 2) Lymphoma should be included in the differential diagnosis of almost any intra-abdominal mass in a patient with HIV infection.[67] Confirmation of diagnosis is optimally done by biopsy, preferably during laparoscopy.

Brief mention needs to be made of a recently found relationship between Kaposi's sarcoma and a new type of lymphoma. Primary body cavity–based, usually AIDS-related lymphoma has been consistently linked to the earlier mentioned KSHV. This type of lymphoma affects the pleural space more often than the peritoneal cavity and presents with serous effusions not associated with tumor masses, adenopathy, ororganomegly.[68] Average survival has been two months. KSHV has also been identified in most AIDS-related or unrelated cases of multicentric Castleman's disease.[69]

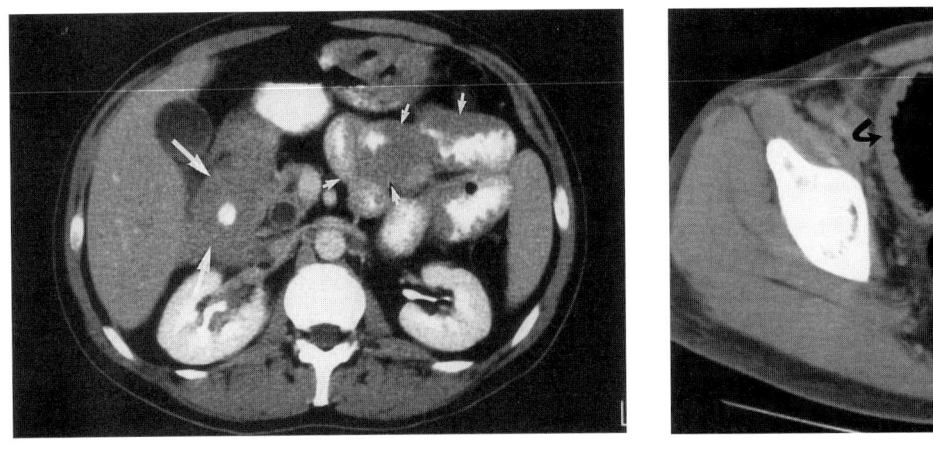
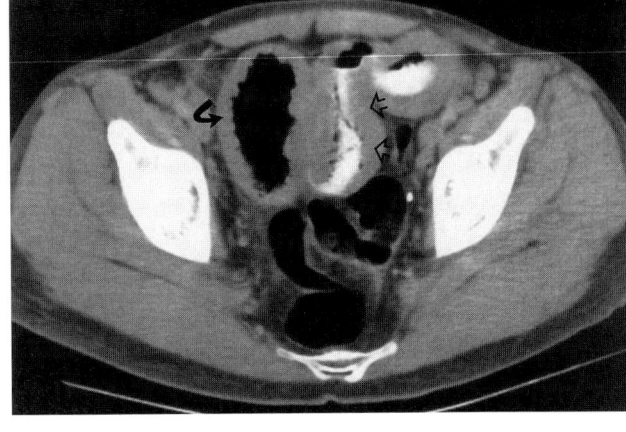

Fig. 17-21. Non-Hodgkin's small bowel lymphoma in AIDS. Large cell lymphoma involving several segments separated by unaffected small bowel.
(a) Uneven annular tumor infiltrate (arrow heads) affects duodenum and proximal jejunum. A segment of ileum is encased by tumor (arrows). (b) A pelvic loop of ileum with annular tumor infiltrate (open arrows) adjoins a cavitary lesion with a thickened wall (curved arrow). (With permission from Balthazar et al.[68])

Secondary Immune Deficiencies

Immune defects can result from many causes, among them underlying disease, advanced age, undernutrition, and a surgical intervention. They are the most frequently encountered form of immune disorders. The reduced levels of the relevant components of the immune system represent the net balance between their synthesis and their loss or destruction.

Protein-losing enteropathy or gastropathy is a significant cause of secondary immune deficiencies. Intestinal lymphangiectasia, Whipple's disease, and extensive inflammatory and ulcerative lesions of the small bowel can be responsible. Cell-mediated immunity is affected to a greater degree than humoral im-

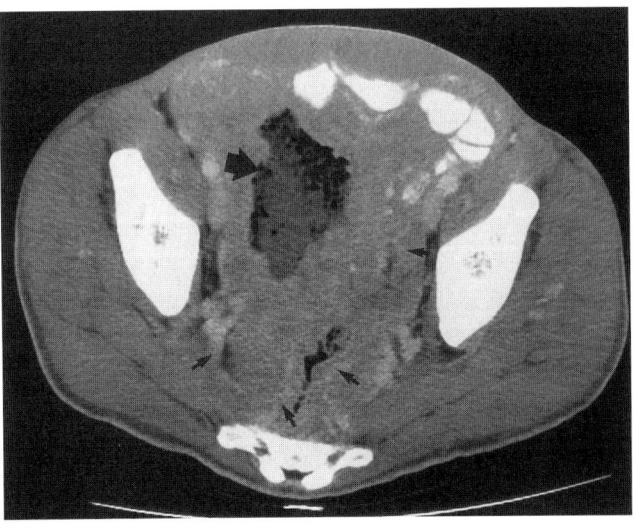
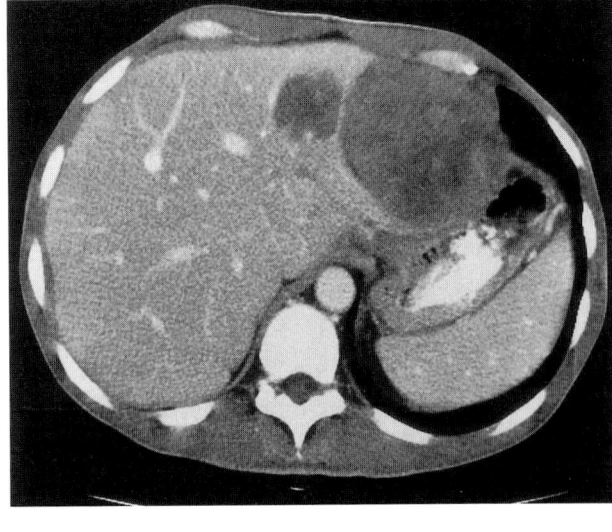

Fig. 17-22. Non-Hodgkin's small bowel lymphoma in AIDS. Ileal lymphoma in a 43-year-old male patient.
(a) Circumferential wall thickening of terminal ileum, which appears engulfed by tumor (arrowheads). The bowel lumen is aneurysmally dilated and contains secretions and gas bubbles (large arrow). (b) Two lymphomatous masses are seen in the enlarged liver.

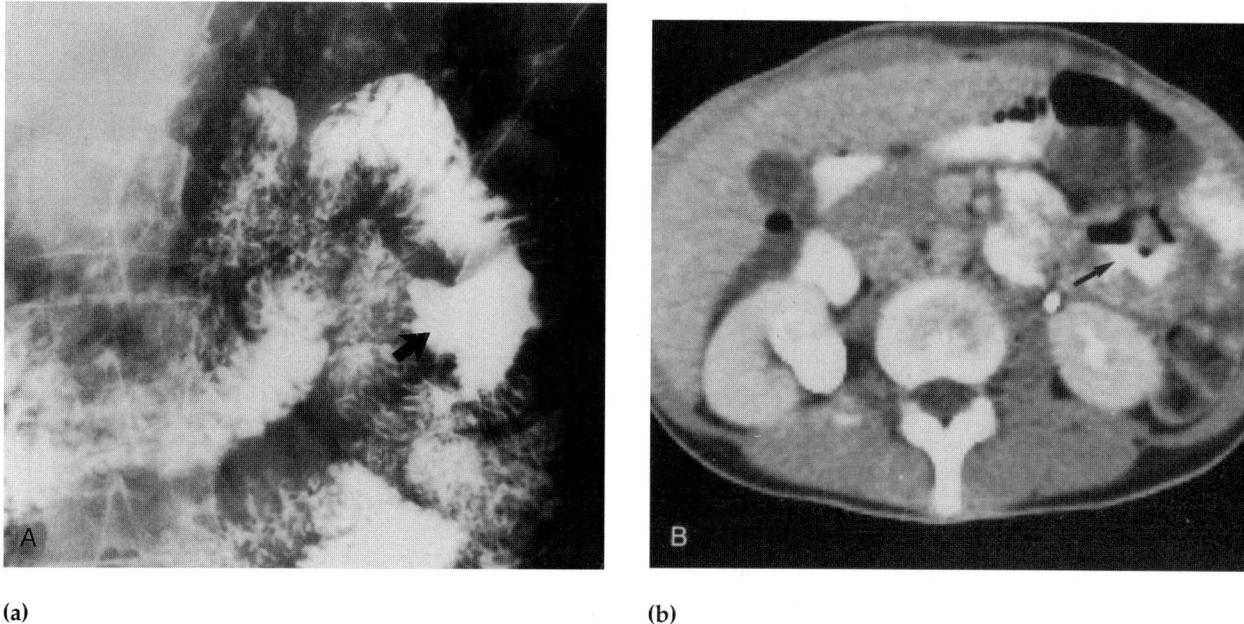

Fig. 17-23. AIDS-related non-Hodgkin's lymphoma of jejunum.
(a) Barium follow-through outlines a cavitary lesion related to the proximal jejunum (arrow). This was a highly aggressive B-cell lymphoma. (b) A CT scan demonstrates the barium- and air-retaining cavitary lesion (arrow). (Courtesy of A. J. Megibow, MD.)

munity. Clinicoradiologic detail of such underlying conditions will be described in Chapter 18.

Solid Organ Transplantation (Immunosuppression)

In recent years there has been a progressive increase in the number of patients immunosuppressed, mostly in relation to organ transplantation. The worldwide increase of solid organ transplantation is based on improvement of surgical techniques and on the increasing avoidance of transplant rejection by the recipient. A major requirement for success has been the judicious suppression of the transplant recipient's ability for a mostly cellular immune response.

Post-Transplant Lymphoproliferative Disorder (PTLD)

A major problem are post-transplant malignancies, among them carcinomas of the skin and lips and the lymphoma-related PTLD. PTLD may result from impaired immune surveillance, chronic antigenic stimulation by the allograft, or oncogenic effects of post-transplant administered immunosuppressive therapy.[70] Epstein-Barr virus (EBV)–driven lymphoproliferation is regarded as the most important causative factor. Patients who were EBV-seronegative at transplantation were found to have acquired an EBV isolate indistinguishable from that of the donor and subsequently developed PTLD.[71] There is preliminary evidence that antiviral prophylaxis can reduce the development of PTLD.[72]

The incidence of PTLD as a complication of transplantation is generally quoted to approximate 8%.[72] The incidence is influenced by the transplanted organ and

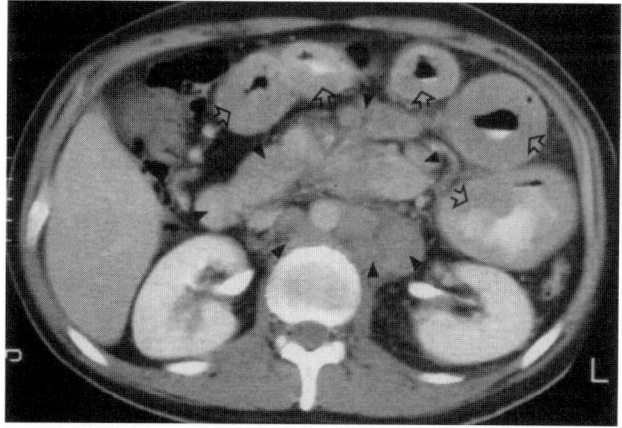

Fig. 17-24. AIDS-related Burkitt's lymphoma in AIDS.
Extensive circumferential bowel wall thickening (open arrows) and large mesenteric and retroperitoneal nodal mass (arrowheads).

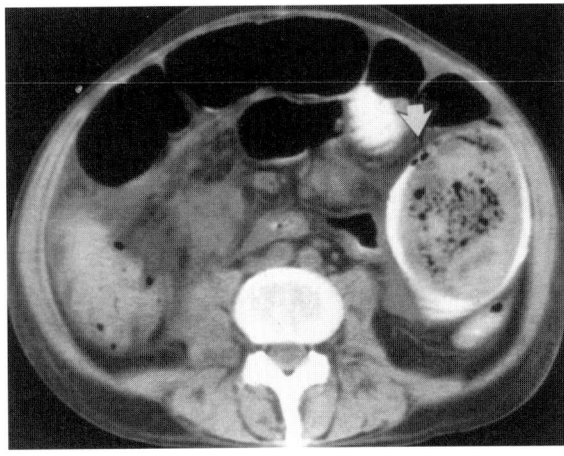
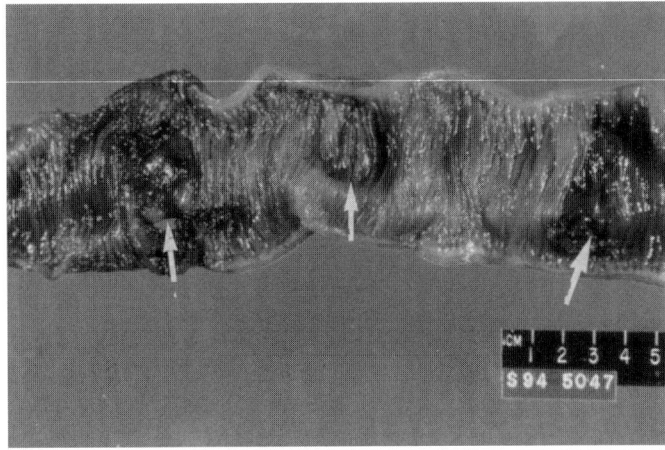

Fig. 17-25. Small bowel localization of PTLD. Following liver transplantation a 54-year-old male patient presented with pyrexia, abdominal pain, partial obstruction, and blood loss.
(a) CT scan demonstrates dilated blood-filled jejunum and indicates tumor extension through a portion of the wall (arrow). Surgery with resection of 82 cm of small bowel demonstrated a perforation, ulcerated tumor nodules, and the entire length of jejunum filled with blood. (b) The surgical specimen contains 2- to 3-cm hemorrhagic tumor nodules (arrows) protruding from the mucosa. (Courtesy of J. L. Chezmar, MD.)

is significantly higher for heart/heart-lung than for renal transplants.[70,73] The primary site of PTLD localization was mostly extralymphoreticular, was brain and lung in over half the cases,[70] and was the oropharynx and the gastrointestinal tract in a smaller number of cases.[70,74] PTLD was diagnosed at a median interval of 80 months post-transplantation.[72] The siting of PTLD can be influenced by the type of immune suppressing agent or agents used. Suppression with cyclosporine was reported to be associated with a higher rate of PTLD localization in the gastrointestinal tract.[75] However, the overall incidence of PTLD relates to the degree and not to the type of immunosuppression used.

PTLD frequently contains a polymorphic distribution of B cells but this may change from poly- to monoclonality. If diagnosed at an early, still polyclonal stage, the reduction or discontinuation of immunosuppression may cause regression of the disease. This can be reinforced by the parenteral administration of high-dose acyclovir.[70] Surgical excision is indicated in localized disease. Radiotherapy and combination chemotherapy are used for nonresponders or for patients diagnosed at a late stage of lymphoma; a high mortality rate exists in this group of patients.[76] Small bowel-related PTLD has usually been a manifestation of more generalized PTLD. In addition to the gastrointestinal tract, PTLD may affect the tonsils, liver, spleen, lungs, kidneys, and the CNS.[76]

The radiologic literature contains very few reports of the diagnostic features of PTLD. A rare example is the report of a renal allograft recipient on cyclosporine suppression who presented acutely with pneumoperitoneum and bleeding. In addition to involvement of the CNS and lungs, there were polypoid changes in the small bowel as shown by a barium follow-through examination.[77] In a recent case report of a post-liver transplant patient who presented similarly with abdominal pain, bleeding, obstruction, and perforation,[77] CT scans outlined dilated, blood-filled jejunum with indications of gas-containing tumor extensions through part of the bowel wall [Fig. 17-25(a)]. Resected bowel revealed numerous ulcerated mural tumor nodules representing PTLD[78] [Fig. 17-25(b)].

References

1. Shanahan FS, Targan SR. Gastrointestinal manifestations of immunologic disorders. In: Yamada, T, ed. *Textbook of Gastroenterology.* Philadelphia, Pa: JB Lippincott Co; 1991:2157–2171.
2. Lederman HM, Winkelstein JA. X-linked agammaglobulinemia: an analysis of 96 patients. *Medicine (Baltimore).* 1985;64:145.
3. Rosen FS, Cooper MD, Wedgewood RJP. The primary immunodeficiencies. *N Engl J Med.* 1984;311:235–242.
4. Wong JT. Case records of the Massachusetts General Hospital, case 7-1995. re: Scully. *N Engl J Med.* 1995;332:663–671.
5. Docke WD, Simon HU, Fietze E, et al. Cytomegalovirus reactivation and tumor necrosis factor. *Lancet.* 1994;343:268–269.

6. Kinlen LJ, Webster AD, Bird AJ, et al. Prospective study of cancer with hypogammaglobulinemia. *Lancet.* 1985;1:263–266.
7. Sander CA, Medeiros LJ, Weiss LM, et al. Lymphoproliferative lesions in patients with common variable immunodeficiency syndrome. *Am J Surg Pathol.* 1992;16:1170–1782.
8. Crooks DJM, Brown WR. The distribution of intestinal nodular hyperplasia in immunoglobulin deficiency. *Clin Radiol.* 1980;31:701–706.
9. Chiaramonte C, Glick SN. Nodular lymphoid hyperplasia of the small bowel complicated by jejunal lymphoma in a patient with common variable immune deficiency syndrome. *AJR.* 1994;163:1118–1119.
10. Castellano G, Moreno D, Galvao O, et al. Malignant lymphoma of the jejunum with common variable hypogammaglobulinemia and diffuse nodular hyperplasia of the small intestine. A case study and literature review. *J Clin Gastroenterol.* 1992;15:128–135.
11. Case records of the Massachusetts General Hospital, case 8-1997, rc: Scully. *N Engl J Med.* 1997;336:786–793.
12. Azar HA. Cancer in Lebanon and the Near East. *Cancer.* 1962;15:66.
13. Blumstein M, Bank S, Greenberg RE, et al. Immunoproliferative small intestinal disease in an American patient with lymphoma and macroamylasemia. *Gastroenterology.* 1992;103:1071–1074.
14. World Health Organization. Report on alpha heavy-chain disease. November 1975; Geneva.
15. Wright DH, Isaacson PG. Mediterranean lymphoma. In: Whitehead R, ed. *Gastrointestinal and Oesophageal Pathology.* Edinburgh, Scotland: Churchill Livingstone; 1989:648–652.
16. Ramos I, Marcos J, Illanas M, et al. Radiological characteristics of primary intestinal lymphoma of the "Mediterranean" type. Observations on twelve cases. *Radiology.* 1978;126:379–385.
17. Matsumoto T, Iida M, Matsui T, et al. The value of double-contrast study of the small intestine in immunoproliferative small intestinal disease. *Gastrointest Radiol.* 1990;15:159–163.
18. Armitage JO. Bone marrow transplantation. Review article. *N Engl J Med.* 1994;330:827–838.
19. Fast LD, Valeri CR, Crowley JP. Immune responses in major histocompatibility complex homozygous lymphoid cells in murine F1 hybrid recipients: implications for transfusion-associated graft-versus-host disease. *Blood.* 1995;86:3090–3096.
20. Jones B, Kramer SS, Saral R, et al. Gastrointestinal inflammation after bone marrow transplantation: graft-versus-host disease or opportunistic infection? *AJR.* 1988;150:277–281.
21. Ma LD, Jones B, Lazenby AJ, et al. Persistent oral contrast lining the intestine in severe mucosal disease: elucidation of radiographic appearance. *Radiology.* 1994;191:747–749.
22. Rosenberg HK, Serota FT, Koch P, et al. Radiographic features of gastrointestinal graft-versus-host disease. *Radiology.* 1981;38:371–374.
23. Jones B, Fishman EK, Kramer SS, et al. Computed tomography of gastrointestinal inflammation after bone marrow transplantation. *AJR.* 1986;146:691–695.
24. Musey L, Hughes J, Schacker T, et al. Cytotoxic T-cell responses, viral load, and disease progression in early human immunodeficiecy virus type 1 infection. *N Eng J Med.* 1997;337:1267–1274.
25. Pantongrag-Brown L, Nelson AM, Brown AE, et al. Gastrointestinal manifestations of acquired immunodeficiency syndrome: radiologic-pathologic correlation. *Radiographics.* 1995;15:1155–1178.
26. Cohn JA. Recent advances—HIV infection I. Clinical review. *Brit Med J.* 1997;314:487–491.
27. Perelson AS, Neuman AU, Markowitz M, et al. HIV-1 dynamics *in vivo*: virion clearance rate, infected cell life span, and viral generation time. *Science.* 1996;271:1582–1586.
28. Smith PD, Mai UEH. Immunopathophysiology of gastrointestinal disease in HIV infection. *Gastroenterol Clin N Am.* 1992;21:331–342.
29. Kotler DP, Reka S, Clayton F. Intestinal mucosal inflammation associated with human immunodeficiency virus infection. *Digest Dis Sci.* 1993;38:1119–1127.
30. Kotler DP, Reka S, Borcich A, Cronin WL. Detection, localization and quantitation of HIV-associated antigens in intestinal biopsies from HIV-infected patients. *Am J Pathol.* 1991;139:823–830.
31. Nelson JA, Wiley CA, Reynolds-Kohler C, et al. Human immunodeficiency virus detected in bowel epithelium from patients with gastrointestinal symptoms. *Lancet.* 1988;2:259–262.
32. Centers for Disease Control. Update—Acquired Immunodeficiency Syndrome—(AIDS)—United States. *MMWR.* 1986;35:221–223.
33. Mehta P, Bentrup KL. Women and HIV infection. *J Fl Med Assoc.* 1996;83:473–478.
34. Solinger AM, Hess AV. Acquired immunodeficiency syndrome—an overview. *Semin Roentgenol.* 1987;22:9–13.
35. Megibow AJ, Balthazar EJ, Hulnick DH. Radiology of nonneoplastic gastrointestinal disorders in the Acquired Immune Deficiency Syndrome. *Semin Roentgenol.* 1987;22:31–41.
36. Nime FA, Burek JD, Page DL, et al. Acute enterocolitis in a human being infected with the protozoan *Cryptosporidium. Gastroenterology.* 1976;70:592–598.
37. Sears CL, Guerrant RL. Cryptosporidiosis: the complexity of intestinal pathophysiology. Editorial. *Gastroenterology.* 1994;106:252–254.
38. Goodgame RW, Kimball K, Ou C-N, et al. Intestinal function and injury in acquired immunodeficiency syndrome-related cryptosporidiosis. *Gastroenterology.* 1995;108:1076–1082.
39. Hicks P, Zwiener RJ, Squires J, Savell V. Azithromycin therapy for *Cryptosporidium parvum* infection in four children infected with human immunodeficiency virus. *J Pediatrics.* 1996;129:297–300.
40. DeHovitz JA, Pape JW, Boncy M, Johnson WD. Clinical manifestations and therapy of *Isospora belli* infection in patients with the acquired immunodeficiency syndrome. *N Engl J Med.* 1986;315:87–90.
41. Kotler DP. Gastrointestinal complications of the acquired immunodeficiency syndrome. In: Yamada T, ed. *Text-

book of *Gastroenterology*. 2nd ed. Philadelphia, Pa: JB Lippincott Co; 1995:2322–2343.
42. Frank D, Raicht RF. Intestinal perforation with CMV infection in patients with acquired immune deficiency syndrome. *Am J Gastroenterol*. 1984;79:201–205.
43. Teixidor HS, Honig CL, Norsoph E, et al. Cytomegalovirus infection of the alimentary canal: radiologic findings with pathologic correlation. *Radiology*. 1987;163:317–323.
44. Sackier JM, Kelly SB, Clarke D, et al. Small bowel haemorrhage due to cytomegalovirus vasculitis. *Gut*. 1991;32:1419–1420.
45. Lai JR, Chen KM, Shun CT, Chen MY. Cytomegalovirus enteritis causing massive bleeding in a person with AIDS. *Hepatogastroenterology*. 1996;43:987–991.
46. Balthazar EJ, Martino JM. Giant ulcers in the ileum and colon caused by cytomegalovirus in patients with AIDS. *AJR*. 1996;166:1275–1276.
47. De Francesco MA, Colombrita D, Pinsi G, et al. Detection and identification of mycobacterium avium in the blood of AIDS patients by the polymerase chain reaction. *Euro J Clin Microbiol & Infect Dis*. 1996;15:551–555.
48. Cappell MS, Philogene C. The endoscopic appearance of severe intestinal mycobacterium avium complex infection as a coarsely granular mucosa due to massive infiltration and expansion of intestinal villi without mucosal exudation. *J Clin Gastroenterol*. 1995;21:323–326.
49. Nightingale SD, Cameron DW, Gordin FM, et al. Two controlled trials of rifabutin prophylaxis against mycobacterium avium complex infection in AIDS. *N Engl J Med*. 1993;329:828–833.
50. Beiser C. HIV infection II. Recent advances. Clinical review. *Brit J Med*. 1997;314:579–582.
51. Bargallo N, Nicolau C, Luburich P, et al. Intestinal tuberculosis in AIDS. *Gastrointest Radiol*. 1992;17:115–118.
52. Snyder DE, Roper WI. The new tuberculosis. Editorial. *N Engl J Med*. 1992;326:703–705.
53. Balthazar E, Gordon R, Hulnick D. Ileocecal tuberculosis: CT and radiologic evaluation. *AJR*. 1990;154:499–503.
54. Moore EH, Russel LA, Klein JS, et al. Bacillary angiomatosis in patients with AIDS: multiorgan imaging findings. *Radiology*. 1995;197:67–72.
55. Tuur SM, Macher AM, Angritt P, et al. AIDS case for diagnosis series, 1988. *Mil Med*. 1988,153:M57–M64.
56. Wall SD, Ominsky S, Altman DF, et al. Multifocal abnormalities of the gastrointestinal tract in AIDS. *AJR*. 1986;145:1–5.
57. Bryk D, Farman J, et al. Kaposi's sarcoma of the intestinal tract: roentgen manifestations. *Gastrointest Radiol*. 1987;3:425–430.
58. Taylor JP, Templeton AC, Vogel CL, et al. Kaposi's sarcoma in Uganda: a clinico-pathologic study. *Int J Cancer*. 1971;8:125–135.
59. Nyberg DA, Federle MP. AIDS-related Kaposi's sarcoma and lymphoma. *Semin Roentgenol*. 1987;22:54–65.
60. Chang Y, Cesarman E, Pessin MS, et al. Identification of herpes virus-like DNA sequences in AIDS-associated Kaposi's sarcoma. *Science*. 1994;266:1865–1869.
61. Rady PL, Yen A, Martin RW, et al. Herpes-like DNA sequences in classic Kaposi's sarcomas. *J Med Virol*. 1995;47:179–183.
62. Miller G, Rigsby MO, Heston L, et al. Antibodies to butyrate-inducible antigens of Kaposi's sarcoma-associated herpesvirus in patients with HIV-1 infection. *N Engl J Med*. 1996;334:1292–1297.
63. Rabkin CS, Janz S, Lash A, et al. Monoclonal origin of multicentric Kaposi's sarcoma lesions. *N Engl J Med*. 1997;336:988–993.
64. Rose HS, Balthazar EJ, Megibow AJ, et al. Alimentary tract involvement in Kaposi's sarcoma: limitations of abdominal CT in acquired immunodeficiency syndrome. *AJR*. 1982;139:661–666.
65. Herts BR, Megibow AJ, Birnbaum BA, et al. High-attenuation lymphadenopathy in AIDS patients: significance of findings at CT. *Radiology*. 1992;185:777–781.
66. Radin DR, Esplin JA, Levine AM, Ralls PW. AIDS-related non-Hodgkin's lymphoma: abdominal CT findings in 112 patients. *AJR*. 1993;160:1133–1139.
67. Balthazar EJ, Noordhoorn M, Megibow AJ, Gordon RB. CT of small-bowel lymphoma in immunocompetent patients and patients with AIDS: comparison of findings. *AJR*. 1997;168:675–680.
68. Jaffe ES. Primary body cavity-based AIDS-related lymphomas. Evolution of a new disease entity. *Am J Clin Pathol*. 1996;105:141–143. (Editorial comment):221–229.
69. Cesarman E, Knowles DM. Kaposi's sarcoma-associated herpesvirus: a lymphotropic human herpesvirus associated with Kaposi's sarcoma, primary effusion lymphoma and multicentric Castleman's disease. *Seminars Diagn Pathol*. 1997;14:54–66.
70. Morrison VA, Dunn DL, Manivel CJ, et al. Clinical characteristics of post-transplant lymphoproliferative disorders (clinical studies). *Am J Med*. 1994;97:14–24.
71. Haque T, Thomas JA, Falk KI, et al. Transmission of donor Epstein-Barr virus (EBV) in transplanted organs causes lymphoproliferative disease in EBV-seronegative recipients. *J Gen Virol*. 1996;77:1169–1172.
72. Davis CL, Harrison KL, McVicar JP, et al. Antiviral prophylaxis and the Epstein Barr virus-related post-transplant lymphoproliferative disorder. *Clin Transplant*. 1995;9:53–59.
73. Mihalov ML, Gattuso B, Abraham K, et al. Incidence of post-transplant malignancy among 674 solid-organ-transplant recipients at a single center. *Clin Transplant*. 1996;10:248–255.
74. Dodd GD, Ledesma-Medina J, Baron RL, Fuhrman CR. Post-transplant lymphoproliferative disorder: intrathoracic manifestations. *Radiology*. 1992;184:65–69.
75. Basgoz N, Preiksaitis JK. Post-transplant lymphoproliferative disorder. *Infect Dis Clin N Am*. 1993;9:901–923.
76. Stone RM, Ferry JA. Case records of the Massachusetts General Hospital, case 31-1997, re: Scully. *N Engl J Med*. 1997;337:1065–1074.
77. Tubman DE, Frick MP, Hanto DW. Lymphoma after organ transplantation: radiologic manifestations in the central nervous system, thorax and abdomen. *Radiology*. 1983;149:623–631.
78. Chezmar JL. Post-transplant lymphoproliferative disorders. In: *Summer Abdominal Imaging Conference Report*, University of Pennsylvania Medical Center, Department of Radiology; 1997; Philadelphia, Pa.

18 Malabsorption States

Hans Herlinger and David C. Metz

Chapter Contents

Introduction
Classification
Celiac Disease (CD)
Tropical Sprue
Bacterial Overgrowth Syndrome
Chronic Intestinal Pseudo-Obstruction
Systemic Sclerosis
Jejunal Diverticulosis
Short Bowel Syndrome
Whipple's Disease
Systemic Mastocytosis
Eosinophilic Gastroenteritis
Abetalipoproteinemia
Zollinger-Ellison Syndrome
Amyloidosis
Endocrine Disorders
Maldigestion
Lactase Deficiency
Crohn's Disease
Lymphangiectasia
Waldenstrom's Macroglobulinemia
Cystic Fibrosis in Adults

Introduction

Malabsorption states comprise a range of grades of diminished uptake of nutrients into the body. Patients may present with only isolated deficiencies, eg, of folate, to more severe manifestations, eg, those associated with frank steatorrhea. Malabsorption may be the dominant clinical feature or be part of a systemic disease, often overshadowed by other abnormalities. Among such systemic diseases are several major and potentially life-threatening disorders. Various other conditions that predominantly present with chronic diarrhea include an element or a major component of malabsorption.

In this labyrinth of many diseases and syndromes, radiology of the small intestine can offer only a limited range of changes from the normal appearance. It would, therefore, be an added disadvantage if pattern recognition were to be the only way to a radiologic diagnosis. To achieve the full potential of diagnostic radiology in these circumstances, the following become the essential tasks of the radiologist:

1. To be able to interpret in pathologic-anatomic terms the radiologic changes revealed by the mucosal surface pattern.
2. To relate altered radiologic appearances to each patient's clinical presentation.

It follows that the radiologist will need to be acquainted with clinical aspects of the malabsorption states and be reasonably up-to-date with the never-ending developments in clinical diagnosis and management. These are not easy tasks since, with the exception of Acquired Immunodeficiency Syndrome (AIDS), systemic sclerosis, bacterial overgrowth syndrome, and celiac disease, the many other malabsorption-related conditions are only rarely seen in the working life of each radiologist.

Classification

Deficient delivery of nutrients into the body can be a result of malfunction at several levels:

1. *Maldigestion* within the small bowel lumen can be due to the deficient secretion of enzymes, especially from the pancreas, or the diminished output of bile with its adverse effect on the solubilization of fat. Maldigestion can also occur at the brush border mainly of the jejunal epithelium, where enzymes normally aid the digestion of carbohydrates and peptides.

2. *Malabsorption* proper refers to a deficient intake and metabolism by the columnar cells that line the mucosa, a complex function discussed in Chapter 2. Many of the diseases to be described below belong to this group of cellular-level malabsorption states.

3. *Malassimilation* refers to malfunction in the transport of absorbed and metabolized nutrients from the intestinal mucosa into the body.

4. *Bacterial overgrowth*, a consequence of intraluminal stasis, lowered defense mechanisms, or increased contamination from outside the small bowel, forms an important part of the malabsorption states, one in which radiology can play a crucial diagnostic function.

5. *Miscellaneous causes* of malabsorption include drugs, alcohol, gastric surgery, endocrinopathy, and malnutrition.

Based on these five divisions, Table 18-1 lists the component diseases grouped according to their type of malabsorption.

Approach to Diagnosis

Clinical Aspects

Weight loss, anorexia, abdominal distention, wasting, and steatorrhea—the passage of bulky, greasy feces—provide an unmistakable indication of an advanced malabsorption state. More often, symptoms and signs will be more subtle and may even be misleading. In a study of celiac disease, for example, almost two thirds of the patients were reported to have presented with trivial and unrelated symptoms, and others with unusual ones, such as lymphadenopathy or gonadal dysfunction.[1] A high degree of alertness by the physician is essential if malabsorption states are to be diagnosed before they become advanced. A careful physical examination needs to be supplemented by special laboratory tests, of which only a few are briefly described.

Fecal Fat Test

With the patient on a normal diet a stool suspension in saline is stained with a drop of Sudan III and acetic acid and examined under the microscope. If positive, it is advisable to confirm steatorrhea by a further quantitative Sudan III study using a sample from a 24-hour or 72-hour stool collection.[2]

D-Xylose Absorption-Excretion Test

D-Xylose is absorbed in the proximal small bowel and incompletely metabolized. About 25% is excreted in the urine. Any abnormality of small bowel absorption will reduce renal excretion. Renal insufficiency is one of the factors leading to a false-positive diagnosis.[3]

Breath Hydrogen Analysis and Culture of Duodenal Aspirates

The former test specifically estimates the metabolic activity of the intestinal flora. Excessive breath hydrogen after the administration of 10 g of lactulose indicates bacterial overgrowth.[4] The peak breath hydrogen level is reached within 2 hours of the intake. This is a noninvasive procedure, not requiring radioisotopes, using an inexpensive gas chromatograph. The breath test can also be used to measure orocecal transit. Results are affected by small bowel and gastric motility and are uninterpretable after gastric and small bowel resection. The gold standard for the diagnosis of bacterial overgrowth is the aerobic and anaerobic culture of more than 10^5 bacterial colonies per milliliter of aspirated duodenal fluid, an invasive procedure.

Table 18-1. Classification of malabsorption

Maldigestion
 Chronic pancreatitis
 Pancreatic resection
 Cholestasis
 Ileitis or ileal resection
 Zollinger-Ellison syndrome
 Disaccharidase deficiencies
 Cystic fibrosis

Malabsorption
 Celiac disease
 Ischemia
 Hypogammaglobulinemic sprue
 Radiation enteropathy
 Tropical sprue
 Short bowel syndrome
 Whipple's disease
 Amyloidosis
 Mastocytosis
 Eosinophilic gastroenteritis
 Parasitoses
 Crohn's disease (extensive)

Malassimilation
 Lymphangiectasia
 Abetalipoproteinemia
 Hypobetalipoproteinemia

Bacterial Overgrowth
 Systemic sclerosis
 Pseudo-obstruction (idiopathic)
 Diverticulosis
 Obstructing lesions
 Fistulae
 Surgical blind loops

Miscellaneous
 Diabetes
 Alcohol
 Gastric surgery
 Endocrinopathy
 Malnutrition
 Drugs

Mucosal Biopsy

Whenever a malabsorption state has been shown to exist, especially with likely cellular level pathology, an endoscopic mucosal biopsy from the descending duodenum or the proximal jejunum should be done. A suction instrument is now only rarely used.

The Normal Mucosa

Villi extend from the duodenal bulb through virtually all the small intestine. Their height is about three times the thickness of the lamina propria. Mature epithelial cells, the columnar-shaped enterocytes with a brush border of microvilli, cover the mucosa, including the villi. These cells develop within crypts that occupy the lamina propria and are formed by undifferentiated pluripotent stem cells anchored in the depth of the crypts. A state of equilibrium exists between intestinal surface cell loss and crypt cell proliferation. Six to 40 lymphocytes are found between every 100 enterocytes. The cellular infiltrate in the lamina propria consists mainly of plasma cells, lymphocytes, and macrophages (Fig. 18-1).

Radiology

In most instances, a diagnosis of malabsorption has already been made on clinical and biochemical grounds before a patient is referred to radiology. In these correctly sequenced circumstances, the purpose of radiology is to determine or confirm a cause for the malabsorption state or to demonstrate its possible complications. Only rarely should radiology alone be expected to provide the primary indications for the existence of malabsorption. Such primary radiologic diagnosis would be possible in circumstances where specific radiologic changes are encountered. Examples would be bacterial overgrowth syndromes and celiac disease. The demonstration of flocculation of a barium suspension within the lumen of the small intestine, although it may be associated with malabsorption, is entirely nonspecific; it can also occur with extensive inflammatory conditions and with any hypersecretory state of gastric or small bowel origin, and in apparently disease-free individuals. The so-called "malabsorption pattern" is a totally misleading term.

Celiac Disease

Definition

Celiac disease of children and adults is virtually identical. Only adult celiac disease is described here. It is a disease in which the proximal small bowel shows a characteristic abnormality of the mucosa and is associated with a variable degree of malabsorption of virtually all nutrients. Withdrawal of gluten-containing cereals promptly leads to improvement of both clinical presentation and, soon also, to normalization of mucosal histology. A reintroduction of gluten into the diet will cause abnormalities to recur after a variable time interval.

The above definition is no longer considered adequate as it comprises only a minority of gluten-sensitized patients. A range of lesser mucosal changes has been observed in dermatitis herpetiformis and in ap-

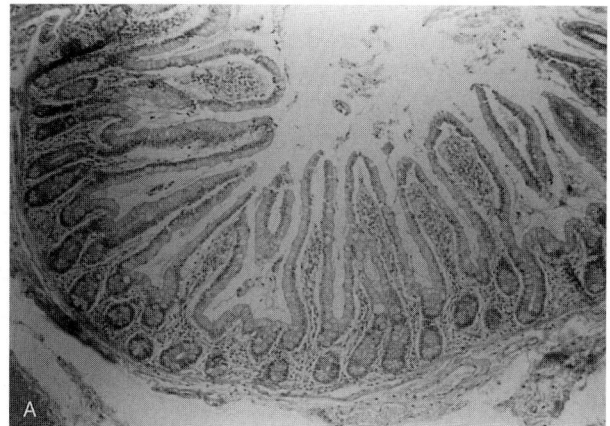
(a)

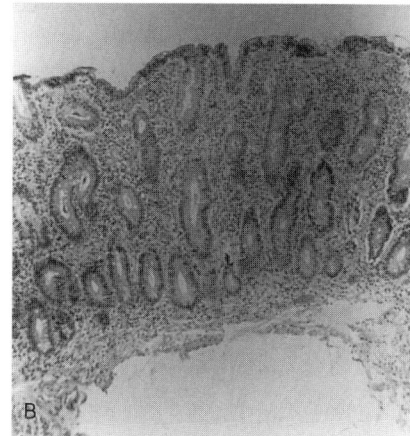
(b)

Fig. 18-1. Histologic sections of jejunal mucosa.
(a) Normal mucosa. More than two thirds of its thickness is taken up by the fingerlike villi. Crypts are seen in the lamina propria. (b) Mucosa in celiac disease. Villi are absent, yet the thickness of the mucosa remains virtually the same. This is caused by widening of the lamina propria due to hypertrophy of the crypts and an increased cellular infiltrate.

parently asymptomatic first-degree relatives of patients with overt celiac disease.[5] Such lesser mucosal changes include marked infiltration by gluten-sensitized intraepithelial lymphocytes covering normal-sized villi, or, at a slightly more advanced stage, also affecting epithelial cells within hypertrophied crypts.[5] It is not clear what proportion of people with these changes develop clinically apparent celiac disease. While an avillous mucosal pattern—the so-called type 3 lesion[5]—characterizes symptomatic celiac disease, the same lesion can also be seen, often without clinically evident small bowel disease, in about 40% of patients with dermatitis herpetiformis and in 10% of first-degree relatives of celiac disease patients.[5] A gluten-sensitized but asymptomatic population extends beyond these two groups and may be large. There are a number of events that may trigger the unmasking of such latency, among them intervening illnesses, surgery,[6] and obstruction.

Epidemiology

Taking Europe as an example, the prevalence of celiac disease is lowest in the southeast and increases in a northwesterly direction to reach its highest level in the west of Ireland, around the old University City of Galway. There, the prevalence has been reported to be 1 in 300 but has declined in recent years.

Clinical Diagnosis

Adult celiac disease occurs with greater frequency in women than in men. A history of childhood celiac disease can be elicited in about a quarter of the adult patients. The classic presentation, as described by Gee in 1888,[7] of bulky stools, muscular weakness, abdominal distention, abdominal discomfort rarely amounting to pain, glossitis, and pigmentation changes, is found in only a minority of patients.[1]

Atypical Presentations

These can take several forms. One of the earliest, very adequate descriptions of the barium radiology now realized to be typical of celiac disease related to a patient then considered to suffer from tetany.[8] Other atypical presentations can include bone pain, iron deficiency, megaloblastic anemia, peripheral neuropathy, and hypokalemia.[9]

Elderly Patients

Patients more than 60 years old seem to show an increasing prevalence for new celiac disease. Of a large group of new celiac disease patients recorded by the Coeliac Disease Society in the United Kingdom, 21% of the patients were aged 60 years or more.[10] Elderly celiac disease patients are particularly likely to present atypically, unexplained anemia being the most frequent presentation.[10,11] Not only does their diagnosis tend to be considerably delayed, they also have a greater likelihood of lymphoma development.[12] In a recent survey the incidence of lymphoma in celiacs aged 51 to 80 years was 3 to 10 times higher than in patients in their 4th and 5th decades.[13]

Diagnostic Delay and Misdiagnoses

These also affect younger patient groups. Of a group of 419 patients with eventually proven celiac disease, 196 (47%) were misdiagnosed at first, leading to a mean delay of the correct diagnosis by 12.9 years; in those patients without initial misdiagnosis the delay amounted to a mean of 8.0 years.[14] Steatorrhea, a frequent feature of the disease, is not necessary for diagnosis.

Positive Diagnosis

While clinical alertness for the possibility of celiac disease as cause in any unexplained deficiency state is desirable, the diagnosis needs to be firmly based since it must lead to long-term and quality-of-life–affecting dietary restrictions. The gold standard for the clinical diagnosis is specific changes in the duodenal or proximal jejunal mucosa, shown by dissecting or transmission microscopy of biopsy material. The celiac disease specificity of these mucosal alterations needs to be supported by a return to at least clinical normality after withdrawal of gluten from the patient's diet. A further diagnostic step, the reintroduction of gluten-containing food, followed by recurrence of clinical and mucosal abnormality, is now rarely taken. The considerable value of radiologic diagnosis or radiologic support of the clinical diagnosis will be discussed below.

Serological Diagnosis

IgA and IgG serum antigliadin antibodies can be found in over 90% of patients with celiac disease. However, such antibodies can also be found in some patients with Crohn's disease. Antigliadin antibodies are best used to confirm compliance with the patient's gluten-free diet. The search for a serology-based diagnosis has presently culminated in the introduction of the IgA-class antiendomysium antibody markers of celiac disease.[15] These antibodies, directed against the extracellular matrix of primate smooth muscle, have become a reliable predictor of celiac disease.[16] A 93.4% sensitivity and 100% specificity have been reported.

Nevertheless, there have yet been no suggestions for the test to replace the distal duodenal biopsy as the gold standard for diagnosis.

The Mucosa in Celiac Disease

In celiac disease there is marked crypt hyperplasia with an accelerated proliferative response to a greatly increased epithelial cell loss into the gut lumen.[17] Villi are absent or almost absent. Enterocytes, no longer columnar shaped, bear stunted, disorganized microvilli. More intraepithelial lymphocytes are seen. The lamina propria is thickened often enough to almost maintain, without the villi, the overall thickness of a normal mucosa. Crypts are considerably hypertrophied. The cellular infiltrate of the lamina propria is markedly increased [Fig. 18-1(b)]. These alterations do not uniformly extend through the affected bowel but show focal variations of intensity and a gradual decrease in the direction of the ileum.[18]

The Mosaic Pattern

Biopsy material of the avillous duodenojejunal mucosa, when viewed under a dissecting microscope, often has a surface pattern of a 1- to 2-mm, almost square area separated by grooves, ie, the mosaic pattern. Numerous openings to groups of crypts can be seen within each mosaic (Fig. 18-2). The same pattern can be identified in the duodenal mucosa by endoscopy, best if accentuated by indigo carmine dye scattering.[19]

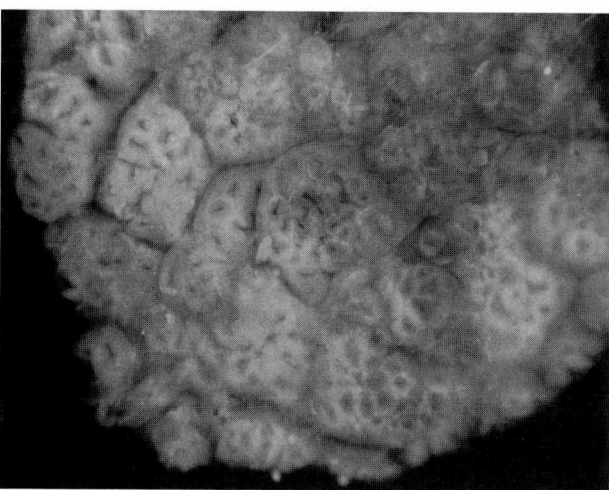

Fig. 18-2. Suction biopsy specimen of jejunal mucosa seen through a dissecting microscope.
Almost rectangular areas separated by grooves contain the openings of multiple crypts and form the so-called mosaic pattern. (Courtesy of Professor M. S. Losowsky, Leeds, England.)

It can occasionally be outlined by enteroclysis. The endoscopic finding of a reduction or loss of folds in the duodenal mucosa should mandate biopsy and could lead to the diagnosis of unsuspected celiac disease.[20]

Mucosal Changes in Differential Diagnosis

Subtotal or partial villous atrophy may be found in other conditions not associated with gluten sensitivity, eg, Whipple's disease, eosinophilic gastroenteritis, ischemia, tropical sprue, and radiation enteropathy. These conditions are more likely to have only partial villous atrophy, without crypt hyperplasia or lymphocytic infiltration of the lamina propria. Parasitic diseases, the small bowel overgrowth syndrome, and some of the immunodeficiency states are also likely to have mucosal alterations resembling those in celiac disease. The nonsteroidal anti-inflammatory drug mefenamic acid (Ponstel) is a known cause of steatorrhea with flattening of the jejunal mucosa.[21] Patients with these conditions will not show improvement after gluten withdrawal, nor will specific radiologic findings be the same as those demonstrated in celiac disease.

Nonspecific Radiologic Findings

1. *Dilatation,* mostly of the jejunum in excess of 30 mm when measured on a follow-through examination, has shown correlation with the elevation of fecal fat and the reduction of red blood cell folate levels.[22,23] It is not specific for celiac disease and can also be found in hypoalbuminemia,[24] obstruction, and scleroderma and after gastric resection. Excess of intraluminal fluid may be seen together with dilatation.

2. *Fold thickening* is *not* a feature of celiac disease. It may occur if hypoalbuminemia supervenes or it may be an artifact, a result of hypersecretion displacing the barium coating from the surface of the folds, producing a gradually widening and blurring outline of folds.

3. *Hypomotility* may correlate with lumen dilatation and may even amount to pseudo-obstruction. Some patients, however, may show normal transit and others may have transit acceleration.

4. *Mucosal changes in the duodenum:* A nodular, "bubbly" pattern of the duodenal bulb has been described as favoring a diagnosis of celiac disease.[25] This pattern can involve much of the descending duodenum [Fig. 18-3(a)]. An identical pattern has been encountered in peptic duodenitis. A review of 49 endoscopic mucosal biopsies taken from the descending duodenum showed acute duodenitis with patchy gastric metaplasia; among this group were four cases of celiac disease with the same surface pattern.[26] It seems that the

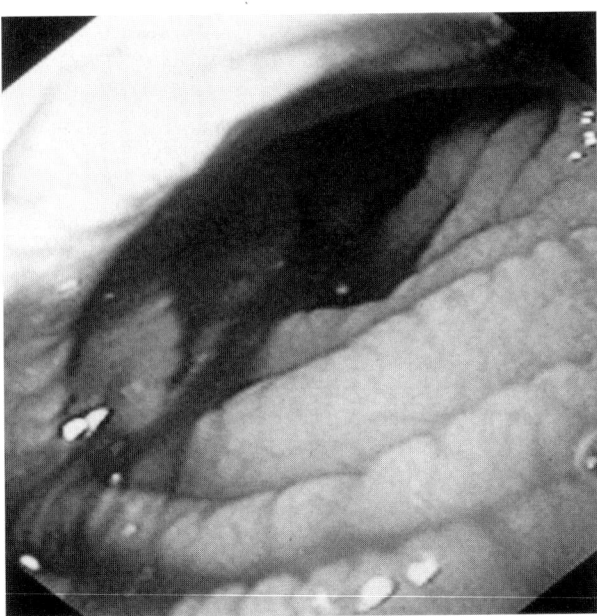

Fig. 18-3. Nodular, descending duodenum in celiac disease. Nodularity is partly due to gastric metaplasia and partly to villous atrophy in an intermittently acid environment. Similar appearances are seen in peptic duodenitis. (a) Barium study showing nodularity with an interspersed mosaic-patternlike appearance (arrows). (b) Endoscopic image of a convoluted nodular pattern; biopsy showed subtotal villous atrophy. (Courtesy of Michael L. Kochman, MD.)

"bubbly duodenum" can be associated with celiac disease without being a specific finding. A "scalloping" of duodenal folds reported to be an endoscopic finding in 12% of celiac disease patients[27] seems to correspond to the radiological "bubbly" duodenum [Fig. 18-3(b)].

5. *Transient intussusceptions:* More than one intussusception may be seen at the same time[28] (Fig. 18-4). They occur without lead point, are nonobstructing and appear to be related to the flaccidity of the bowel wall.[29] Being transient and usually painless, overhead radiographs are unlikely to be exposed at the right time, and examinations that rely on them are prone to miss intussusceptions. The lumen distention associated with a small bowel enema appears to preclude their formation.

Specific Findings by Barium Radiology

Jejunal Folds

Several investigators have reported an increased separation of mucosal folds in the duodenojejunal area in patients with adult celiac disease.[22,30,31] Using the small bowel enema technique, it became possible to obtain accurate measurements of the number of folds

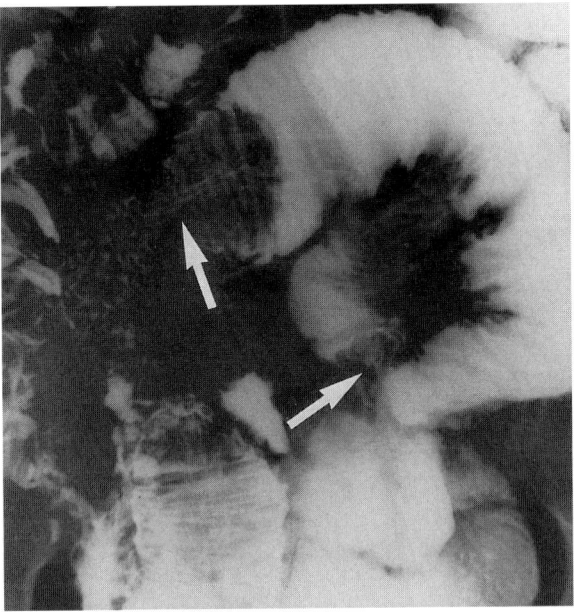

Fig. 18-4. Young patient with untreated celiac disease. Follow-through examination outlines a transient intussusception in the proximal jejunum with an additional intussusception seen distally (arrows). A subsequent enteroclysis did not demonstrate intussusceptions; it would be unusual for intussusceptions to occur during lumen distending enteroclysis. (Courtesy of Charles C. Lu, MD.)

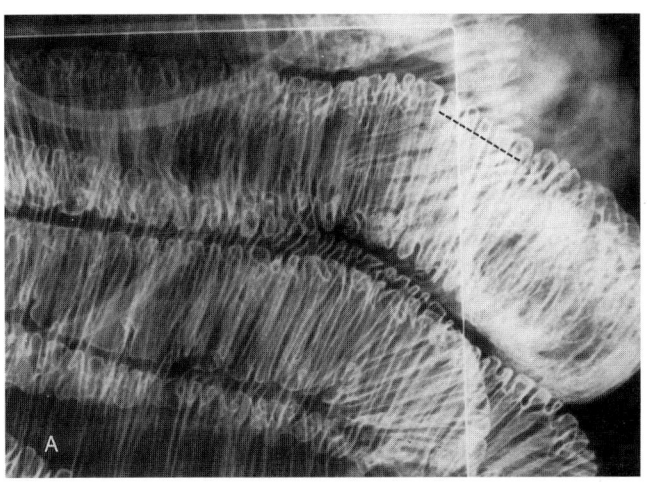

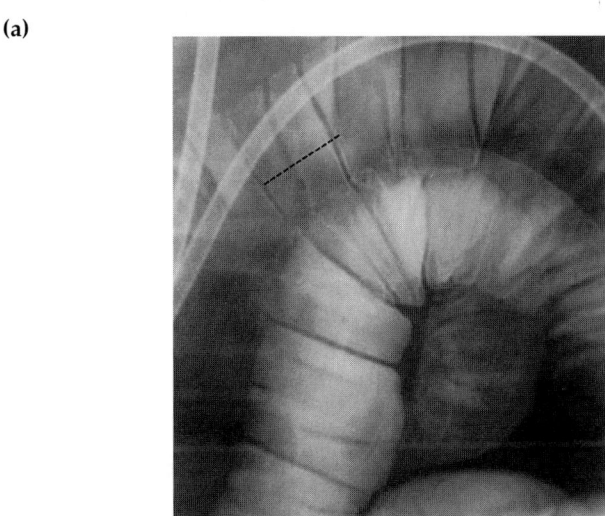

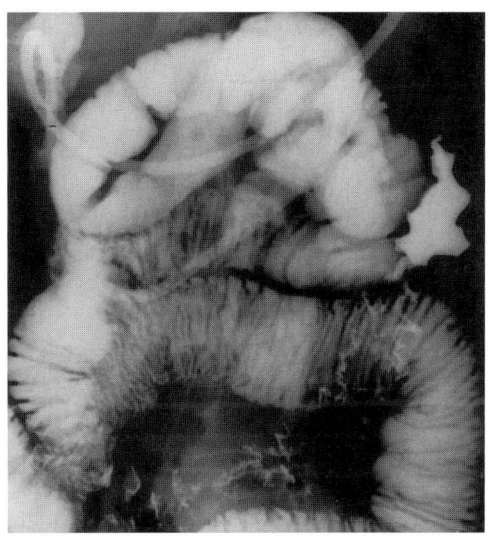

Fig. 18-5. Jejunal fold pattern in untreated celiac disease. (a) For comparison, enteroclysis of a normal proximal jejunum. Six folds are counted over a distance of 1 in (dotted line). (b) The proximal jejunum in celiac disease shown by enteroclysis. Only three folds of normal shape and thickness are seen over a distance of 1 in. (c) Fold pattern typical for celiac disease shown in a patient with dermatitis herpetiformis.

in the distended proximal jejunum in 25 patients who had clinically confirmed, untreated celiac disease. These findings were then compared with an age-compatible group of 25 patients who did not have any known small bowel disease.[32] A further five patients were subsequently added to each group, and the new total number of patients was reanalyzed.[33] It could be shown that the demonstration of three or fewer folds per inch of proximal jejunum (Fig. 18-5) strongly favored the diagnosis of celiac disease occurring in 73% of the 30 patients. Finding five or more folds per inch rendered a diagnosis of celiac disease highly unlikely occurring in 60% of the 30 patients not affected with celiac disease. A reading of four folds per inch of length occurred in both patient groups, in 36% of the controls and in 23% of the patients with celiac disease, and is a nondiagnostic finding (Fig. 18-6).

It is by no means clear why fold separation occurs. Mucosal atrophy is unlikely to be the reason, as mucosal thickness remains almost unchanged (see earlier). The way fold separation is infrequently shown on follow-through studies may provide a clue. Proximal fold separation could be retrospectively identified by us in 5 of 35 follow-through examinations and was associated with loop dilatation and retention of the barium beyond the time when nondilated distal ileum had become opacified (Fig. 18-7). A further indication was given in a case of celiac disease examined only a few weeks after gluten withdrawal. Initially jejunal folds appeared normally spaced but became more widely separated during lumen distention (Fig. 18-8). It seems that reversible flaccidity of the wall of the proximal jejunum favors fold separation and lumen widening during enteroclysis.

As far as we are aware, the increased separation of folds or their total absence in dilated or distensible,

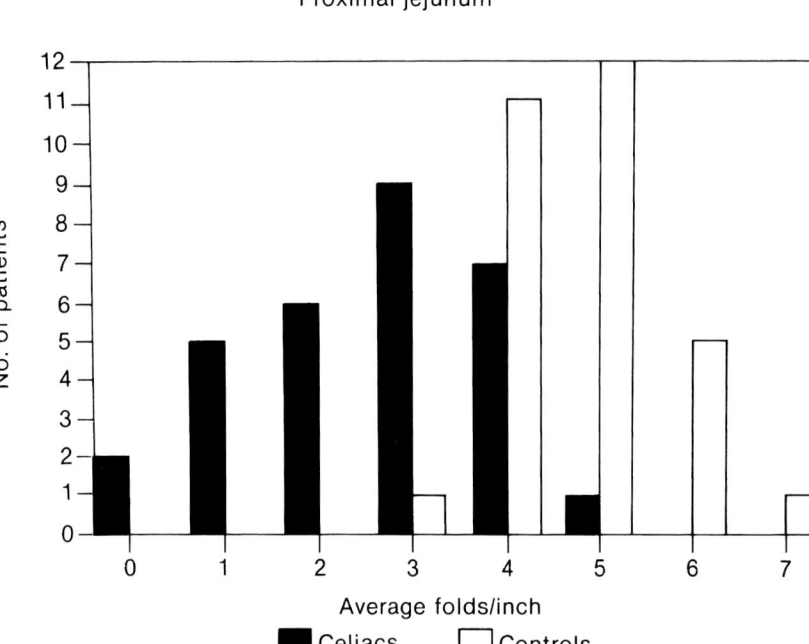

Fig. 18-6. Comparison of the number of folds over 1 in of length of the proximal jejunum in 30 patients with confirmed celiac disease and 30 controls. Four folds per in could be found in both groups of patients.

flaccid loops of proximal jejunum is not found in other conditions. A featureless mucosa in conditions like radiation enteropathy, late-stage ischemia, Crohn's disease, lymphoma, strongyloidiasis, and graft-versus-host disease will be associated with lumen narrowing, ulceration, or short segment involvement, features not seen with uncomplicated celiac disease.

Ileal Folds

Reversal of the normal fold pattern of the jejunum and ileum, their reduced number in the jejunum, and their increase in the ileum ("jejunization" of the ileum) has been considered a feature of celiac disease (Fig. 18-9) and a result of ileal adaptation to the impaired absorptive function of the jejunum.[34] Using films obtained by the small bowel enema technique, the number of ileal folds was measured in the previously mentioned two groups of 30 patients with and without celiac disease. Flocculation, inadequate distention, or loop overlap made it impossible to obtain a sufficiently accurate measurement in nine patients of the celiac disease group.[32] For these reasons, our results have shown these measurements to be of lesser value for diagnosis than those taken in the jejunum (Fig. 18-10). However, an increased thickness of ileal folds above the usual 1 mm is also a result of the adaptation process. Such thickness increase was found in 78% of the patients with celiac disease and in only 20% of the controls (see Fig. 18-9). Fold pattern rearrangement in celiac disease can also be demonstrated by CT scans (Fig. 18-11).

Combining fold changes in jejunum and ileum has increased the rate of positive diagnoses of celiac disease by enteroclysis to 83% This followed a further review of the above-mentioned 30 cases, when it was

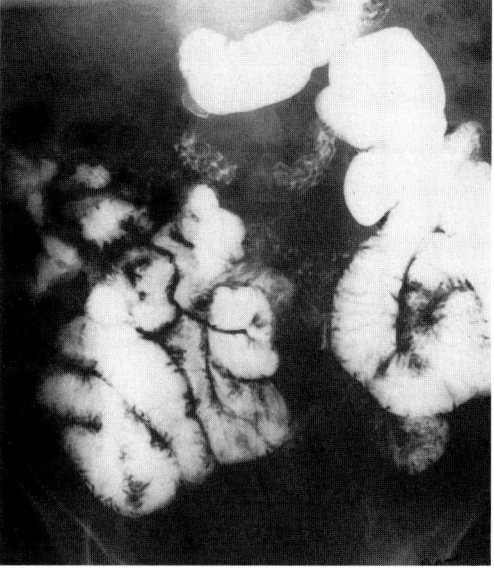

Fig. 18-7. Celiac disease patient examined by follow-through technique.
Barium has already reached the distal ileum but proximal jejunal loops remain dilated and barium-filled, and show only few folds. (Courtesy of Professor C. F. McCarthy, Galway, Ireland.)

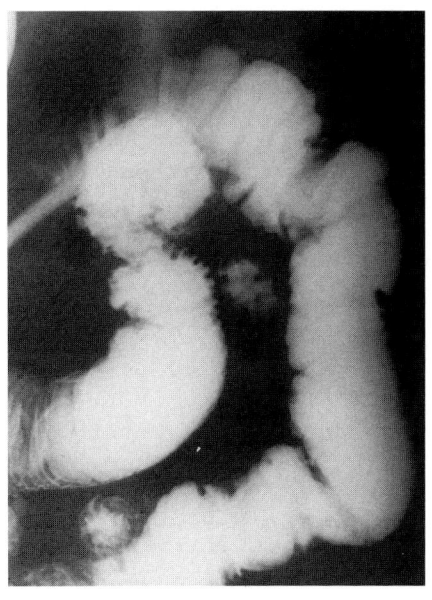 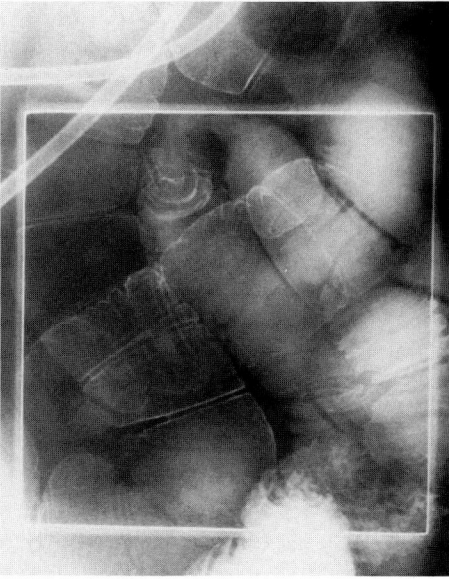

(a)   (b)

Fig. 18-8. Celiac patient with enteroclysis a few weeks after start of diet.
(a) Proximal jejunum is first shown in single contrast before lumen distention. No increase of fold separation is yet seen. (b) Following methylcellulose infusion, now widely separated jejunal folds with only two folds over 1 in of length.

found that in three of seven celiac patients with a nondiagnostic finding of four folds per inch of proximal jejunum, typical changes were present in the ileum. A recent report of small bowel follow-through examinations in 25 celiac patients claimed to have been able to distinguish the jejunoileal appearances from the normal in 75% of the cases.[35]

Mosaic Pattern

The radiologic demonstration of a mosaic pattern in the jejunum (see Fig. 18-2) was not reported until 1986.[33] A network of grooves with a mesh size of 1 to 2 mm could be demonstrated in the jejunum of 3 of the 30 celiac disease patients mentioned earlier (Fig. 18-12). The visualization of this pattern could be improved by digital image adjustment.

Diagnostic Relevance of the Small Bowel Enema

Fold changes in the jejunum, supported by those in the ileum, as described above, are capable of affirming the diagnosis of celiac disease in 83% of patients with active disease or of providing good evidence for its exclusion. Regarding the large group of subclinical or latent celiac disease, which can be detected only in the way mentioned earlier,[5] it must be admitted that there is no radiologic experience of the extent, if any, to which enteroclysis can be diagnostically useful in this group.

Enteroclysis is valuable when dealing with a patient who initially responded favorably to gluten exclusion and then became symptomatic again. The possibility of a complication supervening must then be the first consideration, and this can usually be confirmed or excluded by enteroclysis. A more frequent

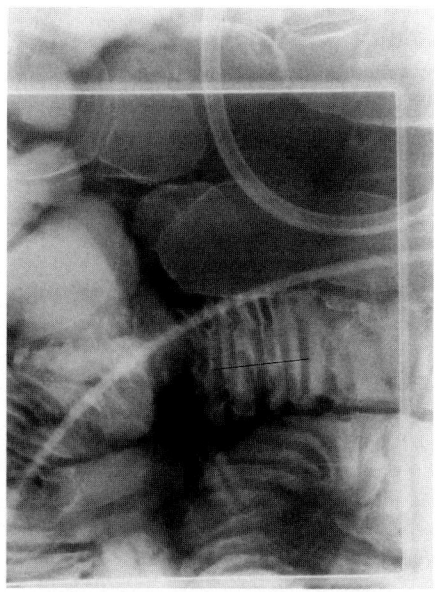

Fig. 18-9. Enteroclysis in celiac disease.
There are two folds per inch in the proximal jejunum and six thickened folds per inch in the "jejunized" ileum (line = 1 inch).

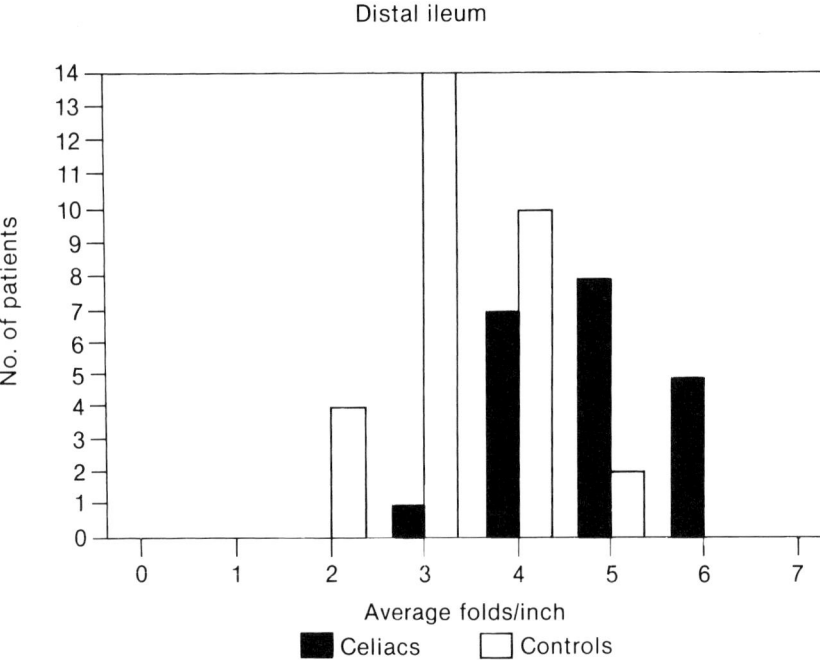

Fig. 18-10. Diagram illustrates the number of folds in the distal ileum over 1 in of length in 30 patients with celiac disease and in 30 controls.
Fold measurement was possible in only 21 celiac patients. There is considerable overlap between the two groups.

cause for clinical relapse is intermittent nonadherence to the diet. Enteroclysis can then demonstrate less obvious features of celiac disease, like a limited area of jejunal fold separation seen only during lumen distention (Fig. 18-13). Images of a patient whose celiac disease was "unmasked" by mesenteric ischemia are an example of diet-driven return to a normal fold pattern (Fig. 18-14).

An interesting recent paper presents a retrospective review of enteroclysis in the follow-up of 15 patients who, it was claimed, adhered to their gluten-free diet. Enteroclysis showed that most patients were unchanged or deteriorated over the years; the authors suggested that follow-up enteroclysis correlated more closely with the clinical situation than did duodenal biopsy.[36] Our own more limited follow-up experience has shown early improvement and eventual normality of fold patterns as long as patients continued their gluten-free diet.

Combining Enteroclysis with Endoscopic Biopsy

Mucosal biopsy specimens are usually obtained from the duodenum during gastroduodenoscopy. It is important that such biopsies are sufficiently large, best

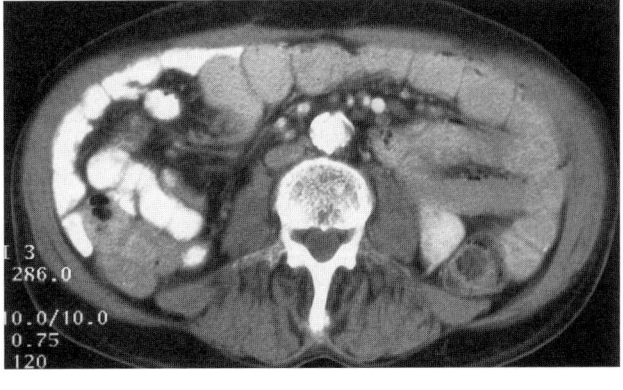

(a)

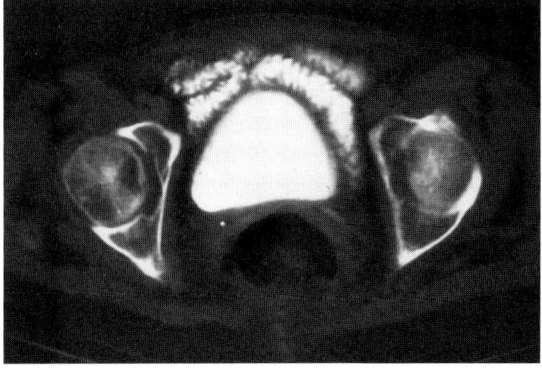

(b)

Fig. 18-11. In a patient with celiac disease CT could demonstrate a greatly reduced number of folds (arrow) in the proximal jejunum (a) and an increased number of thickened folds in the distal ileum (b).

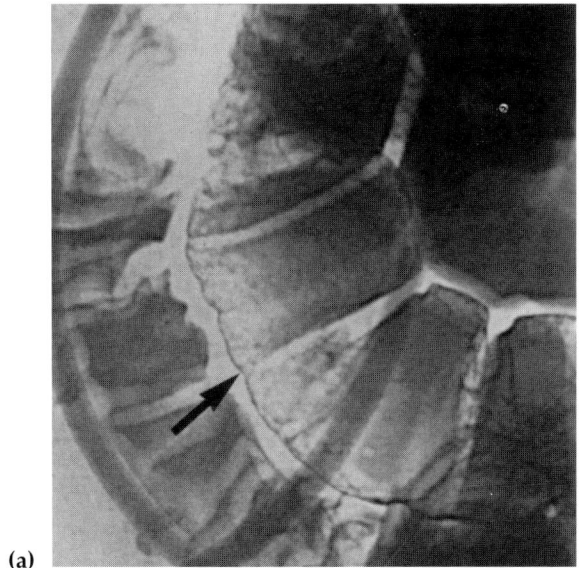 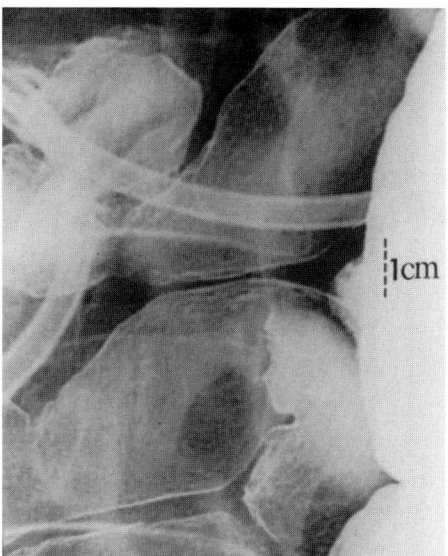

Fig. 18-12. Enteroclysis demonstrates the mosaic pattern.
(a) A reticular pattern of 1- to 2-mm diameter is visible in a segment of proximal jejunum (arrow). (b) In another patient with absent folds in the proximal jejunum, a mosaic pattern is seen throughout the mucosa. (Interrupted line at right = 1 cm.)

taken with a "jumbo" 3.4-mm forceps and then carefully oriented cut side down on a suitable substrate.[37] Suction biopsies are now only rarely used. There are occasions when it may be advantageous to extend duodenoscopic evaluation by the infusion of barium to image to more distal small bowel. To this effect, we have suggested the introduction through the endoscope of a floppy replacement wire and its advance in

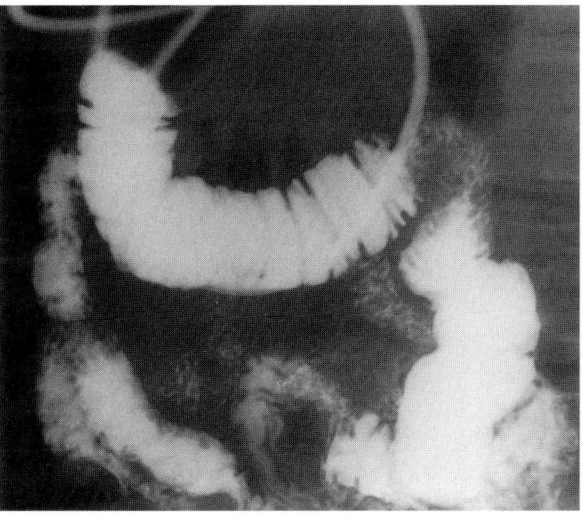 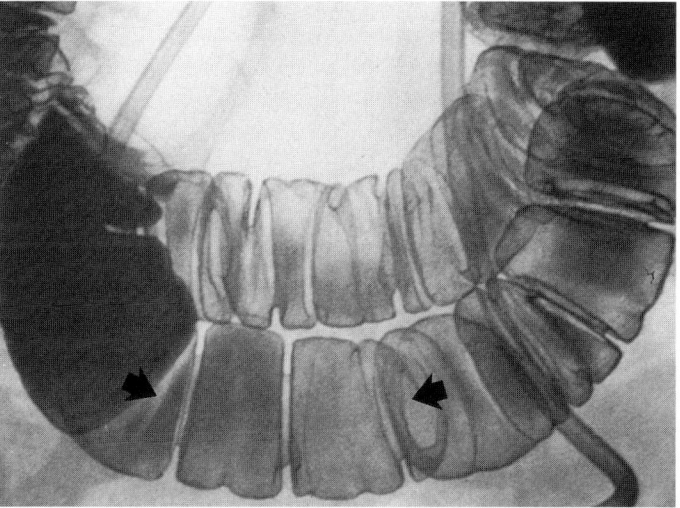

Fig. 18-13. Elderly female who initially did well on a gluten-free diet but developed renewed diarrhea a few months later; enteroclysis was done to rule out malignancy.
(a) Single contrast. (b) Lumen-distended double contrast shows fold separation confined to a short segment of jejunum (between arrows). No malignancy was demonstrated. This enteroclysis appearance is typical for inconstant adherence to the diet.

342 • 18. Malabsorption States

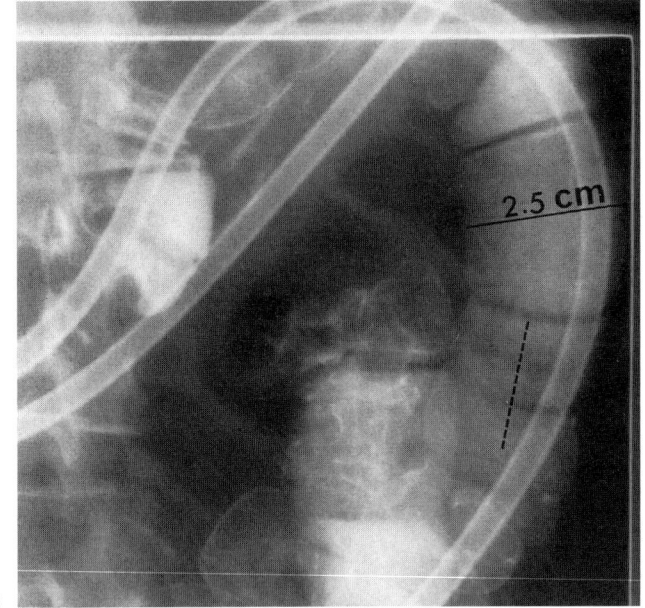

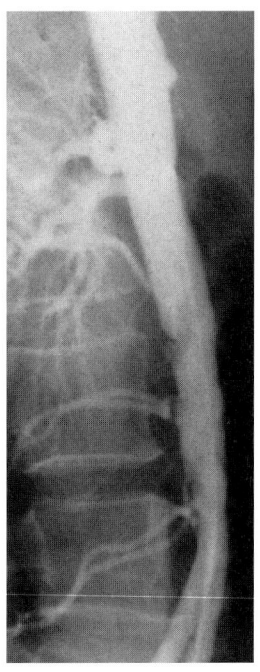

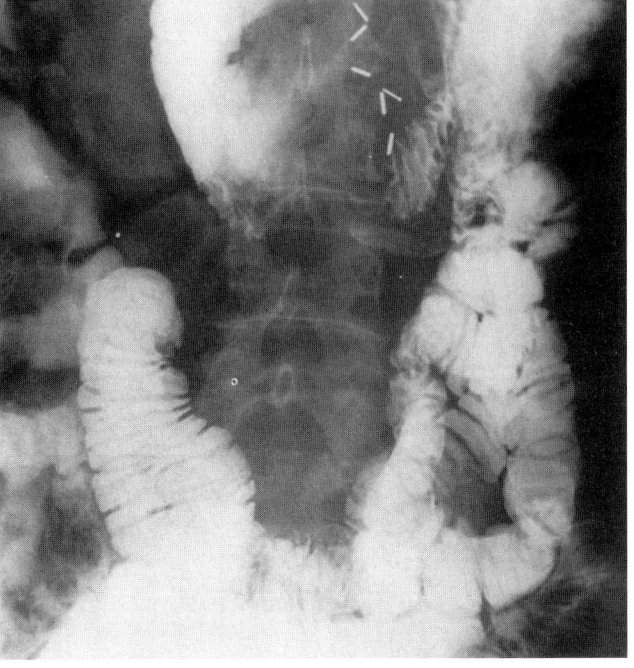

Fig. 18-14. A 54-year-old female patient with a short history suggesting celiac disease and an endoscopic biopsy showing subtotal villous atrophy.
(a) Enteroclysis demonstrates a proximal jejunal fold pattern confirming celiac disease but without lumen widening. The patient was placed on a gluten-free diet but failed to improve. She complained of postprandial pain unexplained by a few erosions shown by a barium meal. (b) Lateral view of an aortogram shows nonfilling of the three major branches. A bypass graft was inserted between aorta and distal superior mesenteric artery. (c) Subsequently, she responded to the gluten-free diet, and a later follow-up barium study confirmed return to a normal fold pattern. The celiac disease is believed to have been "unmasked" by the mesenteric ischemia.

the direction of the jejunum before the endoscope is withdrawn. With the wire secured in position, the patient can then be transferred to the radiology department, where an enteroclysis catheter can be threaded over it, and an enteroclysis is done with the patient still mildly sedated.

A possibly more viable combination study has been reported in 25 patients, almost half of them with sprue.[38] A mucosal biopsy was first carried out by inserting a biopsy cable through an enteroclysis catheter placed in the area of the ligament of Treitz; this was followed by the enteroclysis itself, thus providing two avenues of diagnosis in a single study.

Variants of Celiac Disease

Dermatitis Herpetiformis

This is a relatively rare skin disorder characterized by blisters on elbows, buttocks, and knees. A dermatological diagnosis requires demonstration of deposits of dimeric, intestine-derived IgA in dermal papillary tips.[39] In two-thirds of the patients there is a celiac disease–like enteropathy with villous atrophy. The other patients show features of gluten sensitivity with an increase of intraepithelial lymphocytes.[40] Yet, gastrointestinal symptoms are infrequent in dermatitis herpetiformis. The prevalence of dermatitis herpetiformis is about one fifth of that of celiac disease, with a male rather than a female preponderance. A gluten-free diet reduces the dose requirements used to treat the skin lesions. Skin lesions recur on reintroduction of gluten into the diet. As in celiac disease, there is an increased incidence of autoimmune disorders, like pernicious anemia and insulin-dependent diabetes. There is also a heightened incidence of lymphoma, greatly reduced by a gluten-free diet.[41] The jejunal fold changes shown by the small bowel enema are the same as those described in celiac disease [see Fig. 18-5(c)].

Refractory Sprue

This is rarely a true entity. Patients have all the features of celiac disease yet fail to respond to careful compliance with gluten avoidance. Yet, the likeliest explanation is an incomplete adherence to the diet. Occasionally other offending proteins have been found responsible for the celiac disease, when their elimination from the diet leads to recovery.[42]

Collagenous Sprue

In this condition a deposition of subepithelial collagen has been thought to be responsible for refractoriness. Such collagen deposition, however, has also been found in patients with celiac disease who responded normally to gluten abstinence. It is probably not a true disease entity.[30]

Celiac Disease Unmasked

As mentioned earlier, gastric surgery,[6] pregnancy, and respiratory infection[9] can precipitate activity in hitherto undiagnosed, latent celiac disease. The development of midgut ischemia is another possible precipitating factor that needed to be resolved before a gluten-free diet could be effective (Fig. 18-14).[43]

Other Associations of Celiac Disease

Celiac Disease and Diabetes

Celiac disease patients had insulin-dependent diabetes significantly more often (5.4%) than control patients (1.5%).[44] Or, analyzed differently, 3 of 47 patients with insulin-dependent diabetes tested positive for celiac disease, ie, 6.4% against 0.1% in the general US population.[45] It has been suggested that insulin-dependent diabetes be one of the conditions that merit screening for celiac disease.[45]

Celiac Disease and Anemia

Iron and folate absorption, which normally occur in the proximal small intestine, are significantly decreased in patients with active celiac disease. Iron depletion and megaloblastic changes in the bone marrow are typically present. Occult intestinal bleeding, at least positive Hemoccult tests, have been reported in 47% of patients with total villous atrophy.[46] A recent series of enteroclysis in 128 patients with occult bleeding revealed 1 case of unsuspected celiac disease among 32 positive diagnoses.[47]

Other Diseases

Celiac disease is associated with connective tissue diseases in 7.2% (2.7% in controls), Sjögren's syndrome in 3.3% (0.3% in controls), autoimmune thyroid disease in 5.4% (2.7% in controls), and occasionally lymphocytic colitis.[44]

Pseudo-Obstruction

Intestinal pseudo-obstruction has been a presenting feature of celiac disease in a single case report[48]; the diagnosis was based on mucosal biopsy obtained at laparotomy.

Pneumatosis

There have been few case reports of pneumatosis in celiac disease. In one of the reports[49] it was thought to be caused by obstructing intussusception. In another report[50] pneumatosis cystoides and pneumoperitoneum occurred in an elderly patient who preferred gluten to dieting (Fig. 18-15).

IgA Deficiency

Case reports describe an association of celiac disease with IgA deficiency, at times associated with other immune disorders.[51,52]

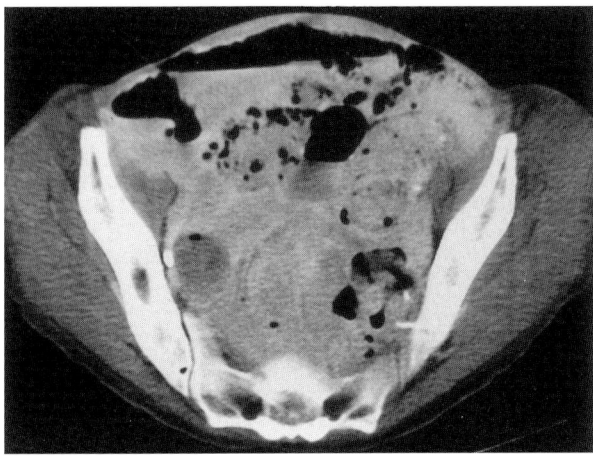

Fig. 18-15. CT demonstration of pneumatosis cystoides in dilated small bowel loops of an elderly patient with known celiac disease.

Complications of Celiac Disease

Hyposplenism

Impairment of splenic function with an intact spleen can occur in sickle cell disease, systemic lupus erythematosus, ulcerative colitis, alcoholic liver disease, long-term parenteral nutrition, and other conditions, including celiac disease.[53] A sensitive method of assessing splenic function in celiac disease is by differential contrast microscopy.[54] Spleen size was found to generally correlate well with splenic function and usefully supplements the diagnosis.[55] Splenic size is best estimated by ultrasound or computed tomography (CT). Evidence of hyposplenism was found in 29% of 41 cases of untreated celiac disease[42]; in a larger group of 177 patients with untreated celiac disease hyposplenism could be diagnosed in 76.2%.[56]

Enlarged Lymph Nodes

Mesenteric and retroperitoneal adenopathy in patients with celiac disease may signify lymphoma (see later). In an uncertain percentage of celiac patients enlarged lymph nodes are found without complicating malignancy and may be an immunologic reaction to gluten.[12] CT or magnetic resonance imaging (MRI) can demonstrate the enlarged nodes[57] but may be unable to distinguish them from the more common malignancy-related adenopathies. However, only in patients with benign adenopathy is there positive response to gluten withdrawal, and possible regression or gradual disappearance of the adenopathy.[58]

Cavitation of Mesenteric Lymph Nodes

This rare complication of long-standing and poorly controlled celiac disease[59,60] is associated with severe splenic atrophy (Fig. 18-16). The nodal cavities contain

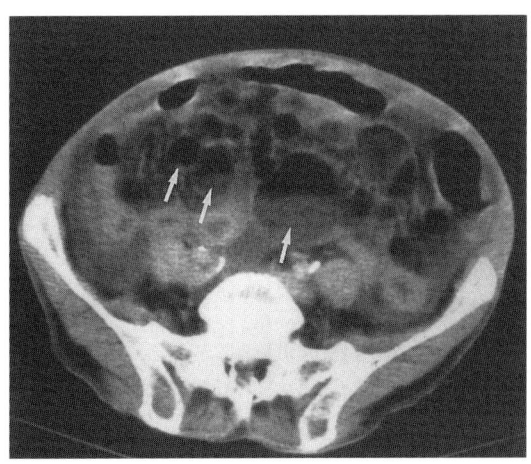
(a)

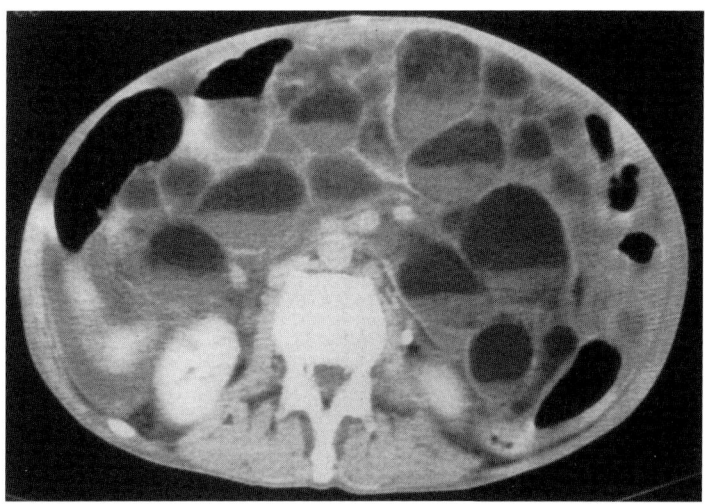
(b)

Fig. 18-16. Male, 63 years old, with a history of weight loss and diarrhea.
A CT scan (a) revealed few smooth, rounded, mesenteric masses containing what seemed to be air-fluid levels (arrows). Laparotomy with resection was followed by a pathology diagnosis of celiac disease–related lymph node cavitation. Duodenal biopsy then confirmed celiac disease. The patient continued to deteriorate despite gluten withdrawal. A further CT scan (b) showed the abdomen filled with thin-walled cavities containing fat/fluid interface levels. A diminutive spleen was outlined. The patient died.

chylous material and show characteristic fat/fluid levels at CT. A more recent report of five cases of lymph node cavitation included two patients who survived.[61]

Chronic Ulcerative Jejunoileitis

Ulcerative jejunoileitis is a rare but serious complication of celiac disease. Ulcers may perforate or bleed or may lead to stricture formation and cause obstruction. Associated with ulceration is nonresponsiveness to gluten exclusion. If not already harboring lymphoma, it is very likely that all cases of ulcerative jejunoileitis will become T-cell lymphomas unless surgery intervenes.[62,63] Early surgical intervention is also recommended to avoid the often fatal complication of ulcer perforation and peritonitis. There are a few cases without demonstrable celiac association, usually called nongranulomatous ulcerative enteritis.

Radiology. Enteroclysis can identify a more rigid segment of bowel, with irregularly thickened or focally flattened folds and shallow ulceration (Fig. 18-17).[64] Although indistinguishable from some cases of lymphoma, this does not change the patients' need for surgical resection; even at surgery the differentiation from lymphoma may have to be left to histology. Patients in the rare chronic stage of the disease may present with multiple, short strictures in a segment of bowel, possibly causing partial obstruction [Fig. 18-17(d)].

Enteropathy Associated T-Cell Lymphoma (EATCL)

EATCL is an infrequent association between lymphoma and malabsorption that has been noted for many years. Ross Golden[65] believed that steatorrhea associated with lymphoma was caused by the infiltration of the bowel wall with tumor cells. It was not until 1962 that Gough and coworkers[66] produced evidence that lymphoma constituted a complication of celiac disease. Immunohistochemical staining has made it possible to identify the pleomorphic tumor cells as T cells.[67] It has been suggested that celiac disease itself may be a low-grade lymphoma of intraepithelial lymphocytes.[68]

Clinical diagnosis. The clinical diagnosis of EATCL can be difficult. Clinical suspicion should be generated when there is a) failure of response to a gluten-free diet after having been in diet-related remission, b) nonresponse to the diet from the start in a newly diagnosed celiac patient, and c) persistent fever, abdominal pain, and profound muscle weakness as part of celiac symptomatology.[13] A diagnosis may be made at or after surgery, especially in cases of ulcerative enteritis or, in up to 30% of cases, at autopsy.[69] The interplay between celiac disease and T-cell lymphoma can take three forms: 1) Celiac disease is diagnosed and treated, later followed by the lymphoma; 2) Lymphoma appears before a diagnosis of celiac disease could be fully established; 3) Infrequently, celiac disease is identified after successful treatment of the lymphoma. This grouping is exemplified in the study of 235 patients with EATCL[70]: 1) Adult celiac disease was followed by lymphoma after a mean of 7.3 years in 66.4% of patients; 2) 18.7% had both diseases simultaneously; 3) in 14.9% the diagnosis of celiac disease followed that of lymphoma. Other studies reported a higher incidence of the concurrent appearance of celiac disease and EATCL. The demonstration by multiple biopsies (endoscopic or suction) of villous atrophy in areas of mucosa unaffected by the discontinuous lymphomatous infiltration has been taken as evidence for celiac disease being the background of the T-cell lymphoma. The celiac disease relationship to the T-cell lymphoma could be confirmed by the demonstration of the same T-cell receptor gene rearrangement in areas of lymphoma and of purely enteropathic bowel.[71] Most of the T-cell–derived enteropathy-associated lymphomas are already widespread at diagnosis, often diffuse with the delayed formation of mass lesions. B-cell–derived lymphomas are infrequent complications of celiac disease.

A recent report of 2 cases of T-cell lymphoma complicating dermatitis herpetiformis[72] increases the total of the known lymphomatous complications of dermatitis herpetiformis to 32 cases.

Unrelated to celiac disease is another "near-lymphomatous" condition in which diarrhea and malabsorption are prominent features; this is the immunoproliferative small intestinal disease often associated with Mediterranean lymphoma. (It is discussed in Chapter 19.)

Aspects of prognosis. EATCL, once developed, has a rapid course and is highly malignant. Celiac disease newly diagnosed at more than 50 years of age has a more than 10% chance of harboring lymphoma, which may become manifest within 4 years.[12] A report from a high incidence area (Galway, Ireland) describes the survival patterns of 31 cases of EATCL among whom the virtually simultaneous appearance of celiac disease and lymphoma accounted for the majority[73]; the 1-year survival was 31%, 5-year survival 11%. In the earlier-mentioned series of 235 patients[70] the 5-year survival was 9.5%.

Radiology. Barium follow-through examinations have been considered unreliable; of 15 patients in whom lymphomas were subsequently confirmed, barium follow-through provided a diagnosis in only 4.[12] Of greater relevance to the clinically oriented function of radiology in situations where an EATCL is suspected is an enteroclysis. This study can rapidly dis-

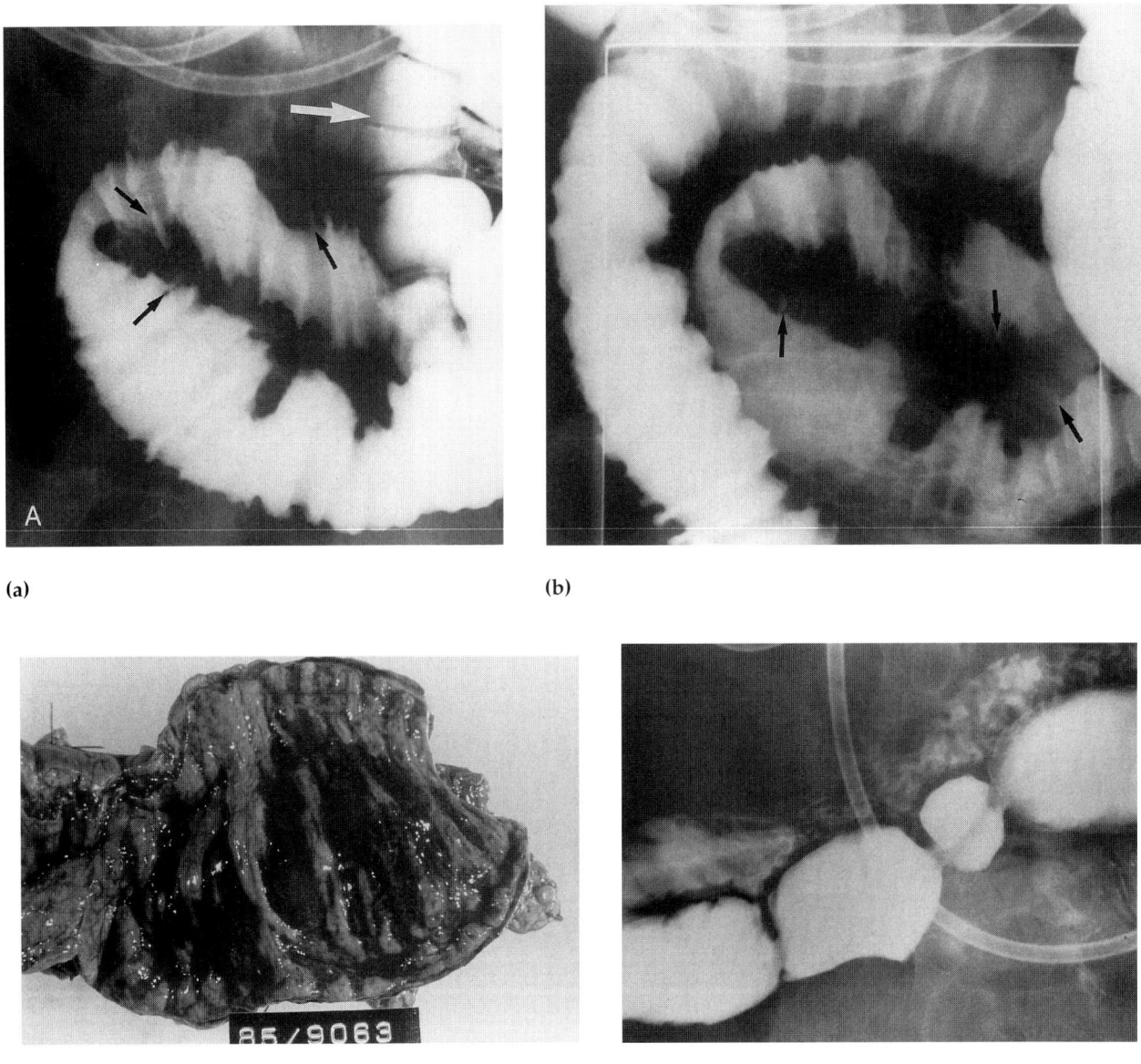

Fig. 18-17. Elderly patient with celiac disease on a gluten-free diet. Recent onset of midabdominal pain and tenderness together with a resumption of diarrhea.
(a) Enteroclysis outlines a loop of jejunum with irregularly thickened folds and several ulcers (arrows to some); the proximal jejunum shows fold separation typical for celiac disease (white arrow). (b) A later view demonstrates wider than normal separation from an adjacent bowel loop indicating wall thickening. The diagnosis must be between lymphoma, ulcerative jejunitis, or a combination of the two. (c) Laparotomy and resection of the abnormal segment followed. The specimen shows extensive ulceration. There was no evidence of lymphoma. During nearly 2 years of follow-up, the patient has remained well on a gluten-free diet. (d) The rare late stage of ulcerative jejunitis. Several short strictures are seen, probably representing scarred annular ulcers. The patient had a history of celiac disease. (Courtesy of Professor M. S. Losowsky, Leeds, England.)

tinguish between a celiac status deterioration caused by dietary noncompliance from other, more serious causes, including lymphoma. T-cell lymphoma can present changes that range from relatively subtle, uneven nodular fold thickening that may be discontinuous (Fig. 18-18) to more extensive nodular infiltration and mucosal ulceration and, occasionally, to mass lesions (Fig. 18-19). Widespread dissemination is common at presentation.[68] CT will demonstrate wall thickening, diffuse or focal, and lymphadenopathy.

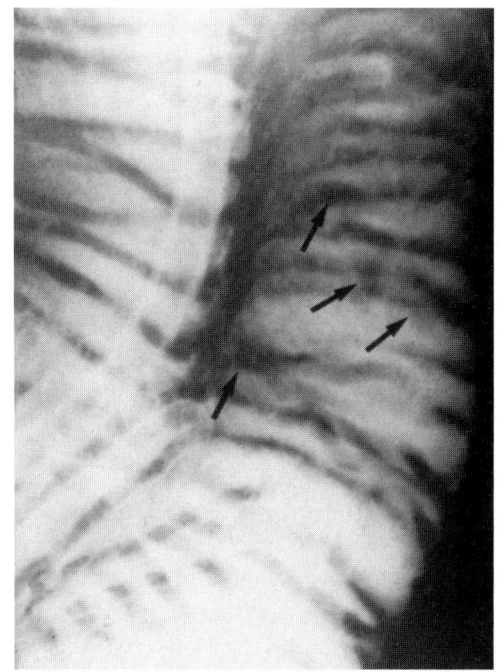
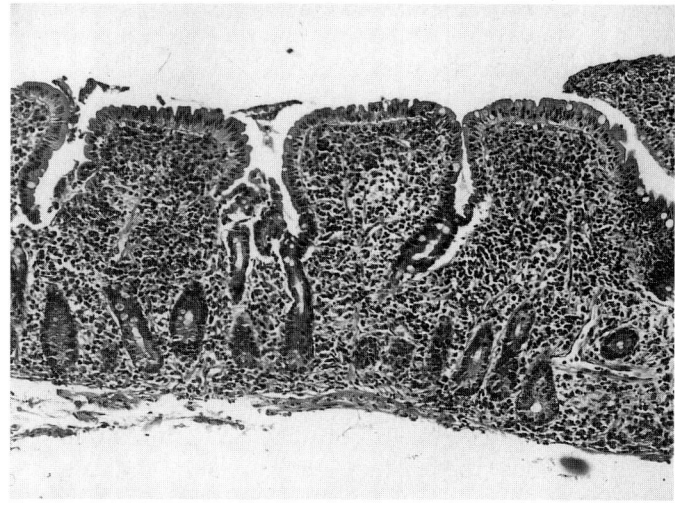

Fig. 18-18. EATCL in a 60-year-old male patient with unconfirmed history of celiac disease.
(a) Enteroclysis shows a segment of proximal jejunum with uneven mucosal fold thickening and several nodular filling defects (arrows). Other small bowel loops showed minor irregularities. (b) Full-thickness biopsy during laparotomy demonstrates villous atrophy and a crowded cellular infiltrate of the lamina propria; a higher magnification showed an increased number of intraepithelial T cells.

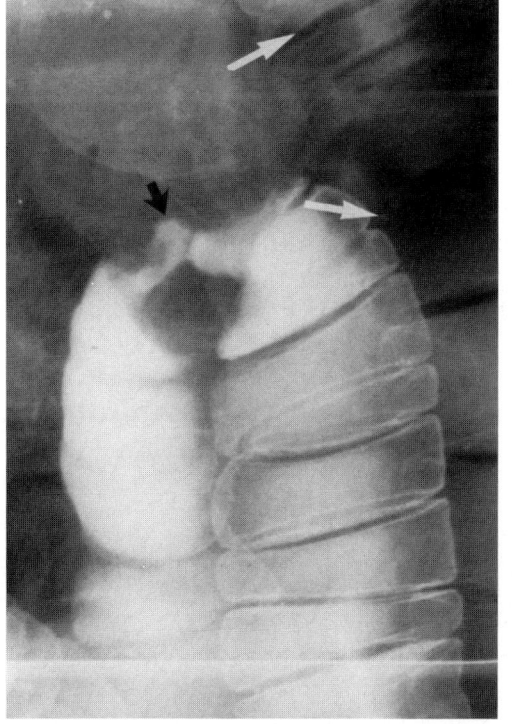
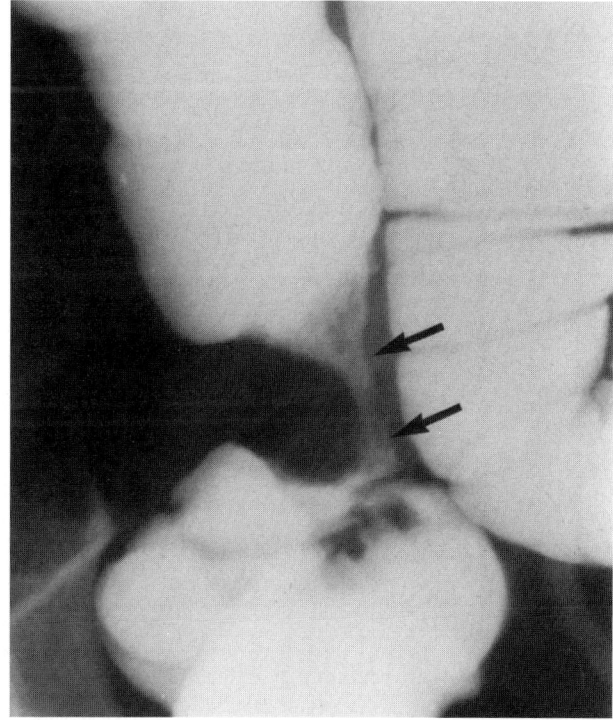

Fig. 18-19. Female patient with long history of celiac disease controlled by diet. Diarrhea, flatulence, and weight loss recurred recently. Enteroclysis was done.
(a) Jejunal fold separation of celiac disease type (long arrows) together with an apple-corelike, ulcerated mass (arrow) thought to be an adenocarcinoma. (b) In the mid small bowel there was another lumen-reducing lesion (arrow), no longer typical for carcinoma. A further lesion, a short, nonobstructing stricture, was seen beyond. The three lesions were resected and were found to be T-cell lymphomas complicating celiac disease.

However, the demonstration of mesenteric node enlargement does not necessarily signify malignancy (see earlier). The definitive diagnosis of the lymphoma is usually based on full thickness biopsies obtained at laparoscopy or laparotomy.

Carcinoma

Carcinoma of the duodenum and upper jejunum can complicate celiac disease and probably occurs with greater frequency than in the general population.[74] More often encountered are carcinomas of the esophagus,[75] pharynx, stomach, or rectum. An association with pancreatic carcinoma has been reported.[76] Men are at increased risk.[30]

A clinical presentation of weight loss and anemia in a patient previously well controlled on a gluten-free diet and without dietary indiscretions should indicate the need to search for a possible malignancy. Later clinical features are due to the local effects of the by then advanced lesion. Occult bleeding can be an early finding.[30] Two metachronous jejunal adenocarcinomas, eight years apart, complicated celiac disease in a male patient; the tumors were demonstrated by enteroclysis and CT and were resectable.[77] Barium radiology, particularly enteroclysis, can be of decisive diagnostic value (Fig. 18-20).

Tropical Sprue

It was formerly believed that tropical sprue and celiac disease were the same, only modified by the geography of their occurrence. However, antibodies to gluten have never been demonstrated in tropical sprue, and the two diseases are now known to be unrelated. Symptoms of tropical sprue can resemble those of celiac disease. Short-term or prolonged residence in an endemic area, tropical or subtropical, is the usual background. Puerto Rico, Cuba, and Indonesia are examples. Villous atrophy is rarely more than partial, and crypt hyperplasia is not severe. A high mixed fecal bacterial load including enterotoxigenic bacteria is usual. Significant differences from celiac disease are the absence of a proximal to distal gradient of disease intensity and the presence of usually pronounced B_{12} deficiency, indicating distal ileal involvement.[78] Proof of the diagnosis of tropical sprue relies on the response, within a few days, to treatment with antibiotics and folate.[79] However, such treatment ought to continue for 3 to 6 months to effect a permanent cure.

Radiology

Barium studies have not been particularly helpful in diagnosis. A report more concerned with a possible relationship of hypoalbuminemia to increased lumen diameter in 35 patients with tropical sprue did not find significant separation of folds in the jejunum in any of the patients but did demonstrate fold thickening.[80]

Bacterial Overgrowth Syndrome

Pathophysiology

The effects of gastric acid, the small bowel's propulsive activity, the mucus cover of its mucosa, and the luminal presence of secretory immunoglobulins normally restrict bacterial growth within the small intestine. Omeprazole inhibition of gastric acid output causes duodenal bacterial overgrowth in about half the patients. However, anaerobic bacteria are usually absent, and clinically evident malabsorption is unusual. In the distal ileum, however, backflow of cecal contents frequently causes an increase of gram-negative and anaerobic organisms. (For other aspects of pathophysiology see Chapter 2.)

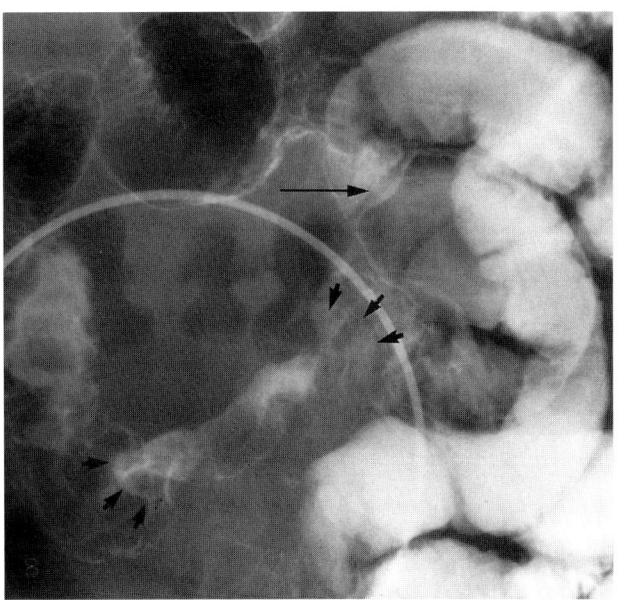

Fig. 18-20. Patient with a history of celiac disease, who generally adhered to a gluten-free diet.
A small bowel meal followed by effervescent granules outlines an annular lesion of the ascending duodenum in which folds are not visible. Arrows indicate shouldering that demarcates the adenocarcinoma. The dilated proximal jejunum demonstrates typical changes of celiac disease (long arrow). Metastases to regional nodes were found at surgery.

Table 18-2. Causes of the bacterial overgrowth syndrome

Increased Entry of Bacteria into the Small Bowel
    Gastrectomy
    Decreased gastric acid output
    Coloenteric or cologastric fistula
    Infected bile

Stasis in the Small Bowel
    Anatomic abnormalities
    Strictures, diverticula, blind loop, blind pouch
    Abnormal motility
    Systemic sclerosis, pseudo-obstruction, diabetic autonomic neuropathy

Defective Defense Mechanism
    Immunodeficiencies

Mucosal injury is an important mechanism in bacterial overgrowth–related malabsorption. Villi are broadened or flattened in a patchy distribution. There is a superficial resemblance to the mucosal changes seen in celiac disease. Conditions that may be responsible for bacterial overgrowth are listed in Table 18-2.

Clinical Aspects

There may be a virtual absence of clinical manifestations over a number of years until an additional event causes malabsorption to become evident. Alternatively, there may be weight loss, diarrhea, anemia, and deficiency of fat-soluble vitamins. The anemia relates to vitamin B_{12} and iron deficiency. Osteomalacia and visual disturbances may be due to vitamin D and A deficiencies. Clinical management may rely on the results of a hydrogen breath test or the effect of an empiric trial of antibiotics. Important would be to relate management to the demonstration of the underlying pathology by barium radiology. Surgically correctable lesions, if responsible for the symptoms, require intervention. Broad-spectrum antibiotics are the standby for most of the other forms of bacterial overgrowth but should be given only intermittently. Nutritional management is important. An associated lactase deficiency is not unusual, and lactose restriction is then indicated as part of the treatment of the diarrhea.

Strictures, especially if multiple, produce stasis and can lead to bacterial overgrowth. Causes may be surgical, postinflammatory, ischemic, or radiation related. Barium radiology can outline the location and number of the strictures and the length of bowel involved (Fig. 18-21) and can serve as a "road map" for treatment by surgery. Surgical blind loops are only rarely created nowadays, but the legacy of earlier years remains. An example is a blind loop about 15 inches in length, a cause of macrocytic anemia and vitamin B_{12} deficiency, requiring intermittent treatment with antibiotics (Fig. 18-22).

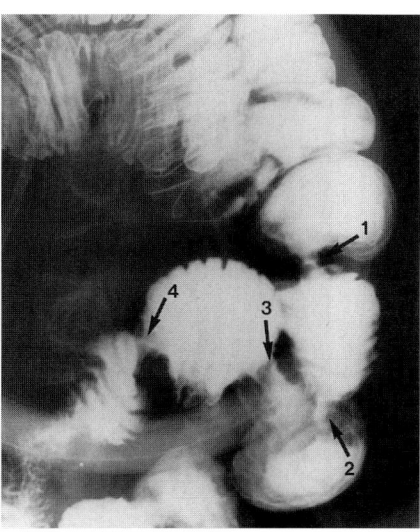

Fig. 18-21. Patient with known Crohn's disease controlled by medical treatment.
Mild malabsorptive features, mostly diarrhea and anemia, were considered to relate to four Crohn's strictures with stasis and bacterial overgrowth; the strictures occupy a short segment of distal jejunum.

Chronic Intestinal Pseudo-Obstruction

Pseudo-obstruction is a clinical entity with the signs and symptoms of an intestinal obstruction, yet without the presence of an intrinsic or extrinsic occlusive process. It may involve only a segment of bowel or most or all of the intestinal tract. Conditions responsible include collagen diseases (systemic sclerosis, dermatomyositis, systemic lupus erythematosus, periarteritis nodosa, mixed connective tissue disease), amyloidosis, endocrine disorders (hypothyroidism, diabetes), neurologic disorders (Parkinson's disease, Chagas' disease, multiple sclerosis, spinal cord injury), drugs (ganglionic blockers, barbiturates, narcotics), and a miscellaneous group. The last group includes celiac disease (ceroidosis), midgut ischemia, cathartic abuse, electrolyte disturbance (hypokalemia of less than 2.5 g/100 ml, hypomagnesemia), strongyloidiasis,[81] and lead poisoning.

Idiopathic chronic intestinal pseudo-obstruction refers to the absence of any discernible extraintestinal cause. It would require electron microscopy of full-thickness biopsy material to identify the neuropathic

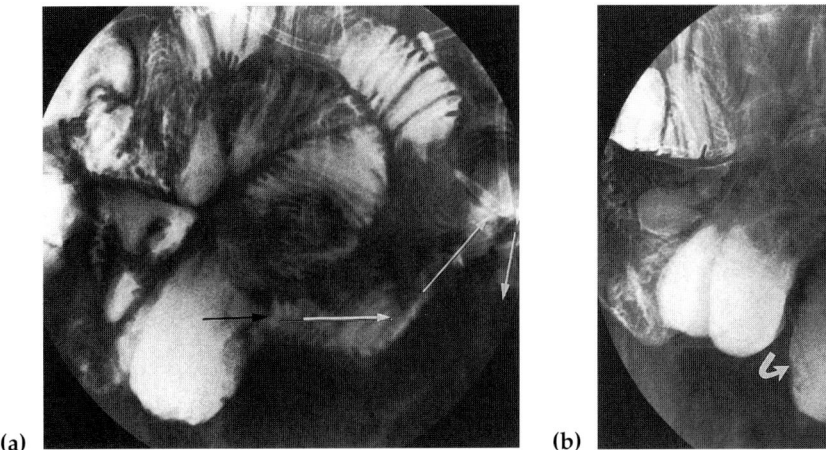

Fig. 18-22. A surgically created blind loop (a,b) arises from an enterostomy in the distal ileum and extends (long arrows) over a length of 15 in to its blind termination (curved arrow). Patient suffers stasis-related malabsorption.

and myopathic subtypes.[82,83] However, the clinical utility of this distinction is questionable. Familial and sporadic cases have been described. Bacterial overgrowth and malabsorption complicate most of the long-standing cases. Whenever possible, treatment should be medical and laparotomy avoided.[84]

Radiology

Esophageal dysmotility—dilatation with aperistalsis, exaggerated tertiary contractions—gastric outflow delay, or duodenal dilatation were often found in association with small bowel dilatation. Patients with visceral myopathy tend to have intestinal aperistalsis, and those with neuropathy an uncoordinated activity. The extent and location of any segmental activity disorder needs to be defined by radiology to assist the occasionally required surgical management, bypass, or resection.

Systemic Sclerosis

Systemic sclerosis is a progressive multisystem disease in which the involvement of the lungs, kidneys, and heart are of major significance to patient survival. Excess of collagen is deposited in a patchy manner in the skin and internal organs. This collagen affects the esophagus in most cases and is associated with hypomotility and a dysfunctional lower esophageal sphincter resulting in gastroesophageal reflux.[85] Small bowel deposition of collagen occurs in over 40% of cases and generally correlates with Raynaud's phenomenon. Malabsorption develops in only a minority of the patients but will occasionally antedate other clinical features of the disease.

Diarrhea and malabsorption, if present, are mostly related to bacterial overgrowth. This is almost invariable with a microbilial concentration in the jejunum of more than 10^5/ml especially with an aerobic content. Anatomic and/or functional disorders cause the disruption of the normal balance between bacterial penetration and control by the host. Stasis is the usual causative background to the bacterial overgrowth. Frequently an associated mucosal atrophy and an accumulation of collagen around small vessels in the submucosa may further impair absorptive capacity. Pseudo-obstruction may be a late complication of systemic sclerosis.

Radiology

Pseudo-obstruction, mostly affecting the small bowel, may be evident on plain radiographs of the abdomen. Barium studies can demonstrate a pathognomonic feature. This is the so-called hidebound bowel sign of dilated segments in which straight folds of normal width are crowded together.[86] In this respect, they differ from bowel loops dilated by obstruction or idiopathic pseudo-obstruction, in which dilatation is always accompanied by elongation and wider separation of folds. The hidebound bowel sign is seen in more than the 60% of cases as suggested in the original study (Fig. 18-23).[86] The crowding of folds in dilated loops is explained by an asymmetric replacement of muscularis propria by collagen, especially the replacement of longitudinal fibers with the resulting restriction of

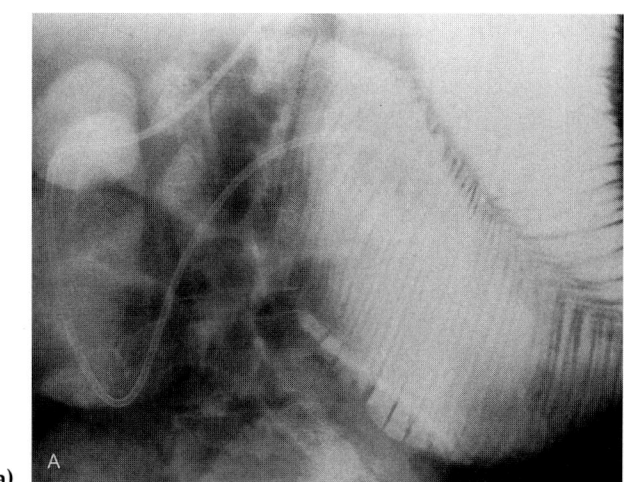 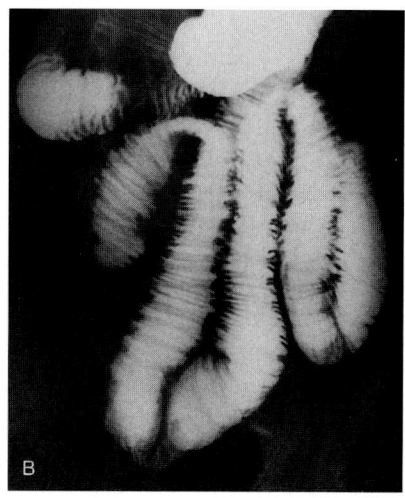

Fig. 18-23. The "hidebound" bowel in systemic sclerosis.
(a) Small bowel enema demonstrates duodenojejunal dilatation with pronounced crowding of stretched mucosal folds. (b) Crowded mucosal folds are seen in the jejunum of another patient with scleroderma whose follow-through examination does not demonstrate lumen dilatation.

elongation without resistance to dilatation. Recognition of this sign allows a diagnosis of systemic sclerosis to be made in the rare cases where this is not already suspected on clinical grounds.

The second portion of the duodenum, at times extending to the ligament of Treitz, may be severely dilated. More distally, a focally more intensive replacement of muscularis propria by collagen can result in the formation of wide-necked outpouchings. These sacculations are more likely to be seen in the colon but have also been demonstrated affecting the antimesenteric aspect of small bowel (Fig. 18-24). Transient, nonobstructing intussusceptions, as in sprue, have been observed[86] and are believed to relate to disordered peristalsis. Pneumatosis cystoides has been reported in a few cases; occasionally there is also an associated pneumoperitoneum.[87]

Jejunal Diverticulosis

The reported prevalence of acquired diverticulosis of the jejunum has changed over the years. Autopsy series have reported a frequency of up to 1.3%[88] and radiology by enteroclysis a frequency of 2.3%.[89]

Pathology

Most diverticula begin as small pouches on the mesenteric border where vasa recta pierce the muscularis propria. The pouches are herniations of mucosa with elements of submucosa and usually pass medially into the subperitoneal fat between the two layers of the mesentery. They are acquired lesions, of pulsion type, exiting through points of diminished resistance. These diverticula have a narrow neck, are devoid of muscularis propria (thus "pseudodiverticula"), flaccid, and unable to expel their contents. The age groups beyond 40 years account for 80% to 90% of persons with diverticulosis. Synchronous colonic diverticula are reported to be found in 30% to 50% of cases.[90] In an unknown proportion of cases the pseudodiverticula pass through abnormal muscularis in association with mural changes consistent with systemic sclerosis, visceral myopathy, or neuropathy.[91] Fabry's disease is another possible association of jejunal diverticulosis (see below).

Jejunal diverticula are found twice as often in males as in females. They are larger and more numerous in the proximal jejunum and decrease in size and number more distally. They are not readily detected at laparotomy, being hidden by often adherent jejunum or buried within the mesentery.[92] They usually involve a continuous and limited length of the jejunum. Diverticula tend to recur in previously uninvolved parts of small bowel after resection of a diverticula-bearing segment.[88]

Unlike pseudodiverticula, true diverticula are formed by all the layers of the bowel wall and are usually congenital. The best known example is the Meckel's diverticulum, which is fully described in Chapter 14.

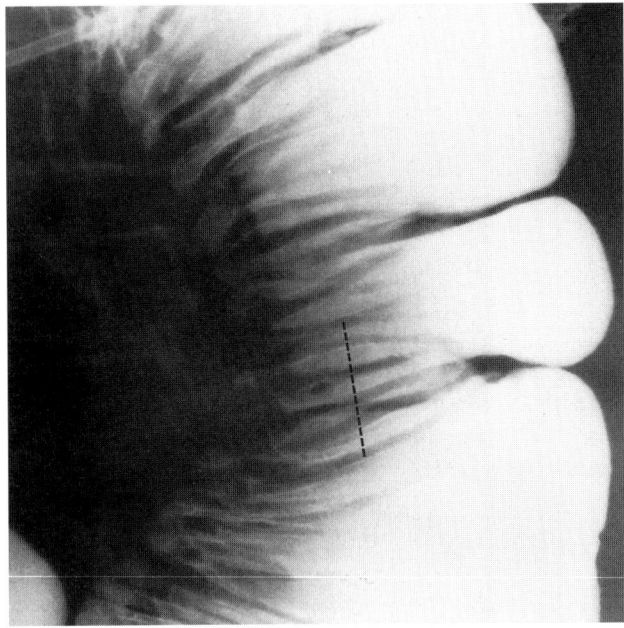

(a)

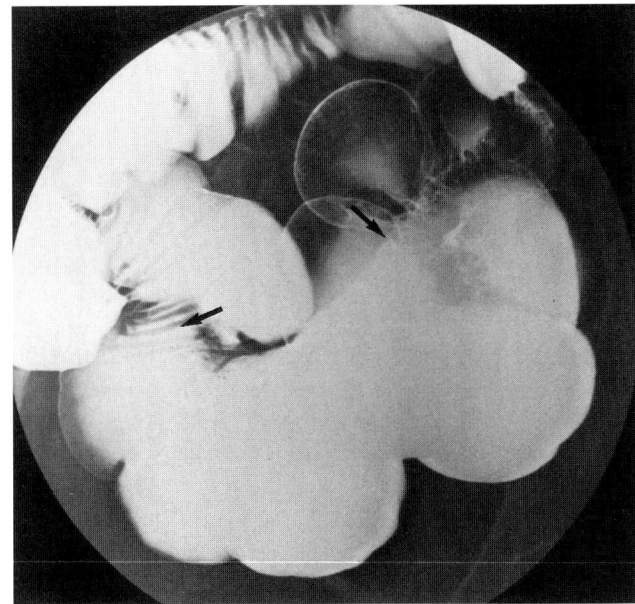

(b)

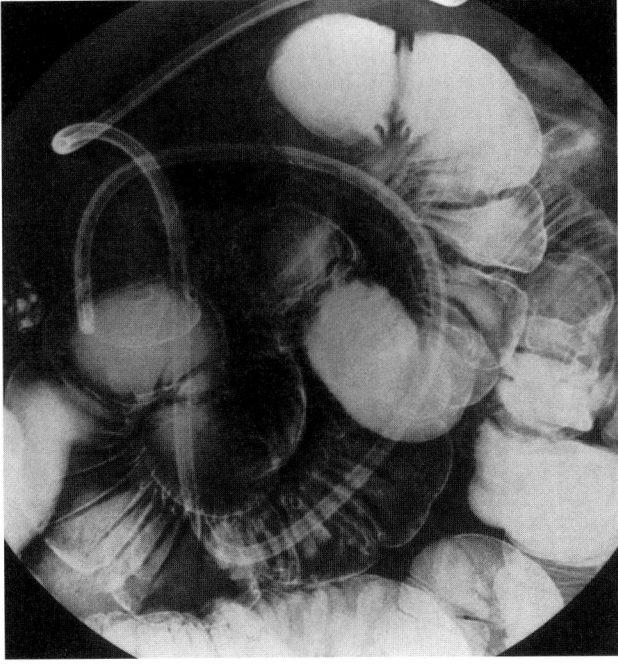

(c)

Fig. 18-24.
Sacculations at the antimesenteric border of the jejunum in a patient with systemic sclerosis (a). Circular folds are crowded to about 7 folds over 1 in of length (dotted line). In another patient (b) gross sacculations virtually obscure the view of crowded folds. Arrows point to segments with hidebound folds at the mesenteric border. Enteroclysis explained the patient's persistent anemia and intermittent diarrhea. (c) Minimal antimesenteric sacculation and crowding of folds in scleroderma.

Clinical Presentation

The literature differs with regard to the clinical presentation of the diverticulosis. Formerly, it was considered to be asymptomatic in the great majority of cases. If searched for, an excessive bacterial population can now be demonstrated in almost all patients and relates to stasis within the diverticula.[93] Malabsorption can be documented in a third of the patients[88] and is associated with reduced uptake of vitamin B_{12} and an increased level of folic acid.[88] Motility disorders associated with diverticulosis range from "jejunal dyskinesia,"[94] which can be observed during radiography, to features of pseudo-obstruction, especially in cases with an abnormal muscularis.[91] There may then be associated motility disturbance in the esophagus, stomach, and colon.

Complications

Possible complications are listed in Table 18-3. The reported incidence of complications requiring surgery varies between 17%[92] and 38%.[90] Indications for surgery include intestinal obstruction, which may be without mechanical cause; diverticulitis possibly with fistula and abscess; hemorrhage; pronounced malabsorption; volvulus; and severe pain. Notably, a diverticulitis-related abscess, whether retroperitoneal or in the mesentery, may remain occult unless the anterior peritoneum is involved.[88] Pneumoperitoneum without peritonitis is another well-described complication.[95] It may be associated with pneumatosis cystoides caused by the subserosal dissection of gas. A massive bleed from a jejunal diverticulum is rare and its preoperative diagnosis rarer still. Of interest is a recent paper reporting diagnosis by enteroclysis in patients referred for obscure bleeding. In addition to a positive diagnosis in 21% of the cases, jejunal diverticulosis was demonstrated in 6% of patients referred for bleeding against a usual 2% incidence in referrals for other indications.[47] A possible causal relationship may have existed.

Table 18-3. Possible Complications of Acquired Jejunoileal Diverticula

Mechanical intestinal obstruction
    Enteroliths, volvulus
        Compression by filled diverticula
        Adhesions following surgery

Inflammatory disturbances
    Diverticulitis, possible abscess formation, peritonitis
    Postinflammatory adhesions, intermittent obstruction

Intestinal stasis causing malabsorption

Rupture of diverticulum
    Spontaneous or due to trauma

Foreign bodies
    Ingested food, parasites, enteroliths

Pneumoperitoneum

Radiology

Large pseudodiverticula retain gas and may appear on plain radiographs as ovoid or rounded collections without visible folds (Fig. 18-25). They may have fluid levels on an erect film. The absence of folds and their shape can distinguish the diverticula from dilated bowel in mechanical obstruction (see Chapter 5). Most

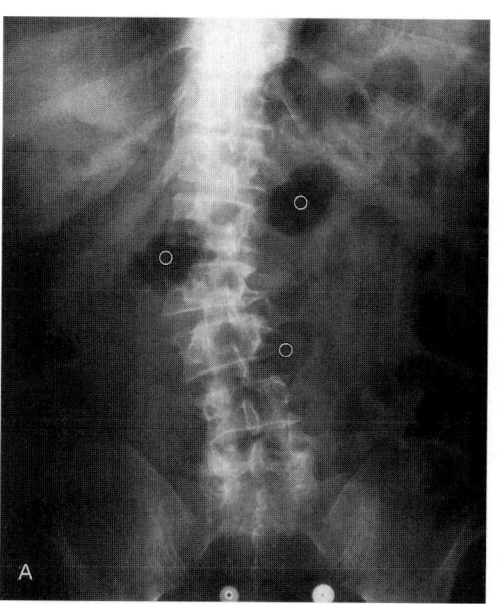 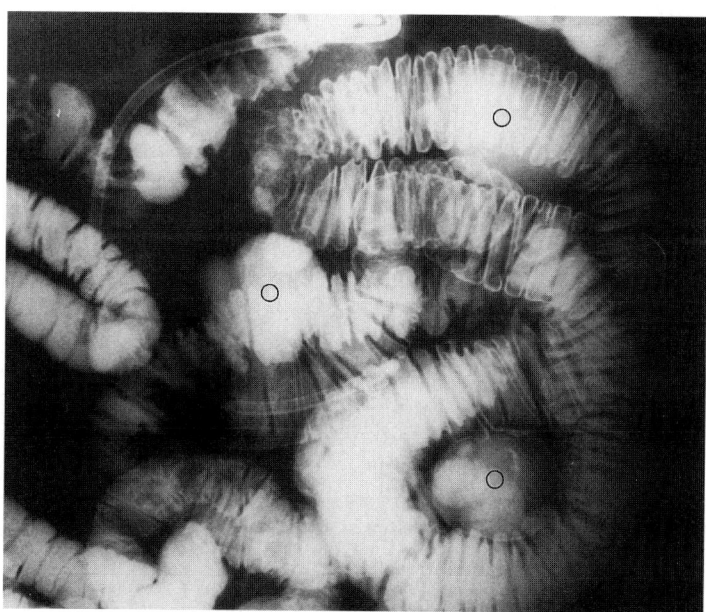

Fig. 18-25. Acquired jejunoileal diverticula.
(a) A plain abdominal radiograph shows ovoid gas collections without fold pattern in the midabdomen (circles). (b) Barium study confirms that the gas collections represent moderate-sized diverticula (circles).

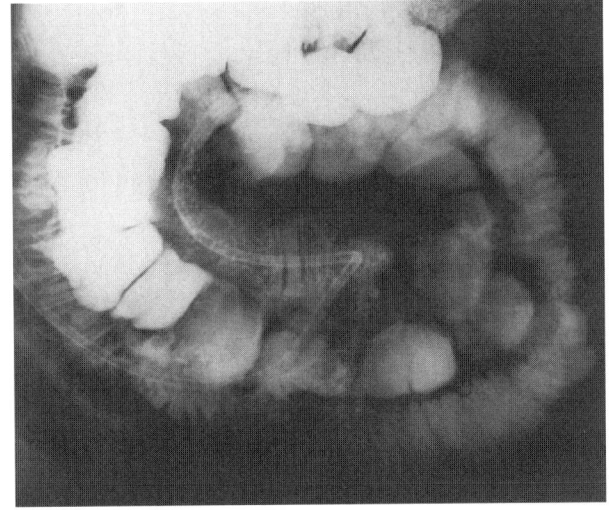
(a)

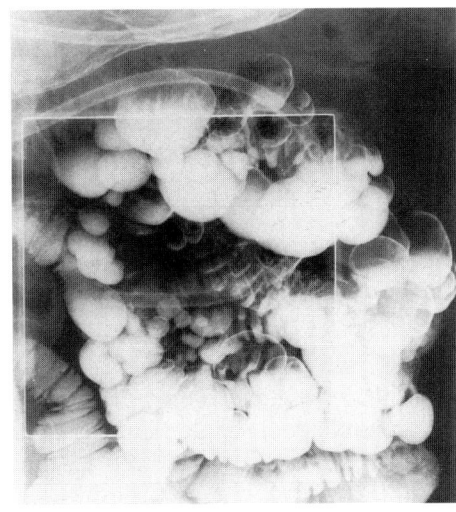
(b)

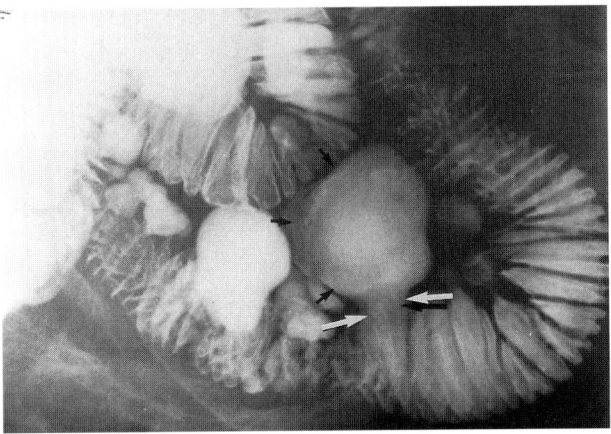
(c)

Fig. 18-26. Patient with numerous jejunoileal diverticula and malabsorption.
The diverticula are largest in the proximal jejunum and decrease in size toward the ileum (a). It can be helpful to identify larger diverticula in the erect view showing their air/fluid levels (b). Folds may be seen in the neck of a pseudodiverticulum at its site of passage through the muscularisis (white arrows); no folds are seen within the pseudodiverticulum itself (c), distinctly different from the junctional fold pattern of a congenital diverticulum.

diverticula may be identified by standard barium examination, although small diverticula may be missed. The luminal distention during enteroclysis outlines all diverticula but, when numerous, they may be more difficult to identify without added compression or in the erect position of the patient (Fig. 18-26). The neck of a diverticulum should have a diameter significantly smaller than the outpouching. This feature distinguishes a diverticulum from a sacculation. Mucosal folds can be identified only in the neck of the diverticulum [Fig. 18-26(c)], the diverticulum itself being without folds.

The barium examination provides an opportunity to evaluate the often associated alterations of motility. There may be pseudo-obstruction, usually only low-grade. Loops are dilated; increased fluid is seen in the lumen and transit is delayed, at times requiring continuation of an enteroclysis into follow-through filming. Interesting is the radiologic observation of "jejunal dyskinesia." Peristalsis, instead of propelling the barium in a normal manner, moves some of it laterally to overdistend a diverticulum that, following the peristaltic contraction, empties the excess of barium back into the bowel lumen. This mechanism can result in significant delay of transit in the presence of continuing peristaltic activity.

The radiologic diagnosis of diverticulitis can be made by barium study and/or CT. Findings on contrast radiography include extravasation into a fistula or an abscess cavity adjacent to the diverticulum, deformity of the normally rounded structure, narrowing, fold thickening, or spasm of the adjacent jejunum.[97] CT may identify thickening of the wall of the diverticulum, peridiverticular edema, or engorged mesenteric vessels.[97] The diagnosis of jejunal diverticulitis largely rests on detection by radiology (Fig. 18-27). Mortality, which can be as high as 40%, can be changed into a favorable prognosis with early diagnosis and aggressive treatment.

The terminal ileum close to the ileocecal valve is a

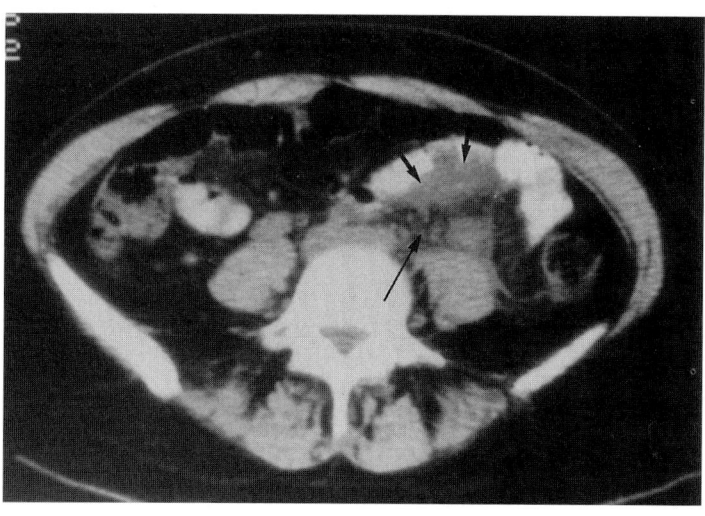 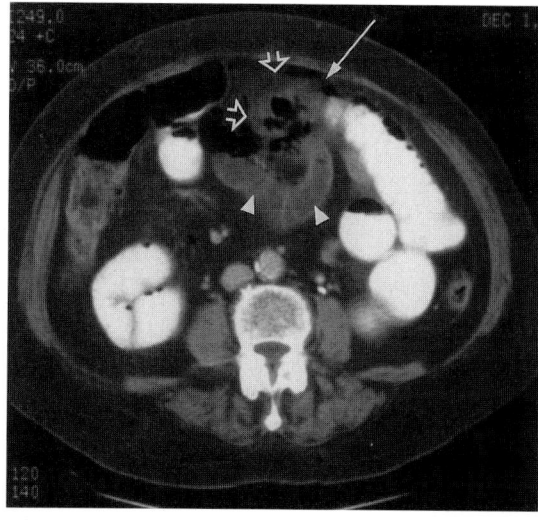

Fig. 18-27. Two examples of jejunal diverticulitis shown by CT.
(a) Demonstration of an inflammatory mass indenting a segment of jejunum (arrows) with increased attenuation in the mesentery (long arrow) (Courtesy of S. E. Rubesin, MD.) (b) Diverticulitis with perforation. A gas-containing abscess (open arrows) occupies the mesenteric side of a loop of jejunum (arrowheads). Free gas is outlined (long arrow). (Courtesy of E. J. Balthazar, MD.)

further site in which mesenteric border pseudodiverticula occur. They are usually no larger than 1 cm in diameter, are found in about 5% of people, and are almost always asymptomatic. Diverticulitis is a very rare complication.[98]

Fabry's disease is a condition in which small bowel diverticula can form as a result of glycolipid deposition in smooth muscle and enteric neurons.[88] Fabry's disease is a rare familial disorder of glycosphingolipid metabolism that affects males and involves kidneys, heart, and other organs but not usually the gastrointestinal tract. When associated with diarrhea and malabsorption, these are due to glycolipid infiltration of Meissner's plexus and impaired jejunal motility with bacterial overgrowth. Radiology is nonspecific, demonstrating thickened folds and diverticula.[99] Diagnosis is by deep biopsy to demonstrate glycolipid deposits in submucosal neurons. Metoclopramide and tetracycline may give symptomatic relief.

Short Bowel Syndrome

Pathophysiology

The consequence of a significant loss of length of small bowel is a reduction of its mucosal surface area and of the contact time available for the absorption and digestion of food. Brush border disaccharidases are normally concentrated in the jejunal mucosa and fade distally. The jejunum is also the important site for the digestion and absorption of fat, protein, minerals, and several vitamins. The ileum can undergo adaptation to compensate for the loss of a large part of the jejunum. However, the specialized ability of the terminal ileum to absorb intrinsic factor/vitamin B_{12} complexes and reabsorb conjugated bile salts cannot be restored after a resection of more than 100 cm of distal ileum. In these circumstances, there will be a reduction of the circulating bile salt pool and an entry of unabsorbed fats and of conjugated bile salts into the colon, where they cause interference with water and electrolyte absorption. This process will cause secretory diarrhea in addition to steatorrhea.[100] Resection of the ileocecal valve leads to ascending bacterial contamination of the small bowel remnant, which hastens transit and further reduces contact time.

Gastric hypersecretion with elevated serum gastrin levels has been found in most patients for a limited time after significant small bowel resection. This effect is possibly a result of decreased gastrin catabolism by the reduced length of the small intestine. Its consequence would be increased gastric acid output and a lowering of the pH in the lumen of the small bowel, adversely affecting digestive processes and possibly causing peptic ulceration in the stomach, duodenum, or small bowel remnant.[101] It may occasionally lead to the

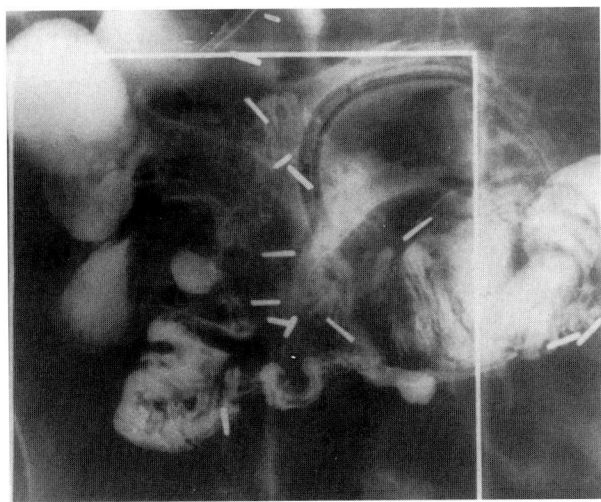

Fig. 18-28. Short bowel syndrome after recent massive resection for vascular occlusion and gangrene.
Breakdown of anastomosis with enterocutaneous fistula, possibly not unrelated to temporary hypergastrinemia and high gastric acid output.

breakdown of surgical anastomoses and the formation of a fistula (Fig. 18-28). Though gastric hypersecretion is usually a time-limited phenomenon, inappropriate hypergastrinemia may continue indefinitely.[102]

Intestinal Adaptation

When much or all of the jejunum has been resected, the loss of absorptive surface stimulates the residual ileum to increase its functional capacity. Cellular proliferation can speed up to three times the normal rate, increasing the height and surface area of villi although not their number.[103] Segments dilate and elongate and folds thicken. In general, the degree of adaptive hyperplasia depends upon the length of gut excised or excluded and on the particular segments involved. The presence or absence of a normal luminal stream of nutrients is also important, as total parenteral nutrition abolishes the compensatory stimulus. In the past, failure to maintain initial weight loss after now defunct jejunoileal bypass surgery has been blamed on excessive compensatory hyperplasia.[104] Patients with both small and large intestinal resection fare much worse than those in whom only small bowel was resected, but massive enterectomy can overwhelm the adaptive capacity of the gut and cause chronic intestinal failure. The adaptive response in children is more favorable than in adults. Their small bowel remnant has potential for linear growth and has been known to sustain normal development by oral nutrition with only 15 to 20 cm of small bowel.[105] Adult patients who have suffered a major loss of small intestine, usually secondary to small bowel infarction, may be unable to survive on ingested food and require at least supplementary parenteral nutrition.

Clinical Aspects

Vascular occlusions and Crohn's disease are the predominant reasons for massive or repeated resections of small bowel. Extensive intraperitoneal malignancy and radiation damage can be further possible indications for massive resections or for the bypass of major portions of small bowel.

Surgical treatment has two purposes, to slow transit and to increase the absorptive area in the shortened bowel. Reversal of a bowel segment into the antiperistaltic direction has had its problems, usually the use of too long a segment leading to obstruction. A recent paper, however, has reported significant success in a single case.[106] Small bowel transplantation has made progress in very recent years and has become a lifesaving option. Using tacrolimus for immunosuppression following intestine plus liver transplantation, graft and patient survival was 64% and 66% at 1 year and 38% and 40% at 3 years.[107]

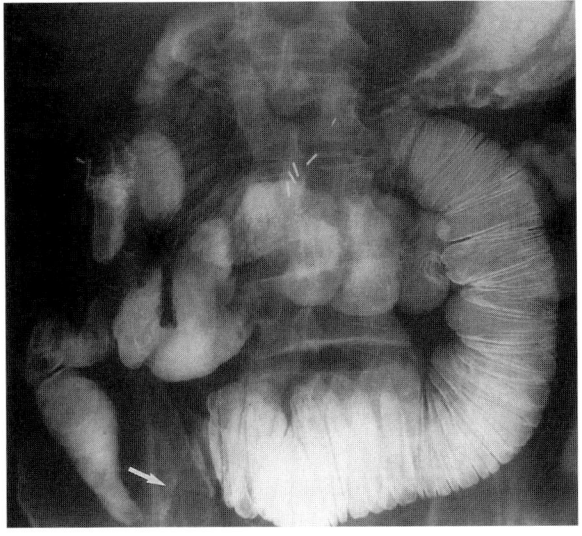

Fig. 18-29. Short bowel syndrome following resection for massive gangrene.
The duodenum and about 2 ft of jejunum show adaptation attempt—dilatation and increased number of folds. However, there is distal ischemic recurrence (arrow).

Radiology

Barium studies provide indications of the length of residual bowel and of the degree of ileal adaptation, as shown by thickening and deepening of an increased number of folds and an increased diameter of the lumen (Fig. 18-29). Barium studies may also demonstrate continuing or recurrent disease for which resections had been undertaken, eg, ischemia (Fig. 18-29) or Crohn's disease with an intense effort at adaptation by a short segment of jejunum [Fig. 18-30(a, b)]. Other findings may relate to the metabolic consequences of the short bowel syndrome. An increased incidence of gallstones occurs, since distal ileal resection renders bile lithogenic. Hyperoxaluria, also following resection of distal ileum, is due to increased oxalate absorption and favors the development of oxalate urinary stones.

Whipple's Disease

This is a rare multisystem disease in which periodic acid-Schiff (PAS)–positive macrophages can be found in most body tissues. There is a strong predisposition for involvement of the lamina propria of the small bowel and its regional lymph nodes, the heart valves, the central nervous system, and joints.[108] The disease is predominantly found in the United States and northern Europe.

Clinical Aspects

The cause of the disease is a bacillus, which has been named after Whipple. Organisms are consistently found at diagnosis and disappear after successful treatment.[109] Yet, they have never been cultured or transmitted to animals. Intestinal biopsy usually finds them in profusion specifically within the lamina propria, mostly within macrophages and in varying stages of digestion. The rod-shaped bacilli can be identified by light microscopy. Electron microscopy shows a thick cell wall surrounded by an outer trilaminar membrane, unique for a gram-positive bacillus (Fig. 18-31).[109] By means of the polymerase chain reaction (PCR) and sequencing of the rRNA gene it has been possible to characterize the bacillus, which has been reclassified and is now named *Tropheryma whippelii*.[110] It has been possible to develop primers specific for the

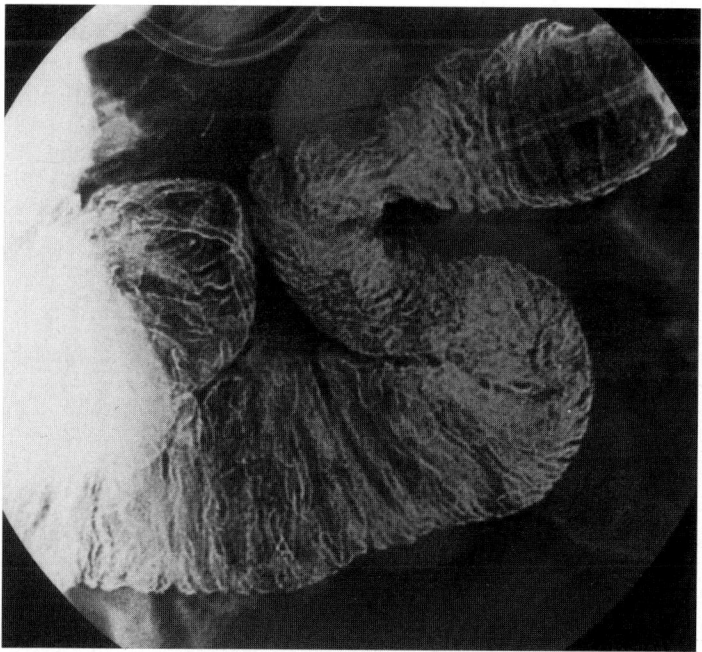
(a)

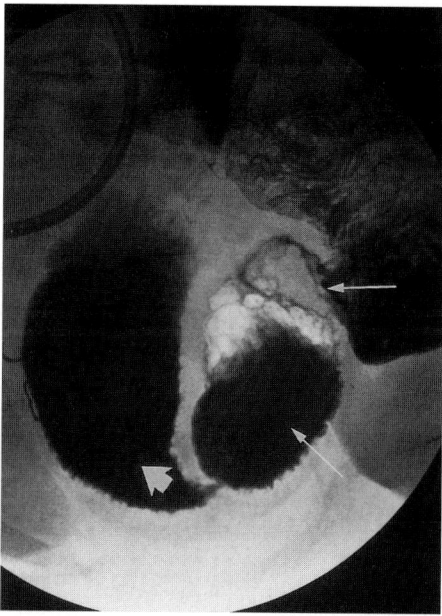
(b)

Fig. 18-30. Short bowel syndrome after small bowel resections for Crohn's disease.
(a) Enteroclysis, balloon just beyond Treitz. Almost 20 in of normal jejunum show maximum possible adaptation; lumen is widened, mucosa shows a crinkled surface in addition to crowded folds. (b) Outlook highly unfavorable because of ulceronodular and strictured Crohn's disease of the neoterminal ileum (arrows) extending far into the hepatic flexure area of the colon (broad arrow).

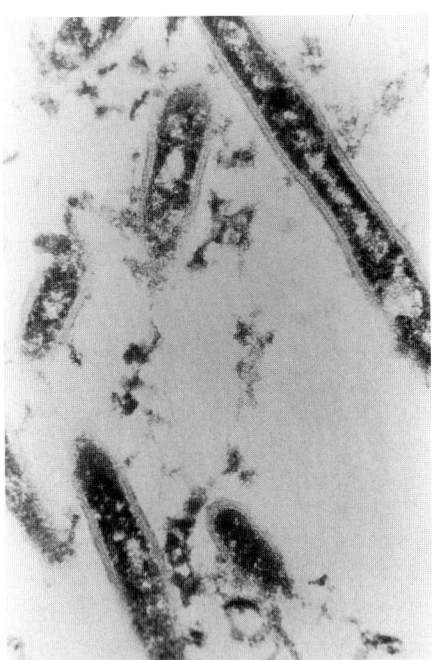

Fig. 18-31. Electron microscopy view of Whipple's bacilli within a macrophage.
Bacilli show typical thick, trilaminar cell walls. Partly digested bacilli and bacillary fragments can be identified.

bacillus and use these in the PCR to amplify the sequences of the bacillary rRNA directly from infected tissue.[111] When applied to formalin-fixed biopsy material, this test was shown to be highly specific and sensitive.[111]

Diagnosis is usually based on endoscopic mucosal biopsy from the duodenum or proximal jejunum.[112] Villi normally contain a core of lamina propria. When Whipple's disease involves the small bowel, biopsies reveal villi distended by the lamina propria, which is filled with bacilli and foamy macrophages. The macrophages contain PAS-positive material derived from the glycoprotein of the cell walls of the Whipple's bacilli. The modified PCR can then confirm the diagnosis of Whipple's disease. When the small bowel is not yet involved, it may be necessary to obtain diagnostic material from other structures, such as lymph nodes, joint capsule, liver, or the central nervous system (CNS).

A review of 114 cases of Whipple's disease found that 22% of patients lacked diarrhea and 40% abdominal pain.[113] Arthritis is a well-documented presentation and may precede gastrointestinal involvement by several years.[114] Usually associated with small bowel involvement is enlargement of mesenteric lymph nodes, at times sufficient to produce a degree of secondary lymphangiectasis. Neurologic abnormalities, including personality changes, may be the initial clinical features or herald relapse after or during treatment.[115] There are a few reports of intestinal bleeding as a feature of Whipple's disease.[116] In the majority of cases, the diagnosis is eventually made by small bowel biopsy. However, the mucosal changes can be patchy and multiple biopsy specimens should be obtained.[117] Steatorrhea is present in over 90% of untreated patients,[115] primarily caused by invasion of the absorptive enterocytes by the bacilli and also by the relative blockage of lymph flow due to macrophage infiltration of the lamina propria and the enlarged mesenteric nodes.

Impaired cellular immunity has been documented before and after successful treatment.[118] Macrophages may take an entire year to become free of bacilli. There is a superficial resemblance to *Mycobacterium avium-intracellulare* (MAI) infection complicating AIDS, which is sometimes referred to as "pseudo Whipple's" (see Chapter 17).

Radiology

Usually normal or, less often, thickened folds with a superimposed impression of surface granularity may be seen on barium follow-through studies. Though not shown in every case, enteroclysis makes it possible to demonstrate a mucosal pattern that can suggest the diagnosis of Whipple's disease in patients presenting with malabsorption.[119] This is the demonstration of a 1- to 2-mm micronodularity of the mucosal surface, usually with folds of normal thickness [Fig. 18-32(a)]. The nodules can be diffusely spread or may congregate into separate patches [Fig. 18-32(b)]. The recognition of these changes can be important in this rare disease, which often presents atypically and may occasionally remain unsuspected until radiologically identified.

Deposits of lipid material in an intercellular location or within macrophages can be sufficient to affect the Hounsfield unit values of mesenteric or retroperitoneal nodal masses shown by CT scans [Fig. 18-32(c)]. Ultrasonography demonstrates such nodal masses as distinctively echogenic structures.[120] CT-guided fine needle aspiration of a nodal mass has demonstrated typical *T whippelii*, confirmed by electron microscopy.[121]

In the radiologic differential diagnosis lymphangiectasia needs to be considered since it has a similar micronodular mucosal pattern. However, there is usually more intraluminal fluid and the folds are more uniformly thickened. CT will also demonstrate mesenteric nodal enlargement in secondary lymphangiectasia from several causes but without the inclusion of

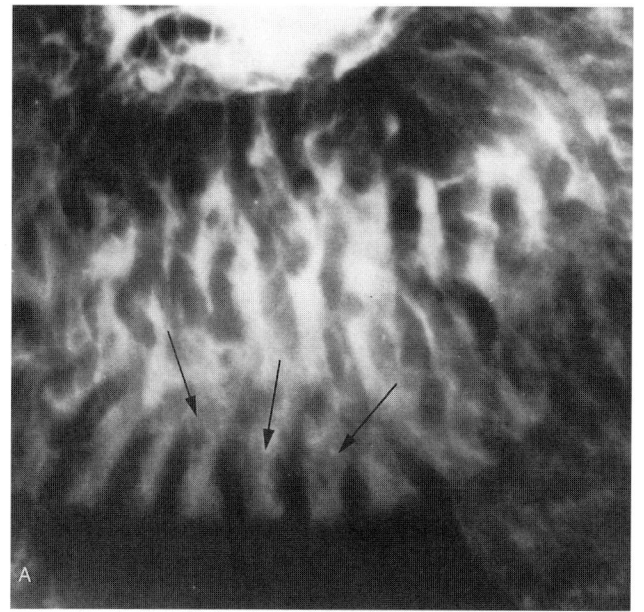
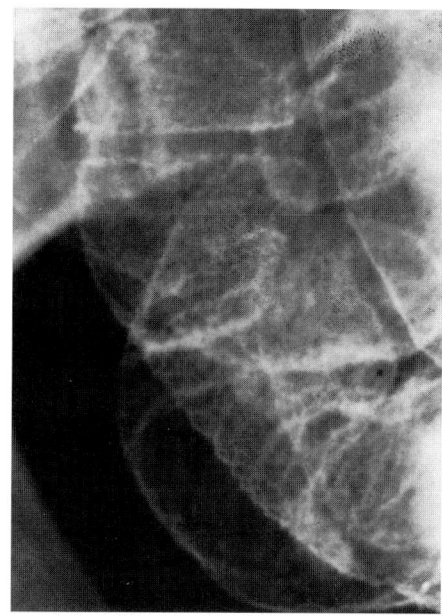
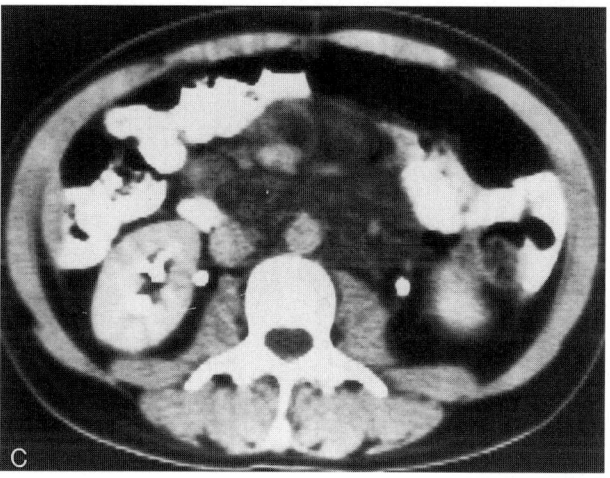

Fig. 18-32. Three cases of Whipple's disease affecting small bowel.
(a) Whipple's disease with scattered micronodules (arrows) demonstrated in the nondistended stage. (Courtesy of Professor D. Brindici, Bari, Italy.) (b) Enteroclysis demonstrates a diffuse micronodular pattern (diameters 1 to 2 mm); fold thickness is within the normal range. (Courtesy of Dr E. Salomonwitz, St. Poelten, Austria.) (c) CT in another case of Whipple's disease shows a typically fat-containing mesenteric and retroperitoneal nodal mass.

fatty material except in cases of infection with MAI complex (see Chapter 17).

Endoscopically, Whipple's disease can be suspected by the visualization of yellowish to white granular material in the mucosa of the descending duodenum; biopsy may confirm the diagnosis.[122]

Treatment

Favorable response to antibiotics is the rule, but relapses have occurred and this mainly involving the CNS. A combination of parenteral penicillin and streptomycin is given initially and is followed for about 1 year by peroral trimethoprim-sulfamethoxazole, which can penetrate the blood-brain barrier.[123] With favorable clinical response, there is no need for invasive surveillance. An enteroclysis might be indicated should intestine-related symptoms recur.

Systemic Mastocytosis

Mast cells, first identified and named by Ehrlich in 1877, are widely distributed and are effective in the body's histamine-induced immediate hypersensitivity reaction. Mastocytosis, the proliferation of mast cells, presents with skin localization (urticaria pigmentosa) in almost 80% of cases. In 20% to 30% of the cases, the disease slowly extends to involve several organs as systemic mastocytosis. These organs include the bone marrow, the liver and spleen, lymph nodes, and the gastrointestinal tract; their involvement is by mast cell infiltration and/or by the release of mediators.[124] The mostly indolent disease presents with attacks of flushing with warmth, hypotension, headache, diarrhea, nausea, and pruritus. These attacks, at times severe enough to be termed crises, are associated with mast cell degranulation and the release of histamine and prostaglandin D2.[125] The gut is frequently involved but obvious malabsorption occurs only rarely. However, careful analysis will demonstrate impairment of absorptive function in most cases. The finding of six or more mastocytes per high-power field in the lamina propria of biopsy material has been considered to support a diagnosis of enteric mast cell infiltration.[126] Systemic mastocytosis can become complicated by a myeloproliferative disorder mostly affecting liver and spleen. In the rare aggressive form of mastocytosis a fatal outcome from mast cell leukemia may occur after only a few years.[127]

Clinical Aspects

Most patients are less than 20 years old. Without urticaria pigmentosa it can be difficult to establish a clinical diagnosis. Urinary excretion of histamine metabolites is usually increased, especially during crises.

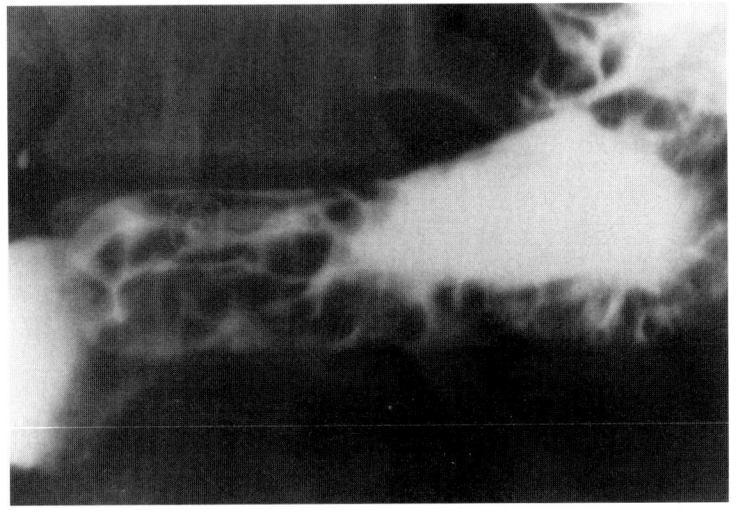

(a)

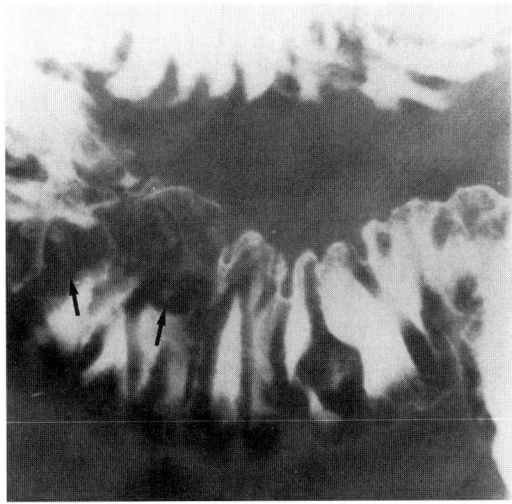

(b)

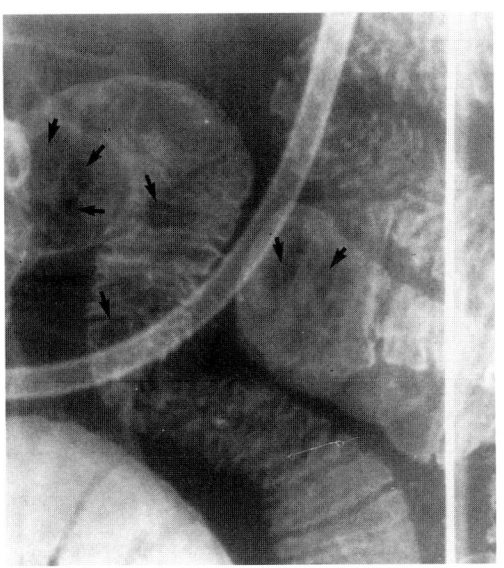

Fig. 18-33. **Patient with known systemic mastocytosis.**
(a) Nodules are present in the gastric antrum. (b) Umbilicated elevations are demonstrated in the distal duodenum (arrows). (c) Numerous groups of smaller nodules (arrows to some of them) are found in the proximal jejunum.

(c)

Alcohol intake precipitates symptoms. Endoscopic findings included erosive gastroduodenitis, and peptic ulceration as a consequence of gastric acid hypersecretion and the presence of nodules in stomach, duodenum, and jejunum.[128]

Radiology

Like the skin, the mucosa of the gastrointestinal tract is a major target of the byproducts of mast cell degranulation.[125] In the stomach and duodenum, fluid excess, swollen folds, and peptic ulceration indicate a high acid output state; 4- to 5-mm nodules are best seen between acute episodes [Fig. 18-33(a, b)]. Similar nodules are infrequently seen in the small bowel, mostly the jejunum [Fig. 18-33(c)].[125,129] There is conflicting input on the histologic composition of the nodules. One report[130] mentions nests of mast cells within the nodules; other reports[128,131] consider the nodules to be urticaria-like lesions.

CT scanning can demonstrate bowel wall thickening, hepatosplenomegaly, and enlargement of mesenteric or retroperitonal nodes. The spleen may contain areas of low attenuation, probably related to myeloproliferative change.

Eosinophilic Gastroenteritis

This is a rare disease; less than 200 cases have been reported since it was first described by Kaijser in 1937. Three criteria should be used to define eosinophilic gastroenteritis: the presence of gastrointestinal symptoms, an eosinophilic infiltrate in part of the gastrointestinal tract, and the exclusion of parasitic or extraintestinal disease. Peripheral eosinophilia is absent in up to 23% of patients. The disease can involve any portion of the gastrointestinal tract from esophagus into colon, but the gastric antrum and proximal small bowel are most often affected.[132] Eosinophilic gastroenteritis can be subclassified according to the part of the bowel wall that is predominantly infiltrated by eosinophils. In mucosal disease, mucosa and submucosa are densely infiltrated resulting in protein-losing enteropathy or malabsorption. In the mural disease type infiltration of the muscularis may cause obstruction. The predominantly subserosal form is usually accompanied by eosinophilic ascites. Abdominal pain is common to all three subgroups. The rare idiopathic hypereosinophilia syndrome differs from eosinophilic gastroenteritis in having a high peripheral eosinophil count, diffuse gastrointestinal involvement, and infiltration of other organs like liver and lungs.

Predominantly Mucosal Disease

Periodic diarrhea, abdominal pain, weight loss, eosinophilia, iron deficiency anemia, mild steatorrhea, and protein loss are usual clinical features. A history of atopy is obtained in half the patients. Microscopically, an eosinophilic infiltrate is seen in the lamina propria and tends to be more dense in the submucosa, where it is associated with a variable degree of fibrosis.[133] Usually, antral endoscopic biopsies are strongly positive for eosinophilic infiltration.

Barium studies of the small bowel show thickened, straightened, and somewhat rigid mucosal folds in affected segments (Fig. 18-34). The gastric antrum often shows mucosal thickening and nodularity [Fig. 18-35(a)]. Bowel involvement may be segmental and interspersed between normal loops with an abrupt change from diseased to normal bowel [Fig. 18-35(b)]. In places, mucosal folds may be blunted or effaced. Increased irritability and spasm are frequent.[134] Part of the colon may be involved, with evidence of edema and interference with its normal haustral architecture [Fig. 18-35(c)]. Return to normality, following corticosteriods or spontaneously, is a useful diagnostic indicator.

The radiological differential diagnosis, in patients showing focal disease, includes intramural hematoma due to trauma or coagulopathy, ischemia, or hereditary angioneurotic edema. Any of these conditions may be followed by return to normality, but the history will usually provide a clue. With extensive involvement, edema, amyloidosis, lymphangiectasia, and some of the immune system disorders have to be

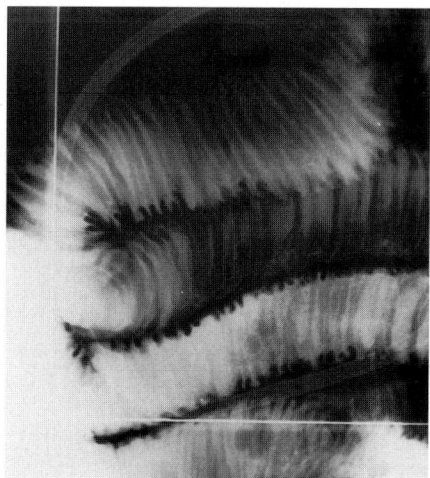

Fig. 18-34. Predominantly mucosal eosinophilic gastroenteritis in a young man with episodic diarrhea, atopic history, and an antral biopsy showing an eosinophilic infiltrate. Crowded, straightened, and mildly thickened folds are seen throughout the jejunum.

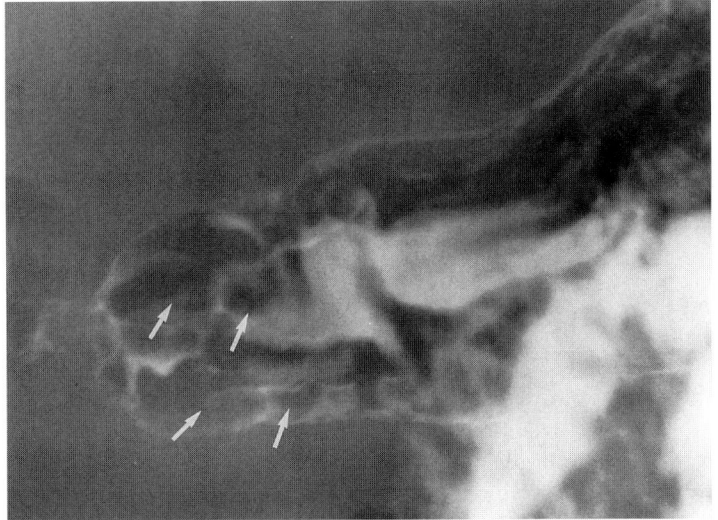
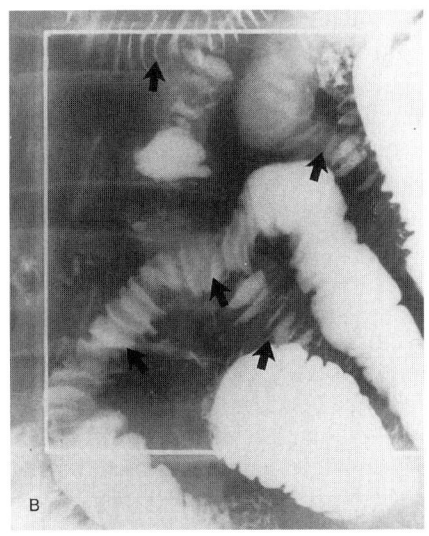
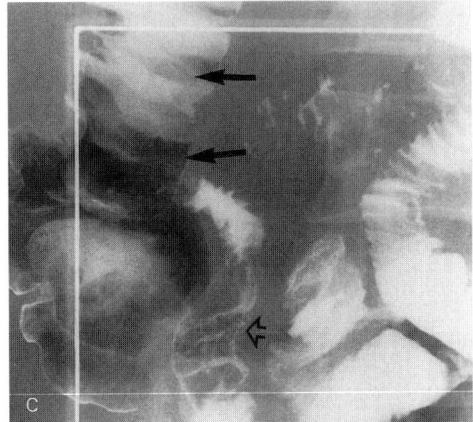

Fig. 18-35. Case of eosinophilic gastroenterocolitis, predominantly mucosal.
(a) Gastric antrum with mucosal nodularity (arrows). (b) Bowel segments with thickened and crowded folds (arrows) are separated by normal-appearing bowel. (c) The terminal ileum shows few straightened folds (arrowhead); extension into the colon is indicated by mucosal edema and thickening of haustra (arrows).

considered in the differential diagnosis. Polyarteritis nodosa, also associated with eosinophilia and known to show gastrointestinal involvement in 25% of cases, may closely resemble eosinophilic gastroenteritis. However, it is likely that systems outside the intestinal tract are also involved, eg, the liver and kidneys. It should be noted that in eosinophilic gastroenteritis ulceration is not a feature.

Predominantly Muscularis Propria Involvement

In this subtype infiltration of the submucosa with sheets of mature eosinophils extends into the muscularis propria. The antrum and involved small bowel are markedly thickened and rigid and show lumen narrowing. Most patients present with partial obstruction, more often of the antrum than the small bowel.[135] Surgery may be resorted to and resection or bypass performed.

Barium examinations may show concentric narrowing of the antrum with polypoid filling defects and with outlet obstruction. Though no mucosal destruction or ulceration is seen, differentiation from carcinoma can be impossible and endoscopy with biopsy may be needed. Involvement of the ileocecal area can resemble Crohn's disease.[135] The absence of ulceration, the associated changes in the gastric antrum, and the eosinophilia can assist in the correct interpretation. CT scans can identify focal or more diffuse fold and wall thickening. There may be a response to the administration of steroids.[136]

Predominantly Serosal Disease

In this subtype patients present with abdominal bloating, pain, and ascites.[137] The eosinophilic infiltrate extends from the muscularis into the subserosa.[132] There is usually no history of allergy. Response to steroids is reported to be dramatic.[137] Unlike in the other forms of eosinophilic enteritis, the majority of the reported patients have been women. Radiology can provide evidence of ascites and, in most of the patients with this rare presentation, can demonstrate features of frequently associated mucosal and submucosal involvement.

Unusual Presentations

Isolated colonic involvement has been reported as a form of eosinophilic gastroenteritis.[138] An association between eosinophilic enteritis and eosinophilic pneumonia has also been recorded.[139]

Although the radiographic findings of the three subtypes are nonspecific, the possible diagnosis of eosinophilic gastroenteritis should be considered in repeatedly symptomatic younger patients in whom an infiltrating lesion is seen in the distal stomach together with nonulcerated, focal, or extensive abnormalities of the small bowel. An atopic history and the presence of peripheral eosinophilia should be sought in support of the diagnosis. There should rarely be a need for diagnostic laparotomy.

Abetalipoproteinemia

Clinical Pathophysiology

Abetalipoproteinemia is a rare, recessively inherited disease that presents from birth. Following entry of lipids into an enterocyte, the mobilization of intracellular apolipoproteins is an essential step in their further transport. Normally, apolipoprotein-coated chylomicrons carry the absorbed fats, fat-soluble vitamins, and cholesterol through the basolateral membrane out of the enterocyte and into the mesenteric lymph and general circulation.[140] Without apoliprotein synthesis chylomicrons accumulate within enterocytes. Diarrhea, steatorrhea, and abdominal distention become evident in the first few months after birth. Acanthosis, a spiky outline of red blood cells, is an early feature. When approaching puberty, later sequelae may appear including retinitis pigmentosa and spinocerebellar degeneration, both as a result of malabsorption of fat-soluble vitamin E. High-dose supplements of vitamin E can avoid these complications. The histologic changes shown by jejunal mucosal biopsy, which must be done in the fasting patient, are typical.[141] The villous architecture is undisturbed, but villous enterocytes are ballooned by foamy globules of fat.

Hypobetalipoproteinemia is a related disease. It is autosomal-codominant, is clinically milder, and has a later onset.

Radiology

Mucosal folds in the duodenum and jejunum show uniform thickening with an added granular surface pattern; thickening extends into ileal folds (Fig. 18-36). There may be a mild increase of intraluminal fluid, moderate lumen dilatation, and increased irritabil-

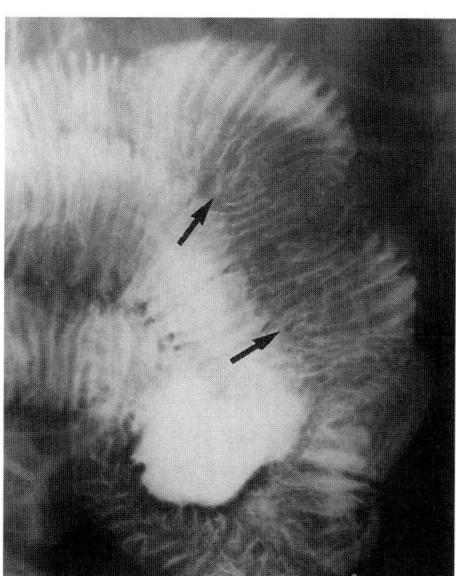
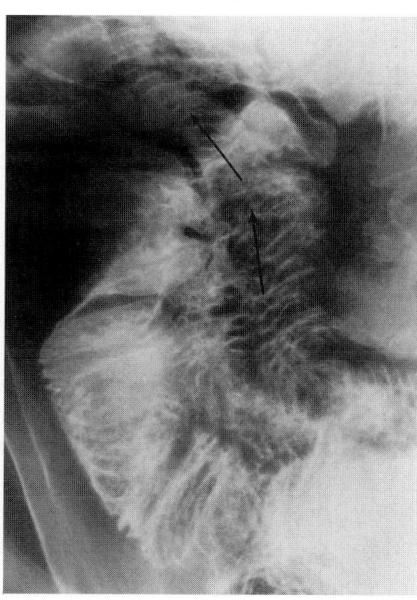

Fig. 18-36. **Underdeveloped young male patient with steatorrhea. Clinical diagnosis of hypobetalipoproteinemia.**
(a) Enteroclysis shows fold thickening of the jejunum together with a fine granular pattern (arrows), presumably due to villous enterocytes dilated by retained globules of fat.
(b) Ileal folds show increased thickening; the course of the terminal ileum is indicated by arrows.

ity.[142] The radiologic picture can resemble that of giardiasis, possibly also of edema in hypoalbuminemia and, in some cases, lymphangiectasia. The patient's age, history, and clinical presentation will usually eliminate the diagnostic alternatives.

Zollinger-Ellison Syndrome (ZES)

Pathophysiology

Gastrin-secreting neuroendocrine tumors are responsible for the syndrome, which typically presents with peptic ulceration and diarrhea. About 80% of gastrinomas occur in the gastrinoma triangle, an area between the confluence of the cystic and common bile ducts, the junction of the second and third portions of the duodenum and the neck and body junction of the pancreas.[143] Sixty percent to 90% of all gastrinomas are malignant.[144] If carefully searched for (endoscopic transillumination during surgery) more gastrinomas are demonstrated in the duodenum than in the pancreas; compared to pancreatic gastrinomas they tend to be smaller (average size 6 mm), are more often multiple, have a higher incidence of metastases, and have a shorter disease-free interval after resection.[144] In up to 25% of cases, the gastrinomas are part of the multiple endocrine neoplasia syndrome type I (MEN I), usually associated with hypercalcemia from parathyroid hyperplasia. The MEN I–related gastrinomas are more likely to be situated in the duodenum. The gastrinoma-produced hypergastrinemia has three effects: 1) overstimulation of gastric parietal cells to secrete acid at near maximum level, 2) an increase of the parietal cell mass, and 3) trophic changes to the pancreas. The clinical results are peptic ulceration and diarrhea.[143] The mucosa of the duodenum bears the brunt of the gastric acid hypersecretion and is frequently edematous, inflamed, and hemorrhagic. Patchy loss of villi, erosions as well as ulcers, may be found. This inflammatory change may extend into the proximal jejunum.

Clinical Features

Most patients are between 30 and 50 years old and the majority are male. Gastroduodenal ulcerations occur in up to 75% of patients. Duodenal ulcers are often found in the postbulbar or more distal duodenum; some 10% of ulcers are found in the jejunum. Ulcers are slow to heal and tend to recur, bleed, or perforate. A basal acid output exceeding 15 mEq per hour is typical for ZES, and the maximum acid output (MAO) is invariably above the normal levels of 48 mEq per hour for men and 30 mEq per hour for women. A fasting serum gastrin level greater than 1000 pg/ml strongly indicates the diagnosis of ZES. Many patients, however, show lesser elevation, and in these a secretin provocation test is indicated. A postinjection rise of serum gastrin by 200 pg/ml is diagnostic[143] and distinguishes ZES from other hypergastrinemic states, such as antral G-cell hyperplasia, the retained gastric antrum, short bowel syndrome, or chronic renal failure. False-positive secretin test results can occur with appropriate hypergastrinemic states (eg, achlorhydria from pernicious anemia) so that it is important to confirm acid production with at least gastric juice pH measurement in all hypergastrinemic patients even if the secretin test is positive. Increased delivery of acid into the duodenum can drop the small bowel lumenal pH to as low as 1.5 and impair digestion by inactivating pancreatic lipase and precipitating bile acids. However, postprandial buffering may allow duodenal pH to return to near normal levels. Steatorrhea in ZES is, therefore, usually mild and inconstant.[143] However, excessive gastric acid output in the interdigestive period may cause watery diarrhea. In about 35% of patients diarrhea may precede peptic ulceration.[145]

Exclusion of MEN I in patients with ZES is clinically relevant. The most frequently associated condition, four gland parathyroid hyperplasia with hyperparathyroidism, can be excluded or confirmed by serum calcium and parathyroid hormone estimations.[146] However, in almost a third of the patients ZES can precede other features of MEN I, and MEN I may become apparent only after gastrinoma surgery.[147]

Management

In earlier years, treatment was symptom-related and targeted the end organ, the stomach. Total gastrectomy could render patients symptom-free until tumor malignancy took over. Gastrectomy could be abandoned with the introduction of H_2 receptor blockers and omeprazole. Curative surgery, requiring resection of the entire primary tumor or tumors, was infrequently attempted because of inadequate, preoperative tumor localization and the belief that complications of surgery would outweigh its benefits. In recent years, diagnostic radiology has taken a giant step forward and results of surgery in ZES have been generally excellent. Surgery for cure should now be considered an option in all cases of ZES except those already with liver metastases or where the gastrinoma is part of MEN I, even when radiology has failed to localize the gastrinoma. An important recent study compared the outcome in 83 metastases-free patients in whom a gastrinoma was resected with 26 comparable patients who did not have surgery.[148] Follow-up was similar for the two groups. During the follow-up period, 23% of the medically treated patients developed liver metastases, against only 3% of those treated surgically. All surgically treated patients survived, only 10% with significant postsurgical complications.

Radiology

Barium studies show features in keeping with high gastric acid output, hyperrugosity, fluid increase, exaggerated areae gastricae, and gastroduodenal erosions. Peptic ulceration may be single or multiple. A feature in support of ZES is a dilated descending duodenum with coarse folds, at times showing nodules with erosions [Fig. 18-37(a)]. In the jejunum, thickened folds, fluid increase, and, occasionally, peptic ulceration may increase the level of suspicion for ZES [Fig. 18-37(b)]. Reflux esophagitis is a frequent finding and is more often severe; 17% of endoscoped patients had a Barrett's esophagus.[149]

The more important function of radiology is the localization of the gastrinoma and the exclusion or demonstration of metastases. An intra-arterial secretin test was reported to have high specificity but low sensitivity and mostly regionalizes rather than localizes the gastrinoma.[150] Although highly selective visceral angiography may surpass the accuracy of other studies[151] it is invasive and out of favor. Imaging techniques are the main radiologic options. Continued improvements in technology and techniques soon render estimates of detection rates out-of-date. Presently, MRI is generally superior to ultrasound and CT in localizing pancreatic gastrinomas [Fig. 18-38(a, b)]. Duodenal endoscopic ultrasonography (EUS) appears to be able to identify more than half the pancreatic gastrinomas in the vicinity of the duodenum and most of the usually small duodenal wall gastrinomas.[145,152] Duodenal microgastrinomas may also occasionally be identified at endoscopy[145] or be demonstrated during surgery by ultrasound or endoscopic transmural illumination.[152] The presently most accurate method for identifying pancreatic and duodenal gastrinomas and

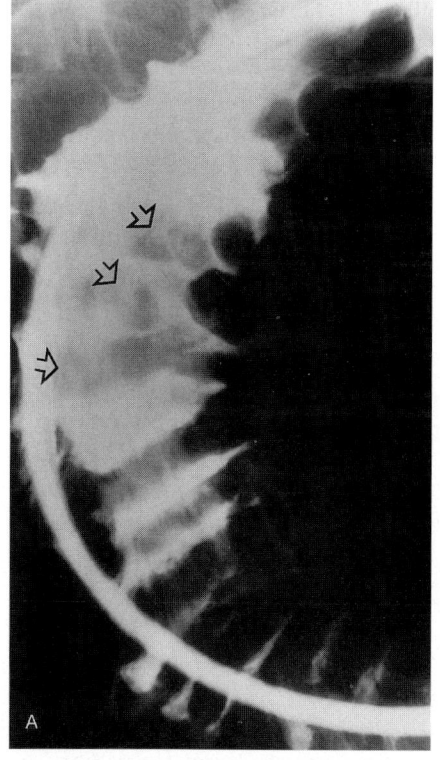
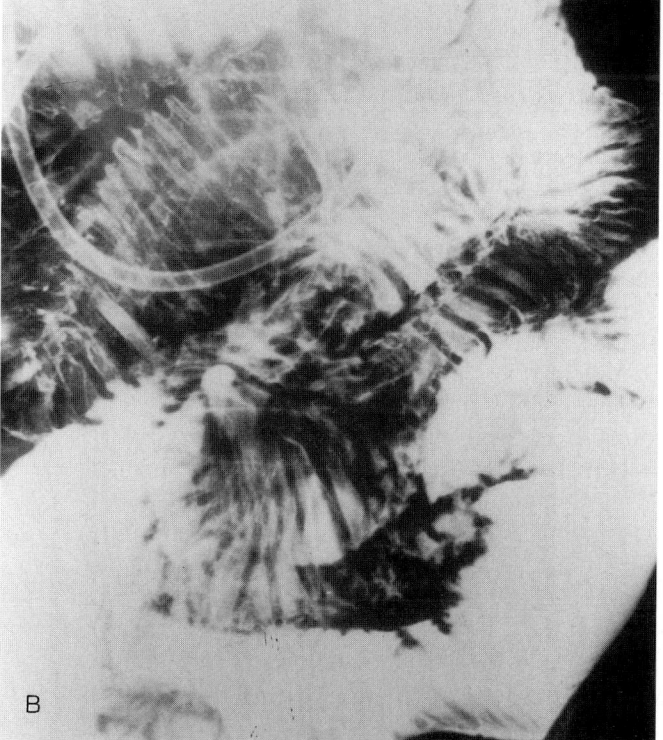

Fig. 18-37. Zollinger-Ellison syndrome.
(a) Barium outlined descending duodenum with thick folds, nodules, and several erosions (arrows). (b) The jejunum shows a lesser degree of fold thickening.

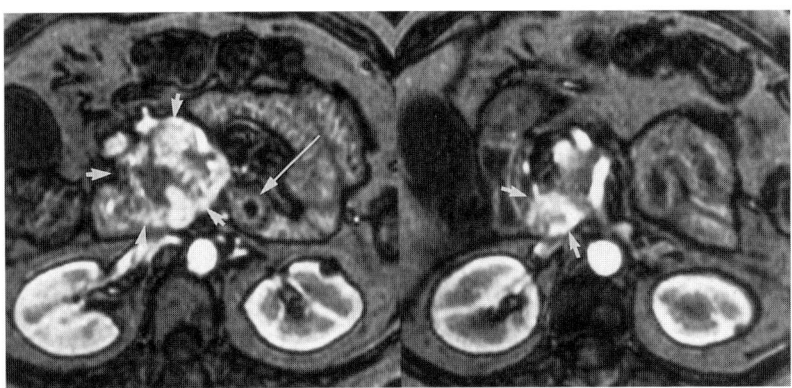 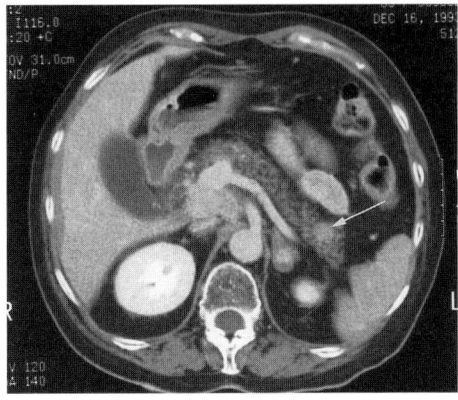

(a) (b)

Fig. 18-38.
(a) Two consecutive contrast-enhanced breath-hold T1-weighted gradient echo images through the low pancreatic head show a heterogeneous hypervascular mass typical for an islet cell neoplasm (short arrows). An enhancing mucosa and mild submucosal edema are indicated in the cross-sectional view of an adjacent segment of jejunum (long arrow) suggesting ZES in this patient with extensive gastrinoma and markedly elevated serum gastrin levels. (b) CT scan demonstrated a further, smaller gastrinoma in the tail of the pancreas (arrow).

their liver metastases is somatostatin receptor scintigraphy[153,154]; it could alter clinical management of 47% of 122 patients evaluated prospectively.[155] (See Chapter 11.)

Amyloidosis

Amyloidosis is a rare systemic disease caused by the extracellular deposition of an insoluble fibrillar protein with a beta-pleated configuration.[156] In *primary or AL amyloidosis*, myeloma-associated amyloidosis, and, occasionally, in Waldenstrom's macroglobulinemia, fragments of monoclonal immunoglobulin light chains form amyloid fibers, probably related to an underlying plasma cell dyscrasia.[157] Deposits of AL amyloid are found in skeletal muscle, heart, tongue, gastrointestinal tract, joints (also causing the carpal tunnel syndrome), liver, and spleen. Of the gastrointestinal tract, the small intestine, including the duodenum, is more frequently affected. The *secondary* or *amyloidosis A* involves the kidneys, liver, spleen, and also the gastrointestinal tract. It is associated with chronic inflammatory disorders, such as rheumatoid arthritis, familial Mediterranean fever,[158] and occasionally Crohn's disease.[159]

Pseudo-obstruction, diarrhea, malabsorption, ischemic changes with ulceration or bleeding, and even perforation are possible features of intestinal amyloidosis. Rectal biopsy allows a diagnosis to be made in 70% of patients; an endoscopic duodenojejunal biopsy would be more rewarding, provided the small bowel is involved. Necropsy in patients who had developed pseudo-obstruction showed an interesting pattern of amyloid deposition. In AL amyloidosis there was extensive amyloid infiltration of the muscularis propria with muscle degeneration; the pseudo-obstruction was unresponsive to treatment.[160] Pseudo-obstruction in amyloidosis A was related to amyloid deposition in the myenteric plexuses but with focal variations of intensity; treatment was more likely to succeed.[160] In both types of amyloidosis, intestinal deposits were most commonly found in the submucosa and in the wall of small vessels. Partial villous atrophy may also be present.

Familial Mediterranean fever is a hereditary disease characterized by attacks of fever and polyserositis with secondary amyloidosis. It tends to affect Sephardic Jews, Armenians, and Arabs and is infrequently found in other nationals around the Mediterranean basin.[161]

Radiology

With amyloidosis the small bowel can be radiologically normal, even in the presence of a positive biopsy.[162] It is important to distinguish bowel distention due to pseudo-obstruction from that caused by mechanical obstruction, as unnecessary surgery should be avoided. Barium studies can show mucosal folds diffusely thickened and the intervalvular distance less than normal[163]; the intensity of these changes parallels the severity of symptoms.

Double-contrast enteroclysis has been able to demonstrate mucosal patterns that relate to the type of amyloidosis. Innumerable fine granular lucencies on irregularly thickened folds were found in 16 patients with amyloidosis A [Fig. 18-39(a)]. Endoscopy with dye scattering confirmed these findings, and a biopsy demonstrated amyloid A deposits in the lamina propria, extending into blunted villi.[164] A follow-through examination in a patient with rheumatoid arthritis showed scattered 2-mm nodules due to amyloidosis A [Fig. 18-39(b)]. Multiple polypoid protrusions, up to 10 mm in diameter, were found in six patients, extending throughout the gut [Fig. 18-40(a)]. Endoscopy showed them as whitish elevations that bled on touch. Biopsy demonstrated amyloid AL deposition in the mucosa and submucosa or in the wall of submucosal vessels.[164] These findings were further analyzed and confirmed in a subsequent publication.[165] A similar appearance of nodularity due to amyloid AL was demonstrated by barium follow-through [Fig. 18-40(b)]; Barium examination in a further patient could demonstrate nodularity later shown to be due to amyloid AL complicating multiple myeloma [Fig. 18-40(c)].

CT scanning in small bowel amyloidosis has demonstrated mural thickening considered to resemble an ischemic change. Ischemia due to amyloid deposition in the wall of submucosal vessels may be responsible for this appearance.[166] An amyloid-associated, serum-derived amyloid P component labeled with iodine-123 can be used for the scintigraphic evaluation of more massive amyloid deposition.[157]

Endocrine Disorders

Diabetes

Diarrhea in long-standing diabetes can be a problem in over 10% of patients. Steatorrhea may occur and may relate to autonomic neuropathy and associated bacterial overgrowth. Other causes of steatorrhea can be exocrine pancreatic insufficiency, inadequate emulsification of triglycerides due to gastroparesis, and, occasionally, coexistent celiac disease. Barium studies show evidence of gastroparesis and thickened folds in a dilated jejunum. Octreotide, the somatostatin analog, has been found useful in the treatment of refractory diabetic diarrhea.[167]

Hypoparathyroidism

Associated hypocalcemia may impair gastrointestinal contractile activity. Bowel loops are then dilated and transit time is prolonged. Ileus and steatorrhea may result and improve with calcium administration.

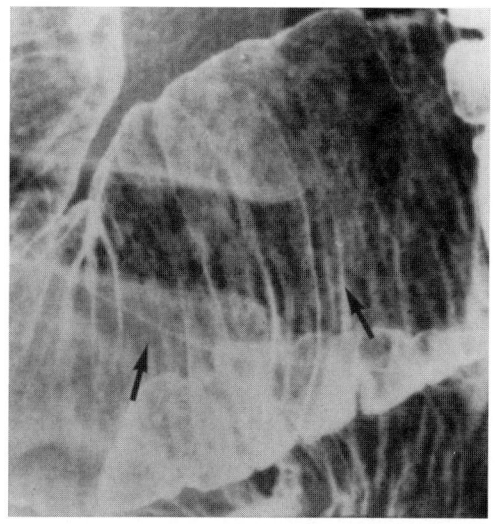
(a)

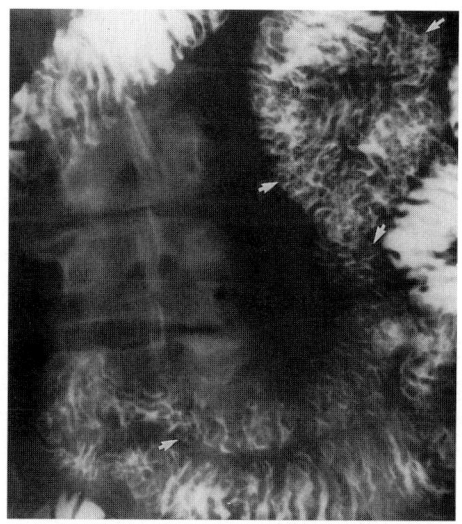
(b)

Fig. 18-39. Barium studies in amyloidosis A.
(a) Enteroclysis demonstrates coarse granularity due to amyloid deposition in the lamina propria, superimposed on slight fold thickening. (Courtesy Professor S. Tada, MD, Fukuoka, Japan.) (b) Patient with rheumatoid arthritis for many years. Follow-through study outlines numerous 1- to 2-mm nodules (arrows).

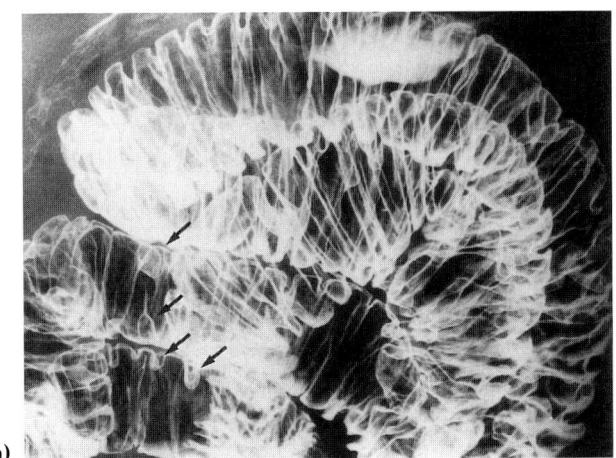
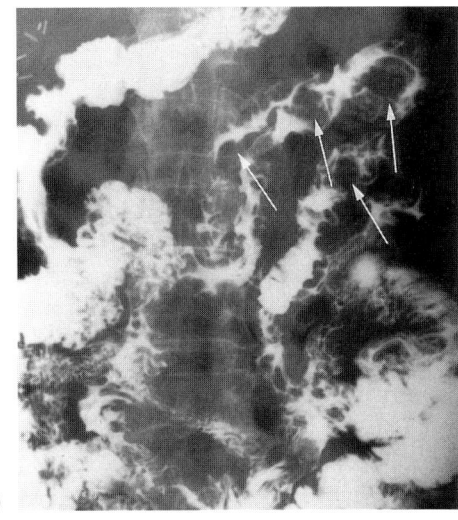
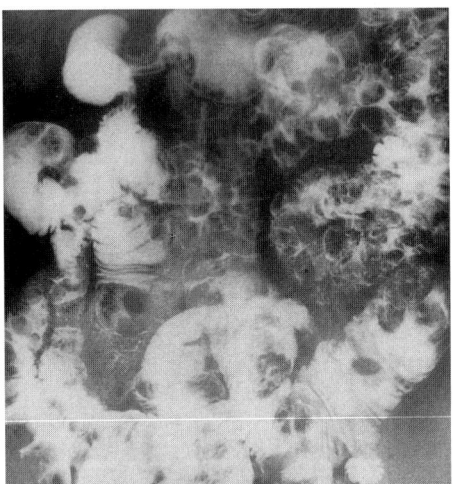

Fig. 18-40. Light chain–derived amyloidosis AL presents a different pattern from the secondary amyloidosis.
(a) Enteroclysis reveals numerous up to 10-mm polypoid protrusions (arrows) on a normal mucosal surface. (Courtesy Professor S. Tada, Fukuoka, Japan.) (b) Amyloidosis AL shown by barium follow-through. Numerous 1-cm nodules (arrows to some), predominate in the jejunum. (Courtesy of Jacqueline A. Brown, MD, Vancouver.) (c) A similar nodular pattern is demonstrated in a barium study of amyloidosis AL complicating multiple myeloma.

Hypothyroidism

Usually the colon is more severely affected than the small bowel. Muco-polysaccharide infiltration causes thickening of the bowel wall and mucosal atrophy. Hypothyroidism can be a cause of general dilatation of the gastrointestinal tract, with emphasis on the colon, and may be associated with steatorrhea and depressed levels of fat-soluble vitamins.[111] Occasionally, the disease may present with myxedema ileus which, if recognized, responds to replacement therapy.

Maldigestion

Pancreatic achylia, whether due to chronic pancreatitis, carcinoma, pancreatectomy, or cystic fibrosis, implies nonsecretion of pancreatic lipase and bicarbonate and leads to an excess of neutral fat in the stool. *Hepatocellular* or *obstructive jaundice* is associated with defective delivery of bile into the duodenum and will also cause steatorrhea. Barium studies of the small bowel usually show normal appearances.

Lactase Deficiency

Disaccharidases required for the digestion of disaccharides are constituents of the microvillous membrane of absorptive cells in the jejunum. Lactase, one of the disaccharidases, develops late during fetal life and reaches high levels during fetal maturity. It persists into adult life, especially in people of northern European origin, but may become totally absent in several population groups, including Arabs, Chinese, Bantus, and Eskimos. Secondary lactase deficiency may develop in patients with celiac disease, Crohn's disease, ulcerative colitis, bacterial overgrowth syndrome, and alcoholism, and in patients following administration of drugs, such as colchicine and neomycin.[168] The diagnosis can be confirmed by the hydrogen breath test (see earlier) or by transoral jejunal biopsy with enzyme assay.

Radiology has been helpful in diagnosis in the past,[169] but is no longer needed.

Crohn's Disease

Malabsorption occurs frequently and its cause can be multifactorial. A reduction of absorbing surface—either due to inflammation or surgery—is the most important factor. Bacterial overgrowth in stagnant segments caused by strictures or bypass (also see Chapter 15), loss of protein and electrolytes into the lumen, and, at times, acceleration of transit are further factors. There is an almost routine elevation of serum amyloid-A protein in patients with Crohn's disease, with higher levels in more advanced disease.[170] Secondary amyloidosis may become an additional cause of malabsorption.

Lymphangiectasia

Lymphangiectasia results from obstruction to the flow of lymph from the small intestine into the mesentery, leading to dilatation of intestinal and serosal lymphatic channels. It occurs as a primary, congenital disease or secondary to retroperitoneal or mesenteric abnormalities. The *primary* form is usually part of a more extensive hypoplasia of lymphatics, often with asymmetric edema of the extremities (Milroy's disease). Although it is based on a congenital defect, symptoms usually become evident in young adults, both sexes being equally affected. Increased pressure in the intestinal lymphatics impairs the absorption of chylomicrons, their transport out of enterocytes, and also the recirculation of intestinal lymphocytes.[171] Lymphoenteric fistulae may form; lymph, lymphocytes, and protein then drain into the bowel lumen. Malabsorption with steatorrhea, hypoalbuminemia, and lymphocytopenia is the result. The loss of T lymphocytes affects cell-mediated immunity. Serum gamma globulins, especially IgG and IgA, are decreased.[172] However, opportunistic infections are uncommon. In the management of primary lymphangiectasia, replacing long-chain dietary triglycerides by short- or medium-chain triglycerides reduces malabsorption and raises serum albumin levels. Chylomicrons in obstructed lymphatics are diminished in this way, and this may reduce lymphatic pressure and loss of lymphocytes.[171]

Secondary lymphangiectasia can be part of numerous conditions associated with lymphatic occlusion at any level between the gut and the thoracic duct. These include nodal involvement by extensive abdominal or retroperitoneal malignancy, mesenteric or retroperitoneal fibrosis, lymphoma, Whipple's disease, radiation damage, chronic pancreatitis, tuberculosis, Crohn's disease, constrictive pericarditis, and congestive cardiac failure.[171]

The *diagnosis* is supported by positive findings during duodenal endoscopy. Villi distended by dilated lacteals are seen as slightly elevated whitish spots. Biopsy, in addition to the dilated lacteals, shows fat-laden lipophages crowding dilated lymphatics or lying free in the lamina propria and edematous submucosa.[141] These changes can be patchy. Similar appearances are seen in cases of secondary lymphangiectasia.

Radiology

Barium follow-through examinations have shown nonspecific appearances, fold thickening, fluid increase, and slight lumen dilatation. The small bowel enema has made it possible to demonstrate finer and more specific abnormalities of the mucosa in some patients. In addition to fold thickening that is more pronounced in the jejunum, there are groups of millimeter-sized nodules that represent individual lacteal distended villi [Fig. 18-41(a–c)]. A few larger nodules may also be seen and have been shown to represent a conglomerate of dilated lymphatics mostly in the submucosa. No ulcers are seen. It is of interest that a recent report of air double-contrast studies in patients with lymphangiectasia of mixed etiologies refers predominantly to the larger, smooth mucosal elevations and barely to the micronodules that represent dilated villi.[173] In patients with secondary lymphangiectasia, CT studies may demonstrate fold thickening, occasionally with evidence of micronodularity in ascites (Fig. 18-42). Retroperitoneal or mesenteric lymph node enlargement may also be shown.

Unexplained hypoalbuminemia should suggest protein-losing enteropathy and, if associated with lymphocytopenia and steatorrhea, lymphangiectasia is likely.[171] A scintigraphic assessment of such protein loss follows the intravenous injection of 99Tc-labeled albumin; radionucleide excretion into small bowel was shown after 45 minutes.[174] The diagnosis was subsequently confirmed by endoscopy and biopsy.

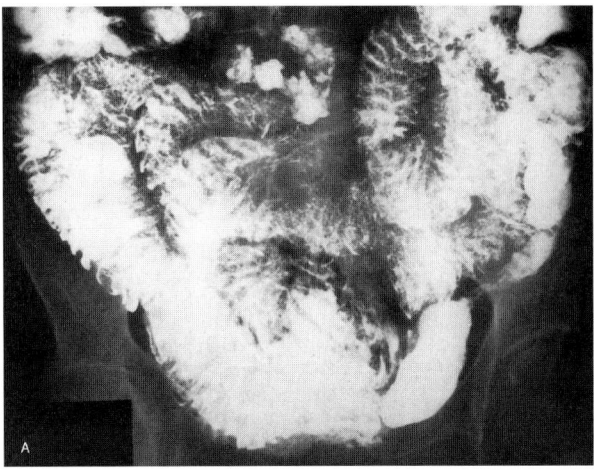
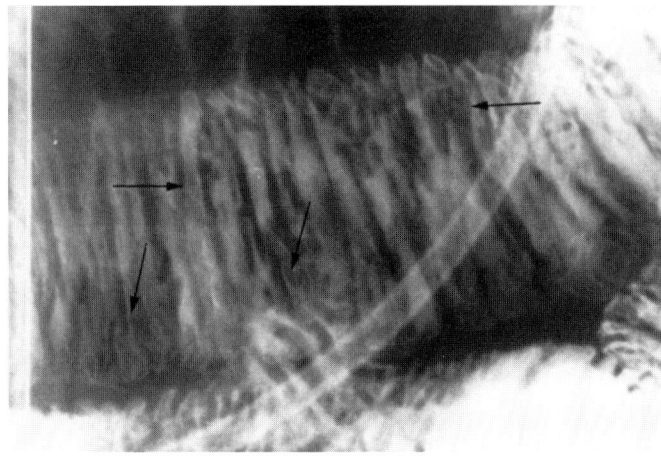
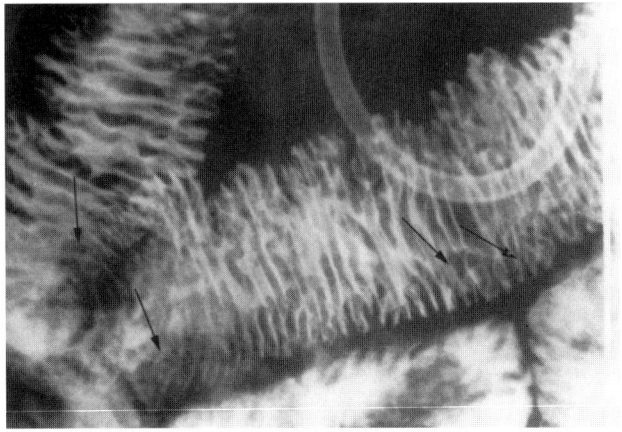

Fig. 18-41. **Two young men with primary lymphangiectasia.** (a) Follow-through film shows thick folds and an indication of fine nodularity. (b) The first enteroclysis of the second patient showed mild fold thickening and groups of up to 2-mm nodules (arrows), representing villi containing dilated lacteals. (c) Enteroclysis was repeated 5 years later, following dietary correction (see text) and with patient doing well. Groups of nodules (arrows) and mild fold thickening persist.

Waldenstrom's Macroglobulinemia

The disease is characterized by the presence in the plasma of monoclonal IgM protein with lymphadenopathy, hepatosplenomegaly, and anemia. With time, most cases progress to a lymphoma, usually of small lymphocytic type. Diarrhea is a possible feature, and can be persistent. Two more recent case reports[175,176] discuss and illustrate the deposition of extracellular PAS-positive monoclonal IgM macroglobulin in the lamina propria and submucosa of the small bowel. Histology shows enlargement of villi caused by this amorphous material, which has extended out of the lamina propria to compress stromal cells and distend lacteals. Small bowel involvement is rare but it accounted for two of the three cases described in Waldenstrom's original paper.[177]

Macroglobulinemia affects mostly elderly patients, males predominating. However, a 2:1 female to male

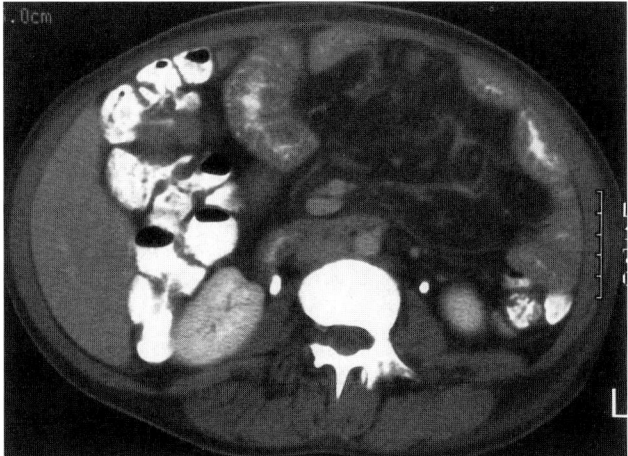

Fig. 18-42. **Secondary lymphangiectasia in a male patient with a history of nonHodgkin's lymphoma.** CT outlined contrast filled loops of pelvic ileum have thickened folds with a superadded pattern of micronodularities. Ascites is outlined by open arrows.

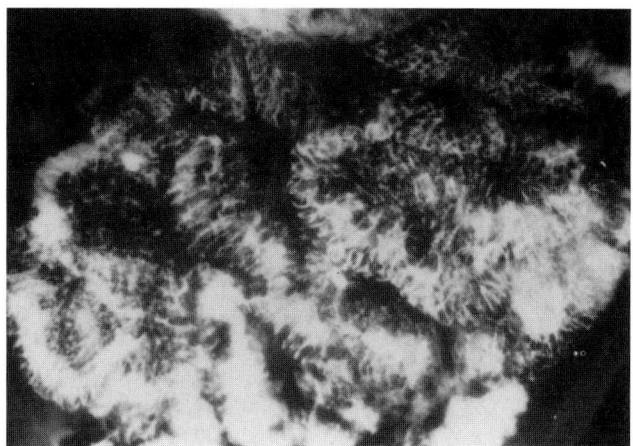

Fig. 18-43. Barium study in patient with known Waldenstrom's macroglobulinemia with malabsorption.
Folds are diffusely thickened with an added pattern of fine nodularity. (Courtesy of MP Capp, MD, Tucson.)

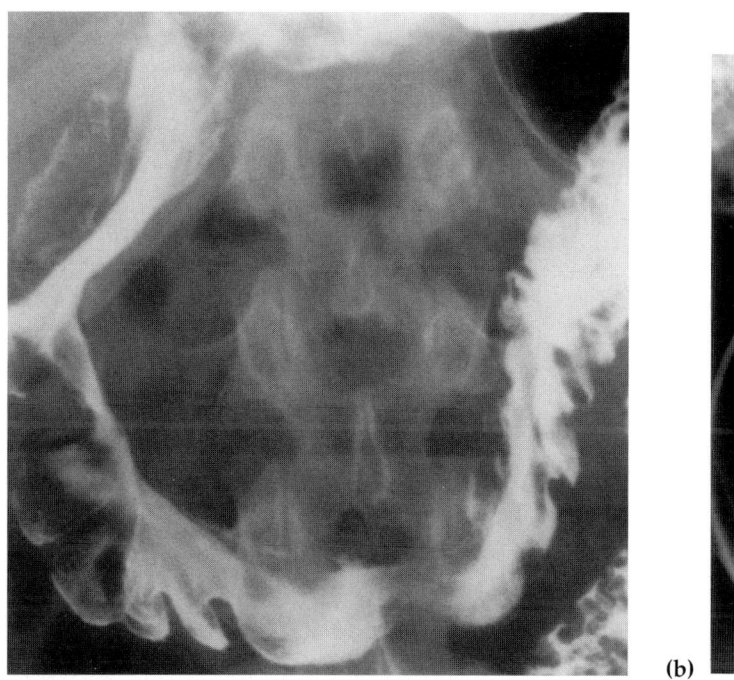

(a)

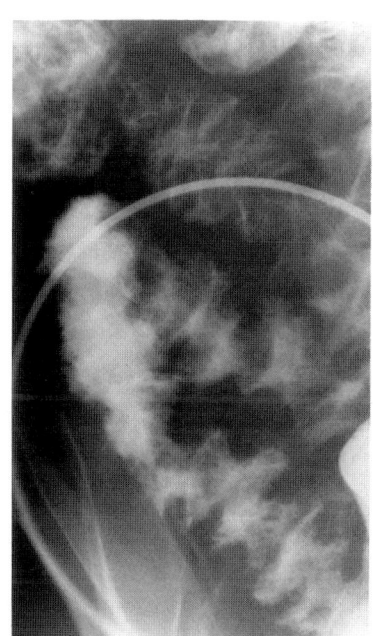

(b)

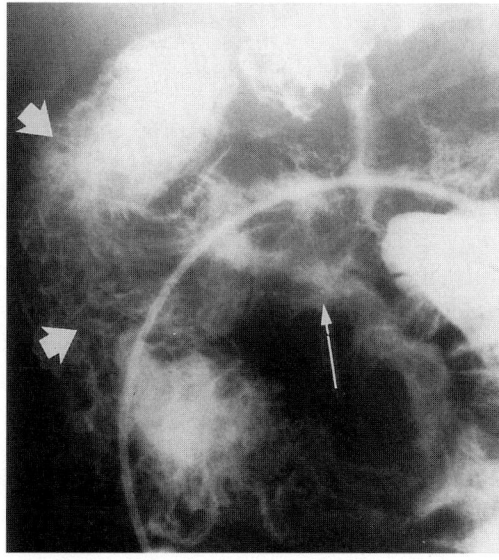

(c)

Fig. 18-44. Adult cystic fibrosis with malabsorption as part of the symptomatology.
(a) Typical changes in duodenum, cause not clear. Flattened medial border, sacculation and nodularity of outer border, without ulceration. (b) Barium follow-through in another young patient. Ileal fold pattern replaced by curving lines and nodules. (c) Similar change in terminal ileum (long arrow) and colon (arrows). Inspissated mucus is believed to be the cause of this pattern.

ratio has been reported for cases complicated by small bowel involvement.[175] The small intestine, including the duodenum, is the only portion of the gastrointestinal tract affected. Duodenal endoscopy can identify villous distention, which can be accentuated by scattering of indigo carmine dye.

Radiology

Diffuse and uniform thickening of mucosal folds is present in most cases. Enteroclysis, occasionally a dedicated barium meal, can show a pattern of 1- to 2-mm micronodules extending over the mucosal surface (Fig. 18-43).[119] It represents the clubbed villi containing IgM macroglobulin and resembles findings in Whipple's disease or lymphangiectasia. When lymphoma supervenes, the uniform thickening of folds is replaced by larger nodules of submucodal origin and by deformities from extrinsic masses.

In uncomplicated macrogobulinemia, CT scans demonstrate mural thickening of the small bowel and hepatosplenomegaly. With the almost inevitably complication of lymphoma, CT scans show mesenteric nodal masses infiltrating bowel loops.

Cystic Fibrosis in Adults

Almost 20% of children afflicted with this congenital disease survive, and in some of them the diagnosis is not made until early adulthood. Recurrent respiratory infections, variable degrees of malabsorption, and episodes of bowel obstruction dominate the adult clinical picture. This brief clinicoradiological note will confine itself to a description of changes shown by a barium study, which may suggest the diagnosis.

An unusual pattern is found in the duodenum.[178] Mostly seen in the descending duodenum are thickened folds, some with nodules; there are also areas of fold flattening and, at times, an appearance of sacculation without ulceration [Fig. 18-44(a)]. More pronounced in the ileum than jejunum are irregular curved lines that replace the normal fold pattern and may extend into the colon. It is likely that these barium lines demarcate blobs of inspissated mucus [Fig. 18-44(b, c)].

References

1. Losowsky MS. The protean clinical manifestations of celiac disease. In: Ferguson A, ed. *Advanced Medicine*. London: Pitman Ltd;1984:48–60.
2. Simko V. Fecal fat microscopy. *Am J Gastroenterol.* 1981;75:204–208.
3. Wright TL, Heyworth MF. Maldigestion and malabsorption, Chapter 18. In: Sleisinger MH, Fordtran JS, eds. *Gastrointestinal Disease.* (4th ed). Philadelphia, Pa.: WB Saunders Co;1989:263–282.
4. Kerlin P, Wong I. Breath hydrogen testing in bacterial overgrowth of the small intestine. *Gastroenterology.* 1988;95:982–988.
5. Marsh MN. Gluten, major histocompatibility complex, and the small intestine. A molecular and immunobiologic approach to the spectrum of gluten sensitivity ("celiac sprue"). *Gastroenterology.* 1992;102:330–354.
6. Bai J, Moran C, Martinez C, et al. Celiac sprue after surgery of the upper gastrointestinal tract. *J Clin Gastroenterol.* 1991;13:521–524.
7. Gee S. On the coeliac affection. *Saint Bartholomew's Hospital Report.* 1888;24:17–20.
8. Comroe B, Pendergrass E. Roentgen study of the gastrointestinal tract in chronic idiopathic adult tetany. *AJR.* 1935;33:647–656.
9. Losowsky MS, Walker BE, Kelleher J. *Malabsorption in Clinical Practice.* Edinburgh, Scotland: Churchill Livingstone; 1974:191–196.
10. Hankey GI, Holmes GKT. Coeliac disease in the elderly. *Gut.* 1994;35:65–67.
11. Brady CE. Occult celiac sprue masquerading as severe iron deficiency anemia. *J Clin Gastroenterol.* 1994;18:130–132.
12. Cooke WT, Holmes GKT. *Coeliac Disease.* Edinburgh, Scotland: Churchill Livingstone; 1984:172–180.
13. Mathus-Vliegen EMH. Lymphoma in coeliac disease. *J Roy Soc Med.* 1995;88:672–677.
14. Corazza GR, Brusco G, Andreani MI, et al. Previous misdiagnosis and diagnostic delay in adult celiac sprue. *J Clin Gastroenterol.* 1996;22:324–326.
15. Chorzelski TP, Sulej J, Tchorzewska M, et al. IgA class endomysium antibodies in dermatitis herpetiformis and coeliac disease. *Ann NY Acad Sci.* 1983;420:325–334.
16. Corrao G, Corazza GR, Andreani ML, et al. The reliability of noninvasive tests for celiac disease. *Gut.* 1994;35:771–775.
17. Savidge TC, Walker-Smith JA, Phillips AD. Intestinal proliferation in coeliac disease: looking into the crypt. *Gut.* 1995;36:321–323.
18. Scott BB, Losowsky MS. Patchiness and duodenal-jejunal variation of the mucosal abnormality in coeliac disease and dermatitis herpetiformis. *Gut.* 1976;17:984–992.
19. Stevens FM, McCarthy CF. The endoscopic demonstration of coeliac disease. *Endoscopy.* 1976;8:177–180.
20. Corazza GR, Brocchi E, Caletti G, Gasbarrini G. Loss of duodenal folds allows diagnosis of unsuspected coeliac disease. *Gut.* 1990;31:1080–1081.
21. Batt M. Non-coeliac flat jejunal mucosa. *Gut Festschrift.* 1989;30:67–68.
22. Marshak RH, Lindner AK. *Radiology of the Small Intestine,* 2nd ed. Philadelphia, Pa: WB Saunders Co; 1976.
23. Kumar P, Bartram CI. Relevance of the barium follow-

through examination in the diagnosis of adult celiac disease. *Gastrointest Radiol.* 1979;14:285–289.
24. Farthing MJG, McLean AM, Batram CI, et al. Radiological features of the jejunum in hypoalbuminemia. *AJR.* 1981;136:883–886.
25. Jones B, Bayless TM, Hamilton SR, Yardley JH. "Bubbly" duodenal bulb in celiac disease radiologic-pathologic correlation. *AJR.* 1984;142:119–122.
26. Jeffers MD, Hourihane DO. Coeliac disease with histological features of peptic duodenitis: value of assessment of intraepithelial lymphocytes. *J Clin Path.* 1993;46:420–424.
27. Maurino E, Capizzano H, Niveloni S, et al. Value of endoscopic markers in celiac disease. *Dig Dis Sci.* 1993;38:2028–2033.
28. Ruoff M, Lindner AE, Marshak RH. Intussusception in sprue. *AJR.* 1968;104:525–528.
29. Cohen MD, Lintott DJ. Transient small bowel intussusception in adult coeliac disease. *Clin Radiol.* 1978;29:529–534.
30. Cooke WT, Holmes GKT. Gluten-induced enteropathy (celiac disease). In: Berk JE, ed. *Bockus Gastroenterology.* 4th ed. Philadelphia, Pa: WB Saunders Co; 1985;1719–1757.
31. Muller WFH. Adult celiac disease. In: Sellink JL, Miller RE, eds. *Radiology of the Small Bowel.* The Hague, the Netherlands: Martinus Nijhoff;1982:369–379.
32. Herlinger H, Maglinte DDT. Fold patterns in celiac disease (abstract). *Gastrointest Radiol.* 1985;10:300.
33. Herlinger H, Maglinte DDT. Jejunal fold separation in adult celiac disease: relevance of enteroclysis. *Radiology.* 1986;158:605–611.
34. Bova JG, Friedman AC, Weser E, et al. Adaptation of the ileum in nontropical sprue: reversal of the jejunoileal fold pattern. *AJR.* 1985;144:299–302.
35. La Seta F, Salerno G, Buccellato A, et al. Radiographic indicants of adult celiac disease assessed by double-contrast small bowel enteroclysis. *European J Radiol.* 1992;15:157–162.
36. Barlow JM, Johnson CD, Stephens DH. Celiac disease. How common is jejunoileal fold pattern reversal found at small-bowel follow-through? *AJR.* 1996;166:575–577.
37. Rubin CE, Haggit RC, Levine DS. Endoscopic mucosal biopsy. In: Yamada, T., ed. *Textbook of Gastroenterology.* Philadelphia, Pa: JB Lippincott Co; 1991;2479–2523.
38. Makuch RS, Bender GN. Proximal small bowel biopsy before enteroclysis. Presented at the 1996 Meeting of the Radiological Society of North America. Scientific program page 146. 1 December 1996; Chicago, IL.
39. Katz SI, Strober W. The pathogenesis of dermatitis herpetiformis. *J Invest Dermatol.* 1978;70:63–75.
40. Fry L. Dermatitis herpetiformis. *Baillieres Clin Gastroenterol.* 1995;9:371–393.
41. Collins P, Pukkala E, Reunala T. Malignancy and survival in dermatitis herpetiformis: a comparison with coeliac disease. *Gut.* 1996;38:529–530.
42. Mike N, Udeshi U, Asquith P, Ferrando J. Small bowel enema in non-responsive coeliac disease. *Gut.* 1990;31:883–885.
43. Upadhyay R, Park RHR, Russel RI, et al. Acute mesenteric ischemia. A presenting feature of coeliac disease? *Br Med J.* 1987;295:958–959.
44. Collins P, Reunala T, Pukkala E et al. Celiac disease associated disorders and survival. *Gut.* 1994;31:1215–1218.
45. Rensch MJ, Merenich JA, Lieberman M, et al. Gluten-sensitive enteropthy in patients with insulin-dependent diabetes mellitus. *Ann Int Med.* 1996;124:564–567.
46. Fine KD. The prevalence of occult gastrointesinal bleeding in celiac sprue. *N Eng J Med.* 1996;334:1163–1167.
47. Moch A, Herlinger H, Kochman ML. Enteroclysis in the evaluation of obscure gastrointestinal bleeding. *AJR.* 1994;163:1381–1384.
48. Dawson DJ, Sciberras CM, Whilwell H. Coeliac disease presenting with intestinal pseudo-obstruction. *Gut.* 1984;25:1003–1008.
49. Gefter WB, Evers KA, Malet PF, Kressel HY. Nontropical sprue with pneumatosis coli. *AJR.* 1981;137:624–625.
50. Khouri MR, Levine MS, Dabezies M, Saul SH. Benign pneumoperitoneum in a patient with celiac sprue. *J Clin Gastoenterol.* 1989;11:70–72.
51. Mawshinney H, Tomkin GH. Gluten enteropathy associated with selective IgA deficiency. *Lancet.* 1971;2:121–124.
52. Quigley EMM, Carmichael HA, Watkinson G. Adult celiac disease (celiac sprue), pernicious anemia and IgA deficiency. *J Clin Gastroenterol.* 1986;8:277–281.
53. Muller AF, Toghill PJ. Hyposplenism in gastrointestinal disease. *Gut.* 1995;36:165–167.
54. Corraza GR, Bullen AW, Hall R, Losowsky MS. A simple method of assessing splenic function in coeliac disease. *Clin Sci.* 1981;60:109–113.
55. Robertson DAF, Swinson CM, Hall R, Losowsky MS. Coeliac disease, splenic function and malignancy. *Gut.* 1982;23:666–669.
56. O'Grady JG, Stevens FM, Harding B, et al. Hyposplenism and gluten sensitive enteropathy. *Gastroenterology.* 1984;87:1326–1331.
57. Deutch SJ, Sandler MA, Alpern MB. Abdominal lymphadenopathy in benign diseases: CT detection. *Radiology.* 1987;163:335–338.
58. deBoer WA, Maas M, Tytgat GNJ. Disappearance of mesenteric lymphadenopathy with gluten-free diet in celiac sprue. *J Clin Gastroenterol.* 1993;16:317–319.
59. Matuchansky C, Colin R, Hemet J, et al. Cavitation of mesenteric lymph nodes, splenic atrophy, and a flat small intestinal mucosa. Report of six cases. *Gastroenterology.* 1984;87:606–614.
60. Holmes GKT. Mesenteric lymph node cavitation in coeliac disease. *Gut.* 1986;27:728–733.
61. Howat AJ, McPhie JL, Smith DA, et al. Cavitation of mesenteric lymph nodes: a rare complication of coeliac disease, associated with poor outcome. *Histopathology.* 1995;27:349–354.
62. Robertson DAF, Dixon MF, Scott BB, et al. Small intestinal ulceration. Diagnostic difficulties in relation to coeliac disease. *Gut.* 1983;24:565–574.
63. Wright DH. The major complications of coeliac disease. *Baillieres Clin Gastroenterol.* 1995;9:351–369.
64. Rubesin SE, Herlinger H, Saul SH, et al. Adult celiac

disease and its complications. *RadioGraphics.* 1989;9: 1045–1066.
65. Golden R. The small intestine and diarrhea. *AJR.* 1936;36:892–901.
66. Gough KR, Read AK, Naish JM. Intestinal reticulosis as a complication of idiopathic steatorrhea. *Gut.* 1962;3: 232–239.
67. Graeme-Cook FM. Pathological discussion. In: Case records of the Massachusetts General Hospital. *N Eng J Med.* 1996;334:1316–1322. Case 15-1996.
68. Wright DH, Jones DB, Clark H, et al. Is adult onset celiac disease due to a low-grade lymphoma of intraepithelial T lymphocytes? *Lancet.* 1991;337:1373–1374.
69. Cooper BT, Holmes GKT, Ferguson R, Cooke WT. Celiac disease and malignancy. *Medicine.* 1980;59: 249–261.
70. Swinson CM, Slavin G, Coles EC, Booth CC. Celiac disease and malignancy. *Lancet.* 1983;1:111–115.
71. Murray A, Cuevas EC, Jones DB, Wright DH. Study of immunohistochemistry and T-cell clonality of enteropathy-associated T cell lymphoma. *Am J Path.* 1995;146:509–519.
72. Bose SK, Lacour JP, Bodokh J, Ortonne JP. Malignant lymphoma and dermatitis herpetiformis. *Dermatology.* 1994;188:177–181.
73. Egan LJ, Walsh SV, Stevens FM, et al. Celiac-associated lymphoma. A single institution experience of 30 cases in the combination chemotherapy era. *J Clin Gastroenterol.* 1995;21:123–129.
74. Holmes GT, Dunn GI, Cockel R, Brookes VS. Adenocarcinoma of the upper small bowel complicating coeliac disease. *Gut.* 1980;21:1010–1016.
75. O'Brien CJ, Saverymuttu S, Hodgson HJF, Evans DJ. Coeliac disease, adenocarcinoma of jejunum and in situ squamous carcinoma of oesophagus. *J Clin Pathol.* 1983;36:62–67.
76. Chessler RK, Scherl ND, Schere BA, et al. Celiac sprue and pancreatic carcinoma. *J Clin Gastroenterol.* 1982;4: 173–175.
77. Begos CD, Kuan S, Dobbins J, Ravikumar S. Metachronous small-bowel adenocarcinoma in celiac sprue. *J Clin Gastroenterol.* 1995;20:233–236.
78. Case records of the Massachusetts General Hospital. *N Eng J Med.* 1990;322:1067–1075. Case 15-1990.
79. Westergaard H. The sprue syndrome. *Am J Med Sci.* 1985;290:249–262.
80. McLean AM, Farthing MJG, Kurian C, Mathan VI. The relationship betwen hypoalbuminaemia and the radiological appearances of the jejunum in tropical sprue. *Br J Radiol.* 1982;5:725–727.
81. Golladay LS, Byrne WJ. Intestinal pseudo-obstruction. *Surg Gyn Obstet.* 1981;153:257–273.
82. Rohrmann CA Jr, Ricci MT, Krishnamurthy S, Schuffler MD. Radiologic and histologic differentiation of neuromuscular disorders of the gastrointestinal tract. Visceral myopathies, visceral neuropathies, and progressive systemic sclerosis. *AJR.* 1981;143:933–941.
83. Schuffler MD, Leon SH, Krishnamurthy S. Intestinal pseudo-obstruction caused by a new form of visceral neuropathy: palliation by radical small bowel resection. *Gastroenterology.* 1985;89:115–1156.
84. Dudley HAF, Paterson-Brown S. Pseudo-obstruction (Editorial). *Br Med J.* 1986;292:1157–1158.
85. Recht MP, Levine MS, Katzka BA. Barrett's esophagus in scleroderma. Increased prevalence and radiographic findings. *Gastrointest Radiol.* 1988;13:1–5.
86. Horowitz AL, Meyers MA. The "hide-bound" small bowel of scleroderma. Characteristic mucosal fold pattern. *AJR.* 1973;119:332–334.
87. Myers MA, Ghahremani GG, Clements JL, Goodman K. Pneumatosis intestinalis. *Gastrointest Radiol.* 1977;2: 91–105.
88. Case records of the Massachusetts General Hospital. *N Eng J Med.* 1990;322:1796–1806. Case 25-1990.
89. Maglinte DDT, Chernish SM, DeWeese R, et al. Acquired jejunoileal diverticular disease. Subject review. *Radiology.* 1986;158:577–580.
90. Palder SB, Frey CB. Jejunal diverticulosis. *Arch Surg.* 1988;123:889–894.
91. Krishnamurthy S, Kelly MM, Rohrman CA, Schuffler MD. Jejunal diveritculosis. A heterogenous disorder caused by a variety of abnormalities of smooth muscle and myenteric plexus. *Gastroenterology.* 1983;85:538–547.
92. Williams RA. Surgical problems of diverticula of the small intestine. *Surg Gynecol Obstet.* 1983;152:621–626.
93. Donaldson RM Jr. Small bowel bacterial overgrowth. *Adv Int Med.* 1970;16:191–212.
94. Altmeier WA, Bryant LR, Wulsin JH. The surgical significance of jejunal diverticulosis. *Arch Surg.* 1963;86: 732–741.
95. Wright FW, Lumsden K. Recurrent pneumoperitoneum due to jejunal diverticulosis. *Clin Radiol.* 1975;26: 327–331.
96. Moch A, Herlinger H, Kochman ML, et al. Enteroclysis in the evaluation of obscure gastrointestinal bleeding. *AJR.* 1994;163:1381–1384.
97. Benya EC, Ghahremani GG, Brosnan JJ. Diverticulitis of the jejunum. Clinical and radiological features. *Gastrointest Radiol.* 1991;16:24–28.
98. Greenstein S, Jones B, Fishman EK, et al. Small-bowel diverticulitis: CT findings. *AJR.* 1986;147:271–274.
99. Friedman LS, Kirkham SE, Thistlethwaite JR, et al. Jejunal diverticulosis with perforation as a complication of Fabry's disease. *Gastroenterology.* 1984;86:558–563.
100. Weser E, Urban E. The short bowel syndrome. In: Berk JE, ed. *Bockus Gastroenterology.* 4th ed. Philadelphia, Pa: WB Saunders Co; 1985:1792–1802.
101. Buxton B. Small bowel resection and gastric hypersecretion. *Gut.* 1974;15:229–238.
102. Williams NS, Evans P, King RFGJ. Gastric acid secretion and gastrin production in the short bowel syndrome. *Gut.* 1985;26:914–919.
103. Bristol JD, Williamson RCN. Postoperative adaptation of the small intestine. *World J Surg.* 1985;9:825–832.
104. Miskowiak J, Andersen B. Intestinal adaptation after jejunoileal bypass for morbid obesity. A possible explanation for inadequate weight loss. *Br J Surg.* 1983;70:27.
105. Klish WJ, Putnam TC. The short gut. *Am J Dis Child.* 1981;135:2056–2061.

106. Pigot F, Messing B, Chaussade S, et al. Severe short bowel syndrome with a surgically reversed small bowel segment. *Digest Dis Sci.* 1990;35:137–144.
107. Frezza EE, Tzakis A, Fung JJ, Van Thiel DH. Small bowel transplantation: current progress and clinical application. *Hepatogastroenterology.* 1996;43:363–376.
108. Dobbins WO III. Current concepts of Whipple's disease (editorial). *J Clin Gastroenterol.* 1982;4:205–208.
109. Dobbins WO III, Kawanishi H. Bacillary characteristics in Whipple's disease. An electron microscopic study. *Gastroenterology.* 1981;80:1468–1475.
110. Relman DA, Schmidt TM, MacDermott RP, Falkow S. Identification of the uncultured bacillus of Whipple's disease. *N Eng J Med.* 1992;327:293–301.
111. vonHerbay A, Ditton H-J, Maiwald M. Diagnostic application of a polymerase chain reaction assay for the Whipple's disease bacterium to intestinal biopsies. *Gastroenterology.* 1996;110:1735–1743.
112. Geboes K, Ectors N, Heidbuchel H, et al. Whipple's disease: the value of upper gastrointestinal endoscopy for the diagnosis and follow-up. *Acta Gastroenterol Belg.* 1992;55:209–219.
113. Maizel H, Ruffin JM, Dobbins WO III. Whipple's disease: a review of 19 patients from one hospital and review of the literature since 1950. *Medicine.* 1970;99:175–205.
114. Winfield J, Dourmashkin RR, Gumpel JM. Diagnostic difficulties in Whipple's disease. *J Roy Soc Med.* 1979;72:859–863.
115. Dobbins WO III. Whipple's disease. In: Berk JE, ed. *Bockus Gastroenterology.* 4th ed. Philadelphia, Pa: WB Saunders Co; 1985:1803–1813.
116. Feldman M, Price G. Intestinal bleeding in patients with Whipple's disease. *Gastroenterology.* 1989;96:1207–1209.
117. Moorthy S, Nolley G, Hermos JA. Whipple's disease with minimal intestinal involvement. *Gut.* 1977;18:152–155.
118. Donaldson RM Jr. Whipple's disease—rare malady with uncommon potential (editorial). *N Eng J Med.* 1992;327:346–347.
119. Herlinger H. Radiology in malabsorption (editorial). *Clin Radiol.* 1992;45:73–78.
120. Davis SJ, Patel A. Case report. Distinctive echogenic lymphadenopathy in Whipple's disease. *Clin Radiol.* 1990;42:60–62.
121. Saleh H, Williams TM, Minda JM, Gupta PK. Whipple's disease involving the mesenteric lymph nodes diagnosed by fine-needle aspiration. *Diagn Cytopathol.* 1992;8:177–180.
122. Mayberry J, Furness P, Austin M, Toghill P. Endoscopic appearances in Whipple's disease. *J Roy Soc Med.* 1986;79:483–486.
123. Dobbins WO III, Klipstein FA. Chronic infections of the small intestine. In: Yamada T, ed. *Textbook of Gastroenterology.* Philadelphia, Pa: JB Lippincott Co; 1991:1472–1485.
124. Case records of the Massachusetts General Hospital. *N Eng J Med.* 1992;326:472–481. Case 7-1992.
125. Johnson AC, Johnson S, Lester PD, et al. Systemic mastocytosis-like syndrome: radiologic features of gastrointestinal manifestations. *Southern Med J.* 1988;81:729–733.
126. Scott BB, Hardy GJ, Losowsky MS. Involvement of the small intestine in systemic mast cell disease. *Gut.* 1975;16:918–924.
127. Stone GC. Case records of the Massachusetts General Hospital. *N Engl J Med.* 1986;315:816–824.
128. Ammann RW, Vetter D, Deyhle P, et al. Gastrointestinal involvement in systemic mastocytosis. *Gut.* 1976;17:107–112.
129. Huang T-Y, Yam LT, Li C-Y. Radiological features of systemic mast-cell disease. *Br J Radiol.* 1987;60:765–770.
130. Janowar ML. Mastocytosis of the gastrointestinal tract: Report of a case. *Acta Radiol.* 1962;57:489–493.
131. Cherner JA, Jensen RT, Dubois A, et al. Gastrointestinal dysfunction in systemic mastocytosis. A prospective study. *Gastroenterology.* 1988;95:657–667.
132. Case records of the Massachusetts General Hospital. *N Eng J Med.* 1993;329:343–349. Case 30-1993.
133. Morson BC, Dawson IMP. Inflammatory disorders. In: Chapter 20, *Gastrointestinal Pathology.* Oxford, England: Blackwell Scientific Publications; 1989:272–336.
134. Schulman A, Morton PCG, Dietrich PE. Eosinophilic gastroenteritis. *Clin Radiol.* 1980;31:101–104.
135. Caldwell JH, Mekhjian HS, Hurtubise PE, Beman FM. Eosinophilic gastroenteritis with obstruction. Immunological studies of seven patients. *Gastroenterology.* 1978;74:825–828.
136. Stallmeyer MJB, Chew FS. Eosinophilic gastroenteritis. *AJR.* 1993;161:296.
137. Talley NJ, Shorter RG, Phillips SF, Zinsmeister AR. Eosinophilic gastroenteritis: a clinicopathological study of patients with disease of the mucosa, muscle layer, and subserosal tissues. *Gut.* 1990;31:54–58.
138. Moore D, Lichtman S, et al. Eosinophilic gastroenteritis presenting in an adolescent with isolated colonic involvement. *Gut.* 1986;27:1219–1222.
139. Marnocha KE, Maglinte DDT, Kelvin FM, et al. Eosinophilic gastroenteritis associated with chronic eosinophilic pneumonia. *Am J Gastroenterol.* 1986;81:1205–1208.
140. Lloyd ML, Olsen WA. Abetalipoproteinemia. In: Yamada T, ed. *Textbook of Gastroenterology.* Philadelphia, Pa: JB Lippincott Co; 1991:1527.
141. Lee FD, Toner PG. *Biopsy Pathology of the Small Intestine.* London, England: Chapman and Hall; 1980.
142. Weinstein MA, Pearson KD, Agus SG. Abetalipoproteinemia. *Radiology.* 1973;108:269–273.
143. Yamada T, Del Valle J. Zollinger-Ellison syndrome. In: Yamada T, ed. *Textbook of Gastroenterology.* Philadelphia, Pa: JB Lippincott Co; 1991:1340–1352.
144. Norton JA, Doppman JL, Jensen RT. Curative resection in Zollinger-Ellison syndrome. Result of a 10-year prospective study. *Annals Surg.* 1992;215:8–18.
145. Zimmer T, Stolzer U, Bader M, et al. Brief report: a duodenal gastrinoma in a patient with diarrhea and normal serum gastrin concentrations. *N Eng J Med.* 1995;333:634–636.
146. Cadiot G, Houillier P, Allouch A, et al. Oral calcium

tolerance test in the early diagnosis of primary hyperparathyroidism and multiple endocrine neoplasia type 1 in patients with the Zollinger-Ellison syndrome. *Gut.* 1996;39:273–278.
147. Benya RV, Metz DC, Venzon DJ, et al. Zollinger-Ellison syndrome can be the initial endocrine manifestation in patients with multiple endocrine neoplasia-type 1. *Am J Med.* 1994;97:436–444.
148. Miller TA. Comment to paper by Fraker DL, Norton JA, Alexander HR, et al. Zollinger-Ellison syndrome. Surgery should still play an important role in its management. *Gastroenterology.* 1996;108:1601–1602.
149. Miller LS, Vinayek R, Frucht H, et al. Reflux esophagitis in patients with Zollinger-Ellison syndrome. *Gastroenterology.* 1990;98:341–346.
150. Gibril F, Doppman JL, Chang R, et al. Metastatic gastrinoma: localization with selective arterial injection of secretin. *Radiology.* 1996;198:77–84.
151. Hammond PJ, Bloom SR. Searching for gastrinomas. Visceral angiography is improving detection. *BMJ.* 1993;307:4–6.
152. Wolfe MM: Localization of gastrinoma using arterial secretin stimulation—worthwhile or passing fancy? *Gastroenterology.* 1991;100:1472–1474.
153. Cadiot G, Lebtahi R, Sarda L, et al. Preoperative detection of duodenal gastrinomas and peripancreatic lymph nodes by somatostatin receptor scintigraphy. *Gastroenterology.* 1996;111:845–854.
154. Gibril F, Reynolds JC, Doppman JL, et al. Somatostatin receptor scintigraphy: its sensitivity compared with that of other imaging methods in detecting primary and metastatic gastrinomas. A prospective study. *Ann Int Med.* 1996;125:26–34.
155. Termanini B, Gibril F, Reynolds JC, et al. Value of somatostatin receptor scintigraphy: a prospective study in gastrinoma of its effect on clinical mangement. *Gastroenterology.* 1997;112:335–347.
156. Scott PP, Scott WW, Siegelman SS. Amyloidosis: an overview. *Seminars Roentgenol.* 1986;21:103–112.
157. Hawkins PN, Lavender JP, Pepys MB. Evaluation of systemic amyloidosis by scintigraphy with 123 I-labeled serum amyloid P component. *N Eng J Med.* 1990;323:508–513.
158. Zerner D. Colchicine in the prevention and treatment of the amyloidosis of familial Mediterranean fever. *N Engl J Med.* 1986;314:1001–1005.
159. Becker SA, Bass D, Nissim F. Crohn's ileitis complicated by amyloidosis. Observations and therapeutic considerations. *J Clin Gastroenterol.* 1985;7:296–300.
160. Tada S, Iida M, Yao T, et al. Intestinal pseudo-obstruction in patients with amyloidosis: clinicopathologic differences between chemical types of amyloid protein. *Gut.* 1993;34:1412–1417.
161. Chilovi F, Dobrilla G. Familial Mediterranean fever: first report from Italy. *Ital J Gastroenterol Hepatol.* 1985;17:275–277.
162. Legge DA, Carlson HC, Wollaeger EE. Roentgenologic appearance of systemic amyloidosis involving gastrointestinal tract. *AJR.* 1970;110:406–412.
163. Tada S, Iida M, Fuchigami T, et al. Barium meal study for amyloidosis of the small intestine: measurements on radiographs. *Gastrointest Radiol.* 1990;15:320–324.
164. Tada S, Iida M, Matsui T, et al. Amyloidosis of the small intestine. Findings on double contrast radiographs. *AJR.* 1991;156:741–744.
165. Tada S, Iida M, Yao T, et al. Gastrointestinal amyloidosis. Radiologic features by chemical types. *Radiology.* 1994;190:37–42.
166. Urban BA, Fishman EK, Goldman SM, et al. CT evaluation of amyloidosis. Spectrum of disease. *Radiographics.* 1993;13:1295–1308.
167. Walker JJ, Kaplan DS. Efficacy of somatostatin analog octreotide in the treatment of two patients with refractory diabetic diarrhea. *Am J Gastroenterol.* 1993;88:765–767.
168. Hammond JB, Littman A. Disaccharide malabsorption. In: Berk JE, ed. *Bockus Gastroenterology.* 4th ed. Philadelphia, Pa: WB Saunders Co; 1985:1703–1718.
169. Laws JW, Neale G. Radiological diagnosis of disaccharidase deficiency. *Lancet.* 1966;2:139–143.
170. DeBeer SC, Mallya RK, Fagan EA, et al. Serum amyloid-A protein concentration in inflammatory diseases and its relationship to the incidence of reactive systemic amyloidosis. *Lancet.* 1982;2:231–233.
171. Rubin W. Lymphangiectasia. In: Yamada T, ed. *Textbook of Gastroenterology.* Philadelphia, Pa: JB Lippincott Co; 1991:1419–1420.
172. Heresbach D, Raoul JL, Genetet N, et al. Immunological study in primary intestinal lymphangiectasia. *Digestion.* 1994;55:59–64.
173. Aoyagi K, Iida M, Yao T, et al. Intestinal lymphangiectasia: value of double-contrast radiographic study. *Clin Radiol.* 1994;49:814–819.
174. Puri AS, Aggarwal R, Gupta RK, et al. Intestinal lymphangiectasia: evaluation by CT and scintigraphy. *Gastrointest Radiol.* 1992;17:119–121.
175. Case records of the Massachusetts General Hospital. *N Eng J Med.* 1990;322:183–192. Case 3-1990.
176. Gad A, Willen R, Carlen B, et al. Duodenal involvement in Waldenstrom's macroglobulinemia. *J Clin Gastroenterol.* 1995;20:174–177.
177. Waldenstrom J. Incipient myelomatosis or "essential" hyperglobulinemia with fibrinogenopenia—a new syndrome? *Acta Med Scand.* 1944;117:216–247.
178. Taussig L, Saldino R, di Sant'Agnese P. Radiographic abnormalities of the duodenum and small bowel in cystic fibrosis of the pancreas (mucoviscidosis). *Radiology.* 1973;106:369–376.

Small Bowel Neoplasms

Dean D.T. Maglinte and Hans Herlinger

Chapter Contents

Introduction
Benign Tumors
Malignant Tumors
Non-Hodgkin's Lymphoma
Hodgkin's Disease
Leiomyosarcoma
Secondary Malignancies

Introduction

The early diagnosis of small bowel neoplasms continues to be a challenge to clinical medicine.[1] Frequent atypical presentations increase the diagnostic difficulty of both malignant and benign small bowel tumors. Particularly with malignant tumors, the main focus of radiologic examination should be to draw attention to their likely presence at a time when curative removal is still possible.[2] Even if a specific radiologic diagnosis is not possible, the unequivocal recognition of a small bowel mass that is likely to represent a neoplasm is of profound importance to the management of a patient, as it will prompt surgical exploration. A continuing significant problem in the radiologic diagnosis of small bowel neoplasms is the false-negative radiographic examination (Fig. 19-1).[3–5] A false-negative examination deflects the clinical work-up away from the small bowel, wasting time and money in eventually reaching a diagnosis. More importantly, delays in diagnosis adversely affect the survival of patients with small bowel malignancies and also result in significant morbidity in patients with benign neoplasms. Clinicians rely on a good-quality small bowel study to find early disease or exclude its presence beyond the range of the endoscope.[4] Because of the low prevalence of small bowel disease, there is a need for a diagnostic examination with a high negative predictive value and proven accuracy.[3,6] The evolving technology of enteroscopy can play a significant role in the diagnosis of small bowel tumors, but predominantly used instruments cover an only limited length of small bowel[7,8] and are no substitute for barium studies.[3] Radiologists, therefore, should assume a major role in the work-up of patients with possible small bowel neoplasms.

Although the small intestine represents 75% of the total length of the gastrointestinal tract and more than 90% of its total mucosal surface, it is a rare site for neoplasms. It is the site of origin of less than 25% of all gastrointestinal neoplasms and of less than 2% of all malignant neoplasms. Precise numbers expressing the prevalence and distribution of the many forms of malignant neoplasms involving the small intestine differ among reports in the medical literature. Some reports confine themselves to the mesenteric small intestine (ie, jejunum and ileum); others include the duodenum. The prevalence of small bowel neoplasms in autopsy reports and clinical reports varies considerably; benign tumors are more common in autopsy reports (74% of lesions), whereas malignant neoplasms account for 75% of symptomatic lesions leading to surgery.[9,10] The reported age-adjusted incidence is 1 per 100,000 population, with a prevalence of 0.6%.[11] Males have a higher incidence of small bowel neoplasms than females. Malignant small bowel tumors account for 1.4% of gastrointestinal cancers. Colonic malignancies are 50 to 60 times more common.[12] Like colon cancer, small bowel malignancies appear to be more prevalent in Western populations.

More than 35 histologic types of small bowel neoplasms have been identified.[13] Leiomyomas are the most common benign lesion, whereas adenocarcinomas are the most frequent primary malignancy. Their incidence appears to increase from duodenum to jejunum, but per unit area the duodenum is still the most common site. Carcinoid tumors occur most frequently in the ileum. Adenomas in the small bowel, similar to their counterparts in the colon, may be premalignant. This is exemplified by patients with familial adenomatous polyposis, more than 50% of whom will develop small bowel polyps that may progress to

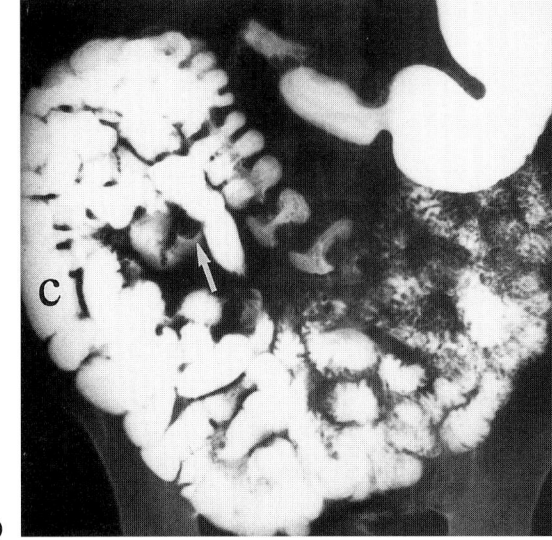 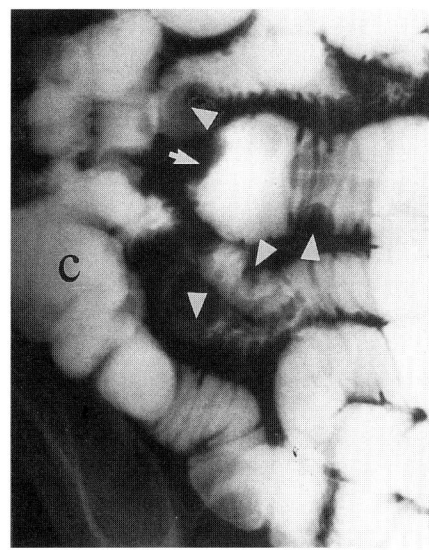

Fig. 19-1. Radiologic delay in diagnosing tumors of the small intestine. False-negative conventional small bowel follow-through (SBFT) in an elderly woman with unexplained recurrent abdominal pain and anemia.
(a) Overhead SBFT radiograph of prone patient was reported without abnormality. In retrospect, there is a small polypoid defect (arrow) in a loop of ileum in the right hemiabdomen. (C = cecum) (b) After referral to a gastroenterologist, enteroclysis was done 6 months later for similar indications. It shows multiple intramural defects (arrowheads) with partial obstruction of one segment by the largest mass (arrow). Surgery revealed multifocal carcinoid with extension to mesenteric nodes. (C = cecum) (From Maglinte and Reyes,[2] with permission.)

adenocarcinoma.[14,15] Other hereditary diseases associated with the development of small bowel tumors include multiple endocrine neoplasia syndrome type I, gastric sarcoma, and von Recklinghausen's disease (paragangliomas).

Etiologic Factors

Despite having cell proliferation rates similar to those of the colon, the small bowel is less susceptible to tumor formation. Several mechanisms are postulated to account for this reduced incidence of neoplastic transformation.[16,17] The contents of the small bowel are liquid and may be less irritating to the mucosa. In addition, the contents of the small bowel are at a neutral or alkaline pH and also contain a high level of benzopyrene hydroxylases, which may inhibit carcinogens.[18] The transit time through the small bowel is much faster than that through the colon, thereby reducing the time of exposure to potential carcinogens.[19] The bacterial flora of the small bowel has fewer anaerobes and far lower total bacterial counts than the colon; bacterial degradation of bile salts to carcinogenic metabolites in the colon is often postulated as a source of colonic carcinogenesis. Immunoproliferative small intestinal disease (Mediterranean lymphoma or α-chain disease), a condition found in the Middle East, is associated with chronic enteric infection by bacteria and parasites, poor sanitation, and low economic status.[20] If untreated, an eventual impairment of normal immunologic and mechanical barriers may relate to its progression to diffuse intestinal lymphoma. The normal small bowel is rich in lymphoid tissue with a high level of surface IgA expression, and this may be protective, whereas the increase in frequency of small bowel tumors in Crohn's disease may indicate a decrease in the surveillance capability of the small bowel.[21] It has been noted that patients with small bowel malignancies experience a higher incidence of tumors at other sites, reinforcing the importance of the immunoprotective role of the small bowel.[22]

Malignant stromal tumors occur with equal infrequency throughout the alimentary tract. With regard to metastases, however, the small intestine has its full share in accordance with its length and larger surface area.

Clinical Presentation

More than 50% of benign lesions remain asymptomatic and are discovered at autopsy. Symptomatic benign neoplasms usually manifest with obstructive features, producing intermittent abdominal pain, or, occasionally, signs of complete bowel obstruction.

Constitutional symptoms such as anorexia, malaise, and weight loss are infrequent, as is the ability to palpate the tumor at clinical examination. Intermittent obstruction can be caused by intussusception; benign tumors are responsible for the majority of adult cases of intussusception.[23]

Bleeding, usually occult, occurs in about 30% to 40% of patients with benign tumors.[23,24] Gastrointestinal bleeding may be due to ulceration of an epithelial adenoma, or from the mucosa overlying an intramural tumor. In reports in which enteroclysis was used to evaluate occult gastrointestinal blood loss, small bowel neoplasms accounted for one half of the positive findings; there was nearly equal detection of benign and malignant tumors.[25,26] Rarely, benign tumors bleed severely and require emergency therapy.[23] An exoenteric benign tumor occasionally induces intestinal volvulus or compromises the lumen by a simple mass effect. Benign small bowel tumors are usually discovered in persons between the ages of 50 and 80 years and occur with equal frequency in men and women.

In patients with histologically confirmed primary malignancies of the small intestine, abdominal pain is the most common (69%) presenting symptom.[27] In this study, gastrointestinal bleeding was noted in 52%, nausea and/or vomiting in 49%, weight loss (more than 5 lb) in 45%, diarrhea in 29%, and a palpable abdominal mass in only 4% In the same review, obstruction was stated to be the presentation in 36% of the patients. At the time of surgery, the majority of patients had local extension of the tumor and/or distant tumor spread. Primary small bowel malignancies are most common between 50 and 70 years of age.

Imaging Considerations

Despite significant improvements in diagnostic technology and operative mortality, the survival of patients with primary malignancies of the small intestine has not changed in four decades. One reason for the failure to improve prognosis has been the considerable delay before the diagnosis is made, resulting in an advanced stage of disease at the time of surgery. An analysis of the contributions to this delay in diagnosis showed that responsibility was shared by patients who failed to report symptoms, physicians who failed to order the appropriate diagnostic tests, and radiologists who did not arrive at a correct diagnosis.[27] This study showed that the major delay in diagnosis occurred after medical help was sought by the patient. The delay before medical contact (patient's delay) was only one seventh of the delay after medical contact (physician's delay). Although radiologists were responsible for a minority of the physicians' errors, radiologic errors caused the longest periods of delay of diagnoses. This report concluded that only greater awareness of the small intestine as a potential source of unexplained abdominal symptoms would lead to more prompt use of sensitive methods of radiologic examination (Fig. 19-2) and thus to improvement of the patient's prognosis.[27]

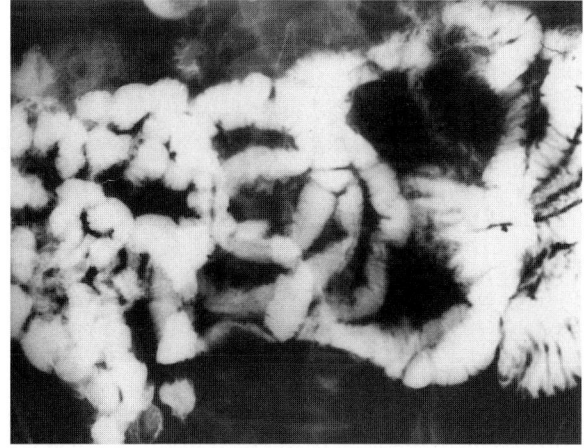
(a)

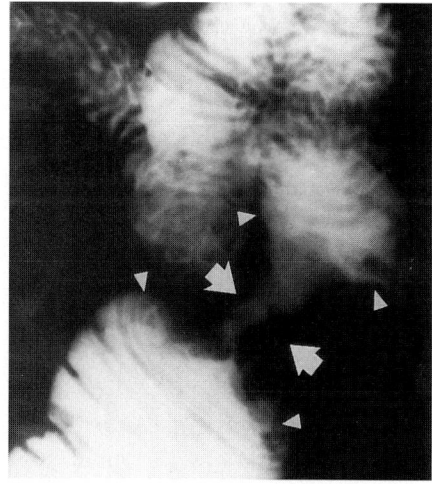
(b)

Fig. 19-2. Unreliable negative predictive value of SBFT in excluding small bowel malignancy.
(a) Representative overhead radiograph of most recent of two SBFTs done in a 1½-year period for anemia in an elderly male. At the last examination the referring physician was asked to rule out malignancy. Both examinations were reported as negative for malignancy. (b) Enteroclysis done following referral to a gastroenterologist 6 months later shows a typical apple-core lesion highly suggestive of an annular adenocarcinoma of the jejunum. Arrows indicate narrowed segment with mucosal destruction, and arrowheads show overhanging edges. (From Maglinte,[27] with permission.)

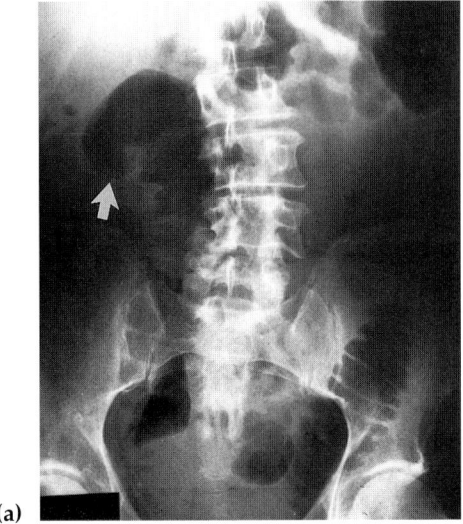 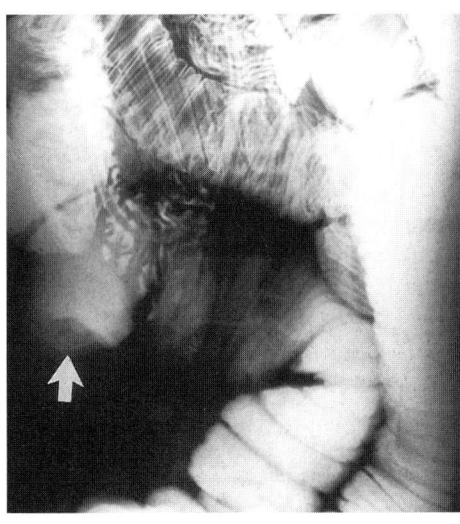

Fig. 19-3. Plain film radiography in small bowel malignancy presenting as possible small bowel obstruction. (a) Supine radiograph of elderly male with diffuse abdominal pain and history of prior appendectomy shows dilated loops of small bowel and normal colon gas distribution suggestive of small bowel obstruction. Abrupt smooth termination of gas column (arrow) was suspected as point of adhesive obstruction. (b) Enteroclysis performed following overnight long tube decompression, to assess severity of obstruction for planned nonsurgical management, confirmed suggested point of obstruction on plain film but revealed a mass (arrow) producing complete obstruction. Surgery revealed carcinoid. Adjacent nodes were involved.

Plain film radiography has a very limited role in diagnosis but may provide diagnostic information if it is performed during an obstructive episode (Fig. 19-3) or if an ulcerating or necrotic tumor has perforated. The soft-tissue outline of a tumor, its displacement of adjacent, gas-filled bowel, or the presence of tumor calcification can be a means of positive identification by plain film radiography.

Except for the proximal jejunum, which can sometimes be reached during upper gastrointestinal (GI) panendoscopy, and the distal part of the terminal ileum, which can often be entered by the colonoscope, the preoperative demonstration of a tumor of the mesenteric small bowel depends on contrast radiology, preferably a barium examination by the enteroclysis method. In the patient evaluated for unexplained gastrointestinal bleeding, the technique of enteroclysis is modified to include the duodenum. The duodenal sweep is examined in detail either simultaneously or after the jejunoileal assessment (Fig. 19-4).

The reported sensitivity for the detection of malignant small bowel tumors by the small bowel follow-through (SBFT) examination, the most commonly used method in most institutions, varies widely. Most studies have accepted indirect as well as direct evidence of a tumor as being diagnostic. An abnormality shown by the SBFT has been reported in 53% to 83% of primary malignant tumors, although direct evidence of a tumor was noted in only 30% to 44% of the cases.[28–30] In a study comparing the sensitivity and tumor detec-

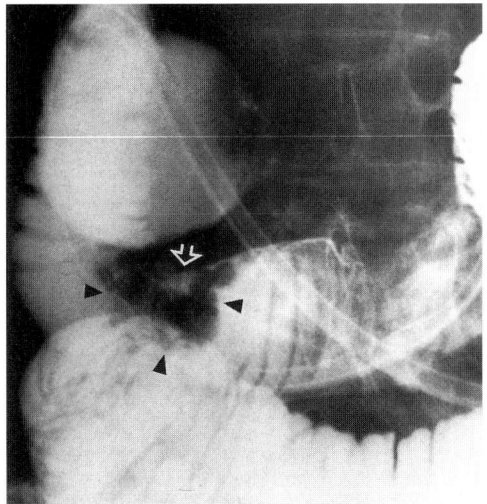

Fig. 19-4. Modification of enteroclysis technique in the patient with unexplained gastrointestinal (GI) bleeding and a negative upper GI panendoscopy.
A lobulated mass (arrowheads) with ulceration (arrow) is shown in the proximal horizontal segment during infusion of barium after the enteroclysis catheter had been retracted into the horizontal segment. The mass did not interfere with antegrade tube passage. Repeat endoscopy and biopsy confirmed presence of a villous adenocarcinoma. This maneuver should be performed routinely in the evaluation of anemia or unexplained GI bleeding because the segment of duodenum distal to the ampulla may not be visualized at an esophagogastroduodenoscopy. (From Maglinte and Reyes,[2] with permission.)

tion rate of the small bowel enema (enteroclysis) and the SBFT, the SBFT showed abnormalities in 11 of 18 patients for a sensitivity of 61% and enteroclysis showed abnormalities in 19 of 20 patients for a sensitivity of 95%.[30] The actual tumor detection rate was 33% (6 of 18 patients) for the SBFT and 90% (18 of 20 patients) for enteroclysis. Four patients had both types of examination, with normal findings on conventional SBFT followed by demonstration of a tumor by enteroclysis.

Radiologists have to assume responsibility for the preoperative imaging and diagnosis of small bowel neoplasms. This requires the use of optimal barium contrast techniques.[31] For this reason, several investigators have advocated enteroclysis, noting that technical factors inherent in small bowel follow-through studies have accounted for frequent false-negative diagnoses.[2,5,30,32] Reported series have shown enteroclysis to be more reliable not only in the demonstration of small bowel tumors, but also in the evaluation of occult gastrointestinal bleeding and of intestinal obstruction.[25,26,32–37] Increasingly, the role of barium studies is complemented by computed tomography (CT), ultrasonography, and magnetic resonance. CT, in particular, is playing an increasingly important role in the detection of small bowel neoplasms.[38] CT is now frequently used for the evaluation of patients with vague abdominal symptoms and may provide the initial opportunity to detect and characterize tumors of the small bowel. The recognition of certain patterns of CT findings now allows a reasonable distinction to be made between benign and malignant small bowel tumors (Fig. 19-5) and, in cases of certain benign tumors, such as lipoma and leiomyoma, may make it possible to suggest the specific diagnosis.[39,40]

A retrospective review of 40 malignant tumors in one institution over 14 years found that barium studies detected 20 of 24 (83%) in patients who underwent small bowel radiography. CT and ultrasonography were less sensitive for jejunal tumors (17% and 31%, respectively) than for duodenal tumors (100% and 50%, respectively) or ileal tumors (70% and 73%, respectively).[41] In a review of CT findings in 35 patients with small bowel neoplasms, CT findings were considered abnormal in 97%, with the neoplasm demonstrated in 80%.[41] Barium studies were interpreted as abnormal in 80% of the patients in whom they were done. In another report, CT was interpreted as showing the tumor in 73% of the cases.[39] Of 17 undetected tumors, all were smaller than 3 cm and most were 2 cm or smaller (Fig. 19-6). CT demonstrates extraluminal extension of malignant tumors, can help stage lym-

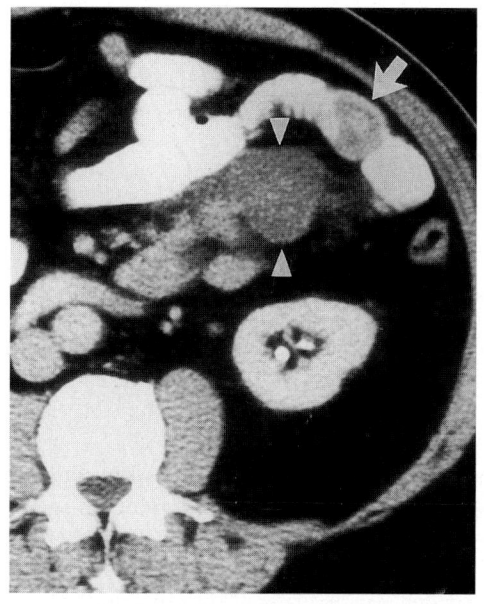
(a)

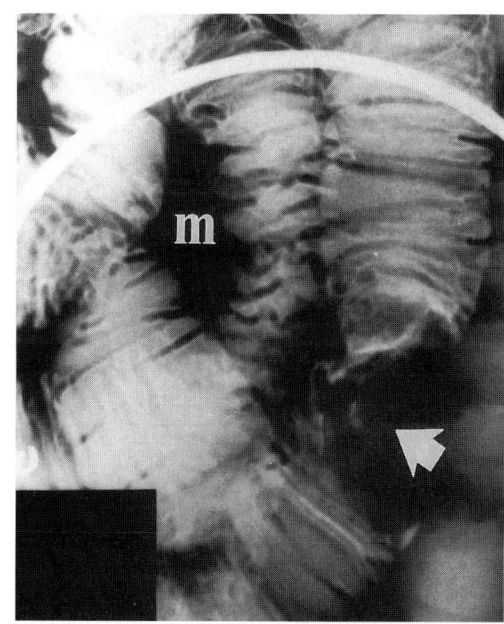
(b)

Fig. 19-5. CT imaging of malignant small bowel tumor.
(a) Section through midabdomen shows an ulcerating annular lesion in jejunum (arrow) with an associated mesenteric mass (arrowheads) in a 54-year-old male with vague abdominal pain. The pattern is suggestive of a malignant small bowel tumor, either a non-Hodgkin's lymphoma or an adenocarcinoma with mesenteric involvement. (b) Enteroclysis done prior to the CT demonstrates a moderately long annular ulcerating lesion in the jejunum (arrow) suggestive of a malignant jejunal tumor. Subtle separation of adjacent loops (m) suggests mass in mesentery but is easier to appreciate on CT. Surgery revealed non-Hodgkin's lymphoma. (Courtesy of Jack Scatarige, MD.)

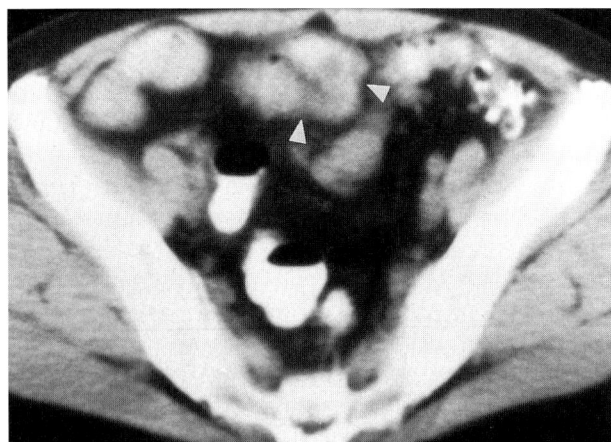
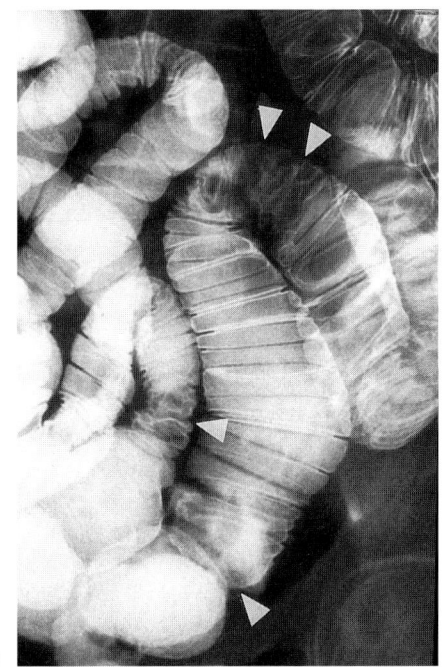

Fig. 19-6. Imaging of focal intramural neoplasm—complementary role of CT and barium examinations. (a) CT section through upper pelvis of 65-year-old patient with weight loss and unexplained anemia. Examination was initially interpreted as unremarkable. Note subtle focal mural nodularity (arrowheads), which is difficult to appreciate because of isoattenuating effect of positive luminal contrast. (b) Enteroclysis done after CT shows nodular thickening (arrowheads) of multiple segments of small bowel in pelvis suggestive of non-Hodgkin's lymphoma. Surgery confirmed preoperative diagnosis.

phomas, and may identify secondary mesenteric and hepatic disease. In cases of acute gastrointestinal hemorrhage arising from benign or malignant neoplasms, angiographic techniques provide precise localization of the bleeding site and allow therapeutic transcatheter control of the hemorrhage. Angiographic demonstration of tumor neovascularity without contrast agent extravasation may also be of diagnostic importance, especially in patients with chronic occult bleeding when other diagnostic studies, endoscopy, and barium contrast have been negative.[42] Scintigraphy with technetium-labeled red blood cells may identify bleeding sites with blood loss rates as low as 0.1 ml/min.[43] In unexplained bleeding, intraoperative enteroscopy may allow visualization of the lesion even if it is nonpalpable.

A small bowel neoplasm diagnosed only at surgical exploration performed as an elective procedure or as an emergency, not uncommon in the past, is currently a rarity with the armamentarium of the investigational methods employed. When the cause of abdominal pain or gastrointestinal bleeding has not been found, empiric treatment should not be a substitute for further diagnostic studies. If no significant disease is identified in the upper gastrointestinal tract or colon, the small bowel should be studied to exclude it as the site of disease.[27]

Benign Tumors

Leiomyomas, adenomas, lipomas, and hemangiomas account for approximately 90% of benign small bowel neoplasms. Reports of benign tumors arising from virtually all other mesenchymal cell types have appeared in the literature.[44] Benign neoplasms commonly display similar morphologic characteristics on barium contrast studies. Because of this, a specific histologic diagnosis is usually not possible, but a useful differential diagnosis can be obtained in most instances by observing the location, the number of lesions, and radiographic features of the tumor. A European study of surgically confirmed benign small bowel tumors diagnosed over a period of 7 years by enteroclysis reported that the average time lapse from the onset of symptoms to diagnosis was 16 months (range = 1 month to 7 years).[45] This report suggested that enteroclysis is an effective means for evaluating patients with unexplained abdominal symptoms when the possibility of a benign small bowel tumor is a clinical consideration.

Leiomyoma

Leiomyoma is the most common symptomatic benign small bowel tumor and occurs predominantly in the fifth decade of life. It has a slightly greater frequency of occurrence in the jejunum than in the ileum.[46] It may arise in a Meckel's diverticulum or in a small bowel blind pouch. On gross examination, four growth patterns are identified: intramural, intraluminal (indicating an endoenteric growth), extraluminal (exoenteric), and dumbbell (bidirectional). Leiomyomas are usually grayish-white, firm, and often umbilicated with a central ulceration secondary to compromise of the vascular supply. Microscopically, they consist of well-differentiated smooth muscle cells with an absence of mitoses. On occasion, the histologic picture is unclear and borderline malignancy can be difficult to exclude.

These tumors generally present with bleeding (67%); obstruction from either luminal compression or intussusception is the next most common presentation (25%).[47] The time interval between the onset of symptoms and radiological diagnosis ranges from a few months to 5 years.[48] Intramural, intraluminal, and bidirectional growth patterns are diagnosed by barium contrast examination as either oval or round defects reflecting their predominant sites of involvement (Fig. 19-7). Extraluminal (exoenteric or subserosal) leiomyomas, unless large, are difficult to diagnose with barium studies. Such lesions may show only displacement of bowel loops by the extrinsic tumor. They are, however, readily demonstrated by cross-sectional imaging methods (Fig. 19-8).

Leiomyomas are responsible for approximately half of the cases of small bowel tumors that present with either an acute or chronic bleeding episode.[23,26] Angiography may demonstrate these lesions, even in the absence of active bleeding.[49] Although the vascularity of smooth muscle tumors is variable, they are usually hypervascular with intense capillary opacification and with early visualization of draining veins (Fig. 19-9). The more hypovascular tumors tend to have prominent vessels in their periphery. If radionuclide scintigraphy with technetium-99m (99mTc)–red blood cells is performed during an episode of gastrointestinal bleeding, leiomyomas may be manifested by a focal area of increased uptake.[50] This finding may be confused with a bleeding Meckel's diverticulum.[51] The CT appearance of leiomyomas is fairly characteristic.[52] They produce sharply defined spheric or ovoid masses, ranging from 1 to 10 cm in size, and display homogeneous tissue density and uniform contrast enhancement. Calcifications are occasionally noted within the tumor.

The malignant potential of leiomyomas is related mainly to the size and biologic behavior of the tumor, rather than their histologic appearances. Large size and extensive tumor cavitation are more common in the presence of malignancy. Experience with CT also suggests that malignant smooth muscle tumors are larger than benign tumors, less uniform in shape, and of variable attenuation.[52]

Adenoma

Small bowel adenomas are probably the most common benign small bowel tumor, but most remain asymptomatic. Review of their histology, however, has shown that many were misinterpreted hamartomas or inflammatory polyps.[53] True adenomas occur mostly in the duodenum. They are similar to their large bowel counterparts in histological type (tubular, villous, tubulovillous). Like large bowel adenomas, they can be premalignant, with villous architecture, increasing size, and atypia being markers of malignant progression; up to one third of villous duodenal adenomas contain invasive elements.[54] They occur predominantly in the periampullary region of the descending duodenum (see Fig. 19-4). Most small bowel adenomas are single, usually in older patients, but occasionally multiple adenomas are present, especially in those with variations of familial adenomatous polyposis or Gardner's syndrome.[55] Small bowel adenomas should be differentiated from Brunner's gland adenomas, which arise from specific mucus-secreting glands. Brunner's gland enlargement is caused by the accumulation of secreted mucin, by diffuse hyperplasia, or by the formation of a discrete polypoid adenoma. These lesions are found most frequently in the duodenum but may also be noted in the proximal jejunum or ileum.[44]

Adenomas are usually asymptomatic. Bleeding and/or obstruction are the usual presentations in adenomas that become symptomatic. Obstruction is secondary to pedunculated tumors that may intussuscept.

Typical adenomas are small (1 to 3 cm), smooth or lobulated polypoid lesions. On barium studies they appear as either sessile or pedunculated intraluminal defects (Fig. 19-10). The stalk of pedunculated adenomas can be several centimeters long so that the polyp may exhibit considerable movement within the bowel lumen.

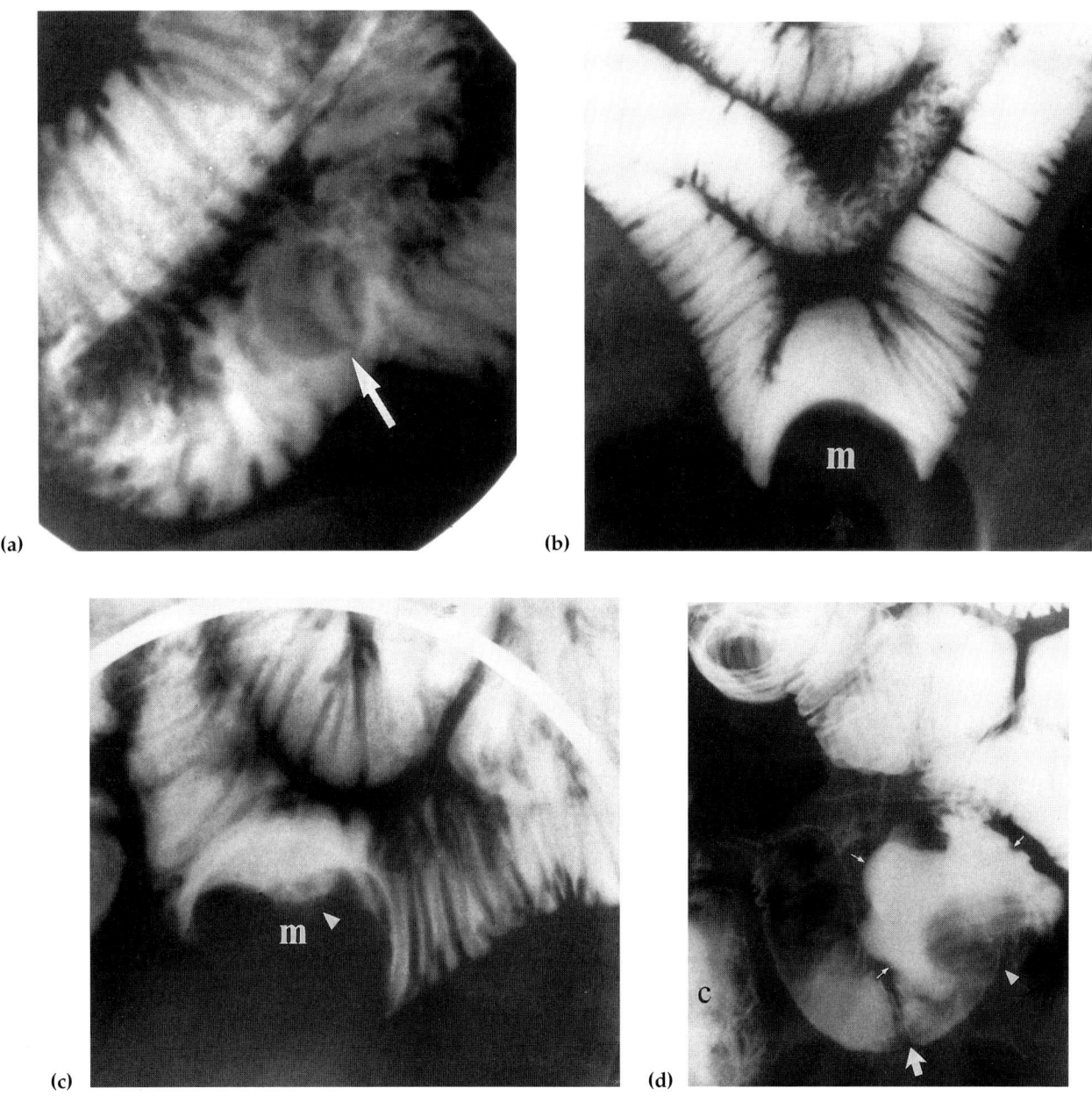

Fig. 19-7. Endoenteric and intramural patterns of small bowel leiomyomas.
(a) A small intraluminal rounded mass (arrow) is seen in the proximal jejunum on enteroclysis of a middle-aged man with unexplained GI bleeding. At surgery, a leiomyoma was found. The intraluminal pattern of a leiomyoma is indistinguishable from that of other benign polypoid neoplasms. (Courtesy of Richard P. Gold, MD.) (b) A rounded intramural (m) mass is shown by enteroclysis in pelvic ileum of a 45-year-old male with recent onset melena. The appearance is highly suggestive of an intramural leiomyoma. (c) An ovoid (arrows) mass is present in the distal ileum on enteroclysis of a middle-aged man with unexplained anemia. Note ulceration (arrowhead) in center of the mass. Prior small bowel follow-through was unremarkable. Surgery revealed ulcerating leiomyoma. (Courtesy of George Harrell, MD.) (d) Leiomyoma in a blind pouch. An intraluminal polypoid mass (arrowhead) is present within a dilated segment (small arrows) of distal ileum proximal to a surgical anastomosis (large arrow) in a patient with unexplained GI bleeding. (C = cecum) At surgery, a leiomyoma was found growing in a blind pouch proximal to an end-to-side ileoileal anastomosis done at birth for intestinal atresia (With permission from Maglinte DDT et al. Leiomyoma in a "blind pouch." *Dig Dis Sci.* 1984;29:376–379).

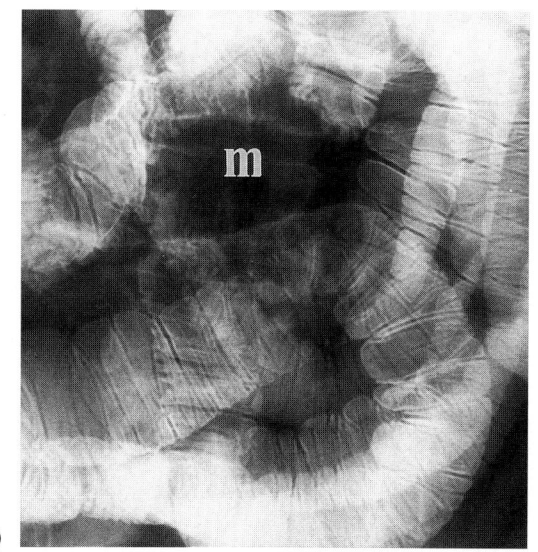 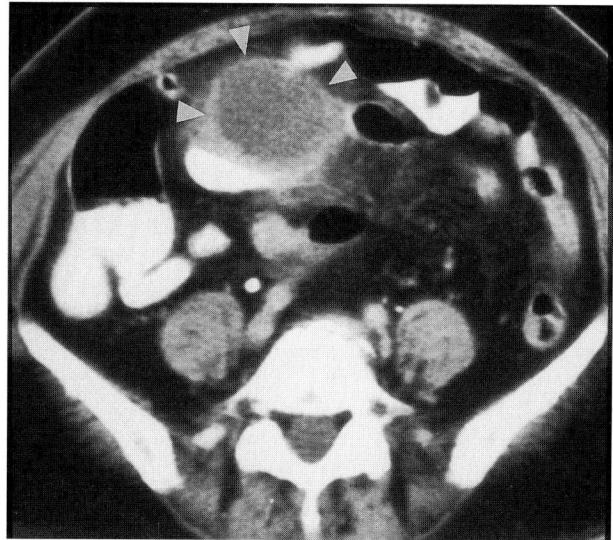

Fig. 19-8. Exoenteric growth pattern of a leiomyoma.
(a) Enteroclysis examination of a 69-year-old man for unexplained abdominal pain shows subtle flattening of walls and separation of loops of small bowel in midabdomen suggestive of a mesenteric mass (m). The folds are normal. (b) CT section through midabdomen shows a large homogeneous mass in mesentery displacing adjacent loops of small bowel (arrowheads). Surgery revealed a necrotic leiomyoma. There was no evidence of malignancy.

Lipoma

Lipomas are variously regarded as the second commonest[24,44,55] or third commonest[48] benign tumor of the small bowel. They usually occur in the distal small bowel, but occasionally are found more proximally. For the most part, they are seen in the sixth and seventh decades of life. Less than one third are symptomatic. The commonest clinical presentation is with obstruction, usually caused by intussusception, or bleeding

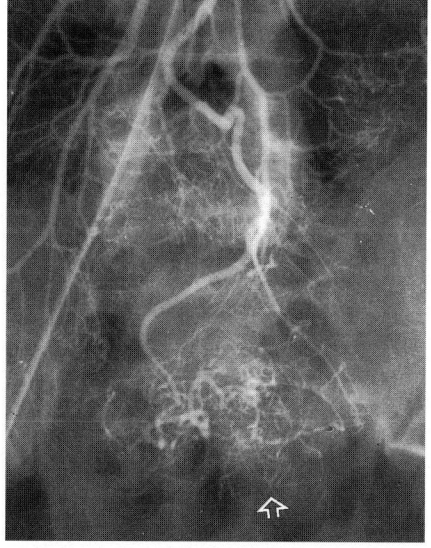 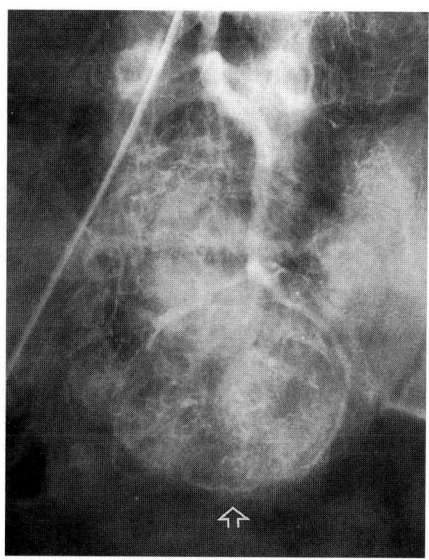

Fig. 19-9. Angiography of a leiomyoma.
(a) Arterial phase. Dilated ileal branches of the superior mesenteric artery supply many tumor vessels to a mass (arrow) in the upper pelvis. (b) Venous phase. There is an increase in contrast accumulation throughout the tumor. Vessels are displaced around the tumor (arrow). Note early and dense venous drainage. An encapsulated hypervascular tumor is suggested by the findings. A leiomyoma of the ileum was found at surgery.

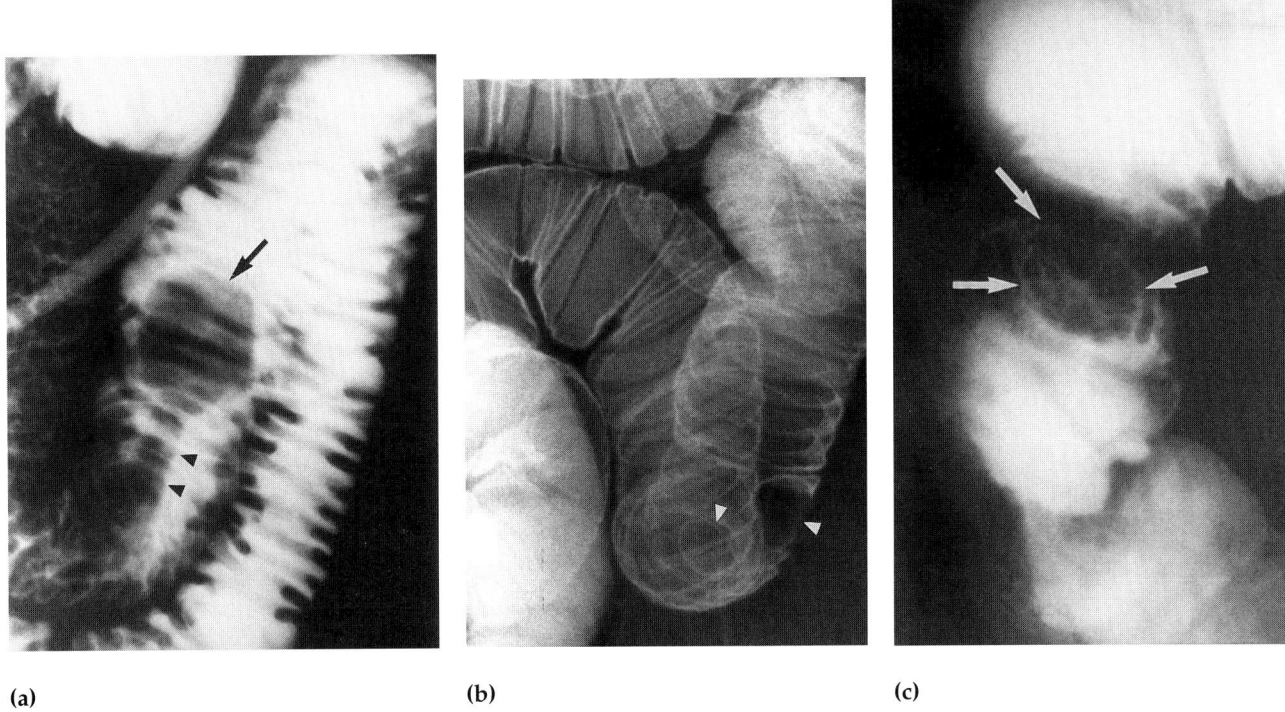

(a)   (b)   (c)

Fig. 19-10. Radiology of adenomatous polyps.
(a) Single-contrast radiograph of an enteroclysis showing an intraluminal polyp (arrow) with a long pedicle (arrowheads) in the jejunum of a 30-year-old female with unexplained recurrent abdominal pain. Surgery revealed a pedunculated polyp, which was partially intussuscepted. (b) Double-contrast radiograph of an enteroclysis done for unexplained GI bleeding shows two intraluminal sessile polypoid defects (arrowheads) in the jejunum. Surgery revealed two adjacent adenomatous polyps. (c) Small rounded intraluminal adenoma with finely lobulated surface (arrows) seen to intussuscept intermittently during the enteroclysis.

secondary to ulceration of the overlying mucosa.[56] Lipomas arise as well-circumscribed submucosal proliferations of fat and usually grow intraluminally, because outward extension is deflected by the firmness of the muscularis propria. They are characteristically solitary, relatively avascular, and of variable size (1 to 6 cm). Malignant change has not been reported.

Barium contrast studies demonstrate a sharply demarcated, often pedunculated tumor that tends to conform to the contour of the small bowel lumen. The configuration of the tumor may change during compression or peristalsis; this finding is an indication of its soft fatty nature (Fig. 19-11).[57] CT can establish the diagnosis of small bowel lipoma by showing its attenuation values to be consistent with fat. A homogeneous mass with Hounsfield units between -80 and -120 is considered pathognomonic (Fig. 19-12).[57] Identification of soft-tissue strands within an otherwise uniform lipoma on CT scans has been attributed to fibrovascular changes associated with ulceration within the tumor.[57] Multiple lipomas are rare. A report of a case of small bowel lipomatosis diagnosed by CT has been published (Fig. 19-13).[58]

Hemangioma

Hemangiomas are benign hamartomatous lesions and may or may not be accompanied by hemangiomas at other sites. They account for 3% to 4% of all small bowel tumors. The age distribution ranges from 6 months to 70 years; males are more frequently affected than females.[53]

In contrast to other benign small bowel tumors, which are more often asymptomatic, 80% of hemangiomas produce significant symptoms.[23] GI bleeding is the usual manifestation. Hemorrhage in association with a hemangioma is often acute, severe, and intermittent in nature. Anemia and occult fecal blood loss are also common clinical presentations. Mechanical obstruction

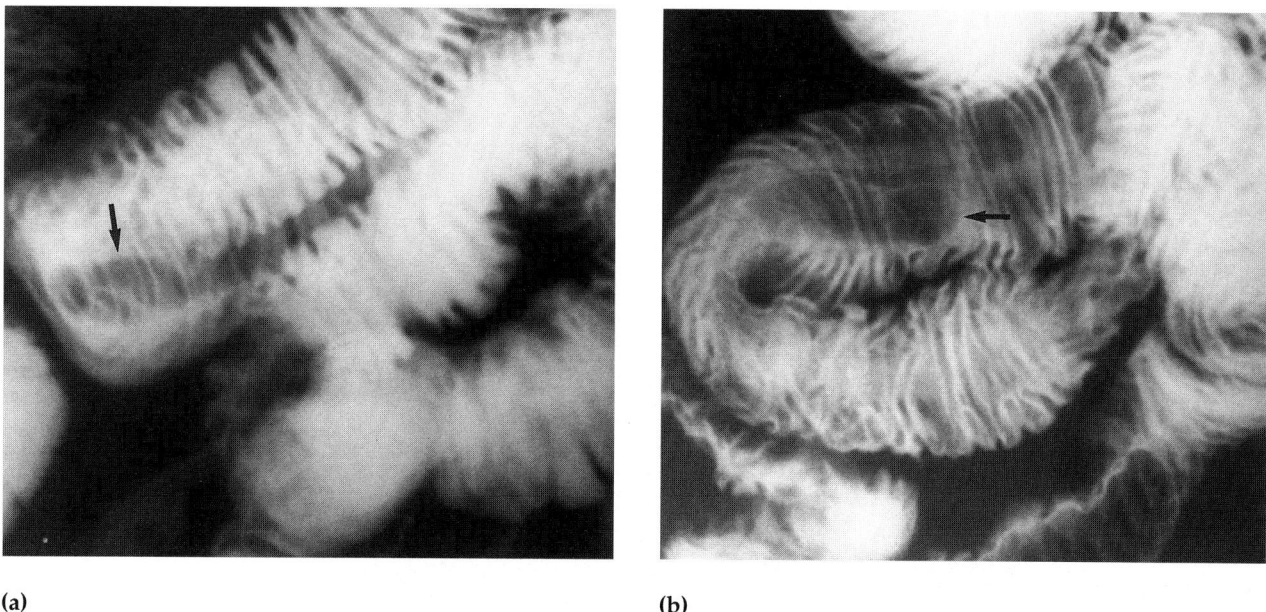

Fig. 19-11. Contrast examination of a lipoma.
(a) Single-contrast radiograph with mild compression shows a long polypoid defect in jejunum (arrow). (b) Double-contrast radiograph without compression shows a long pedunculated polyp (arrow) conforming to the lumen and flow of contrast. Surgery revealed a pedunculated lipoma.

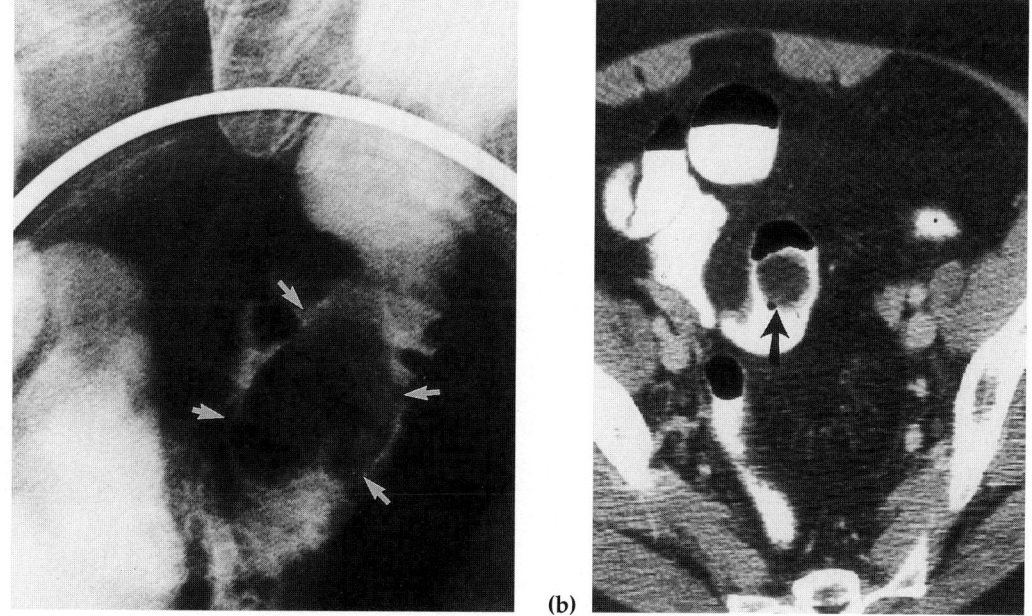

Fig. 19-12. Barium and CT of a lipoma.
(a) Double-contrast enteroclysis of an elderly female with recurrent abdominal pain shows an ovoid intraluminal polypoid mass (arrows), which is partially intussuscepted. (b) CT section through midabdomen shows the intussuscepting mass (arrow) with an attenuation value consistent with fat. Surgery confirmed an intussuscepting lipoma.

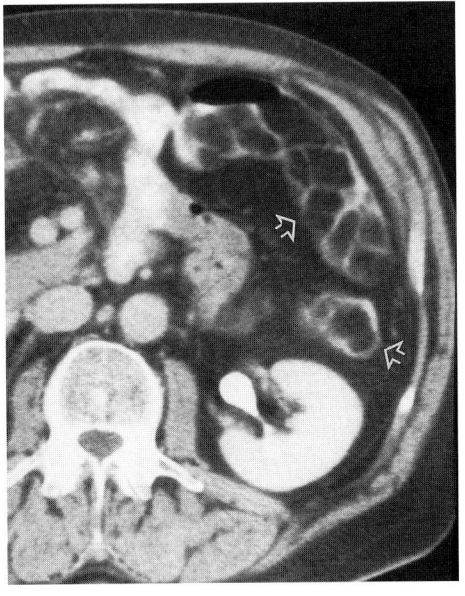 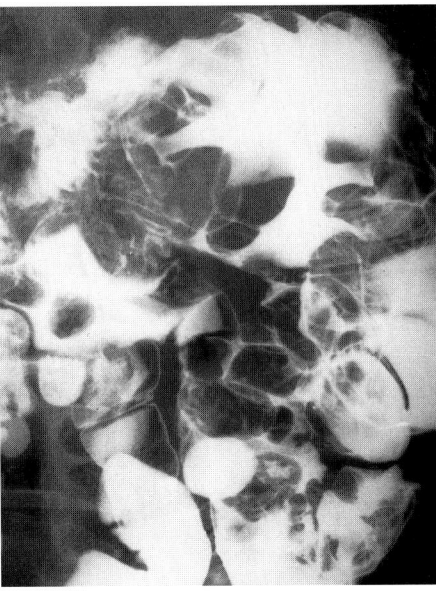

Fig. 19-13. Small bowel lipomatosis.
(a) CT section, through midabdomen of patient with back pain, shows multiple radiolucent ovoid masses outlined by contrast material in intestinal lumen (arrows). The masses are of the same attenuation as normal abdominal fat. (From Ormson MJ et al.[58]) (b) Barium examination of small intestine shows multiple smooth radiolucent masses projecting into lumen of jejunum and upper ileum. The findings are consistent with an asymptomatic lipomatosis.

is a rare presentation, caused either by intussusception or sclerosis that can lead to narrowing of the lumen.

These benign angiomatous tumors include two principal forms: the capillary hemangioma and the cavernous hemangioma. The capillary form occurs in younger patients than the cavernous type. The latter predominates in the small bowel and occurs either as a single polypoid tumor or in a diffusely expansive form.[53]

Microscopically, these submucosal neoplasms consist of variably enlarged vascular channels or sinuses, lined by endothelium and surrounded by minimal stromal tissue. Hemangiomas may be single or multiple and, although usually a few millimeters in size, may enlarge and protrude into the lumen. Direct invasion of the mucosa or penetration beyond the serosa is uncommon. Multiple phlebectasia refers to the small (1 to 5 mm) cav-

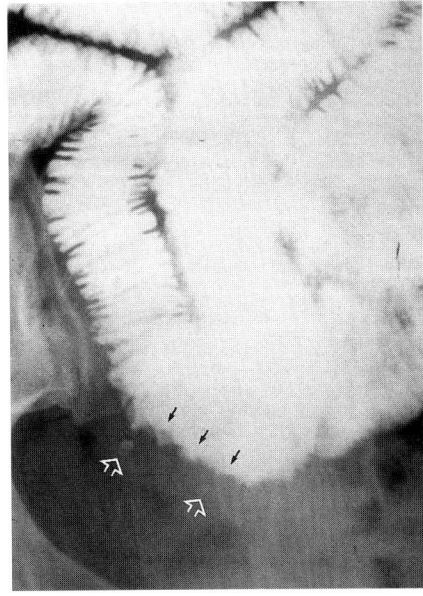 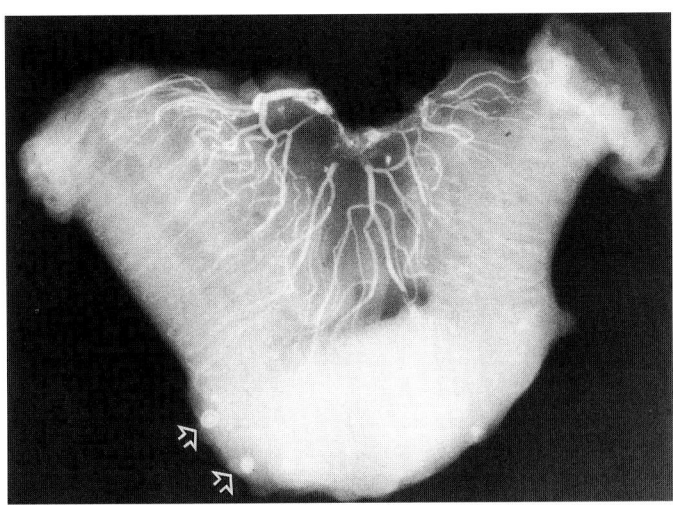

(a) (b)

Fig. 19-14. Phleboliths in hemangioma of small bowel.
(a) The hemangioma causes only moderate outline alteration of bowel margins (small arrow). Calcified phleboliths (open arrows) are in constant relationship to the marginal defect, allowing accurate diagnosis. (b) Specimen radiograph shows location of phleboliths (arrows) within the wall of the small bowel. [(a) and (b) by permission from Shepherd L, Nolan DJ. *Radiologic Atlas of Gastrointestinal Diseases*. New York: John Wiley and Sons.]

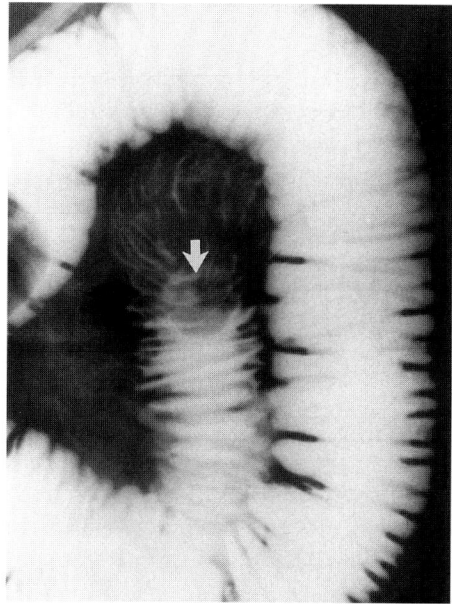 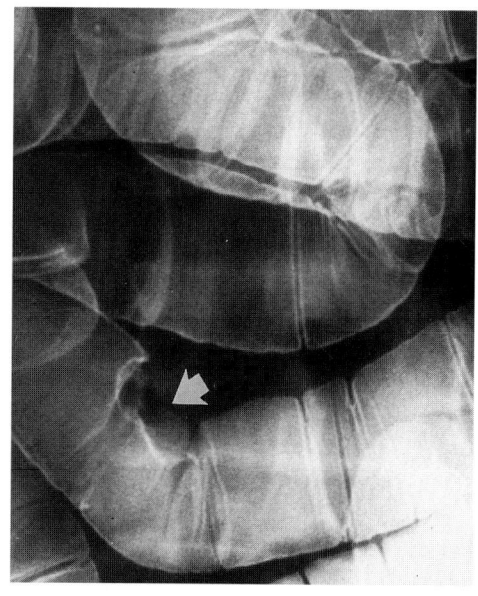

Fig. 19-15. Barium examination of hemangioma of small bowel.
(a) A rounded intraluminal polypoid defect (arrow) is present in the jejunum of a 92-year-old man with unexplained GI bleeding and anemia. (b) Cavernous hemangioma demonstrated as a soft, sessile polypoid tumor (arrow) seen to change shape during abdominal compression. (From Maglinte et al.,[31] with permission.)

ernous hemangiomas that predominate in the jejunum but may occur throughout the gastrointestinal tract.

Plain films of the abdomen occasionally will show calcified phleboliths in different locations in the abdomen, a result of normal positional changes of bowel loops.[59] Barium studies rarely outline hemangiomatous polyps and are likely to miss the usually shallow elevations, unless the presence of phleboliths draws attention to them (Fig. 19-14). Occasionally, a compressible polypoid protrusion of a cavernous hemangioma allows detection by barium examination (Fig. 19-15). These radiographic abnormalities, seen in combination with vascular cutaneous lesions or with syndromes such as tuberous sclerosis, Turner's syndrome, and Osler-Weber-Rendu disease, should increase the level of suspicion for intestinal hemangiomas,[60] as hemangiomas occur with an increased incidence in patients with these disorders. In selected patients, superior mesenteric arteriography can detect an intestinal vascular abnormality, although differentiation from other vascular tumors or malformations is seldom possible.

Neurogenic Tumor

Neurogenic tumors arise from the intramural neural plexus of the small bowel. Neurofibromas are the most frequently encountered nerve tumors and are composed of cell types found in peripheral nerves, including Schwann cells.[61] Neurofibromas may occur as single tumors or, more commonly, as multiple lesions with or without systemic neurofibromatosis. Although rare in the general population, neural tumors of the small bowel are reported in 11% to 25% of patients with neurofibromatosis.[61] Malignant transformation is seen in 10% to 15% of cases of neurofibromatosis. Neurolemmomas consist entirely of Schwann cells, are encapsulated, and almost never become malignant. Diagnosis is important because bleeding can be substantial and sarcomatous degeneration may occur.[49,62] Angiography has been suggested as an effective modality for the diagnosis of small bowel neurofibromas, because they are often exoenteric and are hypervascular with angiographic characteristics similar to those of leiomyomas.[49]

Two types of neurofibromatous involvement of the small bowel exist, each with a different radiographic appearance.[62] The nonplexiform type is subserosally located, mainly on the antimesenteric aspect of the bowel, and, therefore, infrequently presents clinically[61] and is difficult to diagnose on contrast studies. Occasionally this lesion is submucosal, in which case it can grow into the bowel lumen and cause intestinal bleeding, intussusception, or obstruction and may manifest on barium studies as solitary or multiple submucosal polypoid masses with or without ulceration on the antimesenteric border.[63,64] The rarer plexiform variety is diagnostic of von Recklinghausen's disease even if the plexiform neurofibroma is the only manifestation.[65] The findings on barium studies are suggestive; the term "mesenteric small bowel polyposis" has been proposed to describe the appearance of multiple polypoid filling defects along only the mesenteric aspect (concave side) on barium examination (Fig. 19-16).[62,66] With involvement of the adjacent mesentery, CT will show mesenteric nodules in addition to the nodularity along the mesenteric aspect of the small bowel.[67]

Ganglioneuromas are made up of ganglion cells and of cell types seen in neurofibromas. Ganglioneuromatosis forms part of the syndrome of multiple endocrine neoplasia type 2B. These lesions are usually too small to be demonstrated.

Inflammatory Fibroid Polyp

The term inflammatory fibroid polyp (IFP) was first proposed by Helwig and Ranier in 1953 and is now widely accepted as the most appropriate name for this lesion.[68] The small bowel is the second most common site for IFPs (the gastric antrum, the most frequent site). Patients are generally elderly, and the lesions generally occur in the ileum. They are non-neoplastic cellular proliferations originating primarily in the submucosa and composed of fibroblasts, blood vessels, and inflammatory cells within an adenomatous and collagenous stroma. They are usually large and nonencapsulated and may infiltrate through the muscularis propria. Erosions and ulcerations of the polyps are common. They have been incorrectly referred to as eosinophilic granulomatous polyps but are not associated with eosinophilia.[53] They are usually solitary. Their etiology remains uncertain. They have been regarded as an exuberant host response to an unknown injury.[68] Due to the submucosal origin of IFPs, surgical resection of the lesion for both diagnosis and treatment is required.

There are no distinctive features to differentiate IFPs from other mural or intraluminal lesions of the gastrointestinal tract.[69] Contrast studies may demonstrate a smooth, rounded mass in the distal small bowel. They may be pedunculated and may reach a size in excess of 5 cm (Fig. 19-17). In their clinical presentation, IFPs are commonly associated with intussusception. They may also ulcerate and bleed.

Uncommon Tumors

Myoepithelial hamartoma is a rare developmental tumor consisting of varied amounts of pancreatic tissue, smooth muscle, and epithelial structures. Predominance of pancreatic acinar tissue confers the designation ectopic pancreas. Most myoepithelial hamartomas

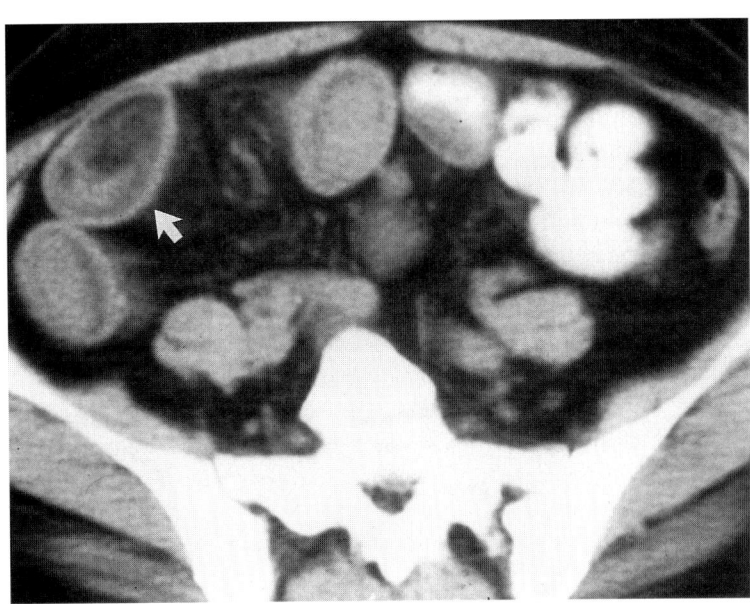
(a)

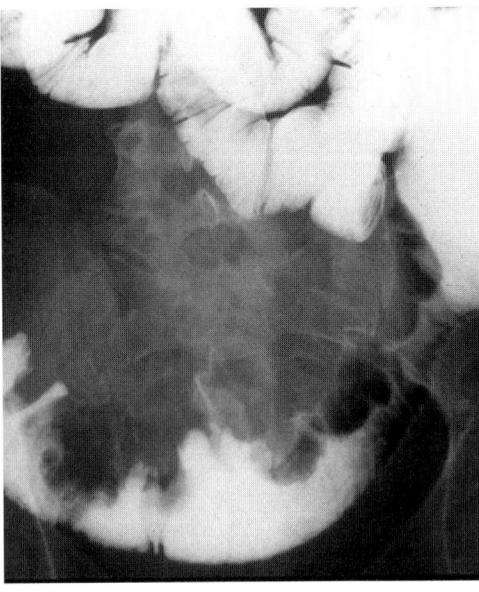
(b)

Fig. 19-16. Imaging of polyposis in mesenteric small bowel.
(a) CT scan of a 42-year-old woman with plexiform neurofibromatosis showing thick-walled ileum with multiple intraluminal soft-tissue masses, one of which contains fat, suggesting intussusception (arrow). (b) Enteroclysis during early filling of ileum reveals multiple polypoid filling defects only along mesenteric aspect (concave side) of small bowel. (Courtesy of Dr R. Seppala with permission.[62])

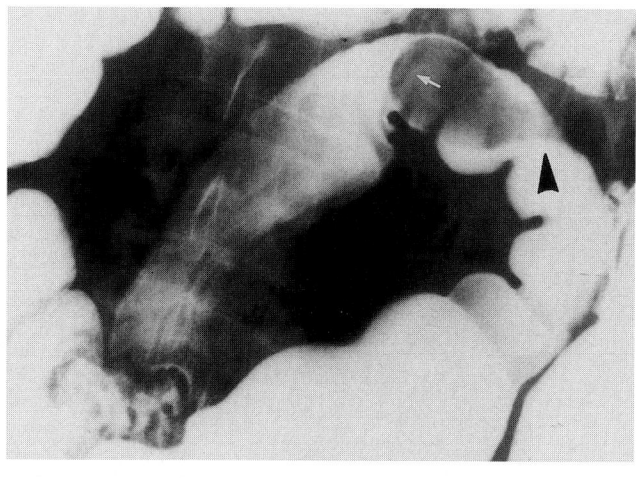
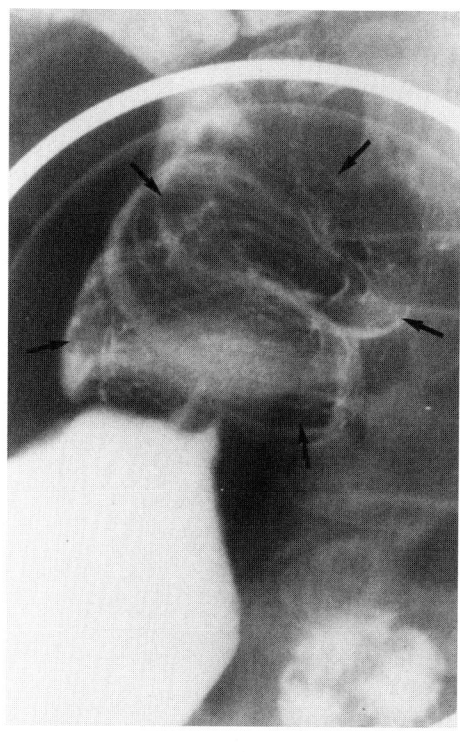

Fig. 19-17. (a) Pedunculated inflammatory fibroid polyp.
An ovoid intraluminal polyp with a short pedicle (arrowhead) is shown in the distal ileum of a patient with unexplained intermittent abdominal pain. During fluoroscopy, the polyp was seen to move in the direction of contrast flow (arrowhead). (C = cecum) Surgery and histology revealed an inflammatory fibroid polyp. (b) A barium study in a different patient revealed an intussuscepted polypoid mass (arrows) causing obstruction. Surgery and histology demonstrated an inflammatory fibroid polyp. (Courtesy of Richard Baron, MD.)

occur in the gastric antrum or duodenum, although some are reported in the mesenteric small bowel.[44] Lesions are solitary and usually under 3 cm in size. A smooth, nonpedunculated mass with occasional central umbilication (similar to the finding when it occurs in the gastric antrum) can be seen radiographically.

Heterotopic gastric mucosa may be found in the mesenteric small bowel, either as isolated lesions or in association with malformations such as Meckel's diverticulum or an enteric duplication. Occasionally, the heterotopic mucosa presents as a polypoid lesion, either sessile or pedunculated.

Fibromas, lymphangiomas, and other benign tumors can also occur in the small bowel. They cannot be differentiated radiographically from other benign tumors.

Hamartomatous Polyposis Syndromes

Peutz-Jeghers Syndrome

This is considered an autosomal dominantly inherited condition, although in about half the patients the disease occurs without a family history.[70] The syndrome consists of multiple hamartomatous polyps of the gastrointestinal tract and of characteristic brown pigmented lesions of the skin, the lips, the buccal mucosa, and sometimes over the palmar aspects of the digits. The polyps present a smooth, lobulated, fronded surface, are sessile or pedunculated, and may be several centimeters in diameter. Histologically, the polyps are benign hamartomas containing a proliferative smooth muscle core and are lined by normal intestinal epithelium.[44] These hamartomas grossly resemble adenomatous polyps except for their variation in size (1 to 5 cm) and their multiplicity. Peutz-Jeghers polyps are more commonly found in the jejunum than the ileum but may also occur in the stomach or colon. In association with Peutz-Jeghers syndrome, there is an increased incidence of carcinoma involving the stomach, duodenum, or colon. Small bowel malignancy is extremely rare.[71] Extraintestinal malignancy, especially of breast, pancreas, and reproductive organs, is significantly increased.[72]

Cutaneous lesions appear in early life, often predating the formation of gastrointestinal polyps. They typically fade during adolescence, with only the buccal lesions persisting into adulthood. Characteristically, the polyps become manifest during the second

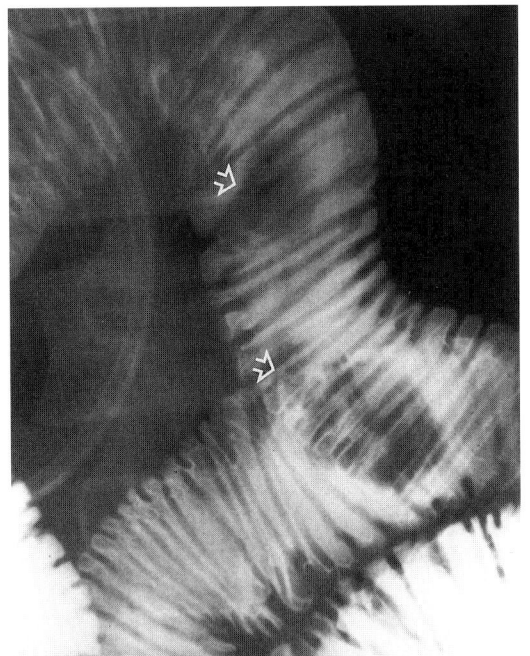

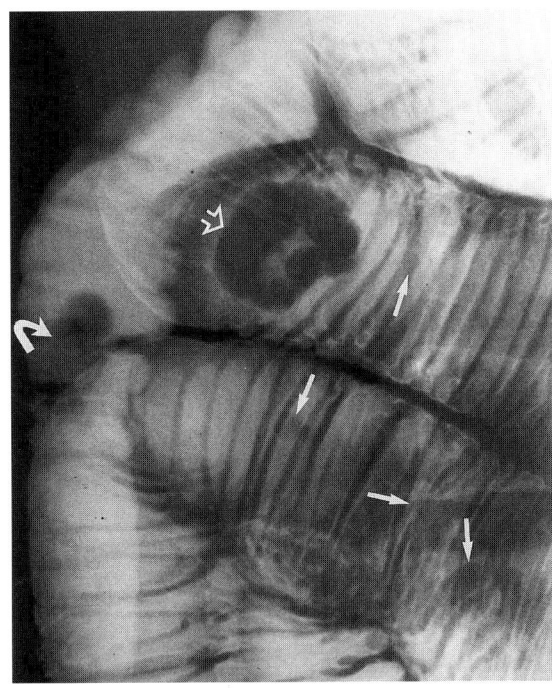

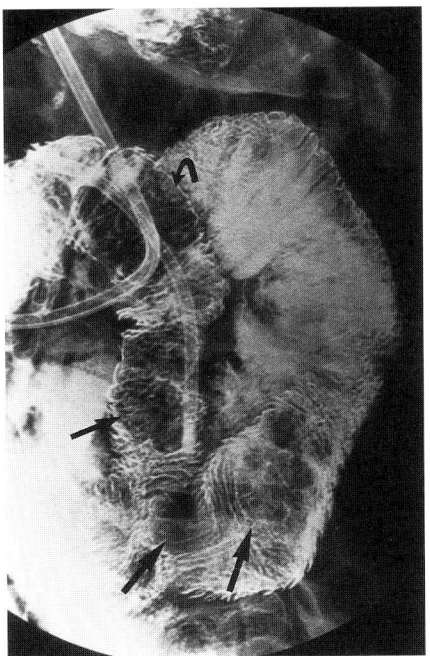

Fig. 19-18. Enteroclysis in Peutz-Jeghers syndrome.
(a, b) Double-contrast enteroclysis radiographs of jejunum and ileum of a 21-year-old patient with oral pigmentation whose mother recently died of a brain tumor. Larger (open arrows) and smaller (arrows) intraluminal polyps are present in the jejunum and ileum; a lobulated polyp is seen in ascending colon (curved arrow). Endoscopic biopsy of colonic polyp revealed hamartoma. (c) Enteroclysis on a 23-year-old medical student with prolonged crampy abdominal pain and episodes of bleeding. Three jejunal tumors (arrows), one of them coarsely lobulated. Histology confirmed hamartomas (curved arrow to catheter balloon).

or third decade. Episodes of intermittent abdominal pain caused by transient intussusception of the small bowel are common. Gastrointestinal bleeding is also a frequent mode of presentation and may be severe. Because Peutz-Jeghers polyps continue to develop throughout the life of the patient, a conservative approach to surgical intervention is recommended.[23] Surgical intervention in this disease is one of the causes of the short bowel syndrome.

Radiographically, barium contrast studies of the small bowel demonstrate luminal polyps of various sizes (Fig. 19-18). Larger polyps typically present a lobulated contour; pedunculated lesions with broad-based attachment may also be detected. Diffuse proliferation of intestinal polyps is atypical for Peutz-Jeghers syndrome. Usually, uninvolved small bowel segments alternate with others that contain several hamartomas. Small bowel polyps discovered in children younger than 10 years old are commonly Peutz-Jeghers hamartomas. On CT scans, single and multiple Peutz-Jeghers polyps can be detected as soft-tissue masses within the contrast medium–filled intestinal loops.[73] Follow-up examinations may demonstrate polyps in segments that had previously been clean.

Juvenile Polyposis

This is a rare familial/sporadic condition characterized by polyps in the colon (>10) and occasionally in the small bowel. The polyps appear before the age of 10 years but may also occur in adults. The polyps are mostly pedunculated, have smoothly rounded surfaces, and often are ulcerated. Commonly they present with rectal bleeding and may prolapse due to their long stalk. An association with colorectal cancer has been observed in the familial form.[74]

Cowden's Disease
(Multiple Hamartoma Syndrome)

This is a rare condition with autosomal dominant inheritance of high penetration. The disease is mostly described in the dermatologic literature because of the characteristic skin lesions with which it usually presents. Multiple facial papules are identified in all patients, in some with oral papillomatosis.[74] The majority of patients have intestinal polyps, which usually remain asymptomatic. Their main clinical relevance is an indicator of likely associated breast lesions, which range from fibrocystic disease to cancer, and of possible thyroid malignancy.[74]

The small bowel is less often involved than the stomach or colon. In a 1987 review of published cases of Cowden's disease, the small bowel was involved in 14 of 32 patients.[75] In addition to hamartomatous polyps, the intestinal tract may contain hyperplastic, lipomatous, juvenile, or inflammatory polyps. Enteroclysis has demonstrated multiple small bowel polyps that produced a nodular mucosal surface pattern in a patient with diffuse gastrointestinal tract disease.[76] A case of Cowden's disease with typical skin lesions and polyps in stomach and jejunum is demonstrated in Fig. 19-19.

Ruvalcaba-Myre-Smith Syndrome

This is an extremely rare form of an autosomal dominant hamartomatous polyposis.[77] The polyps occur anywhere in the alimentary tract including the small bowel. The syndrome comprises macrocephaly, pigmented genital lesions, intestinal polyposis, and other abnormalities.[76]

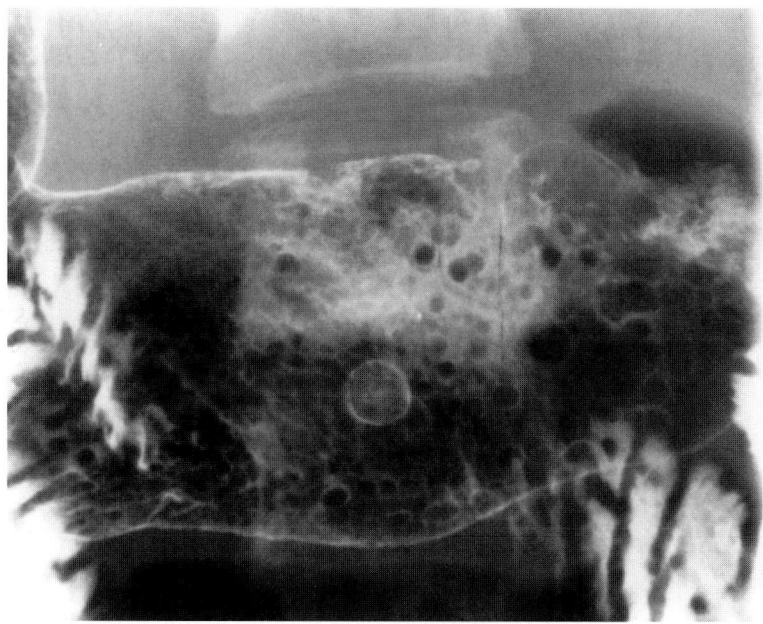
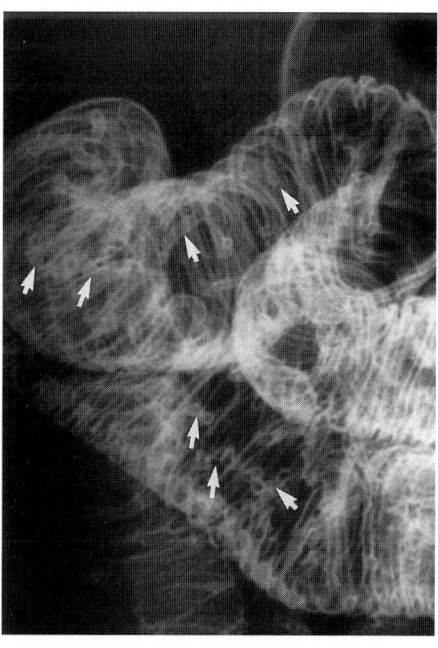

Fig. 19-19. Barium studies in Cowden's disease. A 37-year-old female patient with history of colon carcinoma surgery complained of abdominal discomfort and constipation.
(a) At double-contrast upper GI examination, the gastric antrum was filled with small, rounded polyps. (b) Enteroclysis outlined numerous tiny filiform polyps (arrows) in proximal jejunum. Endoscopic biopsy of antrum and jejunum demonstrated hamartomatous polyps compatible with Cowden's disease. (Courtesy of K. Cho, MD.)

Rare Forms of Polyposis

These polyposes comprising hemangiomatous and neurogenic tumors, have been mentioned previously.

Cronkhite-Canada Syndrome

This syndrome consists of polyposis of an inflammatory type, of ectodermal changes and onset in adulthood with watery diarrhea and protein loss. This rare, not familial polyposis syndrome involves the small bowel in half of the cases, whereas polyps occur in the stomach and colon in virtually all affected patients. The polyps are inflammatory in nature and consist of dilated cystic interstitial glands, closely resembling the hamartoma-like juvenile polyps. The polyps develop after the age of 40 years and no sexual, racial, familial, or geographic distribution has been established.[78] The etiology of the disease is not known.

Symptoms of abdominal pain, diarrhea, and anorexia precede or occur together with the development of the ectodermal changes, alopecia, hyperpigmentation, and dystrophy of nails. The onset is usually gradual, and older adults (mean age of onset is 60 years) are affected. Intestinal malabsorption and protein loss can be severe and the clinical course is potentially fatal.[79] Remissions have been reported, both spontaneous and following treatment with nutritional supplements.[80]

The patterns of involvement can be radiographically classified as follows: 1) innumerable small polyps carpeting large areas (most common), 2) scattered polyps of various sizes, and 3) sparse involvement with few small polyps.[79,81] In addition, small bowel studies may show findings related to malabsorption and hypoproteinemia including thickened folds and increased luminal secretions.

Familial Polyposis Coli (Including Gardner's Syndrome)

Adenomatous polyps in familial polyposis coli typically involve the entire colon. Generally, 100 or more polyps should be identified to establish the diagnosis. Histologically, the polyps are tubular or tubulovillous adenomas. Gardner's syndrome is familial polyposis plus cutaneous lesions with or without bone manifestations. Small bowel polyps may occur in familial polyposis or Gardner's syndrome. Gastric polyps are present in 20% to 60% of patients; 60% to 100% of these patients have duodenal polyps.[82,83] It has been estimated that up to 12% of patients will develop periampullary carcinoma. At least 50% have osseous involvement (osteomas in flat bones and cortical hyperostosis in long bones). Multiple epidermal cysts are present in approximately 65% of patients. There is also increased prevalence of thyroid carcinoma. Turcot syndrome (glioblastoma) and medulloblastoma may be a legitimate expression of the familial adenomatous polyposis syndromes.

Small bowel adenomas have been reported to develop in the ileum after colectomy for familial polyposis coli.[84] Adenomas are dominant in the jejunum, whereas lymphoid hyperplasia is more common in the ileum. Several cases of carcinoma have been reported. These malignant lesions may also occur after colectomy. There is a distinct association between Gardner's syndrome and the finding of intra-abdominal desmoids.

Desmoid tumors (mesenteric fibromatosis) are aggressive fibrous tumors but are usually classified as benign because they do not metastasize, although they have a strong tendency toward local recurrence and focal invasion. They are usually provoked by abdominal surgery and may involve the area of the abdominal scar. Their preferred site, however, is the base of the small bowel mesentery, and this may lead to small bowel obstruction. Most desmoids reported in the radiologic literature have been associated with Gardner's syndrome. However, among a larger number of desmoids reported, only 13% were related to Gardner's syndrome.[85] CT is an ideal imaging method for

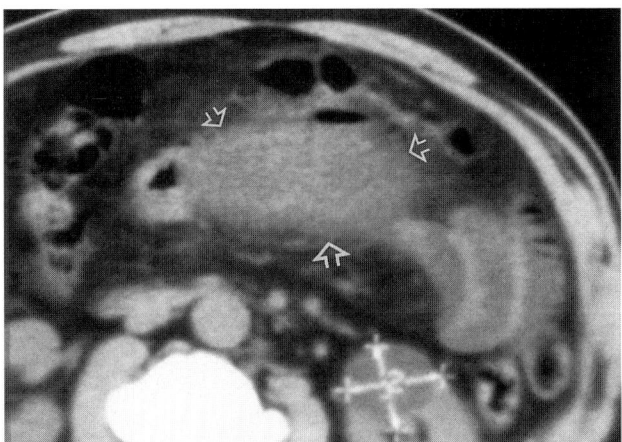

Fig. 19-20. CT of mesenteric desmoid tumor.
Axial section through upper abdomen shows a moderate-size mesenteric mass (arrows). Unenhanced study shows musclelike attenuation of mass with poorly defined margins and adherent adjacent small bowel loops. Surgery disclosed a solid mesenteric tumor attached to small bowel mesentery with adherence of adjacent small bowel loops. Histologic sections revealed a fibromatous mesenteric tumor.

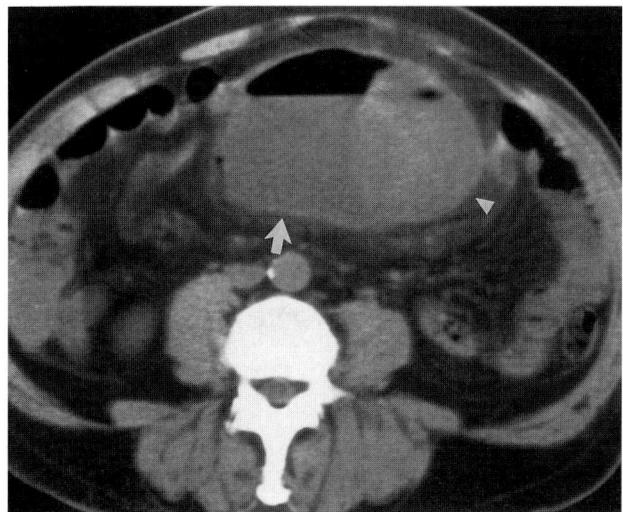

Fig. 19-21. CT of necrotic mesenteric desmoid tumor. Unenhanced CT section through midabdomen shows a large mesenteric mass with musclelike attenuation of part of mass (arrowhead) and a large area of decreased attenuation with a fluid level (arrow) in a 76-year-old previously healthy male who presented with an acute abdomen, sepsis, and hypotension. An intra-abdominal abscess was the interpretation. Four hundred ml of pus was drained percutaneously and the patient improved symptomatically on antibiotics. Abdominal pain and fever recurred; surgery performed revealed a solid mesenteric tumor attached to small bowel mesentery with adherent small bowel loops. Histologic section revealed a necrotic mesenteric desmoid tumor. The patient had neither Gardner's syndrome nor a history of prior abdominal surgery. The CT image is indistinguishable from a large leiomyosarcoma.

the demonstration of desmoids as it can also show the extent of invasion of the mesentery and of the small bowel.[86,87] Mesenteric fibromatosis most often appears as a large, homogeneous, musclelike density on CT scans (Fig. 19-20). Absence of areas of decreased density may occasionally be of help in differentiating desmoids from lymphoma and leiomyosarcoma, which frequently have large areas of necrosis. Angiographically, desmoids are usually hypervascular. Necrosis is rare (Fig. 19-21).

Malignant Tumors

The American Cancer Society estimates that 4,600 persons in the United States will develop cancer of the small bowel in 1996, with 1,140 deaths.[88] This figure approximates the number of deaths from Hodgkin's disease, primary bone tumors, or thyroid cancer. Malignant tumors develop in all histologic components of the small bowel including epithelial cells, lymphoid tissue, lymphatics, blood vessels, nerves, and muscle. The cell type of tumor is often characteristic for the portion of small bowel involved. Table 19-1 lists the distribution of the different histologic types of small bowel tumors. Sixty percent to 75% of all symptomatic small bowel tumors prove to be malignant. There are a number of risk factors associated with the development of small bowel tumors (Table 19-2).[89]

Adenocarcinoma

If the duodenum is included, adenocarcinomas are the most common primary malignancy of the small intestine; the duodenum is the most frequent site.[90] Worldwide, the prevalence of carcinoma of the small intestine is 0.5 to 3 per 100,000 population and is slightly higher for males than for females. Adenocarcinomas of the small intestine are associated with an increased incidence of primary malignant tumors in other locations. A greater than eightfold increase in second malignancy is associated with small bowel adenocarcinoma.[91] Twenty-nine percent are associated with cancers of the colon, rectum, or both.

Adenocarcinoma occurs more frequently in the jejunum than in the ileum.[12] Most jejunal tumors are found in the first 30 cm beyond the ligament of Tre-

Table 19-1. Distribution by histologic type of malignant small bowel tumors

	Duodenum (%)	Jejunum (%)	Ileum (%)
Primary adenocarcinoma (N = 1,138)	40	38	22
Malignant carcinoid (N = 794)	6	10	84
Primary lymphoma (N = 144)	16	48	36
Leiomyosarcoma (N = 98)	10	37	53

Data compiled from eight series.[88]

Table 19-2. Clinical conditions associated with increased risk of small bowel tumors[89]

Associated Condition	Type of Tumor	Usual Site
Celiac sprue	Adenocarcinoma	Duodenum or jejunum
Crohn's disease	Adenocarcinoma	Ileum
Familial adenomatous polyposis	Adenoma Adenocarcinoma	Duodenum
Ileal conduit or ileocystoplasty	Adenocarcinoma	Adjacent to anastomosis
Ileostomy after colectomy	Adenocarcinoma	Ileocutaneous junction
Neurofibromatosis	Adenocarcinoma; leiomyoma	Ileum
Celiac sprue	Non-Hodgkin's lymphoma (T cell)	Jejunum
Immunoproliferative small intestine disease	Non-Hodgkin's lymphoma (B cell)	Jejunum
Nodular lymphoid hyperplasia	Non-Hodgkin's lymphoma	Ileum
Acquired Immunodeficiency Syndrome	Non-Hodgkin's lymphoma; Kaposi's sarcoma	Ileum

itz.[92] Carcinomas of the small intestine seem to be well differentiated even when metastases have developed.[53] A mucin-producing columnar epithelium can frequently be identified.[93] Lymphatic spread to the regional nodes and spread to the liver via the portal venous system are the expected further developments. There may also be peritoneal implants and direct extension into adjacent structures.[94] Multiple adenocarcinomas must be distinguished from metastases. Adenocarcinoma of the small bowel share risk factors with colorectal cancer (see Table 19-2).[95,96] An adenoma-carcinoma sequence can take place in the small intestine just as occurs in the colon.[96] For a tumor to be considered a primary carcinoma, a transition from normal epithelium through severe dysplasia to frank malignancy must be demonstrated at its edge.[95,97]

Precancerous Conditions

Celiac disease. There is evidence that adult celiac disease is associated with a higher than expected incidence of carcinoma of the gastrointestinal tract (especially of the esophagus).[97] The mean duration of symptoms of celiac disease before the diagnosis of carcinoma of the gastrointestinal tract has been calculated to be 38 years. There is also an increased risk of development of adenocarcinomas of the small intestine.[98] A survey in the United Kingdom found 19 celiac disease–related carcinomas of the small intestine, compared with 0.23 carcinomas expected for the same number of patients without celiac disease.[99,100] The cause of the increased malignancy associated with celiac disease is unclear, but loss of immune surveillance and viral oncogenesis are possible explanations. An obvious change in the patient's condition, from being well controlled with a gluten-free diet to rapid clinical deterioration during continued dietary restriction, should raise the possibility of superimposed malignancy. Enteroclysis has been recently established as the method of investigation in the work-up of complications of celiac disease.[101]

Crohn's disease. The first case report of a carcinoma in the jejunum in a patient with Crohn's disease of the small intestine appeared in 1956.[102] There is an increased prevalence of adenocarcinoma of the small intestine in patients with long-standing Crohn's disease, although accurate figures are not available.[103–105] Risk factors include bypassed bowel and male sex.[106,107] Crohn's carcinoma is often diffuse and may not be apparent macroscopically. The diagnosis may only be made following resection and histologic examination. Preoperative clinical suspicion may be aroused when recrudescence of symptoms after prolonged quiescence or development of a mass, stricture, or obstruction is seen.[108] Conventional barium studies have rarely permitted a preoperative diagnosis to be made. Barium examination often shows a smooth and deceptively benign-appearing stricture.[109] Survival from the time of diagnosis is between 7.9 and 11.4 months.[105,110] For further detail see Chapter 15.

Peutz-Jeghers syndrome. An increased incidence of carcinoma in the stomach, jejunum, and colon has been reported in patients with Peutz-Jeghers syndrome.[53] Of the 380 cases of Peutz-Jeghers syndrome in the literature until 1972, 13 were associated with malignancy but only 1 involved the small intestine.[111] In a later report of 72 patients with Peutz-Jeghers syndrome, malignant tumors developed in 16 (22%), of whom all but 1 had died; 9 of the cancers were in the gastrointestinal tract and 7 occurred elsewhere.[112] There is also a report of extraintestinal malignancy developing in 15 of 31 patients with Peutz-Jeghers syndrome,[72] suggesting that the gene locus involved is relevant to the development of malignancy in general.

Radiology

Although CT and sonography are of value in staging, these modalities have a limited role in the initial detection of smaller malignant tumors or in their exclusion. Currently, barium examinations, preferably by enteroclysis, appear to be the best method for the early diagnosis or confident exclusion of adenocarcinomas of the small intestine (Fig. 19-22). (Also see Figs. 19-2 and 19-14.)[2,27,30,39,113] Some authors have reported the sensitivity of a combined upper gastrointestinal study and SBFT for adenocarcinoma to be as high as 85% to 90%.[44,114] These reports, however, included a large percentage of duodenal lesions that were detected during the upper gastrointestinal study. A 1989 report showed that the SBFT had a sensitivity of 61% and enteroclysis had a sensitivity of 95%.[30] Because of the usual location of adenocarcinomas within 25 cm of the duodenojejunal junction, a patient referred for an upper gastrointestinal examination for pain, vomiting, or anemia should have an evaluation not only of the duodenum but also of the proximal loops of jejunum (Fig. 19-23). A dilated proximal jejunum with retrained fluid observed in this extended upper gastrointestinal examination should alert the radiologist to a possible obstructive neoplasm and should be an indication to continue the procedure as a fluoroscopic small bowel study. Suspicion should be particularly high when the dilated distal duodenum or proximal jejunum contains excessive fluid. Seventy percent of tumors in the duodenum are polypoid. Larger duodenal lesions are ulcerative in 20%. Infiltrative lesions (10%) are less frequent in the duodenum.[2] The periampullary region is the most frequent site of duodenal carcinomas.

At the usual time of diagnosis, adenocarcinomas of the mesenteric small intestine are primarily annular (75%), are constricting, and may be partially ulcerated or fungating. The usual radiologic abnormality of a primary adenocarcinoma of the mesenteric small

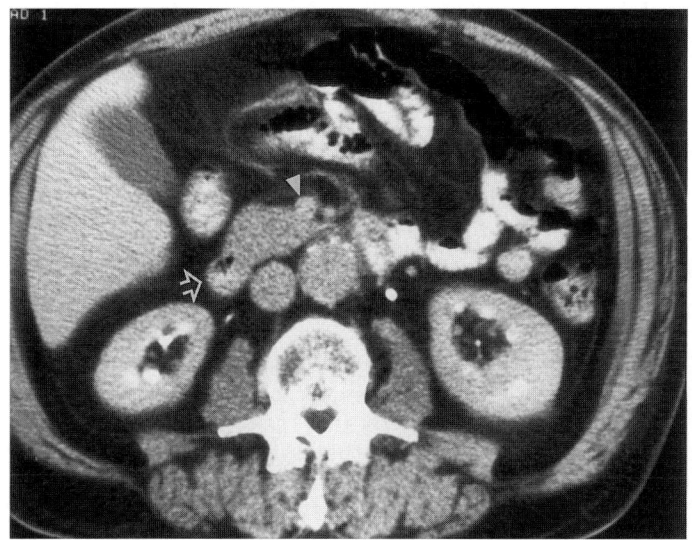
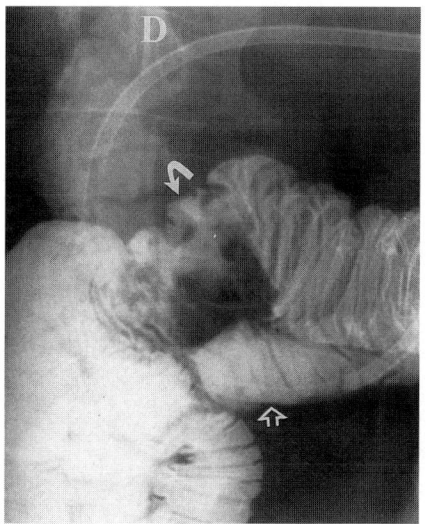

Fig. 19-22. Diagnostic examination to rule out carcinoma.
(a) CT scan through upper abdomen of a 70-year-old male with abdominal pain, nausea, and vomiting, requested to exclude malignancy. No lesion was appreciated at the time of interpretation or in retrospect. Arrowhead points to superior mesenteric vein and arrow to distal descending duodenum. (b) Enteroclysis done 1 week after CT shows a flat ulcerating mass with low-grade obstruction in proximal jejunum (curved arrow). The lesion is at level of distal descending duodenum, slightly cephalad to horizontal segment (open arrow). (D = duodenal cap) Surgery and histology confirmed ulcerating adenocarcinoma of jejunum.

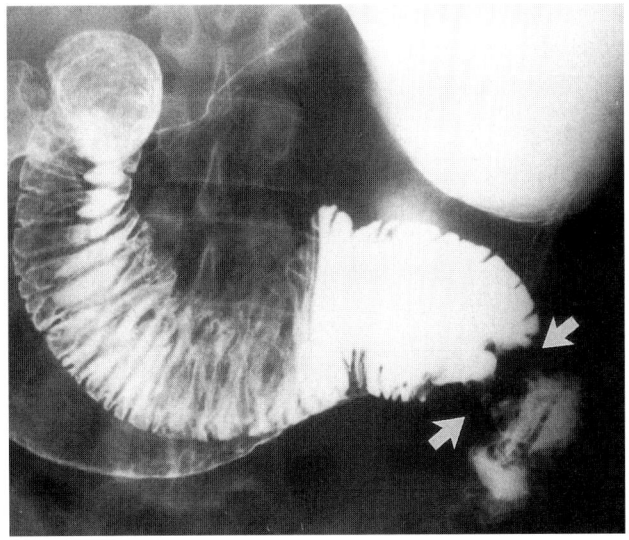

Fig. 19-23. Carcinoma in proximal jejunum shown by hypotonic upper GI examination done for epigastric pain and hemepositive stools.
The annular lesion (arrows) was confirmed at surgery to be an adenocarcinoma. A prior conventional single-contrast upper GI examination was reportedly negative. Note good demonstration of duodenum and the exaggerated effect of hypotonic medication on a minimally obstructing lesion. The duodenojejunal region should be well shown in all upper GI barium examinations. (From Maglinte and Reyes.[2])

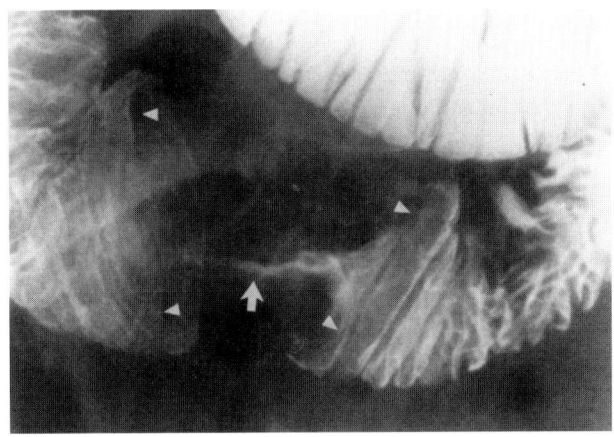

(a)

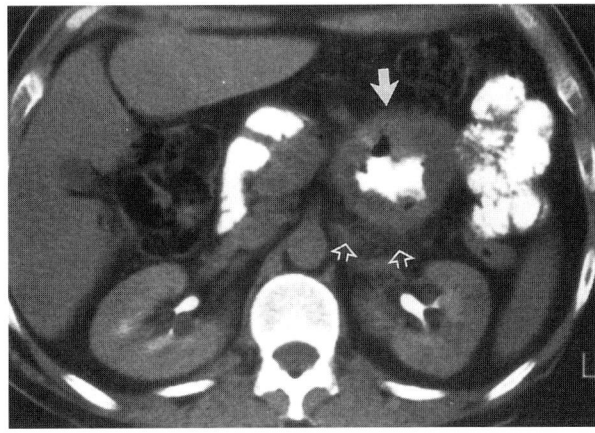

(b)

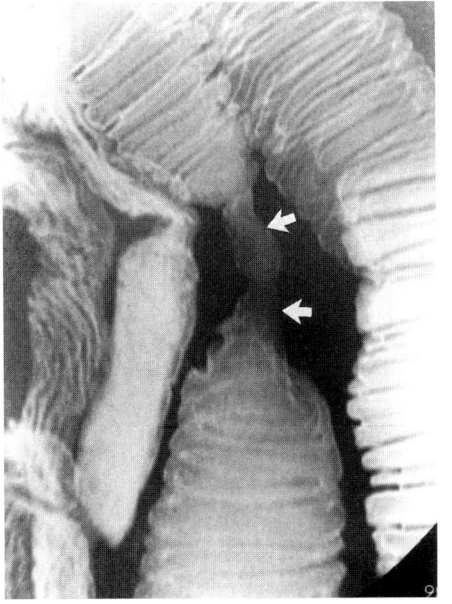

(c)

Fig. 19-24. Jejunal adenocarcinoma.
(a) "Apple core" lesion with circumferential irregular narrowing of lumen (arrow) with features of mucosal destruction. The overhanging edges ("shouldering") at both ends of the lesion (arrowheads) indicate that a circumferential mass causes separation from adjacent normal segment. This is the classic feature of the annular form of adenocarcinoma (see also Fig. 19-2). (b) CT of a similar "apple core" lesion for the purpose of staging. A circumferential mass of slightly heterogeneous density asymmetrically narrows the jejunal lumen (arrow). Increased density and small nodules posterior to mass (open arrows) suggest local spread. No evidence of liver metastases. Surgery confirmed preoperative findings. (c) However, not all adenocarcinomas have abrupt, overhanging margins. This gradually merging lesion is characterized by the absence of folds in its narrowed portion (arrows). (Courtesy of Seth Glick, MD.)

bowel on barium examination is the "apple core" lesion, the same as that found in the rest of the gastrointestinal tract.[2] This is an annular lesion, a somewhat short, circumferentially narrowed segment with features of mucosal destruction, frequently ulcerated and separated from normal bowel above and below it by overhanging edges. The malignant stricture is usually central in position, rigid, and without change of shape during compression (Fig. 19-24).[30,115] On occasion, a lymphoma or leiomyosarcoma has a similar appearance. Both of those tumors, however, show alterations of shape with compression because they are usually softer. Carcinoids only rarely present as annular lesions. It has been reported that 55% of annular, apple core–type lesions of the small bowel are caused by metastases, mostly from a carcinoma of the colon.[116] These lesions are often longer and cause more pronounced narrowing and obstruction because they are frequently associated with desmoplasia. Ulceration of a metastasis tends to produce a more irregular cavity. The ulcerating form of adenoarcinoma appears as a short, narrow lesion, usually with an inconspicuous, mostly central ulcer. Occasionally, a more sizable ulcer is demonstrated (Fig. 19-25). Rarely, adenocarcinoma may present as a polypoid mass that can intussuscept (Fig. 19-26). This cannot be differentiated from other intussuscepting masses. Large polypoid intraluminal masses are difficult to differentiate from a leiomyosarcoma or lymphoma (Fig. 19-27). Small plaquelike adenocarcinomas involving one side of the bowel have been detected by enteroclysis (Fig. 19-28). A patient with several primary adenocarcinomas of the distal ileum manifesting different states of development on small bowel enteroclysis has been reported.[117]

In their CT presentation, adenocarcinomas are proximal solitary soft-tissue masses causing lumen narrowing and obstruction.[38–40,113,114] The narrowed lumen is shown to be either concentric or asymmetric (Fig. 19-29). The lesions may be heterogeneous in attenuation and show moderate enhancement after intravenous contrast medium administration. An intussuscepting polypoid adenocarcinoma can be diagnosed on CT by demonstration of 1) an early target sign, 2) a sausage-shaped mass with alternating high and low attenuation areas, or 3) a reniform mass that suggests vascular compromise.[118] Occasionally, the lesion may be observed as a large, well-defined mass without appreciable bowel obstruction. A mucin-producing adenocarcinoma is then difficult to differentiate from lymphoma if it extends over several centimeters (Fig. 19-30). Forty-five percent of adenocarcinomas have atypical CT appearances, especially when ulcerated or located in the duodenum.[40] The demonstration by CT of large mesenteric mass with heterogeneous attenuation and associated asymmetric

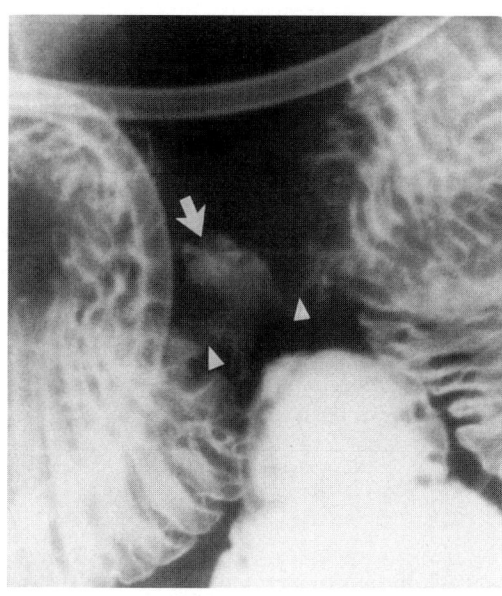

Fig. 19-25. Adenocarcinoma in first segment of jejunum. Short narrowed segment devoid of folds (arrowheads) and larger-than-usual well-demarcated ulcer (arrow). Confirmed by surgery, only local nodes were involved.

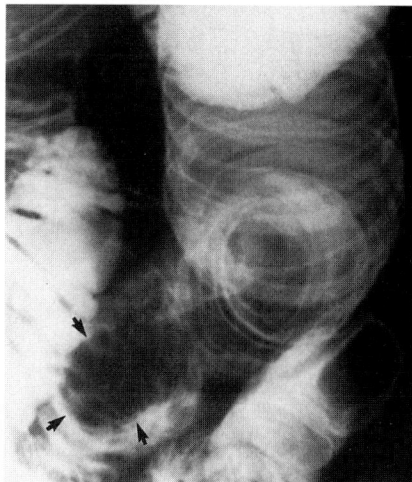

Fig. 19-26. Intussuscepting jejunal adenocarcinoma. The double-contrast radiograph of an enteroclysis shows partial obstruction due to intussusception of a polypoid mass (arrows). Histology revealed adenocarcinoma. Adjacent nodes were not involved. (From Maglinte and Reyes,[2] with permission.)

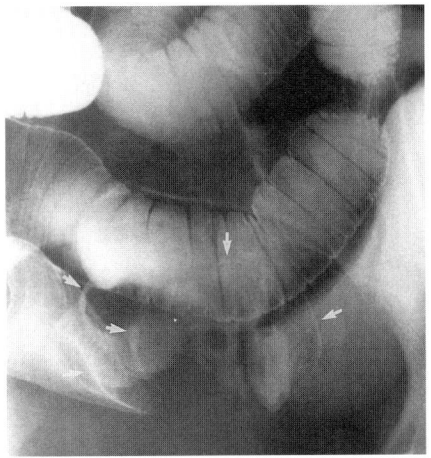
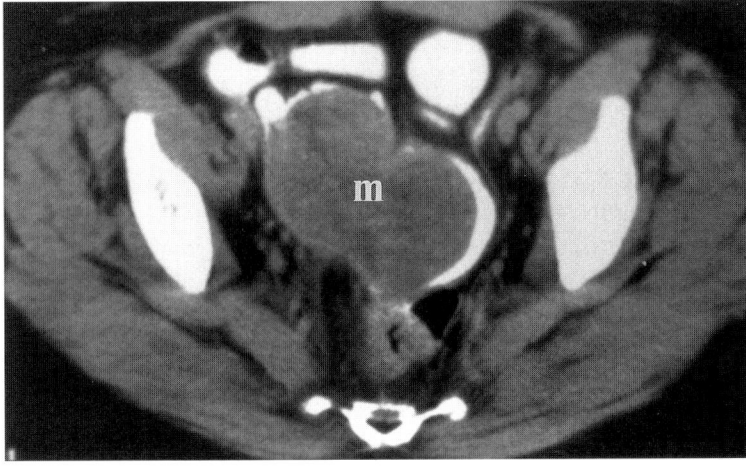

Fig. 19-27. Barium and CT examination of a polypoid adenocarcinoma.
(a) Double-contrast enteroclysis of a 56-year-old female with unexplained lower abdominal pain shows a large lobulated, well-defined mass barely obstructing the pelvic segment of ileum (arrows). A tumor of either connective or lymphoid tissue origin was the primary consideration. (b) CT section through midpelvis of patient shows a large heart-shaped mass (m) displacing intraluminal contrast. Appearances are compatible with the differential diagnosis at enteroclysis, illustrating the difficulty in differentiation of large tumors by either method. Surgery and histology revealed a polypoid adenocarcinoma.

narrowing of small bowel wall should suggest an adenocarcinoma with extension into mesentery (Fig. 19-31). Local lymph nodes, liver, peritoneal surfaces, and ovaries may be involved by mesenteric spread. The lymph node metastasis in adenocarcinoma is usually less bulky than the lymph node replaced by lymphoma.[38] CT has been shown to be helpful to the surgeon in planning the appropriate surgical approach.[118]

Angiography shows carcinomas as mostly hypervascular tumors that displace unencased feeding arteries. The sonographic appearance of small bowel

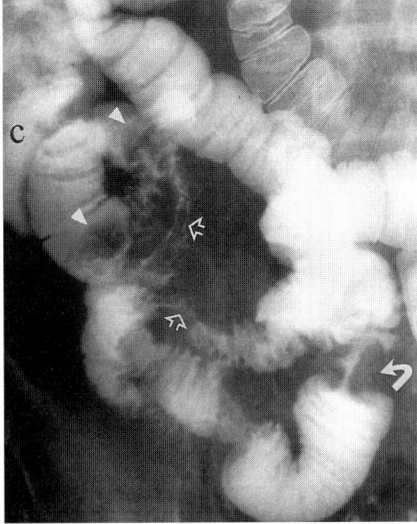

Fig. 19-28. Radiologic diagnosis of a localized ulcerated adenocarcinoma.
A flat eccentric mass (arrowheads) with an irregular ulceration (arrow) is shown by enteroclysis in the proximal jejunum. The balloon (curved arrow) of the enteroclysis catheter is in the distal horizontal duodenum, the catheter tip at the ligament of Treitz. At surgery and histology no nodes were involved. (From Maglinte and Reyes,[2] with permission.)

Fig. 19-29. Multiple primary adenocarcinomas of the small bowel.
Enteroclysis radiograph shows annular (curved arrow), polypoid (arrowheads), and infiltrative (arrow) forms of adenocarcinoma of the ileum. (C = cecum) (Courtesy of Dina F. Caroline, MD.)

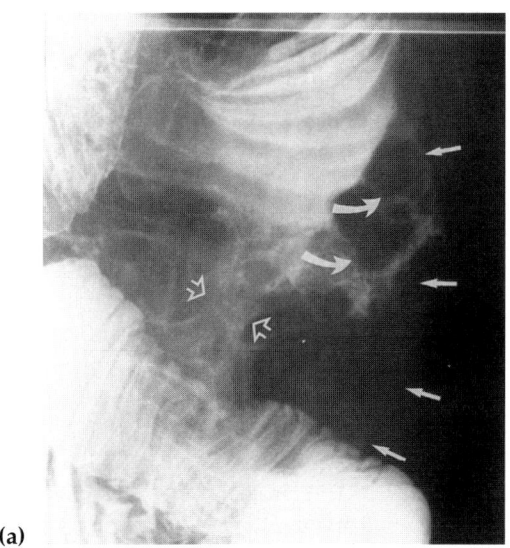 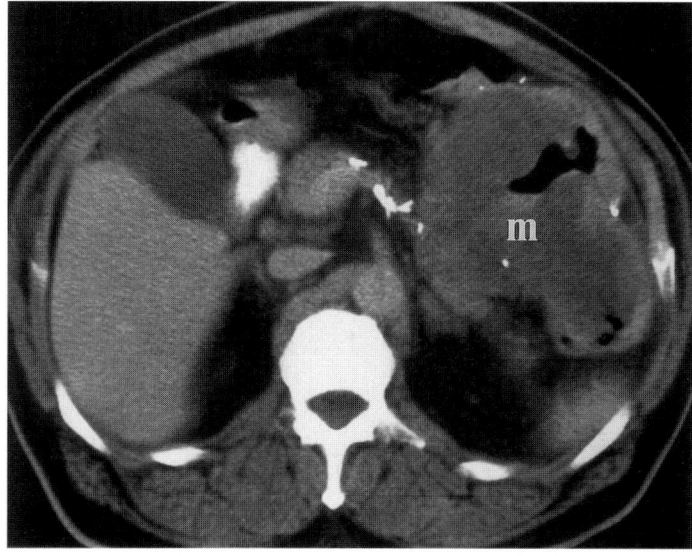

Fig. 19-30. Enteroclysis and CT of two mucin-producing adenocarcinomas.
(a) Enteroclysis demonstrates a narrowed segment of jejunum with its fold pattern destroyed (open arrows). A surrounding soft-tissue mass outline is visible (arrows) and within it, partly barium containing, an area of necrosis (curved arrows). A stromal tumor or lymphoma was the suggested diagnosis. (b) CT scan through upper abdomen of another patient shows a large mass (m) involving the jejunum and extending toward pancreas. Although the attenuation of the mass may appear lower than in a lymphoma or leiomyosarcoma, a precise preoperative differentiation was not possible.

neoplasms is similar to that of thickened bowel wall in other conditions, such as intramural hemorrhage or inflammatory states.[119] (See Chapter 8.)

Differentiation of the annular form of primary adenocarcinoma from benign diseases and secondary malignancies is occasionally difficult.[120] The mostly single and short stricture of the carcinoma is a helpful distinguishing feature but can be mimicked by a Crohn's stricture or other benign conditions. Characteristic radiographic findings in Crohn's disease—"cobblestone" appearance, mesenteric border shortening, ulceration, and lack of significant prestenotic dilatation—are not produced by small bowel carcinoma. Other inflammatory or ischemic strictures do not usually have overhanging edges. Secondary malignancies may be difficult to differentiate radiographically without a clinical history.[2]

Treatment and Prognosis

The survival of patients with adenocarcinoma is stage-dependent; it is favorable when diagnosis is made before lymph node involvement.[121] The only way to cure carcinoma of the small intestine is by early resection. Major advances in surgical and diagnostic imaging techniques in the 40 years before 1986 did not have an impact on the survival of patients with carcinoma of the small intestine.[12,27] Unlike their counterparts in the colon and rectum, small bowel adenocarcinomas do not exhibit a direct relationship between maximal size and invasiveness. Unfortunately, the majority of patients are at an advanced stage at the time of diagnosis. The lateness of diagnosis militates against a fa-

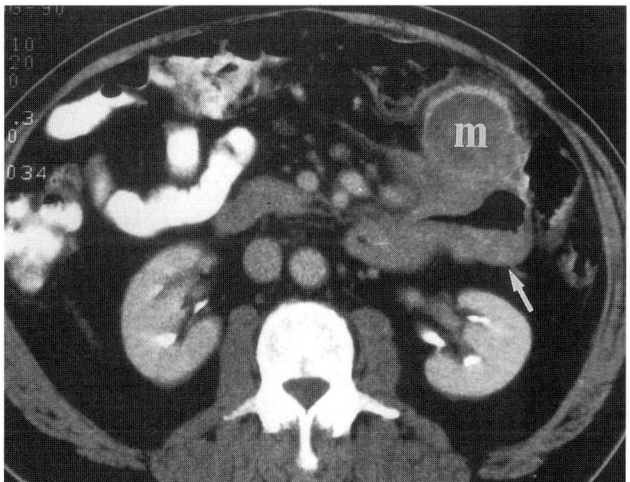

Fig. 19-31. CT of mesenteric extension of adenocarcinoma of the small bowel.
A large mass (m) is seen in the mesentery with associated asymmetric narrowing of the bowel lumen (arrow), suggesting small bowel origin of the mass. Note multiple small involved nodes in mesentery. (From Maglinte,[131] with permission.)

vorable outcome. The proximity of the invaded nodes to major vessels often prevents a truly radical resection. Five-year survival has been reported to be 46% for carcinoma in the jejunum and 20% for carcinoma in the ileum.[121] In comparison, patients with malignant carcinoids have a better overall survival rate of approximately 64%. Radiation therapy has little to offer. The benefits of chemotherapy have not been established.

Carcinoids

Almost 50% of carcinoids occur in the appendix and 33% in the small bowel. Carcinoids account for 25% of all primary small bowel tumors; they are at least 10 times more common in the ileum than in the jejunum. Rarely, they may arise in a Meckel's diverticulum.

Carcinoids are slow-growing tumors that have been thought to arise from enterochromaffin cells at the base of the crypts of Lieberkühn but are more likely to take their origin from undifferentiated progenitor stem cells. Carcinoids, even those in the ileum, are asymptomatic in their early development or may present vague, nonspecific symptoms like abdominal pain or dyspepsia for 5 to 7 years. All carcinoid tumors are potentially malignant and have been called "malignant neoplasms in slow motion."[122] The extent of invasion is a function of time, anatomic location, and size. There are no distinct histologic differences between the benign and malignant stages of carcinoid tumors. Malignant status is confirmed if local invasion or distant metastases are observed.[123] Only 2% of the tumors less than 1 cm in diameter invade and metastasize, whereas 80% of tumors more than 2 cm in diameter are associated with metastatic disease. Between 30% and 67% of ileal carcinoids are found to have extended beyond the bowel wall at the time of diagnosis.[124] Even appendiceal carcinoids, which are considered benign, may show microscopic invasion of the muscularis.

Clinicopathologic Aspects

Carcinoid tumors, together with insulinomas, gastrinomas, nonfunctioning islet cell tumors, vipomas, glucagonomas, and somatostatinomas, are grouped as apudomas (amine precursor uptake and decarboxylation tumors). Apudomas may present with gastrointestinal, metabolic, and/or vasomotor symptoms caused by the production of active amines or peptides. Hormonally active substances such as 5-hydroxytryptamine (serotonin), kallikrein, bradykinin, and histamine are secreted by carcinoid tumors and are generally metabolized in the liver. Serotonin, the major biomedical product of carcinoid tumors, requires dietary tryptophan for its synthesis.[125] Normally, only about 1% of tryptophan is converted to serotonin, but carcinoid tumors can utilize as much as 60% Serotonin released by the tumor is bound to platelets in the plasma. Deamination by monoamine oxidase in liver and lungs converts serotonin to 5-hydroxyindoleacetic acid (5-HIAA), which is excreted in the urine in increased amounts. A normal adult excretes less than 10 mg of 5-HIAA in the urine during 24 hours. Output of 5-HIAA can be mildly increased in patients taking serotonin-containing foods or drugs like phenothiazines and in patients with malabsorption states or prolonged intestinal obstruction. Kallikrein is related to the production of bradykinin, high levels of which appear in the plasma of patients with carcinoid tumors.[125]

Although carcinoids also arise from other parts of the gastrointestinal tract, this chapter concerns itself almost entirely with midgut, ileal carcinoids. Foregut or hindgut carcinoids show very different behavior patterns. Initially, carcinoids grow toward the submucosa as well as the mucosal surface, bulge into the bowel lumen, and may even become semipedunculated and the lead point of an intussusception. The overlying mucosa may ulcerate, and bleeding may be an early manifestation. As soon as further growth has reached the muscularis propria, ileal carcinoids cause a local serotonin-mediated desmoplastic change. Fibrosis may produce fixation and kinking of a bowel loop, sometimes sufficient to cause obstruction. Diarrhea is not usually an early feature. Urinary 5-HIAA levels may be mildly elevated at this stage. In the course of transmural growth, carcinoid cells spread through perivascular lymphatic channels or by direct tissue penetration to produce metastases in mesenteric lymph nodes. These metastases enlarge and tend to fuse to form a mesenteric mass that exceeds the primary tumor in size and in the production of endocrine substances. Fibrosis emanating from the mesenteric mass gradually extends in spoke-wheel fashion toward adjacent bowel loops and causes them to draw closer. The same desmoplastic change also involves mesenteric blood vessels and produces ischemia. This is further compounded by the development of a special form of elastic fibrosis that causes thickening of smaller mesenteric arteries and veins over a wide area and may render bowel ischemia more severe, at times leading to gangrene. The mesenteric mass is not the only carcinoid metastasis in the peritoneal cavity; peritoneal surfaces, other lymph nodes, and the omentum may be additional sites.

Because of the deaminizing capacity of the uninvolved liver, much of the serotonin produced by the mesenteric mass usually fails to reach the systemic circulation. At a mostly much later stage of the disease the carcinoid tumor may spread to the liver via the portal stream to produce further and often numerous metastases. In their presence, vasoactive substances are released directly into the systemic venous flow, giving rise to the carcinoid syndrome. The carcinoid syndrome can occasionally occur without hepatic involvement.[125] This may happen if the primary carcinoid or any of the peritoneal metastases have infiltrated the retroperitoneum or, rarely, if the carcinoid has originated where it can drain directly into the systemic circulation, eg, from ovaries or bronchi.[126] Carcinoids are multiple in about 30% of cases[127] and can be associated with other synchronous or metachronous neoplasms in about 30% of patients.[128]

The carcinoid syndrome is a late and infrequent presentation. Its symptoms are periodic cutaneous flushing,[129] diarrhea, and, less frequently, bronchospasm. The carcinoid syndrome is always associated with elevated blood levels of serotonin and a significant elevation of urinary 5-HIAA. Entry of serotonin into the right side of the heart produces a special form of subendothelial fibrosis. Carcinoid heart disease is manifested by a systolic murmur along the left heart border due to the pulmonic stenosis. Tricuspid insufficiency is suggested by increased pulsations in the liver. The left side of the heart is unaffected, being protected by monoamine oxidase in the lung. The presence of liver metastases need not always be associated with clinical carcinoid syndrome, this usually because of extensive necrosis of liver metastases.

Radiology

With conventional small bowel barium examination, some ileal carcinoids have been incorrectly diagnosed and were treated for other conditions such as Crohn's disease for as long as four years before surgery revealed the correct diagnosis.[130] The radiographic findings by means of barium depend on the stage of the disease and on the technique used. The conventional SBFT, the most frequent examination in the United States, rarely detects primary carcinoid tumors before they reach 2 cm in size.[4] The demonstration by enteroclysis or by a carefully performed fluoroscopic SBFT of a smoothly rounded mucosal elevation of about 5 to 10 mm in diameter, located in the distal ileum, should always place a carcinoid tumor at the top of differential diagnoses, although it lacks radiodiagnostic features characteristic for a carcinoid tumor and is indistinguishable from other lesions, such as a leiomyoma, lipoma, or adenoma (Fig. 19-32). The reason for this emphasis is that such early carcinoids have usually not yet involved mesenteric lymph nodes and their resection can be curative. However, occasionally even very small carcinoids may have produced histologically shown micrometastases in regional lymph nodes, and it is advisable to resect all palpable nodes near early carcinoids (Fig. 19-32). The presence of one or more additional polyps of similar appearance further supports diagnosis of carcinoid.[131] Multiple carcinoids tend to contain at least one more advanced lesion, and it may already be possible to support the barium diagnosis by the CT demonstration of a mesenteric metastasis (Fig. 19-33). The mucosa overlying carcinoids can ulcerate, and bleeding may be an important early manifestation. It may be possible to demonstrate a carcinoid ulcer by enteroclysis (Fig. 19-34).

Occasionally carcinoids can become the lead point of an intussusception and cause high-grade obstruction (Fig. 19-35). More often carcinoid-related obstructions are of lower grade and are caused by tumor growth extending into and through the gut wall, when local serotonin output produces hypertrophy of the muscularis and fibrosis with crowding of folds, outline distortion, and kinking of the lumen. The intraluminal bulk of the tumor, though rarely exceeding 3 cm in size, may add to the obstruction [Fig. 19-36(a–e)]. Sooner or later the fibrosis emanating from the mesenteric metastasis can significantly add to the focal causes of the bowel obstruction. Occasionally, CT can identify the metastasis as being the major cause of obstruction [Fig. 19-36(f, g)]. CT or magnetic resonance imaging (MRI) are essential adjuncts to barium studies because of the truly synergistic quality of this imaging combination. The desmoplastic influence of the mesenteric metastasis may affect the area surrounding the primary carcinoid to the extent that it may no longer be possible to identify it in a sea of fibrosis; CT and/or MRI then make it possible to confirm the association with a carcinoid tumor by the demonstration of the typical metastasis in the mesentery [Fig. 19-37(a–d)]. CT scans of a mesenteric metastasis, in addition to the spoke-wheel arrangement due to the emanating fibrosis, show it to contain calcifications in well over half the cases. Calcifications can be massive, coarse, rounded, or punctate. In other cases, though the primary carcinoid may have been demonstrated by enteroclysis, desmoplasia derived from the mesenteric mass distorts more distal bowel loops so that a possible additional carcinoid tumor can no longer be identified or excluded [Fig. 19-37(e, f)]. The often intense desmoplastic process radiating from the mesenteric metastasis narrows or kinks blood vessels supplying the bowel loops that are being drawn ever closer.

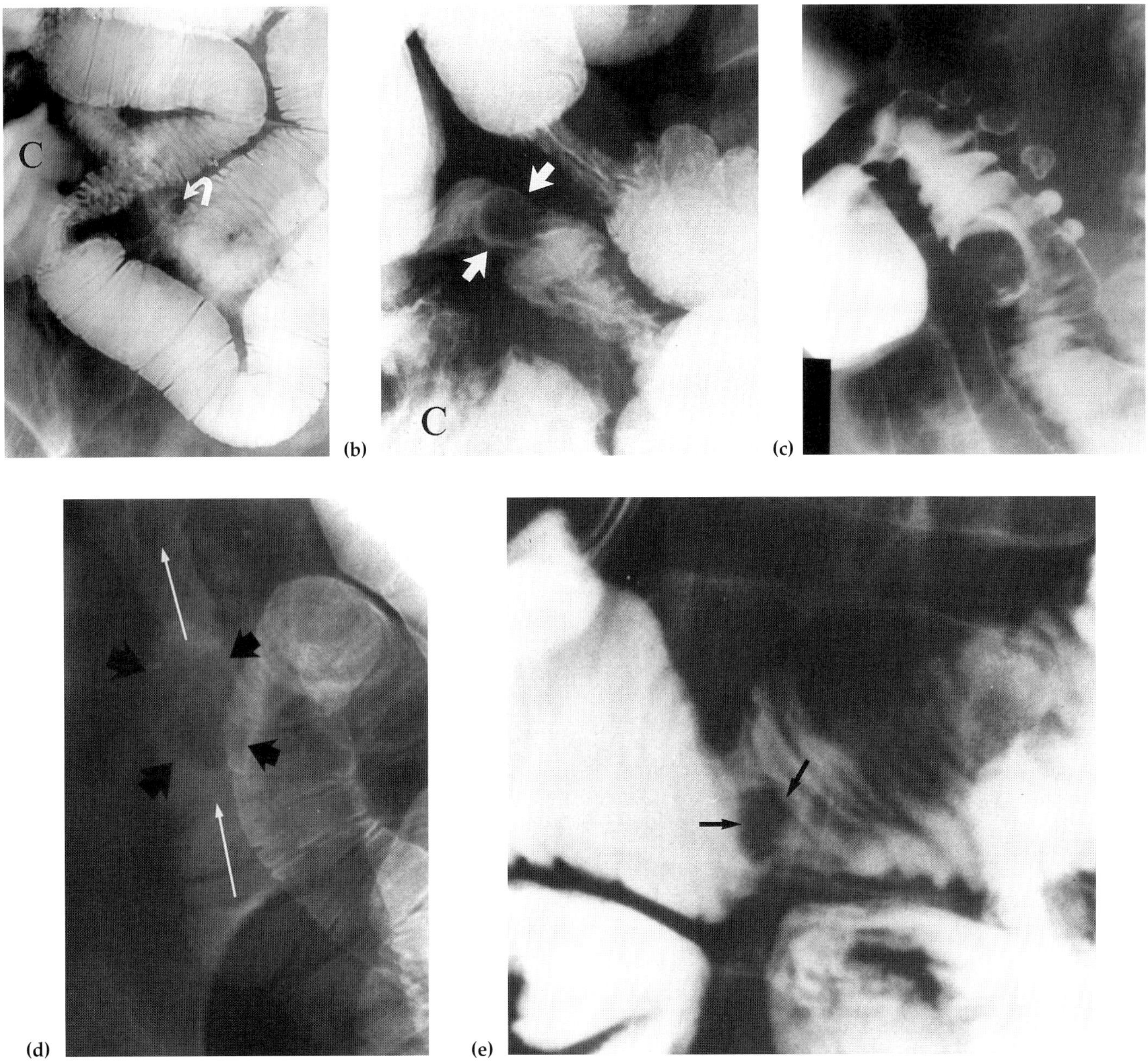

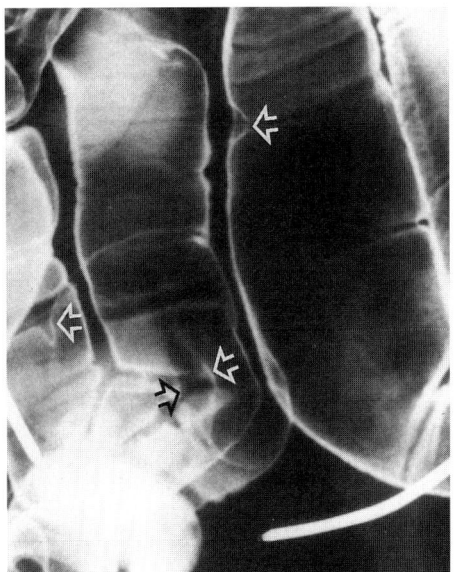

Fig. 19-32. Radiologic diagnosis of small, unsuspected carcinoids.
(a) A 6-mm intramural defect (curved arrow) is shown in the distal ileum by enteroclysis. Surgery disclosed a carcinoid tumor. Adjacent nodes were not involved. (C = cecum) (From Bessette et al.[30]) (b) Enteroclysis compression radiograph shows a 10-mm polypoid mass in the terminal ileum (arrows) of a middle-aged woman with undiagnosed lower GI bleeding. Prior investigations were unrevealing. Surgery and histology showed carcinoid with small ulcer. There were no nodes involved. (From Maglinte et al.[3]). (c) Chance finding of 1-cm polyp in terminal ileum (also pseudodiverticula). Carcinoid had to be at the top of the differential diagnostic list. Surgery confirmed carcinoid. (d) Similar intraluminal 1.2-cm mass (arrows) in terminal ileum (long arrows). Again carcinoid top of list of diagnoses. Surgery disclosed a leiomyoma. However, with such a tumor in the distal ileum radiology must always place a carcinoid as first diagnosis. (e) Enteroclysis disclosed an 8-mm polyp (arrows) in upper ileum in a patient with iron deficiency anemia. Carcinoid with tiny ulcer found at surgery. Microscopic metastases reported in two small local nodes. (f) Patient with obscure bleeds referred for enteroclysis before a renal transplant. One 6-mm polyp and two other tiny polyps were reported. Bowel explored at surgery and altogether eight tiny carcinoids resected. Micrometastases found in small lymph nodes.

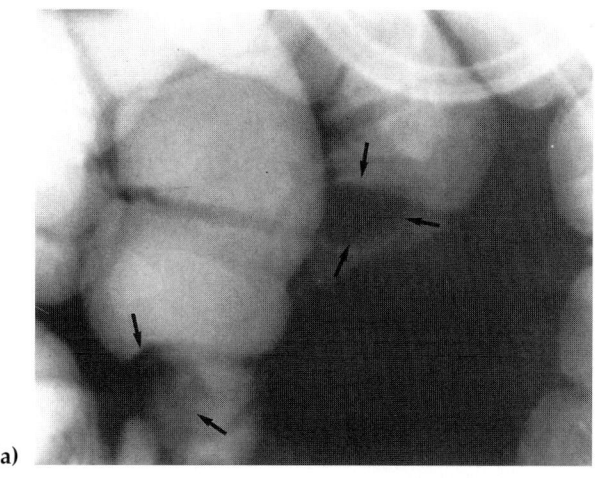
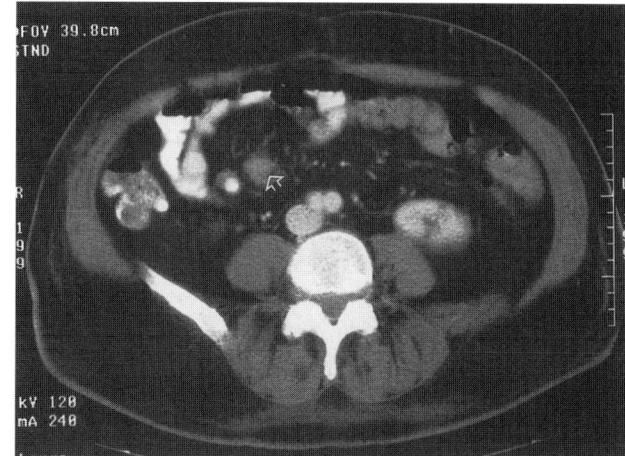
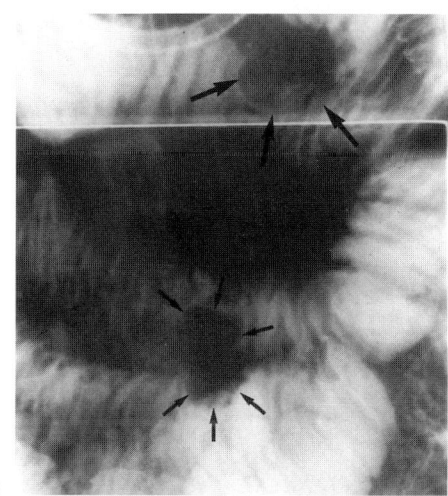
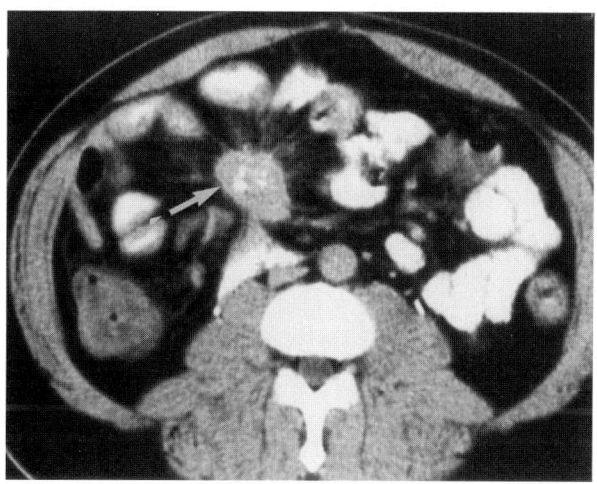
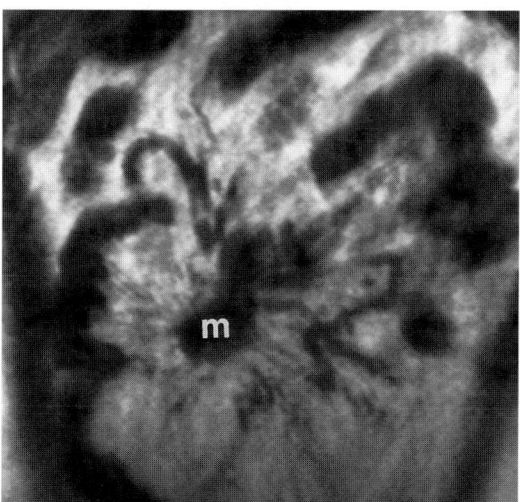

Fig. 19-33. Demonstration of multiple carcinoids.
(a) Enteroclysis in a 71-year-old male 9 years after colon cancer surgery followed by liver metastases. Presented with bleeding seen to exit ileocecal valve at colonoscopy. Two midileal polyps (arrows), each 8-mm diameter, were resected. Diagnosis carcinoids with involvement of one local node. A 2.0-cm firm mass resected in mesentery. (b) Same patient. Earlier CT scan with a mesenteric mass (arrow), a likely extension from ileal carcinoids. No visible desmoplasia as yet. (Courtesy of Marc J. Gollup, MD.) (c) A further patient with diarrhea referred for enteroclysis. Three tumors demonstrated (arrows), carcinoids considered the likely diagnosis. CT recommended. (d) CT scan demonstrates a typical carcinoid mesenteric metastasis (arrow). Mesenteric vascular bundles are accentuated by fibrosis, and adjacent bowel loops show minimal wall thickening. The metastasis contains coarse nodular calcification. (e) Spin-echo T1-weighted coronal MRI of a different patient with ileal carcinoids. It outlines a mesenteric metastatic mass (m) from which accentuated vascular structures radiate and begin to retract surrounding bowel. (Courtesy of Koula Coliadis, MD.)

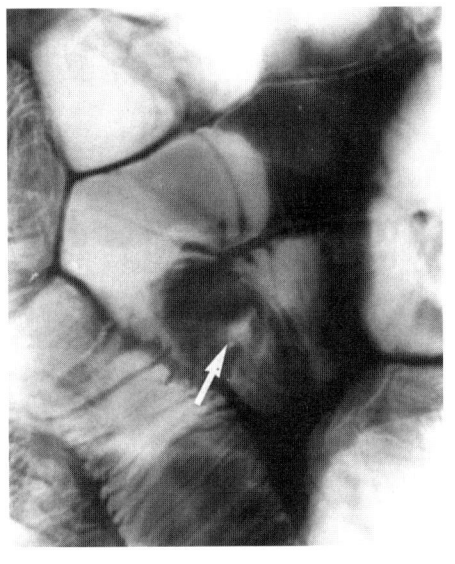
(a)

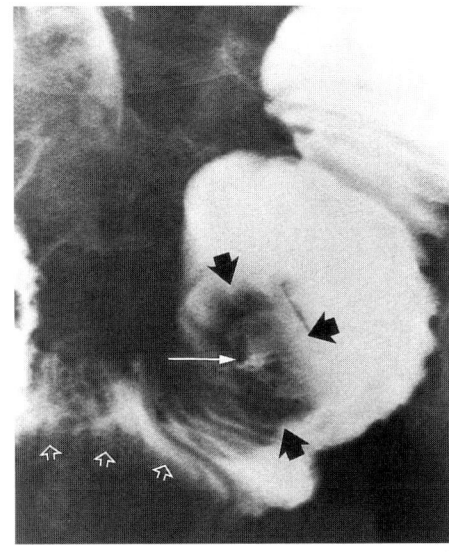
(b)

Fig. 19-34. Ulcers in primary carcinoids, cause of presentation with bleeding.
(a) Male patient, obscure blood loss. Enteroclysis demonstrates 2-cm mass with ulcer (arrow) and typical desmoplasia-related crowding of intact folds. Resected. (b) Female patient with anemia, abdominal pain. Enteroclysis outlines about 2-cm ulcerated (arrow) mass with desmoplastic change of surrounding folds. Low-grade obstruction is due to displacement and infiltration (open arrows) by an endometrial carcinoma.

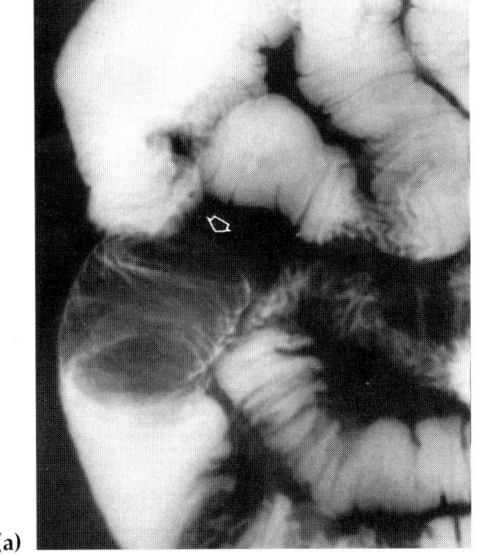
(a)

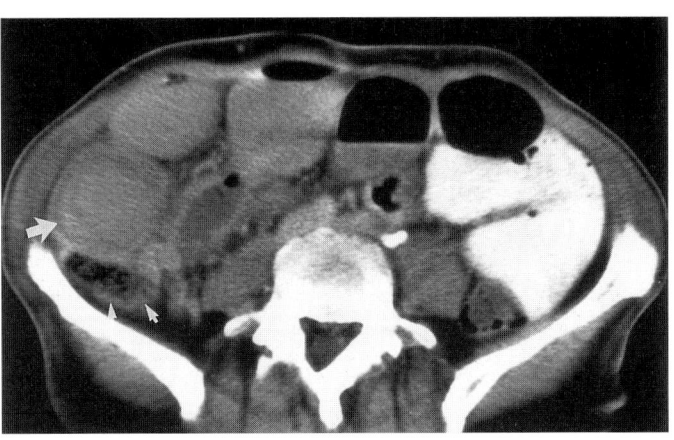
(b)

Fig. 19-35. Intussuscepting carcinoid.
(a) Enteroclysis spot film shows an intussuscepting mass (arrow) in distal ileum in a female patient with intermittent abdominal pain presumed to be from irritable bowel syndrome. Surgical resection of an intussuscepting polypoid mass shown by histology to be a carcinoid. Adjacent nodes were not involved. (From Maglinte and Reyes.[2]) (b) CT scan through midabdomen of a 64-year-old male with weight loss and severe abdominal pain shows a target sign indicating edema of dilated small bowel (arrow). Note markedly dilated loops of small bowel, collapsed distal ileum (arrowheads) indicating obstruction. (c) In same patient, delayed radiograph of an enteroclysis done after initial long tube decompression confirmed presence of a partially intussuscepted mass (arrow) in ileum with high-grade obstruction. (C = cecum) Note collapsed distal ileal loops. Surgery confirmed presence of a 3-cm intussuscepted carcinoid. Adjacent nodes were involved.

(c)

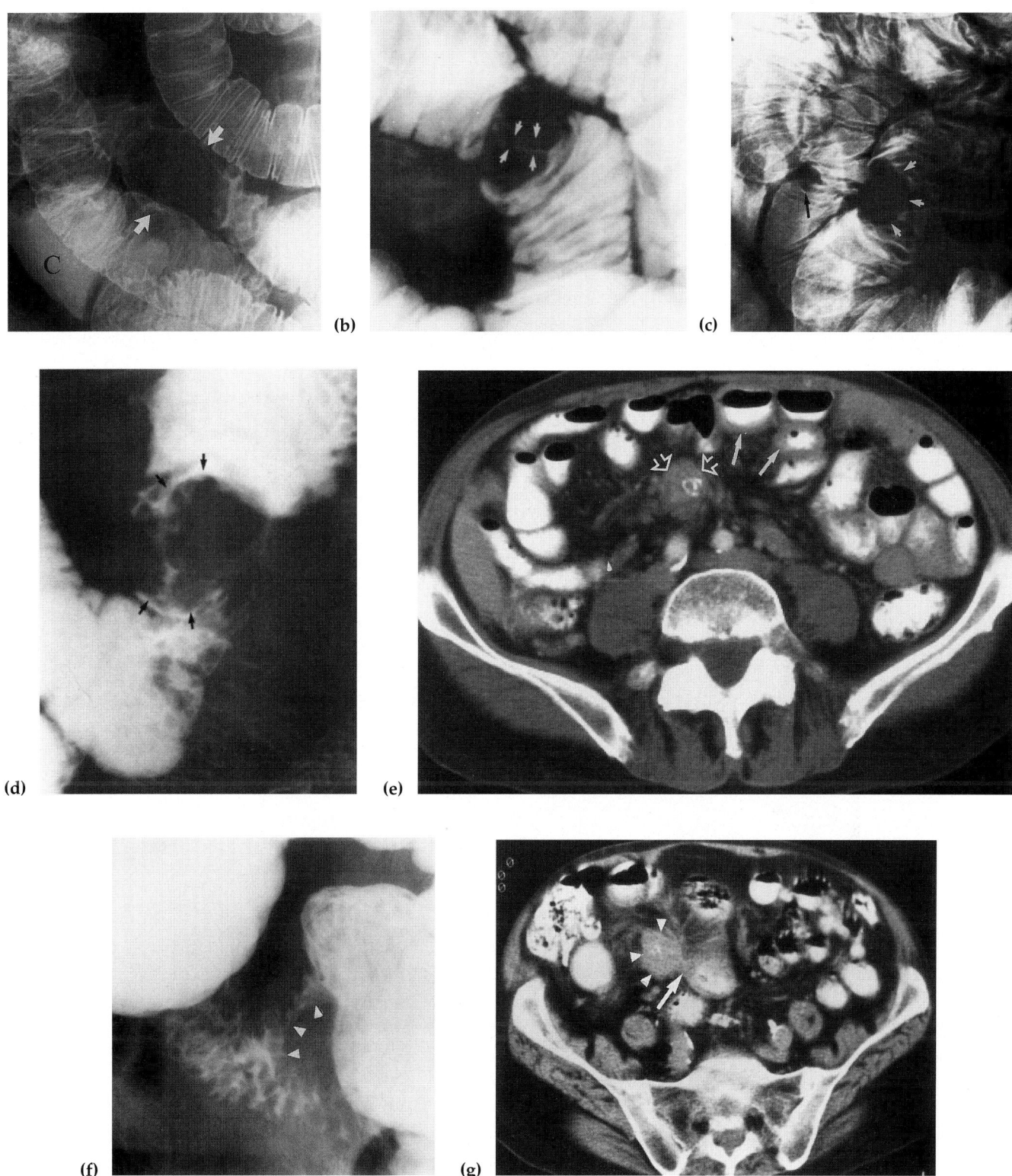

Fig. 19-36. Desmoplasia-related obstruction due to ileal carcinoids.
(a) Bulk of 2.5-cm intramural carcinoid (arrows) contributes to low-grade obstruction mostly caused by fibrotic changes at either end of the lesion (C = cecum.) (b) "Apple core"-like seemingly annular tumor minimally obstructing ileum. (c) More oblique view of above tumor (arrows) shows its appearance to favor carcinoid, this reinforced by the presence of a second smaller tumor (black arrow). Carcinoids were resected. (d) Large, 3-cm tumor of ileum with a suggestion of "shouldering" (arrows) is associated with low-grade obstruction. It might represent an adenocarcinoma. (e) CT scan in above case demonstrates for carcinoid typical mesenteric metastasis with calcification (open arrows) and indication of bowel ischemia (arrows). (f) High-grade small bowel obstruction in a 92-year-old man. Abrupt caliber change with narrowed segment retaining fold pattern (arrowheads). Desmoplasia distally. (g) CT scan in above patient. Obstruction site (arrow) related to calcium-containing mesenteric mass (arrowheads). Primary carcinoid not outlined in (f) or (g).

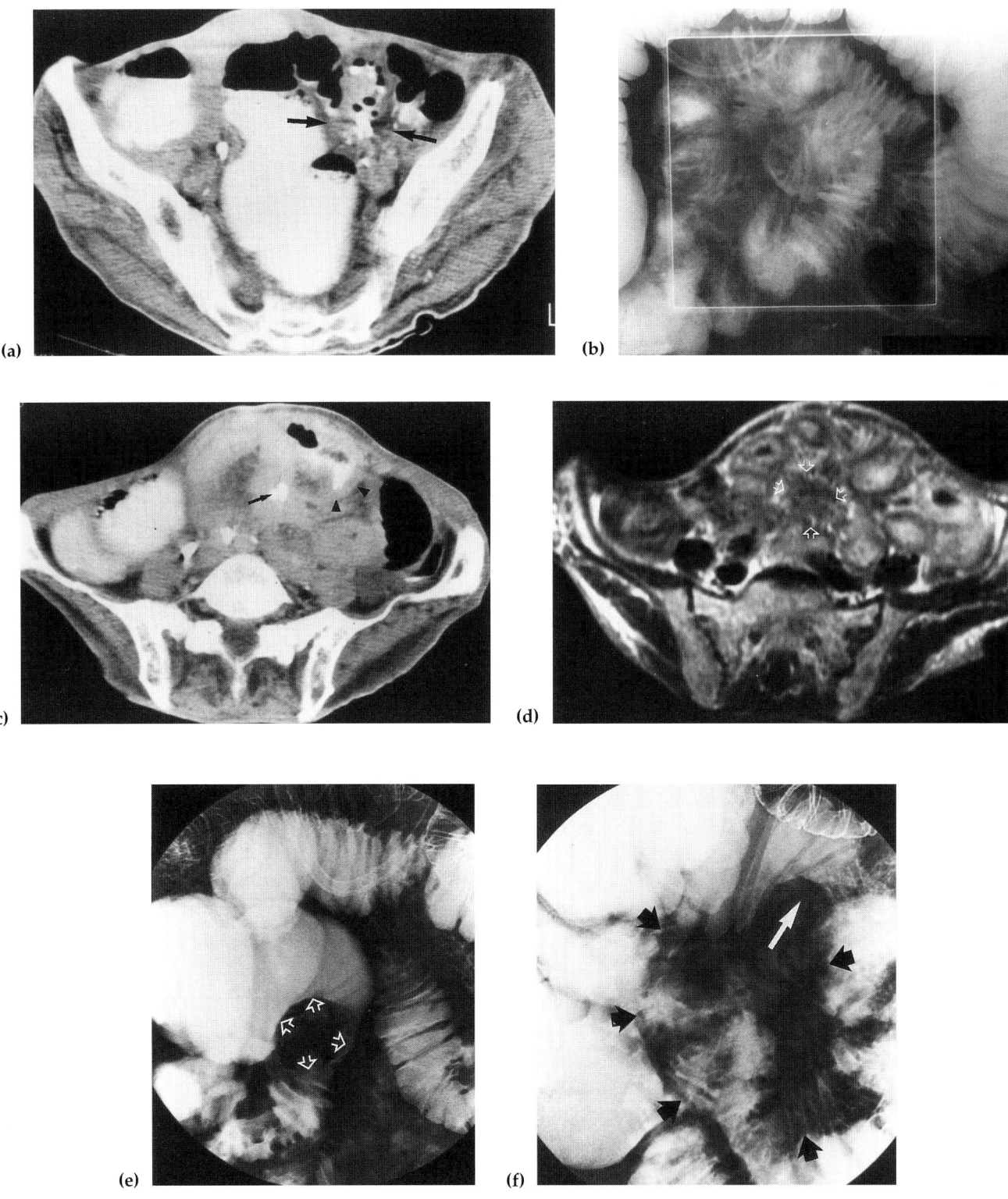

Fig. 19-37. Small bowel obstruction (SBO) in advanced carcinoid.
(a) Clinically obvious SBO in 70-year-old male with likely carcinoid. CT of pelvic area after peroral contrast showed distended ileum near area of irregular narrowing (arrows). (b) Enteroclysis demonstrated, distal to dilated bowel, an area of distorted and kinked loops in which there may or not be one or more carcinoids. (c) CT done in this emaciated patient indicated large mesenteric mass with calcium (arrow), surrounded by dilated bowel loops with wall thickening (arrowheads). (d) MRI T1-weighted spin-echo image indicates mesenteric mass (open arrows) and more clearly demonstrates bowel wall thickening with features of ischemia. (e) In another patient enteroclysis demonstrates a primary carcinoid (arrows) as main cause of SBO. (f) Distal to obstructing carcinoid (long arrow), distortion and displacements extend over an area (arrows) in which it is impossible to distinguish the effect of further carcinoids from desmoplasia extending out of the mesenteric metastasis.

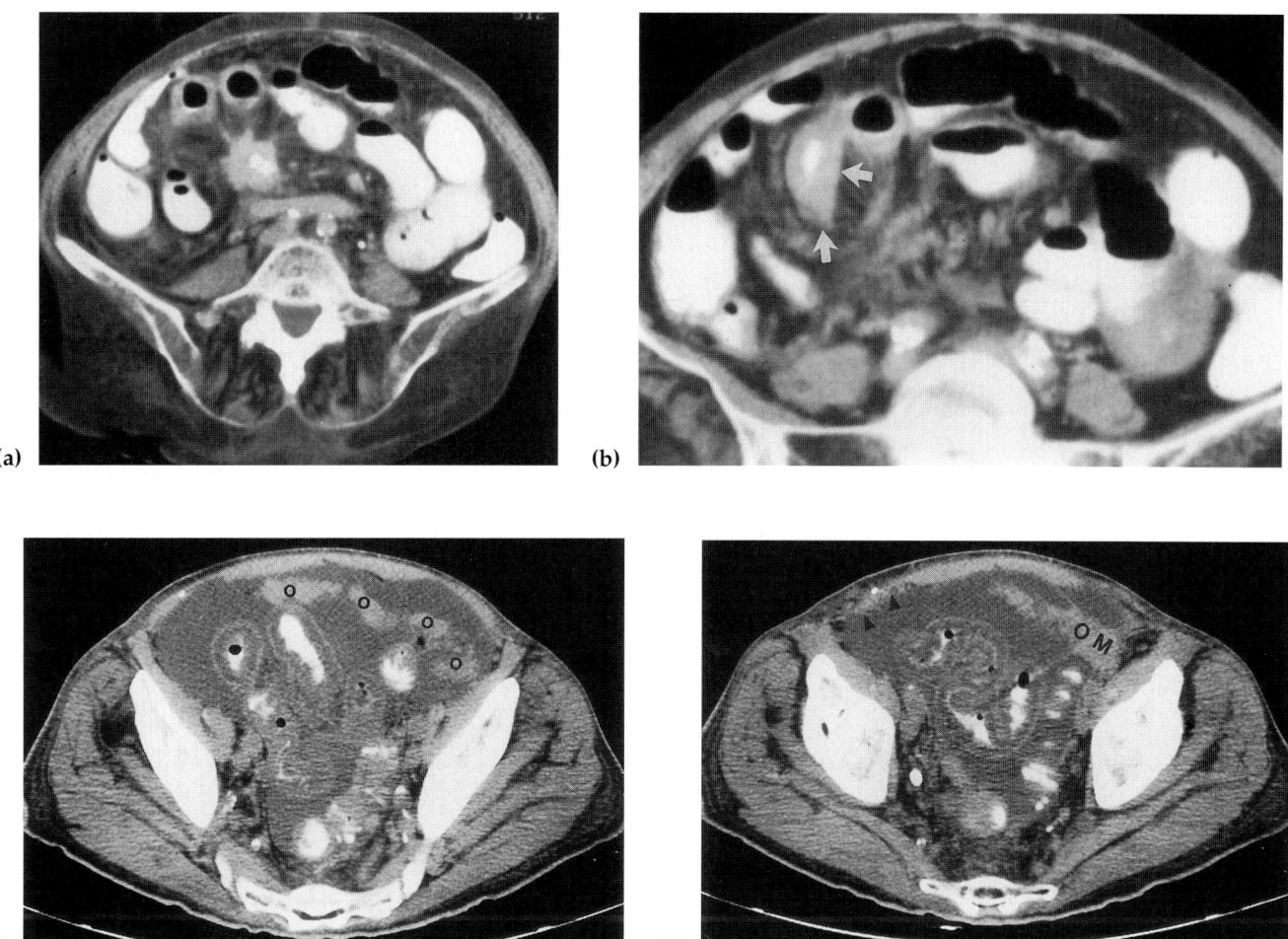

Fig. 19-38. Small bowel ischemia, carcinoid related.
(a) Female, 64 years, with known carcinoid. Recently increasing abdominal pain. CT scan shows typical calcified mesenteric metastatic mass. Bowel loops have been moved close to the mass and show pronounced wall thickening. (b) Mural thickening is grossly increased in a single loop (arrows). Surgery required for severe pain and bleeding. Gangrenous bowel resected, including cecum. (c) Male patient, 77 years, carcinoid syndrome with liver metastases. Recently deteriorated with abdominal pain, anemia, weight loss. CT scan without contrast shows target appearance of ischemic bowel loops surrounded by massive ascites. Omental metastases (o). (d) Identical target appearance of bowel loop. Ascites indicates peritoneal metastases. Omental mass (OM). Irregularly thickened peritoneal surface (arrowheads) due to carcinoid deposits.

Ischemic changes ranging from edema to gangrene have been intensified by elastic sclerosis and can be identified by CT as focally pronounced mural thickening [Fig. 19-38(a, b)] or as the "double halo" sign[132] [Fig. 19-38(c, d)]. Occasionally mesenteric stranding has been demonstrated by CT prior to the development of a dominant nodal mass.[133]

In addition to the metastatic mass in the mesentery, the often extensive metastases within the peritoneal cavity are highly significant for symptomatology and patient survival. There can be multiple peritoneal implants, some miliary, others large enough to be shown on CT scans.[134] Findings include omental caking, thickening of the parietal peritoneum with indistinct borders, adenopathies as in celiac axis and para-aortic regions, and increasing mesenteric stranding indicating further tumor extention in the mesentery. Peritoneal cavity metastases are usually accompanied by ascites, which can be massive [see Fig. 19-38(c, d)].

The patients illustrated in Fig. 19-38 underline the significance of dissemination within the peritoneal cavity in terms of symptoms and survival. Surgical intervention is usually required and rarely adds to the quality of life. Of relatively lesser importance seems to be the development of liver metastases with features of the carcinoid syndrome. Metastases are generally well shown by CT or MRI (Fig. 19-39). MRI, by combining unenhanced spin-echo and dynamic gadolin-

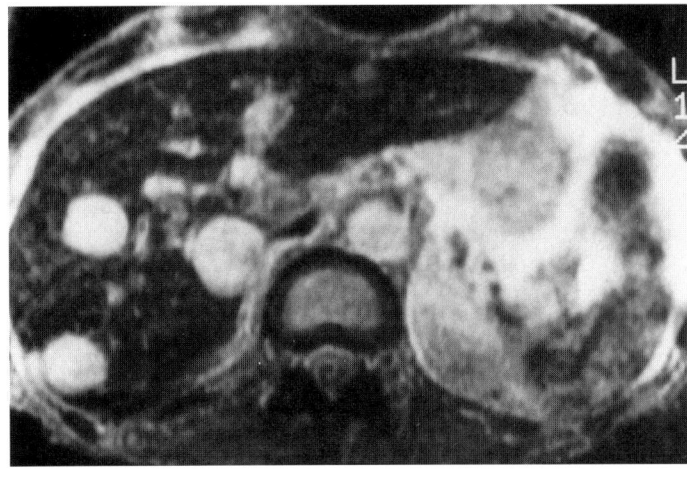

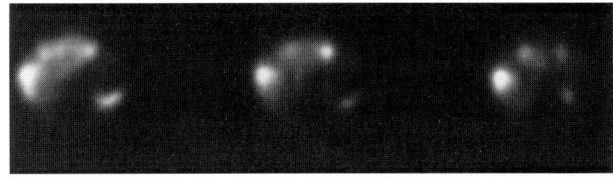

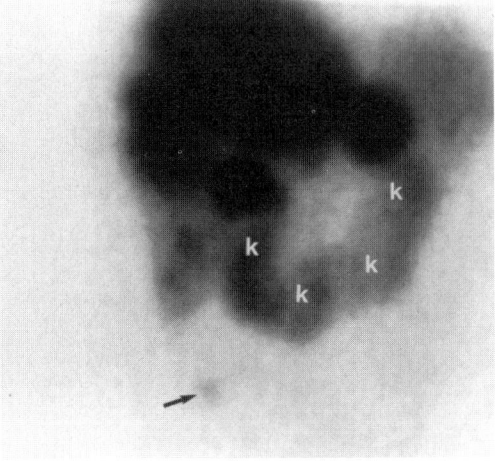

Fig. 19-39. Demonstration of carcinoid metastases to liver. (a) MRI axial view, T2-weighted, with fat suppression, dramatically demonstrates carcinoid metastases. (b) Example of octreotide imaging. SPECT at 24 hours demonstrates liver metastases. (Structure marked "k" represents a horseshoe kidney.) (c) Octreotide scintigram indicates site of primary carcinoid (arrow).

ium chelate-enhanced gradient-recalled echo images, can more accurately distinguish carcinoid metastases from hemangiomas.[135] Somatostatin receptor scintigraphy using indium-111-pentetate-labeled octreotide (pentetreotide) for gut or liver carcinoid tumors has been reported to have 75% sensitivity, 100% specificity, 100% positive predictive value, and 63% negative predictive value.[136,137] Another report considered CT to be more sensitive than somatostatin receptor scanning and regards the two techniques to be complementary.[138] Yet it is claimed that during whole body imaging with a somatostatin analogue the power of resolution could be at or above 1.0 cm in size.[139] Pentetreotide scintigraphy has been considered to be more cost-effective than conventional imaging.[139] Further improvement of the accuracy of somatostatin receptor scintigraphy is achieved by combining it with single positron emission computed tomography (SPECT). Patients with positive indium-111-pentetreotide scans have tumors that express somatostatin receptors and are therefore more likely to respond to octreotide therapy.[140] For this purpose, the octapeptide lanreotide is available in slow release form and can be administered at 14-day intervals.[141] This treatment is particularly effective in the relief of flushing and wheezing and, to a somewhat lesser extent, in the reduction of diarrhea and 5-HIAA concentration. Some tumor regression may occur. The dose of lanreotide may have to be increased over time. The long-term value of lanreotide management of flushing and diarrhea is exemplified in the case of a patient who also illustrated two further aspects of carcinoid tumors. These are the development of carcinoid-syndromelike features in the absence of liver metastases and the catastrophic effect of intraperitoneal spread of the tumor (Fig. 19-40).

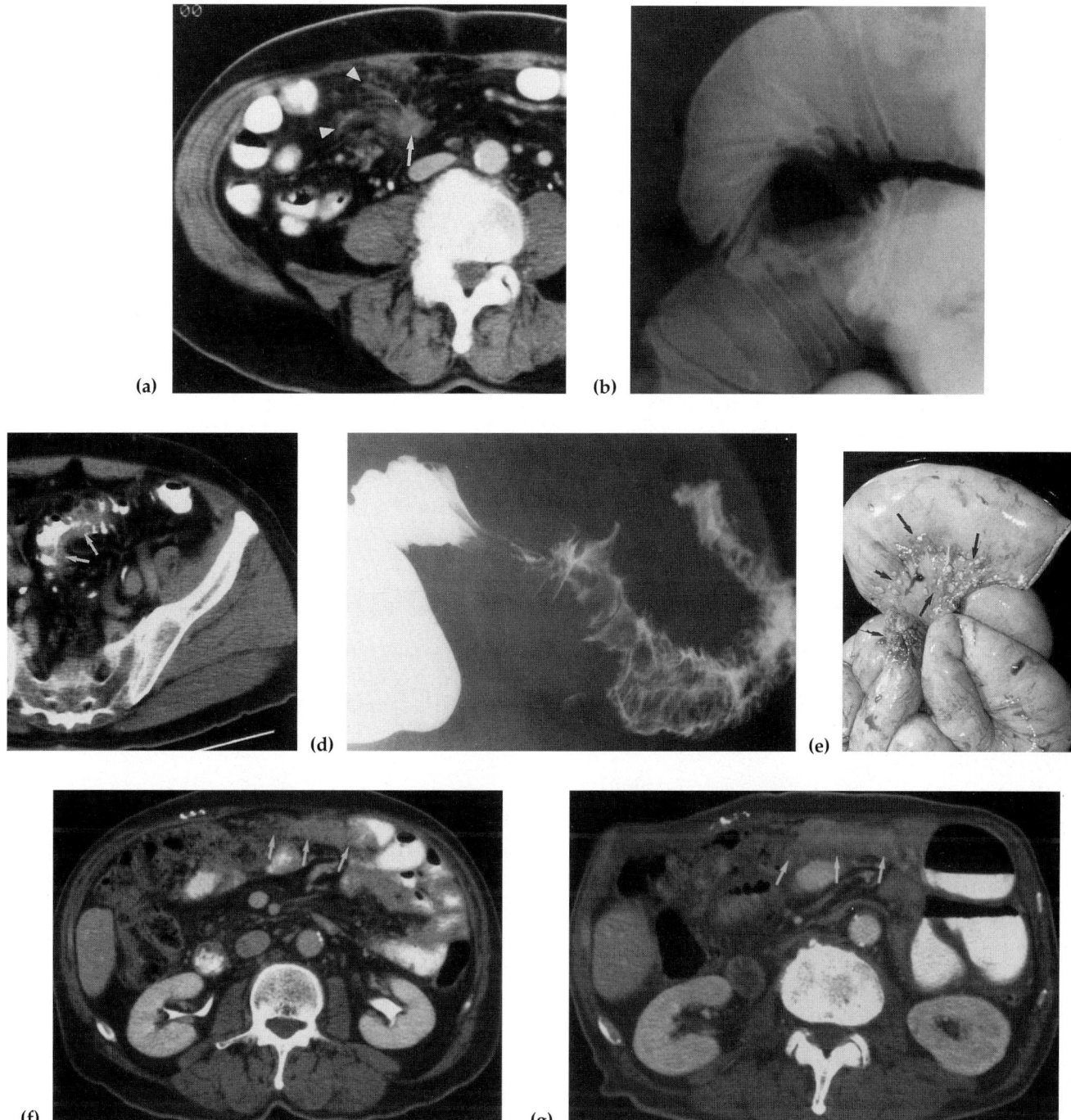

Fig. 19-40. Male physician aged 70 years with history of mesenteric non-Hodgkin's lymphoma that responded to therapy. Several years later, became aware of carcinoid-type flushing, mild diarrhea, and wheezing, and found HIAA to be elevated. He started long-acting sandostatin treatment, which made possible an almost normal lifestyle for the next 2.5 years. His CT liver scans were normal throughout. Began to have increasing abdominal pain, and following investigations were done:

(a) CT scan of the abdomen showed a mesenteric mass (arrow) from which thickened fibrovascular bundles began to radiate (arrowheads). (b) Enteroclysis then demonstrated four typical ileal carcinoids, one illustrated here. (c) Ten days later became increasingly obstructed. CT scan showed a mass lesion extending into mesenteric border of narrowed sigmoid colon (arrows). (d) Barium enema followed and revealed retrograde obstruction by a severely deformed and narrowed sigmoid. Resection of obstructing sigmoid mass; histology diagnosed a carcinoid metastasis. (e) Laparotomy included resection of mesenteric mass with adherent bowel. Specimen showed miliary metastases, all confirmed carcinoids (arrows). (f) Eighteen months later increasing abdominal pain and general deterioration. CT scan shows omental cake (arrows) and some thickening of crowded bowel loops. (g) One year later, after further surgery for bleeding, worsened status, signs of SBO. CT scan shows larger omental mass with smudging of outline (arrows). Haziness of mesenteric structures indicates increased tumor burden. SBO. Further surgery refused, died. At autopsy no evidence of liver metastases.

Liver bypassing entry of serotonin into the systemic circulation can occur when peritoneal metastases find it possible to access extraperitoneal vasculature. In the case of the patient in Fig. 19-40 this may have been facilitated by prior non-Hodgkin's lymphoma that had involved abdominal lymph nodes and did respond to therapy. In another patient [Fig. 19-41(a, b)], a carcinoid of terminal ileal origin infiltrated in retroperitoneal direction, obstructed the right ureter, and caused symptoms of the carcinoid syndrome in the absence of liver metastases. Furthermore, a patient with several ileal carcinoids and multiple necrotic metastases in an otherwise healthy liver did not show features of the carcinoid syndrome [Fig. 19-41(c)].

The angiographic findings of an infiltrating carcinoid are distinctive. Typical findings include a stellate arterial configuration at the tumor periphery, poor to moderate accumulation within the tumor, nonfilling of major draining veins, and irregular narrowing of mesenteric artery branches (Fig. 19-42).[142] Angiography, however, is now rarely used for carcinoid diagnosis. Occasionally, however, there may be problems of interpretation of the CT features of retractile mesenteritis, Hodgkin's disease, extensive radiation damage, and advanced metastatic disease (eg, from the ovaries) with appearances similar to those of carcinoids; angiography has been used in such cases.[142]

Treatment

The 5-year survival rate of patients with appendiceal carcinoids is 99%, 83% for those with carcinoid in the

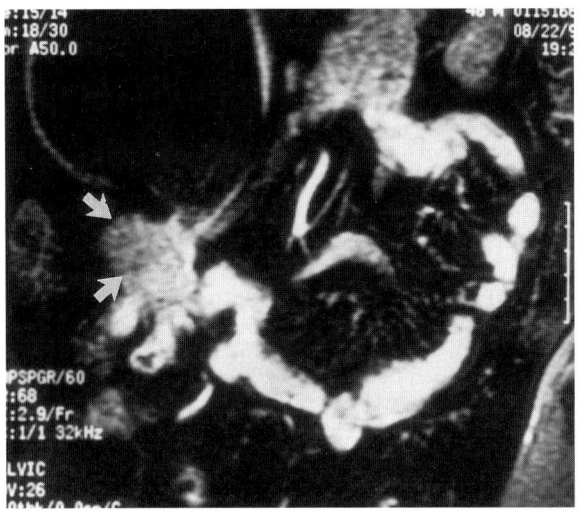

(a)

(b)

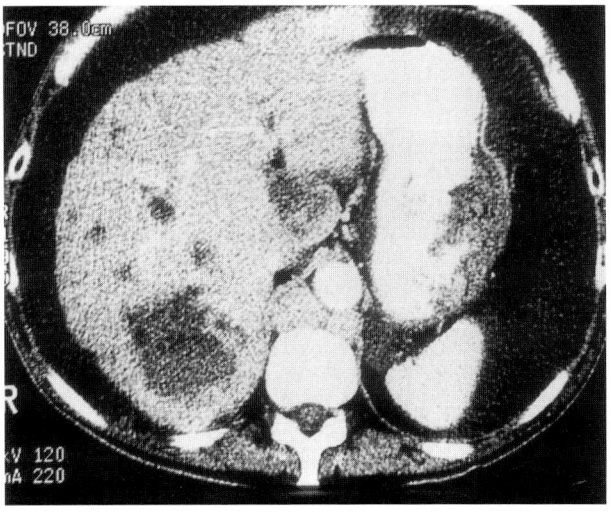

(c)

Fig. 19-41. Further atypical causes of the carcinoid syndrome.
(a) Male patient, 51 years old, with right hydronephrosis and back pain complained of flushing, diarrhea, and wheezing. A T1-weighted, fat-saturated, gradient-echo coronal contrast enhanced MRI demonstrates contrast uptake by a mass (arrows) arising distal ileum. Dorsally directed growth of this poorly differentiated carcinoid penetrated retroperitoneum, obstructed the right ureter, and secreted serotonin and other peptides directly into systemic veins to cause the carcinoid syndrome. (b) The liver of the above patient as shown by T1-weighted, spin-echo sequence MRI is free of carcinoid or other metastases. (c) Male patient, 56 years old complains of intermittent abdominal pain, weight loss, anemia. Two mildly obstructing ileal carcinoids shown by enteroclysis. CT scan outlines numerous liver metastases, all with necrotic centers. Patient without symptoms of a carcinoid syndrome.

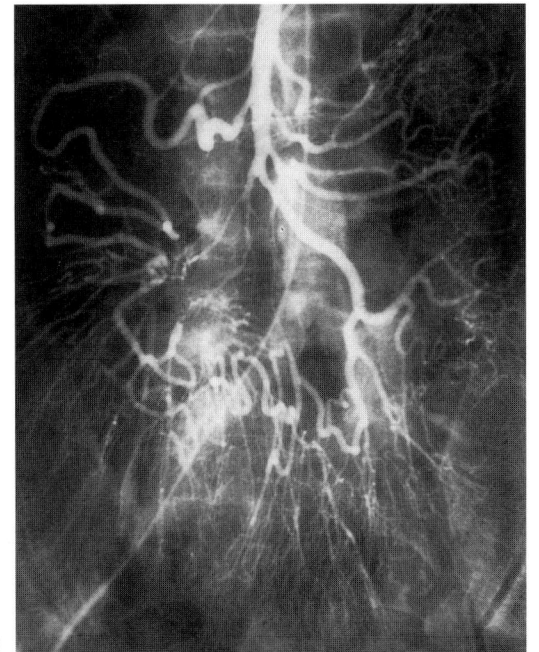 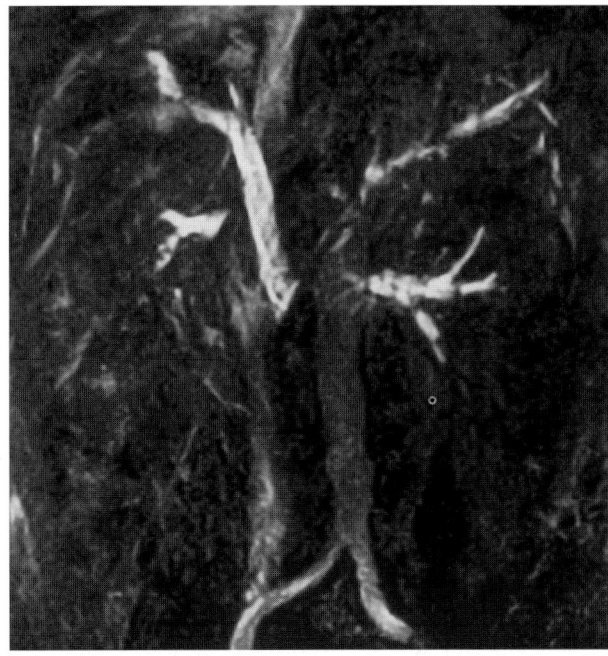

Fig. 19-42. Angiographic features of carcinoid.
(a) Arterial phase. Superior mesenteric artery injection shows irregularly narrowed terminations to the distal ileal and ileocolic areas. A conglomerate of distorted vessels demarcates the peripheral aspect of the mesenteric carcinoid metastasis (arrows). The narrowed branches do not seem to contribute to the mesenteric arcade of the small bowel or colon. (b) Venous phase of a magnetic resonance angiographic sequence in a case of ileal carcinoma shows occlusion of the distal portion of the superior mesenteric vein, indicating mesenteric invasion. (Courtesy of Koula Coliadis, MD.)

colon and rectum, and 54% in those with small bowel carcinoids. With complete resection of a small bowel carcinoid, the survival rate increases to 75% and decreases to 19% in patients with distant metastases.[88] The main reasons for resection of a primary small bowel carcinoid are 1) to achieve a cure in cases diagnosed by serendipity, or 2) in symptomatic patients to prevent or treat the frequently complicating intestinal obstruction. Surgical therapy is the usual option when there is limited spread to regional lymph nodes or when it is unavoidable because of the development of severe ischemia or gangrene.

Patients with the carcinoid syndrome already have widespread metastatic disease. Patients with positive octreotide scans are likely to respond to octreotide therapy. Some 15% to 20% of carcinoids, however, do not express somatostatin receptors. Some of these tumors may be dedifferentiated and may be responsive to combined infusional etoposide and cisplatin.[143] Hepatic artery embolization remains a therapeutic alternative and is possibly preferred to surgery because the vascular approach permits repeated embolization.[144,145] Although there is agreement that embolization improves the quality of life of the patient, its effect on survival is less clear.

Sandostatin, a long-acting form of octreotide, an analog of somatostatin, is capable of inhibiting the release of various intestinal peptides with alleviation of the clinical features of carcinoids (eg, flushing and diarrhea) in about 90% of patients.[140,143] Sandostatin is the presently most useful long-term treatment option for patients with the carcinoid syndrome and liver metastases. It can be used alone or in combination with interferon-alpha.[146] Carcinoid tumors exhibit low-grade radiation sensitivity, but radiation may be helpful in patients with painful bone metastases.[88]

Conclusion

At the present time it is possible to maintain a patient with liver metastases for several years in a state of almost normal activity. With the advent of carcinoid spread within the peritoneal cavity—unfortunately a process that often precedes liver metastases—a combination of ischemic, obstructive, and widespread metastatic changes occurs and intensifies. It is this development, and not what occurs in the liver, that causes real suffering and will very negatively affect the outcome.

Non-Hodgkin's Lymphoma

Lymphoma, the third most common small bowel malignancy, may involve the gastrointestinal tract primarily or as a manifestation of systemic disease.[47] Primary small bowel lymphomas account for approximately 5% of all lymphomas and one third of the gastrointestinal tract lymphomas and are, next to the stomach, the most common of the extranodal sites of origin. The incidence of small bowel lymphoma has been estimated to be 1.6 cases per million per year.

The gastrointestinal tract plays an important role in host immune defenses. Gut-associated lymphoid tissue (GALT) is the largest immunologic organ of the body and the basis of most types of lymphoma. In contrast to adenocarcinoma and leiomyosarcoma, which produce a focal or segmental lesion, lymphoma tends to originate at multiple sites and to extend along the axis of the small intestine.[147] Primary or secondary lymphoma may occur in any portion of the gastrointestinal tract. In general, primary lymphomas have a better prognosis than carcinomas. To make a diagnosis of primary gastrointestinal lymphoma, the following criteria should be fulfilled: 1) no palpable superficial lymph nodes; 2) normal chest roentgenogram (no adenopathy); 3) normal white blood cell count (total and differential); 4) at laparotomy, a predominantly alimentary tract lesion with lymph node involvement, if any, confined to the drainage area of the involved segment of gut; and 5) no involvement of the liver or spleen.[148] A less rigid definition of primary lymphoma requires the main bulk of the tumor to be located in the gastrointestinal tract, with treatment having to be directed there.[149] Secondary gastrointestinal lymphoma usually affects multiple sites; at autopsy, gross or microscopic evidence of gastrointestinal involvement has been found in up to 50% of cases of disseminated lymphoma.[150] In both the primary and secondary forms, the stomach is most commonly involved (51%), followed by the small intestine (33%), the colon (16%), and the esophagus (less than 1%). Small bowel lymphoma varies in frequency with geographic location, constituting 8.7% of all gastrointestinal tumors in the Middle East, compared with 0.9% to 1% in the United States.[151]

Most "Western" intestinal B-cell lymphomas are of GALT type. They are often single lesions; mesenteric lymph nodes are commonly involved, but spread beyond the abdomen is unusual at presentation.[149] Though GALT lymphomas tend to be low grade and composed of small cleaved cells, they are prone to high-grade transformation.

Classification and Staging

Classification refers to the histologic composition of non-Hodgkin's lymphoma. Whereas Hodgkin's disease is a single entity and extends in an orderly manner and by contiguity, non-Hodgkin's lymphoma may comprise several diseases, typically with noncontiguous spread. Histologic classification forms the basis for the identification of the subgroups with their different natural histories and responses to treatment. The modified Rappaport classification of non-Hodgkin's lymphoma has been applied for more than 20 years.[152] Its validity has been questioned for a number of reasons, including the fact that lymphocytes, after histologic classification, can transform into larger and more aggressive cell forms.[153] Several other methods of classification have emerged, and a working formulation for clinical usage has been devised by an international study group sponsored by the National Cancer Institute.[154] Cell types are grouped into categories as low grade, intermediate grade, and high grade indicating their aggressiveness and prognosis. Immunohistochemical methods are increasingly added to purely histologic determination. Most of the non-Hodgkin's lymphomas of the small intestine and about 60% to 70% of those elsewhere in the gastrointestinal tract are now classified as high grade and of the large cell or immunoblastic cell type.[155] Fewer are of the diffuse, small, noncleaved cell type; some of these also considered high grade by the working formulation.[156] With the exception of sprue-related T-cell lymphomas, virtually all other small bowel lymphomas are of B-cell type.[157]

Staging refers to the distribution and extent of lymphoma. The Ann Arbor staging system for Hodgkin's disease has been adapted to the staging of non-Hodgkin's lymphoma.[149] The subscript E is used to designate disease of extranodal sites, in this context the small intestine. Stage I_E means disease confined to a single extranodal site. Stage II_{E1} indicates associated involvement of a group of regional lymph nodes. More extensive subdiaphragmatic node involvement is identified as stage II_{E2}. Stage III_E refers to small intestinal lymphoma with extension to structures below and above the diaphragm. Stage IV implies widespread dissemination.

The histologic classification seems to be of less practical clinical relevance than staging because the majority of non-Hodgkin's lymphomas of the small bowel are known to be of large cell type and high-grade aggressiveness. Staging directly affects treatment options in every patient. Cases of stage I_E small bowel lymphoma are rare; nearly half of the small bowel lymphomas are stage II_E. Of 39 cases of lymphoma in stages I_E and II_E, 28 cases were high-grade (72%) and 11 low-grade (28%). Ten of the 11 low-grade cases were GALT lymphomas.[158] Whether high-grade or low-grade, patients should have surgical resection as far as possible, followed by radiotherapy and/or combination chemotherapy.[159] Surgical staging when compared to thorough noninvasive staging did not improve staging accuracy or final outcome.

Clinical Features

The most frequent clinical presentation is abdominal pain,[149] often associated with nausea or vomiting, bleeding, anemia, weight loss, and pyrexia. A palpable abdominal mass or small bowel obstruction or both may be present. A presentation with bleeding, pyrexia, or obstruction is associated with a reduced life expectancy.[160] Malabsorption and diarrhea are rare presenting features in the so-called Western form of lymphoma.[161] These clinical findings are more common in Mediterranean lymphoma and the lymphoma associated with adult celiac disease.

Patients with systemic lupus erythematosus and with other diffuse connective tissue diseases have a higher than expected incidence of non-Hodgkin's lymphoma. In most of the cases, immunosuppressive drugs have not been administered. A 1990 report describing 25 patients with small bowel lymphoma included 2 associated with lupus erythematosus.[162] The possibility of non-Hodgkin's lymphoma should be considered in any patient with systemic lupus erythematosus who develops an abdominal mass or adenopathy.

Radiology

Small bowel lymphoma can be grouped into four major forms: a primary form, lymphoma associated with celiac disease, a mesenteric nodal form, and a disseminated form.[163,164] The diverse radiologic appearances on barium study reflect the gross morphology of the disease.[163–167] The principal radiologic presentations of small bowel lymphoma are: a) circumferential segmental infiltration; b) endo-exoenteric disease with cavitation; c) aneurysmal dilatation; d) polypoid lesions; e) mesenteric nodal lymphoma with secondary infiltration of small bowel; and f) the possible transformation of diffuse nodular lymphoid hyperplasia into lymphoma. In a study in which 25 cases of non-Hodgkin's lymphoma of the small intestine were evaluated, the infiltrating form was the most frequent radiologic appearance (often with moderate lumen widening), closely followed by the cavitary form.[164]

Circumferentially infiltrating non-Hodgkin's lymphoma [Fig. 19-43(a–e)] involves a usually well demarcated, variable length of small intestine with thickening and later effacement of folds.[165] It may be a single lesion or may affect a few separate segments. The lumen is more often widened than narrowed; rarely, a stricture is formed. Barium studies present mural thickening as increased separation from adjoining bowel loops. Multiple shallow ulcers are not infrequently present but are not well shown by conventional barium examination. On CT scans, single or multiple segments showed circumferential 0.5- to 7.0-cm wall thickening, homogeneous in attenuation[168] [Fig. 19-43(e)]. Contrast enhancement is usually minimal, less than that seen with leiomyosarcomas or carcinomas. The lack of a desmoplastic reaction in non-Hodgkin's lymphoma renders it an unlikely cause of obstruction even though the associated mural mass may be larger than with an adenocarcinoma.

The cavitary form. Focal transmural infiltration may lead to localized perforation into a sealed-off space, usually between the leaves of the mesentery. This cavitary form of non-Hodgkin's lymphoma typifies a primary small bowel origin (Fig. 19-44, Fig. 19-45). The site of extravasation, the so-called "closed perforation," and the separate continuity of the small bowel lumen around it are readily shown by enteroclysis. There may also be additional fistulas into the lymphoma cavity as indicated by focally thickened mucosal folds. The irregular contour of the excavation, its relation to the mesenteric border of a small bowel loop, the fact that it contains air and debris, and the generally thin soft-tissue space separating it from adjacent bowel [Fig. 19-44(c, d)] distinguish cavitary lymphoma from a barium-containing cavity within an exoenteric stromal tumor. An aneurysmal dilatation or sacculation may superficially resemble the lymphomatous cavity (see below). Cavitary lymphoma requires surgical excision, at times of several surrounding bowel loops.

Aneurysmal dilatation (or sacculation). Replacement of the muscularis and destruction of the autonomic nerve plexus by lymphoma may cause the bowel wall to give way and bulge focally, not usually in a circular fashion (Fig. 19-46). Unlike cavities, aneurysmal dilatations involve predominantly the unsupported, antimesenteric side of a small bowel segment and remain in continuity with the bowel lumen. The contour may revert to normal after treatment; however, perforation is a life-threatening complication of radiation or chemotherapy, which should be introduced gradually and at low dosages. For this reason, complete resection should be attempted whenever possible.[159]

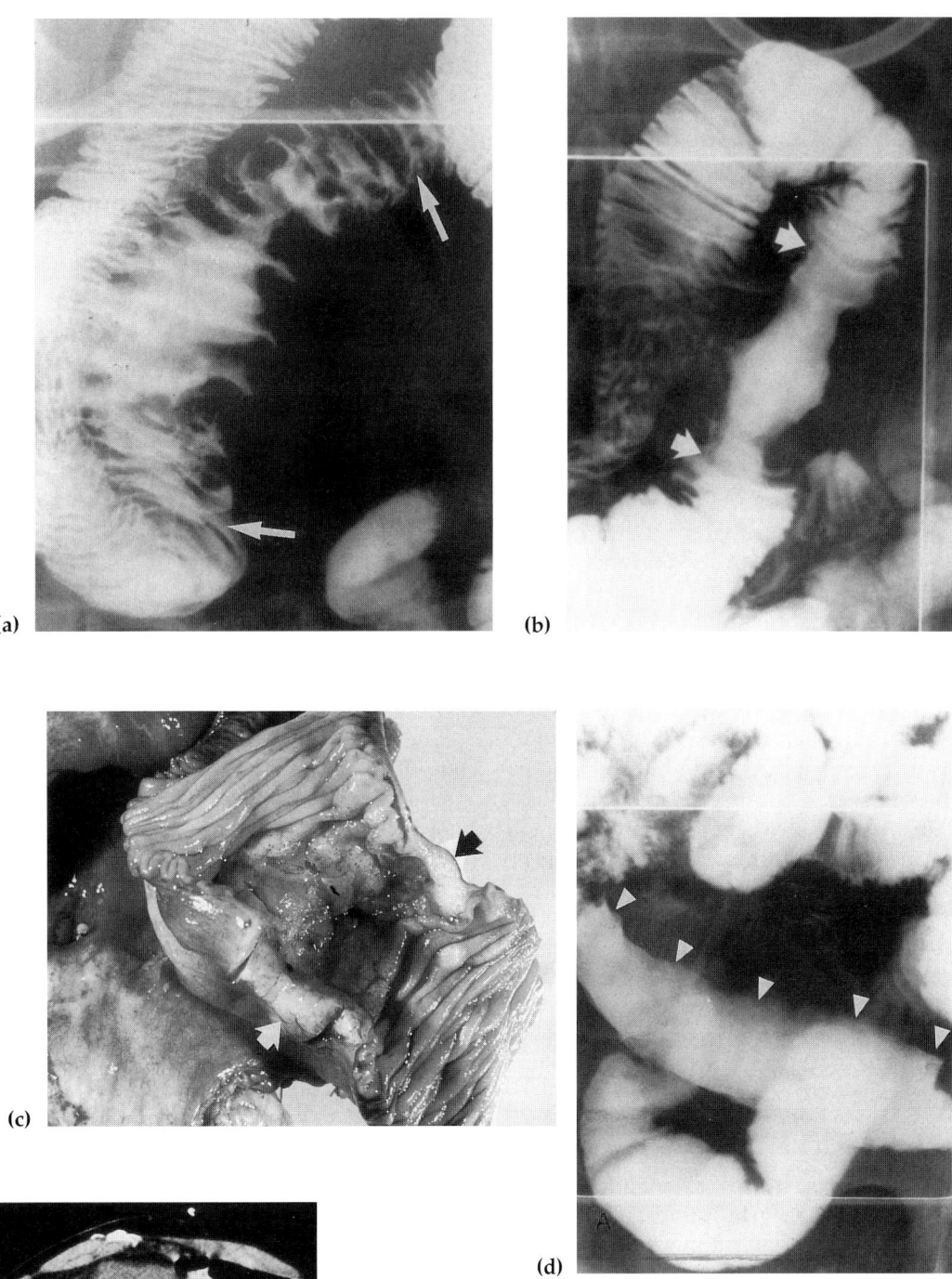

Fig. 19-43. Circumferentially infiltrating primary small bowel non-Hodgkin's lymphoma.
(a) Fold thickening, most pronounced in middle of ileal segment with sharp demarcation against normal folds above and below (arrows). (b) Sharply demarcated segment (arrows) with obliterated folds and lumen widening in center of lesion. (c) Resected specimen (b) shows thickened wall uniformly replaced by lymphoma (arrows). (d) A longer segment terminal ileum diffusely infiltrated by lymphoma (arrowheads). (e) CT scan of above shows lymphomatous thickening of the bowel wall.

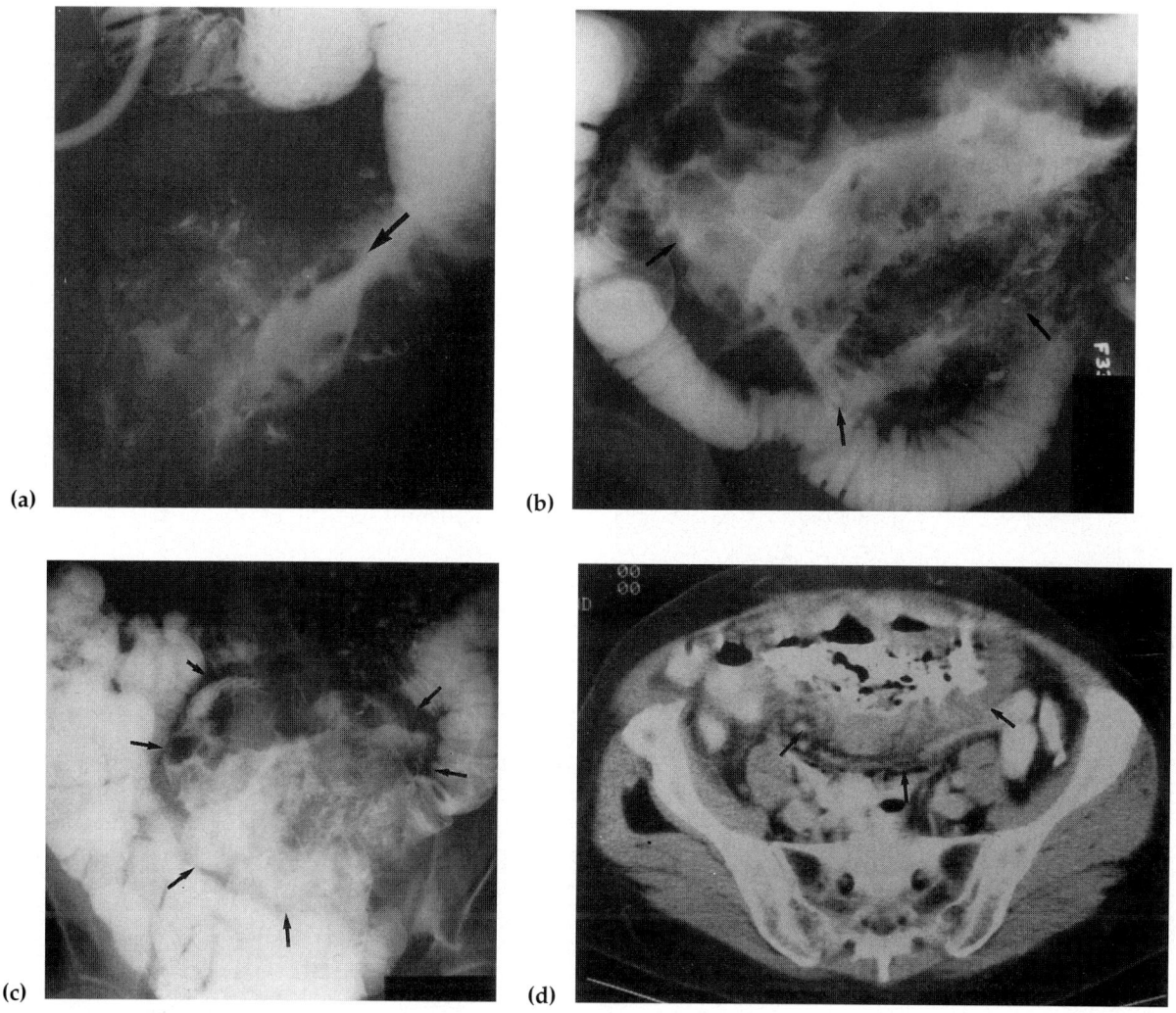

Fig. 19-44. The cavitary form of primary small bowel non-Hodgkin's lymphoma.
(a) Focal perforation (arrow) with escape of barium into a mesenteric border space. (b) Barium gradually spreads through the space, which also contains debris. Surrounding bowel loops unaffected except for possible fistulae (arrows). (c) Late stage of enteroclysis shows barium occupying most of sealed-off space, leaving rim of enclosing lymphoma (arrows). (d) Subsequent CT scan outlines the large barium air- and debris-containing cavity within the mesentery (arrows).

Polypoid disease. There may be one or more lesions that protrude into the lumen, occasionally develop a pseudopedicle, and intussuscept.[169] Dissemination of lymphoma of nongastrointestinal origin can present in the form of scattered nodules in the 0.5- to 2.0-cm range, often ulcerated or umbilicated [Fig. 19-47(a, b)], involving stomach, duodenum, and/or any part of the mesenteric small bowel. A further, somewhat rare condition, known as *malignant lymphomatous polyposis* (MLP) can cause multiple or diffuse nodularities in the small intestine.[170] This rare condition has more recently been classified as a *mantle cell lymphoma* (MCL), predominantly affecting elderly men. It has been subdivided into diffuse, nodular, and mantle zone types, at times with blastic transformation. General lymphadenopathies often precede involvement of bone marrow, spleen, and liver and of the gastrointestinal tract. When the small bowel is affected, polyps can be found in any part of it but are more likely to occur in the distal and terminal ileum where larger and small lesions are interspersed (Fig. 19-48).[171,172] Further clarification of the variant forms of mantle cell lymphoma is awaited. MCL is generally associated with a poor prognosis; the tumors are usually either advanced or too widespread, and surgery is impossible. Radiochemotherapy is not curative at this time.

Mesenteric nodal disease. Non-Hodgkin's lymphoma of nodal origin may develop in the small bowel mesentery. As the tumor enlarges, it first displaces, then gradually infiltrates the walls of adjacent bowel loops.

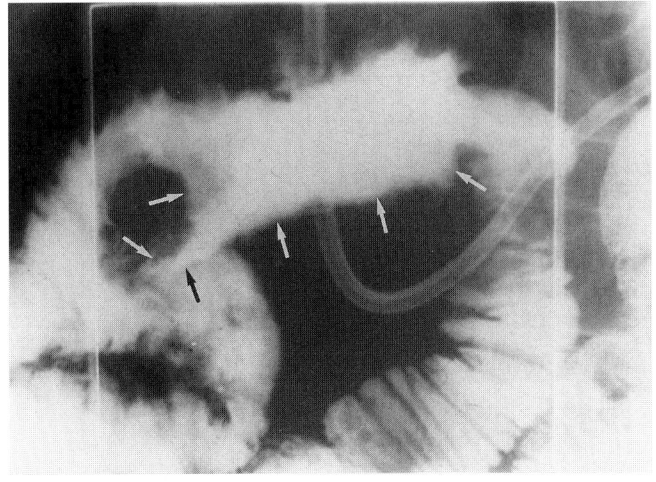
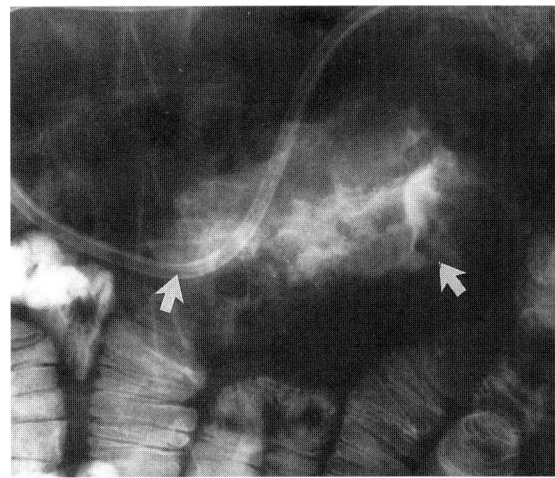
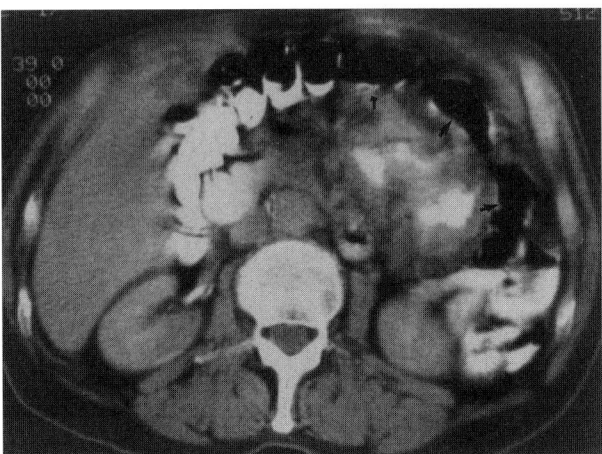

Fig. 19-45. Further cavitary primary non-Hodgkin's lymphoma in 71-year-old male patient referred for enteroclysis with obscure GI bleeding.
(a) A 10-cm-long dilated segment of jejunum with hazy contour (arrows) is sharply demarcated from normal bowel. (b) In the course of the enteroclysis, barium gradually extends into a space (arrows) still separated from adjacent normal bowel loops. (c) Later CT scan shows mostly contrast-containing space anteriorly bordered by colon. At surgery, resection of cavity-related small bowel and colon.

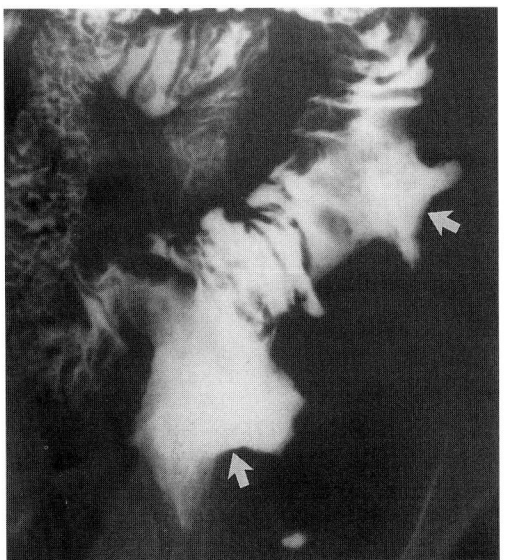

Fig. 19-46. Aneurysmal dilatation in intestinal non-Hodgkin's lymphoma.
Follow-through barium study shows two adjacent antimesenteric sacculations (arrows). A further small bowel lesion more distally. Careful chemotherapy resulted in virtual normalization of the segments.

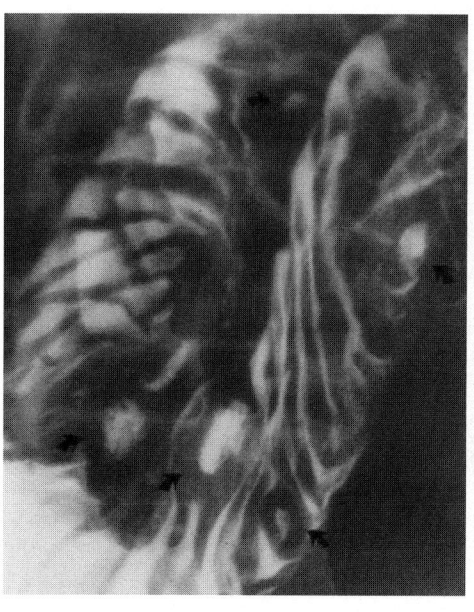 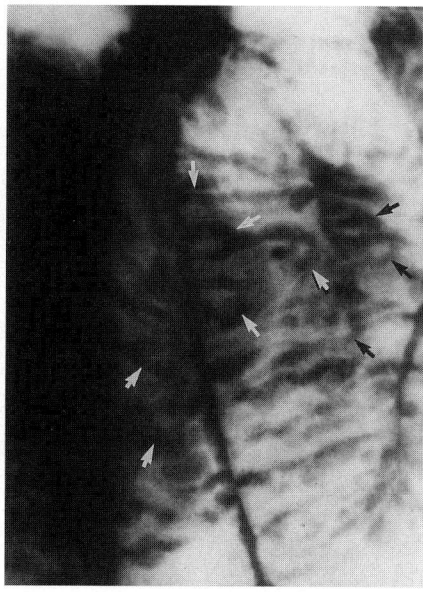

Fig. 19-47. **Metastatic involvement of small bowel in a 54-year-old female patient with widespread nodal non-Hodgkin's lymphoma.** (a) Many ulcerated nodules 1.5 to 2.5 cm in size (arrows) occupy distal duodenum and first segment of jejunum. (b) In same patient, remainder of jejunum is filled with numerous 1.0- to 1.5-cm ulcerated nodules (arrows).

Barium examination can depict the stages from abutment to displacement and compression and to eventual infiltration that may cause obstruction (Fig. 19-49). The mesenteric mass is best outlined by CT when its lobulated contour seems initially to surround adjacent bowel to produce a classic "sandwich" appearance.[173] A similar "sandwich pattern" can be shown by ultrasonography in the relation of a mesenteric nodal lymphoma to unaffected mesenteric vessels. Calcification of the mesenteric lymphomatous tumor is rare and is more likely to occur after radiotherapy or chemotherapy.

Burkitt's Lymphoma (sporadic). Unlike the endemic form, which only rarely affects the gastrointestinal tract, rapidly proliferating tumors of sporadic Burkitt's lymphoma can be found in bowel, especially the ileocecal region (Fig. 19-50). It is a B-cell lymphoma with small noncleaved cells,[149] predominantly affecting children, but infrequently also young adults. Gallium-67 radionucleide studies can define the bulk of the abdominal mass and may outline other sites of involvement, including bone.[174] Treatment has been generally ineffective with a median survival of 14 months.[175] (See also Chapter 17, Burkitt in AIDS.)

Diffuse, nodular lymphoid hyperplasia (NLH) and lymphoma. This condition resembles immunoproliferative small intestinal disease and Mediterranean lymphoma (which has been described in Chapter 17) but is not associated with alpha-heavy chain disease and affects an older age group. Diffuse NLH of the small intestine is also found in patients with acquired hypogammaglobulinemia, but its progression into lymphoma is rare. In nonimmunodeficient adults, however, the finding of diffuse small bowel NLH demands two considerations: 1) whether it already represents a lymphoma and 2) the need for follow-up to identify possible subsequent development into a lymphoma.[156]

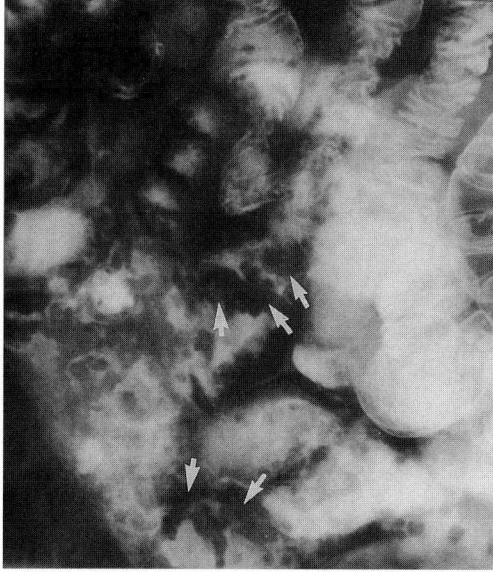

Fig. 19-48. **Case of malignant lymphomatous polyposis.** Enteroclysis outlines normal and distensible bowel short of distal ileum. The latter resists distension and contains numerous up to 1.8-cm polypoid masses in the area of the terminal ileum (arrows). Nodular lymphoid hyperplasia is seen more proximally. The colon is also involved.

19. Small Bowel Neoplasms

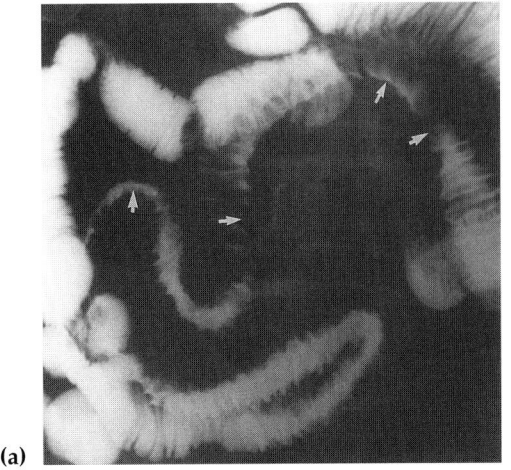
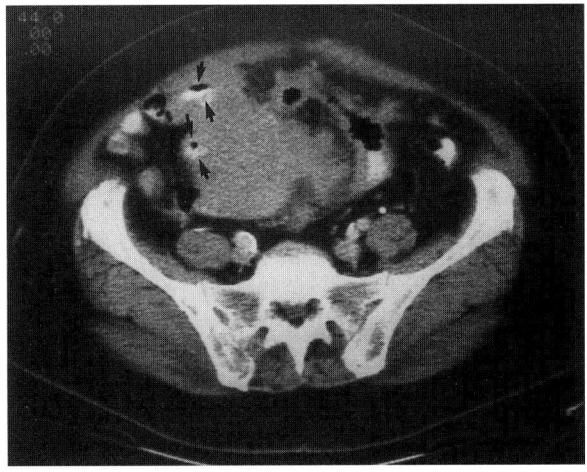
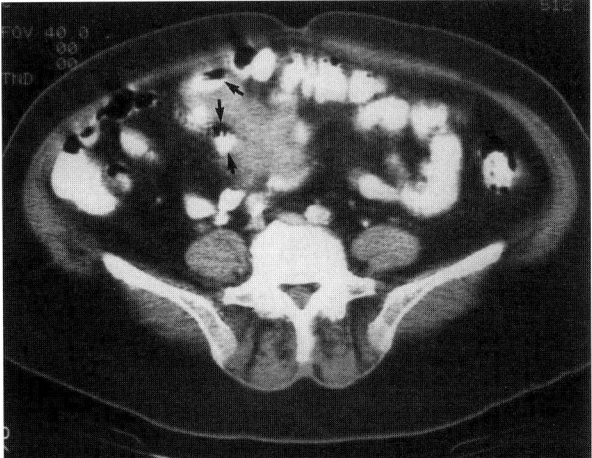

Fig. 19-49. Secondary involvement of small bowel by mesenteric nodal lymphoma.
(a) Areas of mild narrowing (arrows) in widely displaced loop of small bowel. (b) CT scan show large mesenteric nodal mass surrounding two segments of bowel ("sandwich sign" of lymphoma) (arrows). (c) Following therapy 4 months later CT shows reduction in size of mesenteric nodal lymphoma, still with "sandwich sign" (arrows).

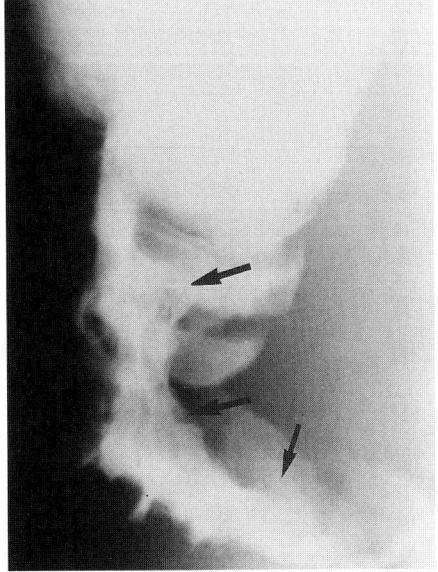

Fig. 19-50. Burkitt's lymphoma in non-HIV-infected 19-year-old male.
Terminal ileum is extensively ulcerated (arrows). Only short-term response to treatment.

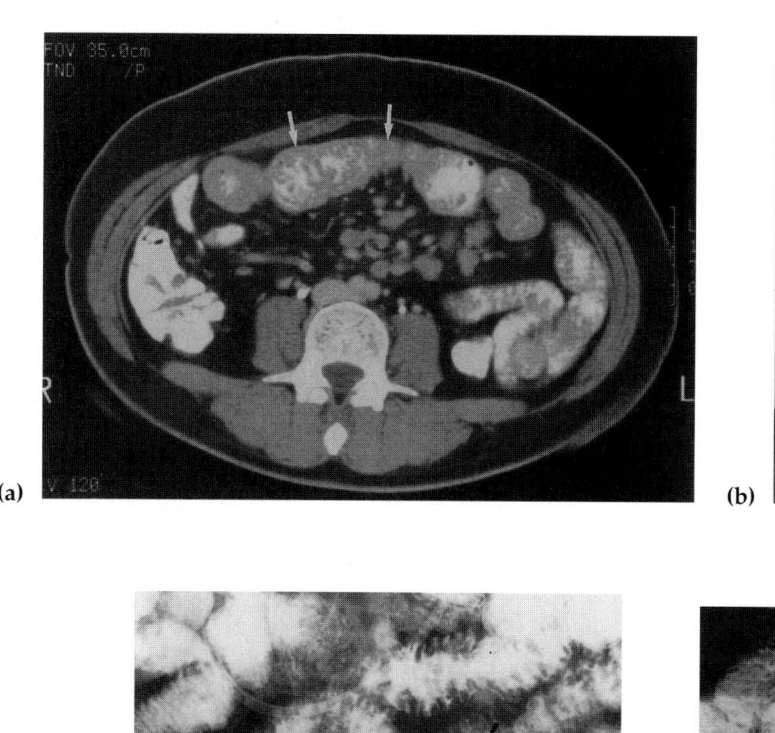
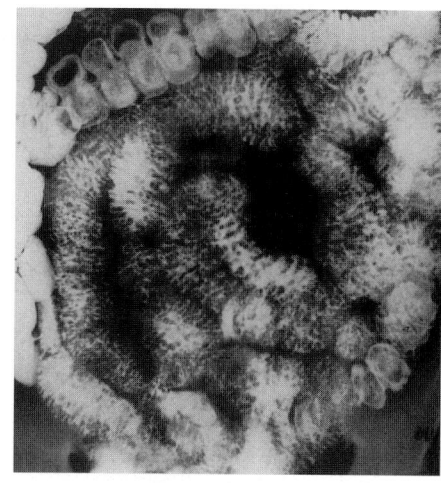
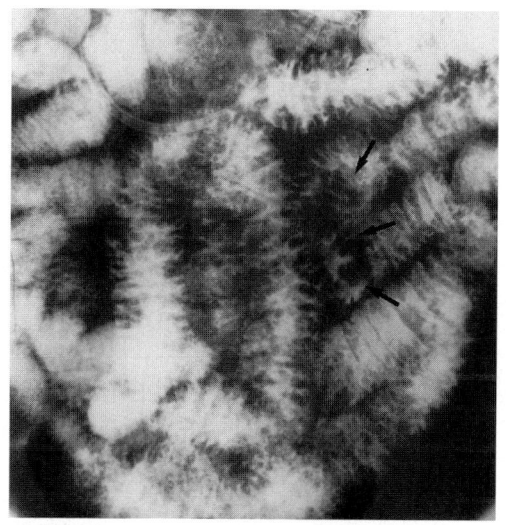
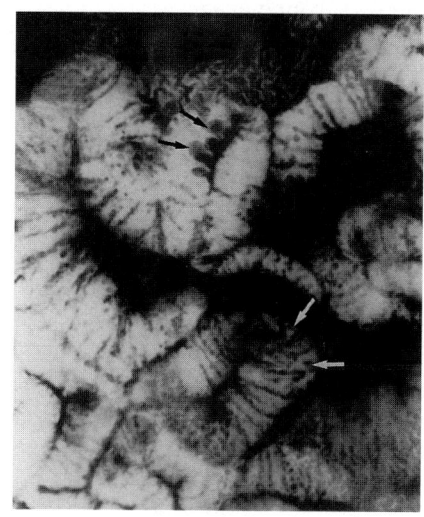
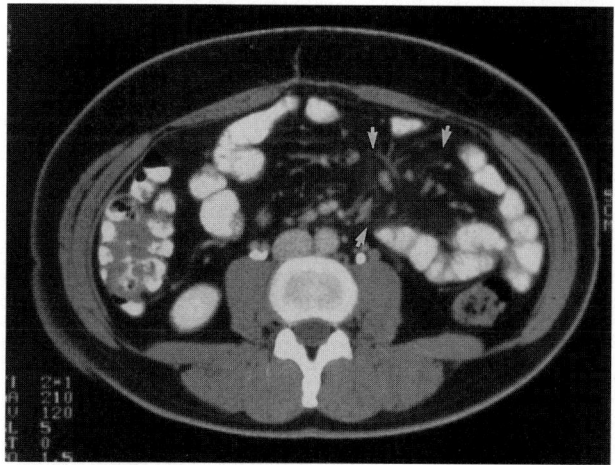

Fig. 19-51. A 44-year-old female with abdominal pain and occasional diarrhea.
(a) CT scan with intraluminal contrast showed small bowel with thickened folds (arrows), mesenteric vessel engorged, nodes enlarged. (b) Barium follow-through 20 days later demonstrated entire small bowel surface filled with nodules, some larger than expected for nodular lymphoid hyperplasia (NLH). (c) Enteroclysis done 4 months later found the small bowel with merging nodules superimposed on thick folds and areas of larger, about 2.0-cm nodularities (arrows). Laparotomy with full-thickness biopsy determined lymphoproliferative disease to be monoclonal, a lymphoma. Chemotherapy followed. (d) Barium follow-through after therapy shows small bowel now filled with nodules of NLH size, except for at least two areas of fused nodules (arrows). (e) CT now showed engorged mesenteric vessels and an area of "misty" mesentery (between arrows) indicating edema. (Courtesy of K. Cho, MD.)

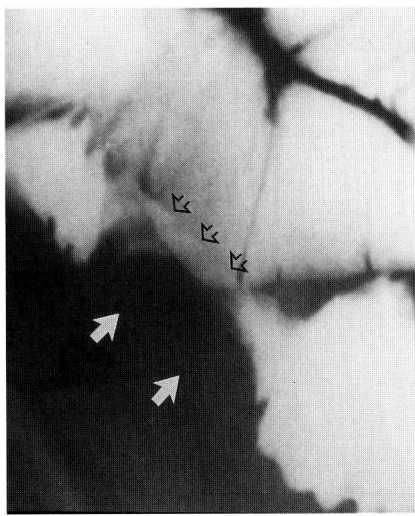

Fig. 19-52. Hodgkin's lymphoma.
A moderately long segment of distal small bowel is narrowed with effaced folds (open arrows). There is a large extramural component (arrows). Surgery disclosed a large mass and adjacent enlarged nodes. (From Maglinte,[133] with permission.)

The lymphoma could be a MALT-type lymphoma with extensive lymphoid proliferation beyond the lamina propria and submucosa. Generally a polyclonal lymphoid proliferation is still benign, and monoclonality indicates lymphoma.[156]

The case of a 44-year-old female without significant past history who presented with abdominal pain and occasional diarrhea illustrates this rare sequence of events (Fig. 19-51). Initial enteroclysis showed diffuse NLH which, within five months, changed into an irregular and larger nodular pattern that was superimposed on thickened folds. Initial endoscopic jejunal biopsy was compatible with a reactive polyclonal hyperplasia. A later full-thickness biopsy was interpreted as monoclonal infiltrate of a multicentric non-Hodgkin's lymphoma with predominantly small cleaved cells. Following adequate therapy, she was last seen 3 years later and was found to be in good health.

Radiologic Differential Diagnosis

As already indicated, barium studies can aid the differentiation between primary and secondary small bowel lymphoma.[176] The segmentally infiltrating and cavitary forms tend to be expressions of primary small intestinal origin, whereas the polypoid and nodular types usually denote dissemination. It needs to be reemphasized that for a more complete radiologic diagnosis of this entity, enteroclysis needs to be supplemented by CT or MRI to define the location and extent of the mass and to guide possible biopsy.

In most cases, with enteroclysis, there is no difficulty in differentiating small bowel lymphoma from Crohn's disease.[177] Fold thickening may be an early feature in both conditions but is rarely the only radiologic abnormality in either. Ulcers in lymphoma are usually more broad-based than the fissures or longitudinal ulcers seen in Crohn's disease.

The apple-core deformity typical of adenocarcinoma is unusual in non-Hodgkin's lymphoma. Should it occur, it tends to involve a longer segment, does not show overhanging edges, and may be multiple. Furthermore, lymphoma produces a softer lesion that may show outline change with abdominal compression. CT demonstration of bulky mesenteric node involvement favors lymphoma.[178]

Needle Biopsy

Percutaneous fine-needle biopsy for a histologic diagnosis of non-Hodgkin's lymphoma can be guided by the barium-outlined lesion.[179] Core biopsies are generally preferred for histologic determination. Use of an 18-gauge biopsy gun allows more accurate placement, fewer crush artifacts, and less discomfort for the patient.[180] However, many surgeons prefer full-thickness biopsy specimens obtained at laparotomy or laparoscopy,[181] in the belief that they are more accurate and supply sufficient material for immunologic characterization.

Staging Improved by Imaging Techniques

Periaortic, celiac, and retrocrural nodes that may be missed during a staging laparotomy can be shown by imaging.[182] Although diffuse enlargement of spleen or liver in a patient with known intestinal lymphoma must raise the possibility of their involvement, CT or MRI provide more specific information, at times needing biopsy confirmation. This is an important determinant considering that abdominal solid organ involvement will change an otherwise I_E or II_E stage into stage IV_E.[183]

Treatment and Prognosis

Misdiagnosis has delayed the start of correct treatment for more than 6 months in nearly half of patients.[184] Deaths may be grouped into those occurring within 6 months of diagnosis and those occurring much later. Early deaths are related to complications of chemotherapy in patients with transmural disease, namely bleeding and perforation. A preference for surgical excision has already been mentioned. Alternatively, cautiously administered, relatively low-dose chemotherapy may have to be employed, always with close observation for any early signs of bleeding or perforation. For advanced disease, after a palliative resection, multidrug chemotherapy appropriate for the histologic type of the non-Hodgkin's lymphoma has been given intermittently for a long time and has been supplemented by radiotherapy for residual disease.[185]

(Lymphoma associated with celiac disease or complicating organ transplantation and Acquired Immunodeficiency Syndrome is described in Chapter 17.)

Hodgkin's Disease (HD)

Hodgkin's disease represents only about 1% of all malgnant lymphomas of the gastrointestinal tract.[186] Involvement in decreasing frequency has been reported for the stomach, jejunum, ileum, and duodenum. Because of the rarity of gastrointestinal localization, radiologic findings suggesting gastrointestinal tract involvement in a patient with known HD need to be interpreted with caution, as a second disease process would be the more likely explanation. Diagnosis of HD should be based on confirmation by histology together with immunohistochemistry.[186] The development of non-Hodgkin's lymphoma after treatment of HD has been fully documented.[187] A correct diagnosis is relevant to clinical management, as non-Hodgkin's lymphoma does not sufficiently respond to the chemotherapeutic combinations used in Hodgkin's disease.

Radiology

Because HD incites fibrosis of the bowel wall, lesions are more likely to be focally stenotic and usually lack an overhanging edge (Fig. 19-52); a few have been ulcerated or lobulated.[186] The most likely appearance, however, would be displacement of uninvolved small bowel by an adjacent nodal mass.

Leiomyosarcoma

Leiomyosarcomas are the fourth most common malignant tumor of the small bowel. They arise from smooth muscle cells. They occur most commonly in the jejunum and least often in the duodenum. They are usually found in the fifth and sixth decades, with a male to female ratio of 3:1.[188] It is not clear whether leiomyosarcomas arise de novo or from preexisting benign smooth muscle tumors. Leiomyosarcomas account for 9% of all primary malignant tumors in the small intestine. Reliable differentiation between a benign leiomyoma and a leiomyosarcoma cannot be made radiographically. However, smooth muscle tumors that are large or show significant ulceration are usually malignant.

Pathology

The determination of tumor malignancy may be a problem for the pathologist. The demonstration of 5 or more mitotic figures per 10 high-power fields may signify malignancy, especially if associated with nuclear atypia or pleomorphism. However, even tumors without mitotic figures have been known to metastasize.[189] A further problem of histology can be the distinction between a neurogenic sarcoma and leiomyosarcoma. The demonstration by immunoperoxidase staining of S-100 protein favors the former diagnosis. Sarcomas grow more slowly than adenocarcinomas. Sixty-five percent of leiomyosarcomas of the small intestine are reported to be of the exoenteric growth type.[190] They can become extremely large and develop central necrotic and cystic changes. A connection between the tumor cavity and the intestinal lumen may not always be identified. Spread is usually via direct extension into the adjacent parts of the peritoneal cavity or via the hematogenous route primarily to the liver.[191] Extension to lymph nodes is infrequent.

Clinical Features

Most of these tumors are slow growing and are associated with a long period of symptoms. Patients are often anemic due to recurrent melena arising from the ulcerated component and may complain of abdominal discomfort or pain. Obstruction is not a frequent presentation, although an endoenteric tumor may intussuscept and a large exoenteric mass may compress the intestinal lumen. A mass, often large, soft, and mobile, may be palpated clinically. These large exocentric tumors may bleed profusely into the bowel lumen or, infrequently, into the peritoneal cavity.

Radiology

Plain films occasionally show a large soft-tissue mass or collections of air representing tumor excavation if in communication with the intestinal lumen. On a con-

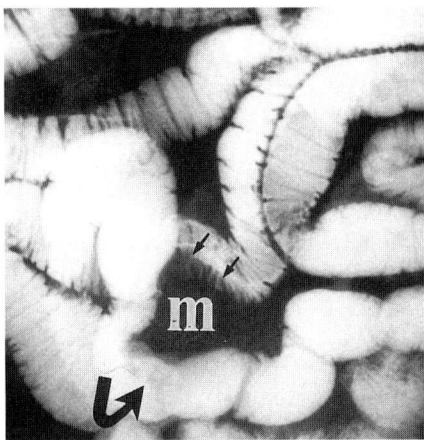

Fig. 19-53. Exoenteric ulcerating leiomyosarcoma.
Enteroclysis done for unexplained GI bleeding reveals a large ulcer (curved arrow) with an extramural component (m) displacing adjacent loop. Note mild thickening of displaced tethered folds (small arrows). Surgery confirmed an ulcerating mass with a large exoenteric component. Histology revealed an ulcerating leiomyoma. (From Maglinte and Reyes,[2] with permission.)

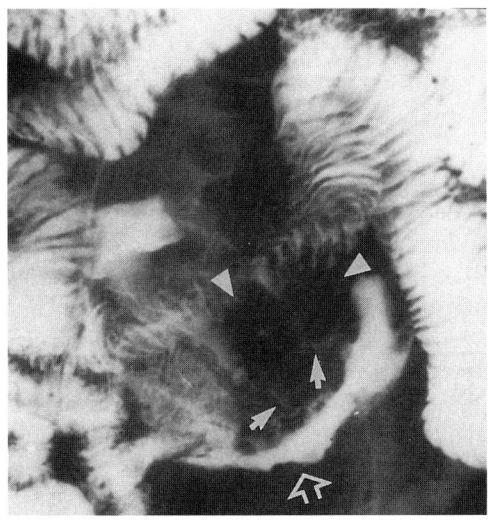

Fig. 19-54. Necrotic leiomyosarcoma.
A large ulcerating (open arrow) gas-containing mesenteric mass (arrowheads) as well as multiple tracts within the mass (small arrows) are shown by enteroclysis on a patient with abdominal pain and anemia. Barium has entered the necrotic portions of the mass and may remain there for more than 24 hours. This "closed perforation" will allow clearing of the retained contrast because of continuity of the small bowel. This should not be confused with a cavitating lymphoma. Surgery and histologic examination revealed leiomyosarcoma. (From Maglinte,[131] with permission.)

trast study, the cavity fills with barium and several tracts may be outlined (Fig. 19-53). Occasionally, calcifications similar to those often seen in uterine fibroids are present.[191] Because of the predominantly extraluminal growth, leiomyosarcomas usually appear as an extrinsic mass displacing small bowel loops. Barium studies demonstrate a deformity of the small bowel segment from which the tumor originates, with flattening, stretching, and possible ulceration of the mucosa (Fig. 19-54). Adjacent loops may adhere to the mass as a result of infiltration or tethering by the considerable saprophytic blood supply. Leiomyosarcomas alter in shape during compression because they are generally soft. Because of the exoenteric growth type of smooth muscle tumors, the manifestations on barium studies tend to be more subtle than the CT findings. On CT scans, smaller lesions have a nondescript appearance of homogeneous density, closely associated with the bowel wall. The more characteristic CT pattern of a leiomyosarcoma is that of a bulky lesion, growing exoenterically and sometimes calcified.[192] The soft-tissue component of the tumor usually shows significant enhancement with intravenous contrast. Necrosis is depicted as a low-density central area rendered more obvious by surrounding contrast enhancement. Local extensions are demonstrated in a minority of cases. Metastatic disease tends to involve the liver, often with cystic or low-density deposits associated with solid tumor nodules. Peritoneal metastatic masses, occasionally accompanied by masses in the omentum, are well outlined by CT. They are discrete lesions with smooth outer margins, at times containing necrotic areas.[193] Bolus injection of contrast medium can usually differentiate a highly vascular leiomyosarcoma from hypovascular lymphoma. Angiography demonstrates characteristic features such as hypervascularity of the sharply demarcated mass of the stromal tumor, outlined tumor vessels, and early venous return.[194]

Treatment

Complete resection is the only effective therapy. It can produce a 5-year survival rate of 50%—27% for tumors >5 cm and 73% for tumors <5 cm. Multiple surgical interventions are associated with a longer survival. Adjuvant therapy has shown no consistent benefit endpoints.

Miscellaneous Tumors

Liposarcoma, angiosarcoma, and fibrosarcoma of the small bowel are among those reported in the literature. They are radiologically indistinguishable from leiomyosarcomas.

Secondary Malignancies

Metastases from melanoma and neoplasms of the breast, lung, and kidney can be responsible for isolated small bowel lesions and may be a cause of diagnostic and therapeutic difficulty. Frequently, they are an incidental finding in a patient with known abdominal carcinomatosis. Tumor cells can spread to the small intestine through different pathways, namely 1) intraperitoneal seeding, 2) hematogenous dissemination, and 3) extension from an adjacent tumor mass either directly or through lymphatic channels.[195–197] A further avenue for the extension of disease is based on the fact that the intraperitoneal and extraperitoneal spaces constitute an anatomic continuum via the subperitoneal space.[198] The mechanism of tumor spread influences its radiographic appearance. Characteristic imaging features can lead to the uncovering of an occult primary tumor site. Intraperitoneal spread occurs more frequently than hematogenous dissemination and is more likely to pose a problem of radiologic differential diagnosis.[199–202]

Intraperitoneal Seeding of Metastases

The natural pattern of flow of ascitic fluid within the peritoneal recesses influences the serosal implantation of cancer cells.[203–204] Areas where ascitic fluid accumulates and stagnates before overflowing to an adjacent space are preferred sites for malignant cell deposition. Such sites are the ileocecal region, the numerous pools within the ruffles of the small bowel mesentery, and the depth of the pelvic cavity.[205]

Malignant cells deposited on serosal surfaces may adhere through fibrinous exudation. Deposits coalesce and grow into metastatic masses implanted on the serosa of a segment of bowel or on the peritoneal surface between loops. The neoplastic implants (most often from tumors of gastrointestinal origin in men and tumors of ovarian or uterine origin in women) typically grow in relation to the concave or mesenteric border of bowel loops and can incite fibrosis.[197]

Clinical Aspects

The primary tumor is known in most cases. A problem for diagnostic radiology and surgical management is the patient whose small bowel obstruction follows surgery for abdominal malignancy, because adhesion, metastases, or radiation enteropathy may be responsible. An enteroclysis-based radiologic differential diagnosis is possible in more than two-thirds of cases.[200]

Seeded metastases cause obstruction by protrusion into the bowel lumen, by associated desmoplasia, or by the combined effect of their multiplicity. Blood loss, other than occult, is unusual in seeded metastases. An additional consideration in patients with obstruction due to multiple metastases is the radiologic demonstration of noninvolved segments of small bowel proximally for possible palliative bypass surgery.

Radiology of Seeded Metastases[201]

Only lesions that are large enough to produce focal alterations of the lumen contour or of the mucosal surface pattern can be recognized by barium contrast studies. Interloop metastases must grow to a larger size before their impingement on a segment of bowel can be recognized by radiology. Enteroclysis excels in demonstrating radiologically identifiable seeded metastases and in determining the degree and sites of obstruction caused by them. Metastases are often multiple. Ascites, minimal or pronounced, is almost always present. CT is of complementary value in determining the full extent of metastatic disease. The various manifestations of intraperitoneally seeded metastases located in the pelvis, the most common site of deposition, are shown on Fig. 19-55.

When metastases are deposited on the serosal surface of a segment of the small bowel, rounded protrusions toward the lumen of lesions at least 1 cm in diameter can be demonstrated by a carefully performed contrast examination. With distention of the small bowel lumen by contrast medium infusion, involvement of a bowel segment becomes more obvious. The folds may assume a curved appearance at the periphery of a metastasis or may seem stretched and "tacked down." When shown predominantly in profile, metastatic infiltration and fixation of folds at the affected bowel edge are accentuated by a divergence of folds toward the unaffected side. Angulation and tethering of folds are features of frequently associated fibrous reaction. Resultant small bowel obstruction can then be of considerable severity. The significance of obstruction can often be better appreciated by delayed imaging. Mucosal ulceration is a late feature.

Loops of small bowel that prolapse into the pelvis after a hysterectomy or pelvic exenteration are frequent sites of seeded metastases. Enteroclysis with films taken in oblique, lateral, or angled projections is the best method for recognition of metastatic involvement of these segments. Interloop peritoneal metastases produce shallow indentations, often with loop fixation and mucosal tethering (Fig. 19-56). They tend to involve the mesenteric border of several small bowel loops, usually in the lowest part of the right infracolic space.[202] Peritoneal and mesenteric carcinomatosis can

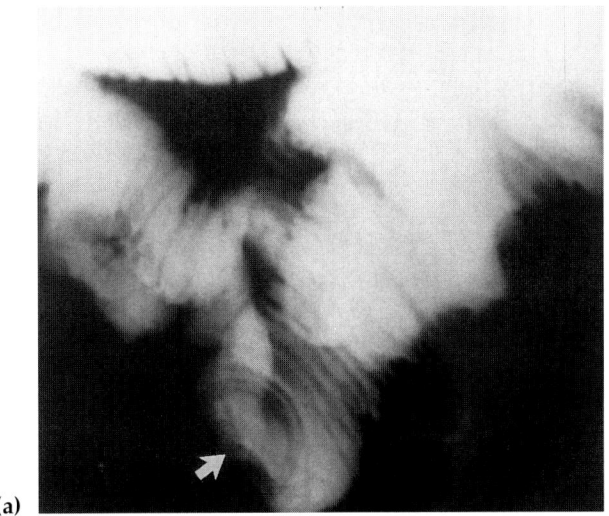
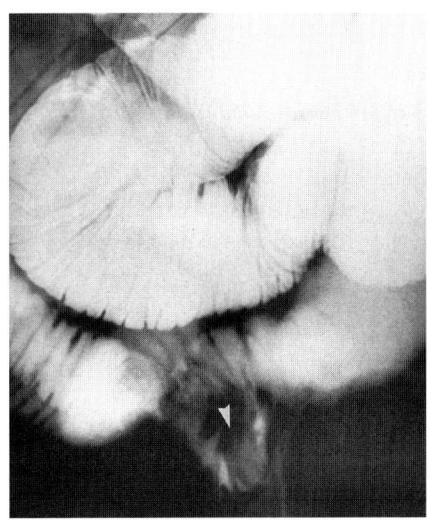

Fig. 19-55. Radiology of intraperitoneal seeded metastases. Seeded metastases from ovarian carcinoma.
(a) Multiple segments of pelvic ileum show decreased distensibility and are fixed. Partial obstruction is caused by an intramural implant (arrow). The folds are transversely stretched but intact. (b) Enteroclysis shows focal obstruction due to fixation and deformity of a segment along its mesenteric margin by a mass (arrowhead).

be associated with multiple metastatic deposits involving adjacent loops of small intestine, producing an appearance termed "palisading" (Fig. 19-57(a)]; ultrasound can also demonstrate associated involvement of the omentum [Fig. 19-57(b)].

CT plays an important role in the radiologic demonstration of metastatic lesions in the mesentery, peritoneal surfaces, and lymph nodes as well as in the bowel wall. With advanced and aggressive metastatic disease, the mesentery is extensively involved in addition to multiple serosal deposits.[192] Barium studies may demonstrate multiple areas of small bowel narrowing, often with intervening distention. Small bowel folds in areas of narrowing appear nodular and distorted but are not destroyed or ulcerated. The desmoplastic effect produces shortening of the mesentery with apparent reduction of the length of small bowel loops, which show crowded folds and an abnormal configuration.[204]

Radiologic Differential Diagnosis

Preoperative radiologic differentiation between adhesions, radiation enteropathy, and metastases was previously considered to be only rarely possible.[204] Adhesive bands cause linear compression defects across the lumen, mostly with straight margins. Multiple adhesions are grouped together and usually fixed anteriorly to an abdominal scar.[199] Neither tethering of folds nor nodular defects are observed. Chronic radiation enteropathy produces diffuse thickening of folds with a decreased distance between them, producing a corrugated outline of the involved segments. The distribution of these changes corresponds to the site of the radiation portal. Advanced forms of radiation damage, however, may be associated with the presence of metastases, and the differential diagnosis by contrast radiography can be difficult or impossible. Only positive cytology of specimens obtained by needle biopsy can then provide a definitive diagnosis be-

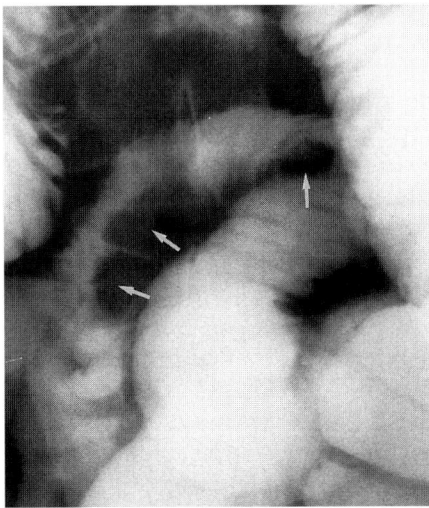

Fig. 19-56. Interloop seeding.
Intramural masses (arrows) with loop fixation and mucosal tethering of a loop of small bowel in the midabdomen in a patient with prior surgery for colon malignancy who presented with small bowel obstruction.

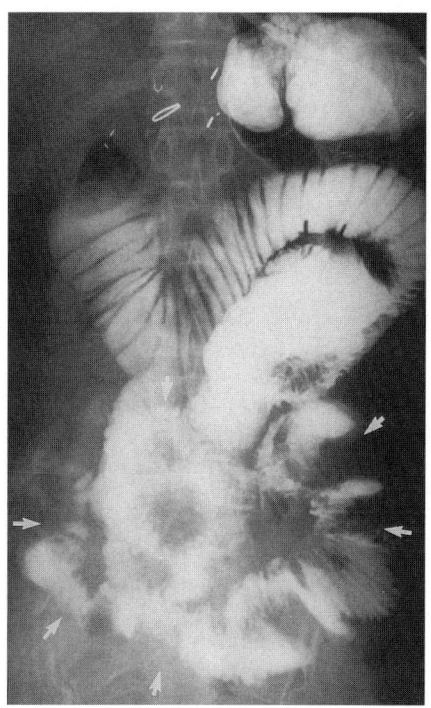 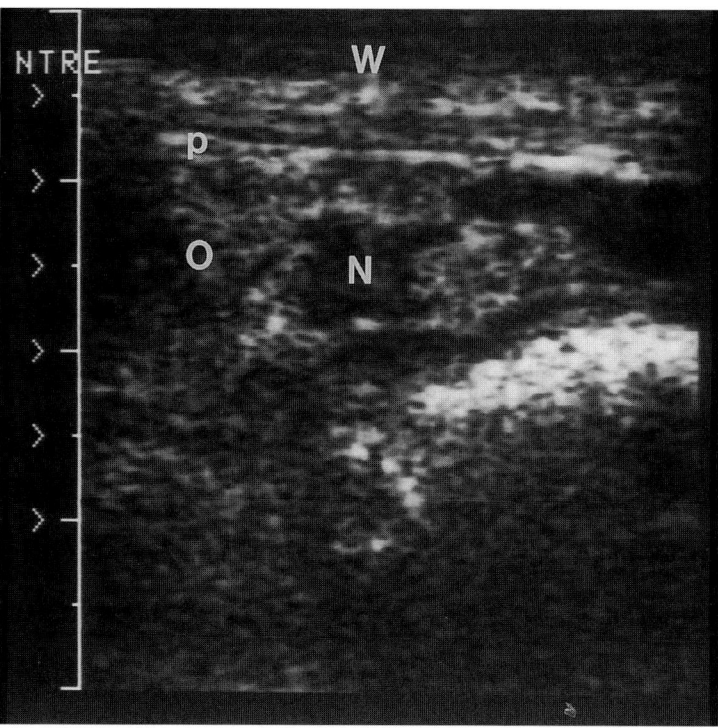

Fig. 19-57. "Palisading" and intraperitoneally seeded carcinomatosis.
(a) Several loops of small bowel in the lower abdomen are centrally positioned and fixed (arrows). The involved folds are tethered. There is low-grade obstruction. Ascites is apparent. Enteroclysis was done for possible bypass surgery. Note the short uninvolved jejunum. The patient had prior gastrectomy for malignancy. (From Maglinte.[133]) (b) Sonography in a patient with colon carcinoma delineates a hypoechoic nodular metastatic deposit (N) in the omentum (O) (W = abdominal wall, p = peritoneum.) (Courtesy of Michel Rioux, MD, Québec.)

fore surgery. Extensive infiltration by metastases in the right lower quadrant can superficially resemble Crohn's disease. Folds involved, whether displaced, distorted, nodular, or angulated, do not show ulceration or a cobblestone pattern, and the presence of fistulas is unusual. Endometrial implants may seed in the lower right quadrant after reflux of endometrial cells through the fallopian tubes. The ectopic endometrium continues to be hormonally responsive and may be a site of intermittent bleeding associated with fibrosis. Plaquelike serosal deposit in the terminal ileum have been shown by enteroclysis.[206] It is frequently seen in association with the more typical radiologic changes affecting the anterior wall of the rectosigmoid.

Hematogenous Dissemination

Malignant melanoma, a tumor of increasing incidence, is the most frequent source of hematogenous metastases to the small intestine. Though a frequent finding at autopsies of melanoma patients, the metastases are discovered in less than 9% of patients during life.[207] The median interval between the initial skin melanoma and the diagnosis of intestinal metastases was reported to be 4.4 years.[208] Although metastases to the liver may occur with somewhat greater frequency than to the small bowel, there are numbers of patients in whom metastases to the small bowel precede those to other organs. Anemia, abdominal pain, obstruction, and bleeding are among their clinical presentations. An early as possible recognition of intestinal metastases and their complete surgical removal can significantly improve patient prognosis.[208] In cases where enteroclysis was able to demonstrate no more than 10 melanoma metastases to the small bowel, their complete resection was reported to have prolonged survival threefold compared to patients in whom larger numbers of metastases had been demonstrated.[209] A more recent report[210] has further analyzed the value of curative resection of all small bowel metastases. Patients who had only partial resection or were without surgical intervention had a median survival on only 5.5 months. Following complete resection of all the metastases, the median survival was 48.9 months, with

41% of the patients surviving more than 5 years. The authors agreed that enteroclysis would be the most accurate method for the preoperative demonstration of the totality of resectable melanoma metastases.[210]

Radiology

The early radiologic changes in hematogenous metastases to small bowel are usually multiple nodules, seen mostly along the antimesenteric border, where the vasa recta arborize into a rich submucosal plexus. The lesions arise at different times and may be grouped into stages of development. Depending on the desmoplastic character or cellularity of the deposits as well as their vascularity, patterns may be recognized that suggest the site of the primary carcinoma.

The radiographic appearance of gastrointestinal malignant melanoma metastases corresponds to its two known pathologic types: 1) polypoid and 2) infiltrating, ulcerating lesions. The polypoid lesions are more common and tend to be large and multiple and have a worse prognosis. Radiographically, smoothly rounded polypoid lesions of different sizes are the usual appearance of early melanoma metastases to the small bowel. "Target" lesions—nodules with central ulcerations that are frequently found in the stomach and duodenum occur less often in the mesenteric small intestine (Fig. 19-58).[210] Larger polypoid masses often

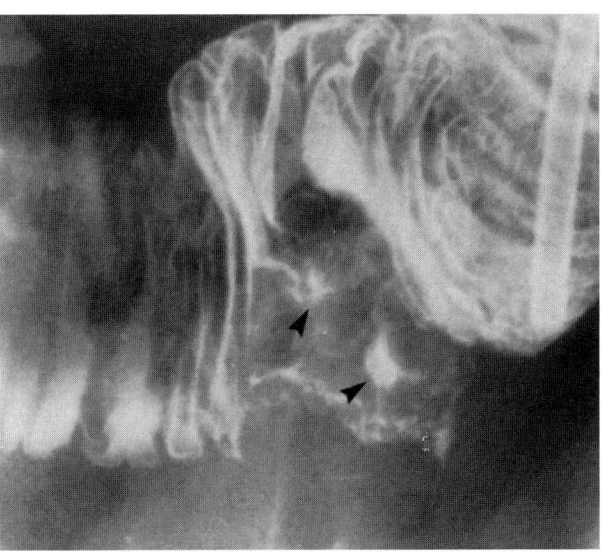

Fig. 19-59. Ulcerating metastasis from melanoma.
A larger polypoid melanoma metastasis contains two ulcers (arrowheads), each with radiating linear ulcerations forming the spoke-wheel pattern of melanoma metastases.

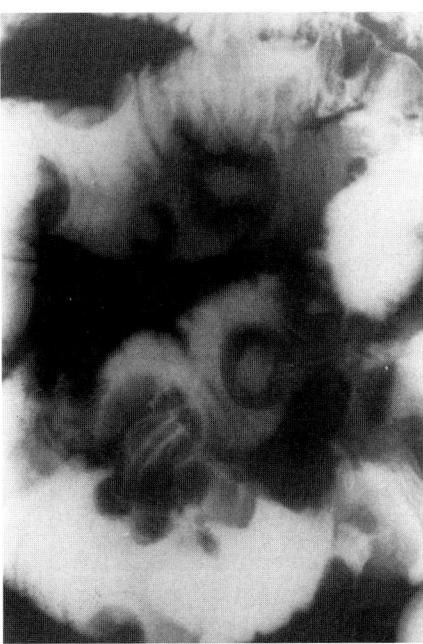

Fig. 19-58. "Target" lesions secondary to metastases from malignant melanoma.
Multiple nodules with central ulcerations are seen in multiple loops of ileum by enteroclysis. (Courtesy of Michael Davis, MD.)

ulcerate and may show a spoke-wheel pattern of fissuring extending from the ulcer edge to the periphery of the mass (Fig. 19-59). The metastases, even when occupying virtually the entire bowel lumen, may not cause significant obstruction. This is due to the softness of the highly cellular mass, which contains little stroma. The demonstration on barium examination of a nonobstructing, fairly large intraluminal mass favors the diagnosis of melanoma metastasis [Fig. 19-60(a)]. Such intraluminal masses of melanoma, however, may cause transient intussusceptions or, less often, a high-grade obstruction caused by complete intussusception [Fig. 19-60(b, c)]. Large melanoma deposits may grow through the small bowel wall, expand into the mesentery, ulcerate, and cavitate.[211] Melanoma deposits in exoenteric locations can enlarge considerably before involving a segment of bowel by displacement or compression. Infiltrative and stenotic lesions have been reported in the ileum, sometimes together with polypoid masses. These variations in appearance have been attributed to varied host reactions to the tumor.[212] Patients with a history of melanoma should have contrast examination if they present with frank or occult bleeding. CT enteroclysis has been successful in outlining melanoma deposits throughout the small bowel (Fig. 19-61); it is the method of choice for demonstrating the total distribution of melanoma throughout the abdominal cavity.[213] Bulky retroperitoneal masses are unusual.

Metastatic Melenoma: Tumor cells shed into the bloodstream by the primary melanoma possess a site-

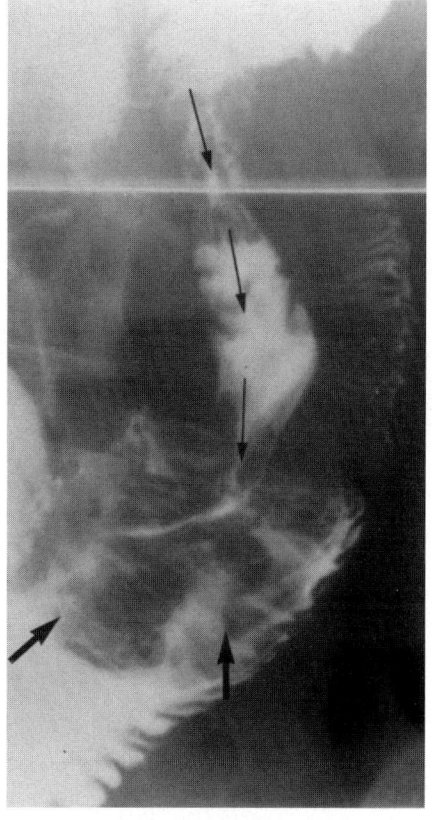
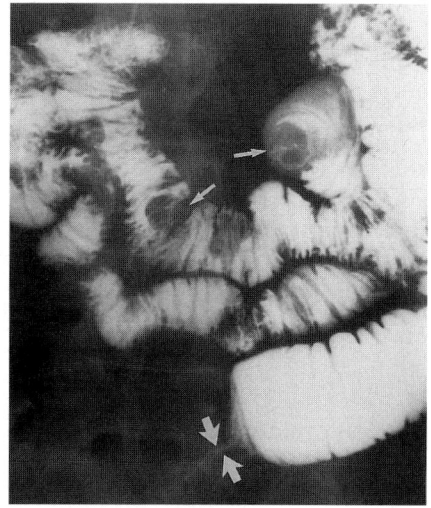
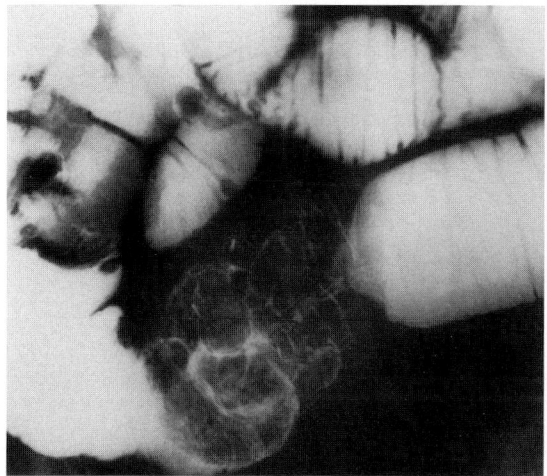

Fig. 19-60. Intussuscepting melanoma metastases usually do not obstruct because of the high cellularity of the soft mass. (a) Intussuscepted melanoma metastasis (thick arrows) not obstructing flow of barium (long arrows). (b) In a different patient enteroclysis demonstrates numerous melanoma metastases (arrows to some). Thick arrows indicate a significant obstruction. (c) Later film demonstrates cause of obstruction, an intussuscepted large melanoma metastasis.

specific adhesion molecule to bind to vascular endothelium and then access the interstitial space for further growth.[210] Small bowel melanoma metastases develop in the submucosa.

Metastases from bronchogenic carcinoma: Symptoms do not usually draw attention to the gastrointestinal tract unless significant bleeding or a perforation occur. The autopsy incidence of metastases to small bowel has been reported to be 11%; it is higher (39%) for a primary large cell bronchial carcinoma.[214] Metastases may be shown as single or multiple discrete intramural lesions, either flat or polypoid. They are frequently ulcerated (Fig. 19-62). An associated desmoplastic effect may cause constriction and obstruction. The pronounced tendency for the metastases to penetrate the bowel wall can lead to localized extravasation, rarely to free perforation.[215]

Metastases from carcinoma of breast: The stomach,

430 • 19. Small Bowel Neoplasms

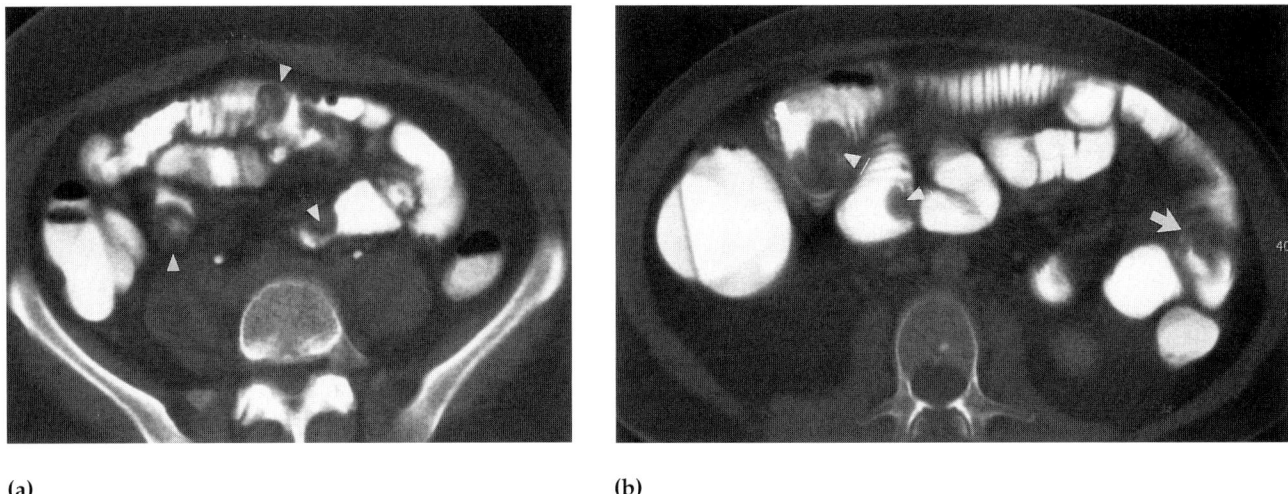

Fig. 19-61. CT enteroclysis of metastatic melanoma to small bowel.
(a, b) The infusion of a low-density water-soluble contrast demonstrates multiple nodules (arrowheads) in the small bowel. Note partial intussusception in left hemiabdomen (arrow) with metastatic deposit as the lead point. (Courtesy of Greg N. Bender, MD.)

duodenum, and colon are more often involved than the mesenteric small bowel. It has been suggested that treatment of the primary tumor with corticosteroids increases the likelihood of metastases.[216] Secondary metastases from breast cancer typically form highly cellular masses that spread through the submucosa. The rare metastases to the small bowel have been described as multiple strictures with intervening dilata-

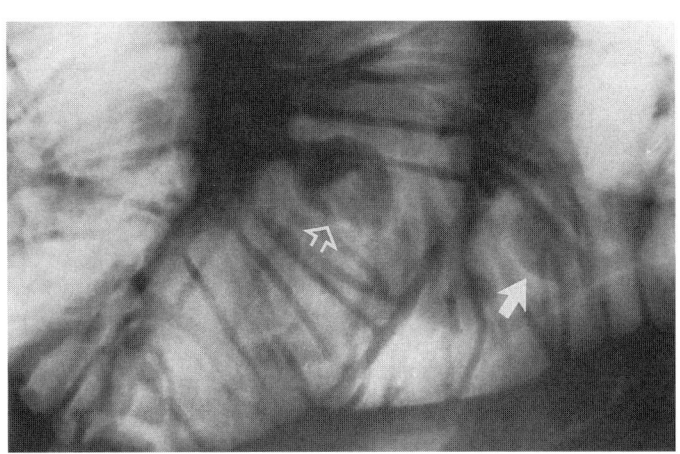
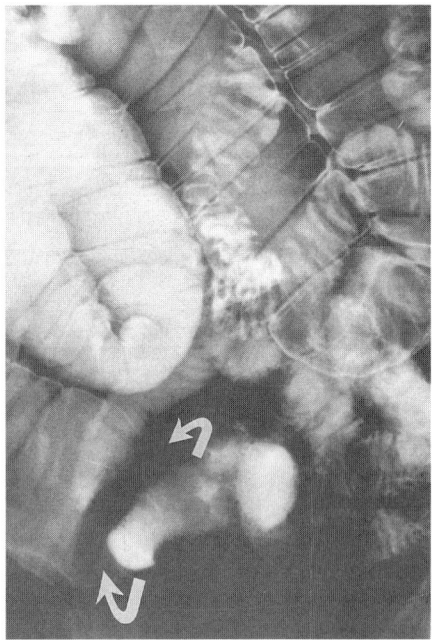

Fig. 19-62. Metastases from bronchogenic malignancy.
(a) Rounded polypoid metastasis with (open arrow) and without (solid arrow) ulceration from lung carcinoma in a patient who presented with unexplained bleeding. (From Maglinte.[131]) (b) Hematogenous metastasis with desmoplastic effect. Enteroclysis shows high-grade obstruction secondary to a short circumferential stricture (curved arrows) from a lung (scar) carcinoma. (From Maglinte and Reyes,[2] with permission.)

tions or as an intussuscepting ulcerated mural lesion (Fig. 19-63).[217]

Noncontiguous Extension and Lymphatic Spread

The subperitoneal space serves as a pathway for the spread of malignancies (and inflammatory processes) between the retroperitoneum and the peritoneal cavity.[218] Potential bidirectional spread through subperitoneal areolar tissue can connect right lower quadrant abdominal malignancies with pelvic organs and female pelvic malignancy with peritoneal structures like the terminal ileum.[219,220] This is also a not infrequent method of involvement of more proximal mesenteric small bowel.

Malignant tumors can utilize lymphatic channels for their spread. For example, the extension of a carcinoma from the splenic flexure area or the descending colon can occur via lymphatic vessels that parallel the arterial supply. Such lymphatics relate to part of the ascending branch of the inferior mesenteric artery, which courses lateral to the fourth portion of the duodenum. The adjacent jejunum can become involved by this mode of spread (Fig. 19-64).

Blockage of a proximal lymph node by tumor may produce retrograde flow of lymph and of tumor em-

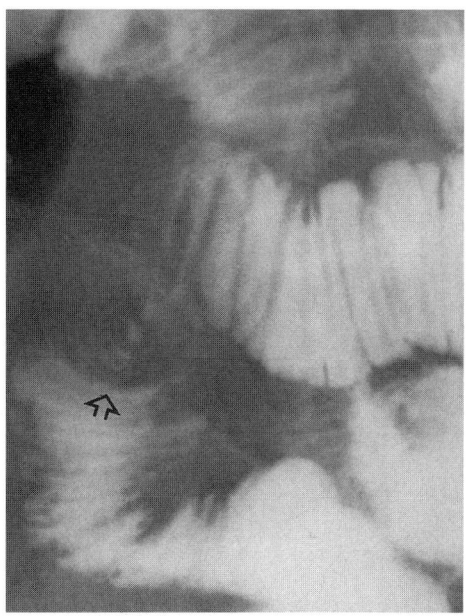

Fig. 19-63. Intussuscepting hematogenous metastasis. Enteroclysis performed for unexplained GI bleeding shows a partially intussuscepted lesion (arrow) without significant obstruction, a metastasis from breast carcinoma. This is an uncommon occurrence.

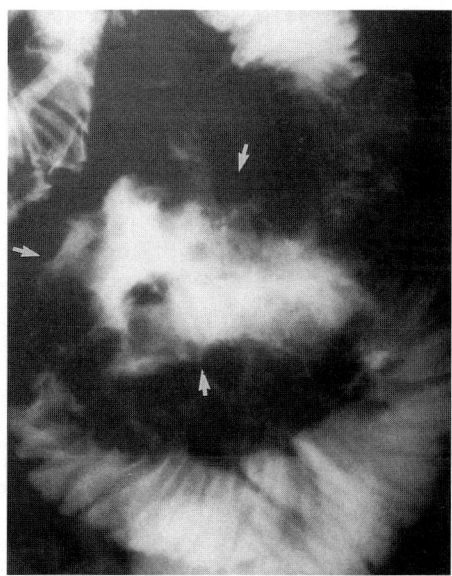
(a)

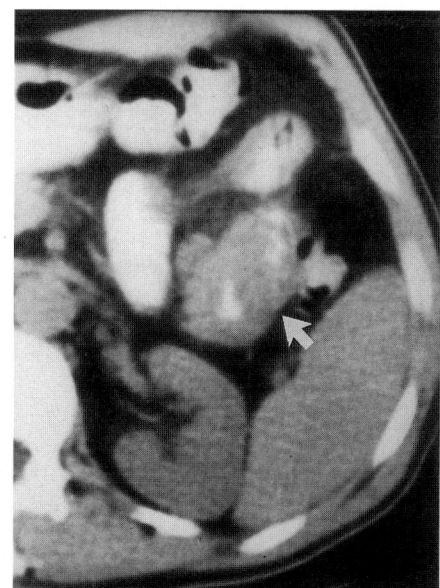
(b)

Fig. 19-64. Metastasis to the jejunum from a carcinoma of the descending colon.
(a) Enteroclysis performed for abdominal pain and GI bleeding shows a large ulcerating mass (arrows) occupying the left upper abdomen involving proximal jejunum. (b) CT scan demonstrates the large mass (arrow) in left upper quadrant. Metastatic disease should be diagnosed when proximal jejunal loops are involved in a patient with a known malignancy of the left colon.

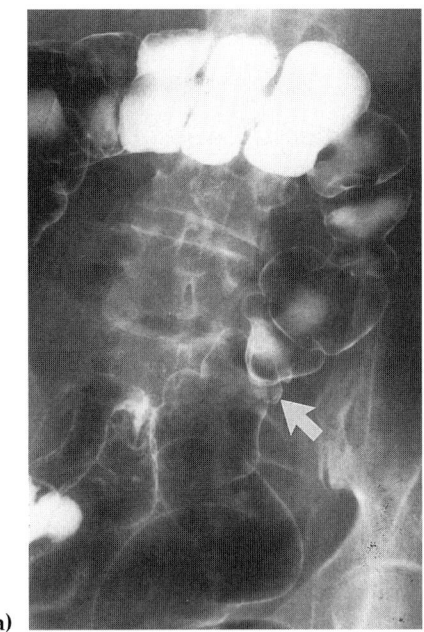 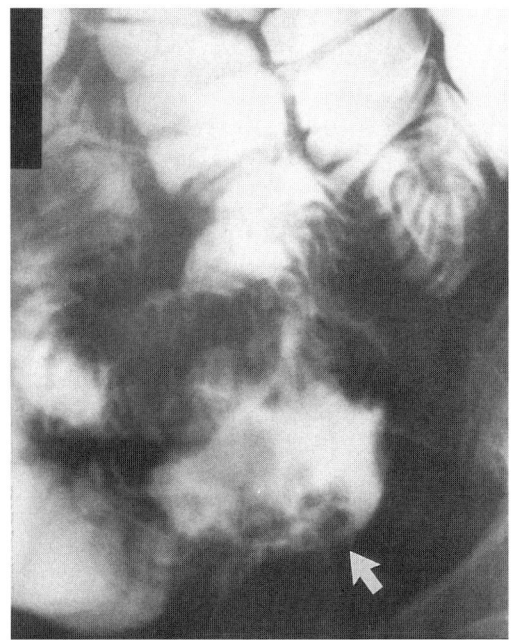

Fig. 19-65. Metastatic involvement of small bowel adjacent to an anastomotic site.
(a) Double-contrast barium enema done because of lower GI bleeding shows end-to-end anastomosis between transverse colon and sigmoid (arrow) after segmental colectomy for carcinoma. (b) Enteroclysis after colon examination shows large ulcerating mass (arrow) in the small bowel adjacent ot the sigmocolic anastomosis. Surgery confirmed metastatic disease.

boli and the involvement of an adjacent segment of bowel.[221] After resection for colon carcinoma, this mechanism may be responsible for the metastatic involvement of small bowel near a colocolic anastomosis (Fig. 19-65).

References

1. Ciresi DL, Scholten DJ. The continuing clinical dilemma of primary tumors of the small intestine. *Am Surg.* 1995;61:698–703.
2. Maglinte DDT, Reyes BL. Small bowel cancer: radiologic diagnosis. *Radiol Clin North Am.* 1997;35:361–380.
3. Maglinte DDT, Kelvin FM, O'Connor K, et al. Current status of small bowel radiography. *Abdom Imag.* 1996;21:247–257.
4. Maglinte DDT, O'Connor K, Bessette J, et al. The role of the physician in the late diagnosis of primary malignant tumors of the small intestine. *Am J Gastroenterol.* 1991;86:304–308.
5. Gurian L, Jendrzejewski S, Katon R, et al. Small bowel enema: an underutilized method of small bowel examination. *Dig Dis Sci.* 1982;27:1101–1108.
6. Dixon PM, Roulston ME, Nolan DJ. The small-bowel enema: a 10 year review. *Clin Radiol.* 1993;47:46–48.
7. Bowden TA Jr. Endoscopy of the small intestine. *Surg Clin North Am.* 1989;69:1237–1247.
8. Lewis BS, Kornbluth A. Small bowel tumours: yield of enteroscopy. *Gut.* 1991;32:763–765.
9. Herbsman H, Wetstein L, Rosen Y, et al. Tumors of the small intestine. *Curr Probl Surg.* 1980;17:121–182.
10. Barclay THC, Schapira DV. Malignant tumors of the small intestine. *Cancer.* 1983;51:878–881.
11. DiSario JA. Small bowel tumors. *Pract Gastroenterol.* 1992;16:24E–24N.
12. Zollinger RM Jr. Primary neoplasms of the small intestine. *Am J Surg.* 1986;151:654–658
13. Mason GR. Tumors of the duodenum and small intestine. In: Sabiston DC Jr, ed. *Textbook of Surgery*. 13th ed. Philadelphia, Pa: WB Saunders Co;1986:868–873.
14. Rodriguez-Bigas M, Penetrante RB, Herrera L, Petrelli NJ. Intraoperative small bowel enteroscopy in familial adenomatous and juvenile polyposis. *Gastrointest Endosc.* 1995;42:560–564.
15. Starke J, Rodriguez-Bigas M, Marshall W, Sohrabi A, Petrelli NJ. Primary adenocarcinoma arising in an ileostomy. *Surgery.* 1993;114:125–128.
16. Lowenfels AB. Why are small bowel tumors so rare? *Lancet.* 1973;1:24–26.
17. Ashley SW, Wells SA Jr. Tumors of the small intestine. *Semin Oncol.* 1988;15:116–128.
18. Wattenberg LW. Studies of polycyclic hydrocarbon hydroxylases of the intestine possibly related to cancer. Effect of diet on benzpyrene hydroxylase activity. *Cancer.* 1971;28:99–102.
19. Calman KC. Why are small bowel tumours rare? An experimental model. *Gut.* 1974;15:552–554.

20. Khojasteh A, Haghshenass M, Haghighi P. Current concepts: immunoproliferative small intestinal disease. A "Third-World lesion." *N Engl J Med*. 1983;308:1401–1405.
21. Lightdale CJ, Sternberg SS, Posner G, Sherlock P. Carcinoma complicating Crohn's disease. Report of seven cases and review of the literature. *Am J Med*. 1975;59:262–268.
22. Alexander JW, Altemeier WA. Association of primary neoplasms of the small intestine with other neoplastic growths. *Ann Surg*. 1968;167:958–964.
23. Dial P, Cohn I Jr. Tumors of the jejunum and ileum. In: Scott HW, Sawyers JL, eds. *Surgery of the Stomach, Duodenum and Small Intestine*. 2nd ed. Boston, Mass: Blackwell Scientific;1992:859–871.
24. Wilson JM, Melvin DB, Gray G, et al. Benign small bowel tumors. *Ann Surg*. 1975;181:247–250.
25. Maglinte DDT, Elmore MF, Chernish SM, et al. Enteroclysis in the diagnosis of chronic unexplained gastrointestinal bleeding. *Dis Colon Rectum*. 1985;28:403–405.
26. Rex DK, Lappas JC, Maglinte DDT, et al. Enteroclysis in the evaluation of suspected small intestinal bleeding. *Gastroenterology*. 1989;97:58–60.
27. Fenoglio-Preiser C, Pascal RR, Perzin KH. *Tumors of the Intestines*. Washington, DC: Armed Forces Institute of Pathology; 1990:175–250.
28. Vuori JV, Vuorio MK. Radiological findings in primary malignant tumors of the small intestine. *Ann Clin Res*. 1971;3:16–21.
29. Ekberg O, Ekholm S. Radiography in primary tumors of the small bowel. *Acta Radiol Diagn (Stockh)*. 1980;21:79–84.
30. Bessette JR, Maglinte DDT, Kelvin FM, et al. Primary malignant tumors in the small bowel: a comparison of the small bowel enema and conventional follow-through examination. *AJR*. 1989;153:741–744.
31. Maglinte DDT, Lappas JC, Kelvin FM, et al. Small bowel radiography: how, when, and why? *Radiology*. 1987;163:297–305.
32. Maglinte DDT, Burney BT, Miller RE. Lesions missed on small bowel follow-through: analysis and recommendations. *Radiology*. 1982;144:737–739.
33. Antes G, Neher M, Hiemeyer V, Burger A. Gastrointestinal bleeding of obscure origin: role of enteroclysis. *Eur Radiol*. 1996;6:851–854.
34. Maglinte DDT, Hall R, Miller RE, et al. Detection of surgical lesions of the small bowel by enteroclysis. *Am J Surg*. 1984;147:225–229.
35. Antes G, Lissner J. Double contrast small bowel examination with barium and methylcellulose: result in 300 cases. *Radiology*. 1983;148:37–40.
36. Nolan DJ, Marks CG. The barium infusion in small intestinal obstruction. *Clin Radiol*. 1981;32:651–655.
37. Maglinte DDT, Peterson LA, Vahey TN, et al. Enteroclysis in partial small bowel obstruction. *Am J Surg*. 1984;147:325–329.
38. Buckley JA, Jones B, Fishman EK. Small bowel cancer: imaging features and staging. *Radiol Clin North Am*. 1997;35:381–402.
39. Dudiak KM, Johnson CD, Stephen DH. Primary tumors of the small intestine: CT evaluation. *AJR*. 1989;152:995–998.
40. Laurent F, Raynaud M, Biset JM, et al. Diagnosis and categorization of small bowel neoplasms: role of computed tomography. *Gastrointest Radiol*. 1991;16:115–119.
41. Kusumoto H, Takahashi I, Yoshida M, et al. Primary malignant tumors of the small intestine: analysis of 40 Japanese patients. *J Surg Oncol*. 1992;50:139–143.
42. Rollins ES, Picus D, Hicks ME, et al. Angiography is useful in detecting the source of chronic gastrointestinal bleeding of obscure origin. *AJR*. 1991;156:385–388.
43. D'Alonzo WA, Alavi A. Scintigraphy. In: Herlinger H, Maglinte D, eds. *Clinical Radiology of the Small Intestine*. Philadelphia, Pa: WB Saunders Co; 1989:201–210.
44. Olmsted WW, Ros PR, Hjermstad BM, et al. Tumors of the small intestine with little or no malignant predisposition: a review of the literature and report of 56 cases. *Gastrointest Radiol*. 1987;12:231–239.
45. Gourtsoyiannis NC, Bays D, Papaioannou N, et al. Benign tumors of the small intestine: preoperative evaluation with a barium infusion technique. *Eur J Radiol*. 1993;16:115–125.
46. Gupta S, Gupta S. Primary tumors of the small bowel: a clinicopathological study of 58 cases. *J Surg Oncol*. 1982;20:161–167.
47. O'Riordan BG, Vilor M, Herrera L. Small bowel tumors: an overview. *Dig Dis*. 1996;14:245–257.
48. Gourtsoyiannis NC, Bays D, Malamas M, et al. Radiological appearances of small intestinal leiomyomas. *Clin Radiol*. 1992;45:94–103.
49. Uflacker R, Alves MA, Diehl JC. Gastrointestinal involvement in neurofibromatosis: angiographic presentation. *Gastrointest Radiol*. 1985;10:163–165.
50. McDonald KL. Technetium-99m RBC scintigraphy in the evaluation of small bowel leiomyoma. *Clin Nucl Med*. 1987;12:131–133.
51. Dunn EK, Farman J, Teitcher J, Smith T. Ileal leiomyosarcoma and leiomyoma: false positive scintiscans for Meckel's diverticulum. *Clin Nucl Med*. 1987;12:440–444.
52. Megibow AJ, Balthazar EJ, Hulnick DH, et al. CT evaluation of gastrointestinal leiomyomas and leiomyosarcomas. *AJR*. 1985;144:727–731.
53. Morson BC, Dawson IMP. *Gastrointestinal Pathology*. 2nd ed. Oxford, England: Blackwell Scientific; 1979:400–432.
54. Bjork KJ, Davis DJ, Nagorney DM, Mucha P Jr. Duodenal villous tumors. *Arch Surg*. 1990;125:961–965.
55. Garvin PJ, Herrmann V, Kaminski DL, Willman DL. Benign and malignant tumors of the small intestine. *Current Problems in Cancer*. 1979:1–46.
56. Ashley SW, Wells SA Jr. Tumors of the small intestine. *Semin Oncol*. 1988;15:116–128.
57. Taylor AJ, Stewart ET, Dodds WJ. Gastrointestinal lipomas: a radiologic and pathologic review. *AJR*. 1990;155:1205–1210.
58. Ormson MJ, Stephens DH, Carlson HC. CT recognition of intestinal lipomatosis. *AJR*. 1985;144:313–314.
59. Herbsman H, Wetstein L, Rosen Y, et al. Tumors of the small intestine. *Curr Probl Surg*. 1980;17:121–182.

60. Schey WL, Emanuel B, Raffensperger J. Benign neoplasia and pseudoneoplasia of the small bowel in children. *Gastrointest Radiol.* 1979;4:47–55.
61. Sivak MV, Sullivan BH, Farmer RG. Neurogenic tumors of the small intestine: review of the literature and report of a case with endoscopic removal. *Gastroenterology.* 1975;68:374–380.
62. Seppala R, Prefontaine M, Mikhael NZ. Mesenteric small-bowel polyposis: a diagnostic radiographic sign of neurofibromatosis. *AJR.* 1997;168:434–436.
63. Marshak RH, Freund S, Maklansky D. Neurofibromatosis of the small bowel. *Am J Dig Dis.* 1963;8:478–483.
64. Reeder MM, Gelford GJ, Robb PL. An exercise in radiologic-pathologic correlation. *Radiology.* 1968;90:1023–1029.
65. Harkin JC, Reed RJ. Tumors of the peripheral nervous system. In: Firminger HI, ed. *Atlas of Tumor Pathology.* 2nd ser, fasc 3. Washington, DC: Armed Forces Institute of Pathology;1969:67–97.
66. Ginsburg LD. Eccentric polyposis of the small bowel. A possible radiologic sign of plexiform neurofibromatosis of the small bowel and its mesentery. *Radiology.* 1975;116:561–562.
67. Fukuya T, Lu CC, Mitros FA. CT findings of plexiform neurofibromatosis involving the ileum and its mesentery. *Clin Imaging.* 1994;18:142–145.
68. Shimer GR, Helwig EB. Inflammatory fibroid polyps of the intestine. *Am J Clin Pathol.* 1984;81:708–714.
69. Harned RK, Buck JL, Shekitka KM. Inflammatory fibroid polyps of the gastrointestinal tract: radiologic evaluation. *Radiology.* 1992;182:863–866.
70. Bussey HJR, Veale AMD, Morson BC. Genetics of gastrointestinal polyposis. *Gastroenterology.* 1978;74:1325–1330.
71. Perzin KH, Bridge MF. Adenomatous and carcinomatous changes in hamartomatous polyps of the small intestine (Peutz-Jeghers syndrome): report of a case and review of the literature. *Cancer.* 1982;49:971–983.
72. Buck JL, Harned RK, Lichtenstein JL, Sobin LH. Peutz-Jegher's syndrome. Review. *Radiographics.* 1992;12:365–378.
73. Sener RN, Kumcuoglu Z, Elmas N, et al. Peutz-Jegher's syndrome: CT and US demonstration of small bowel polyps. *Gastrointest Radiol.* 1991;16:21–23.
74. Radin DR. Hereditary generalized juvenile polyposis: association with arteriovenous malformation and risk of malignancy. *Abdom Imag.* 1994;19:140–142.
75. Chen YM, Ott DJ, Wu WC, et al. Cowden's disease, a case report and literature review. *Gastrointest Radiol.* 1987;12:325–329.
76. Harned RK, Buck JL, Sobin LH. The hamartmatous polyposis syndromes: clinical and radiological features. *AJR.* 1995;164:565–571.
77. Ruvalcaba RHA, Myhre S, Smith DW. Sotos syndrome with intestinal polyposis and pigmentary changes of the genitalia. *Clin Genet.* 1980;18:413–416.
78. Koehler PR, Kyaw MM, Fenlon JW. Diffuse gastrointestinal polyposis with ectodermal changes. *Radiology.* 1972;103:589–594.
79. Freeman K, Anthony PP, Miller DS, Warin AP. Cronkhite-Canada syndrome: a new hypothesis. *Gut.* 1985;26:531–536.
80. Russell DM, Bhathal PS, St John DJB. Complete remission in Cronkhite-Canada syndrome. *Gastroenterology.* 1983;85:180–185.
81. Dachman AH, Buck JL, Burke AP, et al. Cronkhite-Canada syndrome: radiologic features. *Gastrointest Radiol.* 1989;14:285–290.
82. Ushio K, Sasagawa M, Doi H, et al. Lesions associated with familial polyposis coli: studies of lesions of the stomach, duodenum, bones, and teeth. *Gastrointest Radiol.* 1976;1:67–80.
83. Harned RK, Buck JL, Olmsted WW, et al. Extracolonic manifestations of the familial adenomatous polyposis syndromes. *AJR.* 1991;156:481–485.
84. Hamilton SR, Bussey HJR, Mendelsohn G, et al. Ileal adenomas after colectomy in nine patients with adenomatous polyposis coli/Gardner's syndrome. *Gastroenterology.* 1979;77:1252–1257.
85. Burke AP, Sobin LH, Shekitka KM, et al. Intraabdominal fibromatosis: a pathologic analysis of 130 tumors with comparison of clinical subgroups. *Am J Surg Pathol.* 1990;14:335–341.
86. Einstein DM, Tagliabue JR, Desai RK. Abdominal desmoids: CT findings in 25 patients. *AJR.* 1991;157:275–279.
87. Casillas J, Sais GJ, Greve JL, et al. Imaging of intra- and extra-abdominal desmoid tumors. *Radiographics.* 1991;11:959–968.
88. Gore RM. Small bowel cancer. Clinical and pathologic features. *Radiol Clin North Am.* 1997;35:351–360.
89. Lance P. Tumors and other neoplastic diseases of the small bowel. In: Yamada T, ed. *Textbook of Gastroenterology.* 2nd ed. Philadelphia, Pa: JB Lippincott Co; 1995:1696–1713.
90. Brookes VS, Waterhouse JAH, Powell DJ. Malignant lesions of the small intestine. A 10 year survey. *Br J Surg.* 1968;55:405–410.
91. Ripley D, Weinerman BH. Increased incidence of second malignancies associated with small bowel adenocarcinoma. *Can J Gastroenterol.* 1997;11:65–68.
92. Laurent F, Raynaud M, Biset JM, et al. Diagnosis and categorization of small bowel neoplasms: role of computed tomography. *Gastrointest Radiol.* 1991;16:115–119.
93. Wilson JM, Melvin DB, Gray GF, et al. Primary malignancies of the small bowel. A report of 96 cases and review of the literature. *Ann Surg.* 1974;180:175–179.
94. Lightdale CJ, Sherlock P. Small intestinal tumors (other than lymphoma and carcinoid). In: Berk JE, ed. *Bockus Gastroenterology.* 4th ed. Philadelphia, Pa: WB Saunders Co;1985:1887–1899.
95. Neugut AI, Santos J. The association between cancers of the small and large bowel. *Cancer Epidemiol Biomarkers Prev.* 1993;2:551–553.
96. Sellner F. Investigations on the significance of the adenoma-carcinoma sequence in the small bowel. *Cancer.* 1990;66:702–715.
97. Ouriel K, Adams JT. Adenocarcinoma of the small intestine. *Am J Surg.* 1984;147:66–71.

98. Harris OD, Cooke WT, Thomason H, et al. Malignancy in adult celiac disease and idiopathic steatorrhea. *Am J Med.* 1967;42:899–912.
99. Swinson CM, Slavin G, Coles RC, et al. Coeliac disease and malignancy. *Lancet.* 1983;1:111–115.
100. Cooke WT, Homes GKT. *Coeliac Disease.* Edinburgh, Scotland: Churchill Livingstone; 1984:180–183.
101. van den Bosch HC, Tjon a Tham RT, Gooszen AW, et al. Celiac disease: small bowel enteroclysis findings in adult patients treated with a gluten-free diet. *Radiology.* 1996;201:803–808.
102. Ginzberg L, Schneider KM, Drezin DH. Carcinoma of the jejunum occurring in a case of regional enteritis. *Surgery.* 1956;39:347–351.
103. Feczko PJ. Malignancy complicating inflammatory bowel disease. *Radiol Clin North Am.* 1987;25:157–174.
104. Fell J, Snooks S. Small bowel adenocarcinoma complicating Crohn's disease. *J Roy Soc Med.* 1987;80:51–52.
105. Fresko D, Lazarus S, Dotan J, et al. Early presentation of carcinoma of the small bowel in Crohn's disease ("Crohn's carcinoma"). Case reports and review of the literature. *Gastroenterology.* 1982;82:783–789.
106. Lashner BA. Risk factors for small bowel cancer in Crohn's disease. *Dig Dis Sci.* 1992;37:1179–1184.
107. Church JM, Weakley FL, Fazio VW. The relationship between fistulas and Crohn's disease and associated carcinoma. Report of four cases and review of the literature. *Dis Colon Rectum.* 1985;28:361–366.
108. Kerber GW, Frank PH. Carcinoma of the small intestine and colon as a complication of Crohn's disease: radiologic manifestations. *Radiology.* 1984;150:639–645.
109. Miller TL, Skucas J, Gudex D. Bowel cancer characteristics in patients with regional enteritis. *Gastrointest Radiol.* 1987;12:45–52.
110. Hawker PC, Gyde SN, Thompson H, et al. Adenocarcinoma of the small intestine complicating Crohn's disease. *Gut.* 1982;23:188–193.
111. Schier J. Diagnostic and therapeutic aspects of tumors of the small bowel. *Int Surg.* 1972;57:789–792.
112. Spigelman AD, Murday V, Phillips RKS. Cancer and the Peutz-Jeghers syndrome. *Gut.* 1989;30:1588–1590.
113. Hulnick DH, Megibow AJ. Computed tomography of the small bowel. In: Herlinger H, Maglinte D, eds. *Clinical Radiology of the Small Intestine.* Philadelphia, Pa: WB Saunders Co; 1989:161–200.
114. Bruneton JN, Drouillard J, Bourry J, et al. L'adenocarcinome de l'intestin grele. Etat actuel du diagnostic et du traitement. Etude de 27 cas et revue de la litterature. *J Radiol.* 1983;64:117–123.
115. Papadopoulos VD, Nolan DJ. Carcinoma of the small intestine. *Clin Radiol.* 1985;36:409–413.
116. Levine MS, Droos AT, Herlinger H. Annular malignancies of the small bowel. *Gastrointest Radiol.* 1987;12:53–58.
117. Wagner KM, Thompson J, Herlinger H, et al. Thirteen primary adenocarcinomas of the ileum and appendix, a case report. *Cancer.* 1982;49:797–801.
118. Nerine D, Fishman EK, Jones B. CT of the small bowel and mesentery. *Radiol Clin North Am.* 1989;27:707–715.
119. Fleischer AC, Parulekar S, Seibert JJ. Sonography of small bowel. In: Herlinger H, Maglinte D, eds. *Clinical Radiology of the Small Intestine.* Philadelphia, Pa: WB Saunders Co; 1989:153–159.
120. Milman PJ, Gold BM, Bagla S, et al. Primary ileal adenocarcinoma simulating Crohn's disease. *Gastrointest Radiol.* 1980;5:55–58.
121. Johnson AM, Harman PK, Hanks JB. Primary small bowel malignancies. *Am Surg.* 1985;51:31–36.
122. Moertel CG, Sauer WG, Dockerty MB, et al. Life history of the carcinoid tumor of the small intestine. *Cancer.* 1961;14:901–912.
123. Wallace S, Ajani JA, Charnsangavej C, et al. Carcinoid tumors: imaging procedures and interventional radiology. *World J Surg.* 1996;20:147–156.
124. Balthazar EJ. Carcinoid tumors of the alimentary tract. I. Radiographic diagnosis. *Gastrointest Radiol.* 1978;3:47–56.
125. Lightdale CJ, Hornsby-Lewis L. Tumors of the small intestine. In: Berk JE, ed. *Bockus Gastroenterology.* 5th ed. Philadelphia, Pa: WB Saunders Co; 1995:1274–1290.
126. Hossain J, Al-Mofleh I, Tandon R, et al. Carcinoid syndrome without liver metastases. *Postgrad Med J.* 1989;65:597–599.
127. Jeffree MA, Nolan DJ. Multiple ileal carcinoid tumors. *Br J Radiol.* 1987;60:402–403.
128. Kothari T, Mangla JC. Malignant tumors associated with carcinoid tumors of the gastrointestinal tract. *J Clin Gastroenterol.* 1981;3(suppl 1):43–46.
129. Matuchansky C, Launay J-M. Serotonin: catecholamines, and spontaneous midgut flush: plasma studies from flushing and nonflushing sites. *Gastroenterology.* 1995;108:743–751.
130. Mir-Madjlessi SH, Winkelman EI, Davis GA. Carcinoid tumors of the terminal ileum simulating Crohn's disease. *Cleve Clin J Med.* 1988;55:257–262.
131. Maglinte D. Malignant tumors. In: Gore RM, Levine MS, Laufer I, eds. *Textbook of Gastrointestinal Radiology.* Philadelphia, Pa: WB Saunders Co; 1994:900–930.
132. Payne-James JJ, de Gara CJ, Lovell D, et al. Metastatic carcinoid tumour in association with small bowel ischaemia and infarction. *J Roy Soc Med.* 1990;83:54.
133. Woodard PK, Feldman JM, Paine SS, Baker ME. Midgut carcinoid tumors: CT findings and biochemical profiles. *J Comput Assist Tomogr.* 1995;19:400–405.
134. Hulnick DH, Megibow AJ. Computed tomography of the small bowel. In: Herlinger H, Maglinte D, eds. *Clinical Radiology of the Small Intestine.* Philadelphia, Pa: WB Saunders Co; 1989:161–200.
135. Soyer P, Gueye C, Somveille E, et al. MR diagnosis of hepatic metastases from neuroendocrine tumors versus hemangiomas. *AJR.* 1995;165:1407–1413.
136. Modlin M, Cornelius E, Lawton GP. Use of an isotopic somatostatin receptor probe to image gut endocrine tumors. *Arch Surg.* 1995;130:367–374.
137. King CM, Reznek RH, Bomanji J, et al. Imaging neuroendocrine tumours with radiolabelled somatostatin analogues and X-ray computed tomography. *Clin Radiol.* 1993;48:386–391.
138. Modlin IM, Tang LH. Approaches to the diagnosis of gut neuroendocrine tumors: the last word (today). *Gastroenterology.* 1997;112:583–590.

139. Debas HT, Mulvihill SJ. Neuroendocrine gut neoplasms. Important lessons from uncommon tumors. *Arch Surg.* 1994;129:965–972.
140. Kvols LK. Somatostatin receptor imaging of human malignancies: a new era in the localization, staging and treatment of tumors. Editorial. *Gastroenterology.* 1993;105:1909–1914.
141. Ruszniewski P, Ducreux M, Chayvialle J-A, et al. Treatment of the carcinoid syndrome with the longacting somatostatin analogue lanreotide: a prospective study in 39 patients. *Gut.* 1996;39:279–283.
142. Seigel RS, Kuhns LR, Borlaza GS. Computed tomography and angiography in ileal carcinoid tumor and retractile mesenteritis. *Radiology.* 1980;134:437–440.
143. Arnold R. Medical treatment of metastasizing carcinoid tumors (review). *World J Surg.* 1996;20:203–207.
144. Mitty HA, Warner RR, Newman LH, et al. Control of carcinoid syndrome with hepatic artery embolization. *Radiology.* 1985;155:623–626.
145. Coupe MO, Hemingway A, Hodgson HJ, et al. Effect of hepatic artery embolization on survival in carcinoid syndrome. Abstracts of the Jubilee Meeting of the British Society of Gastroenterology. 1987;36.
146. Jammohamed S, Bloom SR. Carcinoid tumors. *Postgrad Med J.* 1997;73:207–214.
147. Marshak RH, Lindner AE. Radiologic features of diagnostic importance. *JAMA.* 1974;229:1498–1499.
148. Dawson IM, Cornes JS, Morson BC. Primary malignant tumors of the intestinal tract. Report of 37 cases with a study of factors influencing prognosis. *Br J Surg.* 1961;49:80–89.
149. Isaacson PG, Wright DH. Gut-associated lymphoid tumors. In: Whitehead R, ed. *Gastrointestinal and Oesophageal Pathology.* 2nd ed. Edinburgh, Scotland: Churchill Livingstone; 1995:755–775.
150. Ehrlich AN, Stalder G, Geller W, et al. Gastrointestinal manifestations of malignant lymphoma. *Gastroenterology.* 1968;54:1115–1118.
151. Berg JW. Primary lymphomas of the human gastrointestinal tract. *Natl Cancer Inst Monogr.* 1969;32:211–215.
152. Rappaport H. The lymphoreticular system. In: *Atlas of Tumor Pathology.* Fasc 8, section 3. Washington, DC: Armed Forces Institute of Pathology; 1966.
153. Jaffe ES. An overview of the classification of non-Hodgkin's lymphomas. In: Jaffe ES, ed. *Surgical Pathology of the Lymph Nodes and Related Organs.* Philadelphia, Pa: WB Saunders Co; 1985:135–145.
154. National Cancer Institute sponsored study of classifications of non-Hodgkin's lymphomas: summary and description of a working formulation for clinical usage. The Non-Hodgkin's Lymphoma Pathologic Classification Project. *Cancer.* 1982;49:2112–2135.
155. Lewin KJ, Ranchod M, Dorfman RF. Lymphomas of the gastrointestinal tract: a study of 117 cases presenting with gastrointestinal disease. *Cancer.* 1978;42:693–707.
156. Fenoglio-Preiser CM, Pascal RR, Perzin KH. Lymphoproliferative lesions. In: *Tumors of the Intestines.* Washington, DC: Armed Forces Institute of Pathology; 1988:371–402.
157. Kojima M, Nakamura S, Kurabayashi Y, et al. Primary malignant lymphoma of the intestine: clinicopathologic and immunohistochemical studies of 39 cases. *Pathol Int.* 1995;45:123–130.
158. d'Amore F, Brincker H, Gronback K, et al. Non-Hodgkin's lymphoma of the gastrointestinal tract: a population-based analysis of incidence, geographic distribution, clinicopathologic presentation, and prognosis. Danish lymphoma study group. *J Clin Oncology.* 1994;12:1673–1684.
159. Baildam AD, Williams GT, Schofield PF. Abdominal lymphoma—the place for surgery. *J Roy Soc Med.* 1989;82:657–660.
160. Randall J, Obeid ML, Blackledge GRP. Hemorrhage and perforation of gastrointestinal neoplasms during chemotherapy. *Ann R Coll Surg Engl.* 1986;68:286–289.
161. Konar A, Brown CB, Hancock BW, et al. Protein-losing enteropathy as a sole manifestation of non-Hodgkin's lymphoma. *Postgrad Med J.* 1986;62:399–400.
162. Agudelo CA, Schumacher HR, Glick JH, et al. Non-Hodgkin's lymphoma in systemic lupus erythematosus. Report of four cases with ultrastructural studies in two. *J Rheumatol.* 1981;8:69–78.
163. Gilchrist AM, Herlinger H, Carr RF, et al. Small bowel lymphoma, a radiologic pathologic correlation. In: Herlinger H, Megibow A, eds. *Gastrointestinal Radiology Review, 1.* New York, NY: Marcel Dekker; 1990:187–211.
164. Rubesin SE, Gilchrist AM, Bronner M, et al. Non-Hodgkin's lymphoma of the small intestine. *Radiographics.* 1990;10:985–998.
165. Levine MS, Rubesin SE, Pantongrag-Brown L, et al. Non-Hodgkin's lymphoma of the gastrointestinal tract: radiographic findings. *AJR.* 1997;168:165–172.
166. Gourtsoyiannis NC, Nolan DJ. Lymphoma of the small intestine: radiological appearances. *Clin Radiol.* 1988;39:639–645.
167. Craig O, Gregson R. Primary lymphoma of the gastrointestinal tract. *Clin Radiol.* 1981;32:63–72.
168. Balthazar EJ, Noordhoorn M, Megibow AJ, Gordon RB. CT of small-bowel lymphoma in immunocompetent patients and patients with AIDS: comparison of findings. *AJR.* 1997;168:675–680.
169. Akcay MN, Polat M, Cadirci M, Gencer B. Tumor-induced ileo-ileal invagination in adults. *Am Surg.* 1994;60:980–982.
170. Smir BN, Pulitzer DR. Multiple lymphomatous polyposis of the gut. A case with unusually widespread distribution. *J Clin Gastroenterol.* 1994;19:139–142.
171. Argatoff LH, Connors JM, Klasa RJ, et al. Mantle cell lymphoma: a clinicopathologic study of 80 cases. *Blood.* 1997;89:2067–2078.
172. Honda K, Mizuno M, Matsumoto T, et al. A case of systemic malignant lymphoma with intestinal involvement of lymphomatous polyposis type. *J Clin Gastroenterol.* 1997;25:362–364.
173. Mueller PR, Ferrucci JT Jr, Harbin WP, et al. Appearance of lymphomatous involvement of the mesentery

by ultrasonography and body computed tomography: the "sandwich" sign. *Radiology.* 1980;134:467–473.
174. Glass RBJ, Fernbach SK, Conway JJ, et al. Gallium scintigraphy in American Burkitt lymphoma: accurate assessment of tumor load and prognosis. *AJR.* 1985; 145:671–676.
175. Vaccher E, Tirelli U. Burkitt's like lymphoma in patients with and without HIV infection. A report of 33 patients from north-east Italy. *Acta Oncol.* 1994;33:507–511.
176. Dodd GD. Lymphoma of the hollow abdominal viscera. *Radiol Clin North Am.* 1990;28:771–783.
177. Sartoris DJ, Harell GS, Anderson MF, et al. Small bowel lymphoma and regional enteritis: radiographic similarities. *Radiology.* 1984;152:291–296.
178. Pagani JJ, Bernardino ME. CT-radiographic correlation of ulcerating small bowel lymphomas. *AJR.* 1981;136: 998–1000.
179. Lunderquist A. Percutaneous biopsy of small bowel lesions. In: Herlinger H, Maglinte D, eds. *Clinical Radiology of the Small Intestine.* Philadelphia, Pa: WB Saunders Co; 1989:235–236.
180. Parker SH, Hopper KD, Yakes WF, et al. Image-directed percutaneous biopsies with a biopsy gun. *Radiology.* 1989;171:663–669.
181. Barr LC, Glees JP, Gazet JC. Diagnostic laparotomy in suspected malignant lymphoma. *Ann R Coll Surg Engl.* 1984;66:402–404.
182. Blackledge G, Best JK, Crowther D. Role of computed tomography in staging and management of gastrointestinal lymphoma. *J Roy Soc Med.* 1979;72:818–822.
183. Bragg DG, Colby TV, Ward JH. New concepts in the non-Hodgkin lymphomas: radiologic implications. *Radiology.* 1986;159:291–304.
184. Back H, Gustavson R, Ridell B, et al. Primary gastrointestinal lymphoma. Incidence, clinical presentation and surgical approach. *J Surg Oncol.* 1986;33:234–238.
185. Brady LW, Asbell SO. Malignant lymphoma of the gastrointestinal tract. *Radiology.* 1980;137:291–298.
186. Libson E, Mapp E, Dachman AH. Hodgkin's disease of the gastrointestinal tract. *Clin Radiol.* 1994;49:166–169.
187. Krikorian JG, Burke JS, Rosenberg SA, et al. The occurrence of non-Hodgkin's lymphoma following therapy for Hodgkin's disease. *N Engl J Med.* 1979;300:452–458.
188. Shiu MH, Farr GH, Egeli RA, Quan SH, Hajdu SI. Myosarcomas of the small and large intestine: a clinicopathological study. *J Surg Oncol.* 1983;24:67–72.
189. Ranchod M, Kempson RL. Smooth muscle tumors of the gastrointestinal tract and retroperitoneum: a pathologic analysis of 100 cases. *Cancer.* 1977;39:255–262.
190. Dodds WJ, Goldberg HI, Margulis AR. Leiomyosarcoma of the small intestine. *AJR.* 1969;107:142–149.
191. Conlon KC, Casler ES, Brennan ME. Primary gastrointestinal sarcomas: analysis of prognostic variables. *Ann Surg Oncology.* 1995;2:26–31.
192. Megibow AJ, Balthazar EJ, Hulnick DH, et al. CT evaluation of gastrointestinal leiomyomas and leiomyosarcomas. *AJR.* 1985;144:727–731.
193. Choi BI, Lee WJ, Chi JG, et al. CT manifestations of peritoneal leiomyosarcomatosis. *AJR.* 1990;155:799–801.
194. Uflacker R, Amaral NM, Lima S, et al. Angiography in primary myomas of the alimentary tract. *Radiology.* 1981;139:361–369.
195. Meyers MA, McSweeney J. Secondary neoplasms of the bowel. *Radiology.* 1972;105:1–11.
196. Meyers MA. Clinical involvement of mesenteric and antromesenteric borders of small bowel loops. I. Normal pattern and relationships. *Gastrointest Radiol.* 1976;1:41–47.
197. Meyers MA. Clinical involvement of mesenteric and antimesenteric borders of small bowel loops. II. Roentgen interpretation of pathologic alterations. *Gastrointest Radiol.* 1976;1:49–58.
198. Oliphant M, Berne AS, Meyers MA. The subperitoneal space of the abdomen and pelvis: planes of continuity. *AJR.* 1996;167:1433–1439.
199. Caroline DF, Herlinger H, Laufer I, et al. Small bowel enema in the diagnosis of adhesive obstructions. *AJR.* 1984;142:1133–1139.
200. Herlinger H, Maglinte D. Small bowel obstruction. In: Herlinger, Maglinte D, eds. *Clinical Radiology of the Small Intestine.* Philadelphia, Pa: WB Saunders Co; 1989:479–507.
201. Meyers MA: Intraperitoneal feeding, In: *Dynamic Radiology of the Abdomen.* 3rd ed. Springer Verlag New York, 1988, pp. 139–178.
202. Zboralske FF, Bessolo RJ. Metastatic carcinoma to the mesentery and gut. *Radiology.* 1967;88:302–310.
203. Marshak RH, Knilnani MT, Eliasoh J, et al. Metastatic carcinoma of the small bowel. *AJR.* 1965;94:385–394.
204. Wittich G, Salomonowitz E, Szepesi T, et al. Small bowel double-contrast enema in stage III ovarian cancer. *AJR.* 1984;142:299–304.
205. Nolan DJ. Secondary Neoplasms, Chapter VI. In: *Imaging of Small Intestinal Tumours.* Elsevier, Amsterdam (publ.), 1997:193–211.
206. Aronchick CA, Brooks FP, Dyson WL, et al. Ileocecal endometriosis presenting with abdominal pain and gastrointestinal bleeding. *Dig Dis Sci.* 1983;28:566–572.
207. McDermott VG, Low VH, Keogan MT, et al. Malignant melanoma metastatic to the gastrointestinal tract. *AJR.* 1996;166:809–813.
208. Krige JE, Nel PN, Hudson DA. Surgical treatment of metastatic melanoma of the small bowel. *Amer Surgeon.* 1996;62:658–663.
209. Branum GD, Seigler MF. Role of surgical intervention in the management of intestinal metastases from malignant melanoma. *Am J Surg.* 1991;126:428–431.
210. Ollila DW, Essner R, Wanek LA, Morton DL. Surgical resection for melanoma metastatic to the gastrointestinal tract. *Arch Surg.* 1996;131:975–980.
211. Goldstein HM, Beydoun MT, Dodd GD. Radiologic spectrum of melanoma metastatic to the gastrointestinal tract. *AJR.* 1977;129:605–612.
212. Zornoza J, Goldstein HM. Cavitating metastases of the small intestine. *AJR.* 1977;129:613–615.
213. Plavsic B, Robinson AE. Variations in gastrointestinal melanoma metastases. *Acta Radiol.* 1990;31:493–495.
214. Fishman EK, Kuhlman JE, Schuchter LM, et al. CT of

malignant melanoma in the chest, abdomen and musculoskeletal system. *Radiographics.* 1990;10:603–620.
215. McNeill PM, Wagman LD, Neifeld JP. Small bowel metastases from primary carcinoma of the lung. *Cancer.* 1987;59:1486–1489.
216. Joffe N. Symptomatic gastrointestinal metastases secondary to bronchogenic carcinoma. *Clin Radiol.* 1978;29:217–225.
217. Hartman WH, Sherlock P. Gastroduodenal metastases from carcinoma of the breast. An adrenal steroid-induced phenomenon. *Cancer.* 1961;14:426–431.
218. Chang SF, Burrell MI, Brand MH, et al. The protean gastrointestinal manifestations of metastatic breast carcinoma. *Radiology.* 1978;126:611–617.
219. Obaro RO, Lata A. Journey through the abdominal underpass: The subperitoneal pathway of disease spread revisited. *J Canad Assoc Radiol.* 1995;46:353–362.
220. Oliphant M, Berne AS, Meyers MA. Imaging the direct bidirectional spread of disease between the abdomen and the female pelvis via the subperitoneal space. *Gastrointest Radiol.* 1988;13:285–298.
221. Szus RA, Turner MA. Gastrointestinal tract involvement by gynecologic diseases. *RadioGrapihcs.* 1996;16:1251–1270.
222. Grinnel RS. Lymphatic block with atypical and retrograde lymphatic metastasis and spread in carcinoma of the colon and rectum. *Ann Surg.* 1966;163:272–280.

Vascular Disorders of the Small Intestine

20

Jill E. Jacobs, Bernard A. Birnbaum, and Dean D.T. Maglinte

Chapter Contents

Introduction
Pathophysiology and Vascular Anatomy
Classification of Mesenteric Vascular Disease

Introduction

Despite continuing advances in gastroenterologic and radiologic diagnostic techniques, early detection and diagnosis of intestinal ischemia remains difficult. A wide range of arterial and venous pathologic processes result in mesenteric ischemia, and the ensuing morbidity and mortality are directly related to the duration and extent of bowel ischemia and infarction. The causes and radiologic appearances of vascular diseases of the small intestine are varied, and will be reviewed in this chapter.

Pathophysiology and Vascular Anatomy

The small intestine derives its blood supply from the celiac artery, which supplies the duodenum, and the superior mesenteric artery (SMA), which supplies the jejunal and ileal segments of the mesenteric small bowel. The jejunal and ileal branches of the SMA form a series of three or four arcades prior to entering the intestinal wall as the arteriae rectae. Although the primary and secondary vascular arcades have the potential to receive collateral flow from branches of the celiac axis and inferior mesenteric artery, the arteriae rectae are end-arteries supplying the intestinal villi. As such, selective occlusion of these arteries, as may occur with low-flow states or vasculitis, may result in segmental intestinal infarction.

Together, the small and large intestine receive approximately 20% of the resting cardiac output. The bowel mucosa is more functionally and metabolically active than the muscularis. This is reflected by the fact that approximately 80% of intestinal flow is directed to the mucosa, while approximately 20% is distributed to the muscularis layer of the bowel wall.[1] As a consequence of its higher metabolic activity and end-artery blood supply, the mucosa is more susceptible to ischemic injury than the muscularis, and bowel necrosis typically begins at the tips of the intestinal villi.

Regardless of etiology, intestinal ischemia is defined as hypoxia of the bowel wall. Adequate intestinal oxygenation depends on numerous factors such as vascular patency, perfusion pressure, arteriolar resistance, arterial oxygen saturation, and tissue oxygen requirements. Multiple factors assist in regulating mesenteric blood flow and maintaining bowel perfusion over a wide range of systemic blood pressures, including splanchnic autoregulation, the cardiovascular system, circulating vasoactive hormones, mesenteric circulation, and intestinal metabolism. As systemic pressures fall, intestinal tissue viability is initially maintained through increased oxygen extraction. This mechanism fails when systemic pressures fall below 40 mm Hg, and anaerobic metabolism replaces aerobic metabolism.[2] This results in progressive bowel ischemia. The resultant intestinal injury depends on many variables, including the state of the systemic circulation, the degree of vascular compromise, the size and number of involved vessels, the vascular bed's response to decreased blood flow, the ability to develop collateral flow, the duration of intestinal ischemia, and the oxygen demands of the affected bowel.[3]

Bowel wall injury may occur during episodes of ischemia and reperfusion. Ischemia stimulates a systemic inflammatory response due to the release of platelet-activating factor, tumor necrosis factor, cytokines, and myocardial depressant factors from activated leukocytes, platelets, mast cells, and endothelial cells in the splanchnic circulation.[4,5] The reduction in blood flow, along with increased expression of adhesion molecules, leads to sequestration of endothelial cells, platelets, and leukocytes in the blood. This may further reduce tissue perfusion, exacerbate tissue acidosis, and potentially result in disseminated intravascular coagulation.[6] Hemoconcentration, increased blood viscosity, and mural and vascular permeability may also develop and contribute to further compromise of tissue perfusion.

Structural changes may be seen within the absorptive cells of the bowel wall within 5 minutes of arterial occlusion.[7-10] Ischemic change begins at the tips of the villi, where the epithelium detaches from the basement membrane and subepithelial blebs develop. The villi become denuded of epithelium within 30 to 60 minutes, and mucosal necrosis and ulceration ensue. The systemic inflammatory response incited by tissue ischemia results in increased capillary permeability followed by loss of capillary integrity. This results in submucosal edema and hemorrhage. The muscular layers of the bowel wall become progressively ischemic, and continued loss of vascular and epithelial integrity results in fluid and protein loss into the bowel lumen, interstitial space, and peritoneal cavity. Transmural infarction occurs within 12 to 24 hours, and may result in peritonitis and sepsis.

The reperfusion phase that follows an episode of intestinal ischemia may cause more tissue damage than the ischemic episode itself. Superoxide anions are formed during reperfusion and lead to the release of free oxygen radicals into the systemic circulation. These free radicals cause local and systemic tissue injury through lipid peroxidation of membranes and denaturation of intracellular macromolecules. This may cause multiorgan failure or cardiac arrest following correction of visceral ischemia.[11,12] As continued tissue ischemia occurs, however, the detrimental effects of the ischemic event outweigh those of tissue reperfusion. With the development of irreversible bowel infarction, outcome is no longer affected by the effects of tissue reperfusion.[13]

Classification of Mesenteric Vascular Disease

Bowel ischemia occurs when oxygen demands of bowel are not met and the bowel becomes hypoxic. Patients' clinical presentations and radiographic findings vary with the etiology and duration of the ischemic event. The onset of abdominal pain may be sudden when bowel ischemia is due to arterial embolism, or it may evolve over hours to days when caused by low flow states, arterial thrombosis, or vasculitis. The following classification of mesenteric vascular disease is useful for correlating the radiographic and clinical findings:

1. Acute intestinal ischemia
   a. Arterial
      —occlusive (thrombosis and embolism)
      —nonocclusive
   b. Venous (thrombosis)
2. Focal ischemia
3. Vasculitis
4. Radiation enteropathy
5. Chronic mesenteric ischemia

Acute Intestinal Ischemia

Classification

Acute intestinal ischemia is predominantly a disease of the elderly, and may result from either occlusive or nonocclusive vascular pathology. Arterial occlusion may be secondary to embolus, thrombus, trauma, compression, or infiltration, whereas mesenteric venous occlusion is usually the result of thrombosis.[14] Although atherosclerotic plaque is the most common cause of narrowing or occlusion of major visceral arteries, other conditions such as aortic dissection, surgical complications from aortic aneurysm repair, obstructing mural thrombus within an aortic aneurysm, and tumor invasion into the visceral vessels (eg, from pancreatic carcinoma) or mesentery (ie, carcinoid tumors) can cause bowel ischemia due to arterial occlusion.[15] Mechanical causes of obstruction include adhesions, strangulating hernias, volvulus, and external trauma. Nonocclusive ischemia is often the result of splanchnic vasoconstriction due to hypovolemic shock.

Despite continued improvements in radiologic diagnosis and surgical technique, the mortality from acute intestinal ischemia remains high, varying with the etiology and extent of bowel ischemia and infarction. Mortality rates are reported to be as high as 95% for patients with thrombotic arterial occlusion, 50% for patients with embolic arterial occlusion, 30% for patients with venous thrombotic occlusion, and 67% for patients with nonocclusive mesenteric ischemia.[16] Even in centers specializing in its diagnosis, reported mortality rates have exceeded 50%.[17-20]

Acute Arterial Thrombosis

Arterial thrombosis is the etiology of acute mesenteric ischemia in approximately 50% of cases. Thrombosis of the SMA usually occurs in elderly patients with atherosclerotic vascular disease, and the vascular thrombosis most commonly occurs within the proximal 2 cm of the artery, at the site of a preexistent ostial lesion. The resultant ischemia affects a larger potion of bowel than does arterial embolism, typically affecting loops from the duodenum to the transverse colon. The devastating effects of this proximal occlusion are reflected in the high mortality associated with this event.

Acute Arterial Embolism

Arterial emboli account for approximately one third of cases of acute mesenteric ischemia. They most commonly originate from the left atrium in patients with atrial fibrillation. Overall, approximately 5% of peripheral emboli lodge in the SMA. The majority (approximately 50%) of these lodge distal to the proximal jejunal and middle colic branches, 35% disintegrate and embolize into more distal branches, and approximately 15% lodge proximally at the ostium.[21] The proximal emboli may be difficult to distinguish radiologically from arterial thrombosis. Because the emboli often lodge within the mid or distal portion of the SMA, the resultant bowel ischemia may involve variable segments of the intestine, typically sparing the duodenum, proximal jejunum, and colon.

Mesenteric Venous Thrombosis

Mesenteric venous thrombosis is an increasingly recognized cause of acute mesenteric ischemia, responsible for up to 30% of cases in some series.[16] Mesenteric venous thrombosis is subdivided into primary, secondary, and idiopathic forms. The majority of cases (60%) are due to the secondary form in which vascular thrombosis results from a combination of hemoconcentration, low-flow states, and endothelial cell damage. Common causes include intra-abdominal sepsis, portal hypertension, inflammatory conditions (pancreatitis, gastroenteritis, inflammatory bowel disease, appendicitis, diverticulitis), abdominal trauma, and intra-abdominal malignancy. Primary thrombosis accounts for 30% of cases and is the result of a primary clotting disorder. Of patients in this category, 15% to 44% will have a history of prior thromboembolic events.[2] Idiopathic causes of mesenteric venous thrombosis represent the remaining 10% of cases. Refinements in diagnostic clotting studies have enabled many of the patients who would have been previously classified as having idiopathic mesenteric venous thrombosis to be more appropriately classified in the primary category.

Pathophysiologically, animal experiments have shown that mesenteric venous thrombosis results in venous dilatation and impaired egress of blood from the intestine.[22,23] Bowel wall congestion and cyanosis result, and intra-arterial pressure increases. As arterial flow decreases, arterial spasm and intestinal ischemia develop, leading to paralytic ileus, intramural hemorrhage, and mesenteric bleeding. Serosanguinous fluid escapes from the bowel wall and mesentery into the peritoneal cavity, and hypovolemia and hemoconcentration result. This process may lead to further arterial thrombosis and/or death due to cardiovascular collapse. As a rule, the amount of bowel and mesenteric hemorrhage is greater with mesenteric venous thrombosis than with arterial occlusions.

Nonocclusive Mesenteric Ischemia

Nonocclusive ischemia is thought to be responsible for approximately 10% to 20% of cases of acute mesenteric ischemia. It represents a low-flow state in which the vasculature is patent, but blood flow is inadequate to provide sufficient oxygenated blood to bowel. This may be due to a combination of low mesenteric flow and secondary reflex mesenteric arterial vasoconstriction. The arterial vasoconstriction may be the result of hypotension, medications (ie, digitalis, pressor agents, and ergots), or drugs (eg, amphetamines and cocaine).[24-30]

Clinical Presentation

Time is of the essence when diagnosing bowel ischemia because patient morbidity and mortality are directly related to the duration and extent of the ischemic event. The clinical diagnosis may be difficult to establish because ischemia can present with variable signs and symptoms. The most important factor in expediting diagnosis is to maintain a high clinical suspicion, as noninvasive laboratory tests lack high diagnostic sensitivity and specificity.

The classic clinical presentation consists of sudden, crampy, periumbilical abdominal pain, followed by diarrhea. Blood and/or mucus may be passed per rectum. The incidence of bloody diarrhea is greatest in patients with arterial embolism compared with arterial thrombosis. The onset of pain is usually sudden when ischemia results from embolic disease; however, it may be intermittent and slowly progressive in patients with thrombotic or nonocclusive disease. Early acute mesenteric ischemia characteristically presents with severe pain that is greatly out of proportion to the patient's physical findings. Pain may be absent in patients who are on steroids or in whom bowel infarction has occurred. Overall, it is estimated that abdominal pain may be absent in 15% to 25% of patients with bowel ischemia, especially those with nonocclusive disease.[2] As a rule, the more complete and abrupt the degree of vascular occlusion, the more likely symptoms of nausea, vomiting, and forceful bowel movements will be present.

Physical examination in patients with early bowel ischemia may reveal intermittent or hyperactive bowel sounds. There may be minimal or absent abdominal tenderness on palpation. In patients with arterial thrombosis, physical examination may reveal absent pulses and bruits. As bowel ischemia progresses, physical examination typically reveals increasing abdominal distention, paucity of bowel sounds, pain on palpation, and rebound tenderness. As bowel infarction develops, peritoneal signs and ascites may become apparent, and patients may develop fever, leukocytosis, and metabolic acidosis. Elevated levels of inorganic phosphate correlate well with the extent of bowel ischemia and, when found in association with leukocytosis and metabolic acidosis, suggest development of intestinal infarction.[31] Although disseminated intravascular coagulation and/or the presence of elevated levels of serum phosphate, lactate, creatinine kinase, lactate dehydrogenase, alkaline phosphatase, diamine oxidase, porcine ileal peptide, and peritoneal fluid amylase are all clues to the diagnosis of acute mesenteric ischemia, they are neither sensitive enough nor specific enough to be reliable indicators.[32,33]

Radiologic Appearances

Plain films. Plain film examination is often normal or nonspecific in patients with mesenteric ischemia. In fact, in a study of 23 patients with proven mesenteric infarction, a mere 30% had plain film findings suggestive of the diagnosis.[34] The plain film findings that are most specific for acute mesenteric ischemia include pneumatosis intestinalis and portal venous gas. Unfortunately, these are present in only a minority of cases and are not specific for the diagnosis. Pneumatosis results when bowel mucosa sloughs and luminal air dissects into the bowel wall. It may be seen in association with a variety of other disorders including steroid use, collagen vascular disease, peptic ulcer disease, and chronic obstructive pulmonary disease. The benign form of pneumatosis is usually cystic or "bubbly" in appearance, whereas the form associated with ischemia and infarction is typically linear or curvilinear in shape. Portal venous air is an ominous finding that is due to ischemic bowel in approximately 75% of cases. It results from gas dissecting from the bowel into the mesenteric and portal venous systems. The portal venous gas lodges peripherally in the liver, and often assumes a finely branching configuration. Left lateral decubitus positioning often facilitates detection of portal venous gas on plain film examination. Besides mesenteric ischemia, portal venous gas may also be seen in association with infection and inflammation (eg, diverticulitis, pancreatitis, inflammatory bowel disease, cholecystitis, pseudomembranous colitis, perforated ulcer disease), gastric emphysema, corrosive ingestion, and multiple types of iatrogenic intervention (ie, air intravasation during barium enema examination, percutaneous abscess drainage, umbilical artery or mesenteric vein catheterization, hepatic artery embolization).[35]

Acute mesenteric ischemia may result in a variety of less specific bowel gas patterns. The earliest physiologic response of bowel to ischemia is muscularis propria spasm. Plain film examination will often be normal within the first several hours of the onset of ischemia. The spasms may persist and cause rapid bowel peristalsis with expulsion of gas and diarrhea. Plain film studies during this period may reveal a gasless abdomen due to the intestine being entirely fluid filled. Continued ischemia eventually leads to loss of normal contractile function of bowel, and cessation of intestinal spasm. Several patterns of dilated, gas-filled bowel loops may result when images are obtained at this time. An ileus pattern may be seen, in which small bowel loops and a portion of the right colon (typically to the level of the hepatic flexure) are distended with gas. A "splenic flexure cut-off" sign may be seen in which small and large bowel loops are dilated and gas-filled to the level of the splenic flexure, and resume a normal caliber distally. A small bowel pseudo-obstruction pattern may also be seen, and is the result of an inability of the proximally functioning small bowel to propel its contents and gas through the ischemic, atonic segment.

During the time when the bowel wall loses its contractile function, mucosal ischemia and necrosis cause increased capillary permeability. This results in submucosal edema and hemorrhage, leading to bowel wall thickening and pinkyprints that may be seen on plain film examination. Rigid, formless bowel loops in fixed position are further plain film findings suggestive of this pathologic process. Pneumoperitoneum may accompany bowel perforation. Plain film findings and correlative computer tomography (CT) and barium examinations are further illustrated in Chapter 5 (section on mesenteric vascular disease).

Barium examination. The administration of oral contrast material may interfere with conventional angiography and CT angiography. Therefore, if there is strong clinical suspicion of acute mesenteric ischemia, barium studies should be deferred, and angiography or cross-sectional imaging with CT or magnetic resonance imaging (MRI) should be ordered. When performed in unsuspected cases, in subacute presentations, or in cases with an atypical clinical presentation, barium examination may demonstrate the bowel dilatation, contour abnormalities, and bowel wall thickening described above. The mucosal folds typically thicken, straighten, and compress the spaces between them, producing a "stack of coins" or "picket fence" appearance. Changes are most pronounced at the mesenteric border where distention of the submucosa may cause adjacent folds to fuse and produce larger or smaller rounded indentations (thumbprints or pinkyprints) [Fig. 20-1(a–f)]. Because it typically results in greater amounts of intramural hemorrhage, mesenteric venous thrombosis generally causes more pronounced mucosal fold thickening than does is-

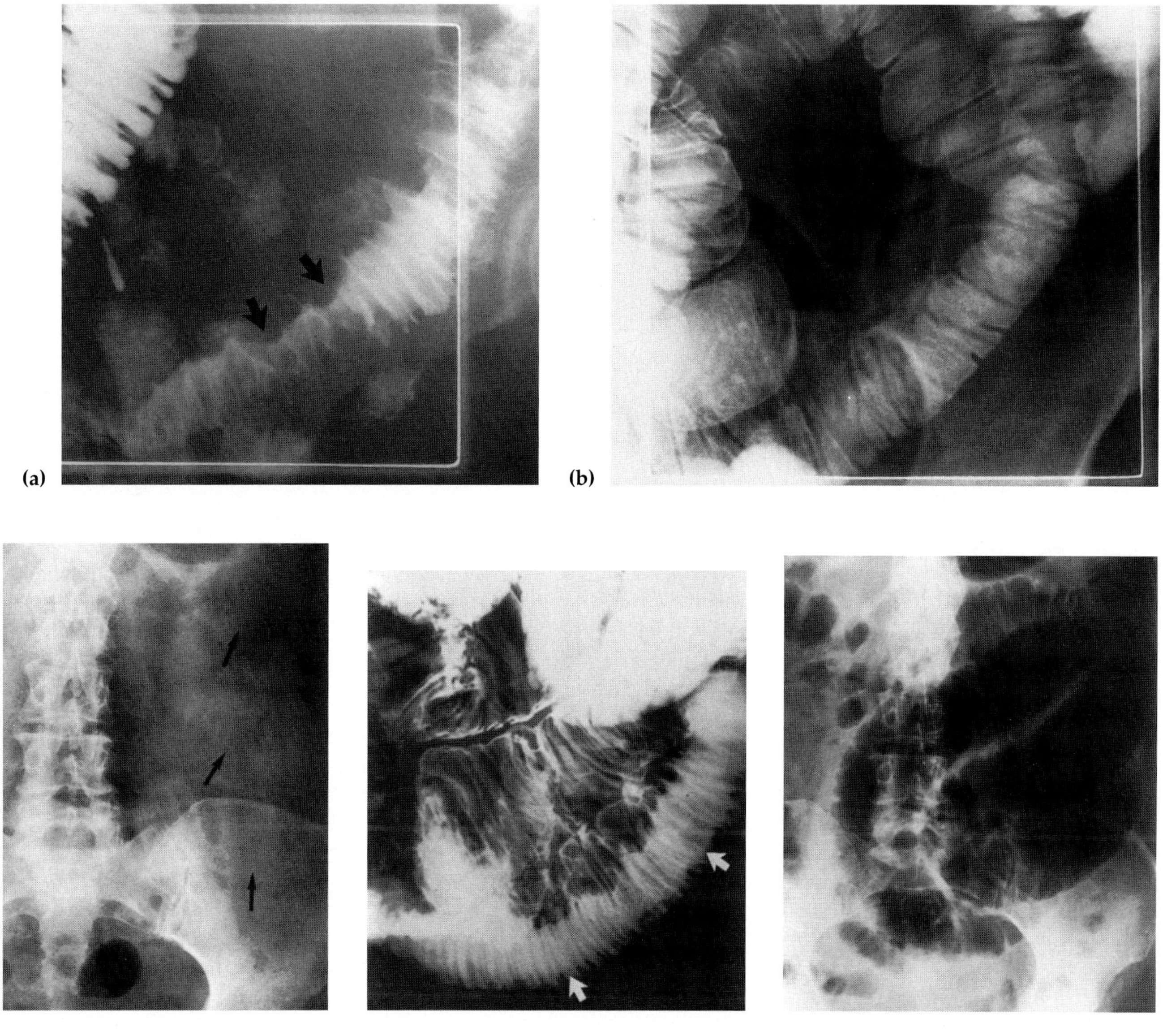

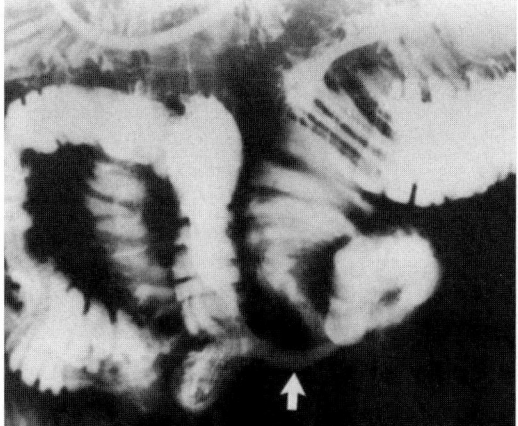

Fig. 20-1. Two patients with subacute mesenteric ischemia. Barium studies demonstrate not only characteristic initial patterns but also the important feature of changed appearances over time-normalization or deterioration.

(a) A 56-year-old male diabetic complained of severe abdominal pain. Enteroclysis demonstrated an ischemic segment of distal jejunum with thickened straight folds and thumbprints (arrows) along part of the mesenteric border. (b) Repeat enteroclysis 2 weeks later shows return to normality. (c) A 59-year-old hypertensive female patient complained of severe pain in the abdomen. A plain film indicated left-sided straight, thickened folds (arrows) in dilated bowel. Ischemia seemed the likely diagnosis, its cause unexplained. (d) Subsequent enteroclysis shows dilatation of proximal jejunum. A long segment of barely peristaltic distal jejunum with straight, thickened folds (arrows) indicates widening of the submucosa. (e) Two months later increasing pain with abdominal distention. A supine film of the abdomen demonstrated a dilated jejunum with pronounced distal caliber reduction. (f) Enteroclysis followed immediately and revealed an about 10-cm-long postischemic annular stricture (arrow) as cause of the partial obstruction.

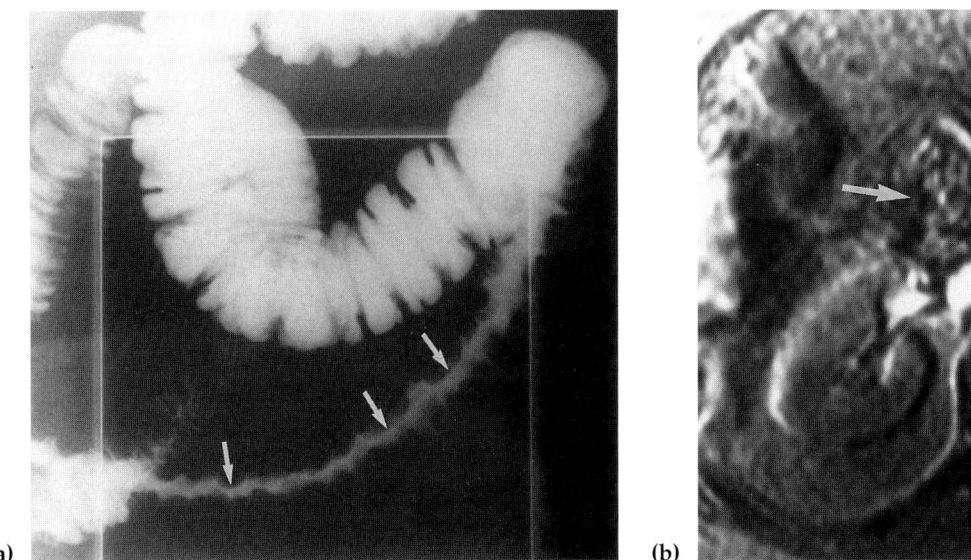

Fig. 20-2. Mesenteric vein thrombosis in a young patient with a hypercoagulability state.
(a) Enteroclysis here demonstrates the most severely altered bowel segment. Accumulations in the submucosa of fluid and blood have caused compression of the lumen with indications of a pinkyprint pattern along the mesenteric border (arrows). (b) MRI indicates (arrow) absence of signal in the thrombosed portal vein, probably of longer duration, with likely more recent extension into the superior mesenteric vein.

chemia due to arterial thrombosis or embolism (Fig. 20-2). Bowel loop separation from mesenteric thickening is also commonly seen. As a rule, mucosal abnormalities are shown to better advantage on barium examinations than on plain film studies. Bowel transit time is typically prolonged because of the atony and compromised contractile ability caused by the ischemia. Bowel strictures, ulcerations, intramural fistulae, and pseudodiverticulae may develop following infarction, and are well demonstrated by barium examination. Bowel viability and depth of bowel wall necrosis correlate poorly with findings on barium examination.[36] In general, spasm and mild fold thickening are good prognostic signs, whereas marked dilatation and stasis with pneumatosis are indicators of strangulation.

When ischemia is reversible, bowel wall recovery usually occurs within 2 to 4 weeks. Barium examinations are useful for monitoring interval disease pro-

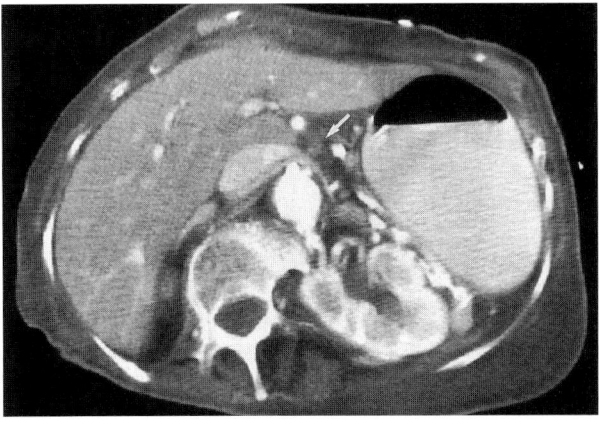
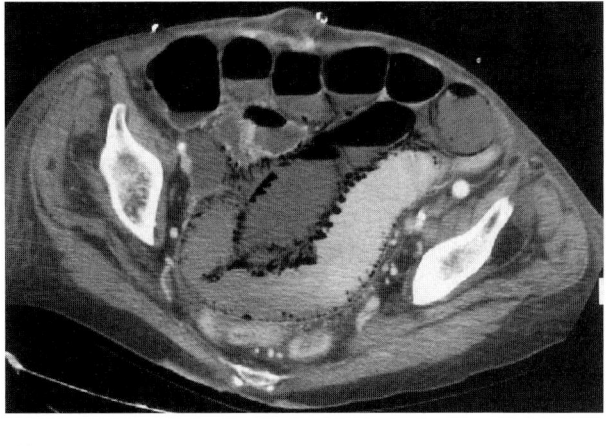

Fig. 20-3. CT in an elderly woman with small bowel ischemia secondary to superior mesenteric artery (SMA) thrombosis.
(a) Contrast-enhanced CT shows occlusion of the SMA (arrow). Note extensive atherosclerotic changes in abdominal aorta and splenic artery. (b) CT scan at level of pelvic inlet demonstrates diffusely dilated small bowel loops with evidence of extensive pneumatosis intestinalis, a likely indication, in this clinical setting, for ischemic change.

gression and improvement. In fact, changes in the intensity of intestinal involvement help to confirm that barium changes are due to ischemia. Ischemic fibrosis may demonstrate unilateral flattening and rigidity of the bowel wall, with plication of the opposing border.[37] Much more typical are annular ischemic strictures with smooth borders and with lumen widening proximally and distally (see Fig. 20-1).

CT and MRI. In contrast to plain film and barium studies, CT and MRI are frequently capable of making a specific diagnosis of acute mesenteric ischemia resulting from primary occlusion or neoplastic infiltration of the mesenteric vasculature by directly demonstrating the occluded mesenteric vessel(s) [Fig. 20-3(a)]. In addition to defining the location and extent of bowel involvement, these modalities can demonstrate the intramural and extraluminal complications of ischemia and infarction such as pneumatosis, pneumoperitoneum, bowel wall and fold thickening, fistulae, mural and mesenteric hemorrhage, ascites, and abscesses [Fig. 20-3(b)].[34,38–47] CT examinations are, in fact, more sensitive than plain film studies for detecting small amounts of pneumoperitoneum and pneumatosis.[34,48–51] The ability to obtain multiplanar reformatted images also aids radiologic diagnosis by allowing better visualization of vessels that, because of their orientation, may not be optimally seen on axial scan planes.

Intraluminal clot appears as a low attenuation central filling defect within a vessel on contrast-enhanced CT (Fig. 20-4). In cases of superior mesenteric venous thrombosis, the vein wall surrounding the clot may

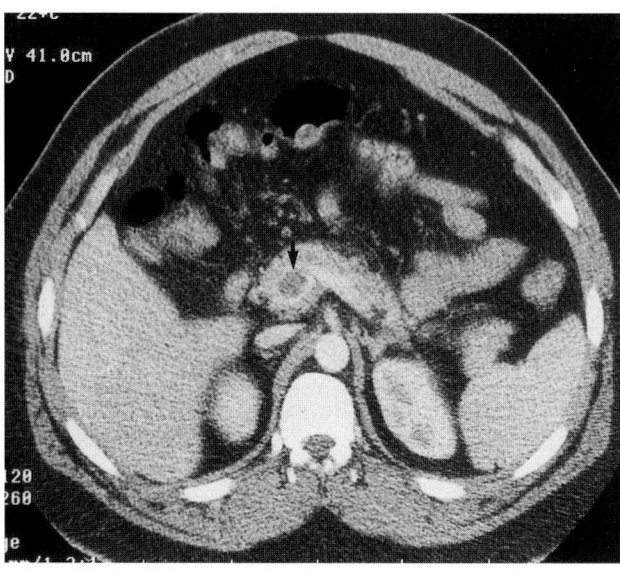

Fig. 20-4. Contrast-enhanced CT demonstration of superior mesenteric vein thrombosis (arrow), presenting as low attenuation compared with that of aorta or inferior vena cava.

demonstrate increased attenuation. This does not represent contrast material flowing around the thrombus, but instead represents enhancement of the arterially supplied vasa vasorum within the vessel wall (Fig. 20-5).[52] On unenhanced CT, occluding emboli and intramural hemorrhage may be hyperattenuating (Fig. 20-6).[53] Additional CT findings of mesenteric ischemia

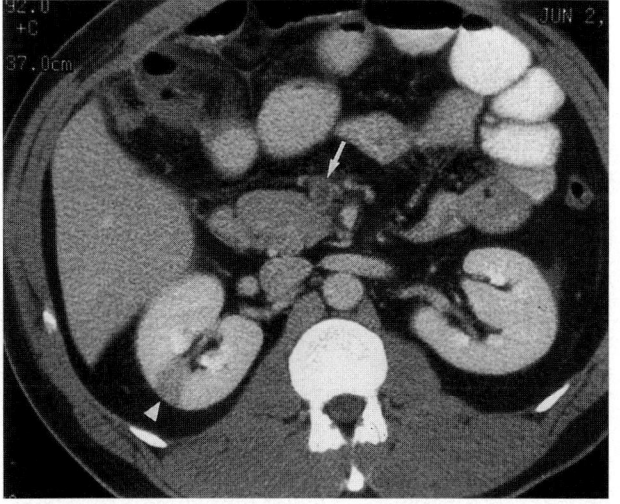

(a)

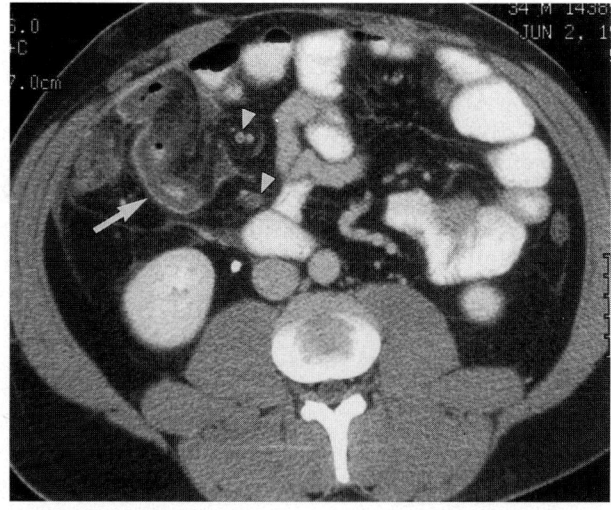

(b)

Fig. 20-5. Superior mesenteric vein (SMV) thrombosis with secondary small bowel ischemia.
(a) Contrast-enhanced CT shows a low-attenuation central filling defect within the SMV representing thrombus (arrow). The high attenuation of the surrounding vessel wall represents enhancement of the vasa vasorum. A small infarct within the interpolar region of the right kidney is identified as a low-attenuation, wedge-shaped cortical defect (arrowhead). (b) Caudal CT image demonstrates thrombus within small branch vessels of the SMV (arrowheads). Associated small bowel ischemia appears as mural thickening with a double-halo enhancement pattern (arrow).

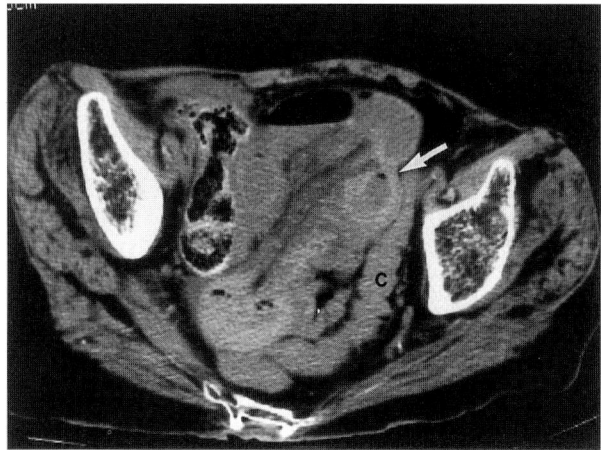

Fig. 20-6. Intramural hemorrhage in an elderly patient with vascular insufficiency.
The unenhanced CT demonstrates thickening and hyperattenuation of the intestinal wall caused by intramural hemorrhage (arrow). Note the higher attenuation of the small bowel wall compared to that of the colon (c).

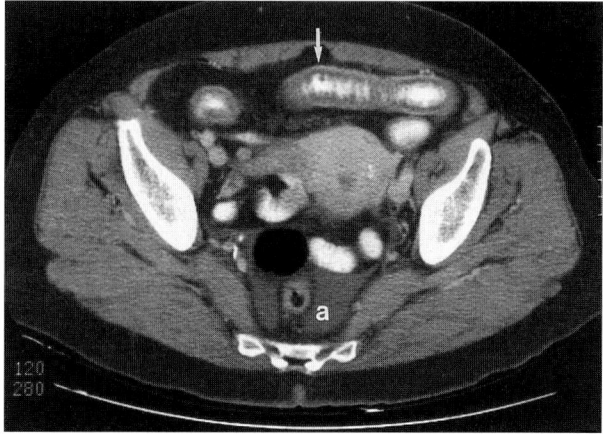

Fig. 20-7. Small bowel ischemia resulting in mural thickening and double-halo sign on contrast-enhanced CT.
This abnormal enhancement pattern consists of two concentric low- and high-attenuation rings due to submucosal edema and adjacent serosal hyperemia (arrow). Ascites is present within the pelvis (a), and a calcified fibroid is incidentally noted within the uterus.

include bowel dilatation, segmental mural thickening, and fold thickening. Ascites and abnormal bowel wall enhancement may also be evident. The abnormal bowel wall enhancement is due to hyperemia and edema, and appears as alternating rings of high and low density (the "target" or "double halo" sign) (Figs. 20-7, 20-8). The aforementioned CT signs are commonly seen in mesenteric ischemia, but are not specific for the diagnosis. Pneumatosis, pneumoperitoneum, and mesenteric and portal venous gas may also be demonstrated on CT examination and are more specific, but not absolutely diagnostic, for ischemia (Figs. 20-9, 20-10).

A retrospective study of 39 patients with surgically proven acute mesenteric ischemia revealed CT sensitivity, specificity, and accuracy values of 64%, 92%, and 75%, respectively.[38] Although this study found that arterial or venous thrombosis, intramural gas, portal venous gas, focal lack of bowel wall enhancement, and hepatic and splenic infarcts each demonstrated specificities of greater than 95% for diagnosing acute mesenteric ischemia (in the proper clinical setting), the sensitivities of each of these signs was determined to be less than 30%. Following administration of intravenous contrast material, approximately one third of the patients in the study demonstrated evidence of arterial or venous occlusion, a fact that underscores the benefits of performing contrast-enhanced CT examinations. Overall, it is estimated that only 26% to 39% of CT examinations will be diagnostic for acute mesenteric ischemia.[34,44] CT appearances in small bowel strangulation and gangrene are further described in Chapter 21.

Advances in radiologic technology have contributed to making cross-sectional imaging techniques increasingly sensitive in diagnosing acute mesenteric ischemia. The introduction of helical CT has made

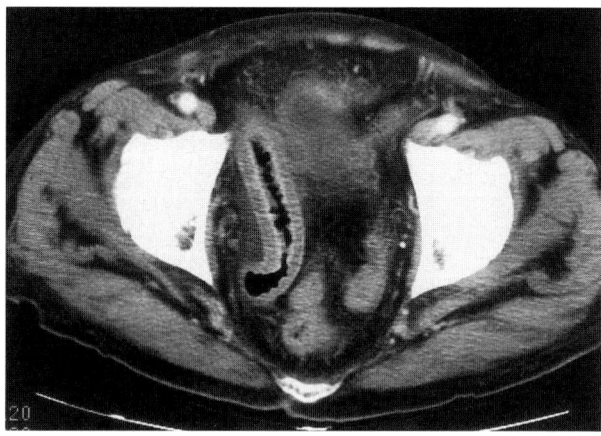

Fig. 20-8. Small bowel ischemia secondary to SMA thrombosis presenting as mural thickening with a target sign pattern.
Three concentric, alternating rings of high, low, and high attenuation are exhibited in the target pattern of bowel enhancement. This abnormal enhancement pattern is caused by hyperemia of the mucosa and serosa with interposed submucosal edema and inflammation.

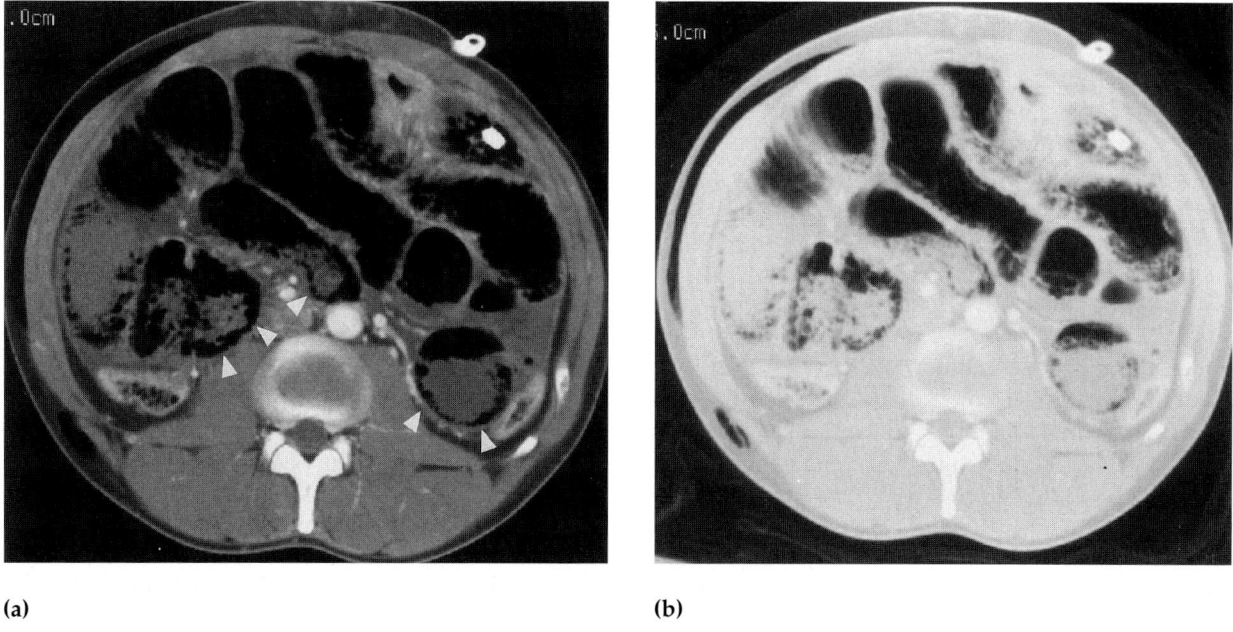

Fig. 20-9. Small bowel pneumatosis secondary to ischemia.
(a) Contrast-enhanced CT demonstrates extensive small bowel pneumatosis with numerous small gas bubbles aligned within the wall of the dilated intestine (arrowheads). Subcutaneous emphysema is noted within the anterior and posterior aspects of the right abdominal wall. (b) When viewed at wider window and level settings, the intramural gas is much more conspicuous, facilitating its differentiation from intraluminal gas. The subcutaneous gas is also easier to identify in the right abdominal wall.

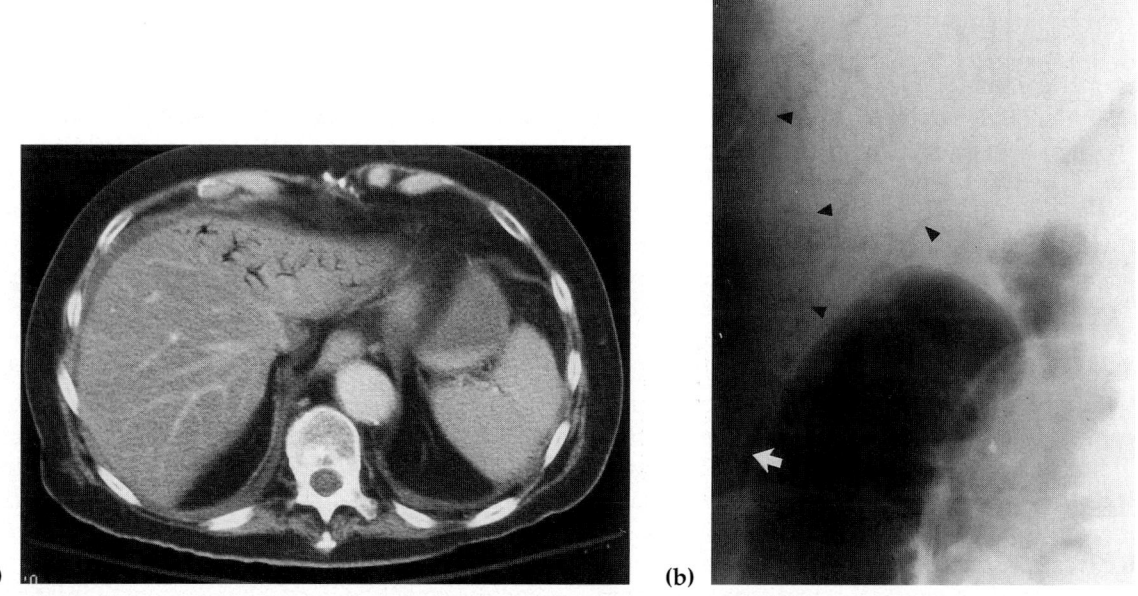

Fig. 20-10. Portal venous gas secondary to bowel infarction.
(a) Note gas within the peripherally located intrahepatic portal venous radicles. The gas is seen as branching tubular lucencies and assumes a "gull-wing" appearance. This may be differentiated from pneumobilia, which is typically centrally located anterior to the portal veins. Perihepatic ascites and small bilateral pleural effusions are also present. (b) In another patient with intestinal gangrene the plain film of the abdomen demonstrates gas in intrahepatic venous radicles (arrowheads). Linear gas collection in wall of dilated bowel (arrow).

possible a rapid acquisition of volumetric data sets during a single breathhold. High-resolution CT images of the mesenteric vessels can now be acquired at levels of peak vascular enhancement, permitting generation of three-dimensional CT angiography data sets. CT angiogram studies corrlelate well with findings on conventional angiography, and have increased helical CT's sensitivity for detecting vascular pathology compared with conventional CT.[54,55]

MR examination is also sensitive in detecting occlusive vascular disease because of its ability to demonstrate and differentiate flowing blood and intravascular thrombus from surrounding soft-tissue structures.[56] Acute thrombus may be hyperintense on both T1- and T2-weighted imaging sequences, whereas older thrombi may be iso- or hypointense on T1-weighted images and hyperintense on T2-weighted images. MRI may also be useful for quantifying mesenteric blood flow.[57] In the past, MRI was inferior to CT examination because of problems related to peristaltic motion. Recent advances in rapid aquisition techniques have reduced problems of bowel motion that previously degraded MR imaging of the mesentery and intestine. Similar to CT, MRI can demonstrate mural thickening, intramural hemorrhage, bowel dilatation, strictures, obstruction, ascites, pneumoperitoneum, and pneumatosis. MRI has the added advantages of acquiring direct multiplanar images and not requiring ionizing radiation. It is limited in detecting small intravascular calcifications. In an experiment in which bowel ischemia was induced in rabbits, MRI findings occurring 45 to 60 minutes after ligation of the mesenteric vasculature included bowel wall thickening, isointense or slightly increased mural signal intensity on T1-weighted images, and hyperintense appearance of the bowel wall on T2-weighted sequences.[47] The MRI findings of mesenteric ischemia are further discussed in Chapter 10.

Angiography. Angiography remains the gold standard for radiologic diagnosis of mesenteric ischemia, and has the added benefit of allowing therapeutic intervention when indicated. Angiography is useful for diagnosing and differentiating occlusive from nonocclusive mesenteric vascular disease, and for assessing patency and perfusion of vessels distal to the site of occlusion. The typical angiographic finding in acute arterial embolism is demonstration of blood clot 3 to 8 cm distal to the origin of the SMA, with patent proximal branch vessels. Conversely, acute arterial thrombosis classically appears as a tapering occlusion located 1 to 3 cm from the origin of the SMA with obstruction of more distal arterial branches.[58] Frequently, collateral filling of the distal SMA via collateral circulation can be demonstrated. The angiographic findings of mesenteric venous thrombosis include a partially or completely occluding thrombus in the superior mesenteric vein (SMV), failure to visualize the SMV or portal vein, absent or diminished filling of mesenteric veins, arterial spasm, failure of arterial arcades to empty, reflux of contrast into the aorta, prolonged blushing involving the affected segment, and presence of collateral flow.[59–61] Nonocclusive mesenteric ischemia is diagnosed when there is angiographic evidence of mesenteric vasoconstriction in a patient who is not in shock or receiving vasopressors, and who has appropriate clinical symptoms. The diagnostic angiographic criteria for nonocclusive mesenteric ischemia include arterial narrowing at the origins of multiple branches of the SMA, irregularity of intestinal branches, arterial spasm in vascular arcades, and impaired filling of intramural vessels.[62,63] A possible radiologic intervention in subacute mesenteric ischemia may be the infusion of urokinase into the SMA,[64] following angiographic assessment. (Further discussion can be found in Chapter 12.)

Sonography. The sonographic evaluation of acute mesenteric ischemia is often difficult. Limiting technical factors include suboptimal vascular visualization due to overlying bowel gas, patient obesity, inadequate depth resolution, and complex and/or postoperative anatomy. Additionally, sonography is very dependent on the skills of the personnel who perform and interpret the examination. Although Doppler sonography has proven useful for evaluating patency of mesenteric vasculature and for determining intravascular flow volumes, it generally plays a limited role in the diagnosis of acute mesenteric ischemia. Its advantages are that it is noninvasive, does not require ionizing radiation, and can be performed portably.

Thrombosed vessels typically appear dilated with sonography. Intraluminal clot, when identified, usually appears echogenic, although its sonographic appearance may range from anechoic to hyperechoic depending on its age. Abnormally reduced or absent intraluminal flow can be detected on both color flow and duplex Doppler examinations. Sonography can detect gas in the walls of bowel segments (Fig. 20-11); also diagnosed is mesenteric or portal venous gas by demonstrating high-amplitude intravenous echoes that move in the direction of blood flow. Intraoperative Doppler sonography has been used, with varying success, to help determine the extent of infarcted, nonviable bowel prior to surgical resection.[65] It remains to be seen whether power Doppler will be more sensitive than color Doppler for determination of bowel ischemia and infarction. (For further information see Chapter 8.)

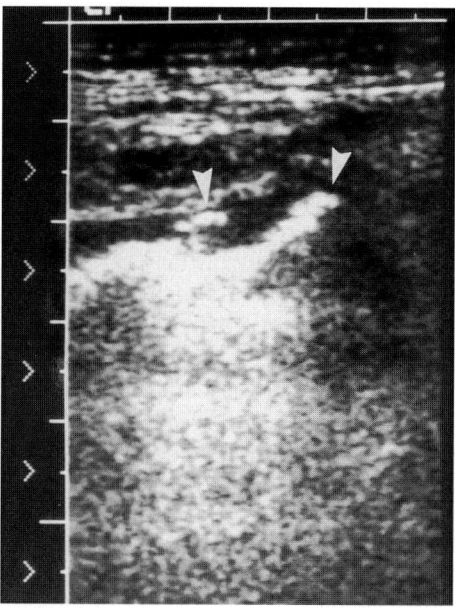

Fig. 20-11. Sonographic demonstration of pneumatosis intestinalis.
In a patient with SMA thrombosis ultrasound demonstrates a fluid-distended bowel wall with numerous intensely hyperechoic dots (arrowheads) fixed in the posterior bowel wall. (Courtesy of Michel Rioux, MD, Québec.)

Treatment

Supportive therapy should be administered to patients with bowel ischemia and infarction. These supportive measures include initiation of nasogastric suction, fluid and electrolyte replacement, and, when warranted, administration of pressor agents and antibiotics. Additional interventional and surgical therapy varies with the etiology of the ischemic event and the clinical status of the patient.

Selective infusion of thrombolytic agents such as streptokinase, urokinase, and recombinant tissue plasminogen activator may obviate the need for surgical intervention in many cases of acute arterial thrombosis, but is contraindicated when bowel infarction is suspected.[2] Definitive treatment of arterial thrombosis typically necessitates arterial revascularization and resection of infarcted bowel. Acute arterial embolism requires laparotomy with embolectomy. Although intravascular infusion of thrombolytic agents and vasodilators has been reported to improve survival rates in patients with arterial embolism, they are considered to be adjuvant forms of therapy and should not replace surgical intervention.[66]

Nonocclusive mesenteric ischemia is usually initially treated by intra-arterial administration of vasodilators through an indwelling catheter. Typically, papaverine is the agent of choice, although tolazoline may also be used. Patients who are refractory to this therapy may require surgical revascularization. Mesenteric venous thrombosis is generally treated by immediate initialization anticoagulant therapy. When necessary, thrombectomy with resection of infarcted segments of bowel can be performed.

Focal Ischemia

Acute focal ischemia occurs when an ischemic insult is limited to a short segment of small intestine. The most common etiologies include strangulating bowel obstruction from an adhesion or volvulus, vasculitis, trauma, distal arterial emboli, or radiation enteritis. Typically, collateral circulation to the intestine prevents ischemia from progressing to transmural infarction. Because of the limited amount of bowel involvement, patients tend to present with fewer symptoms, and their prognosis is much better.

On radiographic studies, focal ischemia may result in a short segment of abnormally thickened bowel. Although in many patients, there is healing without residual evidence of disease, localized ulcers or short, smoothly tapered strictures may develop.[67]

Vasculitis

Mesenteric vasculitis is an uncommon cause of bowel ischemia, accounting for approximately 2% of cases.[68] Vasculitis is defined as inflammatory cell infiltration, at times causing necrosis of blood vessels. A variety of systemic conditions may be associated with the development of this entity. These may all result in inflammatory occlusion of large, medium-size, or small arteries (including the vasa recta and the intramural vessels) that supply blood flow to the intestine. Although their radiographic appearances may be indistinguishable from other causes of acute and focal mesenteric ischemia, the accompanying systemic disease manifestations and laboratory abnormalities, as well as the size and distribution of affected vessels, are important clues to the proper diagnosis (Fig. 20-12).

Polyarteritis Nodosa

Polyarteritis nodosa causes a necrotizing vasculitis affecting medium-sized to smaller arteries in approximately 50% of patients.[69] Angiographically, small aneurysms on branch vessels of the SMA are characteristic of this disease. The extent of bowel involve-

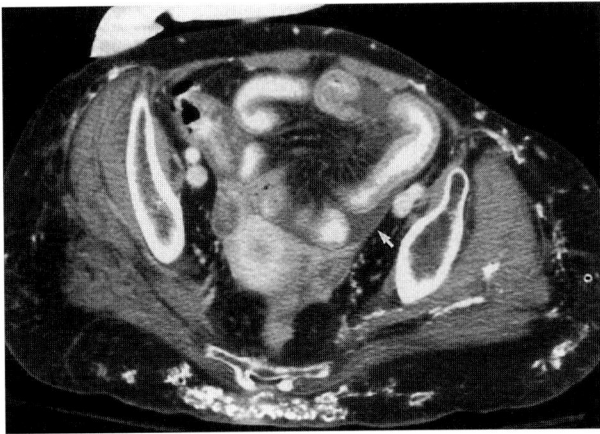

Fig. 20-12. Small bowel ischemia secondary to dermatomyositis vasculitis.
This contrast-enhanced pelvic CT scan reveals a double-halo enhancement pattern due to ischemic change involving thickened distal small bowel loops. A small amount of ascites is also evident (arrow). Note the extensive subcutaneous and intermuscular calcification characteristic of this entity.

ment is variable, but commonly results in segmentally ischemic segments demonstrating penetrating mucosal ulcers and localized hemorrhagic infarcts.[70] Although massive bowel infarction may occur, it is extremely rare. Hypertension, renal involvement, and liver involvement are commonly associated with this entity, and there is evidence of hepatitis B viral infection in approximately 50% of cases.[71]

Rheumatoid Vasculitis

Rheumatoid vasculitis is associated with high titers of rheumatoid factor, and joint involvement and rheumatoid nodules are frequent components of the disease. When it causes vasculitis, rheumatoid arthritis typically affects medium-sized vessels, and results in a form of polyarteritis nodosa. Fibrinoid necrosis affecting the walls of small arteries may cause small arterial thrombosis and segmental infarction. Intestinal strictures may result, but are uncommon.[72]

Systemic Lupus Erythematosus

Lupus erythematosus causes an associated small vessel vasculitis [Fig. 20-13(a–e)] in approximately 10% to 60% of cases.[73,74] Because of its small vessel involvement, massive bowel infarction is rare, although segmental bowel necrosis and perforation may occur. In addition to arterial involvement, this autoimmune disorder may cause a venulitis affecting the submucosa and muscularis.[75]

Henoch-Schönlein Purpura

Henoch-Schönlein purpura, also known as anaphylactoid purpura, causes a postcapillary venulitis affecting the gastrointestinal tract in approximately 50% of patients. Immunoglobulin A is deposited in vessel walls, and can be demonstrated using direct immunofluorescence.[76] The classic clinical triad includes palpable purpura, arthritis, and abdominal pain. Gastrointestinal bleeding, mucosal or submucosal hemorrhage, and segmental ulcers and erosions are common manifestations of the disease. Bowel perforation, massive infarction, and intussusception are rarely reported complications.[77] Typically, the disease is self-limiting and bowel lesions heal without sequelae.

Behçet's Syndrome

Behçet's syndrome is a multisystem disease that commonly affects males 11 to 30 years of age. Although orogenital involvement is a characteristic feature, the skin, joints, central nervous system, and intestinal tract are also affected. The vasculitis associated with this entity preferentially affects the small vessels, and causes gastrointestinal tract involvement in approximately 10% to 15% of cases.[78] Although the ileocecal area is most commonly involved, the esophagus and remainder of the small and large bowel can also be affected. Focal shallow or deep bowel ulcerations are common, and have a propensity to perforate because of associated focal necrosis of the muscularis. Although intervening segments of bowel may be normal in appearance, similar to Crohn's disease, bowel strictures and fistulae are rarely associated with Behçet's syndrome.

Churg-Strauss Syndrome

Churg-Strauss syndrome, also known as allergic granulomatosis angiitis, typically involves large vessels and is characterized by presence of asthma, hypereosinophilia, necrotizing vasculitis, and extravascular granulomas.[79] The gastrointestinal tract is the third most common site of organ involvement in this syndrome, following lung and skin. Gastrointestinal manifestations include small bowel necrosis, multiple colonic ulcers, and ulcerative colitis.[80,81] Although associated bowel perforations (most commonly affecting the small bowel) are commonly reported in the Japanese literature, they are rarely reported in other countries.[81]

Radiation Enteropathy

Radiation enteritis, a complication of radiation therapy, causes an endarteritis obliterans that leads to intestinal ischemia. Overall, the small bowel is the most

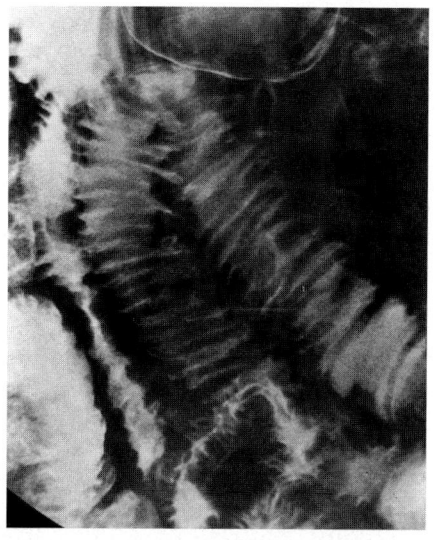
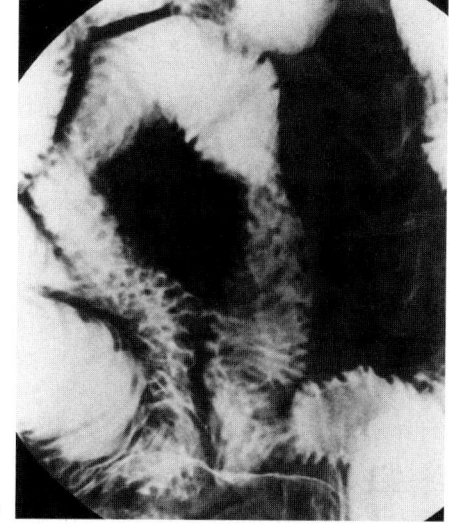
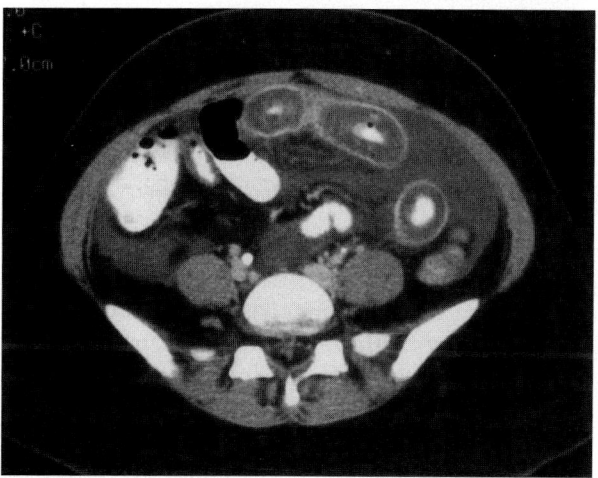

Fig. 20-13. Small bowel ischemia due to systemic lupus erythematosus.
(a) Barium follow-through demonstrates a "stack of coins" pattern typical for segmental ischemia but that could also be seen in Crohn's disease or lymphoma. The diagnosis of ischemia would be confirmed if a follow-up study shows deterioration or, more often, a return to a normal appearance. (b) Repeat examination 12 days later demonstrates a normal jejunum. (c) In another patient, a young female with segmental intestinal ischemia due to lupus vasculitis, CT shows abnormal mural thickening with a double-halo enhancement. Ascites is present.

radiosensitive abdominal organ. Because it is relatively fixed in position, the terminal ileum is particularly susceptible to radiation injury. Although patients may develop radiation enteritis with administered total radiation doses of less than 4000 rads, the incidence of serious intestinal injury significantly rises when the total dosage exceeds 5000 rads. The radiation dose at which 1% to 5% of patients are expected to manifest chronic small bowel damage within 5 years of radiation therapy (the minimal tolerance dosage TD5/5), is approximately 4500 rads, whereas the maximum tolerance radiation dose (the dose at which 25% to 50% of patients will develop damage within 5 years) is estimated to be 6500 rads.[82] These radiation doses are similar to those required for treatment of malignant tumors, clarifying the reason why intestinal injury may occur following radiation therapy.

It is estimated that approximately 2.5% to 25% of patients will develop late complications of radiation enteritis.[83] Several factors are influential in determining whether the persistent complications of radiation injury will occur. These include the radiation dose rate and fractionation schedule, the amount and site of intestinal irradiation, and the presence or absence of predisposing anatomic factors such as intestinal adhesions (due to prior inflammation or surgery) that limit bowel mobility. Chemotherapy and various systemic diseases, including hypertension, vascular disease, and diabetes mellitus, also predispose individuals to a higher incidence of radiation enteritis.[83]

Cellular Radiation Response

Radiation may result in immediate cell death or loss of cellular ability to divide and reproduce. In surviving cells, radiation may cause abnormalities in the genetic program or cellular function. These effects are greatest within the cellular DNA located in the nucleus.

It is well documented that cellular survival is a function of both total radiation dose delivered and rate of dose delivery. Rapid delivery of a radiation dose is more harmful than either slower delivery over a longer time interval or fractionated delivery of separate smaller doses. At low radiation doses, the initial portion of the cell survival curve is nonlinear, demonstrating a threshold region. However, as radiation dosage increases, cellular survival decreases exponentially.[84,85]

The stage of the cell cycle during which radiation exposure occurs and the amount of tissue oxygenation present also directly influence cell survival rates. Cells are most sensitive to injury during mitosis, with resistance peaking in the late S phase.[84–86] Well-oxygenated tissue is more sensitive to harmful effects of radiation than hypoxic tissue. This may be due to free radical production that is potentiated by molecular oxygen during periods of radiation exposure.[84,85]

Pathophysiology

Radiation exposure causes acute, subacute, and chronic changes within the intestine. Acute changes occur during and immediately following radiation exposure, and result in suppression of cellular proliferation and maturation that preferentially affects the crypt stem cells.[83] This may lead to villous shortening and decreased mucosal thickness. Mucosal edema, hyperemia, and inflammatory cell infiltration occur. Crypt abscesses may form, and diffuse or localized mucosal ulceration may also develop due to inadequate epithelial regeneration. Dose fractionation, by allowing a rest period between radiation doses, permits greater epithelial regeneration, thereby reducing these complications.

The subacute phase occurs 2 to 12 months after radiation, and results from obliterative changes within submucosal arterioles that lead to progressive intestinal ischemia. During this phase, the endothelial cells within the submucosal arterioles swell, detach from their basement membranes, and degenerate.[87,88] Fibrin plugs form within the arteriole lumen and lead to vascular thrombosis. The subsequent progressive ischemic change may cause mucosal ischemia, ulceration, necrosis, and bacterial invasion. Submucosal edema and fibrosis result, and focal dilatation of the venous and lymphatic system may develop.

The late phase of radiation damage usually occurs 6 months to 25 years after receiving a total radiation dose exceeding 5000 rads. Whereas damage to the mucosa and submucosa occur early in the course of radiation enteritis, serosal damage occurs in later stages. Fistulae, abscesses, and strictures may develop during this time, and small bowel obstruction may result. Malnutrition may occur due to impaired intestinal absorption of proteins, fats, and carbohydrates. Ileal involvement may result in disturbed bile salt and carbohydrate reabsorption, thereby leading to production of watery diarrhea.

Radiologic Appearances

The radiologic changes of radiation enteritis are nonspecific in appearance, and are usually indistinguishable from other causes of acute intestinal ischemia. Therefore, knowledge of the appropriate clinical history of radiation exposure is crucial for proper diagnosis.

In a very early, acute but short-lived reaction to radiation, CT has shown diffuse bowel edema that had disappeared when enteroclysis was done few days later (Fig. 20-14). In a more usual early, acute phase of radiation enteritis, plain film examination may demonstrate an ileus pattern, whereas barium studies will frequently show dilated, hypotonic loops, local intestinal hypermotility due to anoxia, and/or mucosal edema. During the subacute phase of radiation enteritis, edematous and fibrotic changes occurring in the mucosa and submucosa result in bowel wall and fold thickening on barium and CT examinations. The symmetrically thickened folds frequently align in parallel arrangements, resembling the "stack of coins" or "picket fence" appearance seen with ischemia and mural hemorrhage.[89] Asymmetric submucosal involvement may cause a more localized eccentric thickening of the bowel wall and may disrupt the fold pattern, resulting in thumbprinting. Mucosal ulcerations may also be apparent.

During the chronic phase of radiation enteritis, progressive fibrosis may lead to fixed, narrowed, and poorly distensible small bowel segments. Ulcerations, adhesions, strictures, fistulas, and stenosis may develop [Figs. 20-15(a–d), 20-16, 20-17]. The strictures typically demonstrate smooth borders, and are optimally detected and demonstrated with small bowel enteroclysis.[90] In addition to bowel loop angulation and fixation, the adhesions may cause a characteristic mucosal pattern described as mucosal tacking. The mucosal tacking pattern results in angulation, spiking, and mucosal fold distortion on the antimesenteric side of the intestine in contrast to the perpendicular, regular thickened fold pattern that occurs with subacute radiation enteritis.[91] Small bowel obstruction may re-

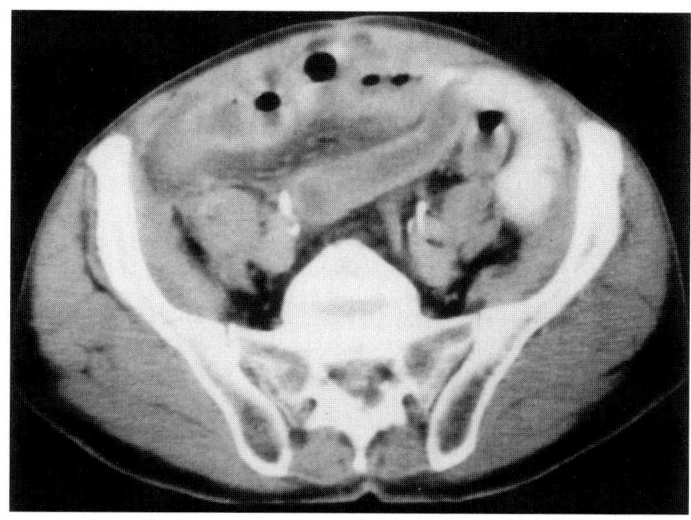 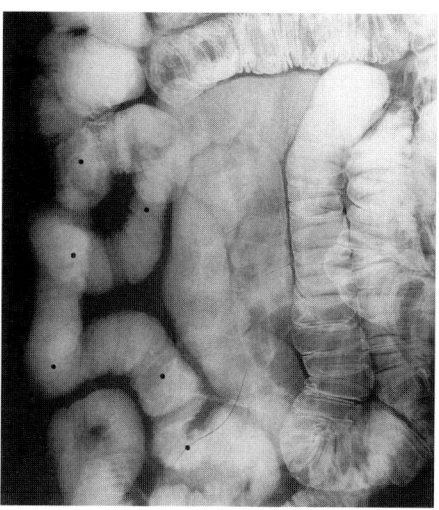

Fig. 20-14. Case of acute, short-lasting postradiation symptomatology.
(a) CT demonstrates diffuse enhancement of the thickened bowel walls and stranding of the mesentery. (b) Enteroclysis, done 5 days later, revealed normal small bowel morphology. (Dots mark the course of terminal ileum.)

sult from the strictures and adhesions, and bowel loop separation may also occur due to associated mesenteric edema and fibrosis. Barium studies and CT examinations during this stage may reveal bowel wall and fold thickening, bowel obstruction, and bowel angulation. Contrast-enhanced CT examination may demonstrate the abnormal "target sign" or "double halo" patterns of bowel wall enhancement (Fig. 20-17). Compared to barium studies, CT examinations may demonstrate the extraluminal complications of radiation enteritis to better advantage. These include the presence of abscesses, small extraluminal fluid collections, and pneumatosis or pneumoperitoneum. In addition, CT is useful for detecting malignant disease recurrence and associated adenopathy. Various radiologic features of radiation enteropathy are also illustrated in Chapter 21 (section on radiation enteropathy).

Chronic Mesenteric Ischemia

Chronic mesenteric ischemia is due to long-standing arterial insufficiency, which results in intestinal ischemia. Although two of the three major vessels supplying the bowel must be shown to be affected before this diagnosis can be made, not all patients with occlusion of these vessels will be clinically symptomatic. Classically, the disease occurs in elderly patients (female preponderance of 3:1) with atherosclerotic vascular disease.

Clinical Presentation

Patients often initially present with nonspecific abdominal pain. The diagnosis of chronic mesenteric ischemia is most frequently one of exclusion, and more common abdominal abnormalities such as gastritis, pancreatitis, cholecystitis, peptic ulcer disease, and irritable bowel syndrome should be eliminated as etiologic factors prior to performing an evaluation for this entity.

Chronic intestinal ischemia may cause a syndrome of intestinal angina characterized by crampy epigastric or periumbilical pain, which may radiate to the back. The pain typically begins 10 to 15 minutes after food ingestion, increases in severity, and may persist for as long as 3 hours. This postprandial pain is thought to result as a sequela of increased metabolic oxygen demands required by bowel during digestion. The discrepancy between oxygen supply and demand results in reduction in bowel wall tissue oxygenation, and leads to muscular spasm. Because of the induced pain, patients develop a food aversion, eating infrequent, small meals. Progressive weight loss, diarrhea, and steatorrhea frequently develop. Interestingly, studies have been unable to demonstrate a correlation between the degree of intestinal arterial occlusion seen at postmortem examination and patients' gastrointestinal symptoms.[92]

Evidence of vascular disease is typically present on physical examination. Diminished peripheral pulses or bruits may be evident, but are nonspecific findings.

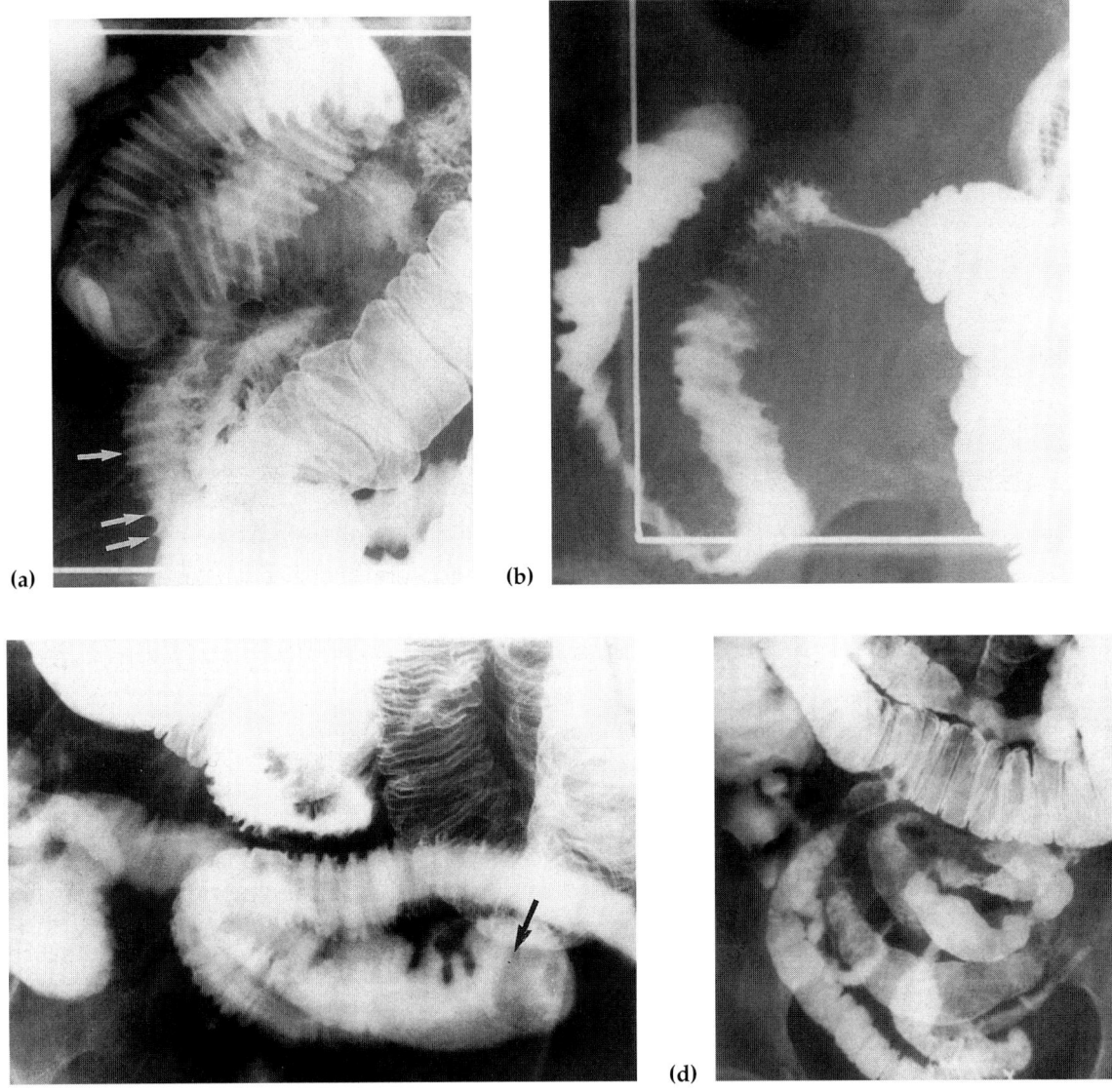

Fig. 20-15. Barium studies in patients with chronic radiation enteropathy.
(a) Radiotherapy for ovarian carcinoma. Radiation-damaged bowel loops seen in double contrast. Unlike a normal pattern, the thickness of folds (dark stripes) exceeds that of the spaces between them (white lines). This is pronounced in radiation enteropathy to produce a spiky outline of the white spaces at the edge of loops (arrows to some). (b) Several years later features of small bowel obstruction. Enteroclysis showed a smooth radiation stricture at edge of radiation portal, a not unusual location. (c) History of radiotherapy for cervix carcinoma. Uneven distribution of radiation damage through the distal ileum (arrow to an uninvolved segment in the midst of disease). Note spiky contour of damaged bowel. (d) Following radiotherapy for endometrial carcinoma several years earlier, a 59-year-old patient presented with obstruction and occasional blood loss. Ileal segments are narrowed slightly, fixed, aperistaltic, and devoid of folds. Mucosa was atrophic with several telangiectases.

Demonstration of a postprandial drop in jejunal intramucosal pH, measured via tonometry, is helpful for diagnosing this entity.[93]

Radiologic Findings

Selective angiography of the three major splanchnic arteries (the celiac axis, SMA, and inferior mesenteric artery) is considered to be the gold standard for radiologic diagnosis of this entity. Angiographic findings include demonstration of at least two-thirds reduction in blood flow within at least two of these three major vessels supplying the bowel. Both anterior and lateral projections are essential for complete angiographic evaluation of the vessels. In addition to defining the location and extent of arterial occlusion, angiography

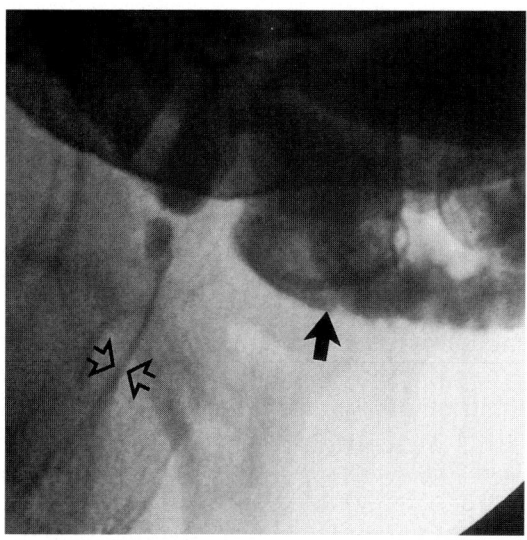

Fig. 20-16. Enterovaginal fistula (open arrows) arising in radiation-damaged ileum (large arrow). (This is best shown in inverted state.)

has the advantage of demonstrating collateral vessels and assessing the aorta and iliac arteries prior to bypass graft placement.

Noninvasive imaging modalities have become increasingly useful in the diagnosis of chronic mesenteric ischemia. Duplex Doppler ultrasound, when

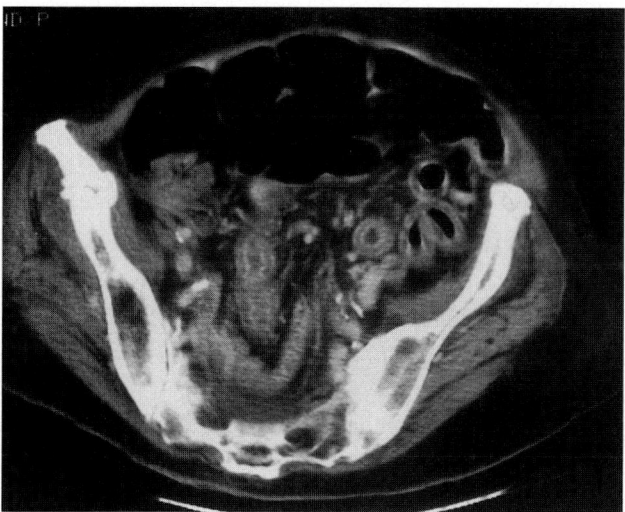

Fig. 20-17. Radiation enteritis in a 63-year-old woman treated for endometrial carcinoma.
Pelvic small bowel loops appear abnormally thickened with a target sign enhancement pattern. This abnormal appearance to the bowel is nonspecific, and differentiation from bowel ischemia and other inflammatory conditions is possible only with knowledge of prior radiation exposure.

technically feasible, may demonstrate arterial narrowing and significant arterial stenosis, and can be performed both prior to and following food ingestion to document responsive blood flow.[94] CT and MR angiography are becoming increasingly successful at demonstrating significant vascular stenosis in the major visceral vessels. In addition, phase-contrast cine MRI can measure SMA blood flow in both fasting and postprandial states, and may discriminate healthy responses from inadequate ones by evaluating percentage change.[95]

Treatment

Although arterial reconstructive surgery was the preferred therapy in the past, transluminal angioplasty is currently assuming an increasingly important therapeutic role.[96] The disadvantage of percutaneous transluminal angioplasty is that recurrent disease, estimated to occur in 10% to 50% of patients within 4 to 28 months, is more common than that which occurs following surgery.[2] Recognized complications of angioplasty include distal embolization, intimal injury, and hemorrhage. Total occlusions and/or long stenoses that are not amenable to angioplasty necessitate operative revascularization with endarterectomy, reimplantation, and/or bypass procedures.

Celiac Axis Compression Syndrome

This is a controversial entity in which compression of the celiac trunk by either the median arcuate ligament of the diaphragm or the celiac ganglion results in chronic mesenteric ischemia. Affected patients are typically women (younger than those who usually present with chronic mesenteric ischemia due to atherosclerotic disease) who manifest symptoms of intestinal angina. One of the reasons this entity remains controversial is that in most cases, the pancreaticoduodenal arcades provide adequate routes for collateral blood flow to the celiac axis. Although compression of the celiac axis by the median arcuate ligament is a common anatomic variant, documented to occur to a variable degree in 10% to 24% of the population,[97] the majority of individuals remain clinically asymptomatic.

Angiographic findings indicative of this abnormality include eccentric stenosis of the proximal celiac trunk, delayed filling of celiac branches via collateral flow, and lack of atherosclerotic change in other vessels.[98]

On CT examination, characteristic findings include a soft-tissue band anterior to the celiac artery, occasionally accompanied by poststenotic arterial dilatation distal to the band, and peripancreatic collateral vessels.[99] However, a CT study of clinically asymptomatic individuals demonstrated that the isolated CT finding of celiac axis effacement or obscuration occurred frequently enough to be insufficient for establishing the diagnosis of celiac axis compression syndrome in the absence of other clinical evidence of chronic mesenteric ischemia.[99]

Vascular Malformations

Vascular malformations may occur as either congenital or acquired abnormalities. When acquired, they may develop in association with a variety of disorders, including the Osler-Weber-Rendu syndrome (hereditary hemorrhagic telangiectasia), the CREST syndrome (calcinosis, Raynaud's phenomenon, esophageal hypomotility, sclerodactyly, telangiectasia), the blue rubber bleb nevus syndrome,[100] Turner's syndrome,[101] and Maffucci's syndrome.

Angiodysplasias/Vascular Ectasias

These terms have been used synonymously to describe ectatic, tortuous submucosal veins and overlying mucosal capillaries. They are frequently multiple, and approximately 80% occur within the colon, preferentially affecting the right side. Gastric and small bowel involvement also occurs. Small bowel angiodysplasia most commonly involves the duodenum, and is thought to be responsible for 1.2% to 8% of cases of upper gastrointestinal tract hemorrhage.[102] Although their etiology remains uncertain, proposed theories include development from chronic or recurrent low-grade submucosal venous obstruction or chronic mucosal edema. Alternatively, they may result from true congenital arteriovenous malformations (AVMs).[103] AVMs are thought to be the most common cause of obscure bleeding from the small intestine, accounting for 30% to 40% of cases.[104,105] Although angiodysplasias have been professed to occur with higher frequencies in patients with aortic stenosis, cirrhosis, renal failure, pulmonary disease, and von Willebrand's disease, there does not appear to be a strong association in most cases.[102] Moore and colleagues separated vascular ectasias into three categories.[106]

Type I lesions are acquired and usually occur in individuals more than 55 years old, and are most commonly located within the right colon. Evidence of hemorrhage is identified in only 50% of these lesions.

Type II lesions are felt to represent congenital arteriovenous malformations, and they occur most frequently within the small bowel and stomach. The lesions are larger than type I lesions, and affect younger individuals (typically 30 to 50 years of age). They are a common cause of obscure gastrointestinal bleeding, and may lead to anemia.

Type III lesions demonstrate an autosomal dominant inheritance pattern, and therefore occur in families. Angiectasias throughout the bowel and within the liver are commonly associated, along with telangiectasias of the skin and mucous membrane. These lesions have a propensity to hemorrhage.

Vascular ectasias are typically located on the antimesenteric bowel wall, and are frequently difficult to diagnose. Endoscopy and colonoscopy are the most sensitive diagnostic tests, but are unrevealing in a significant number of cases. Single contrast barium studies have been reported to detect gastroduodenal bleeding sites in only 30% to 50% of patients.[107] Enteroclysis may aid in diagnosis of the etiology of obscure gastrointestinal bleeding. In one study, it was able to diagnose the etiology of the bleeding in 21% of patients.[108] Most of the causes of obscure bleeding demonstrated by enteroclysis were tumors, malignant, benign, or metastatic. In a very small number of patients features in favor of AVMs were demonstrated, to be later confirmed by enteroscopy or surgery (Fig. 20-18). Although large vascular ectasias may be demonstrated angiographically, smaller lesions are not usually seen, especially if of mainly venous composition. When positive, angiographic findings include demonstration of an early filling vein; presence of a capillary stain, localized blush, or vascular tuft; and visualization of a slowly draining vein after the remainder of the mesenteric veins have emptied.[103,109] Luminal contrast extravasation is seen only with significant bleeding. Recently, a case was reported in which a helical CT examination performed immediately following angiography was able to detect an arteriovenous malformation missed by the diagnostic angiogram.[110] Research has shown that helical CT angiography and biphasic helical CT examination of the intestine may be useful for demonstrating small bowel AVMs and sites of gastrointestinal hemorrhage of obscure origin.[111,112]

Hemangiomas

Hemangiomas are benign hamartomatous lesions. Small bowel hemangiomas are rare, accounting for 7% to 10% of all benign small bowel tumors. The most commonly affected small bowel segment is the jejunum.[113] Two types of hemangiomas are recognized: *capillary hemangiomas*, in which vascular channels are tightly packed, and *cavernous hemangiomas*, containing larger vascular spaces. Capillary hemangiomas arise in the submucosa, resulting in shallow elevations of the mucosal surface. They may occur as solitary or multiple lesions. Cavernous hemangiomas usually occur as solitary lesions. Although they also arise in the submucosa, they project into the intestinal lumen as

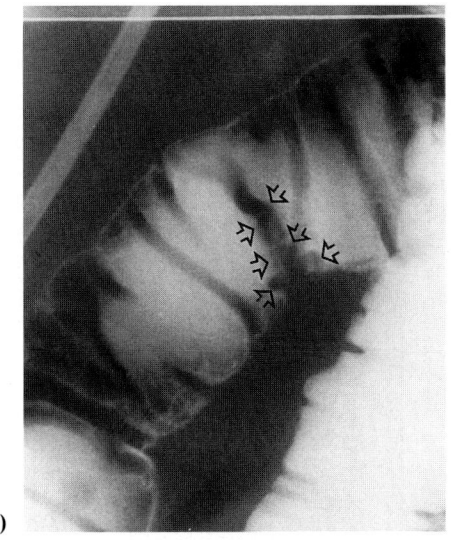

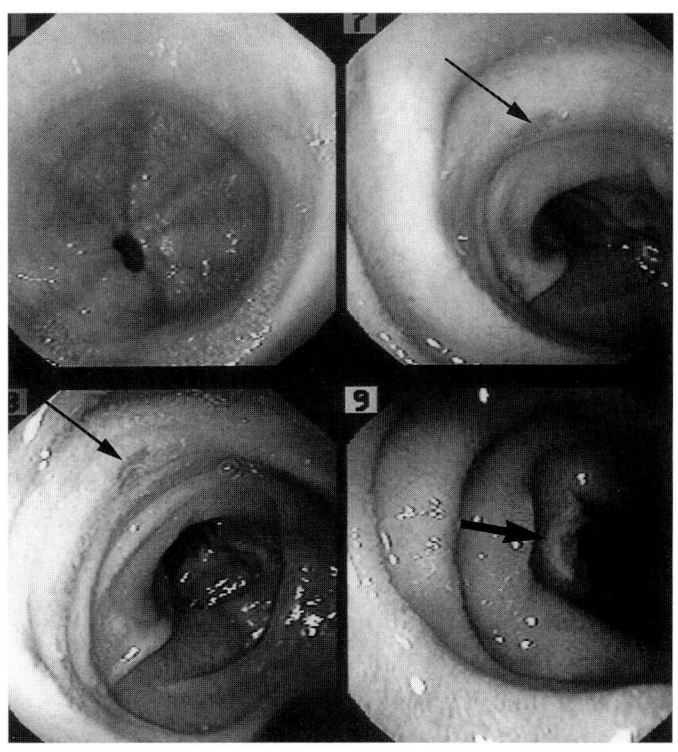

Fig. 20-18. A 62-year-old general practitioner with intermittent low-grade bleeding. No cause was found after routine barium and endoscopic examinations. (a) Enteroclysis drew attention to a single widened fold in the proximal jejunum. Its outline is scalloped (open arrows). An AVM arising in the submucosa and growing through the submucosal core of that fold would produce this appearance (never diagnose this kind of appearance on the inner border of a bend!). (b) AVM was confirmed by enteroscopy (slim arrows) and fulgarized (wider arrow).

polyps. Bleeding invariably occurs from hemangiomas, although it may be occult. There is a relationship between these malformations and cutaneous syndromes (eg, blue rubber bleb nevus syndrome and Klippel-Trénaunay syndrome).

Abdominal plain film examination may reveal calcified phleboliths associated with intestinal lesions. Because of the normal variability in the position of bowel loops, the phleboliths may change location on subsequent examinations. Hemangiomas are infrequently visible on barium studies. Typically, the polypoid projections of cavernous hemangiomas have a higher detection rate than the shallower projections of capillary hemangiomas. The radiologic features are illustrated in Chapter 19 (see section on benign tumors—hemangioma). They may occasionally be demonstrated on MRI or contrast-enhanced CT examinations, but are most reliably demonstrated angiographically.[114]

Mesenteric Varices

Mesenteric varices are acquired vascular malformations that result in marked dilatation and tortuosity of submucosal veins. They most commonly result from portal hypertension leading to development of portosystemic venous collaterals between small tributaries of mesenteric veins on the parietal surface of the viscera and systemic veins in the abdominal wall and retroperitoneum. Common predisposing causes include hepatic cirrhosis, abdominal adhesions between bowel and abdominal wall from prior abdominal surgery, venous occlusion from neoplastic infiltration, and idiopathic thrombosis of the superior mesenteric vein.[115,116] Mesenteric varices may cause significant gastrointestinal hemorrhage.

Superior mesenteric angiography is the most reliable radiologic study for diagnosing the presence and location of varices, although dilated, tortuous veins and collateral vessels may also be demonstrated on CT or MRI examination. On barium studies, varices appear as serpiginous filling defects traversing the bowel mucosa [Figs. 20-19(a,b)], or as nodular, undulating intramural defects.[116,117] Nuclear medicine examinations with 99m Tc-RBC scintigraphy may be useful for diagnosis, as varices appear as persistent abnormal foci of activity during the venous phase of the examination.[118]

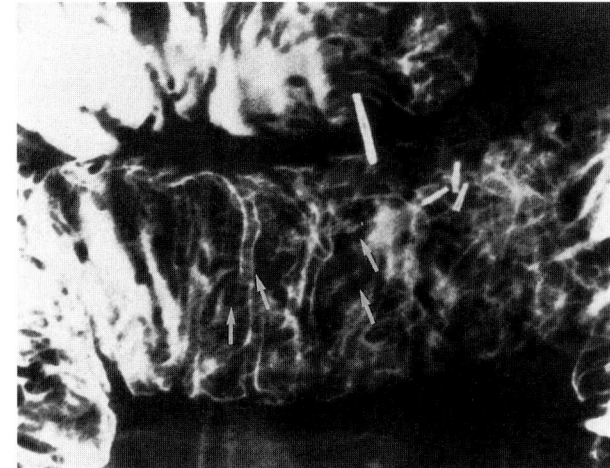
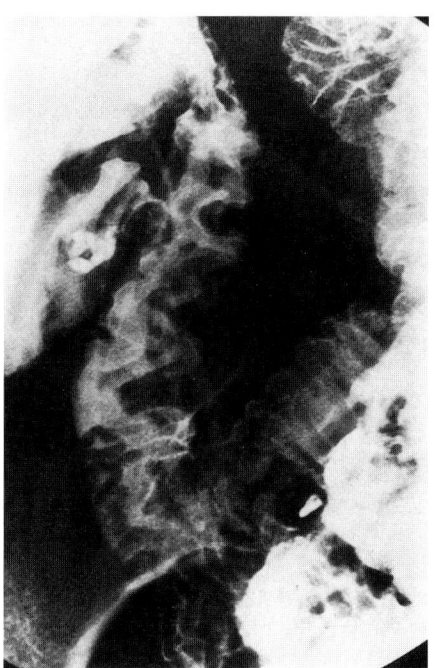

Fig. 20-19. Small bowel varices in two patients with portal hypertension.
(a) Varices in proximal jejunum (arrows to a few of them).
(b) Varices in the terminal ileum.

Intramural Hemorrhage

Intramural hemorrhage may be caused by intestinal ischemia, but is also associated with traumatic injury, anticoagulant therapy, coagulation disorders, and less common etiologies such as pancreatitis, collagen vascular disease, hepatic cirrhosis, and malignancy (eg, leukemia, lymphoma, myeloma, and metastatic carcinoma).

On CT examination, acute intramural hematoma often appears as a focal region of symmetric, homogeneous wall thickening that is frequently of higher attenuation than the adjacent normal bowel wall (Fig. 20-20). Alternatively, focal hematomas may demonstrate eccentric mural thickening with a mass-like appearance (Fig. 20-21). Typically, the hematoma will have density measurements of 40 to 60 Hounsfield units (HU), and will decrease in density as clot lysis occurs. Resolution may be complete within days or weeks.

On barium examination, the mucosal folds may be thickened and arranged in parallel, causing a "picket fence" or "stack of coins" appearance similar to the findings in ischemia. More typically, the bowel lumen may appear to be compressed, the folds less clearly defined and displaced at their mesenteric aspect, indicating a hematoma at its often mesenteric border intramural site [Fig. 20-22(a)]; this was confirmed by MRI [Fig. 20-22(b–d)]. Alternatively, the valvulae conniventes may be completely effaced, resulting in smooth or slightly scalloped narrowing of a longer segment of the intestine.[119]

Small Bowel Injury in Blunt Abdominal Trauma

Blunt abdominal trauma may cause intramural hemorrhage within the small bowel or mesentery, and may also result in bowel perforation (Fig. 20-23). Intra-

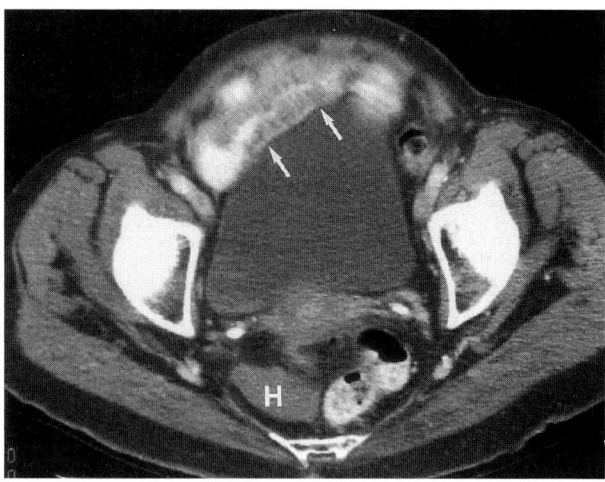

Fig. 20-20. Intramural hemorrhage in an elderly woman following coumadin overdose.
Contrast-enhanced CT scan demonstrates symmetric, homogeneous thickening of the wall of the distal ileum representing intramural hemorrhage (arrows). The intestinal hemorrhage resulted in proximal partial small bowel obstruction (not shown). High-density free blood (hemoperitoneum) was identified within the pelvis (H).

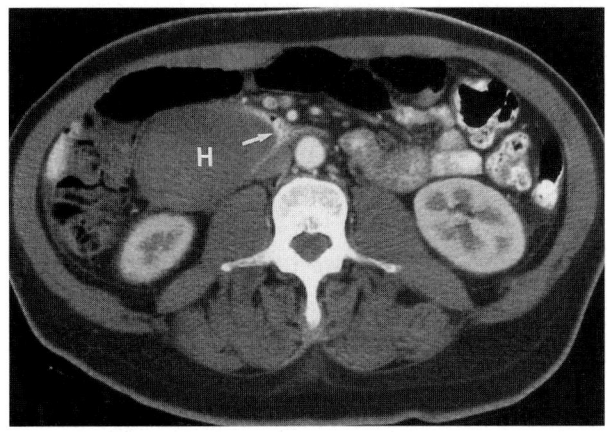

Fig. 20-21. **Intramural duodenal hematoma resulting from endoscopic retrograde cholangiopancreatography.**
This contrast-enhanced CT scan demonstrates an eccentric intramural hematoma (H), which medially displaces and compresses the lumen of the second portion of the duodenum (arrow).

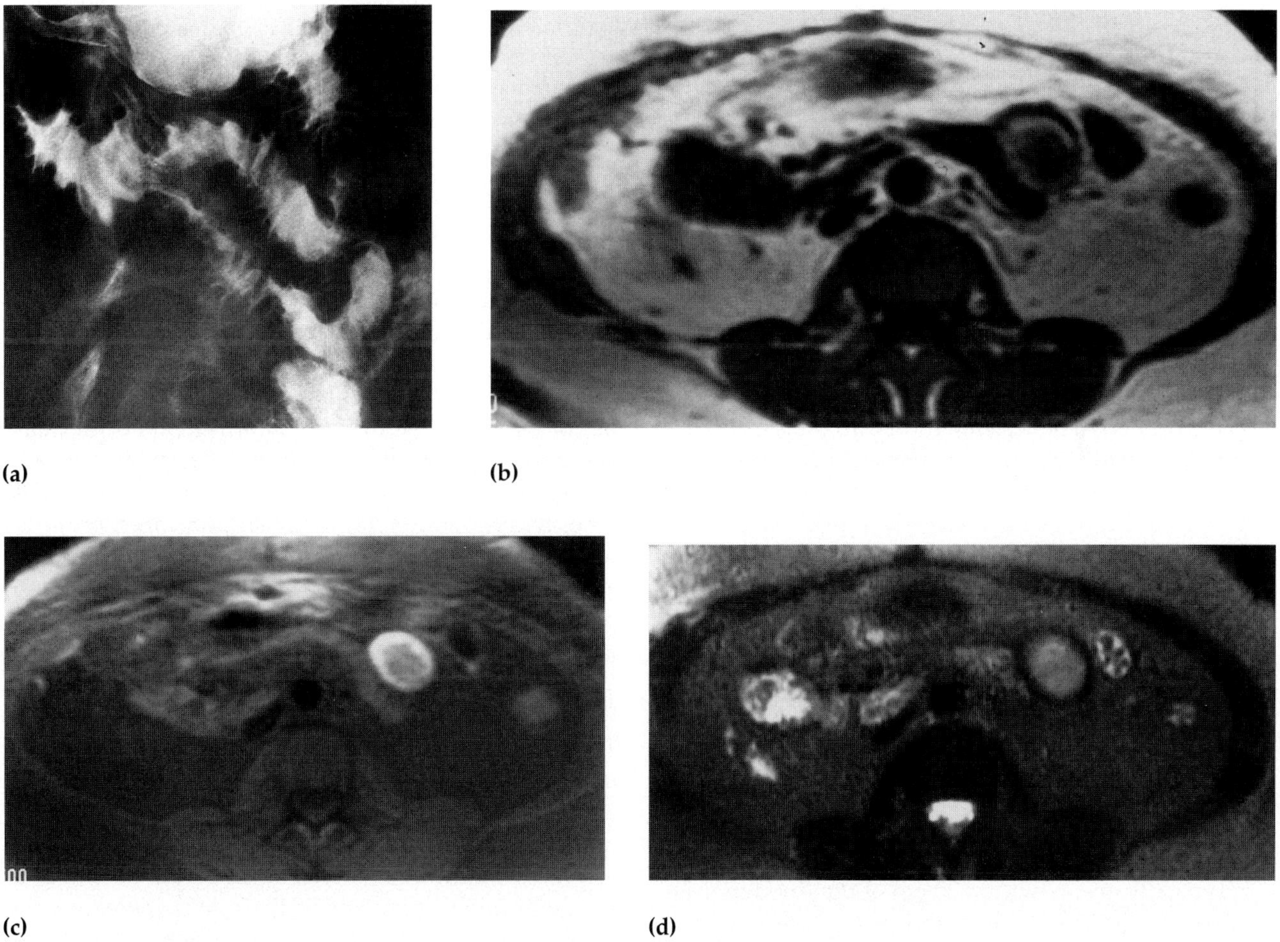

(a)

(b)

(c)

(d)

Fig. 20-22. **A patient with a long history of lupus with renal involvement and recent kidney transplantation developed acute pain in the epigastrium.**
(a) A barium follow-through demonstrated features of ischemia with likely hematoma in the duodeno-jejunal area. (b) Axial T1-weighted spin-echo image shows a well-circumscribed mass along the mesenteric border of a proximal segment of jejunum. (c) Axial T1-weighted spin-echo image repeated with fat saturation shows persistent high signal intensity suggesting the presence of subacute blood. (d) Axial fat-suppressed T2-weighted image shows a low signal rim to the mass, suggestive of hemosiderin within macrophages at the margin of the hematoma.

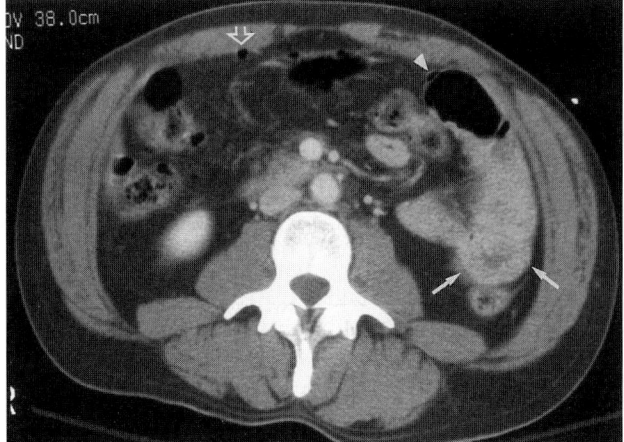

Fig. 20-23. Jejunal perforation and intramural hematoma in a construction worker who fell 40 ft from a roof.
Contrast-enhanced CT reveals jejunal wall thickening (arrows) and pneumatosis (arrowhead). The attenuation of the jejunal wall appears greater than that of adjacent small bowel. A small focus of pneumoperitoneum is present (open arrow), and resulted from a tiny perforation in the jejunal wall. No extravasation of oral contrast material was noted.

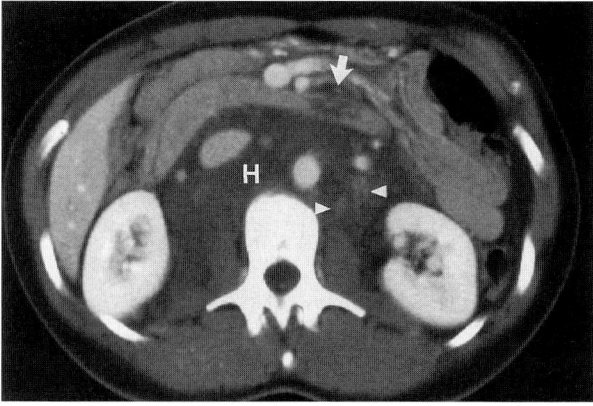

Fig. 20-24. Intestinal transection resulting from motor vehicle accident.
Contrast-enhanced CT shows disruption of the wall of the distal duodenum at the ligament of Treitz (arrow). Amorphous high-attenuation hemorrhage is identified along a branch of the SMA, representing active mesenteric bleeding (arrowheads). Note the large amount of hemorrhage surrounding the aorta, inferior vena cava, and psoas muscles (H).

mural hemorrhages resulting from trauma typically produce more discrete intramural masses and shorter segmental intestinal involvement than those that result from nontraumatic causes.[120] The use of seat belts has contributed to decreasing mortality rates from motor vehicle accidents, but has increased the number of intestinal injuries to the small intestine and its mesentery.[121] Varying types of seat belt injuries have been described, and the resulting injury varies with the causative force involved.[122]

Deceleration Injuries

These are caused by a sudden forward propulsion of small bowel. Because the ligament of Treitz restricts this forward movement of the proximal jejunum, a shearing force is created between the proximally fixed and distally mobile segments, and may result in complete proximal jejunal transection. The site of transection typically occurs within 20 cm of the duodenojejunal flexure (Fig. 20-24). Mesenteric tears, splenic injury, and transverse and proximal descending colonic injuries are commonly associated.

Impact Injuries

These can take the form of a crush injury to the small bowel and its mesentery, which become caught between the vertebral column and seat belt. When these injuries occur, the lap belt has typically been improperly worn above the level of the pelvic brim, causing the protective forces of the iliac crest to be lost. Relatively fixed small bowel loops, including the terminal ileum, or bowel entrapped by adhesions or hernias, and bowel with limited mobility due to an abnormally shortened mesentery as can occur with Crohn's disease, lymphoma, or tuberculosis, are more prone to injury in this scenario. Transverse mesenteric tears and mesenteric hematomas may result, and can cause delayed small bowel infarction.[123]

Transmitted Forces

These are the cause of bowel perforation secondary to intraluminal pressure elevations reaching 120 to 140 mm Hg 1.[24] Solitary or multiple intestinal ruptures may occur, and are due to transmitted abdominal forces acting on a functional small bowel obstruction. As the luminal diameter of the bowel increases, the pressure required to cause bowel rupture diminishes. Thus, conditions that cause bowel distention (eg, postprandial states, ileus, obstruction, or intestinal pathology such as Crohn's disease) predispose the bowel to perforation during this type of blunt trauma. In general, the mesenteric side of the bowel is more prone to rupture, whereas the antimesenteric side more commonly perforates.[125]

Diagnosis by CT

CT is the most useful radiologic study for diagnosing visceral injury in clinically stable patients who have sustained abdominal trauma. Intravenous contrast material should be administered (via a power injector if possible), as visceral injuries may not be apparent on unenhanced examinations. Water-soluble oral contrast material should also be given prior to the examination, so that optimal bowel opacification can be achieved. This will help to detect bowel wall thickening and the presence of bowel perforation.

Bowel and mesenteric injuries may be subtle and difficult to diagnose on CT examination, but detection of hemoperitoneum without evidence of solid organ injury should raise suspicion for their presence. The CT attenuation values of hemoperitoneum vary depending on the size and age of the collection. Overall, most hemorrhagic collections have attenuation values greater than 30 HU. Because of its greater hemoglobin content, clotted blood has a higher attenuation than free-flowing blood or lysed clot, and generally measures more than 60 HU. In general, the attenuation value of blood is highest the closer it is to its organ of origin. This fact is underscored by the usefulness of the *sentinel clot sign*. The sentinel clot represents a focal collection of high-density clotted blood, which is identified on CT examinations to lie adjacent to the injured abdominal organ. Orwig and Federle retrospectively studied 116 patients with documented acute visceral injuries and found that the sentinel clot sign, present in 84% of cases, was the only indicator for the source of hemorrhage in 14% of patients.[126] Arterial extravasations typically appear as focal high-attenuation collections (80 to 130 HU) surrounded by lower-density hematomas.[127] Actively extravasating arterial collections demonstrate the highest CT attenuation values (120 to 170 HU), typically measuring within 15 HU of the aorta or major adjacent arterial structures on the same CT slice.[127]

In addition to hemoperitoneum, focal bowel wall thickening, localized intramural hematoma, and mesenteric fluid may be identified on CT examinations in 75% to 88% of patients with intestinal injury.[125,126,128] Pneumoperitoneum, pneumatosis, and extravasation of oral contrast material are important additional ancillary clues (Fig. 20-23). Although they are more specific for a diagnosis of bowel injury, they are unfortunately absent in approximately 50% of patients.[128–130] The presence of pneumoperitoneum is not diagnostic for bowel rupture. In a study of 18 patients who had blunt trauma and CT evidence of pneumoperitoneum, only 22% of patients had bowel rupture.[131] In the remaining cases, pneumoperitoneum frequently resulted from associated chest trauma, pneumothorax, pneumomediastinum, or mechanical ventilation.

Mesenteric injury can be very subtle, and may be even more challenging to detect than bowel injuries. Hemoperitoneum is the most common CT finding, and blood often assumes a triangular shape as it insinuates between intestinal loops. Associated disruption of mesenteric vessels may be shown as high-density collections of extravasated intravenous contrast media located adjacent to injured vasculature (Fig. 20-25). CT may also demonstrate evidence of bowel ischemia and infarction if the mesenteric injury compromises the bowel's blood supply. Maintaining a high level of suspicion facilitates this diagnosis.

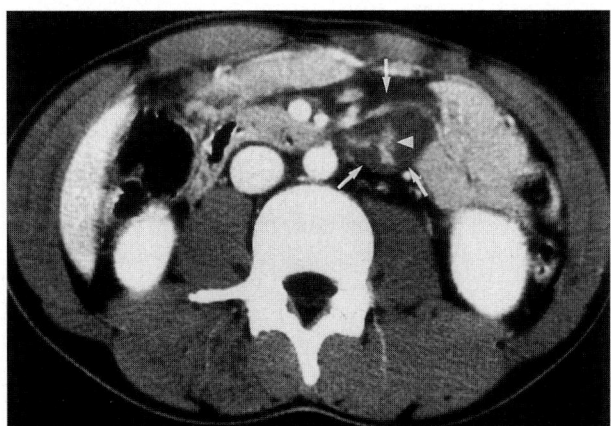

Fig. 20-25. Active mesenteric bleeding in a patient following a motor vehicle accident.
On this contrast-enhanced CT scan, a mesenteric hematoma presents as an interloop fluid collection (arrows). Active mesenteric bleeding appears as amorphous, higher attenuation region within the hematoma, adjacent to branches of the SMA (arrowhead). Note that this actively extravasated blood has attenuation values similar to the adjacent SMA and its branches.

References

1. Schwaiger M, Fondacaro JD, Jacobson ED: Effects of glucagon, histamine, and perhexiline on the ischemic canine mesenteric circulation. *Gastroenterology.* 1979;77:730–735.
2. Bradbury AW, Brittenden J, McBride K, et al. Mesenteric ischaemia: a multidisciplinary approach. *Br J Surg.* 1995;82:1446–1459.
3. Kaleya RN, Sammartano RJ, Boley SJ. Aggressive approach to acute mesenteric ischemia. *Surg Clin North Am.* 1992;72:157–182.
4. Bradbury AW, Murie JA, Ruckley CV. Role of the leukocyte in the pathogenesis of vascular disease. *Br J Surg.* 1993;80:1503–1512.

5. Kuroda T, Shiohara E, Homma T, et al. Effects of leukocyte and platelet depletion on ischemia-reperfusion injury to dog pancreas. *Gastroenterology*. 1994;107:1125–1134.
6. Harward TR, Brooks DL, Flynn TC, et al. Multiple organ dysfunction after mesenteric artery revascularization. *J Vasc Surg*. 1993;18:459–467.
7. Brown, RA, Chiu CJ, Scott HJ, et al. Ultrastructural changes in the canine ileal mucosal cell after mesenteric arterial occlusion. *Arch Surg*. 1970;101(2):290–297.
8. Whitehead R. The pathology of ischemia of the intestines. *Pathol Annual*. 1976;11:1–52.
9. Yamamoto M, Plessow B, Koch HK, et al. Electron microscopic studies on the small intestinal mucosa of rats after mechanical intestinal obstruction and ischemia. *Virchows Arch*. 1980;32(2):157–164.
10. Robinson JW, Mirkovitch V, Winistorfer B, et al. Response of the intestinal mucosa to ischaemia. *Gut*. 1981;22(6):512–527.
11. Wang JH, Chen HS, Wang T, et al. Role of oxygen-derived free radicals in superior mesenteric artery occlusion shock in rats. *Chin Med J (Engl)*. 1990;103:278–282.
12. Fullerton DA, Hahn AR, Koike K, et al. Intracellular mechanisms of pulmonary vasomotor dysfunction in acute lung injury caused by mesenteric ischemia-reperfusion. *Surgery*. 1993;114:360–366.
13. Weixiong H, Aneman A, Nilsson U, et al. Quantification of tissue damage in the feline small intestine during ischaemia-reperfusion: the importance of free radicals. *Acta Physiol Scand*. 1994;150:241–250.
14. Hildebrand HD, Zierler RE. Mesenteric vascular disease. *Am J Surg*. 1980;139:188–192.
15. Scholz FJ. Ischemic bowel disease. *Radiol Clin North Am*. 1993;31(6):1197–1218.
16. Inderbitzi R, Wagner HE, Seiler C, et al. Acute mesenteric ischaemia. *Eur J Surg*. 1992;158:123–126.
17. Brandt LJ, Boley SJ. Ischemic and vascular lesions of the bowel. In: Sleisenger M, Fordtran J, eds. *Gastrointestinal Disease*. 5th ed. Philadelphia, Pa: WB Saunders Co; 1993:1927–1961.
18. Zan S, Giustetto A, Mastroianni V, et al. Acute intestinal ischemia. Diagnosis and surgical treatment. *Minerva Chir*. 1993;48:543–548.
19. Allen KB, Salam AA, Lumsden AB, et al. Acute mesenteric ischemia after cardiopulmonary bypass. *J Vasc Surg*. 1992;16:391–395.
20. Desai MH, Herndon DN, Rutan RL, et al. Ischemic intestinal complications in patients with burns. *Surg Gynecol Obstet*. 1991;172:257–261.
21. Batellier J, Kieny R. Superior mesenteric artery embolism: eighty-two cases. *Ann Vasc Surg*. 1990;4:112–116.
22. Friedenberg MJ, Polk HC, McAlister WH, et al. Superior mesenteric arteriography in experimental mesenteric venous thrombosis. *Radiology*. 1965;85:38–45.
23. Polk HC. Studies in experimental mesenteric venous occlusion I: the experimental system and its parameters. *Surgery*. 1964;108:693–698.
24. Reilly PM, MacGowan S, Miyachi M, et al. Mesenteric vasoconstriction in cardiogenic shock in pigs. *Gastroenterology*. 1992;102:1968–1979.
25. Lambert M, dePeyer R, Muller AF. Reversible ischemic colitis after intavenous vasopressin therapy. *JAMA*. 1982;247:666–667.
26. Beyer KL, Bickel JT, Butt JH. Ischemic colitis associated with dextroamphetamine use. *J Clin Gastroenterol*. 1991;13:198–201.
27. Johnson TD, Berenson MM. Methamphetamine-induced ischemic colitis. *J Clin Gastroenterol*. 1991;13:687–689.
28. Freudenberger RS, Cappell MS, Hutt DA. Intestinal infarction after intravenous cocaine administration. *Ann Intern Med*. 1990;113:715–716.
29. Lee HS, La Maute HR, Pizzi WF, et al. Acute gastroduodenal perforations associated with use of crack. *Ann Surg*. 1990;211:15–17.
30. Nalbandian H, Sheth N, Dietrich R, et al. Intestinal ischemia caused by cocaine ingestion: report of two cases. *Surgery*. 1985;97:374–376.
31. Jamieson WG, Marchuk S, Rowsom J, et al. The early diagnosis of acute massive intestinal ischaemia. *Br J Surg*. 1982;69:552–553.
32. Lange H, Jackel R. Usefulness of plasma lactate concentration in the diagnosis of acute abdominal disease. *Eur J Surg*. 1994;160:381–384.
33. Jonas J, Bottger T. Diagnosis and prognosis of mesenterial infarct. *Med Klin*. 1994;89:68–72.
34. Smerud MJ, Johnson CD, Stephens DH. Diagnosis of bowel infarction: a comparison of plain films and CT scans in 23 cases. *AJR*. 1990;154:99–103.
35. Gore RM. The liver: differential diagnosis. In: Gore RM, Levine MS, Laufer I, eds. *Textbook of Gastrointestinal Radiology*. Philadelphia, Pa: WB Saunders Co; 1994: 2078–2093.
36. Joffe N, Goldman H, Antonioli DA. Barium studies in small bowel infarction. *Radiology*. 1977;123:303–309.
37. Marshak RH, Lindner AE, Maklansky D. Ischemia of the small intestine. *Am J Gastroenterol*. 1976;66:390–400.
38. Taourel PG, Deneuville M, Pradel JA, et al. Acute mesenteric ishemia: diagnosis with contrast-enhanced CT. *Radiology*. 1996;199:632–636.
39. Pérez C, Llauger J, Puig J, et al. Computed tomographic findings in bowel ischemia. *Gastrointest Radiol*. 1989;14:241–245.
40. Clark RA. Computed tomography of bowel infarction. *J Comput Assist Tomogr*. 1987;11(5):757–762.
41. Klein HM, Klosterhalfen B, Kinzel S, et al. CT and MRI of experimentally induced mesenteric ischemia in a porcine model. *J Comput Assist Tomogr*. 1996;20(2):254–261.
42. Frager D, Baer JW, Medwid SW, et al. Detection of intestinal ischemia in patients with acute small-bowel obstruction due to adhesions or hernia: efficacy of CT. *AJR*. 1996;166:67–71.
43. Jones B, Fishman EK, Siegelman SS. Ischemic colitis demonstrated by computed tomography. *J Comput Assist Tomogr*. 1982;6(6):1120–1123.
44. Alpern MB, Glazer GM, Francis IR. Ischemic or infarcted bowel: CT findings. *Radiology*. 1988;166:149–152.
45. Klein HM, Lensing R, Klosterhalfen B, et al. Diagnostic imaging of mesenteric infarction. *Radiology*. 1995;197:79–82.

46. Federle MP, Chun G, Jeffrey RB, et al. Computed tomographic findings in bowel infarction. *AJR.* 1984;142: 91–95.
47. Kaufman AJ, Tarr RW, Holburn GE, et al. Magnetic resonance imaging of ischemic bowel in rabbit model. *Invest Radiol.* 1988;23(2):93–97.
48. Connor R, Jones B, Fishman EK, et al. Pneumatosis intestinalis: role of computed tomography in diagnosis and management. *J Comput Assist Tomogr.* 1984;8(2): 269–275.
49. Kelvin FM, Korobkin M, Rauch RF, et al. Computed tomography of pneumatosis intestinalis. *J Comput Assist Tomogr.* 1984;8(2):276–280.
50. Earls JP, Dachman AH, Colon E, et al. Prevalence and duration of postoperative pneumoperitoneum: sensitivity of CT vs left lateral decubitus radiography. *AJR.* 1993;161(4):781–785.
51. Stapakis JC, Thickman D. Diagnosis of pneumoperitoneum: abdominal CT vs. upright chest film. *J Comput Assist Tomogr.* 1992;16(5):713–716.
52. Rosen A, Korobkin M, Silverman P, et al. Mesenteric venous thrombosis: CT identification. *AJR.* 1984;143(1): 83–86.
53. Nozaki E, Kohno A, Narimatsu A, et al. Superior mesenteric artery occlusion: an unenhanced CT fnding. *J Comput Assist Tomogr.* 1991;15:866–867.
54. Napel S, Marks MP, Rubin GD, et al. CT angiography with spiral CT and maximum intensity projection. *Radiology.* 1992;185:607–610.
55. Rubin GD, Dake MD, Napel SA, et al. Three-dimensional spiral CT angiography of the abdomen: initial clinical experience. *Radiology.* 1993;186:147–152.
56. Hricak H, Amparo I, Fisher MR, et al. Abdominal venous system: assessment using MR. *Radiology.* 1985;156:415–422.
57. Pavone P, Scipioni A, Catalano C, et al. Quantification of mesenteric flow with magnetic resonance imaging before and after a meal: results in healthy volunteers. *Radiol Med (Torino).* 1996;92(4):386–389.
58. Bakal CW, Sprayregen S, Wolf EL. Radiology in intestinal ischemia. Angiographic diagnosis and management. *Surg Clin North Am.* 1992;72:125–141.
59. Clark RA, Gallant TE. Acute mesenteric ischemia: angiographic spectrum. *AJR.* 1984;142(3):555–562.
60. Clavien PA, Durig M, Harder F. Venous mesenteric infarction: a particular entity. *Br J Surg.* 1988;75(3): 252–255.
61. Polk HC. Experimental mesenteric venous occlusion: 3. Diagnosis and treatment of induced mesenteric venous thrombosis. *Ann Surg.* 1966;163(3):432–444.
62. Aakhus T, Evensen A. Angiography in acute mesenteric arterial insufficiency. *Acta Radiol.* 1978;19(6): 945–951.
63. Siegelman SS, Sprayregen S, Boley SJ. Angiographic diagnosis of mesenteric arterial vasoconstriction. *Radiology.* 1974;112(3):533–542.
64. Regan F, Karlstad RR, Magnuson JH. Minimally invasive management of acute superior mesenteric artery occlusion by combined urokinase and laparoscopic therapy. *Am J Gastroenterol.* 1996;97:1019–1021.
65. Shah S, Anderson C. Prediction of small bowel viability using Doppler ultrasound. Clinical and experimental evaluation. *Ann Surg.* 1981;194:97–99.
66. Levine JS, Jacobson ED. Intestinal ischemic disorders. *Digestive Diseases.* 1995;13:3–24.
67. Ginai AZ, Hussain SM, Hordijk ML, et al. Case report: solitary ischaemic small bowel stenosis. *Br J Radiol.* 1994;67:405–407.
68. Mosley JG, Marston A. In: Marston A, Buckley GB, Fiddian-Green RG, Haglund UH, eds. *Splanchnic Ischaemia and Multiple Organ Failure.* London, England: Arnold; 1989.
69. Gorton M, John JF Jr. Polyarteritis overlap syndrome with extensive bowel infarction. *Am J Gastroenterol.* 1980;74:153–156.
70. Cabal E, Holtz S. Polyarteritis as a cause of intestinal hemorrhage. *Gastroenterology.* 1971;61(1):99–105.
71. Duffy J, Lidsky MD, Sharp JT, et al. Polyarthritis, polyarteritis, and hepatitis B. *Medicine.* 1976;55(1):19–37.
72. Kuehne SE, Gauvin GP, Shortsleeve MD. Small bowel stricture caused by rheumatoid vasculitis. *Radiology.* 1992;184:215–216.
73. Fauci AS, Haynes BF, Katz P. The spectrum of vasculitis: clinical, pathologic, immunologic, and therapeutic considerations. *Ann Intern Med.* 1978;89:660–676.
74. Mendeloff AI, Shulman LE. Gastrointestinal responses in connective tissue diseases. In: Gamble JR, Wilber DL, eds. *Current Concepts of Clinical Gastroenterology.* Boston, Mass: Little, Brown and Co; 1965:107–123.
75. Weiser MM, Andries GA, Brentjens JR, et al. Systemic lupus erythematosis and intestinal venulitis. *Gastroenterology.* 1981;81(3):570–579.
76. Kelsey PB, Compton CC. Case records of the Massachusetts General Hospital, case 35-1991. *N Engl J Med.* 1991;325:643–651.
77. Rodriguez-Erdmann F, Levitan R. Gastrointestinal and roentgenological manifestations of Henoch-Schönlein purpura. *Gastroenterology.* 1968;54(2):260–264.
78. Rosenberger A, Adler OB, Haim S. Radiological aspects of Behçet disease. *Radiology.* 1982;144:261–264.
79. Churg J, Strauss L. Allergic granulomatosis, allergic angiitis, and periarteritis nodosa. *Am J Pathol.* 1951;27: 277–301.
80. Schoretsanitis GN, Wakley DM, Maddox T, et al. A case of Churg-Strauss vasculitis complicated by small bowel necrosis. *Postgrad Med J.* 1993;69:828–831.
81. Sharma MC, Safaya R, Sidhu BS. Perforation of small intestine caused by Churg-Strauss syndrome. *J Clin Gastroenterol.* 1996;23(3):232–235.
82. Rubin P, Casarette G. A direction for clinical radiation pathology. In: Vaeth JN, ed. *Frontiers of Radiation Therapy and Oncology, 6.* Baltimore, Md: University Park Press; 1972:1–16.
83. Earnest DL, Trier JS. Radiation enteritis and colitis. In: Sleisenger MH, Fordtran JS, eds. *Gastrointestinal Disease.* 4th ed. Philadelphia, Pa: WB Saunders Co; 1989:1369–1382.
84. Anderson RE. Radiation injury. In: Kissane JM, ed. *Anderson's Pathology.* St. Louis, Mo: CV Mosby Co; 1985:239–277.

85. Painter RB. The role of DNA damage and repair in cell killing by ionizing radiation. In: Meyer RE, Withers HR, eds. *Radiation Biology in Cancer Research*. New York, NY: Raven Press; 1980:59–68.
86. Hagemann RF, Sigdestad CP, Lesher S. Intestinal crypt survival and total and per crypt levels of proliferative cellularity following irradiation: fractionated X-ray exposures. *Radiat Res*. 1971;47(1):149–158.
87. White DC. *An Atlas of Radiation Histopathology*. Technical Information Center, Office of Public Affairs, U.S. Energy Research and Development Administration, TID-26676, 1975:141–160.
88. Ackerman LV. The pathology of radiation effect of normal and neoplastic tissue. *AJR*. 1972;114(3):447–459.
89. Khilnani MT, Marshak RH, Eliasoph J, et al. Intramural intestinal hemorrhage. *AJR*. 1964;92:1061–1071.
90. Mendelson RM, Nolan DJ. The radiological features of chronic radiation enteritis. *Clin Radiol*. 1985;36:141–148.
91. Nolan DJ, Herlinger H. Vascular disorders. In: Gore RM, Levine MS, Laufer I, eds. *Textbook of Gastrointestinal Radiology*. Philadelphia, Pa: WB Saunders Co; 1994:967–983.
92. Marston A, Clarke JMF, Garcia JG, et al. Intestinal function and intestinal blood supply: a 20 year surgical study. *Gut*. 1985;26:656–666.
93. Boley S, Brandt LJ, Veith FJ, et al. A new provocative test for chronic mesenteric ischemia. *Am J Gastroenterol*. 1991;86(7): 888–891.
94. Gentile AT, Moneta GL, Lee RW, et al. Usefulness of fasting and postprandial duplex ultrasound examinations for predicting high-grade superior mesenteric artery stenosis. *Am J Surg*. 1995;169:476–479.
95. Li KCP, Whitney WS, McDonnell CH, et al. Chronic mesenteric ischemia: evaluation with phase-contrast cine MR imaging. *Radiology*. 1994;190:175–179.
96. Boley SJ, Brandt LJ. Mesenteric ischemia. In: Baum S, ed. *Abrams' Angiography*. 4th ed. Boston, Mass: Little, Brown and Co; 1997:1615–1635.
97. Lindner HH, Kemprud E. A clinicoanatomic study of the arcuate ligament of the diaphragm. *Arch Surg*. 1971;103: 600–605.
98. Dunbar JD, Molnar W, Beman FF, et al. Compression of the celiac trunk and abdominal angina. *AJR*. 1965;95:731–743.
99. Patten RM, Coldwell DM, Ben-Menachem YB. Ligamentous compression of the celiac axis: CT findings in five patients. *AJR*. 1991;156:1101–1103.
100. Travis RC. Case of the month. An unusual cause of gastrointestinal haemorrhage. *Br J Radiol*. 1987;60:933–934.
101. Salomonowitz E, Staffen A, Potzi R, et al. Angiographic demonstration of phlebectasia in a case of Turner's syndrome. *Gastrointest Radiol*. 1983;8(3):279–281.
102. Foutch PG. Angiodysplasia of the gastrointestinal tract. *Am J Gastroenterol*. 1993;88(6):807–818.
103. Richardson JD, Max MH, Flint LM, et al. Bleeding vascular malformations of the intestine. *Surgery*. 1978: 84(3):430–436.
104. Lewis BS, Kornbluth A, Waye JD. Small bowel tumours: yield of enteroscopy. *Gut*. 1991;32:763–765.
105. Thompson JN, Hemingway AP, McPherson GAD, et al. Obscure gastrointestinal haemorrhage of small-bowel origin. *Br Med J*. 1984;288:1663–1665.
106. Moore JD, Thompson NW, Appelman HD, et al. Arteriovenous malformations of the gastrointestinal tract. *Arch Surg*. 1976;111:381–389.
107. Katon RM, Smith RW. Panendoscopy in the early diagnosis of acute upper gastrointestinal bleeding. *Gastroenterology*. 1973:65:728–734.
108. Moch A, Herlinger H, Kochman ML, et al. Enteroclysis in the evaluation of obscure gastrointestinal bleeding. *AJR*. 1994;163:1381–1384.
109. Boley SJ, Sprayregen S, Sammartano RJ, et al. The pathophysiologic basis for the angiographic signs of vascular ectasias of the colon. *Radiology*. 1977;125:615–621.
110. Singer AA. Value of CT in localizing site of gastrointestinal hemorrhage following negative angiography. *Abdom Imaging*. 1995;20:31–32.
111. Mindelzun RE, Beaulieu CF. Using biphasic CT to reveal gastrointestinal arteriovenous malformations. *AJR*. 1997;168:437–438.
112. Ettorre GC, Francioso G, Garribba AP. Helical CT angiography in gastrointestinal bleeding of obscure origin. *AJR*. 1997;168:727–730.
113. Ramanujam PS, Venkatesh KS, Bettinger L, et al. Hemangioma of the small intestine: case report and literature review. *Am J Gastroenterol*. 1995;90(11):2063–2064.
114. Sutton D, Murfitt J, Howarth F. Gastrointestinal bleeding from large angiomas. *Clin Radiol*. 1981;32(6):629–632.
115. Raden DR, Siskind BN, Alpert S, et al. Small bowel varices due to mesenteric metastasis. *Gastrointest Radiol*. 1986;11:183–184.
116. Agarwal D, Scholz FJ. Small bowel varices demonstrated by enteroclysis. *Radiology*. 1981;140(2):350.
117. Fleming RJ, Seaman WB. Roentgenographic demonstration of unusual extraesophageal varices. *AJR*. 1968;103:281–290.
118. Hansen ME, Coleman RE. Scintigraphic demonstration of gastrointestinal bleeding due to mesenteric varices. *Clin Nucl Med*. 1990;15(7):488–490.
119. Balthazar EJ, Einhorn R. Intramural gastrointestinal hemorrhage. Clinical and radiographic manifestations. *Gastrointest Radiol*. 1976;1:229–239.
120. Griffin PH, Schnure FW, Chopra S, et al. Intramural gastrointestinal hemorrhage. *J Clin Gastroenterol*. 1986; 8(3):389–394.
121. Cox EF. Blunt abdominal trauma. A 5-year analysis of 870 patients requiring celiotomy. *Ann Surg*. 1984;199: 467–474.
122. Christophi C, McDermott FT, McVey I, et al. Seat belt induced trauma to the small bowel. *World J Surg*. 1985;9:794–797.
123. Winton TL, Girotti MJ, Manley PN, et al. Delayed intestinal perforation after nonpenetrating abdominal trauma. *Can J Surg*. 1985;28:437–439.
124. Andrews EW. Pneumatic rupture of the intestine, a new type of industrial accident. *Surg Gynecol Obstet*. 1911;12:63–74.
125. Raptopoulos V. Abdominal trauma. Emphasis on computed tomography. *Radiol Clin North Am*. 1994;32(5): 969–987.

126. Orwig D, Federle MP. Localized clotted blood as evidence of visceral trauma on CT: the sentinel clot sign. *AJR*. 1989;153:747–749.
127. Jeffrey RB, Cardoza JD, Olcott EW. Detection of active intraabdominal arterial hemorrhage: value of dynamic contrast-enhanced CT. *AJR*. 1991;156:725–729.
128. Nghiem HV, Jeffrey RB, Mindelzun RE. CT of blunt trauma to the bowel and mesentery. *AJR*. 1993;160:53–58.
129. Mirvis SE, Gens DR, Shanmuganathan K. Rupture of the bowel after blunt abdominal trauma: diagnosis with CT. *AJR*. 1992;159(6):1217–1221.
130. Rizzo MJ, Federle MP, Griffiths BG. Bowel and mesenteric injury following blunt abdominal trauma: evaluation with CT. *Radiology*. 1989;173(1):143–148.
131. Kane NM, Francis IR, Burney RE, et al. Traumatic pneumoperitoneum. Implications of computed tomographic diagnosis. *Invest Radiol*. 1991;26(6):574–578.

Small Bowel Obstruction

Bernard A. Birnbaum and Dean D.T. Maglinte

Chapter Contents

Introduction
Classification
Clinical Presentation
Clinical Considerations
Plain Film Radiography
Barium Studies
Computed Tomography
Major Causes of Small Bowel Obstruction
Other Causes of Small Bowel Obstruction
Imaging Recommendations

Introduction

Intestinal obstruction is a common clinical entity that often presents with signs and symptoms similar to those seen in other acute abdominal conditions. It is diagnosed in approximately 20% of patients admitted to surgical services with acute abdominal pain.[1,2] The usual site of obstruction is the small bowel, which may be involved in 60% to 80% of cases.[3] The most common causes of small bowel obstruction (SBO) include adhesions, hernias, and neoplasms.[4,5] In past years hernias outnumbered adhesions as causes of obstruction.[6] In contrast, more recent studies have shown that adhesions are responsible for at least 50% to 75% of cases of SBO.[5,7] The relative and absolute increase in the number of cases of adhesive obstruction is due to the increased number of patients undergoing abdominal surgery and early hernia repair in developed countries. This shift in the relative role played by hernias and adhesions is not universal, however, as hernias remain the predominant cause of intestinal obstruction in some underdeveloped countries.[4]

Classification

Intestinal obstruction may be classified into two major categories on the basis of the associated pathophysiology, simple obstruction or closed loop obstruction.[8]

Simple obstruction refers to bowel occlusion at one or more points causing interference with the passage of luminal contents. The blood supply is not directly affected. Luminal distention occurs secondary to continued intestinal secretion, impaired intestinal absorption, and the presence of swallowed air proximal to the point of obstruction. Loops of bowel proximal to the site of obstruction contain more gas than fluid in the early stages of obstruction; dilated bowel is predominantly fluid-filled in later stages of obstruction. The degree of distention will vary depending on the severity, level, and duration of obstruction. Pronounced intestinal distention can occur in acute simple obstruction without vascular compromise. The degree of distention and intraluminal pressure may reach critical levels, however, when obstruction is severe and prolonged. Immediate gastrointestinal tube decompression or surgery may be needed in these cases to prevent ischemic change.

Closed loop or incarcerated intestinal obstruction describes a loop of bowel occluded at two adjacent points along its course, resulting in occlusion of both its afferent and efferent limbs.[8,9] The obstructed loop may be partially or completely isolated from the remainder of the intestinal tract depending on the degree of compression caused by the constricting lesion. The obstructive process characteristically involves both the bowel and its supporting mesentery. Ischemia results from constriction of mesenteric vessels supplying the involved loop and/or the continuous outpouring of fluid into the occluded space, which raises the intraluminal pressure and may rapidly lead to deprivation of blood supply to that segment of bowel. Common etiologies of closed loop obstruction include adhesive bands and both internal and external hernias. These conditions share the ability to constrict the intestine in localized fashion. If the entrapped bowel remains mobile with respect to its fixed obstructed pedicle, it may twist along its long axis and produce a small bowel volvulus. This usually exacerbates the degree of mechanical obstruction and mesenteric ischemia present.[8] Although the term "closed loop obstruction" is construed by most surgeons as indicating a complete, acute obstruction, a closed loop can be only partially obstructed, may not be associated with strangulation, and can resolve spontaneously.[10]

Strangulated obstruction refers to a closed loop obstruction complicated by intestinal ischemia. The obstructing process initially affects the mesenteric venous system, resulting in vascular congestion of the bowel wall and its subtended mesentery. If the obstruction is not relieved, the increased venous pressure is ultimately transmitted to the capillary and arterial beds. The ensuing vascular complications include intramural and mesenteric hemorrhage, intestinal ischemia, infarction, and perforation.[8]

Partial low-grade, partial high-grade, and complete obstructions are terms used to classify the clinical and radiologic severity of SBO in a somewhat subjective fashion. Objective radiologic criteria have recently been defined to help gauge the severity of SBO.[11] These criteria are reviewed in the Enteroclysis section of this chapter.

Clinical Presentation

The classic presenting features of SBO include crampy abdominal pain, distention, vomiting, and obstipation. Abdominal pain occurs early and is typically intermittent and colicky. The pain may subside over time as progressive bowel distention inhibits motility. Constant, severe abdominal pain suggests strangulation.[12] The onset of vomiting and obstipation relate to the location of the obstruction. Vomiting is an early symptom of proximal SBO and occurs later with distal obstruction. In contrast, obstipation may be delayed with proximal obstruction as residual bowel contents may be present distal to the level of obstruction. The degree of obstipation parallels the severity of obstruction, and is most severe in cases of complete SBO.

Acute simple mechanical SBO is typified by abdominal distention with hyperactive, peristaltic bowel sounds detected at abdominal auscultation. Although a silent abdomen may be found in cases of long-standing SBO where dilated loops contain little or no air, absent bowel sounds may also occur with adynamic ileus and infarction.[13] Physical and laboratory evidence of dehydration and electrolyte imbalance may be seen because secreted fluid within the obstructed bowel is unavailable to the circulation.[14] Abdominal tenderness, guarding, and a palpable mass raise the suspicion of strangulating closed loop obstruction. Strangulation is also suggested by the presence of fever, tachycardia, leukocytosis, metabolic acidosis, hyperamylasemia, and signs of peritoneal irritation.[8]

Clinical Considerations

Diagnostic imaging plays a crucial role in the evaluation of patients with suspected intestinal obstruction because of its ability to answer key questions relevant to clinical management.[9] These questions include 1) Is the small bowel obstructed? 2) What is the level, cause, and severity of obstruction? and 3) Is strangulation likely to be present? Once these issues are addressed, the clinician is then able to determine whether medical or surgical management is appropriate.

An important goal of radiologic imaging is to help separate patients with simple mechanical SBO from those with strangulation. Strangulating obstruction occurs in approximately 10% of patients with SBO.[7,8,15] Clinical experience has shown that it is not possible to reliably differentiate between simple and strangulating obstruction on the basis of clinical, laboratory, and plain film findings.[7,8,15–19] In fact, the preoperative diagnosis may be unreliable in 50% to 85% of patients with surgically proved strangulation.[7,15,20–24] Most patients with simple mechanical obstruction do not have complications. Those with incomplete adhesive obstruction can usually be managed conservatively with a trial of intestinal decompression with the knowledge that delay in surgical intervention is acceptable and that the overall mortality rate of adhesive obstruction has been reduced to 1% to 2%.[25–28] The management of patients with suspected complete adhesive obstruction remains controversial.[29] Some surgeons advocate early surgical intervention in these patients based on the high complication rate associated with delayed surgery and fear of missing strangulation.[15,17] These concerns are highlighted by the fact that the morbidity and mortality of strangulating obstruction is markedly higher than that of simple obstruction, with a mortality rate approaching 25%.[1]

Another problem faced by clinicians is the early

recognition of strangulation developing in patients with incomplete SBO.[30,31] It must be emphasized that closed loop obstruction and strangulation are related phenomena but distinct pathologic entities. Clinical differentiation between incomplete adhesive obstruction and the prestrangulation stage of partial closed loop obstruction is rarely possible, and only radiologic imaging can provide a diagnosis at this stage.[3,30–34]

Radiologic imaging also plays a significant role in preoperatively assessing the cause of SBO in patients previously operated on for abdominal malignancy.[9,35] Etiologies for SBO in this patient population include disease progression by residual tumor growth or metastatic seeding, radiation enteropathy, postoperative adhesions, or a combination of these factors. Surgical treatment of SBO caused by metastases is usually palliative in nature. Patient survival is limited by metastatic disease burden; however, quality of life may be improved if obstruction is relieved. Malignant SBO may be due to a single, potentially resectable metastasis, or to carcinomatosis, where only bypass surgery is feasible. The mortality of hospitalized patients who undergo surgery for malignancy-related SBO is considerably higher than that found for lysis of adhesions.[5] Studies have shown that 21% to 38% of patients with a prior history of abdominal malignancy develop adhesive rather than malignant obstruction.[5,36,37] If diagnostic imaging can provide a correct preoperative diagnosis of the cause of SBO in these patients, patient management can be individualized. This enables the surgeon to triage those patients who benefit most from surgery from those who would incur significant operative risk and be better served by conservative management.[3]

Plain Film Radiography

Plain film examination remains the most cost-effective means of initiating the radiologic evaluation of patients with suspected intestinal obstruction.[3] The plain film findings of SBO are reviewed in Chapter 5. The clinical accuracy of diagnosing intestinal obstruction is excellent when patients present with classic symptoms and plain films demonstrate small bowel dilatation with multiple air-fluid levels and paucity of colonic gas and fecal material.[4] The diagnosis becomes problematic when symptoms are not typical and/or the film findings are ambiguous. It has been estimated that plain film findings are diagnostic in 50% to 60% of cases, "equivocal" in about 20% to 30%, and "normal," "nonspecific," or "misleading" in 10% to 20% of cases.[5,8,11,16–18,38]

Diagnostic confusion can also occur due to a lack of clear terminology used in reporting the intestinal gas pattern.[39,40] This is exemplified by the phrase "nonspecific abdominal bowel gas pattern," which a recent survey showed was used by 70% of radiologists.[39] Though most emergency physicians define this term to mean "normal," only 65% of radiologists shared this interpretation.[40] Twenty-two percent of radiologists defined this as "cannot tell if normal or abnormal," while 13% interpreted this as "abnormal but cannot tell if it represents mechanical obstruction or adynamic ileus." A study of plain film radiography of SBO documented that there is a bowel gas pattern that is not "normal" and does not fit the categories of "probable" or "definite" small bowel obstruction.[11,41] This pattern, termed "abnormal but nonspecific," appeared to have clinical implications, as it was identified in 13% of patients with low-grade and 9% of patients with high-grade obstruction. The term "mild small bowel stasis" has recently been proposed to describe this clinically significant intestinal gas pattern.[41]

The role of plain film radiography in the assessment of varying severities of SBO was recently evaluated in a blinded, retrospective study where enteroclysis and clinical outcomes were used as standards of reference.[38] The overall sensitivity and specificity of plain film examination for diagnosing obstruction was found to be 69% and 57%, respectively. The false-positive diagnosis rate was 44% When classified according to severity, plain film radiography correctly identified 86% of high-grade and 56% of low-grade partial obstructions.

The low diagnostic sensitivity of plain film radiography is related to multiple factors. Plain film findings of low-grade partial obstruction may be subtle and nonspecific. High-grade obstruction may be mistaken for a severe "generalized ileus" pattern or missed completely if obstructed loops are predominantly fluid-filled. Interpretive errors are more likely to occur when only subtle evidence of fluid-filled bowel is present (eg, "string of pearls" or pseudotumor sign).[38] In addition, localization of the site of obstruction may be problematic, as both mechanical and functional colonic obstruction can present with small bowel distention and air-fluid levels suggesting SBO.[42,43] The low negative predictive value of a "normal" or "abnormal but nonspecific" bowel gas pattern must be recognized when evaluating patients with suspected intestinal obstruction. A minority of these patients will have high-grade obstruction and, at times, strangulating closed loop obstruction.[3,31,44] If plain film findings do not explain the patient's clinical presentation, additional diagnostic imaging is advised.

Barium Studies

Accumulated experience has shown that barium does not inspissate proximal to the level of a small bowel obstruction and can be safely used to evaluate the level, cause, and severity of obstruction.[44,45] If barium is retained proximal to an obstruction at laparotomy, it can be easily aspirated in its noninspissated state through a small enterotomy. Performance of barium studies through long tubes that can also be used for decompression has made this concern unimportant.[46] Water-soluble iodinated contrast agents are not advocated for evaluating SBO unless bowel perforation is suspected. In this regard, computed tomography (CT) is preferred and water-soluble contrast examination is usually not necessary. Barium is superior to water-soluble contrast media because it adheres to the mucosa, enabling improved assessment of mucosal detail and the cause of obstruction. Moreover, water-soluble agents are hyperosmolar and stimulate outpouring of fluid into the distended bowel lumen. This may aggravate preexisting fluid and electrolyte imbalance, and further compromise radiographic detail by diluting intraluminal contrast.[47] It should be noted that if both barium and CT studies are to be performed, barium should not be administered prior to CT examination, as retained barium in the small bowel will significantly degrade the quality of the CT study. Hence, CT should be performed first, especially in the acute setting.[3]

Barium evaluation of SBO can be performed using either nonintubation or intubation infusion techniques.[9] Nonintubation methods include the retrograde small bowel enema, per ileostomy small bowel enema, and the small bowel follow-through (SBFT). These techniques are described in Chapter 6. The refinements and accuracy of enteroclysis in the diagnosis of small bowel obstruction have made these techniques secondary. The retrograde small bowel enema is a single-contrast technique used to differentiate distal SBO from both intestinal pseudo-obstruction and right-sided colonic obstruction. Per ileostomy small bowel enema is the preferred method for investigating disease suspected to involve the prestomal and neodistal ileum.[9,30] This technique is capable of demonstrating high-grade distal ileal obstruction, but may miss low-grade obstructing lesions due to its inability to adequately distend the bowel lumen proximal to the site of obstruction. The SBFT method is a useful technique when performed with meticulous fluoroscopy, but has known limitations in the setting of SBO.[48–50] In high-grade obstruction, there is often retention of contrast in the stomach with incomplete small bowel opacification. Mucosal detail is usually inadequate because intestinal contrast is diluted by fluid present within dilated bowel proximal to the point of obstruction. Moreover, the duration of an SBFT procedure is directly related to small bowel transit time, and both may be markedly prolonged in cases of high-grade obstruction.

All nonintubation barium methods are inherently limited in their ability to assess bowel distensibility and fixation.[49] As a result, they may not detect partially obstructing lesions, which may produce only fleeting and inconspicuous prestenotic dilatations even when done with the intermittent fluoroscopic method (Fig. 21-1). These limitations are overcome with the intubation infusion technique of examining the small bowel (enteroclysis or the small bowel enema). Enteroclysis is the barium method of choice in SBO because of its ability to challenge the distensibility of the bowel wall and to exaggerate the effect of minimal or subclinical obstructions. Intubation effectively bypasses the stomach, enabling a nondiluted barium bolus to be delivered to the jejunum. Infusion of barium and methylcellulose allows contrast to be propelled in antegrade fashion toward the obstruction despite the presence of diminished bowel peristalsis. The resulting luminal distention facilitates detection of both fixed and nondistensible bowel segments. Even subtle findings, such as the flattening effect of a minimally obstructing adhesive band, appear more pronounced with this technique. Enteroclysis is capable of accurately demonstrating the level and etiology of SBO. In a recent study, enteroclysis correctly predicted the presence of obstruction in 100%, the absence of obstruction in 88%, the level of obstruction in 89%, and the cause of obstruction in 86% of patients.[11]

Enteroclysis Technique in SBO

Details of the enteroclysis technique are provided in Chapter 7. This section reviews the modifications in technique that are made in patients with SBO in order to ensure patient safety and confront the problem of retained fluid present within obstructed bowel.

No bowel preparation is required, though it is generally useful to aspirate as much retained fluid from the bowel as is possible prior to contrast infusion. Premedication with a single dose of metoclopromide (10 to 20 mg IV) for transgastric intubation even in patients with SBO is safe.[51] Preliminary supine and erect plain films are reviewed for an indication of the level and severity of obstruction, and are checked for possible evidence of strangulation or pneumoperitoneum. If plain film radiography suggests high-grade obstruction or the possibility of strangulation is entertained, CT should instead be done if further diagnos-

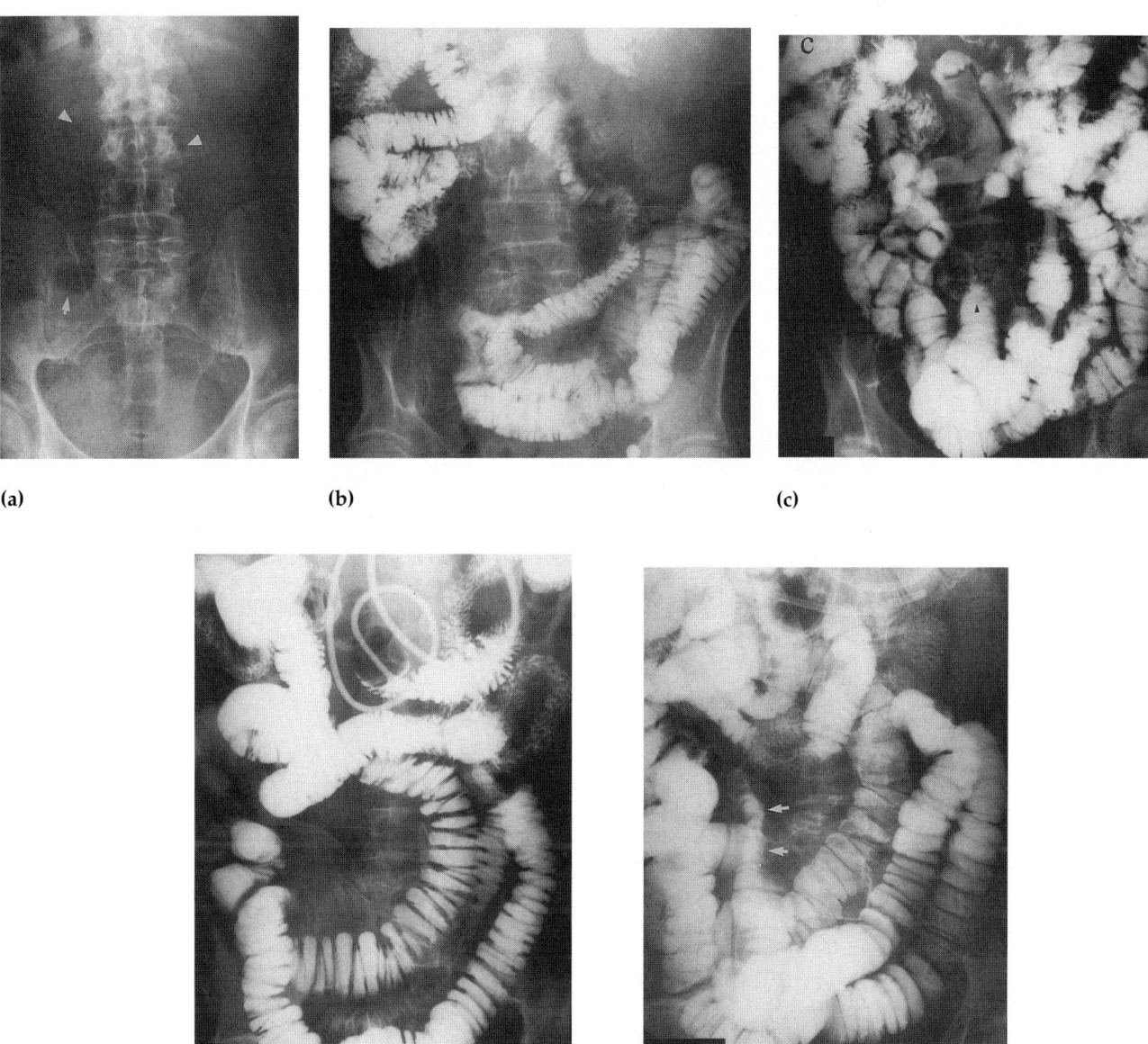

Fig. 21-1. Limitation of nonintubation methods of contrast examination for small bowel obstruction.
(a) Plain film radiography obtained on an elderly male with a history of remote surgery for abdominal aortic aneurysm shows an abnormal but nonspecific gas pattern. Note subtle evidence of fluid-filled small bowel loops ("string of pearls") in upper abdomen obscured by the spine (arrowheads) and mild distention of a loop of small bowel in the right lower abdomen (arrow). (b) Thirty-minute and (c) 60-minute radiograph of a "fluoroscopic" small bowel follow-through was interpreted as unremarkable for obstruction. Fluoroscopy done twice during the 1-hour examination did not show significant obstruction. C = cecum. (d) Single-contrast phase of enteroclysis reveals beginning distention of loops of proximal ileum. Peristalsis of jejunal loops was noted. (e) The point of obstruction was shown to be a long segment of fixed and poorly distensible loop of midileum (arrows). In retrospect, the prestenotic loop can be appreciated in (c) (arrowhead). Prospectively, it was not diagnosed by an experienced fluoroscopist. At surgery, diffuse adhesions with fixation of a loop of ileum to the posterior parietal peritoneum were found.

tic imaging is necessary. The plain film findings suggestive of high-grade obstruction and possible strangulation are described in Chapter 5.

An indwelling Miller-Abbott or Cantor tube can be used for infusion of barium and methylcellulose if the side holes are positioned beyond the duodenojejunal flexure. However, reflux into the stomach occurs because of lack of an antireflux mechanism, and therefore contrast infusion is limited by the amount of gastric reflux (Fig. 21-2). The pressure generated is also

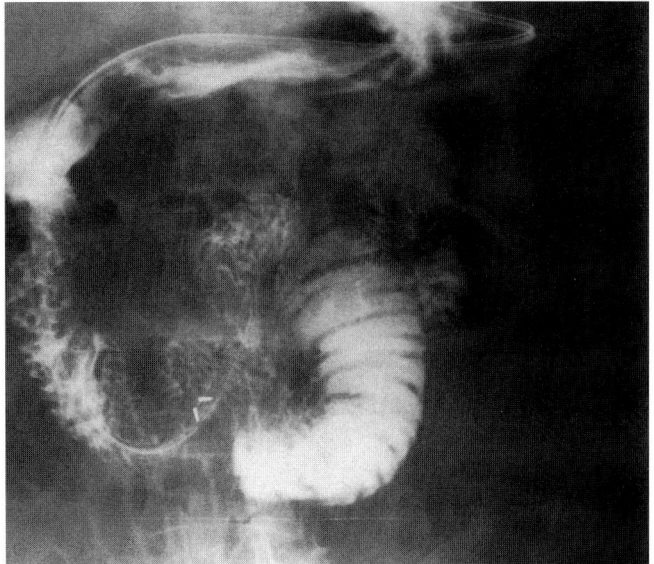 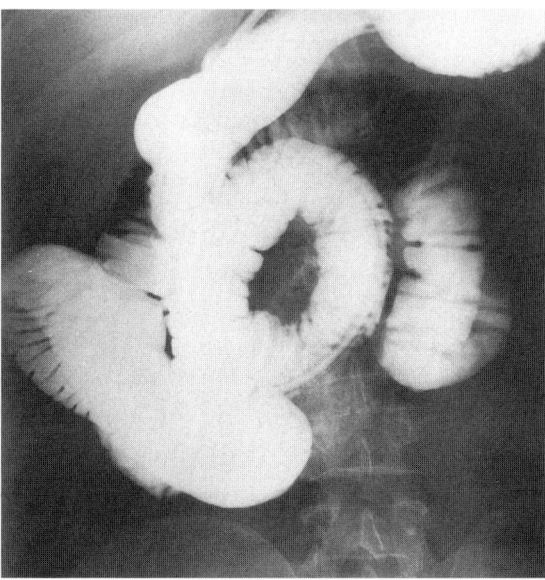

Fig. 21-2. Enteroclysis performed for small bowel obstruction with the use of decompression tubes without an antireflux mechanism.
(a) Infusion of contrast through a nasogastric tube with the tip in the distal horizontal duodenum shows beginning reflux into the stomach. (b) Enteroclysis through a long decompression tube with the tip in the proximal jejunum shows massive reflux into the stomach. This predisposes to aspiration.

suboptimal for adequate distention of the intestinal lumen. A triple-lumen, 14 French, 155-cm-long multipurpose catheter for nasogastric and/or nasoenteric decompression is available for use in patients with SBO (MDEC, Cook Inc., Bloomington, IN), which overcomes the disadvantages of older long tubes for small bowel decompression[46,51] (Fig. 21-3). The initial use of this catheter for gastric decompression instead of the standard 18F Salem sump nasogastric tube spares the patient the trauma of reintubation with the larger standard Salem sump nasogastric tube if further gastric decompression is needed after an enteroclysis is performed or if additional long tube decompression is desired for adhesive obstruction. This tube is better tolerated by patients and, as opposed to other long tubes, can be positioned in the proximal jejunum without difficulty. The main channel is used for either decompression or contrast infusion. The second channel functions as a sump, while the third is used for inflation of a silicone balloon. If fluid is present in the stomach, gastric suction should be done 3 to 12 hours before placement in the jejunum.[51] Proper catheter placement is important, as is frequent monitoring of potential methylcellulose reflux into the stomach, in order to avoid the complications of vomiting and aspiration. Retrograde reflux of contrast may occur in the setting of an inflated enteroclysis balloon if the distended proximal bowel is incompletely occluded. Constant adjustments of the rate of flow are important in the demonstration of low-grade points of obstruction. The aim of adjusting the flow rate is to ensure that the degree of distention of the entire small intestine from jejunum to ileum is uniform. This will ensure that a constant push of the head of the contrast column is present so that mild degrees of luminal narrowing are challenged and prestenotic dilatation or minimal changes in caliber are recognized.[52] A lack of understanding of how the small bowel reacts to varying rates of infusion and luminal distention is usually manifested by an enteroclysis study showing an overly distended jejunum with excessive reflux into the stomach even with a balloon catheter in place and an incompletely distended distal ileum. Obstruction of distal segments of small bowel or of multiple points of obstruction may not be demonstrated when flow rates are inappropriate.

In high-grade obstructions where distended bowel contains a large amount of retained fluid, initial decompression of the stomach and proximal small bowel should be performed. The amount of barium infused will depend on the length of decompressed proximal small bowel. The more peristalsing segments of small bowel are present, the more barium can be infused (250 to 400 ml). Methylcellulose infusion follows unless the amount of retained fluid encountered is excessive. Enteroclysis infusion can usually overcome mild to moderate degrees of bowel hypotonia. In long-stand-

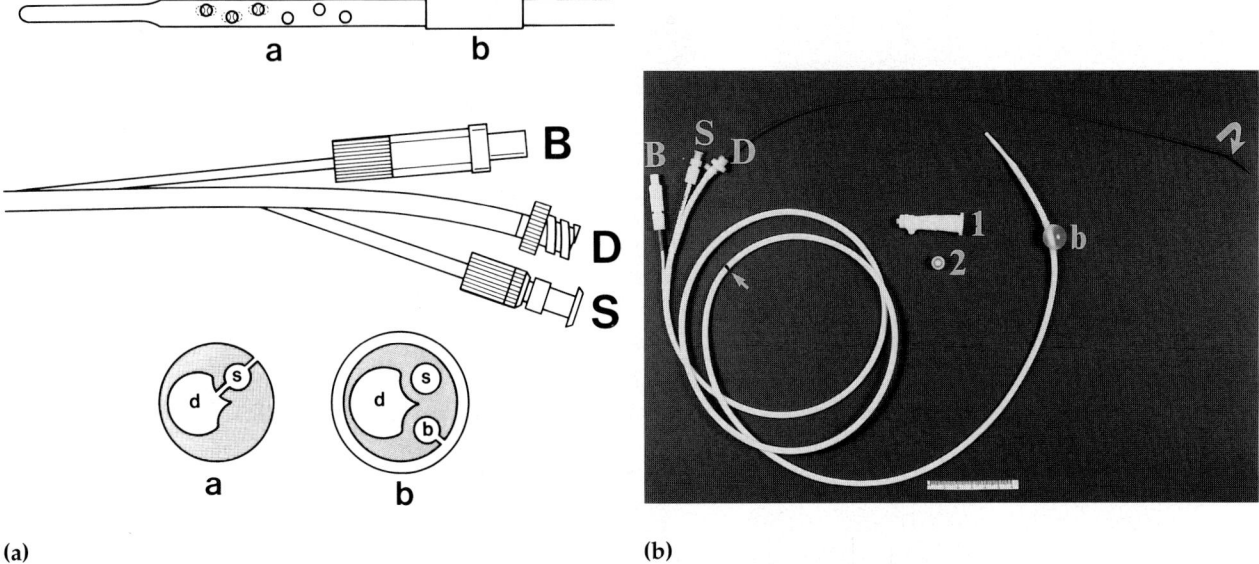

Fig. 21-3. Design and construction of nasogastric/nasoenteric decompression/enteroclysis catheter.
(a) Diagram of internal construction. The uppermost drawing shows the distal end, and the proximal end, and the bottom diagrams are cross sections at levels of distal side ports (a) and at level of balloon attachment (b). The distal side ports (a) in the uppermost drawing connect the intestinal lumen with the sump lumen (s), which in turn communicates with the decompression (suction) lumen (d). The most distal ports (a) are diagrammed to show the longitudinal communication between the sump and decompression (suction) lumina. The side ports communicating with the sump and suction lumina allow flushing from proximal attachment S to clear any blockage of the side ports during decompression. The staggered position of the side ports also helps prevent tissue blockage of the ports during suction. The tapered end results in less nasal mucosal irritation during intubation. The sump lumen (s) is connected externally at S, and the suction lumen is connected at D. The balloon lumen (b), which is provided with a one-way check valve proximally (B), communicates with the circularly disposed silicone balloon (arrow) at level 2. (b) Construction of catheter. The rubber adapter (1) allows connection of decompression lumen (D) to existing suction devices. A small plastic cap (2) prevents fluid from leaking out of the sump port (S) when suction is disconnected. The small external connection to the sump port is labeled "distal air." The balloon shown partially inflated (b) is inflated by first pressing in the balloon inflation opening attachment (B) by the straight tip of a plastic syringe to release the one-way valve in the assembly. The black marker (arrow) indicates the tube tip position in the body of the stomach, which allows the tube to be positioned at bedside, without fluoroscopic guidance. Torque and directional control is provided by a Teflon-coated stainless steel braided torquable guide wire introduced into the suction lumen of the catheter prior to transnasal intubation. The 45-degree angle proximal to the tip (curved arrow) of the 195-cm-long guide wire allows the operator to change the direction of the tube when necessary. (From Maglinte et al[46] with permission.)

ing SBO, however, peristalsis may virtually cease, and the antegrade propulsion of contrast toward the site of obstruction may become very slow. Rates of flow should be slower in higher grades of obstruction, as higher rates will decrease peristalsis further. If this occurs, the study is continued as an intermittent fluoroscopic follow-through.[30] Diagnostic films and/or fluoroscopy may need to be performed 3 to 24 hours later in these patients[30,49] (Fig. 21-4). The long time required to complete the examination in patients with high-grade obstruction is a known limitation of the enteroclysis technique.[3] Residual barium and retained fluid proximal to the obstruction can be decompressed through the decompression/enteroclysis catheter.[51]

Enteroclysis Criteria for Diagnosing SBO

The diagnosis of mechanical small bowel obstruction is made with enteroclysis by demonstrating a transition zone, which is defined as a change in the caliber of the intestinal lumen from a distended segment proximal to the site of obstruction to a segment that is either collapsed or decreased in caliber distal to the obstruction.[3,9,11,30,53] (Fig. 21-5). The level of obstruction is identified during the single-contrast phase of the examination. The cause of obstruction is best seen during the double-contrast phase of the study, when mucosal detail at and above the level of obstruction is optimized. Obstruction is excluded if unimpeded flow of barium

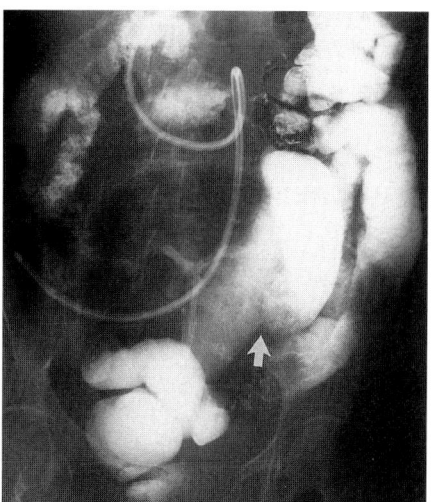

Fig. 21-4. Enteroclysis in high-grade obstruction and the complementary role of CT and enteroclysis.
(a) Supine abdominal radiograph of an elderly female patient who had a history of prior colon surgery for malignancy and recently finished a course of chemotherapy and was referred to our institution for persistent abdominal pain shows distention of small bowel loops (arrows). The plain film findings are consistent with mechanical small bowel obstruction. The nasogastric tube had been in place for 48 hours. (b) CT scan obtained after (a) shows no evidence of a mass at the site of obstruction. The presence of two distended adjacent loops with abrupt transition (arrows) raised the possibility of a closed loop adhesive obstruction. (c) Because the patient refused surgery and physical examination did not show peritoneal signs, an enteroclysis was performed to gauge the severity of obstruction and exclude closed loop obstruction. A long tube replaced the nasogastric tube and additional suction was done for 6 hours to decompress dilated fluid-filled proximal small bowel. Initial infusion of contrast at 50 ml/min shows peristalsis restored in the proximal small bowel. Infusion was stopped when contrast started to reflux proximal to the balloon (arrow). Note contrast diluted by retained fluid in more distal loops (open arrow). (d) Follow-up radiograph at 3 hours demonstrates the point of obstruction (arrow) with no contrast distal to it. (e) Delayed radiograph at 18 hours shows only a small amount of contrast beyond the point of obstruction (arrow) and persistent distention of small bowel despite long tube decompression. Surgery confirmed single-band adhesive obstruction. There was no closed loop.

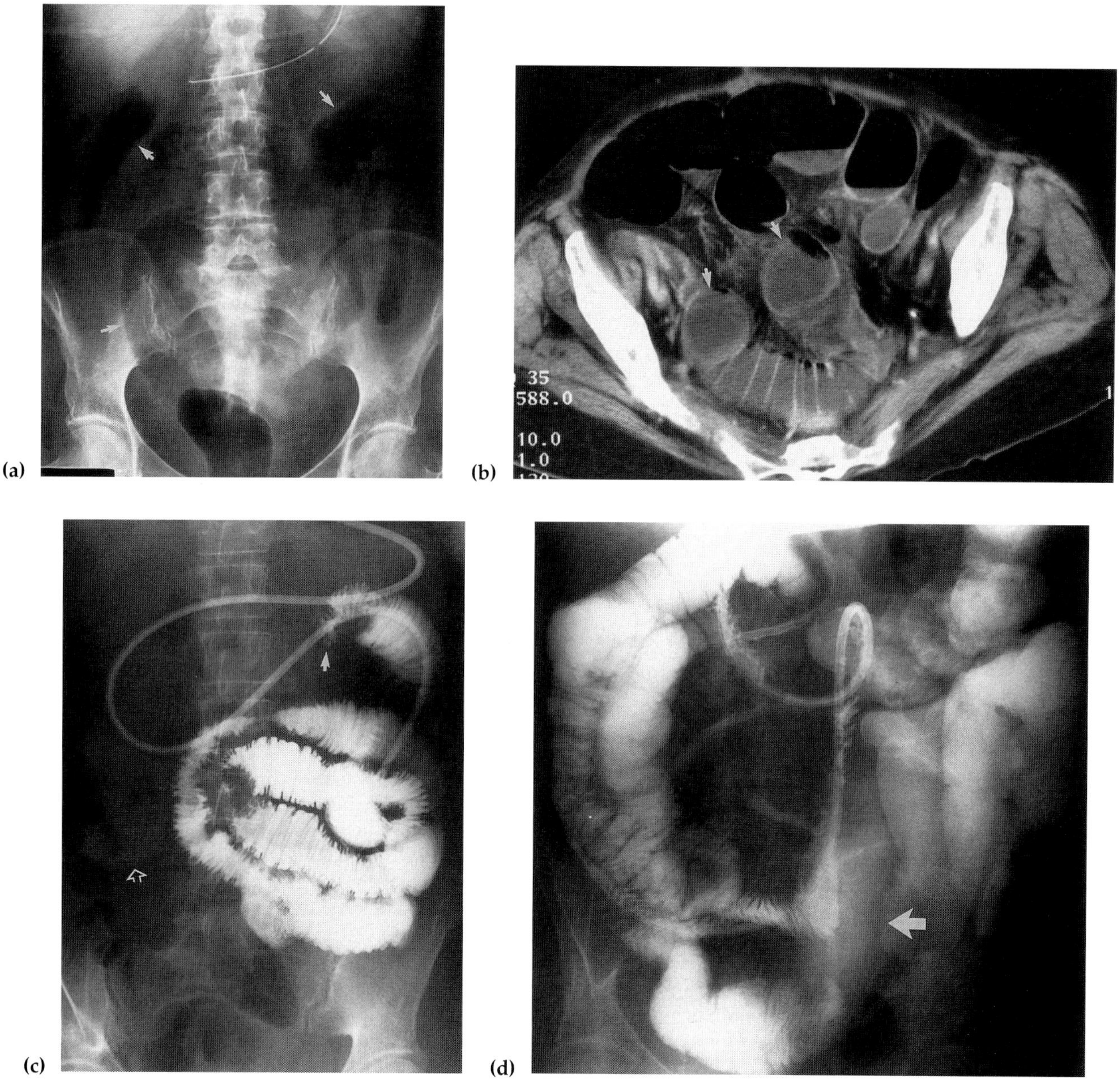

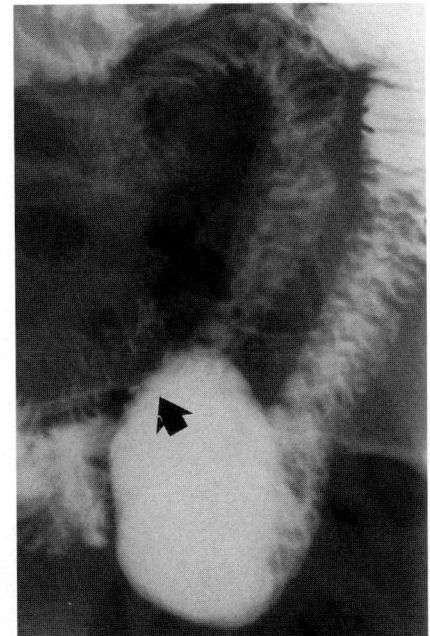 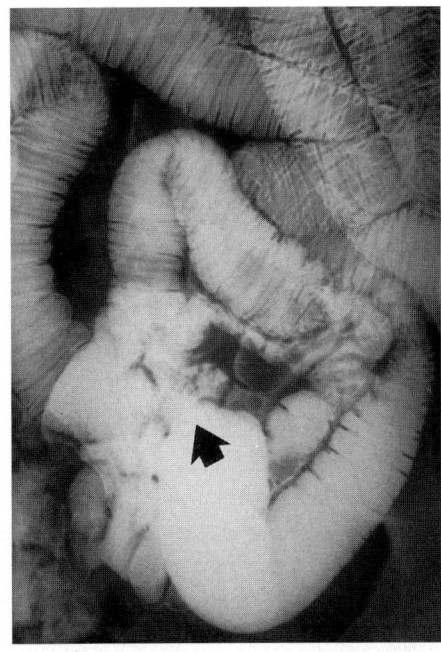

Fig. 21-5. Transition zone.
(a) An abrupt change in caliber (arrow) is seen at the point of obstruction. The distal segment is poorly distended. Note peristalsis of more proximal segments during single-contrast infusion at 55 to 65 ml/min. Arrow indicates direction of flow. (b) Infusion of methylcellulose at a higher rate (70 to 85 ml/min) abolishes peristalsis of proximal segments. The transition point (arrow) remains fixed.

is observed fluoroscopically from the duodenojejunal junction to the ileocecal valve, and if the caliber of the mesenteric small bowel is normal (Fig. 21-6). By enteroclysis criteria, 3 to 4 cm is used as the upper limit for caliber of the jejunal lumen and 2.5 to 3 cm for the ileal lumen.[49] It must be remembered that obstructions can occur synchronously at multiple levels. If dilated, fluid- or gas-filled small bowel loops are encountered distal to a transition zone, additional "downstream" obstructions need to be assessed (Fig. 21-7).

An important advantage of enteroclysis is its ability to objectively gauge the severity of obstruction.[3,11,53] Low-grade partial SBO is diagnosed when there is no delay in the arrival of contrast material at the site of the transition zone and sufficient flow of contrast material occurs through the point of obstruction into the postobstructive loops to enable visualization of the intestinal fold pattern. High-grade partial SBO is diagnosed when there is stasis and delay in the arrival of contrast material at the site of obstruction. This is associated with dilution of contrast material within the distended prestenotic loop and minimal passage of contrast into collapsed postobstructive loops, making it difficult to define the fold pattern. Complete obstruction is diagnosed when there is no passage of contrast material beyond the point of obstruction as shown on delayed radiographs obtained up to 24 hours after the start of the examination.[11,53]

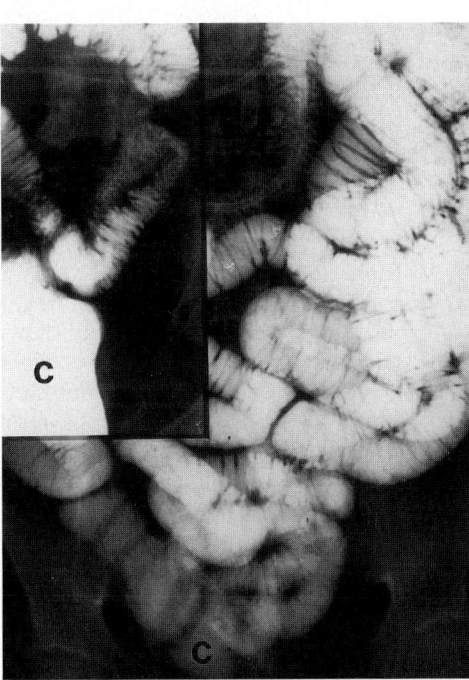

Fig. 21-6. Enteroclysis exclusion of mechanical small bowel obstruction.
There is unimpeded flow of contrast from jejunum to cecum (C). This is best done during single-contrast infusion. Angled compression (inset) radiograph of pelvic segments shows movable pelvic segments of ileum, which excludes nonobstructive pelvic adhesions.

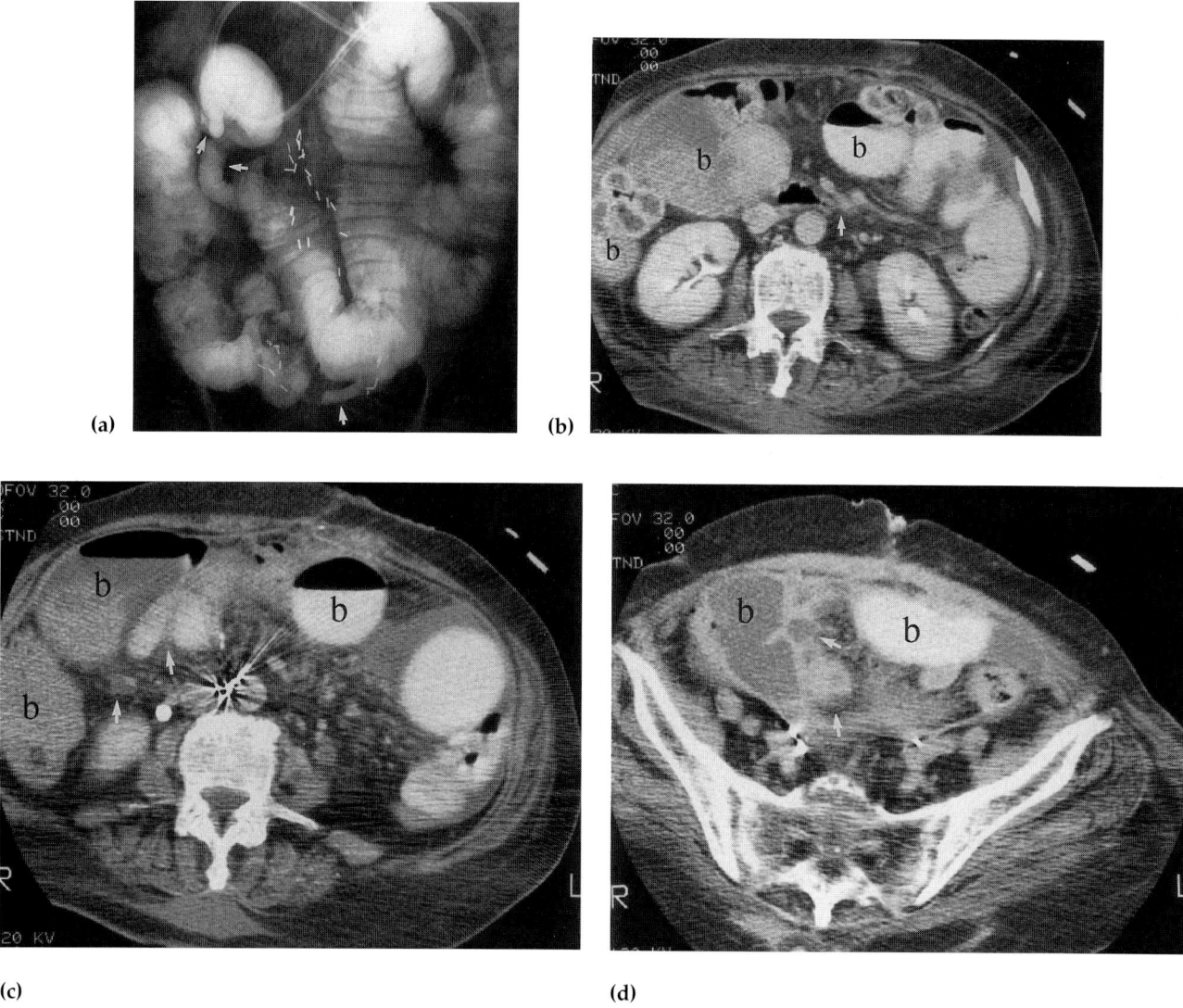

Fig. 21-7. Multiple sites of obstruction.
(a) Enteroclysis of an elderly female with recurrent small bowel obstruction shows multiple radiation strictures (arrowheads). The first obstructing stricture is better shown than the more distal strictures in the pelvis. Note dilated segments distal to the strictures suggesting the presence of multiple points of obstruction. (b) Midabdominal, (c) lower abdominal, and (d) pelvic CT scans demonstrate CT features of multiple points of obstruction. Presence of normal caliber or collapsed loops (arrow) between distended loops of small bowel (b) should suggest the possibility of multiple sites of obstruction. Note contrast-filled more proximal distended small bowel and fluid-filled distal distended loops separated by normal-caliber contrast or fluid-filled intervening loops.

Computed Tomography

Clinical experience over the past decade has shown the importance of CT in the evaluation of patients with suspected intestinal obstruction. CT has several inherent advantages over enteroclysis in this clinical setting: 1) it is readily available; 2) it does not require the technical expertise needed for enteroclysis intubation and interpretation; 3) the examination is not limited in cases of complete or high-grade obstruction because it does not depend on propulsion by small bowel peristalsis; 4) it is noninvasive; and 5) it provides a global assessment of the entire abdomen in addition to the gastrointestinal tract.[3]

The ability of CT to diagnose SBO is related to the severity of obstruction. Initial CT studies revealed sensitivities of 90% to 96%, a specificity of 96%, and accuracy of 95%.[54,55] These promising results were due, in part, to selection bias, as the study cohorts were composed mostly of patients with high-grade obstruction. In a study of patients with varying severity of obstruction, CT showed a sensitivity of 81% for high-grade SBO but only 48% for low-grade SBO.[53] CT had an overall sensitivity of 63%, a specificity of 78%, and an accuracy of 65% in this report.

Studies have demonstrated that CT is able to correctly predict the cause of obstruction in 73% to 95% of cases.[3,53–56] The potential of CT to differentiate SBO from other causes of bowel distention has also been explored. Recent investigations have shown that CT correctly distinguished intestinal obstruction from postoperative ileus or other causes of small bowel dilatation in 84% to 100% of cases.[57,58] CT is now accepted as the imaging modality of choice in the acute clinical setting because of its ability to define the presence and etiology of SBO, and to reliably diagnose other acute abdominal conditions that can mimic obstruction.[3]

CT Technique in SBO

The principles of CT scanning are reviewed in Chapter 9. Preliminary plain films and CT scout radiographs should be carefully reviewed to localize the possible site of obstruction. Contrast-enhanced, thin-section images (4 to 5-mm collimation) should be prospectively acquired through the level of obstruction. Helical scan acquisition is suggested, as this will allow generation of high-resolution reformatted images from overlapping image data sets. Reformatted images may be particularly useful in visualizing the transition zone and analyzing complicated cases of closed loop obstruction. If the transition zone is poorly seen, delayed thin-section images should be acquired through its suspected location. This may allow demonstration of subtle stenoses and serosal implants that may have been initially overlooked.

The need for small bowel opacification remains controversial in patients with high-grade SBO. Retained intestinal fluid proximal to the site of obstruction serves as an inherent contrast agent in these patients.[3] Furthermore, diminished bowel peristalsis may make it impractical to wait for contrast to reach the level of obstruction. Oral contrast is advised in lesser grades of obstruction. Contrast media may be administered via a decompression tube when oral administration is not feasible. Water-soluble iodinated solutions should be used if the possibility of perforation exists.

As a nonintubation technique, CT is limited in its ability to assess bowel distensibility and fixation. CT enteroclysis is a new imaging method that was recently developed to overcome these limitations and to improve the sensitivity of CT for detecting low-grade intestinal obstruction[59] (Fig. 21-8). In this technique, dilute water-soluble contrast is infused first fluoroscopically and then under CT guidance. Preliminary results appear promising, with a site-specific sensitivity and specificity of 82% and 88%, respectively, for low-grade partial SBO. Additional clinical experience is needed to validate these results and to define the potential role of this new technique.

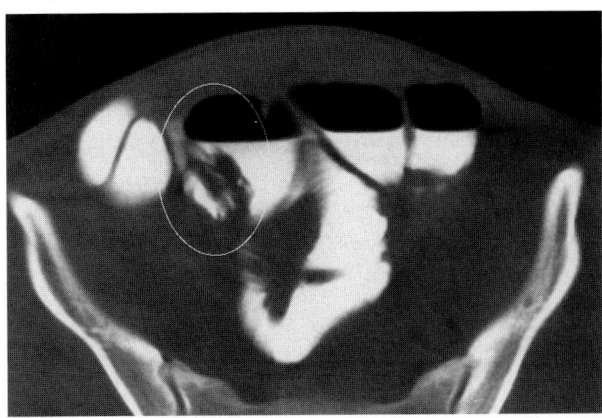

Fig. 21-8. CT enteroclysis in low-grade partial mechanical small bowel obstruction.
The effect of infusion is shown by the clear demonstration of the transition point (encircled). The dilated loops proximally stand out compared to the collapsed distal segment. (Courtesy of Greg Bender, MD.)

CT Criteria for Diagnosing SBO

The CT diagnosis of small bowel obstruction is based on the detection of a definite transition zone between dilated fluid- and/or air-filled small bowel loops located proximally and collapsed loops of small bowel or colon located distal to the site of obstruction[44,53–55] (Fig. 21-9). Collapsed small bowel loops should always be present distally except in cases of obstruction that occur at the ileocecal valve. The distended proximal bowel and collapsed distal bowel should appear as continuous segments when viewed on sequential images.[57] The degree of small bowel dilatation is an unreliable criterion for obstruction. Marked small bowel distention can be present in cases of nonobstructive ileus. The distal small bowel may be of a narrower caliber in pseudo-obstruction of the small bowel. The most important finding is the presence of a transition zone. The greater the discrepancy in size between the dilated proximal bowel and collapsed distal bowel, the more reliable the CT diagnosis.[44]

No objective CT criteria presently exist to gauge the severity of SBO. If oral contrast is present within collapsed loops distal to the site of obstruction, the obstruction is presumed to be partial. Absence of contrast in collapsed distal bowel does not imply that obstruction is complete. Contrast may not have reached, or passed beyond, the transition zone at the time the study was performed in cases of high-grade partial obstruc-

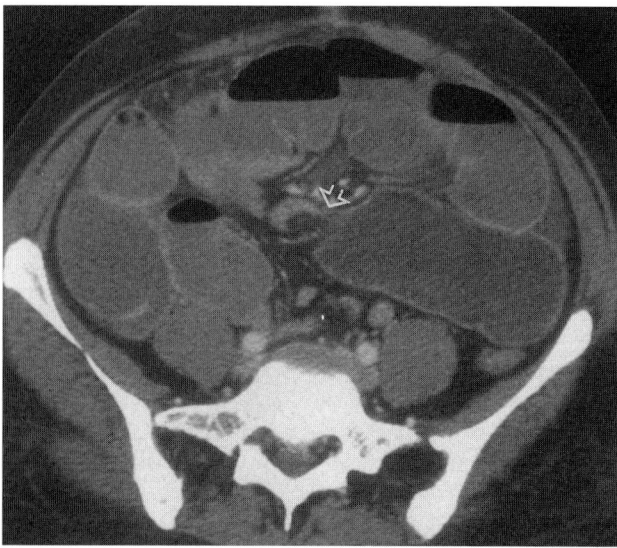

Fig. 21-9. High-grade small bowel obstruction due to surgically proved adhesive band.
CT scan shows dilated, fluid-filled small bowel extending to the transition zone (arrow). No obstructing mass is seen at the site of obstruction. Note the abrupt change in luminal caliber from dilated to collapsed bowel.

Limitations of CT in diagnosing small bowel obstruction relate to multiple factors.[3,44,53–58] CT is relatively insensitive in diagnosing low-grade partial SBO. Identifying the transition zone can be difficult as a result of confusion in following bowel loops in and out of the axial plane.[60] Cine paging may be helpful.[61] The diagnosis of obstruction is more difficult to make in patients who have a gradual rather than an abrupt transition zone. This is particularly true in patients who have undergone prior intestinal decompression. Patients with obstruction at the level of the ileocecal valve who have residual fecal contents in the colon may be mistakenly diagnosed as having nonobstructive ileus. Moreover, the level of obstruction may be incorrectly diagnosed if one erroneously assumes that distal small bowel loops are always displayed on pelvic scans.[54] Obstructed intestinal loops often align themselves in a linear fashion parallel to the long axis of the small bowel mesentery. Proximal jejunal loops may be displaced into the pelvis, while distal ileal loops may be present within the upper abdomen.

Major Causes of Small Bowel Obstruction

The causes of SBO are multiple and can be classified in three major categories: extrinsic, intrinsic, and intraluminal.[30] A representative list of these causes is presented in Table 21-1. Many of these conditions are discussed elsewhere in the text. Some of the most common and important etiologies of small bowel obstruction are reviewed below.

tion. On occasion, semisolid particulate matter that resembles the appearance of fecal material may be present within an obstructed small bowel loop immediately proximal to the transition zone. This finding is usually only seen in high-grade or complete obstructions and is helpful in identifying the site of obstruction.

Table 21-1. Small bowel obstruction in adults

Extrinsic lesions		Intrinsic lesions	
Adhesions	Diaphragmatic (traumatic)	Tumors infiltrating	Hematoma
Hernias	Transomental	intestinal wall	Post-traumatic
External	Iliac fossa	Adenocarcinoma	Anticoagulants
Inguinal	Mesenteric tumor masses	Carcinoid	Henoch-Schönlein purpura
Femoral	Peritoneal metastasis	Lymphoma (rare)	Intraluminal causes
Incisional	Carcinoid	Leiomyosarcoma (rare)	Intussusception
Umbilical	Desmoid	Inflammatory conditions	Tumor
Spigellian	Lymphoma	Crohn's disease	Adhesions
Sciatic	Abscess	Tuberculosis	Duplication
Perineal	Appendicitis	Potassium chloride	Inverted Meckel's
Obturator	Diverticulitis	stricture	diverticulum
Supravesical	Pelvic inflammatory	Eosinophilic	Jejunostomy tube
Lumbar	disease	gastroenteritis	Obturation
Internal	Crohn's disease	Vascular	Gallstone
Transmesenteric	Aneurysm	Radiation enteropathy	Bezoar
Paraduodenal	Hematoma	Ischemia	Foreign body
Epiploic foramen	Endometriosis	Vasculitis	Ascaris
			Meconium

Source: From Herlinger and Rubesin,[30] with permission.

Adhesive Obstruction

Adhesions now account for the majority of cases of intestinal obstruction. Approximately 80% to 90% of adhesions arise after laparotomy, 10% to 15% are due to inflammation, and the remainder are believed due to congenital or unexplained causes.[62] Adhesive obstructions may be classified into those caused by single bands, those caused by multiple bands, and extensive adhesions.[9,35] The clinical relevance of this classification system is that single band obstruction is associated with higher grades of SBO, is more likely to lead to closed loop obstruction, and is associated with strangulation or focal necrosis from band necrosis. Multiple band adhesive obstruction is most likely to respond to conservative intestinal tube decompression.

The characteristic enteroclysis findings of single band obstruction include: 1) an abrupt change in caliber from dilated proximal bowel to collapsed distal bowel occurring at the site of the adhesion, 2) normal or stretched mucosal folds within the proximal, prestenotic segment, and 3) a well-marginated, straight or curvilinear edge at the site where the fibrous band crosses the bowel lumen. If the intestine is well opacified, a narrow bandlike lucency may be seen crossing the bowel, representing the compressed segment with flattened or crowded folds[9,35] (Fig. 21-10). The bowel typically appears fixated at the site of ob-

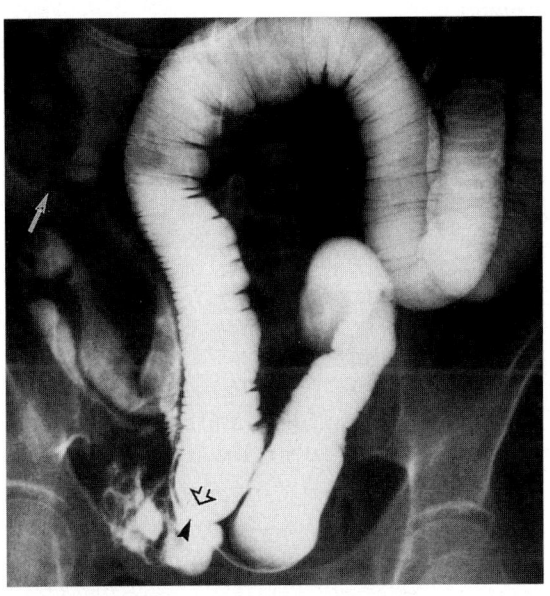

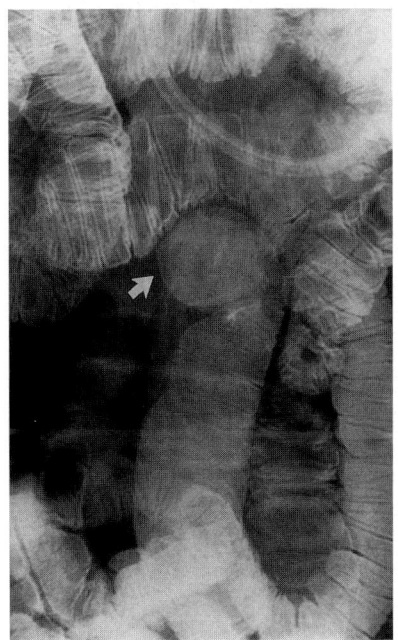

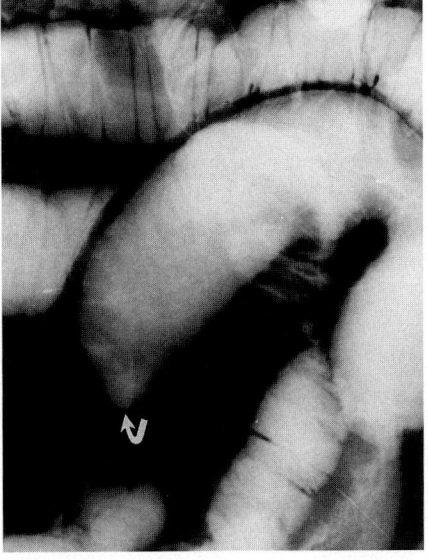

Fig. 21-10. Single-band adhesive obstruction.
(a) Typical smooth well-defined transition point (arrowhead) secondary to an adhesive band with low-grade partial obstruction in a patient with a history of possible recurrent Crohn's disease. Arrow indicates site of ileocolic anastomosis from prior surgery. Open arrow indicates direction of flow. (b) High-grade obstruction secondary to a single-band adhesion showing characteristic smooth transition point (arrow). Note retained fluid proximal to obstruction making folds poorly discernible. (From Maglinte et al,[38] with permission.) (c) "Cobra head" shape of adhesive band obstruction (curved arrow). This usually denotes an attempt by peristalsis to overcome the point of obstruction.

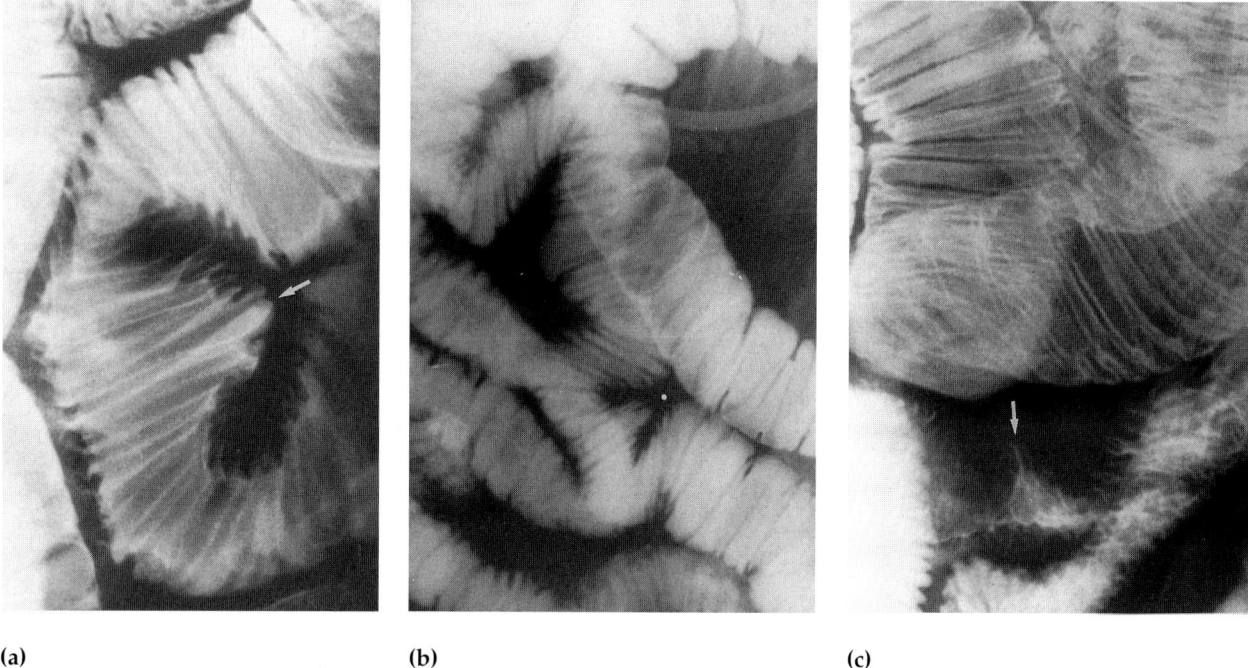

Fig. 21-11. Mesenteric or interloop adhesions.
(a) Compression radiograph of a loop of jejunum involved by mesenteric adhesions shows pseudosacculation (arrow) and tethering of folds along the mesenteric border. (b) Nonobstructive mesenteric adhesion manifested as fixation of mesenteric margins to a central point (.). (c) Mesenteric adhesion with low-grade partial obstruction. There is fixation and decreased distensibility of a loop of bowel with tethering of folds (arrow) along the mesenteric margin. The small bowel proximally is distended. This can mimic a mesenteric mass with a desmoplastic response.

struction. If the obstruction is complete, the bandlike lucency will not be appreciated and only the proximal dilated bowel can be seen extending to the straight or curvilinear edge cutoff. Diagnostic sensitivity for detecting adhesions is maximized with enteroclysis, as this is the only radiologic technique that can demonstrate the compressive effect of minimally obstructing adhesive bands.[63] Interloop or mesenteric adhesions are shown to best advantage by enteroclysis technique (Fig. 21-11).

The findings of multiple band obstruction are related to adhesion formation at the undersurface of an abdominal incision (Fig. 21-12). The enteroclysis findings consist of several narrow constrictions that are often close together. The affected segment has normal intestinal folds and approximates the anterior abdominal wall.[9,35] In contrast, patients with extensive adhesion formation typically have a history of aortic or retroperitoneal nodal surgery and develop posteriorly located adhesions that affect a longer segment of bowel. Several appearances may be seen. The bowel may appear flattened against the posterior abdomen, may be deformed and posteriorly located, or may demonstrate asymmetric involvement where lumen distensibility and fold separation are smoothly but unilaterally restricted.[9,35] This may also develop anteriorly following abdominal surgery or in the pelvis following gynecologic operations (Fig. 21-13).

The CT diagnosis of adhesive obstruction is a diagnosis of exclusion, as adhesive bands are usually inapparent with cross-sectional imaging.[3,53–58] Scans may demonstrate a focal region of beaklike or circular narrowing at the transition zone; however, the actual adhesion is rarely seen. Most commonly, scans reveal evidence of SBO without a causative lesion at the site of obstruction (see Fig. 21-9). In studies where adhesions were presumed to be the etiology of obstruction when an obstructive lesion was not identified, CT correctly predicted the cause of obstruction in 73% to 95% of cases.[3,53–56] The CT differential diagnosis of SBO without apparent cause includes obstruction due to adhesions (most common), small primary tumors, minimal tumor recurrence, and short inflammatory or ischemic strictures. Enteroclysis is complementary to CT in this setting and is indicated if the severity or exact etiology of obstruction must be determined[3] (see Fig. 21-14).

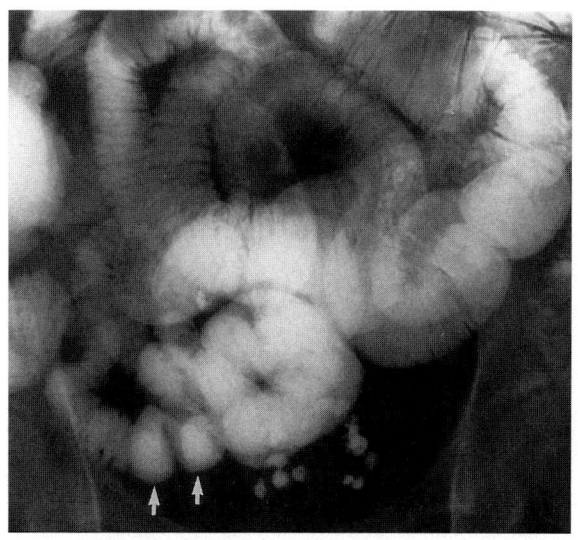 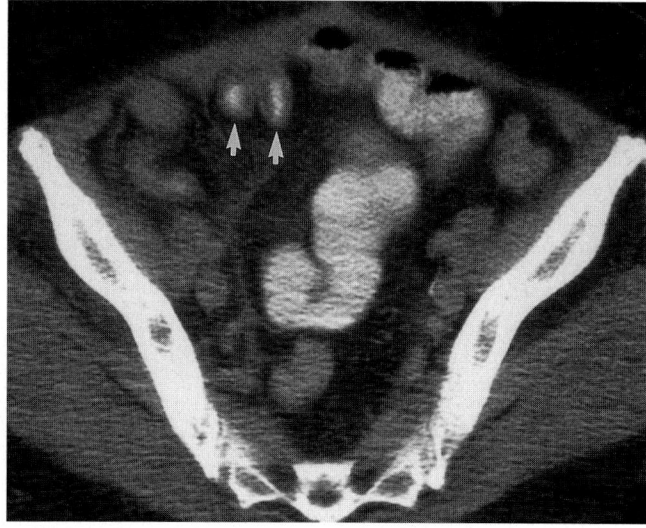

Fig. 21-12. Multiple band adhesion.
(a) Enteroclysis shows low-grade partial obstruction secondary to fixed, kinked loops of small bowel (arrow) in right hemipelvis. (b) CT shows the fixed loops of small bowel with decreased caliber and slightly thickened walls (arrowheads) to be adhesive disease to the anterior parietal peritoneum below an abdominal incision site from prior pelvic surgery. (From Maglinte et al,[38] with permission.)

Obstruction by Peritoneal Metastases

Enteroclysis plays an important role in the evaluation of intestinal obstruction in patients previously operated on for abdominal malignancy. In a study of such patients who presented with symptoms of partial SBO, enteroclysis was approximately 85% accurate in distinguishing adhesions from metastases, tumor recurrence, and radiation enteropathy.[35] The differentiation of metastases from adhesions in the setting of SBO is based on an understanding of the pathophysiologic features of seeded peritoneal metastases.

Seeded peritoneal metastases preferentially implant on the serosal surface of bowel loops that are located in the dependent parts of the mesentery and peritoneal cavity or are related to the ruffles of the mesentery.[64] This pattern of serosal implantation is determined by the natural flow of ascitic fluid within the peritoneal recesses. Serosal metastases most frequently occur in the right lower quadrant, along the mesenteric border of distal ileal loops and the medial wall of the cecum, and in the pelvis. Seeded metastases may cause obstruction by desmoplastic reaction, by intraluminal protrusion, or by the combined effect of their multiplicity.[65,66]

The enteroclysis features of seeded metastases are presented in greater detail in Chapter 19. Metastases that cause SBO typically demonstrate extrinsic mass effect with tethering of mucosal folds in and near the narrowed segment. The infiltrated folds may appear stretched or "tacked down." When viewed in profile, metastatic infiltration and fixation of folds at the affected bowel surface are accentuated by a divergence of folds toward the unaffected side.[9,65,66] In contrast to the well-marginated, smooth, straight proximal edge seen with adhesive obstruction (Fig. 21-14), obstructions by metastases tend to show a more rounded, angular, and somewhat irregular demarcation against the proximal dilated segment (Fig. 21-15). The stenotic segment is often longer than that seen with adhesive bands, and its mucosal folds may be narrowed by apparent mass effect along the mesenteric border. In contrast to the ill-defined distal demarcation of an adhesive obstruction, the distal margin in a metastatic obstruction is usually clearly defined, rounded, and associated with tethered folds.[30] Advanced cases of bowel infiltration may eventually produce tight, annular lesions with narrow, stringlike channels that are associated with desmoplastic kinking and angulation.[9,30,65,67] Invasion of the mucosa is a late feature that presents as ulceration or irregular distortion of the mucosal pattern.

Enteroclysis differentiation of multiple band obstruction from obstruction due to multiple metastases is usually not a problem. The multiple bands will appear grouped together adherent to the anterior abdominal wall, while the metastatic implants will appear loosely clustered in the ileocecal region and demonstrate the typical findings of mesenteric serosal

482 • 21. Small Bowel Obstruction

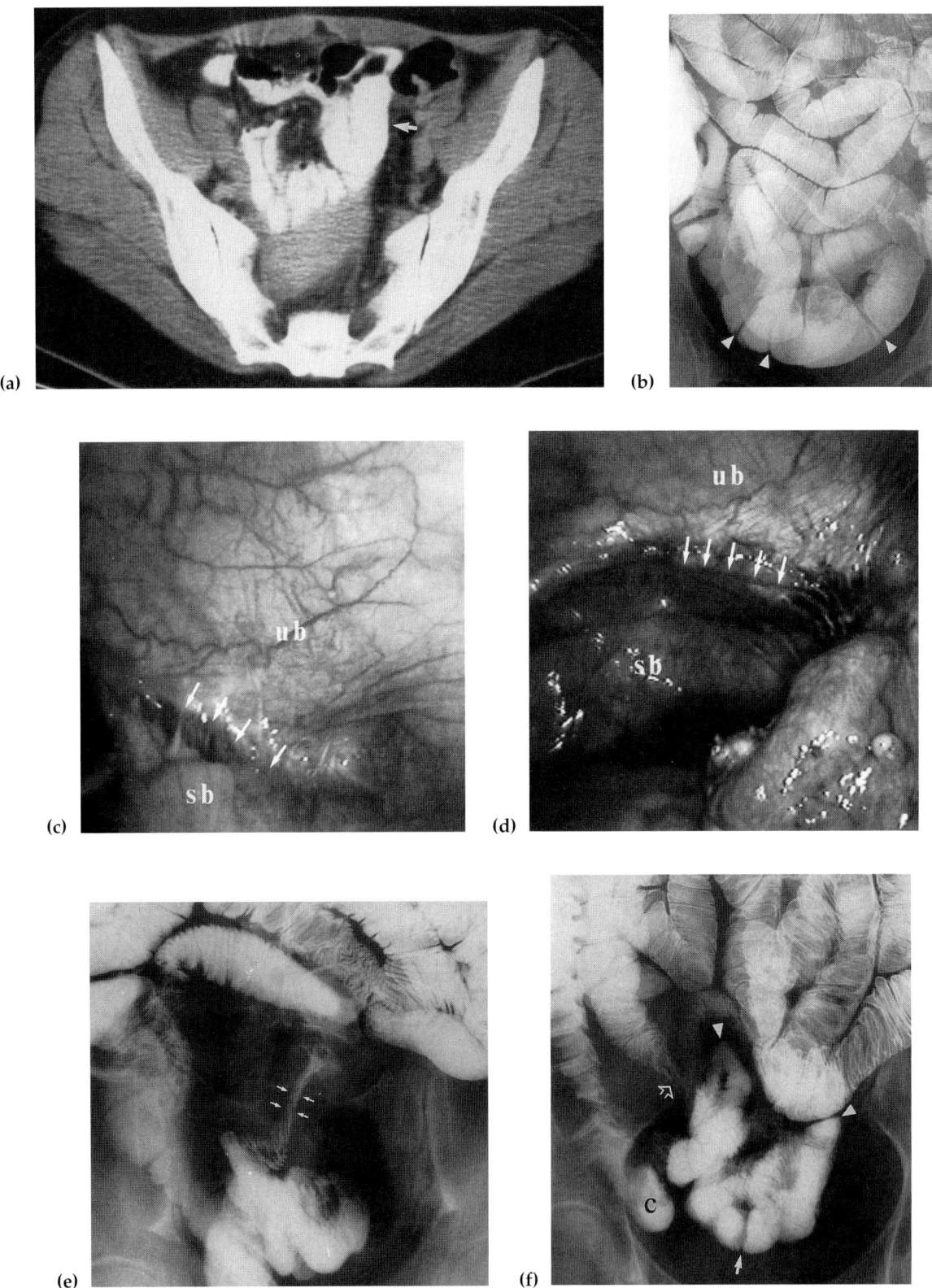

Fig. 21-13. Diffuse adhesive disease.
(a) CT image at the level of the dome of the urinary bladder of a middle-aged woman with prior hysterectomy who presented with unexplained recurrent abdominal pain shows multiple loops of pelvic ileum crowded at the bladder dome. A slightly dilated proximal loop (arrow) is present. (b) At enteroclysis, the pelvic segments were not movable using angled (cephalad) compression during fluoroscopy done in the single-contrast phase of the study. Note scattered areas of peritoneal adhesions manifested during double-contrast enteroclysis as multiple linear defects (arrowheads) secondary to adhesive band fixation. (c) Print obtained during laparoscopy shows small bowel (sb) fixed to vaginal cuff and posterior wall of urinary bladder (arrows) by diffuse adhesions. (ub = urinary bladder.) (d) Following laparoscopic lysis of adhesions, the small bowel (sb) has dropped away from the vaginal cuff and urinary bladder. The cul-de-sac (arrow) can now be seen. The ovaries and Fallopian tube are seen to the right of the small bowel. (From Maglinte et al,[50] with permission.) (e) Low-grade partial obstruction secondary to diffuse anterior peritoneal adhesions involving a long segment of small bowel (arrows). The patient had a history of recent ventral herniorrhaphy. (f) Low-grade partial obstruction secondary to diffuse pelvic adhesions. There is fixation and diminished caliber of pelvic segments with minimal distention of proximal loops. The point of obstruction is marked by the open arrow. Abrupt angulations are noted (arrowheads) and an adhesive band (arrow) is seen in the inferior aspect. C = cecum.

---

implantation.[9] It may be difficult for enteroclysis to differentiate obstruction due to extensive adhesion formation from malignant obstruction. CT is complementary to enteroclysis in these cases because of the ability of CT to directly visualize the serosal surface of the bowel as well as the extraintestinal disease components (Fig. 21-16).

Metastatic obstruction is diagnosed with CT when a solid or cystic mass is evident along the serosa of the bowel at the transition zone[54] (Fig. 21-17). Mural thickening may be seen adjacent to the peritoneal nodule. Secondary findings include loculated ascites, soft-tissue studding along the surface of the mesentery, peritoneal and omental implants, focal thickening of the peritoneal surfaces, adenopathy, and metastases to the solid abdominal organs.[68]

Radiation Enteropathy

Chronic radiation enteritis develops in approximately 5% of patients treated with doses of radiation in the range of 4500 to 5000 cGy.[69] Symptoms may begin months to decades after therapy and are often initially confused with tumor recurrence or adhesive obstruction. The underlying pathologic process is an endarteritis obliterans with secondary compromise to the microvascular circulation of the bowel.[70] The pelvic ileal loops are most commonly affected because the terminal ileum is relatively fixed by its short mesentery and pelvic loops are often within, or in close proximity to, pelvic radiation ports. SBO in these patients may result from either luminal narrowing and dysmotility, or adhesions related to radiation serositis.[70]

Imaging abnormalities may be observed within a few weeks, even in patients without symptoms. Plain abdominal radiographs will often show an ileus pattern, and thickened folds may be apparent (Fig. 21-18). Local hypermotility secondary to anoxia is the earliest finding on contrast examination. This may be the only finding in mild cases of radiation enteropathy (Fig. 21-19). Later hyperemia and edema that are localized mainly to the mucosa and submucosa are shown on contrast examination as thickened, straight folds separated by narrow, compressed-looking interfold spaces.[70] Associated with the fold thickening and part of the same process is thickening of the bowel wall in excess of the 2-mm norm. Straight, thick folds imply a submucosal process, caused by fibrosis and edema (Fig. 21-20). This pattern is not often totally symmetric. Areas of more intense submucosal change

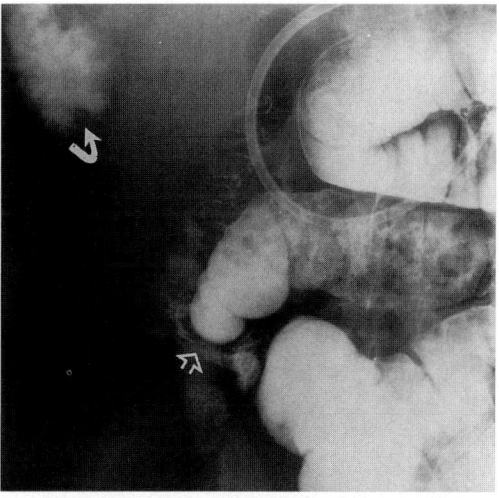

Fig. 21-14. Adhesive band obstruction in a patient with known abdominal carcinomatosis from ovarian malignancy.
The enteroclysis appearance (open arrow) is typical of an adhesive band. Note calcified metastasis (curved arrow) in liver. (From Maglinte et al,[102] with permission.)

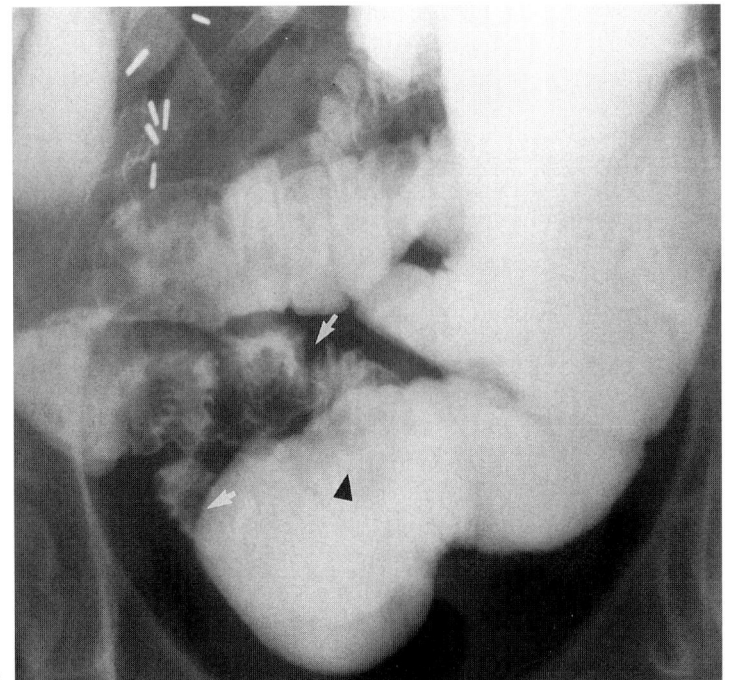
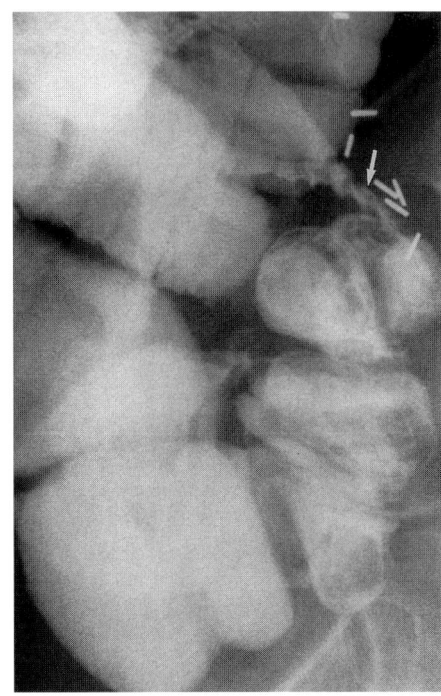
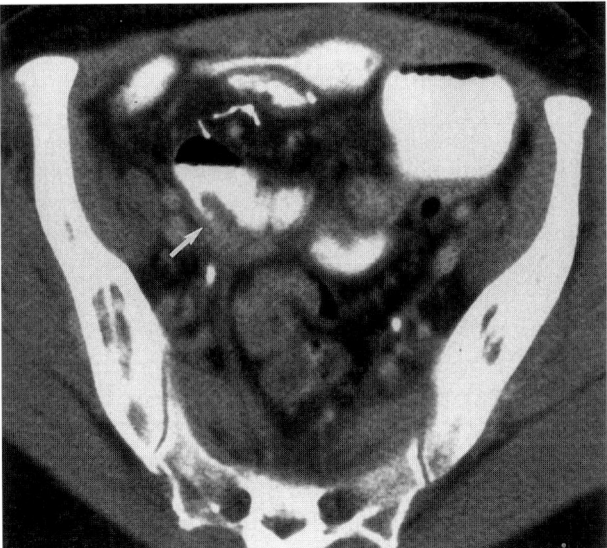

Fig. 21-15. Seeded ovarian metastases with secondary obstruction.
(a) Frontal radiograph during enteroclysis infusion shows partial obstruction (arrow) of ileum in pelvis. The obstructing stricture (arrowhead) is obscured by overlapped dilated bowel. Subtle nodules (arrow) are seen along mesenteric margin of pelvic segments. (b) Lateral radiograph of pelvic ileum shows fixed irregular narrowed channel (arrow) with intact mucosal folds. Note long stenotic segment and clearly defined distal demarcation. (c) CT following enteroclysis shows area of narrowing (arrow) and poorly defined fold thickening. Soft-tissue studding of the mesentery is present. Surgery confirmed the seeded metastases as well as diffuse adhesions.

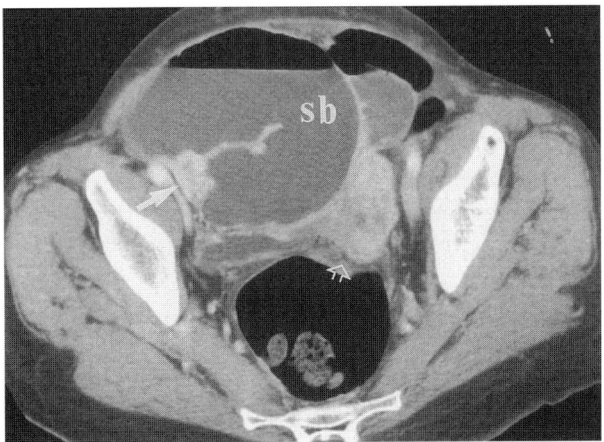

Fig. 21-16. Small bowel obstruction in a patient with metastatic colon carcinoma.
CT scan shows that the small bowel (sb) is markedly distended with fluid and air secondary to an obstructing serosal implant at the transition zone (arrow). A second peritoneal implant is present anterior to the rectum (open arrow). Rectal distention is iatrogenic due to air insufflation technique.

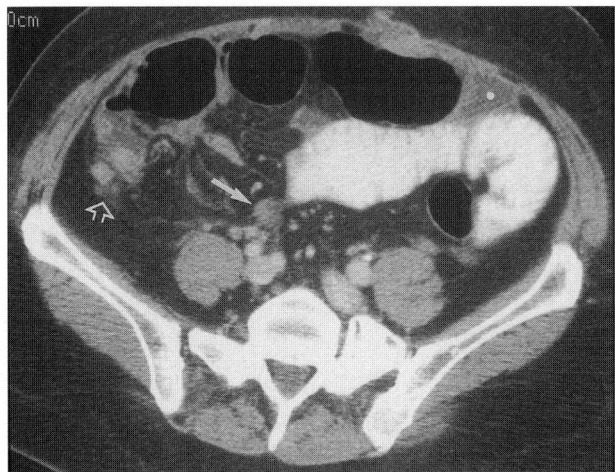

Fig. 21-17. Small bowel obstruction due to ovarian carcinoma metastasis.
CT scan at the transition zone shows a dilated barium-filled jejunal loop in the immediate proximity of a collapsed loop of distal small bowel. A surgically proved serosal implant is identified at the site of obstruction (arrow). Note presence of loculated ascites (.) and additional pericecal peritoneal implants (open arrow).

cause focal disruption of the fold pattern, shown as thumbprinting (Fig. 21-21). In both these respects, this appearance resembles the "picket fence" pattern described in ischemia and mural hemorrhage. At this late stage of radiation enteropathy, however, affected segments show diminished or absent peristalsis and are firmly embedded in adhesions[69–71] (Fig. 21-22). These findings and the permanence of the alternations distinguish them from findings of ischemia or intramural hemorrhage. Tapered strictures may be seen and can be a cause of intestinal obstruction (Fig. 21-23). Mucosal ulceration, fistulae, and sinus tracts may be seen in severe cases. Differentiation from peritoneal metastases becomes difficult when radiation injury causes distortion and kinking of narrowed bowel loops with spiculation of luminal contour.[9] CT is useful in establishing the presence or absence of peritoneal disease in these patients. The CT findings of radiation enteritis are nonspecific, and usually consist of concentric mural thickening involving a mild to moderately long segment of pelvic small bowel. A "target sign" is often appreciated on contrast-enhanced scans indicative of the non-neoplastic nature of bowel wall thickening. The affected bowel may demonstrate a masslike appearance due to confluence of adherent small bowel loops, and increased density to the mesenteric fat may be appreciated.[72] Radiation enteropathy most often causes mild to moderate SBO. If obstruction is present, CT will reveal dilated bowel proximal to the transition zone, circumferential bowel wall thickening with luminal narrowing at the transition zone, and collapsed or normal-appearing bowel distal to the diseased small bowel segment (Fig. 21-24).

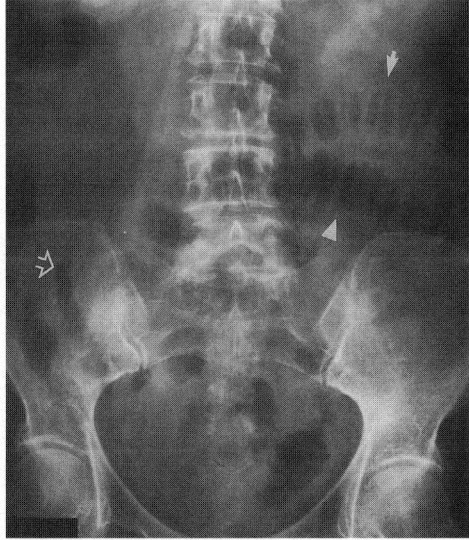
(a)

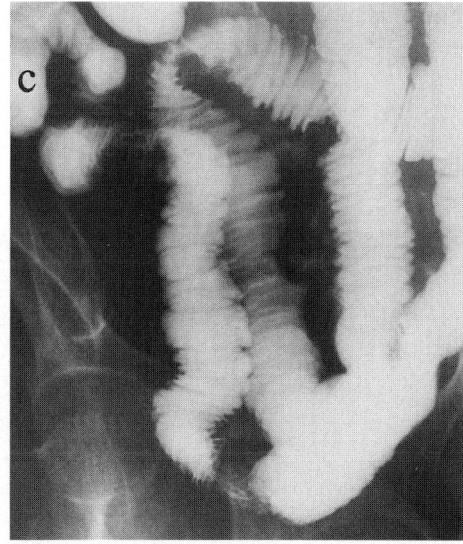
(b)

Fig. 21-18. An 83-year-old female with recent external radiation for carcinoma of the cervix presented with abdominal pain and diarrhea.
(a) Plain film examination shows moderate distention of small bowel loops in the left hemiabdomen. Retained fluid (arrow) and fold thickening (arrowhead) are noted. Distal segment appears narrowed with thickened walls (open arrow). (b) Enteroclysis performed following (a) shows hyperperistalsis, thickened folds, and lumen narrowing in loops of ileum within radiation port. C = cecum.

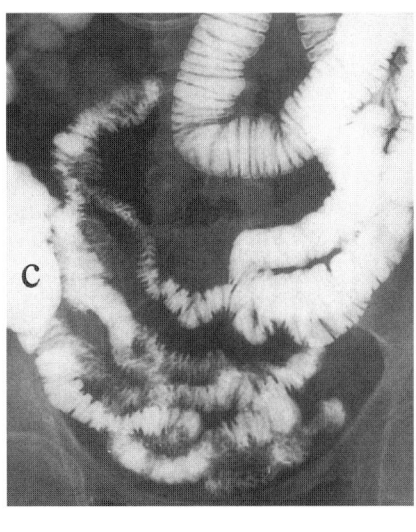 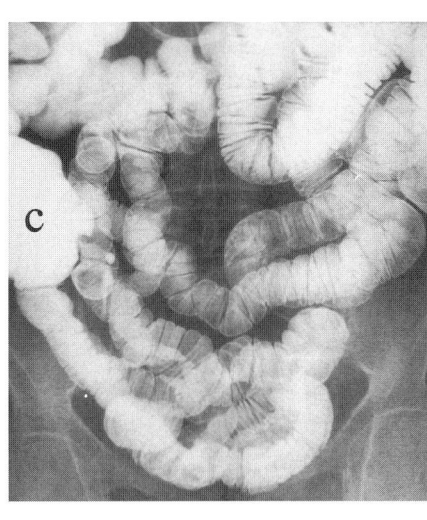

(a) (b) (c)

Fig. 21-19. Focal hyperperistalsis as a manifestation of anoxia in radiation enteropathy in a 69-year-old female with external radiation and implants 12 years earlier for carcinoma of the cervix who now complains of recurrent crampy abdominal pain.
(a) Early enteroclysis radiograph shows diffuse contraction of pelvic segments of ileum. This finding localized to the pelvic ileum persisted throughout the single-contrast phase of enteroclysis. (b) Contraction and increased peristalsis continued into the early part of methylcellulose infusion. C = cecum. (c) Increased flow rate during the double-contrast phase overcomes hyperperistalsis and shows absence of strictures. The pelvic segments were fixed by adhesive disease on compression radiography.

External and Internal Hernias

The majority of cases of SBO are due to extrinsic causes. After adhesions, hernias compete with neoplasms as the second most common cause of acute SBO.[73] External hernias are characterized by prolapse of an intestinal loop through a defect in the wall of the abdomen or pelvis. Those that involve the anterior abdominal wall or groin are often visible or palpable.

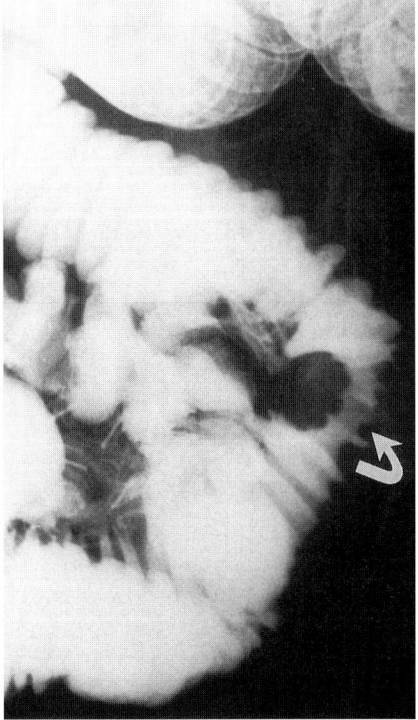

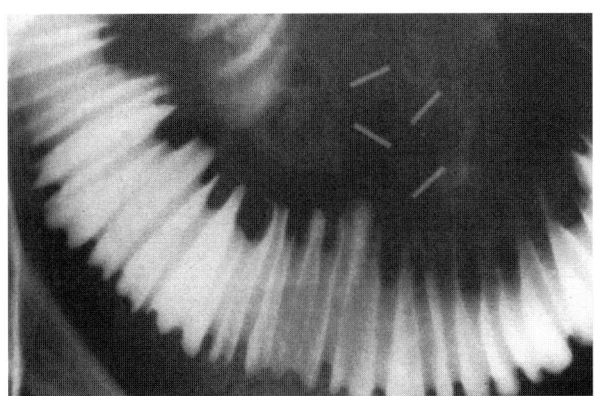

Fig. 21-20. Radiation damage in a 53-year-old female who underwent radiation therapy for ovarian carcinoma.
Coned view of affected pelvic loop shows thickened, straight folds with narrowed interfold spaces.

Fig. 21-21. Patient with a history of external radiation treatment for rectal carcinoma.
A short, narrowed segment in an area with the features of radiation enteropathy shows focal thumbprinting and disruption of folds (curved arrow).

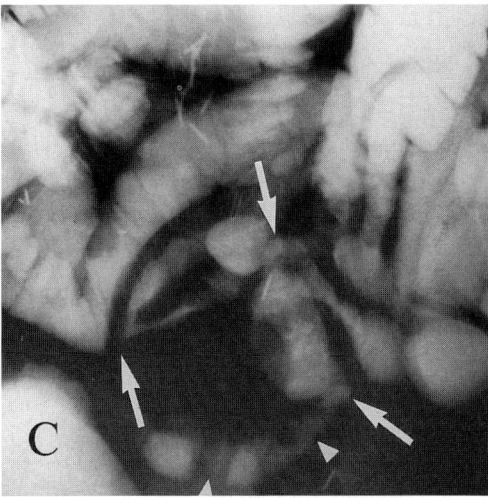

Fig. 21-22. Small bowel obstruction in a patient who had external radiation for cervix carcinoma 7 years ago, now presenting with small bowel obstruction.
The pelvic segments are kinked, angulated, and fixed (arrows) with areas of lumen narrowing and fold thickening (arrowheads). C = cecum. Adhesive obstruction, involving segments of radiation-damaged ileum, was confirmed at surgery. (From Maglinte and Reyes,[65] with permission.)

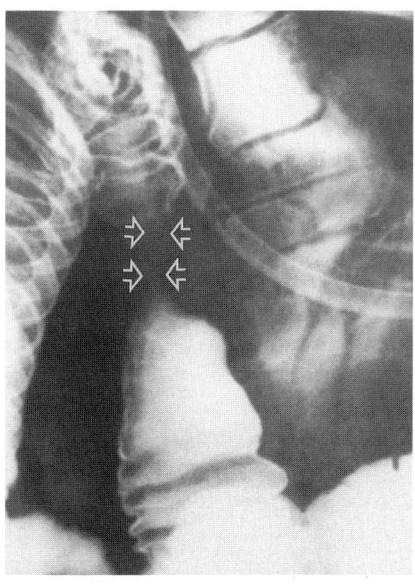

Fig. 21-23. Moderately long stricture (arrows) without overhanging margins secondary to chronic radiation enteropathy.
There is atrophy of the folds proximally suggesting a chronic process. Surgery confirmed presence of a benign stricture. Histology revealed radiation enteropathy. The patient had a history of radiation therapy for carcinoma of the cervix. (From Maglinte and Reyes,[65] with permission.)

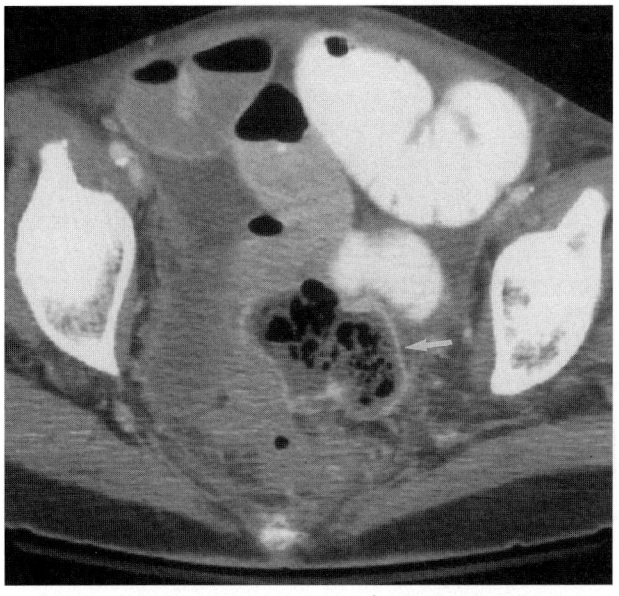

(a)

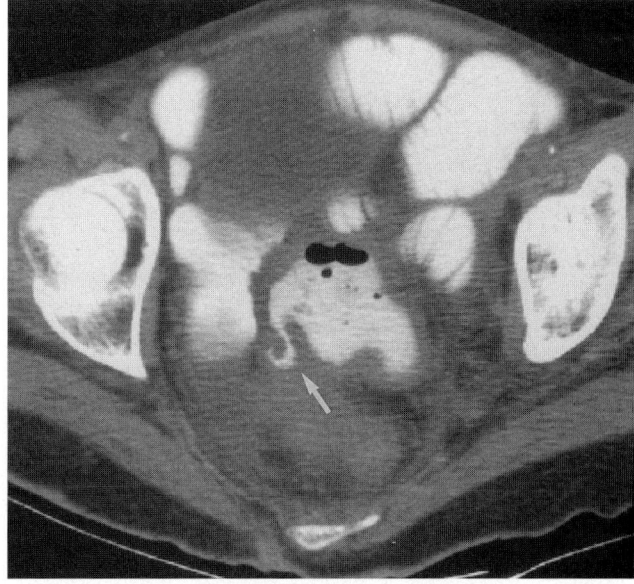

(b)

Fig. 21-24. Small bowel obstruction due to radiation enteropathy.
(a) CT scan of a 55-year-old woman with cervical cancer treated with pelvic radiation shows a peripherally enhanced, tubular structure containing fluid and gas concerning for pelvic abscess (arrow). (b) Delayed CT scan acquired using 5-mm collimation demonstrates that the "pseudocollection" in fact represents a dilated, partially obstructed bowel segment located proximal to a short, ischemic stricture of the ileum (arrow).

External hernias account for the overwhelming majority of obstructing hernias. They develop in approximately 1.5% of the population and most commonly occur in the inguinal and femoral canals, the periumbilical region, and sites of previous surgical incision.[9] Internal hernias are confined within the abdominal cavity, and arise secondary to either intestinal protrusion through a developmental or surgical defect in the peritoneum or mesentery, or prolapse of bowel under an adhesive band. The autopsy incidence of internal hernias ranges from 0.2% to 0.9%.[74] Most remain clinically silent and go undetected. Large internal hernias that are not easily reducible may cause intermittent abdominal pain and recurrent episodes of intestinal obstruction. Small symptomatic hernias may be missed by clinical examination in obese patients or in patients with extensive abdominal scars. These hernias can also be missed radiologically if provocative maneuvers and appropriate positioning are not done during the examination.[75] At the end of the enteroclysis infusion, the patient is positioned lateral and asked to strain or cough. These hernias then protrude

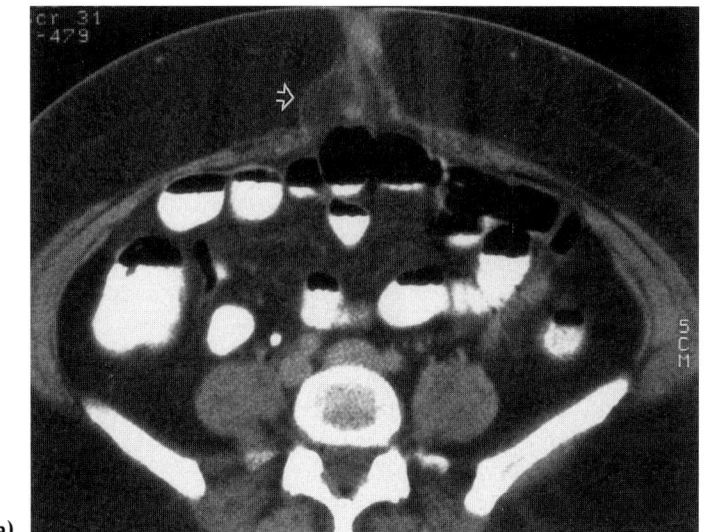

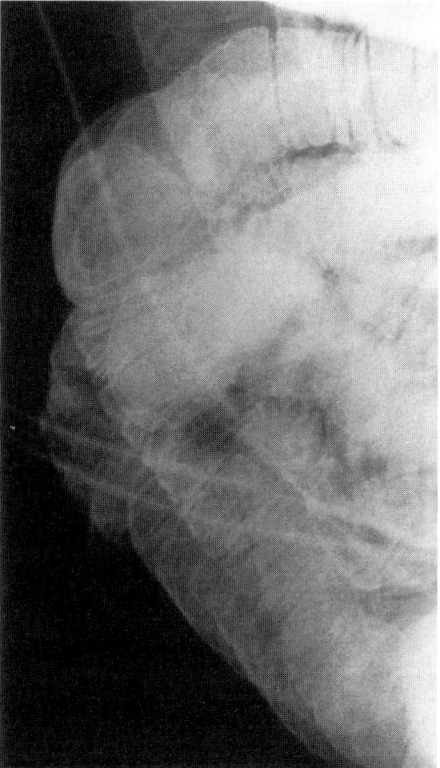

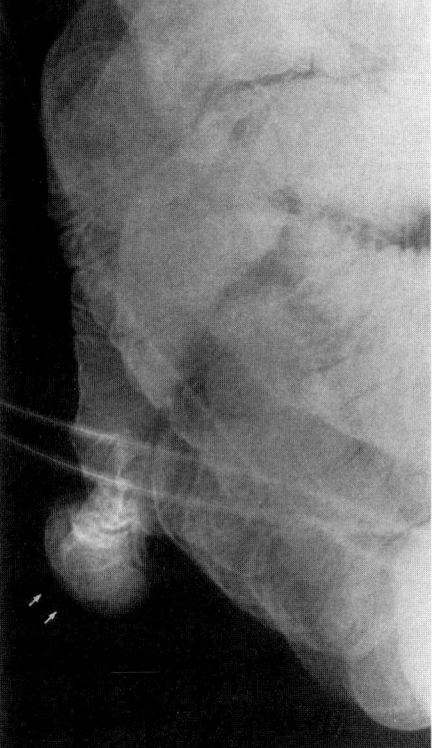

Fig. 21-25. Occult incisional hernia clinically unsuspected in an obese patient.
(a) CT scan done for recurrent unexplained abdominal pain and distention shows intraperitoneal fat (open arrow) herniating through midline incision. Although no loop of herniated bowel is seen, demonstration of herniated intraperitoneal fat is evidence for an incisional hernia. (b) Herniation of bowel is not seen in the lateral position at enteroclysis with the patient in normal respiration during contrast infusion. (c) A small hernia is demonstrated during straining or coughing following cessation of infusion. The arrows mark the skin surface to show the thickness of the subcutaneous fat layer well shown on CT.

Major Causes of Small Bowel Obstruction • 489

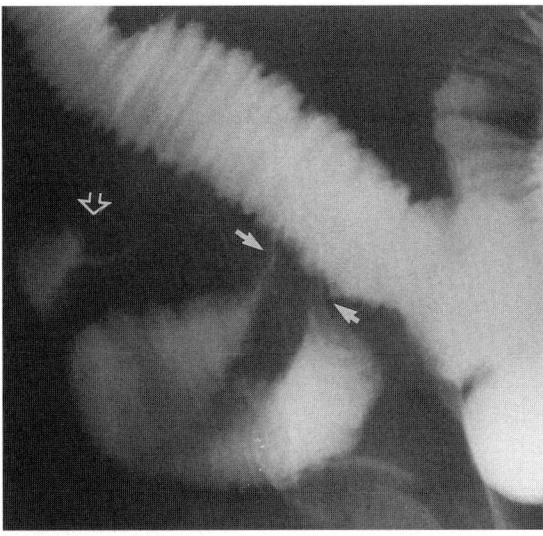

Fig. 21-26. Paraileostomy hernia.
A partial obstruction is produced at the neck of the hernia (arrows) below the prestomal ileum (open arrow). Note thickened folds in the herniated segment and in bowel proximal to the hernia consistent with edema. No vascular compromise was found at laparotomy. (From Maglinte et al,[10] with permission.)

and are recognized. They may, however, reduce during contrast infusion (Fig. 21-25).

The radiologic features of a specific type of hernia will vary depending on the contents of the hernia and the site of herniation. Internal (see next section) and external hernias causing SBO share several radiologic features, which are often apparent on barium studies and cross-sectional imaging. The herniated bowel loops usually appear encapsulated, crowded together, and fixed in an abnormal location (Fig. 21-26). In mild to moderate SBO, barium studies will demonstrate the dilated afferent and collapsed efferent bowel segments leading to and from the hernial orifice, respectively. These segments typically show smooth, symmetric, and tapered narrowing at the neck of the hernia[30] (Fig. 21-27). Delayed emptying of barium from the herniated bowel may be seen depending on the degree of anatomic constriction present. Barium studies may not show the efferent limb in cases of high-grade or complete obstruction. CT is advantageous because it reliably demonstrates the dilated afferent and collapsed efferent limbs in SBO of all grades of severity. Characterization of the hernia is facilitated with CT because it can directly visualize the aberrantly positioned bowel and its relation to surrounding viscera, mesentery, and abdominal wall (Fig. 21-28). When a hernia is

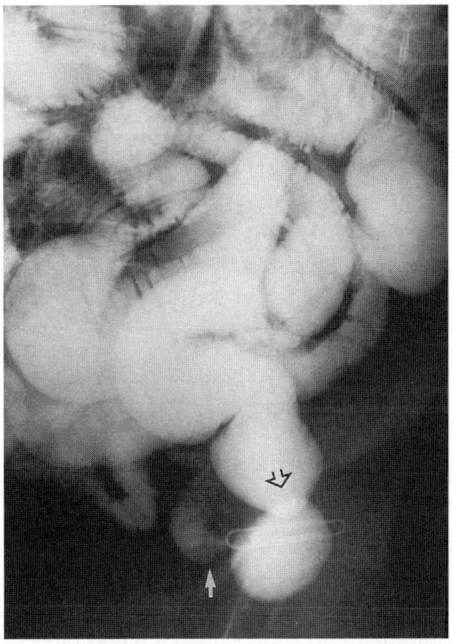

Fig. 21-27. Low-grade obstruction in a reducible external hernia.
Enteroclysis was performed to determine etiology of recurrent abdominal pain. The afferent (entering) limb (open arrow) of a left inguinal hernia is dilated. The herniated segment is also dilated (marked by clip) but the efferent (exiting) limb (arrow) is collapsed, indicating that the point of obstruction involves only one limb, a nonclosed loop adhesive obstruction. The finding was confirmed at surgery.

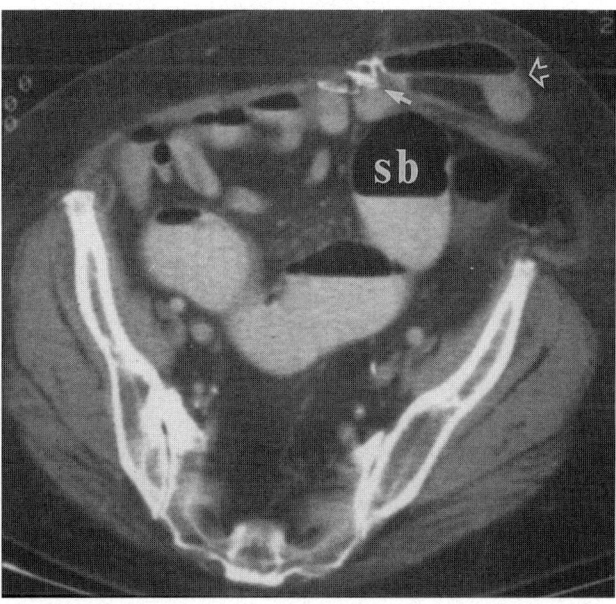

Fig. 21-28. CT of external hernia with high-grade obstruction.
CT of obese patient with recurrent severe abdominal pain shows marked distention of small bowel (sb) proximal to neck of incisional hernia (arrow) indicating high-grade obstruction involving afferent limb immediately proximal to neck of hernia. The herniated segment (open arrow) as well as more distal loops are of normal caliber. Note diffuse adhesive disease fixing small bowel loops to anterior parietal peritoneum.

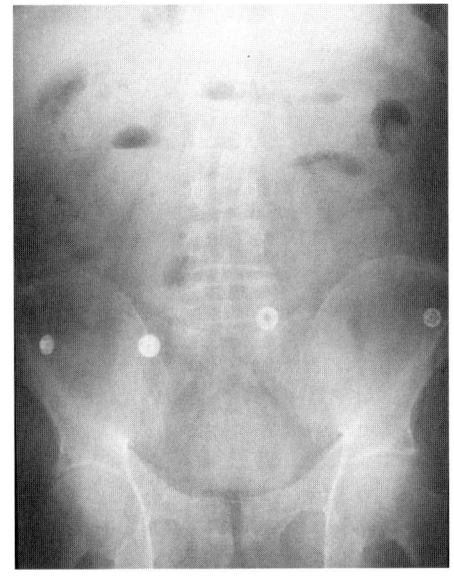 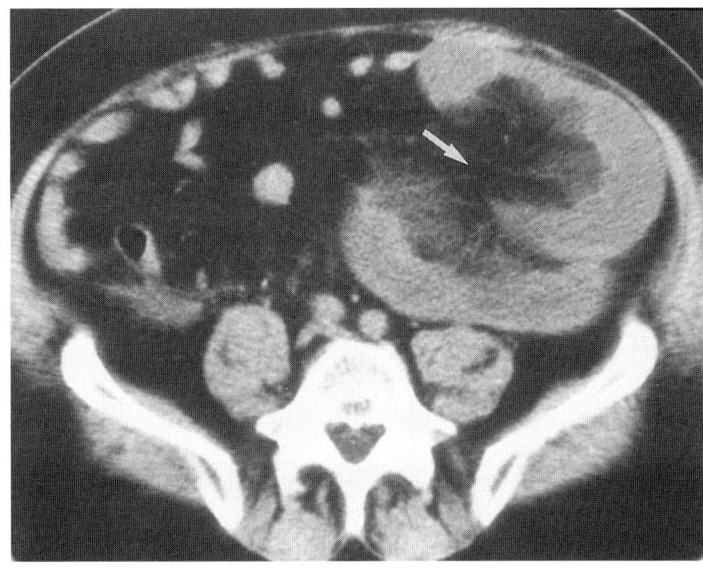

Fig. 21-29. Imaging of acute closed loop obstruction.
(a) Plain film radiography demonstrates findings consistent with mechanical small bowel obstruction. There are no findings to suggest closed loop obstruction. The dilated small bowel, however, is predominantly fluid-filled, a common finding in closed loop obstruction. (b) CT done in the Emergency Radiology Section immediately following plain film to evaluate for other causes of an acute abdomen shows obstructed dilated fluid-filled small bowel loop in a characteristic c-shaped configuration (arrow) suggestive of closed loop obstruction. The diagnosis was confirmed at surgery.

reducible, CT will show the abdominal wall defect but the hernia may not be apparent.

Closed Loop Obstruction

Most closed loop obstructions result from entrapment of a small bowel loop by a single adhesive band. Less common etiologies include bowel incarceration within an internal or external hernia.[34] Preoperative recognition of closed loop obstruction and its differentiation from strangulation remains a difficult clinical problem. The diagnosis is often only established at laparotomy.[22,24] The necessity for accurate and early detection of strangulation is emphasized by the fact that delayed surgical intervention significantly affects patient prognosis.[76,77] Plain film findings are potentially useful in helping to establish the diagnosis if the classic "pseudotumor" or "coffee bean" sign is present.[78] Unfortunately, plain film radiography is often nonspecific and unreliable, and the diagnosis is best established by CT or enteroclysis. CT is the imaging modality of choice for evaluating closed loop obstruction in the acute setting (Fig. 21-29). Enteroclysis is complementary, and may be used to establish the presence of incomplete closed loop obstruction or to help clarify the etiology of obstruction[3] (Fig. 21-30).

Diagnosis by Enteroclysis

The enteroclysis findings of closed loop obstruction are similar to those seen in single band adhesive ob-

Fig. 21-30. Imaging of incomplete closed loop obstruction. Complementary role of CT and enteroclysis.
(a) Supine abdominal radiograph of a 72-year-old female with severe abdominal pain shows dilated small bowel with retained fluid or thickened folds. She had a prior history of appendectomy and recent laparotomy for small bowel adhesions. Note clips (arrow) over right upper sacrum. (b) CT done for further assessment above level of clips, (c) at level of clips, and (d) below level of clips CT shows minimally dilated fluid-filled loops of small bowel and edema of bowel wall. There are no findings to suggest closed loop obstruction. (e) Plain film obtained 18 hours after CT shows successful decompression of distended small bowel by long tube in proximal jejunum. (f) Enteroclysis done through long tube prior to planned discharge shows incomplete closed loop obstruction (arrows) near site of clips. Open arrow points to the site of obstruction of entering limb. Black arrowhead points to site of obstruction of exiting limb. Note collapsed loops distal to efferent limb. White arrowhead points to terminal ileum. Surgery confirmed incomplete closed loop secondary to an adhesive band. (From Maglinte et al,[102] with permission.)

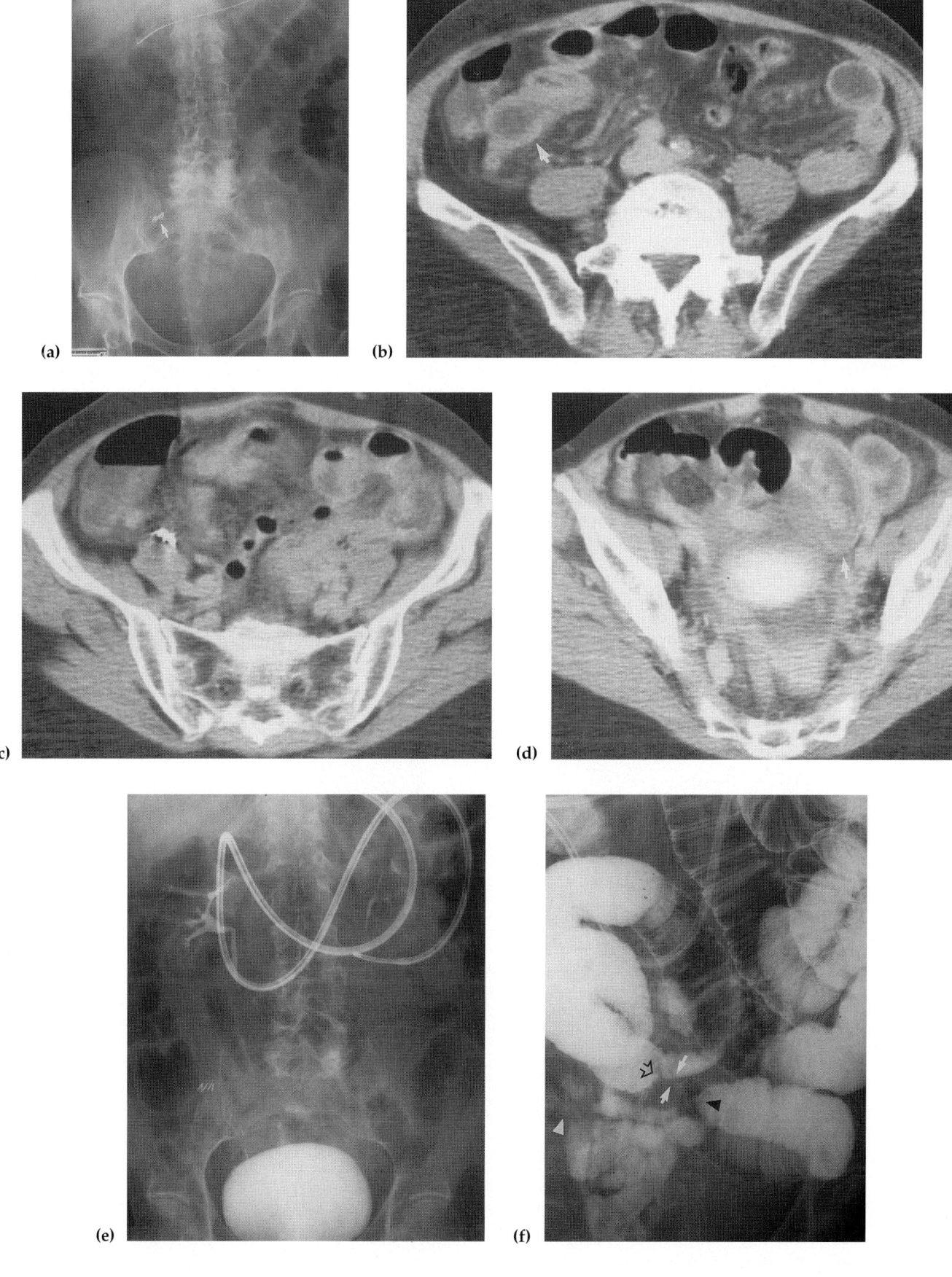

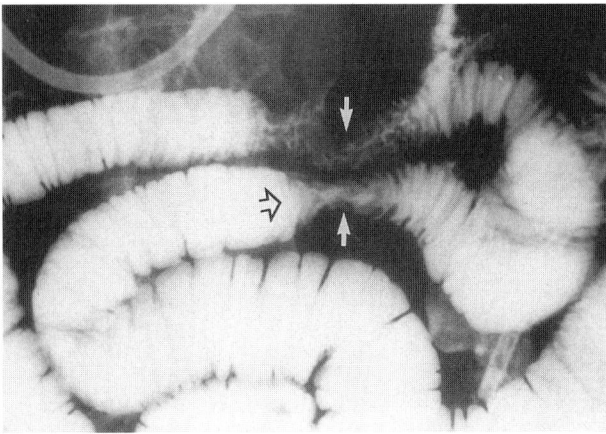

Fig. 21-31. Adhesions (arrows) cross the two limbs of a loop of bowel and produce a partially closed loop with low-grade obstruction.
Open arrow indicates direction of flow and entering limb. The tip of the enteroclysis tube is in the proximal jejunum. Surgery confirmed enteroclysis findings. (From Maglinte et al,[10] with permission.)

of the obstructed segment are located at the base of the closed loop (Fig. 21-31). The length of obstructed bowel is variable. When obstruction is incomplete, fluoroscopy can identify the direction of flow of contrast material entering and exiting the closed loop. Volvulus is diagnosed if the afferent and efferent limbs appear to cross or intertwine with twisting of the folds at the point of obstruction (Fig. 21-32). A separation between the two obstructed limbs excludes the presence of volvulus. In patients with moderate to high-grade obstruction, it may be difficult to exclude volvulus if the involved limbs appear closely approximated, tightly compressed, and angulated at the point of obstruction.[34] It may be difficult to differentiate between a closed loop obstruction caused by an internal hernia through a defect in the mesentery from that due to prolapse of a loop of bowel under an adhesive band[30] (Fig. 21-33). If the constriction is tight, there is usually delayed filling as well as delayed emptying of contrast from the incarcerated loop.[34]

Diagnosis by CT

CT is a valuable diagnostic tool because it can preoperatively establish the diagnosis of both closed loop obstruction and strangulation.[31,33,56,79–85] The CT findings of closed loop obstruction are directly related to

struction, except that the crossing defect traverses two adjacent segments of a single loop of bowel.[10,34] The fixed, adjacent points of the afferent and efferent limbs

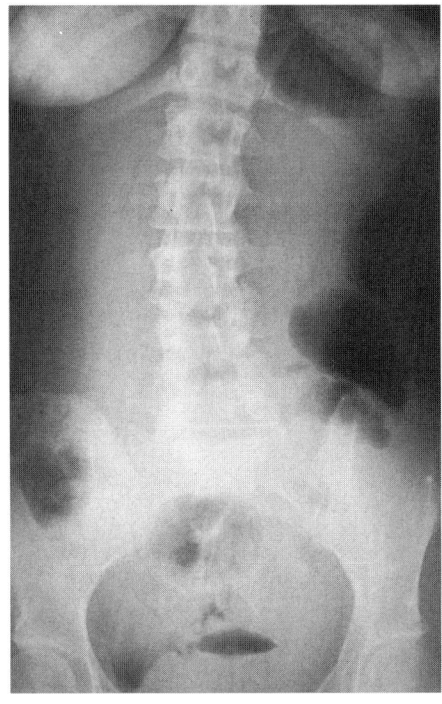
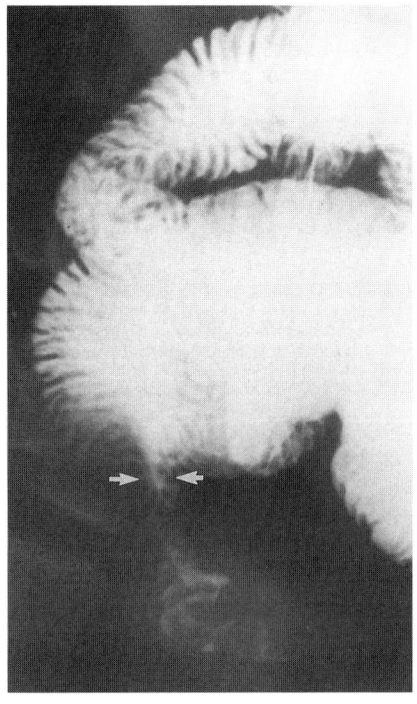

(a) (b)

Fig. 21-32. Contrast radiography of volvulus.
(a) Plain film radiography of middle-aged female patient with recurrent abdominal pain and postprandial vomiting is unremarkable. (b) Enteroclysis shows twisting of folds (arrows) at point of obstruction. Surgery confirmed diagnosis of volvulus involving proximal jejunum.

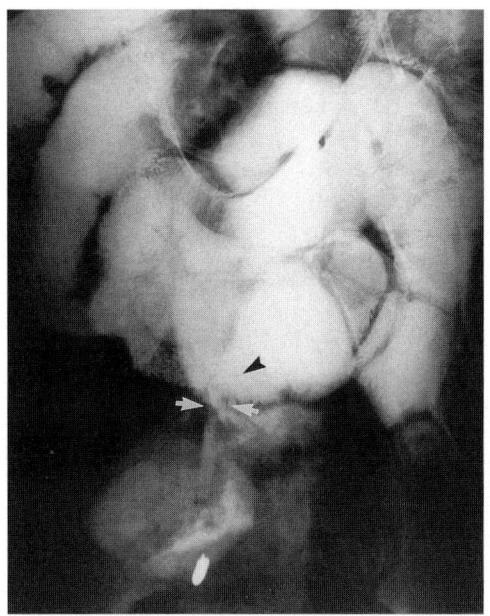 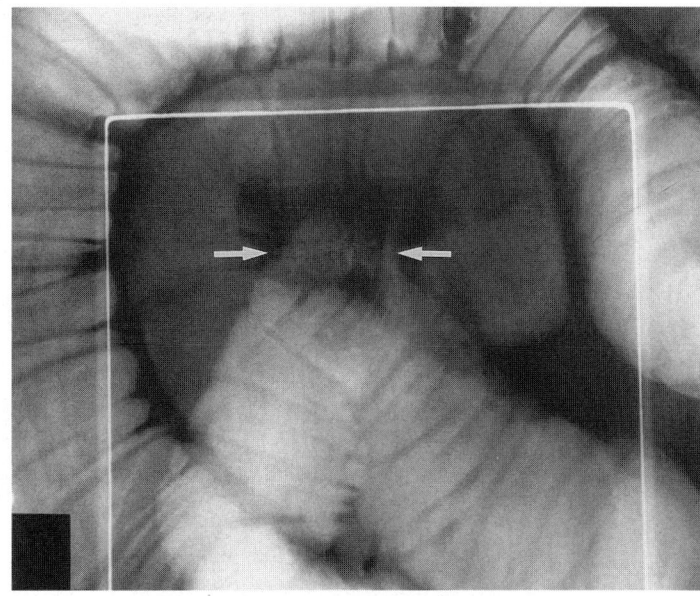

Fig. 21-33. Closed loop obstruction secondary to internal hernia.
(a) Herniation of small intestine through a mesenteric defect (arrows) causing tight closed loop obstruction. Arrowhead in entering limb indicates direction of flow. The herniated segment is only partially filled with contrast. Note bullet fragment near internal hernia. Patient had emergency repair of right external iliac artery, which was damaged by gunshot.
Surgery confirmed enteroclysis findings. (b) Closed loop obstruction secondary to herniation of small bowel underneath an adhesive band (arrows). Note dilution of contrast by retained fluid in closed loop. The involved bowel was viable at surgery. Adhesiolysis was performed. (From Maglinte et al,[10] with permission.)

the length of the closed loop, the degree of bowel distention, and the three-dimensional orientation of the closed loop with respect to the axial imaging plane[31,33] (Fig. 21-34). If the incarcerated loop is horizontally oriented, it will appear U-shaped or C-shaped in the axial plane. If an elongated segment of bowel is involved, sequential axial images demonstrate a characteristic radial distribution of dilated bowel loops with stretched and thickened mesenteric vessels converging to the point of obstruction. The incarcerated segment appears almost entirely fluid-filled. In contrast, bowel loops proximal to the site of obstruction contain greater amounts of air. Images obtained near the site of torsion demonstrate progressive, fusiform tapering of the afferent and efferent limbs. This is manifested as the "beak" sign when imaged in longitudinal section. If a volvulus is present, the "whirl" sign of a tightly twisted mesentery may be seen[83] (Fig. 21-35).

CT signs of strangulation are related to the appearance of the incarcerated bowel wall and its mesentery.[31,33] Ischemia is suggested by the presence of circumferential wall thickening, increased mural attenuation, and the "target" or "double halo" sign seen on contrast-enhanced examination. In unenhanced examination, increased bowel wall attenuation is suggestive of ischemia. Pneumatosis intestinalis may be seen with advanced ischemia and infarction. Mesenteric congestion and hemorrhage are important findings whose presence increase the specificity of the CT diagnosis of strangulation. The presence of ascites is not specific for ischemia. Though often present with strangulating obstruction, ascites may also be seen with simple mechanical obstruction and cases of closed loop obstruction not complicated by ischemic change.[31,84] Mesenteric fluid, bowel wall thickening, and in some instances abnormally increased bowel wall enhancement (hyperemia) can be seen in other entities such as malignant obstruction, inflammatory bowel disease, or peritonitis, in which no vascular compromise is involved.

In a prospective study, contrast-enhanced CT demonstrated a sensitivity of 100% and a negative predictive value of 61% for the diagnosis of SBO-related intestinal ischemia.[85] This study suggested that CT is sensitive but not highly specific in making the diagnosis of intestinal ischemia (Fig. 21-36). Ha et al recently performed a retrospective analysis of 84 cases of simple and strangulated SBO to identify the most useful CT criteria for diagnosing strangulated obstruction.[84] Using logistic regression analysis, these

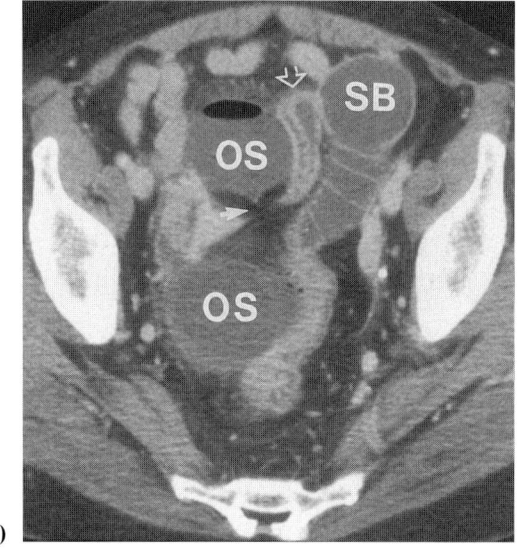
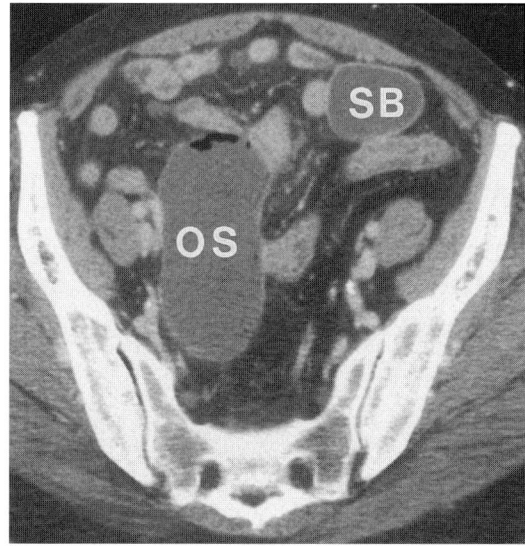
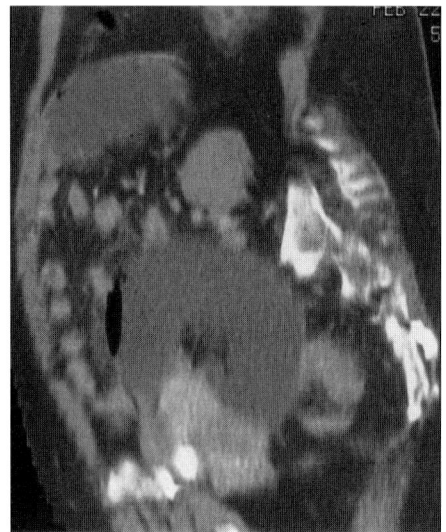

Fig. 21-34. CT of closed loop obstruction produced by adhesive band.
(a) Axial pelvic CT scan shows a dilated, fluid-filled bowel loop (SB) leading to the site of torsion (arrow). Adjacent limbs of the obstructed segment (OS) approximate each other at the base of the closed loop. The collapsed efferent loop exits the site of torsion anteriorly (open arrow). (b) CT scan at midpelvis shows obstructed proximal bowel (SB) and cross-sectional appearance to apex of incarcerated loop (OS). (c) Reformatted sagittal helical CT image best demonstrates the C-shaped configuration to the closed loop.

authors determined that the most specific CT findings for strangulated obstruction included poor or no enhancement of the bowel wall and a serrated beak appearance to the obstructed loop (specificity 100%). Additional findings of importance included a large amount of ascites, an unusual course of the mesenteric vasculature, diffuse engorgement of the mesenteric vasculature, and mesenteric haziness (specificity ≥95%).

Intussusception

Enteroenteric intussusception may result in either partial or complete SBO. Surgical intervention is often required, as benign and malignant polypoid tumors represent the most common causes of intestinal intussusception in adults. The radiologic findings reflect the underlying pathophysiology of the intussusception complex. The essential components consist of the central, invaginating proximal small bowel loop and its mesentery (intussusceptum) and the outer, receiving distal small bowel segment (intussuscipiens).

With antegrade administration of barium, the lumen of the intussusceptum appears as a narrow, tapered, tubular structure that is lined by intact mucosal folds that often assume a twisted appearance. If barium is able to reflux in retrograde fashion into the lumen of the intussuscipiens, a characteristic "coiled-spring" sign may be seen.[86] This appearance is due to barium coating the thickened, edematous folds that line the mucosal surface of the intussuscipiens. Bar-

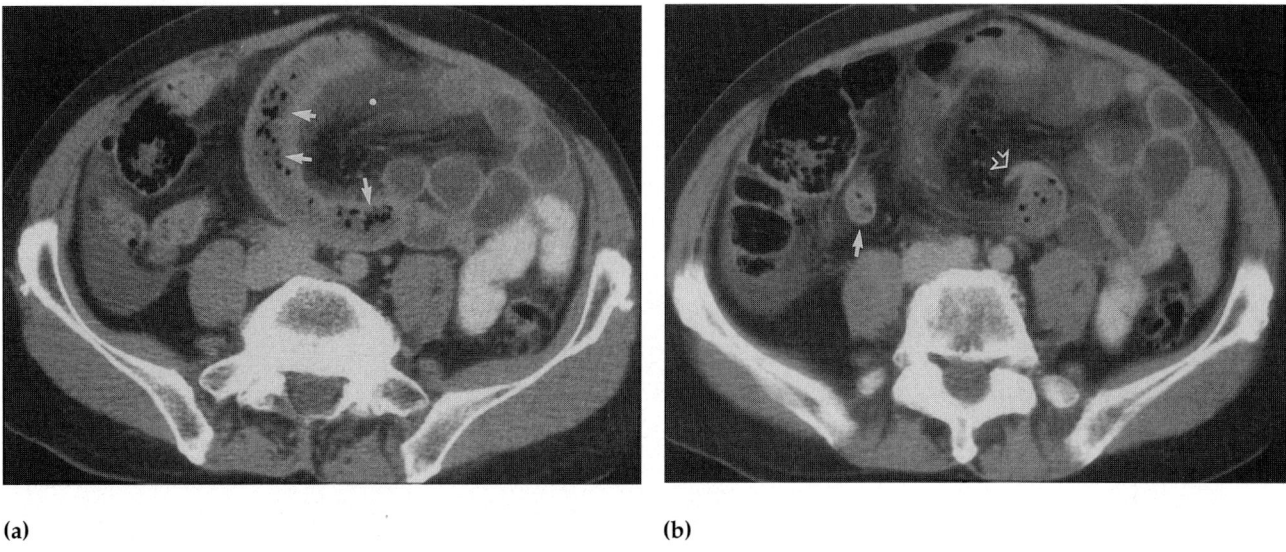

Fig. 21-35. The "beak" sign of torsion at the site of closed loop obstruction.
(a) Incarcerated small bowel loop appears C-shaped and contains both fluid and particulate matter (arrows). Fluid is seen in the mesentery with partial obliteration of the mesenteric fat and vascular structures (.). (b) CT scan at the level of the transition zone shows beaklike tapering to the obstructed small bowel loop (open arrow). Note presence of collapsed distal ileum (arrow). At surgery strangulated small bowel obstruction due to adhesions was found.

ium studies are useful in their ability to demonstrate the intussusception's lead point and to help narrow the differential diagnosis (Fig. 21-37). The polypoid mass causing the intussusception may be outlined with barium immediately distal to the tapered lumen of the intussusceptum. Mucosal lesions, such as a Peutz-Jeghers polyp or an adenoma, are suggested if barium is seen to fill the surface interstices of a lesion.[30] Submucosal lesions, such as a leiomyoma or metastatic melanoma, should be considered if the

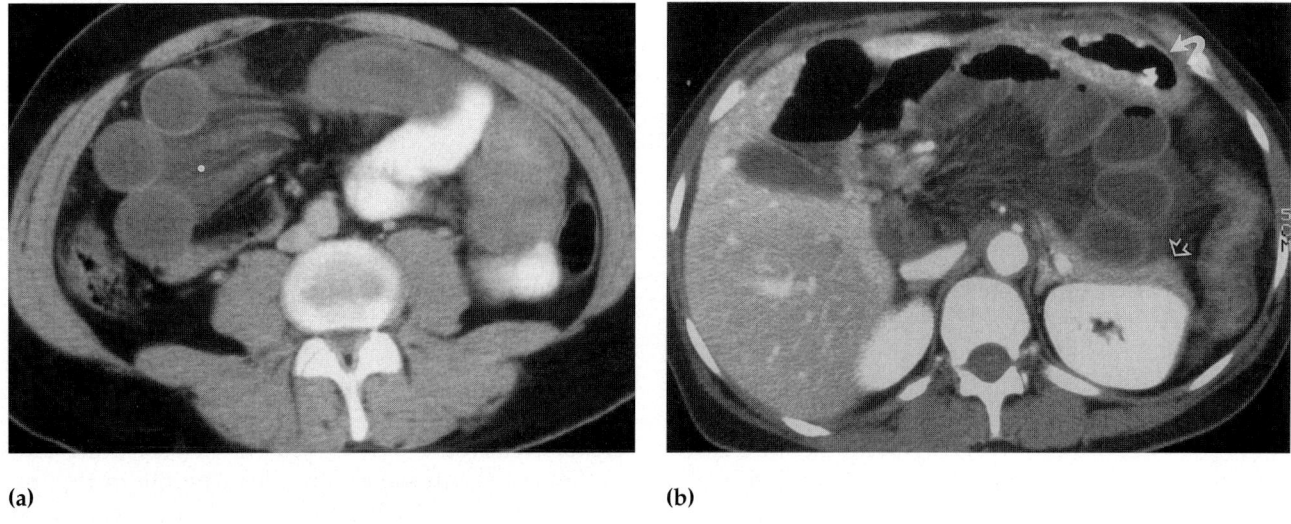

Fig. 21-36. CT of strangulated obstruction.
(a) Strangulated small bowel obstruction due to adhesions. CT scan reveals a fixed radial distribution of dilated small bowel loops. The subtended mesentery is hemorrhagic and shows high attenuation fluid, which obscures the mesenteric vessels. (b) Strangulated small bowel obstruction due to internal hernia. CT scan shows abnormally positioned, thick-walled, jejunal small bowel loops crowded together within the lesser sac. Mesenteric hemorrhage is present with partial obliteration of the vascular markings. Curved arrow points to anteriorly displaced stomach, open arrow points to pancreas. (Courtesy of Jay Heiken, MD.)

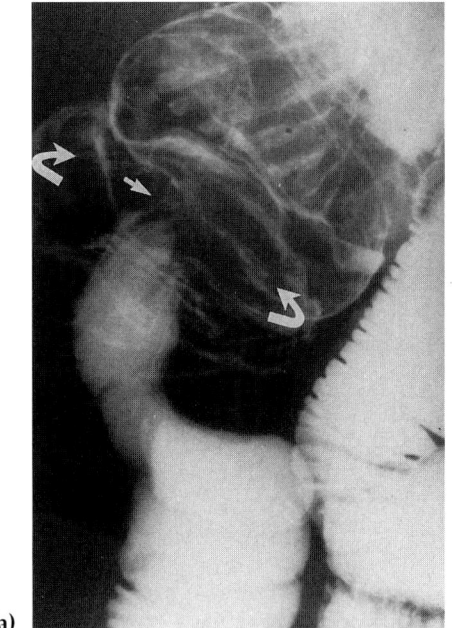 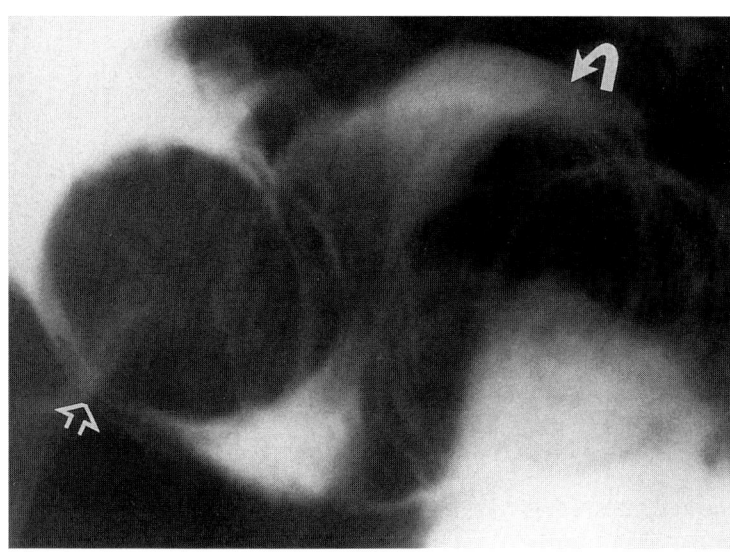

Fig. 21-37. Barium examination in intussusception.
(a) Ileocolic intussusception with the lead point a granuloma of the appendix stump. The narrow channel through the intussusception (arrow) is surrounded by a typical coiled spring pattern (curved arrows), made possible by the reflux of barium into the space between intussusceptum and intussuscipiens. (b) Ileoileal intussusception with the lead point a polypoid mass (open arrow). The lumen of the intussuscipiens is outlined by refluxed barium (curved arrow). An ulcerating lipoma was found at surgery to be the lead point. There is no distinguishing feature on barium examination to identify different polypoid leading masses.

leading mass appears centrally umbilicated or ulcerated. Metastatic lesions will be multiple, and demonstration of mural lesions allows a precise diagnosis. Inflammatory fibroid polyps, lipomas, or an invaginated Meckel's diverticulum should be excluded if the intussusception is due to a pedunculated polyp with a long stalk.[87,88] In some cases, however, no specific radiologic features exist to enable reliable differentiation of benign from malignant causes of intussusception.[65]

The CT features of intestinal intussusception are virtually pathognomonic.[89–91] The most common CT finding is a targetlike mass that represents the earliest stage of intussusception. The "target lesion" consists of a central soft-tissue density mass (intussuscepting intestine), an adjacent eccentric fat-attenuation component (intussuscepting mesentery), and a well-defined, peripheral outer border (intussuscipiens) (Fig. 21-38). If the intussusception complex is oriented in the axial plane, a sausage-shaped mass with alternating layers of high and low attenuation can be seen. Luminal contrast may outline the intussusceptum in cases of incomplete obstruction (Fig. 21-39). As the obstruction proceeds, the intussuscipiens demonstrates progressive mural thickening and edema. This is typically manifested as a reniform pattern that reflects the presence of invaginated intussusceptum surrounded by thickened bowel wall. Recognition of this appearance is important as this pattern has been described in cases of intussusception complicated by ischemia.[90,92] Proximal bowel dilatation is invariably present in symptomatic patients who present with obstruction. Collapsed bowel is noted distal to the intussusception complex, which represents the actual transition zone.

The cause of intussusception may or may not be visualized on CT depending on the size and attenuation features of the lead point. The incidence of adult intussusception has increased due to the increased risk of intussusception in patients with human immunodeficiency virus (HIV)–and Acquired Immunodeficiency Syndrome (AIDS)–associated gastrointestinal pathology.[93] Intussusception lead points in this patient population include primary tumors (eg, B-cell lymphoma and Kaposi's sarcoma), mesenteric adenopathy secondary to infection or neoplasia, and lymphoid hyperplasia associated with hypersecretory infectious enteritides. AIDS-associated intussusception may also occur without a demonstrable lead point when caused by neuroendocrine-mediated intestinal dysmotility.[94]

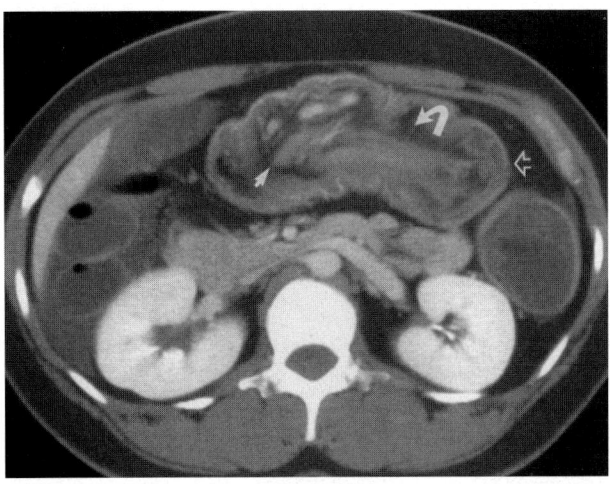

Fig. 21-38. Small bowel obstruction due to ileocolic intussusception.
CT scan shows terminal ileum (arrow) with its mesenteric fat (curved arrow) within dilated intussuscipiens of transverse colon (open arrow). No lead point was identified at surgery.

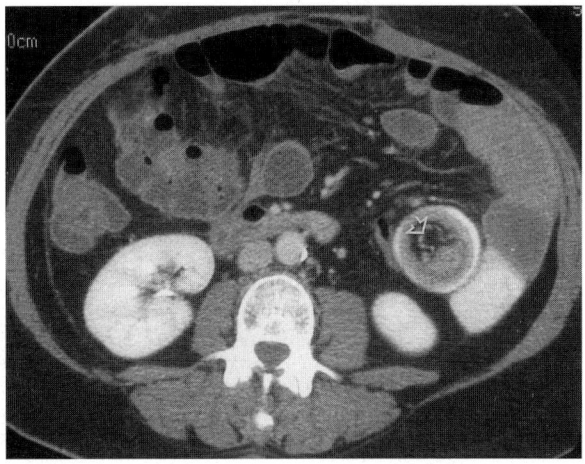

Fig. 21-39. Small bowel intussusception.
CT scan demonstrates eccentric invaginated mesenteric fat (open arrow) characteristic of intussusception. Obstruction is incomplete, as luminal contrast is able to surround the intussusceptum.

Other Causes of Small Bowel Obstruction

Crohn's disease, developmental anomalies, tumors, gallstone ileus, foreign bodies, bezoars, and the effects of trauma are discussed in other chapters. The occasional iatrogenic obturation SBO caused by the inflated balloon of a feeding tube[95] and the self-distending balloon of a Cantor tube,[96] which may cause focal pressure necrosis, can be readily diagnosed by imaging. If deflation does not occur by opening the port, percutaneous transenteric fine-needle deflation of the distended balloon should be done. Obturation of the ileum by an impacted Garren gastric bubble has been reported.[97]

Imaging Recommendations

The diagnostic evaluation of patients with suspected intestinal obstruction is based on an integrated assessment of patient history, clinical presentation, and abdominal plain film findings. Contrast enema, small bowel barium, and CT examinations are complementary procedures that may be used to confirm or exclude the diagnosis of obstruction and its complications. A diagnostic algorithm for triaging patients to a specific imaging modality has recently been proposed as a means of providing cost-effective patient care (Fig. 21-40).[3] These guidelines are illustrated below and are presented according to commonly encountered clinical scenarios.

Scenario one: A definite SBO pattern is detected on plain film radiographs, which serves to confirm the clinical diagnosis of intestinal obstruction. Immediate laparotomy without additional imaging may be considered in patients who have not had prior abdominal surgery or in patients with suspected complete obstruction, incarcerated hernia, or strangulation. Surgery may be delayed or obviated in patients with history of adhesive obstruction, partial obstruction, resected abdominal neoplasm, or inflammatory bowel disease. Patients with adhesive or partial obstruction should undergo CT if their clinical symptoms and plain film findings do not resolve with conservative management (Fig. 21-41). CT should be performed in any patient with a clinical suspicion of strangulation, and is intended to stage the presence and extent of neoplastic or inflammatory disease whenever suspected. Enteroclysis is reserved for those cases where management issues are not resolved by CT.

Scenario two: Plain film radiographs demonstrate both small and large bowel dilatation. If positional maneuvers (lateral, decubitus, or prone views) fail to demonstrate gas in the rectum on plain film radiography, contrast enema examination is advised to differentiate colonic ileus from a distal colonic obstruction associated with an incompetent ileocecal valve (Fig. 21-42). CT is reserved for patients with poor anal sphincter tone. CT should be the initial imaging modality in postoperative and septic patients with suspected intraabdominal inflammation (Fig. 21-43).

Fig. 21-40. Diagram shows algorithm for diagnostic triage of patients with suspected intestinal obstruction. SBO = small bowel obstruction. (Reprinted with permission from Maglinte et al.[3])

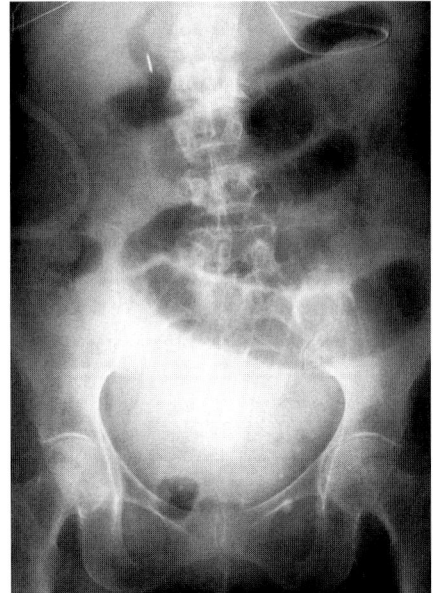

Fig. 21-41. A 66-six-year old woman with abdominal pain and vomiting with history of hysterectomy 10 years earlier and recent mitral valve surgery.
(a) Supine abdominal radiograph following 24 hours of nasogastric suction reveals findings unequivocal for small bowel obstruction. Enteroclysis was requested by attending physicians to gauge severity of presumed adhesive obstruction. CT was instead recommended by radiologist prior to placement of long tube for further decompression. Note coiled tip of tube in fundus of stomach. (b, c) CT sections through upper and lower pelvis show fluid-filled dilated small bowel (sb) and collapsed colon (c). Small bowel dilatation terminated at incarcerated obturator hernia [arrow, (c)]. Demonstration of internal hernia changed planned medical regime to urgent surgical intervention. Findings were confirmed at surgery. No strangulation was present. (From Maglinte et al,[3] with permission.)

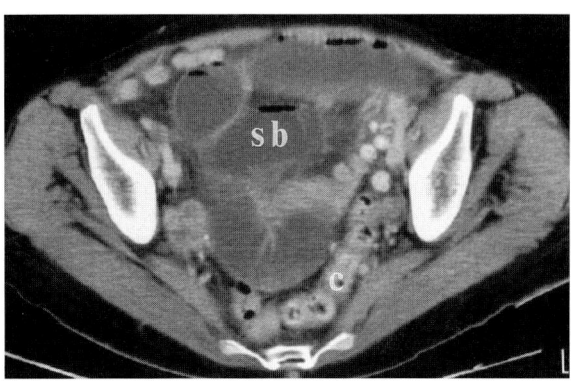

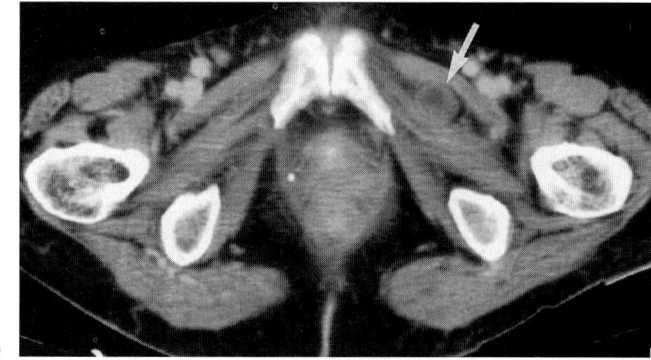

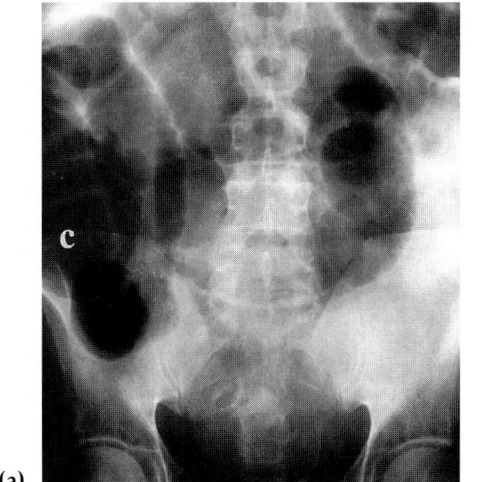 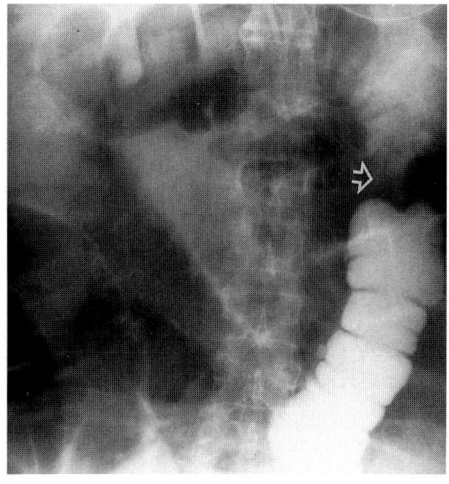

Fig. 21-42. Imaging of patient suspected of intestinal obstruction with plain film findings of dilated small bowel and colon. Use of contrast enema for intestinal obstruction in a 65-year-old man with abdominal distention, pain, and constipation and prior sigmoid resection for diverticulitis.
(a) Supine abdominal radiograph shows gas-distended cecum (C) in addition to small bowel distention. (b) Single-contrast barium enema shows obstructing carcinoma (open arrow) in proximal descending colon. (From Maglinte et al,[3] with permission.)

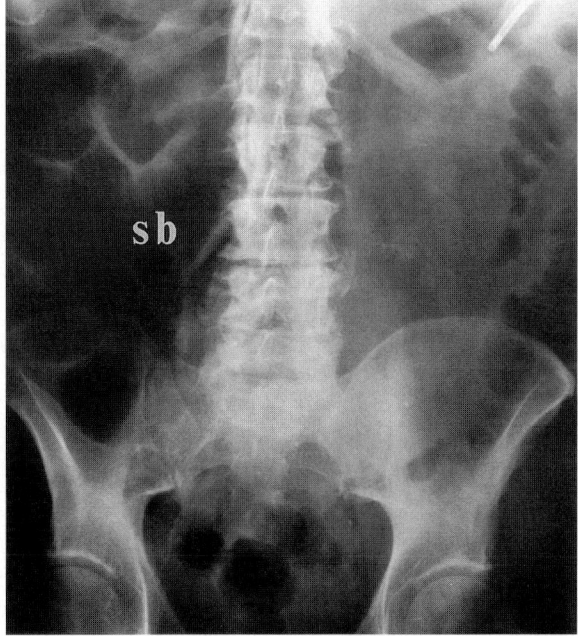 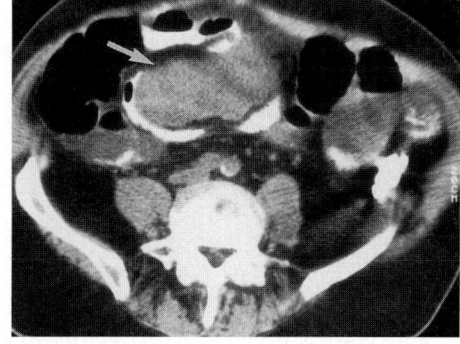

Fig. 21-43. Imaging of postoperative patient with possible ileus.
(a) Supine abdominal radiograph in postoperative patient (recent partial transverse colectomy for malignancy) with possible ileus. Note distention of distal small bowel (sb) with gas seen in rectosigmoid region. A soft tissue density (.) was suspected in left hemiabdomen. Tip of long decompression tube is in proximal jejunum. (b) CT scan shows a large interloop hematoma in anterior peritoneal cavity (arrow) displacing segments of adjacent bowel. (From Maglinte et al,[102] with permission.)

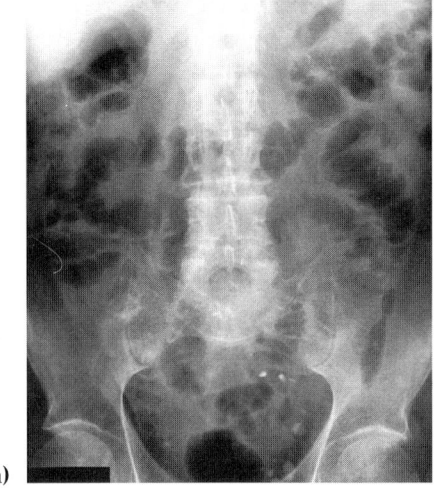 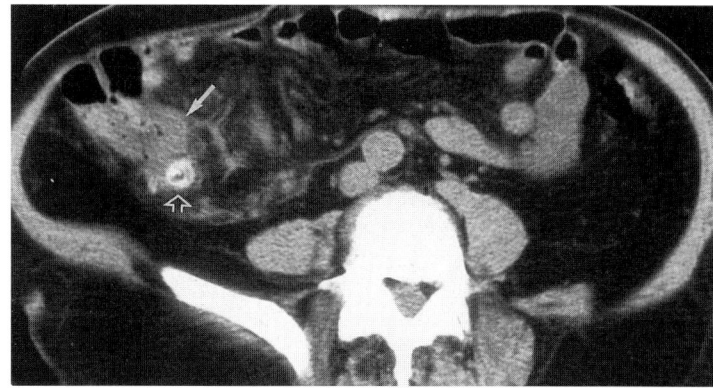

Fig. 21-44. Imaging of patient suspected of intestinal obstruction with plain film findings equivocal for small bowel obstruction: acute setting.
(a) Supine abdominal film in an 82-year-old patient with diffuse lower abdominal pain shows disproportionate distention of small bowel relative to colon, suspicious for mechanical small bowel obstruction. (b) CT scan of lower abdomen shows fluid collection (arrow) adjacent to cecum and proximal ascending colon with gas bubbles indicating abscess. Appendicolith (open arrow) not appreciated on abdominal plain film is seen within abscess. Note presence of distended segments of small bowel. (From Maglinte et al,[102] with permission.)

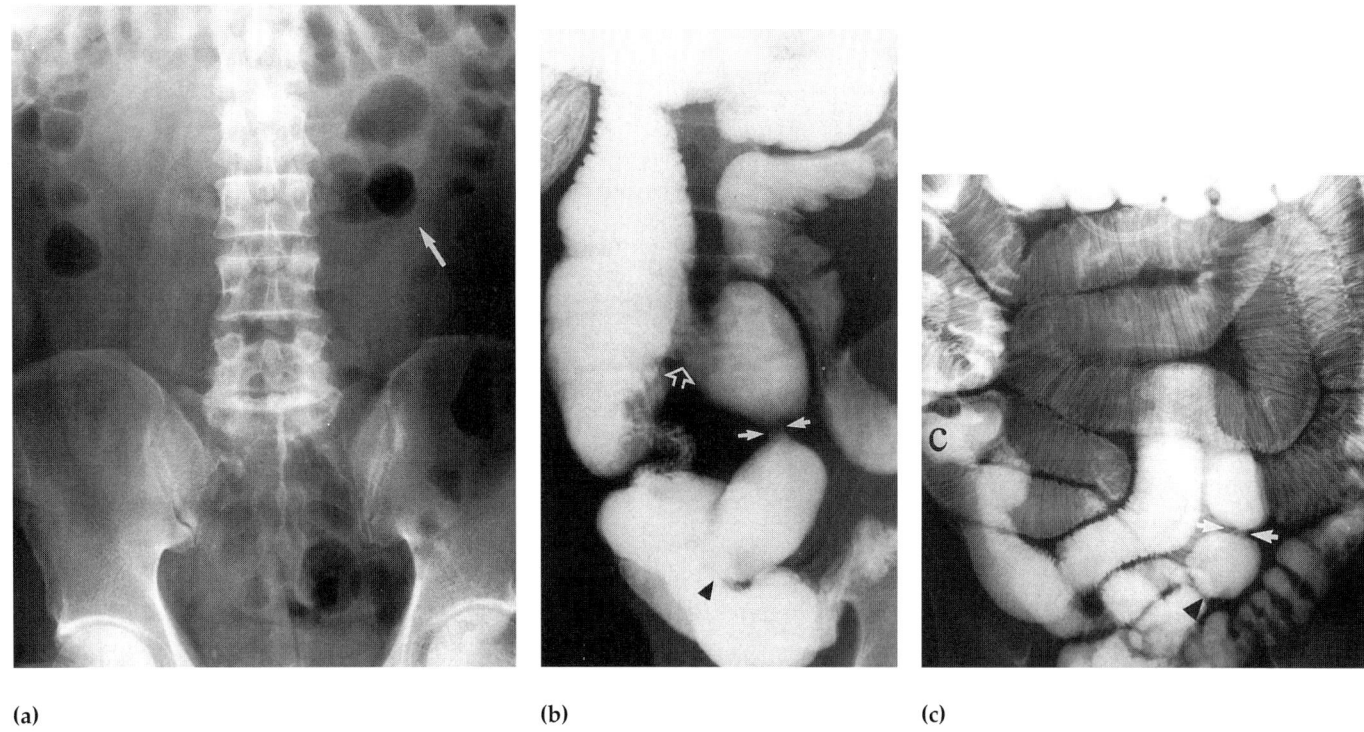

Fig. 21-45. Imaging of patient suspected of intestinal obstruction with normal or "abnormal but nonspecific" plain film findings—the patient with intermittent or nonacute symptoms.
(a) Plain film examination shows variably shaped, gas-filled, slightly distended small bowel in left upper abdomen (arrow) in a 50-year-old man with recurrent abdominal pain and vomiting. (b) Single-contrast enteroclysis demonstrated a Meckel's diverticulum (open arrow points to its attachment to ileum) with a constricted midportion (arrowhead). Arrowhead points to fundus of diverticulum. (c) Double-contrast enteroclysis shows no evidence for small bowel obstruction. At surgery, a fibrous cord was found attaching narrowed segment of diverticulum to lower abdomen, probably acting as fulcrum for intermittent volvulus. Arrowhead point to fundus of diverticulum, arrows point to constricted mid segment where fibrous cord was attached. C = cecum. (From Maglinte et al,[102] with permission.)

Scenario three: Plain film radiographs demonstrate "normal", "equivocal," or "abnormal but nonspecific" SBO patterns. CT is advised in all patients presenting with acute abdominal symptoms (emergency room patients) because of its high sensitivity for diagnosing high-grade or complete SBO, its ability to diagnose closed loop and strangulating obstruction, and its proven role in diagnosing acute abdominal conditions that can mimic intestinal obstruction (Fig. 21-44). Enteroclysis or fluoroscopy-based SBFT studies are used in the acute setting only if CT is not diagnostic. In contrast, a barium study is advocated as the initial imaging procedure in patients who present with mild, intermittent abdominal pain or other chronic, nonacute symptoms (outpatients or clinic patients) (Fig. 21-45).

Enteroclysis is exquisitely sensitive for diagnosing low-grade or partial obstructions, small intraluminal tumors, and subtle mucosal inflammatory changes that may be present in this patient population. CT may be performed as a complementary procedure if barium studies are not diagnostic.[3]

Pseudo-Obstruction of the Small Bowel

Intestinal pseudo-obstruction is defined as a syndrome in which there are signs and symptoms of intestinal obstruction without an actual obstructing lesion. In many cases it is associated with other entities but may be idiopathic. Faulk et al in a review paper described

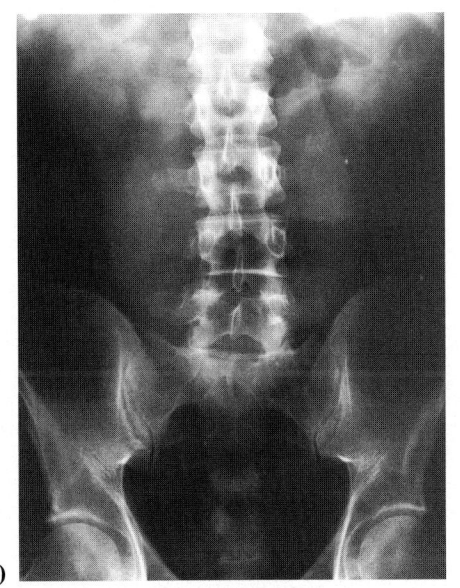

(a)

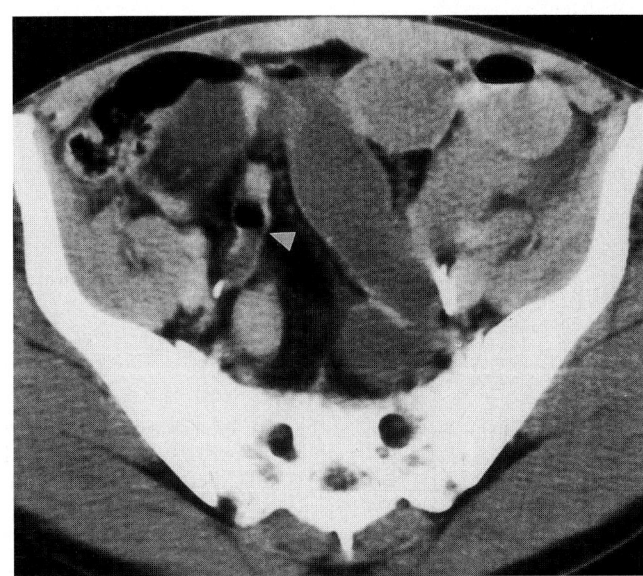

(b)

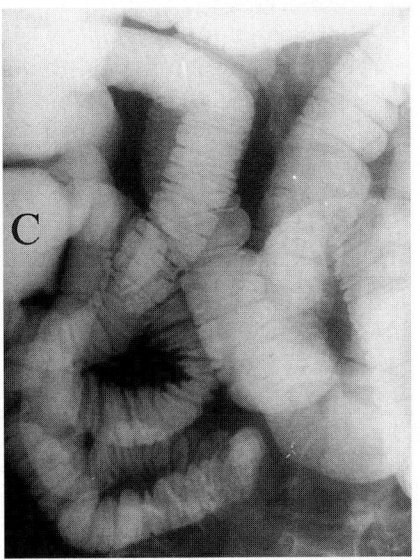

(c)

Fig. 21-46. Pseudo-obstruction of small bowel.
(a) Supine abdominal radiograph of an elderly diabetic patient complaining of abdominal pain and vomiting shows minimally dilated loops of small bowel in upper abdomen and no gas in colon suspicious for mechanical small bowel obstruction. (b) CT scan through lower abdomen following plain film examination shows slightly dilated fluid-filled loops of small bowel and fluid-filled but smaller-caliber distal small bowel (arrowhead) also concerning for mechanical obstruction. (c) Enteroclysis radiograph of right lower abdomen shows no point of obstruction. At fluoroscopy, flow was unimpeded but transit was prolonged. Compression radiography revealed no focal segment of fixation or stenosis. Note caliber of more proximal small bowel compared to narrower distal ileum. The findings are consistent with intestinal pseudo-obstruction secondary to diabetic neuropathy. C = cecum.

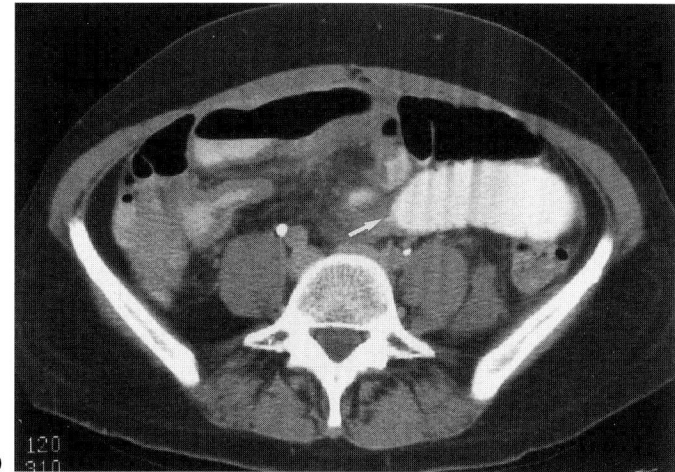
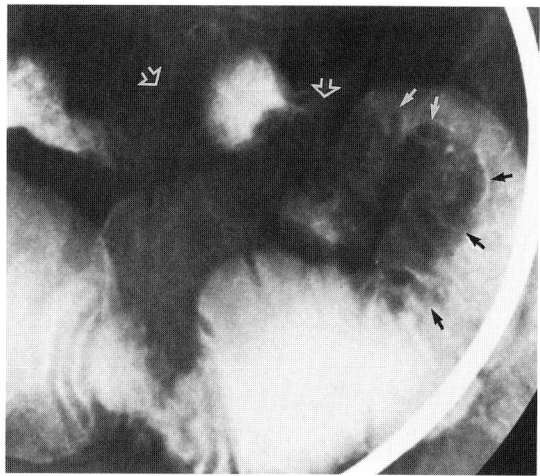
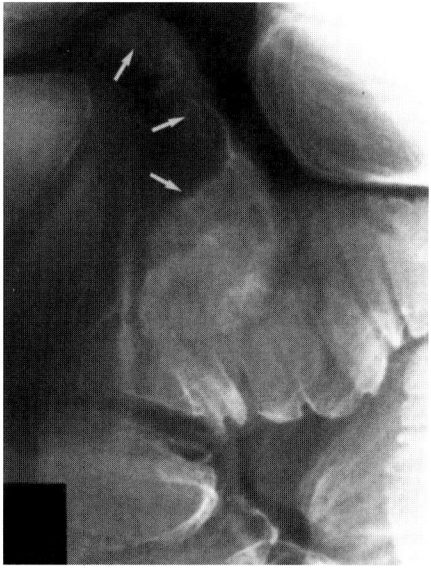

Fig. 21-47. Endometrial implants causing partial obstruction of the distal ileum.
(a) CT scan with intraluminal contrast shows dilated ileum narrowing abruptly (arrow). (b) En face view of multiple plaquelike deposits that reduce bowel lumen to reveal intact but thickened and distorted mucosal folds (short arrrows). Several further plaques seen more distally (open arrows) increase the obstructive effect. (c) Enteroclysis in a patient with known history of endometriosis. In terminal ileum close to ileocecal valve an endometrial plaque (arrows) causes low-grade obstruction.

26 different causes of pseudo-obstruction under five headings: diseases involving the intestinal smooth muscle (eg, collagen vascular disease, amyloidosis), endocrine disorders (eg, diabetes mellitus, hypoparathyroidism), neurological diseases (eg, Parkinson's disease, Hirschprung's disease), pharmacological (eg, phenothiozines, tricyclic antidepressants), and miscellaneous (eg, jejunoileal bypass, psychosis, cathartic colon).[98] It may also result from a prior side-to-side or end-to-end small bowel anastomosis.[99] Division of circular muscles results in disturbance of peristalsis resulting in stasis with dilatation of the proximal segment and formation of a blind pouch (see Chapter 29). Intestinal pseudo-obstruction may be acute (transient), which has been described mainly in the old or chronically ill.[100] It may involve the small or large bowel or both. The small bowel is dilated but in some cases the distal ileum may be of normal caliber.[101]

Differentiation from mechanical obstruction is very difficult. The role of radiology is to exclude mechanical causes of obstruction. Plain film demonstration of dilated small bowel with air-fluid levels is unhelpful. Conventional small bowel follow-through is also not informative, with delayed transit resulting in segmentation of the barium column and poor coating of distal segments. The delineation of the transition point at CT may be difficult and can be misleading. Enteroclysis is clinically of value in excluding a mechanical cause of obstruction (Fig. 21-46).

Miscellaneous Causes

Endometrial Implants

Endometriosis is defined as the implantation of endometrial tissue outside the uterus. Pelvic structures,

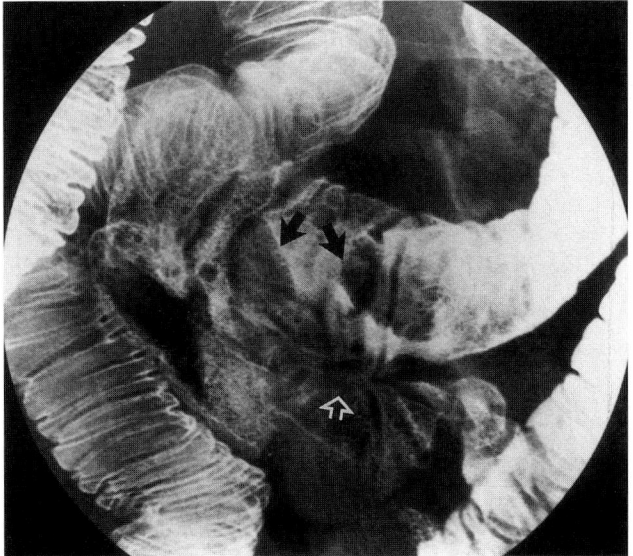

Fig. 21-48. Low-grade obturation of small bowel.
(a) Two enteroliths (arrows) are held up above a side-to-side anastomosis (open arrow) causing mild obstruction. (b) A coin is arrested above a stricture in the distal ileum and bowel above is slightly dilated. (c) A large number of Procardia (nifedipine) sustained-release tablets have accumulated in the terminal ileum short of the ileocecal valve and partially obstruct transit into the colon. (Courtesy of KC Cho, MD.)

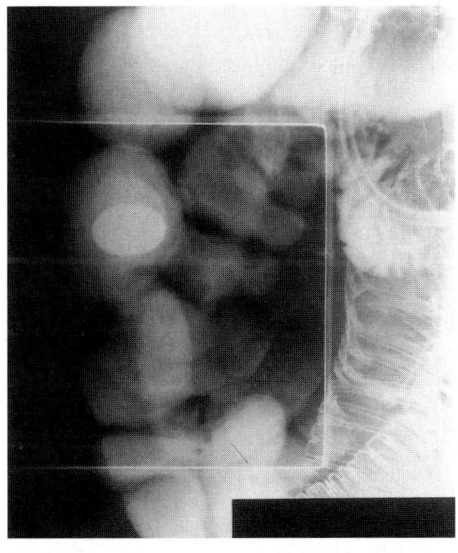

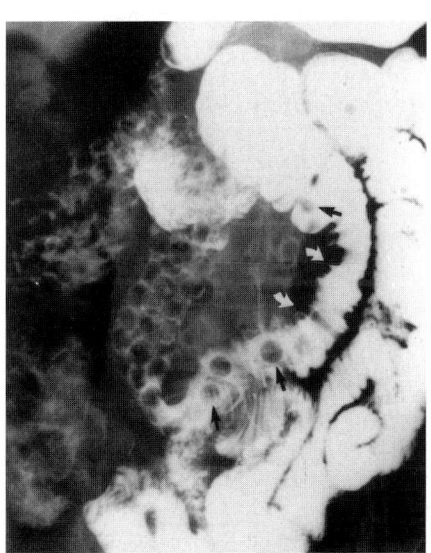

mostly rectum and sigmoid, are the more frequent sites. The small bowel is implanted in only 2% to 7% of cases. Multiple endometrial deposits in distal ileum have been the cause of obstruction in a 38-year-old patient; a CT scan was interpreted as showing partial obstruction by adhesions [Fig. 21-47(a)]. Enteroclysis [Fig. 21-47(b)] demonstrated features that suggested endometrial implants as the cause of obstruction. In another patient an endometrial plaque reduced the lumen of the terminal ileum to cause low-grade obstruction [Fig. 21-47(c)].

Obturation

Obturation refers to blockage by an intraluminal structure that did not originate at that site. Two examples are provided [Fig. 21-48(a, b)], enteroliths above a side-to-side anastomosis and a coin arrested above a stricture in the distal ileum. Another rare cause of partial obturation can be the accumulation of Procardia (nifediine) extended-release tablets above a narrowed segment of the intestinal tract [Fig. 21-48(c)].

Nonsteroidal Anti-Inflammatory Drug (NSAID)–Related Diaphragm Disease

This represents a rare complication of this potentially gastrointestinal tract ulceration–producing medication. Multiple postulcer diaphragms may occur in small bowel or even colon after prolonged use of these anti-inflammatory medications like diclofenac (Fig. 21-49).

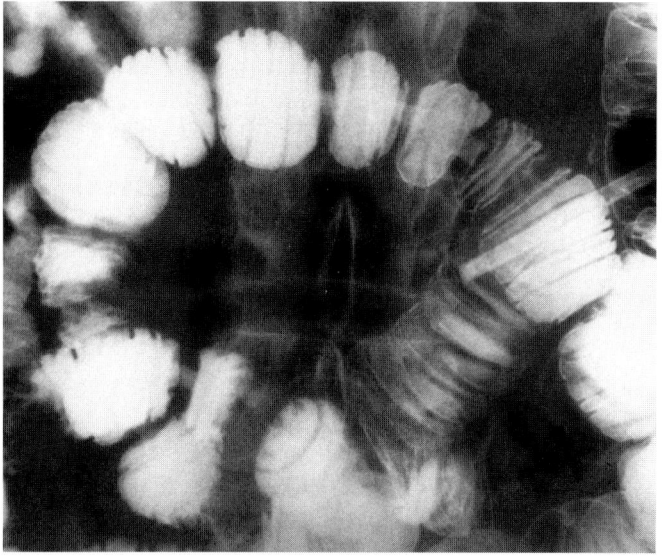 (a)
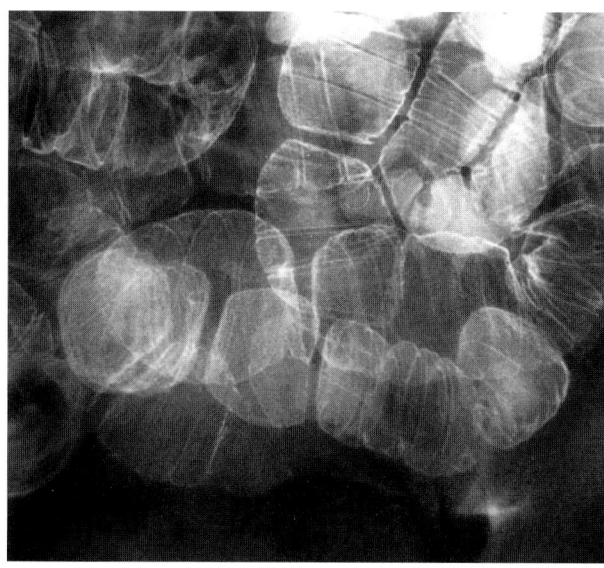 (b)

Fig. 21-49. Prolonged NSAID use for rheumatoid disease.
(a, b) A long loop of mid-jejunum shows typical "diaphragm disease," a mildly obstructing condition consisting of numerous diaphragms with central lumen narrowing; this was best shown during the late single-contrast phase of enteroclysis. Confirmed by surgery. (Courtesy of Arunas Gasparaitis, MD.)

References

1. Welch JP. General consideration and mortality in bowel obstruction. In: Welch JP, ed. *Bowel Obstruction: Differential Diagnosis and Clinical Management.* Philadelphia, Pa: WB Saunders Co; 1990:59–95.
2. Schwartz SI, Storer EH. Manifestations of gastrointestinal diseases. In: Schwartz SI, Shires GT, Spencer FC, et al, eds. *Principles of Surgery.* New York, NY: McGraw-Hill, 1978:1039–1079.
3. Maglinte DDT, Balthazar EJ, Kelvin FM, Megibow AJ. The role of radiology in the diagnosis of small bowel obstruction. *AJR.* 1997;168:1171–1180.
4. Ellis H. *Intestinal Obstruction.* New York, NY: Appleton-Century-Crofts; 1982.
5. Mucha P Jr. Small intestinal obstruction. *Surg Clin North Am.* 1987;67:597–620.
6. Vick RM. Statistics of acute intestinal obstruction. *Br Med J.* 1932;2:546–548.
7. Bizer LS, Liebling RW, Delany HM, et al. Small bowel obstruction: the role of nonoperative treatment in simple intestinal obstruction and predictive criteria for strangulation obstruction. *Surgery.* 1981;89:407–413.
8. Lefall LD, Syphax B. Clinical aids in strangulation intestinal obstruction. *Am J Surg.* 1970;120:756–759.
9. Herlinger H, Maglinte DDT. Small bowel obstruction. In: Herlinger H, Maglinte DDT, eds. *Clinical Radiology of the Small Intestine.* Philadelphia, Pa: WB Saunders Co; 1989:479–507.
10. Maglinte DDT, Nolan DJ, Herlinger H. Preoperative diagnosis by enteroclysis of unsuspected closed loop obstruction in medically managed patients. *J Clin Gastroenterol.* 1991;13(3):308–312.
11. Shrake PD, Rex DK, Lappas JC, et al. Radiographic evaluation of suspected small bowel obstruction. *Am J Gastroenterol.* 1991;86:175–178.
12. Glotzer DJ, Compton CC. Case records of the Massachusetts General Hospital. *N Engl J Med.* 1987;316:394–403.
13. Cohn I Jr. Intestinal obstruction. In: Berk JE, Haubrich WS, Kalser MH, et al, eds. *Bockus Gastroenterology.* 4th ed. Philadelphia, Pa: WB Saunders Co; 1985:2056–2080.
14. Wangensteen OH. Understanding the bowel obstruction problem. *Am Surg.* 1978;135:131–149.
15. Sarr MG, Bulkley GB, Zuidema GD. Preoperative recognition of intestinal strangulation obstruction: prospective evaluation of diagnostic capability. *Am J Surg.* 1983;145:176–182.
16. Laws HL, Aldrete JS. Small bowel obstruction: a review of 465 cases. *South Med J.* 1976;69:733–734.
17. Silen W, Hein MF, Goldman L. Strangulation obstruction of the small intestine. *Arch Surg.* 1962;85:137–145.
18. Barnett WO, Petro AB, Williamson JW. A current appraisal of problems with gangrenous bowel. *Ann Surg.* 1976;183:653–659.
19. Nadrowski LF. Pathophysiology and current treatment of intestinal obstruction. *Rev Surg.* 1974;31:381–407.
20. Shatila AH, Chamberlain BE, Webb WR. Current status of diagnosis and management of strangulation obstruction of the small bowel. *Am J Surg.* 1976;132:299–303.

21. Davis SE, Sperling L. Obstruction of the small intestine. *Arch Surg.* 1969;99:424–426.
22. Snyder EN, McCranie D. Closed loop obstruction of the small bowel. *Am J Surg.* 1965;111:398–402.
23. Frazee RC, Mucha P Jr, Farnell MB, et al. Volvulus of the small intestine. *Ann Surg.* 1988;208:565–568.
24. Otamiri T, Sjodahl R, Ihse I. Intestinal obstruction with strangulation of the small bowel. *Acta Chir Scand.* 1987;153:307–310.
25. Brolin RE, Krasna MJ, Mast BA. Use of tubes and radiographs in the management of small bowel obstruction. *Ann Surg.* 1987;206:126–133.
26. Hofstetter SR. Acute adhesive obstruction in the small intestine. *Surg Gynecol Obstet.* 1981;152:141–144.
27. Snyder CL, Ferrell KL, Goodale RL, et al. Nonoperative management of small bowel obstruction with endoscopic long intestinal tube placement. *Am Surg.* 1990;56:587–592.
28. Peetz DJ Jr, Gamelli RL, Pilcher DB. Intestinal intubation in acute mechanical small bowel obstruction. *Arch Surg.* 1982;117:334–336.
29. Seror D, Feigin E, Szold A, et al. How conservatively can postoperative small bowel obstruction be treated? *Am J Surg.* 1993;165:121–126.
30. Herlinger H, Rubesin SE. Obstruction. In: Gore RM, Levine MS, Laufer I, eds. *Textbook of Gastrointestinal Radiology.* Philadelphia, Pa: WB Saunders Co; 1993:931–966.
31. Balthazar EJ, Birnbaum BA, Megibow AJ, et al. Closed-loop and strangulating intestinal obstruction: CT signs. *Radiology.* 1992;185:769–775.
32. Price J, Nolan DJ. Post-loop obstruction: diagnosis by enteroclysis. *Gastrointest Radiol.* 1989;14:251–254.
33. Balthazar EJ. CT of small bowel obstruction. *AJR.* 1994;162:255–261.
34. Maglinte DDT, Herlinger H, Nolan DJ. Radiologic features of closed loop obstruction: analysis of 25 confirmed cases. *Radiology.* 1991;179:383–387.
35. Caroline DF, Herlinger H, Laufer I, et al. Small bowel enema in the diagnosis of adhesive obstruction. *AJR.* 1984;143:1133–1139.
36. Osteen RT, Guyton S, Steele G Jr, et al. Malignant intestinal obstruction. *Surgery.* 1980;87:611–615.
37. Ketcham AS, Hoye RC, Pilch YH, et al. Delayed intestinal obstruction following treatment for cancer. *Cancer.* 1970;25:406–410.
38. Maglinte DDT, Reyes BL, Harmon BH, et al. Reliability and role of plain film radiography and CT in the diagnosis of small bowel obstruction. *AJR.* 1996;167:1451–1455.
39. Patel NH, Lauber PR. The meaning of a nonspecific abdominal gas pattern. *Acad Radiol.* 1995;2:667–669.
40. Suh RS, Maglinte DDT, Lavonas EJ, et al. Emergency abdominal radiography: discrepancies of preliminary and final interpretation and management relevance. *Emerg Radiol.* 1995;2:1–4.
41. Maglinte DDT. Nonspecific abdominal gas pattern: an interpretation whose time is gone (editorial). *Emerg Radiol.* 1996;3:93–95.
42. Welch J, Donaldson G. Management of severe obstruction of large bowel due to malignant disease. *Am J Surg.* 1977;112:809–812.
43. Chapman AH, McNamara M, Porter G. The acute contrast enema in suspected large bowel obstruction: value and technique. *Clin Radiol.* 1992;46:273–278.
44. Frimann-Dahl J. The administration of barium only in acute obstruction. Advantages and results. *Acta Radiol.* 1954;42:285–295.
45. Nelson SW, Christoforides AJ. The use of barium sulfate suspensions in the study of suspected mechanical obstruction of the small intestine. *AJR.* 1967;101:367–378.
46. Maglinte DDT, Steven SH, Hall RC, et al. Dual purpose tube for enteroclysis and nasogastric/nasoenteric decompression. *Radiology.* 1992;185:281–282.
47. Nelson SW, Christoforides AJ, Roenigh DVM. Dangers and fallibilities of iodinated radiopaque media in obstruction of the small bowel. *Am J Surg.* 1965;109:546–559.
48. Taverne PP, van der Jagt EJ. Small bowel radiography: a prospective comparative study of three techniques in 200 patients. *Fortschr Röntgenstr.* 1985;143:293–297.
49. Maglinte DDT, Lappas JC, Kelvin FM, et al. Small bowel radiography: how, when, and why? *Radiology.* 1987;163:297–305.
50. Maglinte DDT, Kelvin FM, O'Connor K, et al. Review: current status of small bowel radiography. *Abdom Imaging.* 1996;21:247–257.
51. Maglinte DDT, Kelvin FM, Micon LT, et al. Nasointestinal tube for decompression or enteroclysis: experience with 150 patients. *Abdom Imaging.* 1994;19:108–112.
52. Maglinte DDT. Biphasic enteroclysis with methylcellulose. In: Freeny PC, Stevenson GW, eds. *Margulis and Burhennes Alimentary Tract Radiology.* 5th ed. St. Louis, Mo: CV Mosby; 1994:533–547.
53. Maglinte DDT, Gage SN, Harmon BH, et al. Obstruction of the small intestine: accuracy and role of CT in diagnosis. *Radiology.* 1993;186:61–64.
54. Megibow AJ, Balthazar EJ, Cho KC, et al. Bowel obstruction: evaluation with CT. *Radiology.* 1991;180:313–318.
55. Fukuya T, Hawes DR, Lu CC, et al. CT diagnosis of small bowel obstruction: efficacy in 60 patients. *AJR.* 1992;158:765–769.
56. Taourel PG, Fabre VM, Pradel JA, et al. Value of CT in diagnosis and management of patients with suspected acute small bowel obstruction. *AJR.* 1995;165:1187–1192.
57. Gazelle GS, Goldberg MA, Wittenberg J, et al. Efficacy of CT in distinguishing small bowel obstruction from other causes of small bowel dilatation. *AJR.* 1994;162:43–47.
58. Frager DH, Baer JW, Rothpearl A, et al. Distinction between postoperative ileus and mechanical small bowel obstruction: value of CT compared with clinical and other radiographic findings. *AJR.* 1995;164:891–894.
59. Bender GN, Timmons JH, Williard WC, et al. Computed tomographic enteroclysis—one methodology. *Invest Radiol.* 1996;31:43–49.
60. Maglinte DDT, Reyes BL. Computed tomographic diagnosis of partial small bowel obstruction secondary to

anterior peritoneal adhesions: relevance to laparoscopic cholecystectomy. *Emerg Radiol.* 1996;3:84–86.
61. Memel DS, Berland LL. CT of bowel obstruction: interpretation using cine paging (letter). *AJR.* 1995;164:766–767.
62. Menzies D, Ellis H. Intestinal obstruction from adhesions—how big is the problem? *Ann R Coll Surg Engl.* 1990;72:60–63.
63. Maglinte DDT, Peterson LA, Vahey TN, et al. Enteroclysis in partial small bowel obstruction. *Am J Surg.* 1984;147:325–329.
64. Meyers MA. *Dynamic Radiology of the Abdomen. Normal and Pathologic Anatomy.* 3rd ed. New York, NY: Springer-Verlag; 1988:376–377.
65. Maglinte DDT, Reyes BL. Small bowel cancer: radiologic diagnosis. *Radiol Clin North Am.* 1997;35:361–380.
66. Zboralske FF, Bessolo RJ. Metastatic carcinoma to the mesentery and gut. *Radiology.* 1967;88:302–310.
67. Marshak RH, Khilnani MT, Eliasoph J, et al. Metastatic carcinoma of the small bowel. *AJR.* 1965;94:385–394.
68. Walkey MM, Friedman AC, Sohotra P, et al. CT manifestations of peritoneal carcinomatosis. *AJR.* 1988;150:1035–1041.
69. Scholz FJ. Gastrointestinal complications of radiation therapy. In: Gore RM, Levine MS, Laufer I, eds. *Textbook of Gastrointestinal Radiology.* Philadelphia, Pa: WB Saunders Co; 1993:2707–2716.
70. Maglinte DDT, Herlinger H. Vascular disorders of the small intestine. In: Herlinger H, Maglinte DDT, eds. *Clinical Radiology of the Small Intestine.* Philadelphia, Pa: WB Saunders Co; 1989:466–472.
71. Mendelson RM, Nolan DJ. The radiological features of radiation enteritis. *Clin Radiol.* 1985;36:141–148.
72. Fishman EJ, Zinreich ES, Jones B, et al. Computed tomographic diagnosis of radiation ileitis. *Gastrointest Radiol.* 1984;9:149–152.
73. Sufian S, Matsumoto T. Intestinal obstruction. *Am J Surg.* 1975;130:9–14.
74. Ghahremani GG. Internal abdominal hernias. *Surg Clin North Am.* 1984;64:393–406.
75. Maglinte DDT, Miller RE, Lappas JC. Radiologic diagnosis of occult incisional hernias of the small intestine. *AJR.* 1984;142:931–932.
76. Cheadle WG, Garr EE, Richardson JD. The importance of early diagnosis of small bowel obstruction. *Ann Surg.* 1988;54:565–569.
77. Asbun HJ, Halasz NA. Small intestinal obstruction: an update. *Probl Gen Surg.* 1989;6:93–98.
78. Mellins HZ, Rigler LG. The roentgen findings in strangulating obstructions of the small intestine. *AJR.* 1954;71:404–415.
79. Fisher JK. Computed tomographic diagnosis of volvulus in intestinal malrotation. *Radiology.* 1981;140:145–146.
80. Balthazar EJ, Bauman JS, Megibow AJ. CT diagnosis of closed loop obstruction. *J Comput Assist Tomogr.* 1985;9:953–955.
81. Jaramillo D, Raval B. CT diagnosis of primary small bowel volvulus. *AJR.* 1986;147:941–942.
82. Cho KC, Hoffman-Trentin JC, Alterman DD. Closed-loop obstruction of the small bowel: CT and sonographic appearance. *J Comput Assist Tomogr.* 1989;13:256–258.
83. Shaff MI, Himmelfarb E, Sacks GA, et al. The whirl sign: a CT finding in volvulus of the large bowel. *J Comput Assist Tomogr.* 1985;9:410.
84. Ha HK, Kim SK, Lee MS, et al. Differentiation of simple and strangulated small-bowel obstructions: usefulness of known CT criteria. *Radiology.* 1997;204:507–512.
85. Frager D, Baer JW, Medwid SW. Detection of intestinal ischemia in patients with acute small bowel obstruction due to adhesions or hernia: efficacy of CT. *AJR.* 1996;166:67–71.
86. Wiot JF, Spitz HB. Small bowel intussusception demonstrated by oral barium. *Radiology.* 1970;97:361–366.
87. Ghahremani GG. Radiology of Meckel's diverticulum. *Crit Rev Diagn Imaging.* 1986;26:1–43.
88. Rubesin SE, Herlinger H, DeGaeta L. Interlude: test your skills. *Radiology.* 1990;178:636–644.
89. Curcio CM, Feinstein RS, Humphrey RL, et al. Computed tomography of entero-enteric intussusception. *J Comput Assist Tomogr.* 1982;6:969–974.
90. Merine D, Fishman EK, Jones F, et al. Enteroenteric intussusception: CT findings in nine patients. *AJR.* 1987;148:1129–1132.
91. Balthazar EJ. CT of the gastrointestinal tract: principles and interpretation. *AJR.* 1991;156:23–32.
92. Weber A, Nadel S. CT appearance of retrograde jejunoduodenogastric intussusception: a rare complication of gastrostomy tubes. *AJR.* 1991;156:957–959.
93. Wood GJ, Kumar PN, Cooper C, et al. AIDS-associated intussusception in young adults. *J Clin Gastroenterol.* 1995;21:158–162.
94. Sharkey KA, Sutherland LR, Davison JS, et al. Peptides in the gastrointestinal tract in human immunodeficiency virus infection. *Gastroenterology.* 1992;103:18–28.
95. Sato Y, Frey E, Foderaro A, Prinzle KC. Small bowel obstruction due to an intestinal balloon: treatment by percutaneous needle puncture. *AJR.* 1986;147:1019–1020.
96. Smoger BR, Rosen RJ, Teplik SK, et al. Small bowel obstruction caused by gaseous distention of the Cantor tube balloon. *AJR.* 1980;135:612–613.
97. Boyle TM, Agus SG, Bauer JJ. Small intestinal obstruction secondary to obturation by a Garren gastric bubble. *Am J Gastroenterol.* 1987;82:51–53.
98. Faulk DL, Anura S, Christensen J. Chronic intestinal pseudo-obstruction. *Gastroenterology.* 1978;74:922–931.
99. Schlegel DM, Maglinte DDT. The blind pouch syndrome. *Surg Gynecol Obstet.* 1982;155:541–544.
100. Melamed M, Kuhian E. Relationship of the autonomic nervous system to "functional obstruction" of the intestinal tract: report of four cases, one with perforation. *Radiology.* 1963;80:22–29.
101. Maldonado JE, Gregg JA, Green PA, et al. Chronic idiopathic intestinal pseudo-obstruction. *Am J Med.* 1970;49:203–212.
102. Maglinte DDT, Herlinger H, Turner WW Jr, Kelvin FM. Radiologic management of small bowel obstruction: a practical approach. *Emerg Radiol.* 1994;1:138–149.

Postsurgical Small Bowel

22

John C. Lappas and William L. Campbell

Chapter Contents

Introduction
Small Bowel After Gastric Surgery
Enterectomy and Small Bowel Anastomosis
Enterostomy
Ileal Reservoirs
Small Bowel Transplantation

Introduction

Surgical treatment of disease of the small bowel requires the use of relatively few operative techniques, and most of these surgical interventions are applicable to any segment of the jejunum and ileum. Primarily they include enterotomy for removal of polyps or foreign bodies; enteroplasty to resolve a short segmental stricture; enterectomy for resection of obstructed, traumatized, neoplastic, or necrotic segments; plication to prevent intestinal obstruction; and creation of ostomies or mucous fistulas for feeding or drainage purposes.[1] In addition, the small bowel is used for the surgical construction of reservoirs after gastrectomy and proctocolectomy, and for the reconstitution of biliary and pancreatic flow with the gastrointestinal tract. Surgical bypass of the small bowel has also been performed in an attempt to control morbid obesity or lower serum cholesterol. Of most recent development is the surgical option of small bowel transplantation for the treatment of selected patients with short-bowel syndrome and intestinal failure.

Radiological studies are seldom performed as routine follow-up of the surgical procedure; rather they are done to assess the integrity of the small bowel or to investigate postoperative complications. In patients with a prior history of small bowel surgery who present with gastrointestinal symptoms, the postoperative anatomy and site of any anastomosis should be evaluated by carefully performed small bowel studies (Figs. 22-1, 22-2).

Small Bowel After Gastric Surgery

Significant alterations may occur in gastrointestinal physiology after operations on the stomach. Often grouped together as the postgastrectomy syndrome, various pathophysiologic disorders result from interruption of the pyloric sphincter mechanism or from sequelae of truncal vagotomy. Rapid influx of hyperosmotic gastric contents into the small bowel may manifest clinically as the dumping syndrome with symptoms of postprandial cramping and urgent diarrhea. Mild dilatation of the efferent jejunum can be observed. Serotonin, bradykinin, and enteroglucagon are also released systemically by the small intestine in response to luminal distension and are in part responsible for the vasomotor component of dumping.[2,3] In postvagotomy diarrhea, small bowel dysmotility and impaired pancreatic and biliary function are noted. Malabsorption with intestinal mucosal changes and bacterial colonization in the proximal small bowel are also contributing factors.[3,4] Cases of latent celiac disease have become active after gastric surgery, presumably because of more direct contact with gluten.[5] Vagotomy may also render evident previously asymptomatic adult celiac disease.[6]

Afferent Loop Syndrome

Afferent loop obstruction is an uncommon complication of subtotal gastrectomy with Billroth II gastrojejunostomy and occurs with variable clinical severity, acuteness, and chronicity. Causes include internal hernia, kinking of the anastomosis, adhesive band, stomal stenosis, neoplasms, and inflammatory disease.[7,8] Internal hernia is commonly responsible for the onset of an acute syndrome in the immediate postoperative period. Improved surgical techniques incorporating use of a short afferent loop and closure of the retroanastomotic space have reduced the incidence of afferent loop syndrome to 0.3%.[8]

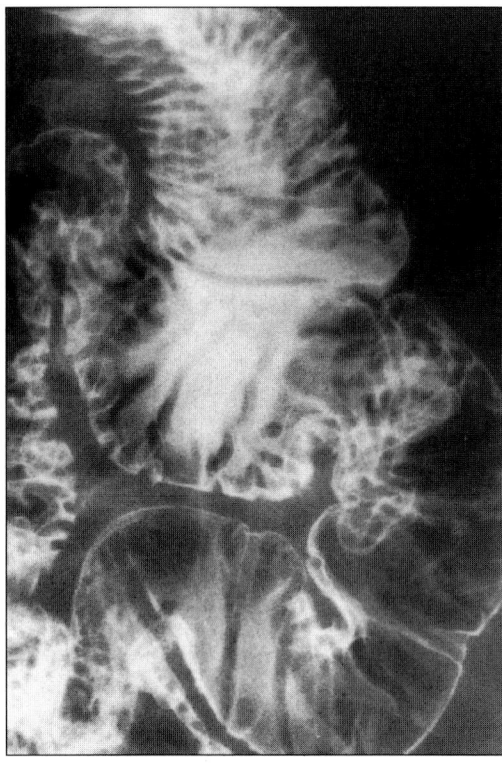

Fig. 22-1. Enteroenteric anastomosis.
End-to-side jejunal anastomosis demonstrated during small bowel enteroclysis. Control of intestinal distension achieved by enteroclysis infusion facilitates the radiographic delineation of the postsurgical small bowel anatomy and is an optimal examination technique.

Clinically the diagnosis may be difficult to establish. Patients may present vague symptoms of nausea, cramps, and postprandial fullness or classic features of bilious vomiting with relief of abdominal pain. Acute obstruction of the afferent loop with elevation in serum amylase can mimic acute pancreatitis. Chronic progression of the syndrome can result in malabsorption, intestinal hemorrhage, or perforation.

Abdominal radiographs are often normal since the afferent loop is fluid-filled and gasless due to distal obstruction. Barium contrast studies may suggest the diagnosis by either nonfilling of the afferent loop or preferential filling of a distended proximal loop in association with stasis and delayed emptying (Fig. 22-3). The efficacy of barium studies is controversial, however, because the afferent loop can remain unopacified during the examination in 20% of normal patients.[9] Radionuclide studies with 99mTc-DISIDA may show persistent activity in the abnormal afferent loop.[10] Computed tomography (CT) and ultrasonography permit direct visualization of the obstructed afferent loop and are the preferred imaging methods for establishing the diagnosis.[11–13] CT demonstrates two or more thinly marginated round cystic masses that are adjacent to the pancreas, and that on sequential scans can be traced to form the distended U-shaped afferent loop (Fig. 22-4). Transmitted pressure from the obstruction may be sufficient to secondarily distend the gallbladder and bile ducts and create additional cystic masses on CT.[12] Ultrasonography similarly demonstrates the dilated afferent loop as a cystic tubular structure in continuity with the gastric anas-

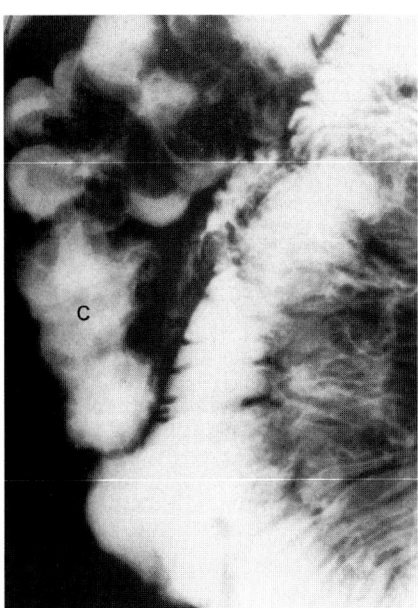

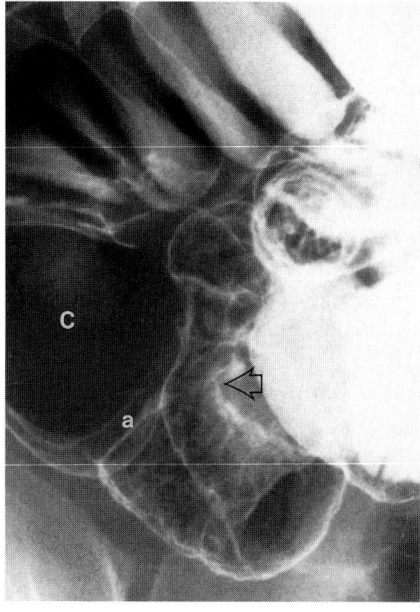

(a) (b)

Fig. 22-2. Ileocolic anastomosis.
(a) Evaluation of the distal ileum in a symptomatic patient with prior ileocolic resection for Crohn's disease is difficult on this small bowel series due to inadequate bowel distention. C = colon. (b) Performance of the peroral pneuomocolon technique, which utilizes retrograde air insufflation and glucagon-induced hypotonia, improves distention of the area of interest. The end-to-end anastomosis (a) is patent but the nodular mucosal surface and mild narrowing of the ileal lumen (arrow) indicate recurrent disease. C = colon.

differentiating afferent loop syndrome from confusing pancreatic pseudocysts.[12,13]

Jejunogastric Intussusception

Jejunogastric intussusception is a rare but potentially lethal complication following simple gastrojejunostomy or after any of the modifications of Billroth II surgery. Intussusception may occur early after operation but is generally a late complication, occurring on the average of 6 years postoperatively. Retrograde peristalsis without other associated abnormality is the most widely mentioned causative factor.[14] Invagination of the efferent jejunal loop accounts for 75% of jejunogastric intussusceptions, and the afferent loop, alone or in combination with the efferent loop, constitutes the remainder.

Clinically, the acute form is associated with the findings of proximal intestinal obstruction, left upper quadrant abdominal mass, and hematemesis. Chronic intussusception is more difficult to diagnose because of its intermittent nature and vague symptoms.

Radiographically, the diagnosis is typically made on barium studies, as abdominal plain films are usually unremarkable. Contrast characteristically outlines concentric stretched and edematous jejunal folds that are associated with the mass defect of the intussusceptum within the gastric remnant (Fig. 22-5). Distinction between anatomic types of intussusception is suggested by normal opacification of one postsurgical limb, implying abnormality of the other. Examination

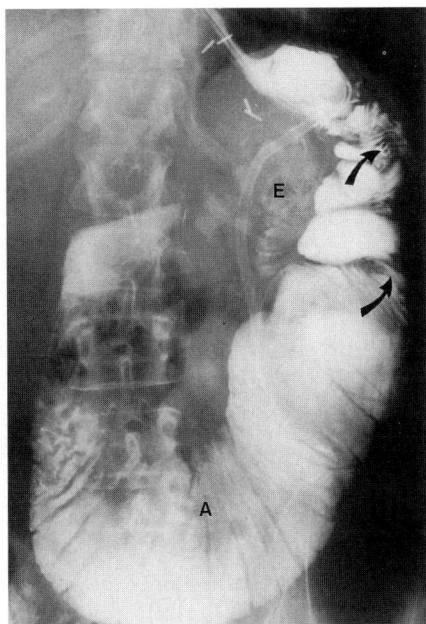

Fig. 22-3. Afferent loop obstruction.
Barium injection into a small gastric remnant results in preferential filling of a distended afferent loop (A) as only minimal contrast enters the efferent (E) segment. Note the distorted bowel margins due to kinking and tethering from multiple adhesive bands (arrows).

tomosis and biliary system.[13] Uniform size of the obstructed afferent loop and anterior displacement of the superior mesenteric artery may be useful clues in

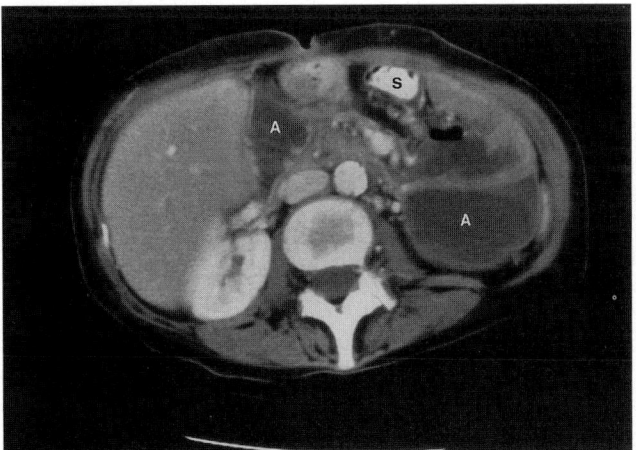

(a)

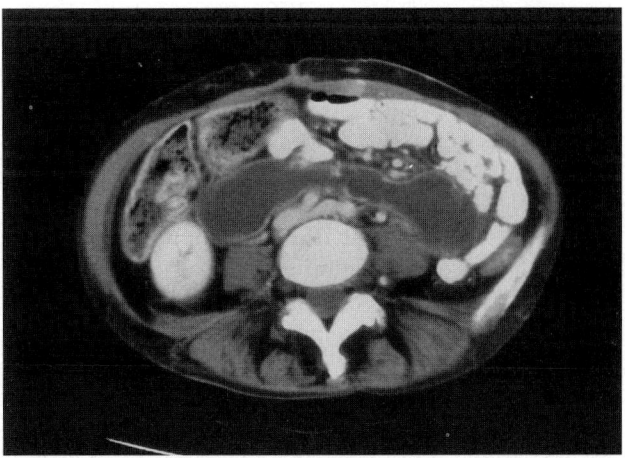

(b)

Fig. 22-4. Computed tomography (CT) of afferent loop obstruction.
(a) Abnormally dilated afferent loop (A) represented by multiple thin-rim cystic masses seen in the retrogastric and peripancreatic regions. Oral contrast opacifies the gastric remnant (S). (b) Caudal scan verifies the characteristic U-shape of the obstructed loop, which remains nonopacified as the normal efferent small bowel loops fill with contrast medium.

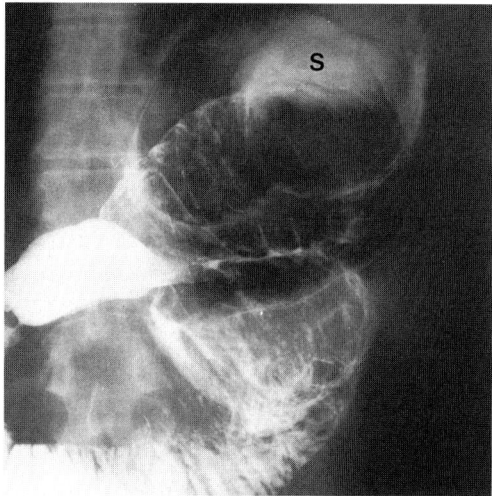

Fig. 22-5. Jejunogastric intussusception.
Retrograde intussusception of the efferent loop into the gastric remnant (S) creates a characteristic coil-spring mass defect and obstruction of the efferent loop.

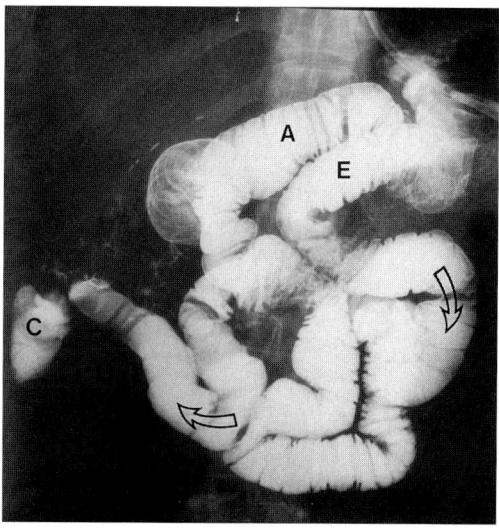

Fig. 22-6. Inadvertent gastroileostomy after subtotal gastric resection and planned Billroth II gastroenterostomy. Enteroclysis infusion into the distal efferent loop (E) demonstrates its abnormal shortened course (arrows) to the right lower quadrant with prompt filing of cecum (C). Progressive barium reflux into the elongated proximal afferent loop (A) became increasingly apparent during the course of examination.

during symptomatic intervals optimizes the diagnosis of chronic intermittent forms of jejunogastric intussusception.

Inadvertent Gastroileostomy

Gastroileostomy represents a surgical misadventure in which an inadvertent anastomosis is performed between the stomach and ileum instead of the jejunum. It usually occurs during a difficult operation complicated by the presence of dense adhesions, and is the result of improper identification of the ligament of Treitz. Intestinal malrotation and obesity may also be contributing factors. Symptoms of diarrhea and weight loss, often extreme, occur shortly after operation. Varying degrees of malabsorption with anemia and electrolyte imbalance result from the short-circuiting of the small bowel. The symptoms of gastroileostomy frequently mimic those associated with postgastrectomy diarrhea or gastrojejunocolic fistula.

Correct diagnosis requires an accurate interpretation of the radiographic contrast studies.[15] The essential diagnostic feature is recognition of a distal efferent loop that crosses from the left upper quadrant of the abdomen directly to the right lower quadrant and rapidly opacifies the normal cecum (Fig. 22-6). In gastroileostomy without prior partial gastric resection, recycling of intestinal barium through the stomach, although potentially confusing, is also a diagnostic sign.[15]

Enterectomy and Small Bowel Anastomosis

Enterectomy refers to surgical excision of intestine and its corresponding mesentery as indicated by a wide variety of clinical conditions. Segmental resection of the small bowel is generally followed by some form of primary anastomosis, although in some instances an external ostomy is created in conjunction with either closure of the distal bowel segment or formation of a mucous fistula.

Anastomosis of the small bowel is one of the most commonly performed gastrointestinal surgical procedures, as it is required for reconstituting continuity of the intestine after resection, bypassing an obstructed intestinal segment, and forming an enteric reservoir. Intestinal anastomoses can be constructed end to end, end to side, or side to side. End-to-end anastomosis is preferred whenever possible in order to avoid small bowel stasis syndromes. An end-to-side anastomosis is used to compensate for disproportionate proximal and distal luminal sizes, and side-to-side anastomosis is indicated in unusual clinical situations that require expeditious bypass of an intestinal obstruction, as with extensive neoplastic disease of the small bowel. When an end-to-side anastomosis is performed, the end of

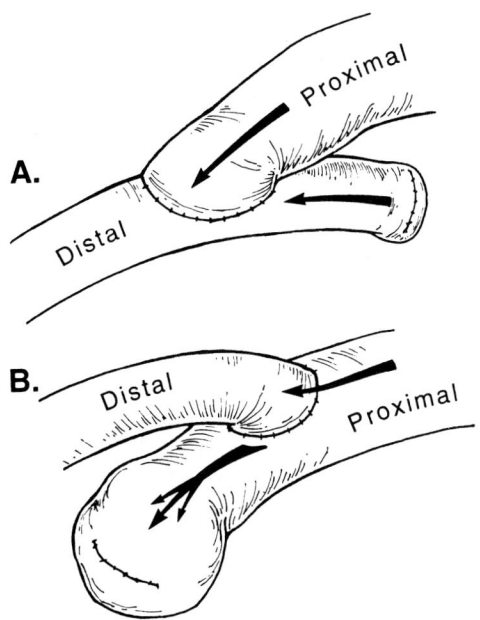

Fig. 22-7. End-to-side anastomosis.
(a) In correct surgical technique the end of the proximal small bowel is anastomosed to the side of the distal small bowel segment, allowing intestinal contents to flow in a normal peristaltic direction (arrows) through a patent bowel lumen. (b) An improper anastomosis, with the side of the proximal bowel segment sutured to the end of the distal bowel segment, allows the direction of intestinal peristalsis (arrows) to be directed into the blind segment and contributes to the complication of lumen dilatation (pouch formation) and stasis of intestinal contents.

the proximal lumen is anastomosed to the side of the distal intestinal segment. This arrangement ensures that peristalsis within the blind (distal) segment is directed antegrade toward and beyond the anastomotic opening, thereby preventing stasis (Fig. 22-7).[1]

Dehiscence of small bowel anastomoses can occur despite careful preoperative patient preparation and meticulous surgical technique. Aside from technical considerations, several factors may adversely affect the success of an anastomosis, including sepsis, tissue hypoxia, malignancy, and advanced patient age. Intestinal perforation from an anastomotic dehiscence may be detected by the presence of free intraperitoneal air on abdominal plain films. Contrast studies performed with water-soluble media may demonstrate an intestinal leak, although similar findings are detectable on CT, which also has the advantage of localizing contaminated peritoneal fluid and imaging the complication of abscess formation (Fig. 22-8). Localized perianastomotic inflammation arising from suture dehiscence can result in partial intestinal obstruction (Fig. 22-9).

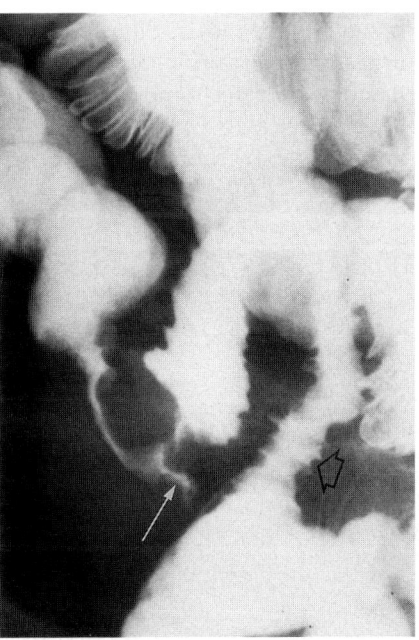

Fig. 22-9. Perianastomotic phlegmon with intestinal narrowing.
Symptoms of mild obstruction developed in this patient shortly after a segmental ileal resection with primary end-to-end anastomosis performed for benign disease. Enteroclysis shows short segment of luminal narrowing with small contained leak (arrow). Note mild narrowing and thickened folds (arrowhead) of proximal ileal loop. At surgery, ischemic dehiscence of the anastomosis was associated with a localized circumferential inflammatory reaction (phlegmon) and submucosal edema of the proximal bowel segment.

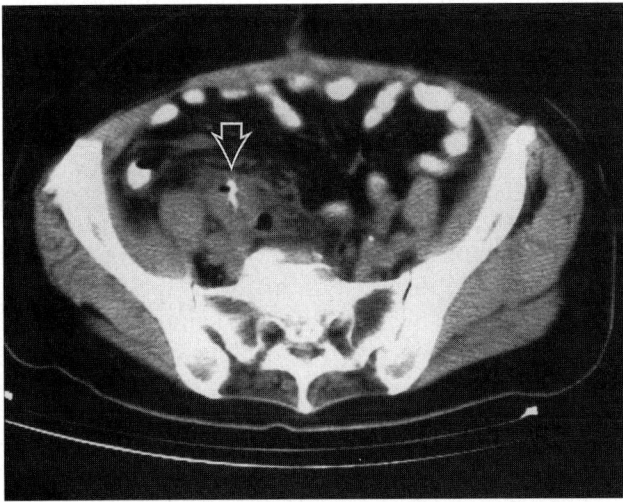

Fig. 22-8. Perianastomotic abscess.
Breakdown of an enteric anastomosis results in a right lower quadrant abscess depicted on CT as a heterogeneous mass (arrow) with extraluminal gas and a focal collection of extravasated contrast media. Note the inflammatory stranding of the adjacent mesentery.

Blind Pouch Syndrome

Although end-to-end surgical anastomoses have essentially replaced side-to-side anastomoses to restore bowel continuity, the latter procedure was once popular, and blind pouches may occasionally be encountered. Dilatation of blind intestinal segments develops late in the postoperative course, some 5 to 15 years after surgery. Division of the circular muscle during side-to-side anastomosis results in stasis secondary to motility disturbances with subsequent dilatation of the proximal segment and formation of a blind pouch. The condition occurs with either enteroenteric or enterocolic anastomoses and, although infrequent, focal dilatation of both proximal and distal bowel segments is reported.[16] An incorrectly performed end-to-side anastomosis (side of the proximal segment of intestine sutured to the end of the distal intestine) creates a similar anatomic abnormality.

Hypertrophy of the pouch with inflammation and ulceration may occur in addition to the intestinal stasis. Symptoms of episodic diarrhea, abdominal pain, weight loss, and a history of previous intestinal anastomosis suggest the diagnosis. Blind pouches may be a source of gastrointestinal bleeding.[17] Segmental resection and end-to-end anastomosis are corrective and eliminate late complications.

Radiographically, blind pouches may appear on abdominal films as either fluid-filled soft-tissue masses or gas-filled structures of variable size and shape. Small bowel contrast studies, particularly enteroclysis, will demonstrate the pouches and their anastomotic location (Fig. 22-10).

Blind Loop Syndrome

In classic blind loop syndrome, a segment of small intestine has been completely bypassed by an enteroanastomosis. Stagnation of small bowel contents leads to bacterial overgrowth, which in the most severely affected patients can approximate the composition of normal colonic flora in both quantity and complexity of organisms. Bacterial overgrowth in the small intestine may result in profound disturbances of absorptive function, malabsorption of lipids and vitamin B_{12} being most notable.[18] Symptoms and clinical signs of the syndrome are those of malabsorption and include diarrhea, steatorrhea, anemia, abdominal pain, and vitamin deficiencies. Although some clinical features are in common with the blind pouch syndrome, the anatomic abnormality associated with the blind loop syndrome is distinctly different. In addition to surgically created blind loops, other anatomic variants may contribute to development of the syndrome. Chronic small bowel strictures with intervening areas of dilatation as may occur in Crohn's disease or radiation enteritis, enteric duplications, jejunoileal diverticulosis, and intestinal scleroderma are among the other causative pathologic conditions. In each case, barium contrast studies accurately demonstrate the associated anatomic abnormality.

Short-Bowel Syndrome

The short-bowel syndrome is characterized by the malnutrition, steatorrhea, and massive acidic diarrhea that result from surgical resection of large portions of the small intestine. Recognition of the metabolic consequences of massive intestinal resection and the aggressive correction of fluid and electrolyte deficits have decreased the mortality in the immediate postoperative period.[19,20] This subject is further discussed in Chapter 18.

Jejunoileal Bypass

Although small intestinal bypass is most often performed for palliation of obstructing nonresectable gastrointestinal cancer, the surgical procedure has also been applied in the treatment of morbid obesity and

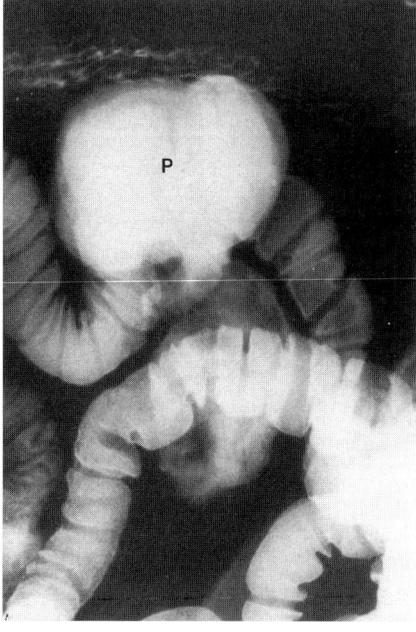

Fig. 22-10. Blind pouch.
Enteroclysis demonstrates saccular blind pouch (P) formation associated with a prior side-to-side jejunal anastomosis.

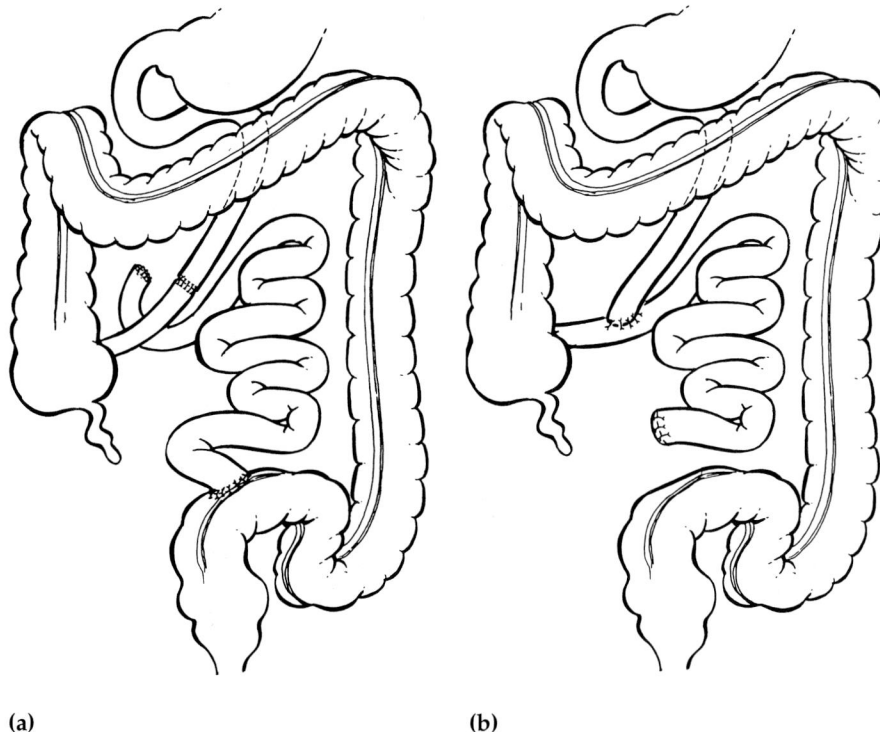

Fig. 22-11. Variations in small bowel bypass procedure for morbid obesity.
(a) Scott's adaptation with end-to-end jejunoileal anastomosis and decompression of the bypassed small bowel into the sigmoid colon. (b) Small bowel bypass with end-to-side jejunoileostomy (Payne's procedure).

control of hyperlipidemia. The rationale supporting jejunoileal bypass for morbid obesity is that weight loss derived from nutrient malabsorption can be achieved by reducing the effective amount of intestinal mucosa available for digestion and decreasing the transit time of food within the gastrointestinal tract. In effect, the operation produces an obligatory short-bowel, malabsorptive state through bypassing the small intestine. Initially proposed by Payne et al[21] and modified by Scott and colleagues,[22] jejunoileal bypass connects various lengths of jejunum (20 to 35 cm) to ileum (10 to 30 cm) as an end-to-end or end-to-side anastomosis (Fig. 22-11). The end-to-end procedures require decompression of the bypassed small intestine into the transverse or sigmoid colon.

The jejunoileal bypass is associated with numerous early and late complications, despite the production of initial weight loss and other beneficial effects.[23,24] Chronic diarrhea, metabolic acidosis, fluid and electrolyte imbalances, calcium and magnesium deficiencies, anemia, hyperoxaluria with renal calculi, cholelithiasis, and progressive liver failure develop to a distressing degree postoperatively. These complications are related to an unpredictable absorption of nutrients by the surgically shortened gut and to the toxic side effects of bacterial overgrowth in the bypassed bowel segments. Mechanical complications include small bowel obstruction and intussusception of the bypassed intestine. Obstruction of bypassed segments may also occur by herniation of bowel through mesenteric defects or by volvulus at the ileocolic anastomosis.

Radiologic evaluation of the abdomen after jejunoileal bypass can often be difficult due to the confusing abdominal plain film patterns and to residual obesity in some patients. Multiple air-fluid levels with varying degrees of distension in the mainstream small bowel are common postoperative radiographic observations. Bypass enteritis, characterized clinically by episodic abdominal distension with tenderness and fever, also presents multiple gas-distended loops of the bypassed intestine on abdominal radiographs.[25] Pneumatosis intestinalis may occur in conjunction with bypass enteritis. Differentiating such complications as enteritis or mechanical bowel obstruction generally requires barium examination, performed either from an antegrade direction for evaluation of the functional small bowel or by retrograde barium enema for study of the bypassed intestinal segment and ileocolic anastomosis. Depending on the specific operation performed, bypassed segments of bowel may not be visualized on contrast studies, and ultrasonography or CT scanning are required. Ultrasonography has been shown to diagnose intussusception of the bypassed segment by demonstrating the pattern of a mass containing strong central echoes surrounded by a sonolucent rim.[26] CT, with its ability to evaluate abdominal pathology without interference by gas, is a more reliable modality. On CT, a concentric target or doughnutlike mass indicates intussusception of the bypassed intestine.[27]

The inevitable complications accompanying jejunoileal bypass, the frequent need to revise or disassemble an intestinal bypass because of progressive liver disease, and excessive mortality gradually made the surgical procedure unacceptable in the management of morbid obesity.[24] Gastric restrictive operations have replaced jejunoileal bypass procedures.

Partial ileal bypass is performed to manage cases of severe or drug-resistant hyperlipidemia. In this procedure the small bowel is transected 200 cm proximal to the ileocecal valve and anastomosed end-to-side to the cecum, resulting in exclusion of the distal one-third of the small bowel. Surgical bypass of the distal ileum disrupts the preferential intestinal absorption of dietary cholesterol and the enterohepatic bile acid cycle. Partial ileal bypass is not associated with the excessive weight loss, metabolic disturbances, or hepatic failure as seen with jejunoileal bypass for morbid obesity. In hyperlipidemia, partial ileal bypass produces a significant and sustained reduction of total and low-density lipoprotein cholesterol levels.[28] The surgical procedure, as utilized in patients with familial hypercholesterolemia and monitored in the Program on the Surgical Control of the Hyperlipidemias (POSCH), has been an effective intervention in reducing atherosclerotic risk and associated adverse coronary events.[29]

Enterostomy

Enterostomy refers to an intestinal opening that is surgically designed to communicate with the skin, in essence an intentional enterocutaneous fistula, and function either temporarily or permanently. In order to prevent intra-abdominal leak from the intestinal lumen, an enterostomy is made in those small bowel segments that are sufficiently mobile to be brought in contact with the anterior abdominal wall.

Jejunostomy

Jejunostomy, while occasionally useful for small bowel decompression, is an ideal route for administering nutritional support.[1] Advantages of a feeding jejunostomy over gastrostomy include reductions of nausea, vomiting, and risk of pulmonary aspiration via gastroesophageal reflux. Surgical feeding jejunostomies are performed in malnourished surgical patients with an anticipated lengthy postoperative course; in patients with pathology of the upper gastrointestinal tract including unresectable malignancy, fistula, or anastomotic leaks proximal to the potential jejunostomy site; and in patients who are not candidates for endoscopic, fluoroscopic, or laparoscopic insertion of feeding jejunostomies or who have failed these approaches. Direct intubated jejunostomies (Witzel or Stamm technique) satisfy temporary nutritional requirements, whereas long-term jejunal feeding is best accomplished by a Roux-en-Y type jejunostomy.

Surgical placement of the jejunostomy at least 70 cm from the duodenojejunal junction and fixation of the jejunal loop to the peritoneum are common precautions employed during jejunostomy construction. Injection of the jejunostomy catheter with water-soluble contrast media before initiating enteric feeding is advocated by some surgeons in order to ascertain proper catheter position and avoid potential misdirected infusion (Fig. 22-12).

Various complications can be associated with any of the surgical jejunostomy methods. Enterogastric reflux of the alimentation fluid, stomal necrosis, dislodgment of the catheter with subsequent intra-abdominal leak, and small bowel obstruction at or near the jejunostomy site are reported (Fig. 22-13).[1,30]

Ileostomy

A distal enterostomy or ileostomy is primarily used for evacuation of intestinal contents in clinical situations that preclude normal use of the colon or require its surgical removal. Typical conditions include familial adenomatous polyposis and inflammatory bowel disease. Conventional (end) ileostomy with total proctocolectomy provides a relatively simplistic and often curative surgical approach that mitigates the future risks of recurrent inflammation or malignant degeneration with these diseases. The loss of fecal continence and its attendant physical and psychological effects remain significant drawbacks of ileostomy surgery. Since the development of the ileoanal reservoir procedures, the use of conventional ileostomy is more selective and seen in patients with extensive Crohn's proctocolitis, anal sphincter dysfunction, or reservoir failure, or in the elderly.[31]

Another form of distal enterostomy, the loop (double-barrel) ileostomy, is performed in situations to permit temporary intestinal diversion. Circumstances include Crohn's disease complicated by abscess or extensive fistulae, emergency intervention for intestinal obstruction, or as an adjunct to complex operations that require the protection of a distal enteric anastomosis in order to promote healing.

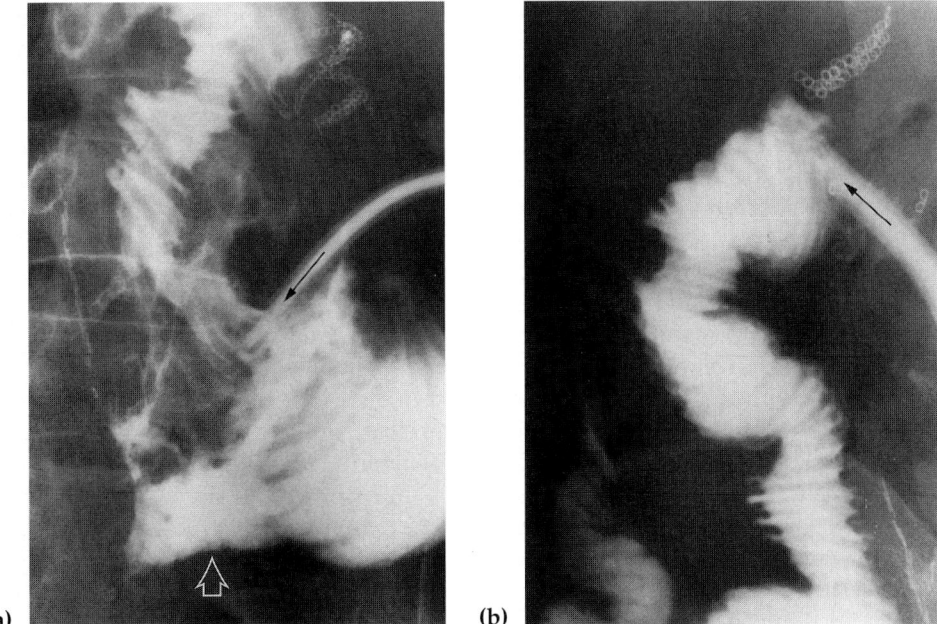

Fig. 22-12. Jejunostomy catheter injection.
(a) Injection of water-soluble contrast media (arrow) demonstrates an incomplete purchase of the jejunal catheter within the bowel lumen and results in tracking of contrast to a focal extraluminal collection (open arrow). (b) Although successful repositioning may be accomplished by catheter manipulations performed under fluoroscopic guidance, an operative repositioning was required in this patient. Postprocedure catheter injection (arrow) shows good jejunostomy tube position and no abnormal extravasation of contrast media.

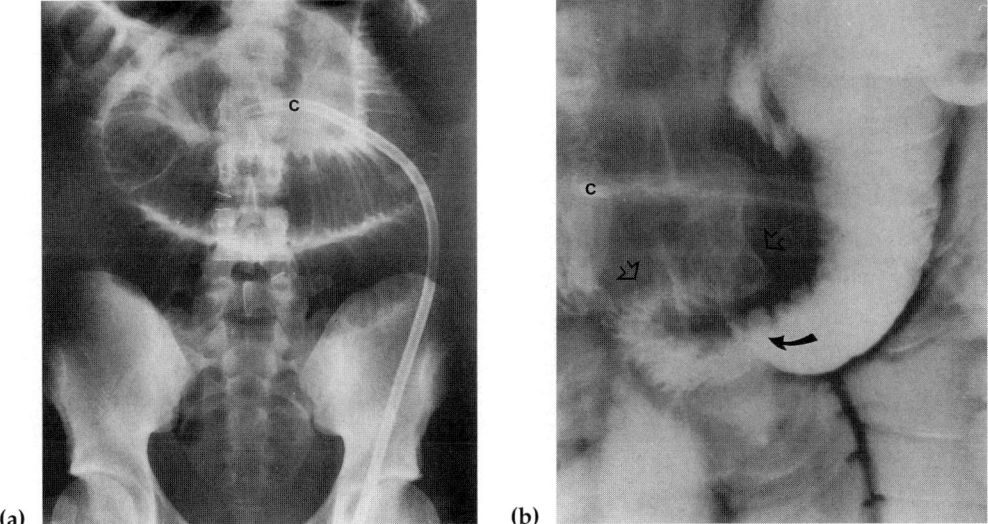

Fig. 22-13. Small bowel obstruction after jejunostomy.
(a) Abdominal plain film shows jejunostomy catheter (C) positioned in the upper midabdomen and abnormal distention of several gas-filled small bowel loops. (b) Enteroclysis demonstrates high-grade luminal obstruction (arrow) with tethering and distortion of the postobstructive loops (open arrows) near the jejunostomy catheter (C). At surgery, multiple adhesions adjacent to the jejunostomy site were responsible for the more distal small bowel obstruction.

Creation of a conventional Brooke or everting end ileostomy involves transection of the ileum with mobilization of a 5-cm ileal segment through an abdominal wall defect and specific suturing technique to allow for ileostomy maturation.[31] Malfunction of a Brooke ileostomy may occur for a variety of reasons, including adhesions, prestomal narrowing of the ileal lumen, paraileostomy herniation, and recurrent inflammatory bowel disease. These abnormalities can present early or late after operation and usually occur at or near the ileostomy site. Symptoms often produced are diarrhea or those of small bowel obstruction.

Management of patients with an ileostomy and suspected complication or ileostomy dysfunction requires good radiologic evaluation of the small bowel. Barium contrast examinations including enteroclysis infusion can be safely performed in retrograde fashion in patients with an ileostomy.[32,33] Specific techniques for adapting enteroclysis catheters, small Foley catheters, and externally applied ostomy cones for ileostomy intubation have been described.[33] Glucagon may be given to abolish intestinal peristalsis and promote the retrograde flow of contrast media. While per ileostomy infusion is well tolerated by patients and the preferred approach for a diagnostic examination, good results are also reported with an antegrade small bowel enteroclysis.[34] Retrograde examination, however, allows greater control over visualization of the distal small bowel, where most abnormalities occur.

On barium studies, indentation or abrupt angulation of the bowel contour, lumen caliber change, or fixation of bowel segments to the abdominal wall or other loops indicates the presence of postoperative adhesions. In cases of partial small bowel obstruction, antegrade enteroclysis infusion may be needed to accurately demonstrate the presence of functionally significant adhesions.[32] Fascial scarring with narrowing of the prestomal segment of ileum as it passes through the abdominal wall may be a cause of partial intestinal obstruction and resulting ileostomy dysfunction.[33] Recurrent Crohn's disease in the distal small bowel can result in symptoms and radiological findings similar to those of obstructive ileostomy dysfunction.

In cases of parastomal herniation, contrast studies can demonstrate the herniated bowel and any associated obstruction provided that lateral radiographs are obtained (Fig. 22-14). Compared to clinical examination, CT demonstrates a higher incidence of paraileostomy herniation in patients with conventional ileostomy, 10% versus 36% respectively.[35] On CT, herniation is often associated with large (>3 cm) defects in the anterior abdominal wall at the stomal site and is common lateral to the stoma (Fig. 22-15).[35] Since CT accurately detects paraileostomy hernia, it is recommended for evaluation of patients with unexplained persistent stomal related or abdominal symptoms and negative clinical findings.

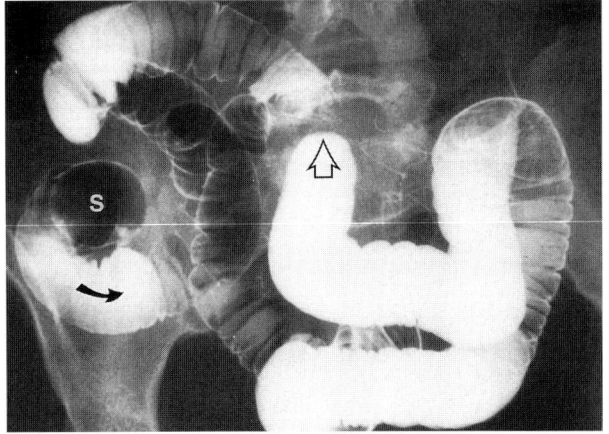
(a)

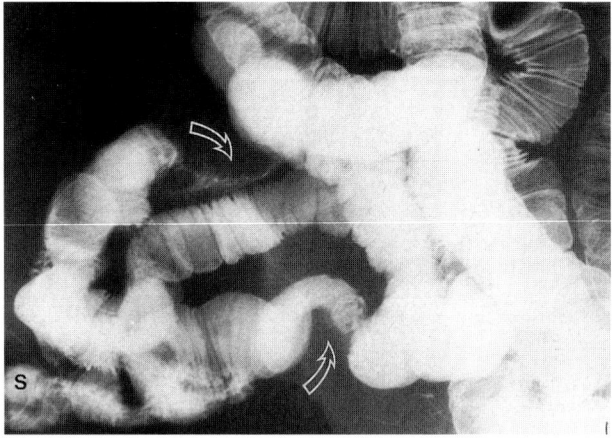
(b)

Fig. 22-14. Paraileostomy hernia.
(a) Enteroclysis infusion (arrow), retrograde per ileostomy, suggests complete intestinal obstruction (open arrow) in this symptomatic patient. (b) Subsequent antegrade study shows several herniated small bowel loops with mild compression (arrows) at the site of the abdominal wall defect. Antegrade examination more accurately depicts the functional degree of obstruction associated with the paraileostomy hernia as clearly demonstrated on this lateral view during enteroclysis. S = ileostomy stoma.

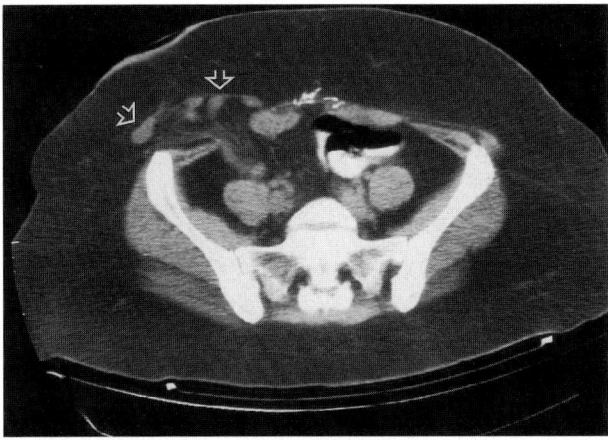

Fig. 22-15. CT of paraileostomy hernia.
CT demonstrates large anterior abdominal wall defect and herniation of multiple small bowel loops and mesentery (arrows). Diagnosis requires review of several scan slices, since herniated loops and cutaneous ileostomy stoma are often in different axial planes.

Ileal Reservoirs

The concept of an internal reservoir associated with a postcolectomy ileostomy was introduced by Kock in 1969, who demonstrated that the terminal ileum could function as a low-pressure, highly compliant reservoir.[36] Later, Parks et al[37] and Utsunomiya and coworkers[38] independently introduced the ileoanal anastomosis with an interposed ileal reservoir for patients after colectomy and mucosal proctectomy. These continence-preserving surgical procedures offer patients the advantage of an improved body image and active lifestyle. Most surgeons consider the presence of Crohn's disease a contraindication to the construction of an ileal reservoir, since the reservoir and proximal bowel are at increased risk for recurrent inflammation and further small bowel resection presents additional problems.[31]

Continent Ileostomy Reservoir

Successful continent ileostomy or Kock pouch procedure obviates the use of an external ileostomy appliance, since the contents of the ileal reservoir are evacuated by stomal intubation several times per day. Patient satisfaction with the continent ileostomy is remarkable considering that complications are frequent and often require major surgical intervention. The complexity of Kock pouch construction and function essentially limits the efficacy of the procedure. Now seldom performed, the surgery is reserved for patients with a prior colectomy and conventional ileostomy or a failed or contraindicated ileoanal pouch.[31,39]

Creation of a Kock pouch involves use of the distal 45 cm of ileum, with the most proximal 30-cm ileal segment fashioned into a spherical reservoir by complex suturing techniques. By design, opposing directions of peristalsis on each wall of the pouch serves to prevent propulsive activity from emptying the pouch. Continence is further maintained by intussusception of the efferent ileal segment into the pouch to form the valve mechanism, while the end of the ileum creates the abdominal wall stoma. Suturing of the Kock pouch to the anterior abdominal wall provides stability and prevents volvulus of the pouch and peripouch herniation.

Complications of the Kock pouch usually occur months after surgery and include various forms of valve dysfunction, nonspecific inflammation of the reservoir or the afferent ileal segment (pouch ileitis), and fistulas. Surgical revision of the Kock pouch is eventually required in almost 25% of patients and long-term continence is achieved in 75% of cases.[40] Based on extensive experience with the operation in Sweden, Lycke et al report a detailed description of the examination technique and the normal radiographic appearance of the Kock pouch.[41] Retrograde double-contrast barium examination following cleansing irrigation of the reservoir is the recommended method for standard evaluation of the Kock pouch. Radiography in a steep oblique or lateral view is required to adequately visualize the efferent ileal segment and ileostomy stoma. Suspicion of suture dehiscence in the immediate postoperative period or pouch perforation after intubation should be evaluated using water-soluble rather than barium contrast media.

On barium studies of the normal mature reservoir, typical small bowel fold patterns are observed and interrupted by a linear mucosal ridge that represents the suture line between the two anastomosed ileal segments.[41] Surface granularity is seen with mild pouchitis, while ulceration and mucosal fold distortion occur with severe pouch inflammation.[42] The intact continence valve appears as a tubular or round lobular structure invaginated within the confines of the reservoir and usually associated with an array of stabilizing surgical clips. Sliding and eversion of the valve from the pouch results in valve shortening with progressive lengthening and tortuosity of the efferent ileal segment to the stoma.[42] Difficulty in pouch intubation, chronic outflow obstruction, and incontinence ensue [Fig. 22-16(a)]. Rarely, adenomas may occur in the continent ileostomy and therefore surveillance of

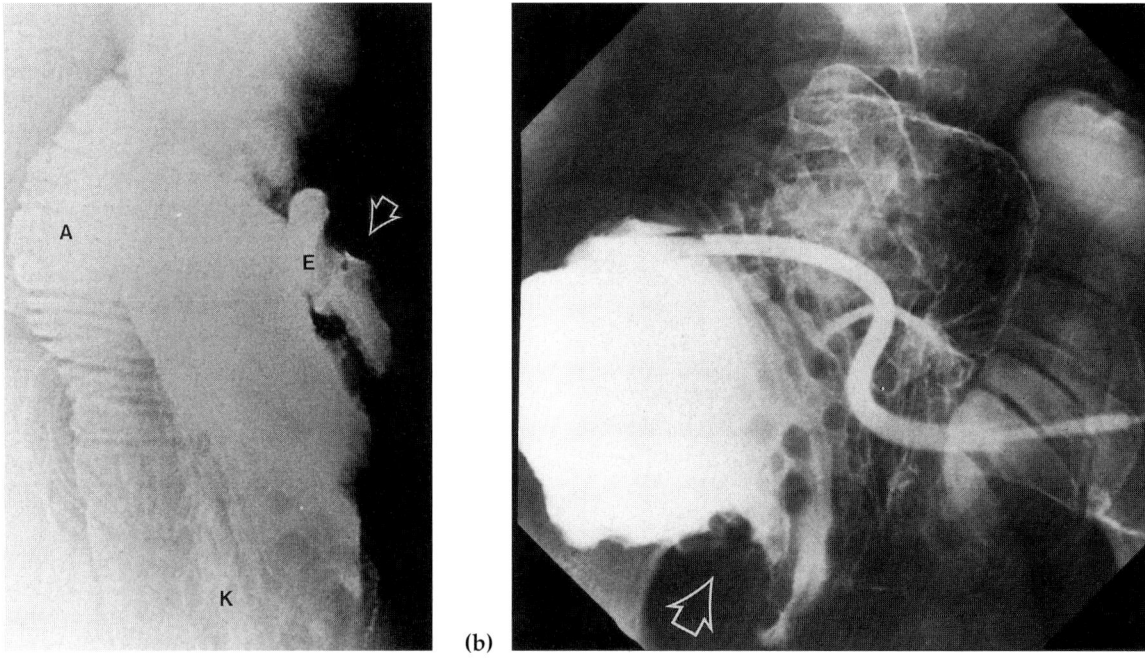

Fig. 22-16. Kock pouch in a patient presenting with symptoms of pouch dysfunction and intubation difficulty. (a) Lateral view of retrograde Kock pouch (K) study shows an irregular and tortuous (arrow) efferent segment (E) and no sign of an intact intussusception valve. A = afferent ileal segment. (b) Multiple round mucosal defects represent recurrent adenomas involving the Kock pouch in this same patient with history of familial adenomatous polyposis and prior colectomy. An irregular mass (arrow) suggests malignant degeneration.

the reservoir in patients with a history of familial polyposis is required [Fig. 22-16(b)].[43]

Ileoanal Pouch

Creation of an ileal reservoir with ileoanal anastomosis following colectomy and rectal mucosectomy has become an important surgical alternative for patients requiring total proctocolectomy. In primary colonic mucosal disease, including ulcerative colitis and the polyposis syndromes, this innovative operation removes potential disease-bearing mucosa while preserving anal continence and the normal defecatory pathway.

Two principal forms of pouch construction for restorative proctocolectomy are used: the smaller J-shaped pouch and the S-shaped pouch.[37,38] An ileal J-pouch is constructed from the distal 20 to 25 cm of ileum, fashioned into a J-shape and secured by side-to-side anastomosis of the two adjacent loops (Fig. 22-17). Construction of an S-shaped pouch requires the folding of a 50-cm segment of ileum into an S configuration, with the distal end allowed to protrude to form an efferent conduit. The folded loops are opened and sutured to create a wide, single ovoid pouch (Fig. 22-18). Alternatively, a W-shaped pouch may be created by incorporating four folded segments of distal ileum. After anorectal mucosectomy and careful rectal transection that spares the integrity of the anal sphincter, the constructed ileal pouch is brought down endorectally and anastomosed to the dentate line of the rectal cuff. Regardless of the method of pouch construction, a proximal diverting ileostomy is usually established for 8 to 12 weeks to allow for healing of the extensive anastomoses. Closure of the protective ileostomy results in functionalization of the ileoanal pouch. Currently, the J-pouch configuration is preferred because of the simplicity of its construction, adequate reservoir capacity, ease of emptying, and absence of a potentially obstructing efferent limb.[31,38]

Although excellent functional results can be achieved in patients with an ileoanal reservoir, the procedure may be associated with significant complications.[44] Common problems include pouchitis, small bowel obstruction, anastomosis dehiscence or stricture, fistula, and pelvic abscess. Most complications are adequately managed with antibiotic therapy and prolonged ileostomy diversion, but ileoanal pouch failure occurs in about 10% of patients.[44] Radiographic evaluation of the ileoanal reservoir is required to assess its function and to exclude anastomotic leakage

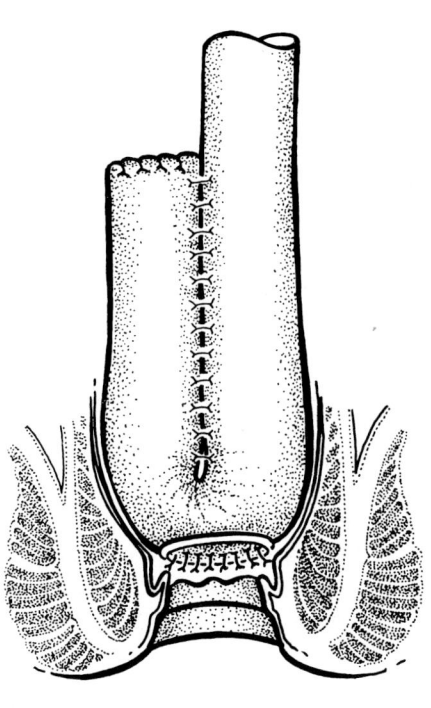
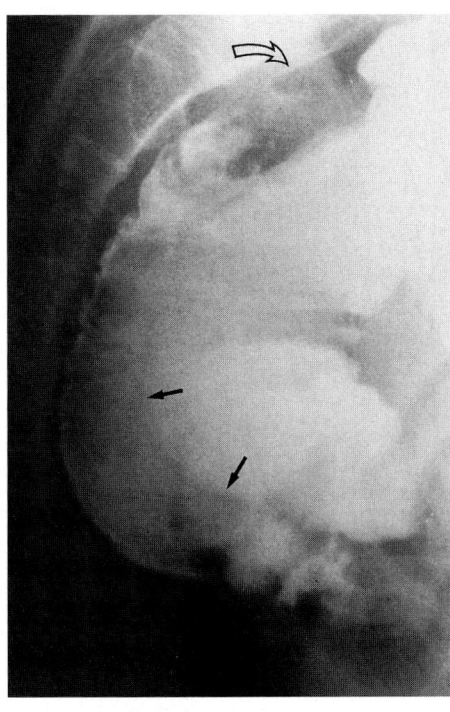

(a)   (b)

Fig. 22-17. J-shaped ileoanal pouch.
(a) Schematic representation showing side-to-side anastomosis of the adjacent ileal loop and direct anastomosis of the inferior apex of the reservoir to the dentate line. (b) Normal single-contrast pouchogram with characteristic vertical raphe (arrows) from the anastomotic line. Traces of contrast (open arrow) may enter a small apical appendage that is variably formed during surgical construction of the reservoir and should not be confused with an abnormal anastomotic leak.[42]

from the reservoir and other potential postoperative complications.[45–47] In the few centers performing restorative proctocolectomy as a single-stage operation, postoperative imaging of the ileoanal pouch and anastomosis is not routine but reserved for the investigation of clinically suspected complications.[48]

Contrast ileograms (pouchograms) can be performed either antegrade through the ileostomy stoma after selecting its efferent limb or retrograde via soft balloon catheter to visualize the ileoanal pouch and anastomosis.[45–47] With demonstration of an intact anastomosis and no sign of pelvic inflammation or fistula, the diverting ileostomy can be closed and intestinal continuity reestablished at a second operation. Careful positioning of the retrograde catheter is necessary to avoid obscuring the ileoanal anastomosis and any evidence of complication.[45] Water-soluble contrast media is appropriate if there is a prior abnormal clinical examination of the pouch; otherwise barium is used for routine asymptomatic evaluations. On normal contrast studies the J-pouch has distinctive vertical raphes corresponding to the side-to-side anastomoses, whereas the globular reservoir and recognizable efferent limb typify the larger capacity S-pouch. Postevacuation films document pouch function, for which there is considerable variation in the degree of emptying on contrast examination.

In patients with anastomotic dehiscence and pelvis sepsis, ileograms may demonstrate abnormal findings

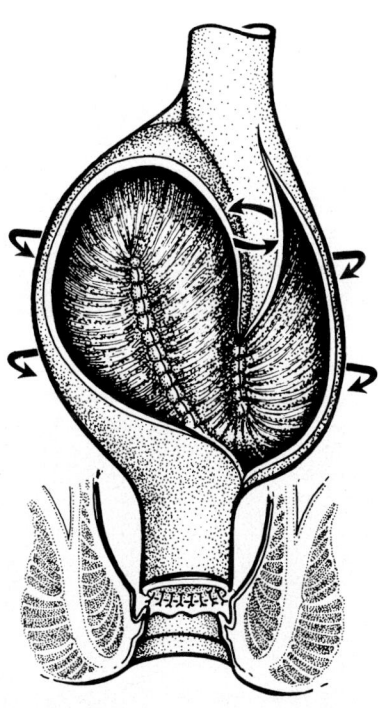

Fig. 22-18. Schematic representation of S-shaped ileoanal pouch.
S-shaped ileal loop is used to create reservoir opposing three segments of terminal ileum (arrows). S-pouch has relatively elongated efferent limb sutured to the dentate line.

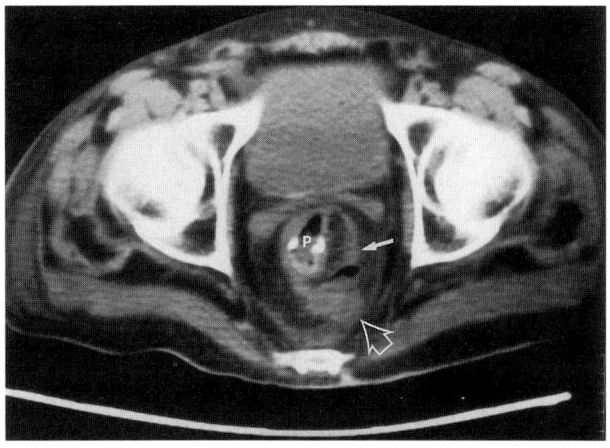

Fig. 22-19. CT of peripouch abscess.
Abscess (open arrow) seen as an abnormal fluid collection containing a small amount of gas, posterior to the ileoanal pouch (P). A thickened rectal cuff wall (arrow) surrounds the pouch mesentery. Abscess arises from the peripouch region and extends to involve the rectal wall and adjacent perirectal fat.

such as contrast extravasation, extraluminal gas, abnormal thickening and spiculation of pouch folds, or extrinsic mass effect. On CT, patients with infections demonstrate abnormal pouch and rectal wall thickness in addition to inflammatory infiltration of the peripouch and perirectal fat.[46] Abscesses are identified on CT, characteristically in the peripouch region between the ileal mesenteric fat and the adjacent rectal muscularis (Fig. 22-19). Some reports indicate that in patients with infectious complications after ileoanal pouch surgery, the ileographic findings are often nonspecific, whereas CT more accurately delineates the inflammatory process and can also direct therapeutic intervention (Fig. 22-20).[46,47]

Pouchitis or mucosal inflammation of the ileoanal pouch occurs in nearly 50% of patients undergoing the procedure and presents as a clinically evident syndrome of fever, abdominal cramping, and diarrhea. Contrast pouchograms are nonspecific but may demonstrate spasm and thickened ileal-pouch folds. Radionuclide scintigraphy showing increased pouch

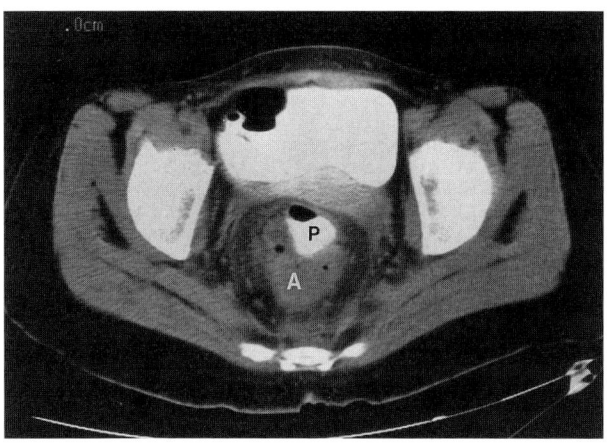

(a)

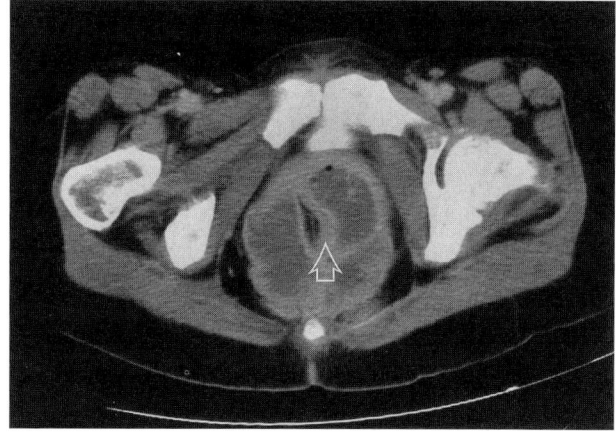

(b)

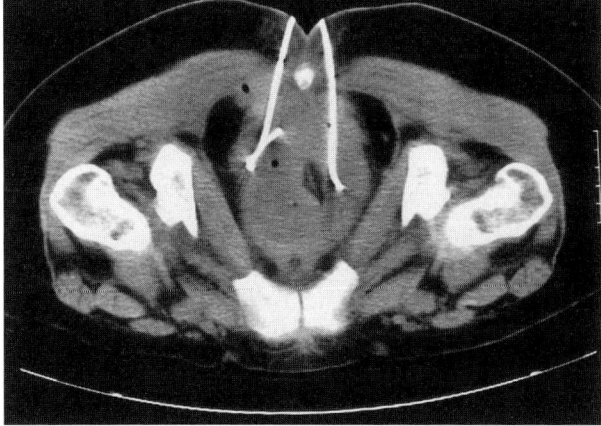

(c)

Fig. 22-20. Peripouch abscess.
(a) Anastomotic breakdown of an ileoanal pouch (P) resulting in formation of a peripouch abscess (A) and inflammatory stranding extending from the abscess into the perirectal fat. (b) Caudal scan shows large low-density abscess encircling the collapsed pouch lumen and its associated fat-density mesentery (arrow). (c) Prone scan after percutaneous placement of abscess drainage catheters.

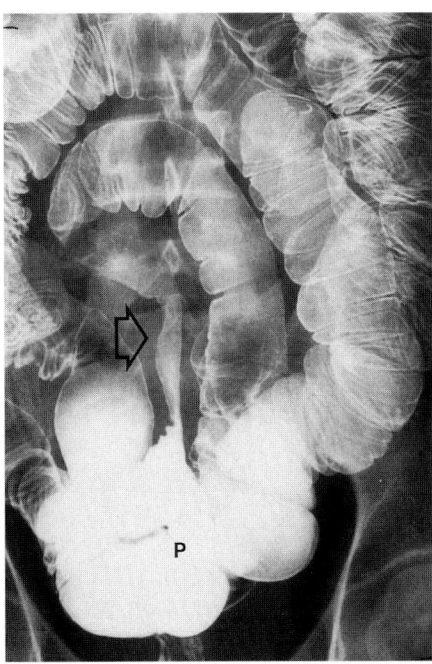

Fig. 22-21. Partial intestinal obstruction in a patient with ileoanal J-pouch (P) and prior diverting ileostomy.
Enteroclysis demonstrates narrowing of the distal ileal lumen (arrow), which was adherent to the anterior abdominal peritoneum following closure of the loop ileostomy.

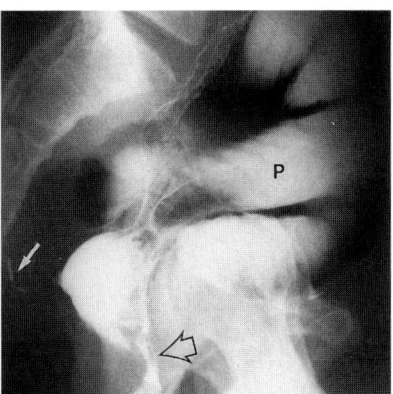

Fig. 22-22. S-shaped ileoanal pouch with abnormal efferent limb.
Pouchogram demonstrates S-shaped pouch (P) with stenotic segment (open arrow) proximal to the anal anastomosis. A small sinus tract (arrow) extends posteriorly from the efferent limb into a thickened presacral space, the site of chronically indurated tissue from prior peripouch abscess.

uptake of 111Indium-labeled leukocytes can be particularly sensitive for the diagnosis.[47]

Intestinal obstruction usually manifests after closure of the ileostomy and commonly affects the closure site or the more distal small bowel (Fig. 22-21).[44,45] Adhesions, associated volvulus, and stricture are problematic and due to the extensive surgical resection and bowel manipulations. Other complications encountered less frequently are stricture of the ileoanal anastomosis and obstruction of the efferent segment, especially with an S-shape pouch construction (Fig. 22-22). Some patients may develop abdominal distension and mild dilatation of small bowel loops on abdominal plain films. Small bowel studies are normal, and stasis due to neuromuscular dysmotility in the perianastomotic region, similar to the motor disturbances in blind pouch syndrome, is suspected.

Small Bowel Transplantation

Intestinal transplantation has emerged as a treatment for patients with short bowel syndrome and irreversible intestinal failure who can no longer tolerate total parenteral nutrition (TPN). Although intestinal transplantation developed more slowly than other types of organ grafting because of problems with rejection and infection, the introduction of the potent immunosuppressive agent tacrolimus has made clinical bowel transplantation feasible. As of June 1995, 180 transplantations had been performed worldwide, with short-term survival rates comparable to lung transplantation.[49]

Intestinal failure may result from surgical or anatomical loss of intestine (short bowel syndrome) or from a functional abnormality. Conditions treated by bowel transplantation include volvulus, gastroschisis, necrotizing enterocolitis, and intestinal atresia in children, and thrombotic disorders, Crohn's disease, desmoid tumors, and intestinal trauma in adults. TPN, the primary treatment for most patients with intestinal failure, can lead to serious, sometimes life-threatening, complications such as venous thrombosis and hepatic failure. These may influence the decision to transplant and the kind of transplant procedure utilized.[50]

Three types of transplant operation are performed (Fig. 22-23). Isolated intestinal transplantation is employed in patients who maintain good hepatic function. Combined intestinal and liver transplantation is done in those with TPN-related or inborn hepatic dysfunction. Abdominal multivisceral grafts (intestine, liver, stomach, duodenum, and pancreas) are reserved for patients with extensive gastrointestinal tract abnormalities caused by vascular, absorptive, or motility disorders. Colon can be transplanted with any of the

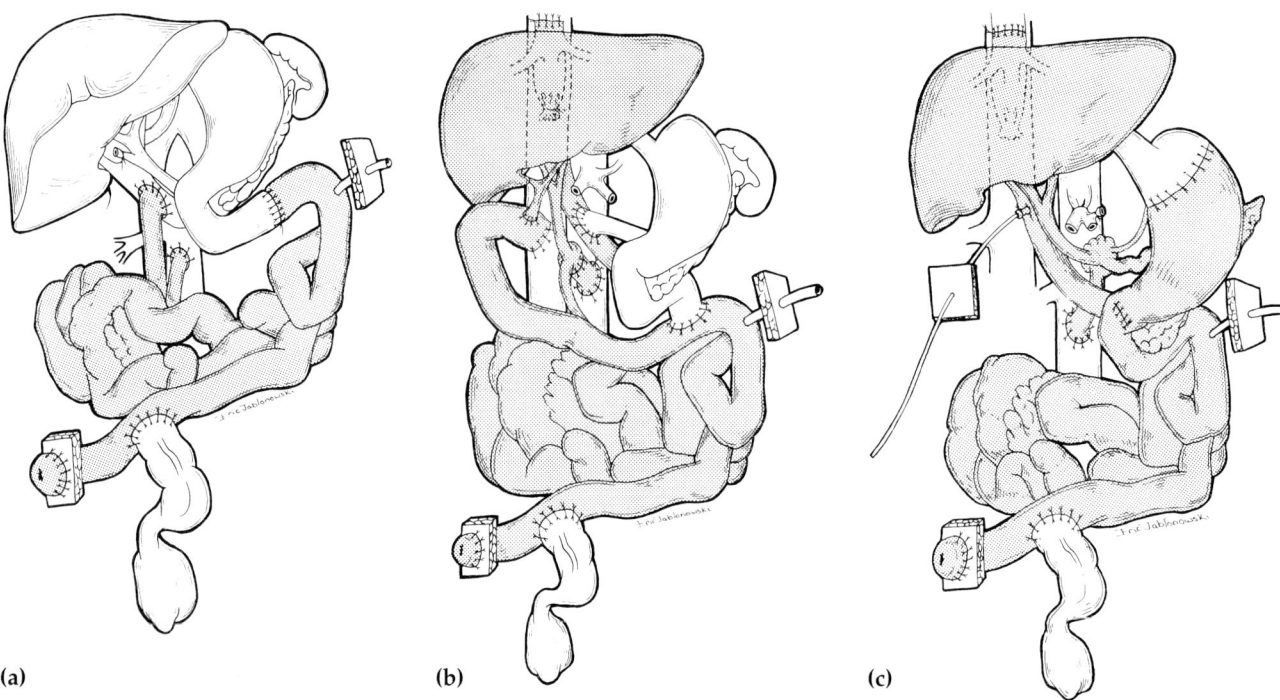

Fig. 22-23. Schematic drawings of three types of intestinal transplantation. Shaded areas are donor organs.
(a) Isolated intestinal transplantation. (b) Combined intestinal-liver transplantation. (c) Multivisceral transplantation of stomach, duodenum, jejunum, ileum, liver, and pancreas.

operations, although current practice is to exclude colon from intestinal allografts.[51]

Before transplantation, gastrointestinal contrast examinations are used to assess the nature and extent of bowel abnormality and, in patients with short gut syndrome, to map the amount and location of the remaining intestine. Abdominal CT provides complementary information on the bowel, and can define masses, inflammatory processes, and fluid collections. If liver transplantation is planned, CT can show hepatic parenchymal and vascular abnormalities.[52–54]

After transplantation, gastrointestinal contrast studies are used to evaluate anastomoses, gastric emptying, intestinal transit, and small bowel mucosal pattern. Usual postsurgical anatomy includes a native-to-donor jejunojejunal, duodenojejunal, or gastrogastric anastomosis and a donor-to-native ileocolic anastomosis with end ileostomy. If colon is included in the graft, a colocolic anastomosis or colostomy is present. Healthy allografts show normal bowel caliber and mucosal pattern, active peristalsis, and normal transit times.[52,53]

Abnormalities on early postoperative contrast studies include gastric atony with delayed emptying, and slow small bowel transit with varying degrees of dilatation. Diffuse thickening of graft mucosal folds may be present soon after operation due to edema related to harvesting injury. Fold thickening encountered later in the postoperative period raises the suspicion of infection, rejection, or ischemia (Figs. 22-24, 22-25,

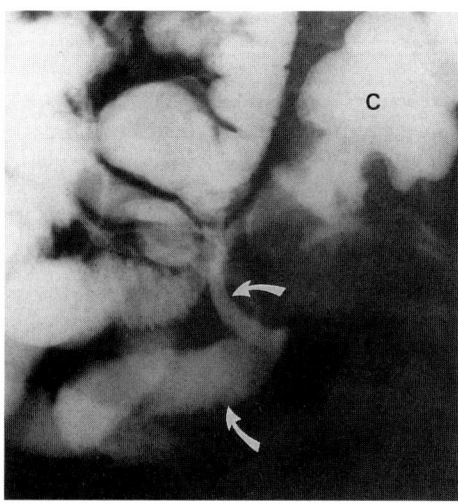

Fig. 22-24. Cytomegalovirus ileitis.
Small bowel series performed 569 days after isolated small bowel transplantation. The allograft ileum (arrows) proximal to the ileo-transverse colon anastomosis shows mucosal irregularity and nodularity with narrowing of the lumen. C = native transverse colon.

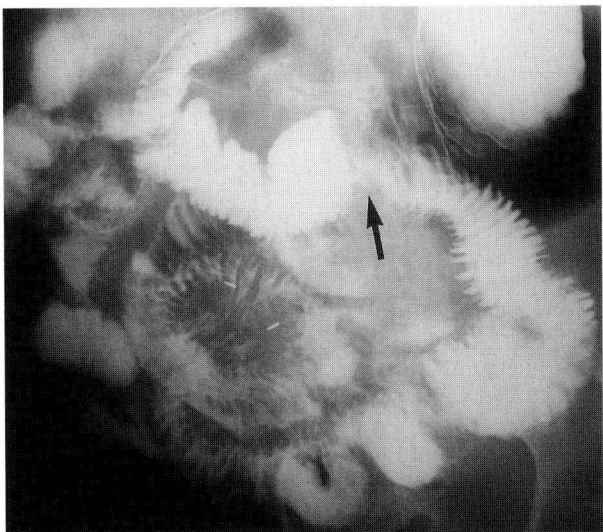

Fig. 22-25. Post-transplantation edema and acute rejection.
Small bowel series performed 21 days after isolated small bowel transplantation shows diffuse thickening of allograft jejunal and ileal folds. The end-to-end duodenojejunal anastomosis (arrow) is edematous. Jejunal biopsy and clinical findings were consistent with acute rejection. Changes resolved after treatment with steroids and increased doses of tacrolimus.

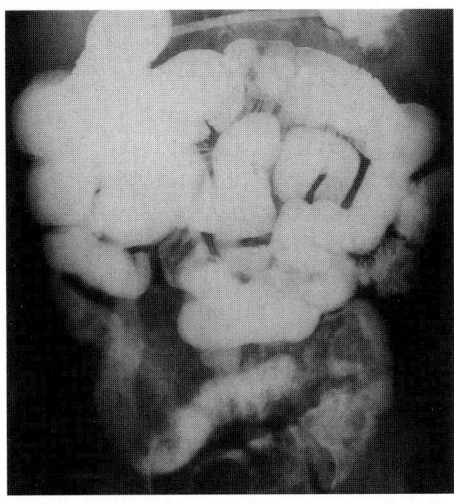

Fig. 22-27. Chronic and acute rejection and infection.
Small bowel enteroclysis performed 570 days after isolated intestinal transplantation. There is loss of the normal mucosal fold pattern, nodularity distally, with relative sparing of the proximal jejunum. The graft failed and was removed 667 days after transplantation.

22-26). Loss of the normal fold pattern resulting in a tubular featureless appearance of the graft may be caused by acute and chronic rejection and infection, usually cytomegalovirus (Fig. 22-27). Bowel caliber in such cases may be increased, normal, or decreased, and strictures may develop. Other abnormalities may include obstruction, ileus, anastomotic leaks, and fistulas. Plain films may reveal obstruction, ileus, and pneumatosis in donor or native bowel. Imaging studies are insensitive for the detection of early acute rejection or infection, which are typically diagnosed using frequent ileoscopy and biopsy.[52,53]

Common indications for cross-sectional imaging are suspected abdominal infection, hemorrhage, hepatic abnormality, or post-transplantation lympho-

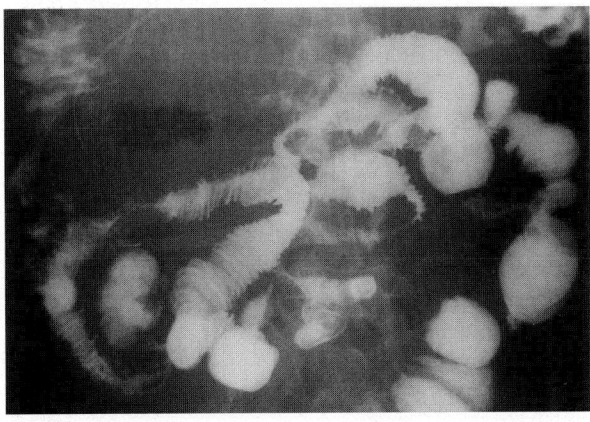

Fig. 22-26. Ischemia of small bowel graft.
Small bowel series done 17 days after combined intestinal-liver transplantation. Intestinal graft shows diffuse fold thickening and multiple areas of narrowing.

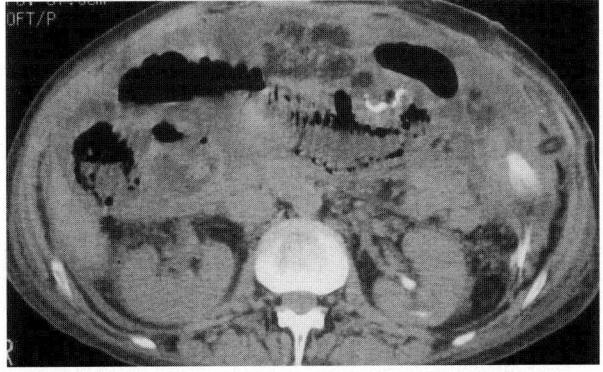

Fig. 22-28. Ischemic necrosis of small bowel graft.
CT done 21 days after intestinal-liver transplantation shows small bowel pneumatosis and wall thickening. There is infiltration of the mesentery and mild ascites. At surgery, a 35-cm segment of necrotic and perforated jejunum was resected. Same patient as Fig. 22-26.

proliferative disorder (PTLD). On CT, uncomplicated intestinal grafts exhibit nondilated loops with normal-thickness walls and mucosal folds. Bowel anastomoses can usually be identified. Donor blood vessels such as interposition arterial grafts can be demonstrated on contrast-enhanced scans. Other abnormalities on CT include bowel wall thickening caused by preservation injury, rejection, infection, ischemia, or PTLD, and bowel dilatation associated with ileus or obstruction. Allograft loops often appear matted together. The mesentery may appear infiltrated, especially in diseased transplants. Interloop fluid and other abdominal fluid collections may occur. Pneumatosis may be seen in infected, rejecting, or ischemic grafts (Fig. 22-28), and sporadically in normal bowel. Other abnormalities detectable by CT include anastomotic leaks, fistulas, thrombosis of arterial or venous grafts, PTLD, and complications of liver transplantation.[54,55]

References

1. Lui KJM, Walker FW. Surgical procedures on the small intestine. In: Zuidema GD, ed. *Surgery of the Alimentary Tract*. 4th ed. Philadelphia, Pa: WB Saunders Co; 1996.
2. Wang PY, Talamo RC, Babior BM, Raymond GG, Coleman RW. Kallikrein-kinin system in postgastrectomy dumping syndrome. *Ann Intern Med*. 1974;80:577–581
3. Sawyers JL, Scott HI. Postgastrectomy sequelae and remedial operations. In: Scott HJ, Sawyers JL, eds. *Surgery of the Stomach, Duodenum, and Small Intestine*. Boston, Mass: Blackwell Scientific Publications; 1987.
4. Ballinger WF. Postvagotomy changes in the small intestine. *Am J Surg*. 1967;114:382–387.
5. Hedburg CA, Melnyk CS, Johnson CF. Glutenopathy appearing after gastric surgery. *Gastroenterology*. 1966;50:79–804.
6. Moss AA. Postvagotomy unmasking of nontropical spree. *Gastrointest Radiol*. 1976;1:173–175.
7. Mitty WF Jr, Grossi C, Nealon TF Jr. Chronic afferent loop syndrome. *Ann Surg*. 1970;172:99–1001.
8. Jordan GL. Surgical management of postgastrectomy problems. *Arch Surg*. 1971;102:251–259.
9. Op Den Orth JO. Tubeless hypotonic examination of the afferent loop of the Billroth II stomach. *Gastrointest Radiol*. 1977;2:1–5.
10. Thomas JL, Cowan RJ, Maynard CD, Wu W. Radionuclide demonstration of small bowel anatomy in the efferent loop syndrome. *J Nucl Med*. 1977;18:89–97.
11. Gale ME, Gerzof SG, Kisler LC, et al. CT appearance of afferent loop obstruction. *AJR*. 1982;138:1085–1088.
12. Swayne LC, Love MB. Computed tomography of chronic afferent loop obstruction: a case report and review. *Gastrointest Radiol*. 1985;10:39–41.
13. Lee DH, Lim JH, Ko YT. Afferent loop syndrome: sonographic findings in seven cases. *AJR*. 1991;157:41–43.
14. Waits JO, Baert PW, Charboneau JW. Jejunogastric intussusception. *Arch Surg*. 1980;115:1449–1452.
15. Katz I, Karp FL. Inadvertent gastroileostomy. *AJR*. 1967;99:162–174.
16. Schlegel DM, Maglinte DDT. The blind pouch syndrome. *Surg Gynecol Obstet*. 1982;155:541–544.
17. Maglinte DDT. Blind pouch syndrome: a cause of gastrointestinal bleeding. *Radiology*. 1979;132:314.
18. Goldstein F. Bacterial populations of the gut in health and disease: clinical aspects. In: Bockus HL, ed. *Gastroenterology*. 3rd ed. Philadelphia, Pa: WB Saunders Co; 1976.
19. Imbembo AL, Bohrer S, Loeff DS. Small-intestinal insufficiency and the short bowel syndrome. In: Zuidema GD, ed. *Surgery of the Alimentary Tract*. 3rd ed. Philadelphia, Pa: WB Saunders Co; 1991.
20. Nightingale JMD, Bartram CI, Lennard-Jones JE. Length of residual small bowel after partial resection: correlation between radiographic and surgical measurements. *Gastrointest Radiol*. 1991;16:305–306.
21. Payne JH, DeWind L, Schwab CE, Kern NH. Surgical treatment of morbid obesity: sixteen years of experience. *Arch Surg*. 1973;106:432–437.
22. Scott HW, Dean R, Shull HJ, et al. New considerations in use of jejunoileal bypass in patients with morbid obesity. *Ann Surg*. 1973;177:723–735.
23. Hocking MP, Duerson MC, O'Leary JP, Woodward ER. Jejunoileal bypass for morbid obesity: late follow-up in 100 cases. *N Engl J Med*. 1983;308:995–999.
24. McFarland RJ, Gaze JC, Pilkington RE. A 13-year review of jejunoileal bypass. *Br J Surg*. 1985;72:81–87.
25. Moss AA, Goldberg HI, Koehler RE. Radiographic evaluation of complications after jejunoleal bypass surgery. *AJR*. 1976;127:737–741.
26. Sarti DA, Zablen MA. The ultrasonic findings in intussusception of the blind loop in jejunoileal bypass for morbid obesity. *J Clin Ultrasound*. 1979;7:50–52.
27. Lo G, Fish AK, Brodey PA. CT of the intussuscepted excluded loop after intestinal bypass. *AJR*. 1981;137:157–159.
28. Campos CT, Matts JP, Fitch LL, et al. Predictors of total and low-density lipoprotein cholesterol change after partial ileal bypass. *Am J Surg*. 1988;155:138–146.
29. Buchwald H, Varco RL, Matts JP, et al. Effect of partial ileal bypass surgery on mortality and morbidity from coronary heart disease in patients with hypercholesterolemia. Report of the Program on the Surgical Control of the Hyperlipidemias (POSCH). *N Engl J Med*. 1990;323:946–955.
30. McGonigal MD, Lucas CE, Ledgerwood AM. Feeding jejunostomy in patients who are critically ill. *Surg Gynecol Obstet*. 1989;168:275–277.
31. Fleschner PR, Baert RW Jr. Ileostomy and its alternatives. In: Zuidema GD, ed. *Surgery of the Alimentary Tract*. 4th ed. Philadelphia, Pa: WB Saunders Co; 1996.
32. Maglinte DDT, Lappas JC, Kelvin FM, Rex D, Chernish SM. Small bowel radiography: how, when, and why? *Radiology*. 1987;163:297–305.
33. Zagoria RJ, Gelfand DW, Ott DJ. Retrograde examina-

tion of the small bowel in patients with an ileostomy. *Gastrointest Radiol.* 1986;11:97–101.
34. Kay VJ, Nolan DJ. The small bowel enema in the patient with an ileostomy. *Clin Radiol.* 1988;39:418–422.
35. Etherington RJ, Williams JG, Hayward MWJ, Hughes LE. Demonstration of paraileostomy herniation using computed tomogography. *Clin Radiol.* 1990;41:333–336.
36. Kock NG. Continent ileostomy. *Progr Surg.* 1973;12:18–201.
37. Parks AG, Nicholls RJ, Bellieveau P. Proctocolectomy with ileal reservoir and anal anastomosis. *Br J Surg.* 1980;67:533–538.
38. Utsunomiya J, Iwama T, Imajo M, et al. Total colectomy, mucosal proctectomy and ileoanal anastomosis. *Dis Colon Rectum.* 1980;23:459–466.
39. Sakier JM, Woods CB. Ulcerative colitis and polyposis coli: surgical options. *Surg Clin North Am.* 1988;68:1319.
40. Dozois RR, Kelly KA, Beart RW, Bealers OH. Continent ileostomy: the Mayo Clinic experience in alternatives to conventional ileostomy. In: Dozois RR, ed. *Alternatives to Conventional Ileostomy.* Chicago, Ill: Year Book Medical Publishers, 1985.
41. Lycke KG, Göthlin JH, Jensen JK, Philipson BM, Kock NG. Radiology of the continent ileostomy reservoir: method of examination and normal findings. *Abdom Imaging.* 1994;19:116–123.
42. Lycke KG, Göthlin JH, Jensen JK, Philipson BM, Kock NG. Radiology of the continent ileostomy reservoir: findings in patients with late complications. *Abdom Imaging.* 1994;19:124–131.
43. Baert RW Jr, Fleming CR, Banks PM. Tubulovillous adenoma in a continent ileostomy after proctocolectomy for familial polyposis. *Dig Dis Sci.* 1982;27(6):553–556.
44. Marcello PW, Roberts PL, Schoetz DJ Jr, Coller JA, Murray JJ, Veidenheimer MC. Long-term results of the ileoanal pouch procedure. *Arch Surg.* 1993;128:500–504.
45. Alfisher MM, Scholz FJ, Roberts PL, Counihan T. Radiology of the ileal pouch-anal anastomosis: normal findings, examination pitfalls, and complications. *Radiographics.* 1997;17:81–98.
46. Brown JJ, Balfe DM, Heiken JP, Becker JM, Soper NJ. Ileal J pouch: radiologic evaluation in patients with and without postoperative infectious complications. *Radiology.* 1990;174:115–120.
47. Thoeni RF, Fell SC, Engelstad B, Schrock TB. Ileoanal pouches: comparison of CT, scintigraphy, and contrast enemas for diagnosing postsurgical complications. *AJR.* 1990;154:73–78.
48. Mowschenson PM, Critshlow JF. Outcome of early surgical complications following ileoanal pouch operation without diverting ileostomy. *Am J Surg.* 1995;169:1143–1145.
49. Grant D. Current results of intestinal transplantation. *Lancet.* 1996;347:1801–1803.
50. Fung JJ, Abu-Elmagd K, Todo S. Intestinal and multivisceral transplantation. In: Bell RHJ, Rikkers LF, Mulholland MW, eds. *Digestive Tract Surgery: A Text and Atlas.* Philadelphia, Pa: Lippincott-Raven; 1996:1229–1261.
51. Todo S, Reyes J, Furukawa H, et al. Outcome analysis of 71 clinical intestinal transplantations. *Ann Surg.* 1995;222:270–280.
52. Bach DB, Hurlbut DJ, Romano WM, et al. Human orthotopic small intestine transplantation: radiologic assessment. *Radiology.* 1991;180:37–41.
53. Campbell WL, Abu-Elmagd K, Federle MP, et al. Contrast examination of the small bowel in patients with small-bowel transplants: findings in 16 patients. *AJR.* 1993;161:969–974.
54. Campbell WL, Abu-Elmagd K, Furukawa H, Todo S. Intestinal and multivisceral transplantation. *Radiol Clin North Am.* 1995;33:595–614.
55. Bach DB, Levin MF, Vellet AD, et al. CT findings in patients with small-bowel transplants. *AJR.* 1992;159:311–315.

Differential Diagnosis of Small Intestinal Abnormalities with Radiologic-Pathologic Explanation

Stephen E. Rubesin and Emma E. Furth

Chapter Contents

Introduction
Normal Anatomy of the Mesenteric Small Bowel
Differential Diagnosis of Focal Mass Lesions
Contour Distortions of Extrinsic Origin: Differential Diagnostic Considerations
Dilated Lumen, Normal Fold Thickness
Thick, Undulating, or Nodular Folds and Mucosal Nodularity
Tubular Bowel
Site Predilection of Diseases

Introduction

When radiologists look at an image, they compare it with a template of normal. In effect, the radiologist subtracts the normal template and perceives what is different, a normal variant or an abnormality. The radiologist determines the size, location, distribution, and radiographic characteristics of the abnormality. A knowledge of the patient's demographics (such as age, race, and location), of the clinical history, and of the gross pathology characterizing compatible diseases may enable the radiologist to construct a list of possible diagnoses.[1] A further step would be to provide a graded differential diagnosis, or even arrive at a specific diagnosis.

Radiologists can apply more complex insight into differential diagnosis if they have a working knowledge of the pathologic basis of disease. An aim of this chapter, therefore, is to teach differential diagnosis based on both pathologic and radiologic findings. The text and tables concerning the differential diagnoses are exhaustive. They present a way of thinking about the most common causes of various radiographic findings.

Normal Anatomy of the Mesenteric Small Bowel (See also Chapter 1)

The macroscopic, gross architecture of the small intestine is characterized by the plicae circulares (valvulae conniventes, folds of Kerckring), which are circumferential folds composed of mucosa and submucosa (Fig. 23-1). The plicae are more numerous, thicker, and protrude further into the lumen in the jejunum than in the ileum (Table 23-1).[2] The greater number, height, and width of the jejunal valvulae conniventes reflect the need for a larger absorptive surface area in the jejunum. The transition from jejunum to ileum is gradual. The jejunum is arbitrarily defined as the first 40% of the mesenteric small intestine, the ileum as the last 60%.

The mucosal surface of the small intestine is organized into villi, which are projections of epithelium surrounding a central core of lamina propria containing penetrating arterioles and a relatively large central lymphatic (Fig. 23-2).[3] The villi are 1 mm in height in the jejunum, a size that is at the limits of resolution of barium radiography. Villi are taller and thinner in the jejunum and broader and flatter in the ileum. Thus, applying our knowledge of anatomy to pathology, a radiographic abnormality in the plicae circulares may be caused by changes in either the mucosa or submucosa. Enlargement of a villus may indicate an abnormality in either the epithelium or the lamina propria.

Conglomerates of lymphoid cells form nodules and patches that distort the mucosal surface contour (Fig. 23-3). Many lymphoid aggregates appear as 1- to 2-

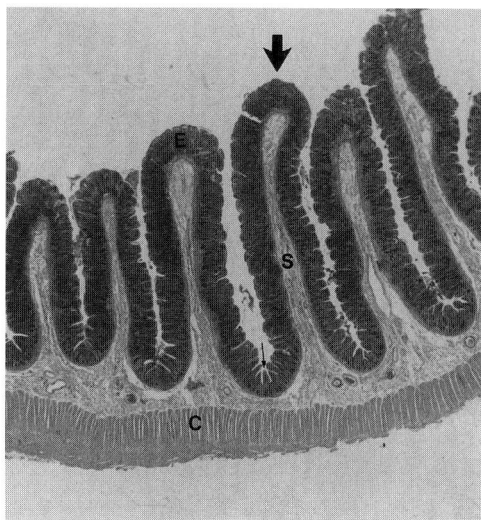

Fig. 23-1. Low-power microscopic view of the jejunum shows six normal small bowel folds.
The valvulae conniventes (plicae circulares) are composed of a central tongue of submucosa (S) covered by the epithelial layer. The circular muscle layer (C) of the muscularis propria is also identified. One villus is identified (arrow). (Hematoxylin and eosin, original magnification ×1.)

mm, smooth-surfaced elevations of the epithelium.[4] In the ileum, these larger aggregates of lymphoid tissue have been termed Peyer's patches. In some areas, the lymphoid tissue spans the mucosa and submucosa.

Normal Radiographic Appearance

The appearance of the small intestine varies greatly depending on the degree of lumen distention. During a small bowel meal, collapsed loops show undulating folds in either a longitudinal or disorganized pattern. This has been described as "feathering" (Fig. 23-4).

With lumen distention, either during a small bowel meal or a small bowel enema, the folds are seen to be either perpendicular or slightly angled to the long axis of the bowel (Fig. 23-5).[5] The fold thickness can dra-

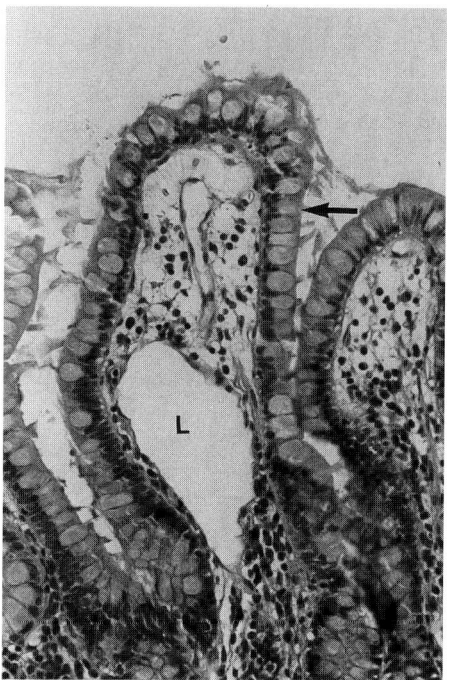

Fig. 23-2. Normal villus with central lymphatic.
The small bowel mucosa is made up of fingerlike projections termed villi. The surface of these villi is lined by epithelial cells, some of which are goblet cells (arrow). Goblet cells secrete acidic mucin. The lamina propria is the area below the epithelial cells and contains a central lymphatic space, termed the lacteal (L), which serves to carry chylomicrons to the portal circulation. (Hematoxylin and eosin, original magnification ×400.)

matically change by factors of 2 or 3 in response to degrees of lumen distention (Fig. 23-6). Thus, one of the advantages of enteroclysis is that, with full distention of the bowel lumen, the plicae circulares are straightened, presenting a reproducible thickness, and the mucosal surface can be studied en face (Table 23-1).

Differential Diagnosis of Focal Mass Lesions

Solitary Polyp

A polyp is defined as a lesion that protrudes into the lumen of bowel. The term polyp has no specific histologic connotation and does not imply a benign or malignant process, a mucosal or submucosal origin. The demarcation between a polyp and a solitary mass is arbitrary. In general, we refer to polyps as lesions less than 2 cm in their greatest dimension and to polypoid masses as larger protrusions.

When polyps are small, the radiologist finds it difficult to distinguish a mucosal from an extramucosal ori-

Table 23-1. Enteroclysis: Normal parameters

	Jejunum	Ileum
Folds per inch	4 to 7	2 to 4
Fold thickness	1 to 2 mm	1 to 1.5 mm
Fold height	3 to 7 mm	1 to 3 mm
Luminal diameter	<4 cm	<3 cm
Wall thickness	1 to 1.5 mm	1 to 1.5 mm

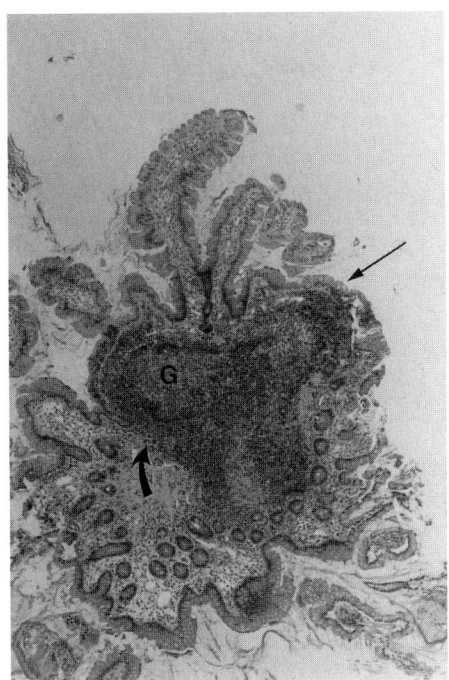

Fig. 23-3. Normal lymphoid aggregate in ileum.
The ileum is rich in mucosa-associated lymphoid tissue (curved arrow). The slightly clear area in the center of the lymphoid follicle is the germinal center (G). The overlying villi (straight arrow) may become slightly blunted as the lymphoid aggregate extends into the lamina propria. (Hematoxlyin and eosin, original magnification ×50.)

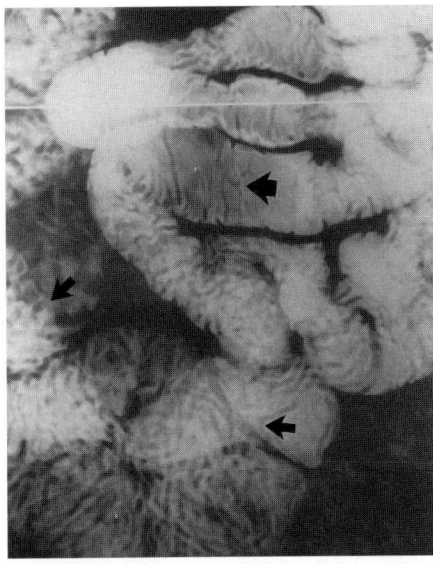

Fig. 23-4. Normal small bowel folds on spot radiograph from small bowel meal.
When small bowel loops are distended and splayed apart, small bowel folds are seen as well as during enteroclysis (large arrow). When loops overlie one another or are not fully distended, assessment of small bowel fold size is difficult (smaller arrows).

gin (arising in the submucosa or muscularis propria). When about 1.5 to 2 cm in size, it should be possible for a radiologist to determine the origin of the lesion. A sufficiently large mucosal lesion presents a nodular or lobulated surface texture (Fig. 23-7). In profile view an extramucosal mass has a smooth protruding surface, with abrupt margins against the surrounding mucosa (Fig. 23-8). Seen en face, the extramucosal lesion is round or ovoid and sharply circumscribed; focal ulceration or umbilication can be seen in about half the cases.

The most common polypoid lesions in the duodenum are different from those in the mesenteric small intestine (Table 23-2). Solitary or multiple polypoid tumors in the duodenal bulb or proximal second part of the duodenum are frequently proliferations of Brunner's glands, so-called Brunner gland hamartomas, "adenomas," or hyperplasias (Fig. 23-9).[6]

Heterotopic gastric mucosa may form a polypoid tumor in the proximal duodenum. The more common form of gastric type mucosa seen in the duodenum, however, is a metaplastic response to peptic disease,[7] and is termed gastric metaplasia. It is manifested as clusters of small, 2- to 3-mm, slightly raised, polygonal islands of mucosa in the juxtapyloric duodenal

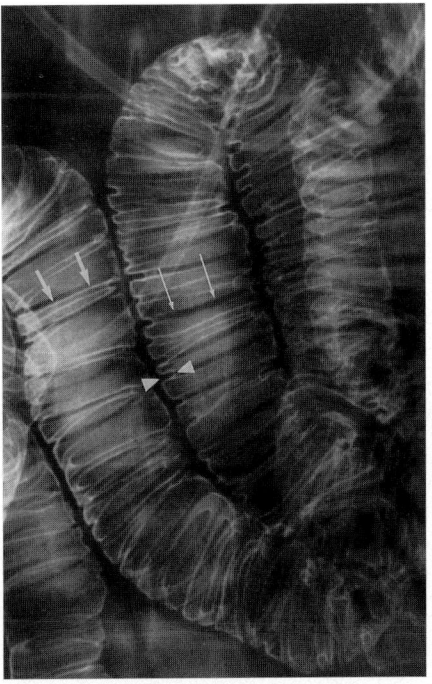

Fig. 23-5. Normal small bowel during enteroclysis.
Close-up of the jejunum shows normal plicae circulares as smooth, straight, 1 mm in thickness, tubular radiolucent filling defects (thin arrows), often etched in white by barium (thick arrows). Fold height is measured from the edge of the expected luminal contour to the edge of the fold seen in profile (arrowheads). (Reproduced with permission from Rubesin et al.[2])

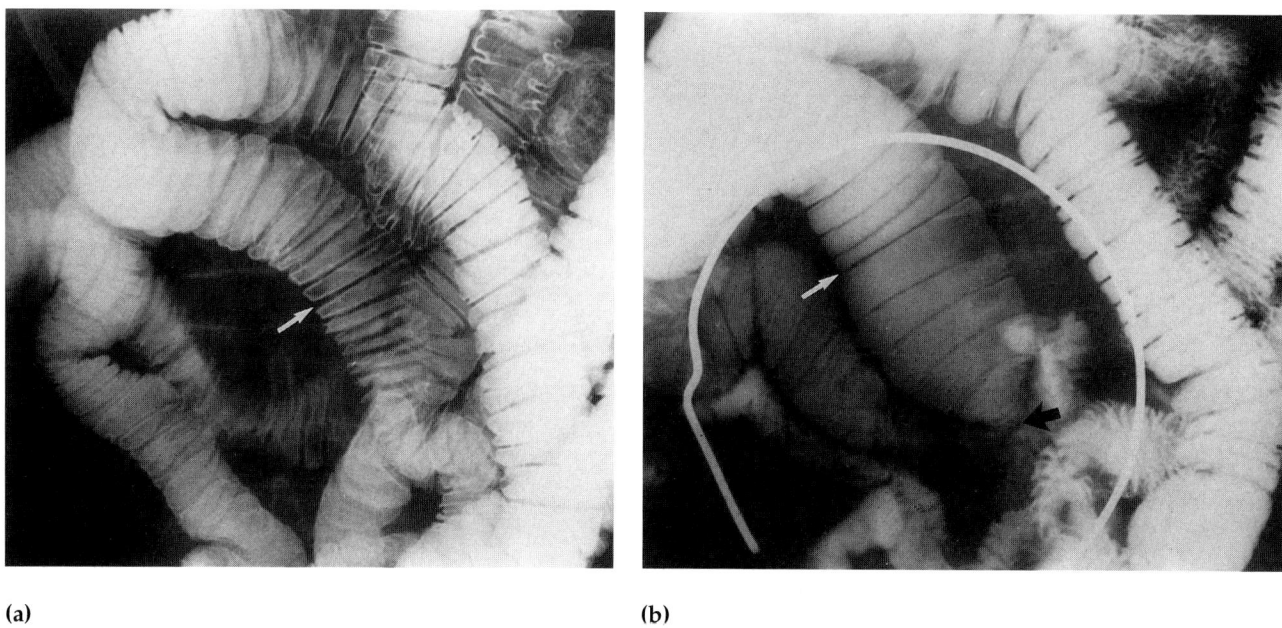

Fig. 23-6. Changing width of valvulae conniventes during enteroclysis.
(a) Spot radiograph of loop of proximal jejunum shows small bowel folds (white arrow). (b) With continued infusion of methycellulose, an adhesive band is better demonstrated (black arrow). The adhesion causes low-grade obstruction manifested as luminal dilatation of the loop shown in (a). The folds in the same, but now-dilated, loop of small intestine (white arrow) appear thinner and of diminished height.

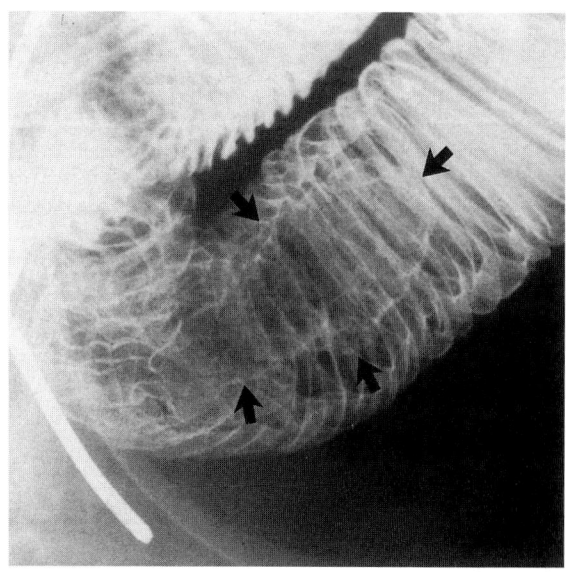

Fig. 23-7. Mucosal lesion with nodular surface.
Spot radiograph of jejunum during the methylcellulose phase of a small bowel enema demonstrates a 3.5-cm polypoid mass with a lobulated edge (arrows). The surface pattern is often better seen during the single-contrast phase of enteroclysis. This was a hamartoma in a patient with Peutz-Jeghers syndrome.

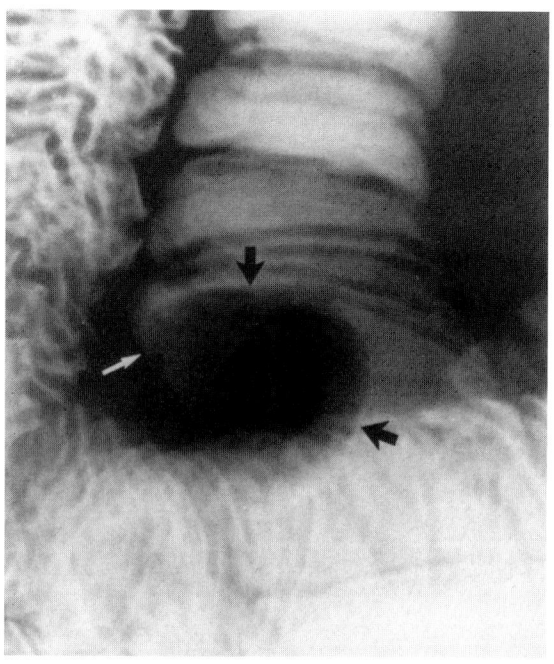

Fig. 23-8. Submucosal mass with smooth surface.
A 2.5-cm-diameter smooth-surfaced mass (black arrows) protrudes into the lumen of the jejunum. Note abrupt angulation with the lumenal contour (white arrow). This was a lipoma.

Table 23-2(a). Solitary polyp

Tumor	Comment
Carcinoid	Ileum:jejunum:duodenum:Meckel's 45:3:1:1
	Size of metastases exceed size of primary tumor
Adenoma	Ampulla of Vater, distal duodenum
	Duodenum:jejunum:ileum 9:1:1
Brunner gland hamartoma	1st, 2nd part duodenum
Ectopic gastric mucosa	Duodenum, occasionally jejunum
Ectopic pancreas	Duodenum:jejunum:ileum 10:6:1
Hemangioma	Evenly distributed in jejunum/ileum
Hamartoma	Peutz-Jeghers type, predominantly proximal
Nerve cell tumors	
Gangliocytic paraganglioma	Near papilla of Vater
Neurofibroma	Most common nerve cell tumor
	Associated with neurofibromatosis
Leiomyoma/Undifferentiated benign	Gastrointestinal stromal tumor
Lipoma	Anywhere, pseudopedicle, compressible

Numbers in ratio form indicate proportion of lesions in bowel.

bulb (Fig. 23-10).[8] Small polypoid lesions of the prepapillary region of the second part of the duodenum are frequently ectopic pancreas or neuroendocrine tumors ("carcinoid," "islet cell tumors").[9] Adenomas arising in or distal to the papilla of Vater may be polypoid or carpetlike lesions (Fig. 23-11).[10]

If a solitary lesion is seen in the mid small bowel or ileum, especially the terminal ileum, the radiologist must first of all consider a carcinoid tumor, a tumor with malignant potential, even when small (Fig. 23-12). Although there are many histologic types of solitary polypoid lesions in the small bowel (Table 23-2a), a solitary nodule or polyp in the terminal ileum must elicit the radiologic diagnosis of "possible carcinoid tumor." Carcinoid tumors arise in undifferentiated cells in the basal layer of the epithelium or neuroendocrine cells in the epithelium or lamina propria.[6,11] Therefore, some of these tumors may appear to be small submucosal masses, rather than nodular mucosal elevations. The other small polyps (Fig. 23-6) that arise from the various tissues in the small intestine—epithelial cells, fat, nerve tissue, lymphoid tissue, blood vessels, and smooth muscle of the muscularis mucosae or muscularis propria—are, in general, less serious lesions.[6,12–15]

Long, soft, changeable lesions are composed of tissue that is pliable, such as fat and fluid. The most common causes of a long, pliable, polypoid lesion in the distal ileum are an inverted Meckel's diverticulum,[16] a lipoma, or a fibroepithelial polyp (Table 23-3) (Fig. 23-13).

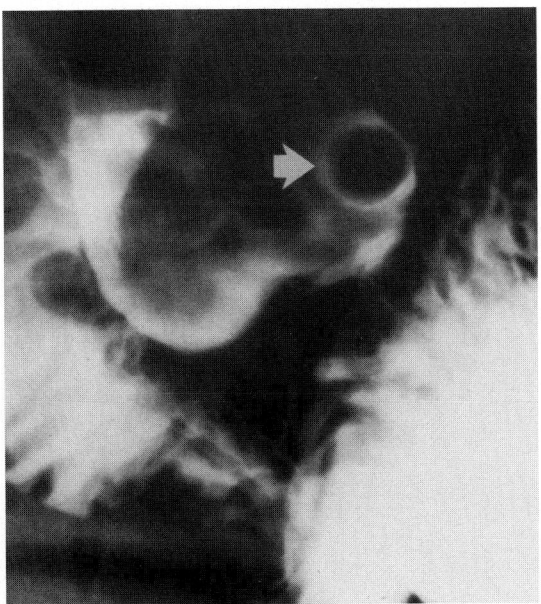

Fig. 23-9. Brunner gland hamartoma.
Spot radiograph of duodenal bulb shows a round, slightly lobulated filling defect (arrow) in the barium pool.

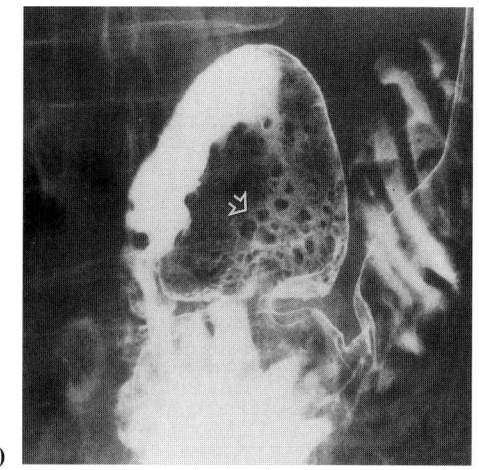
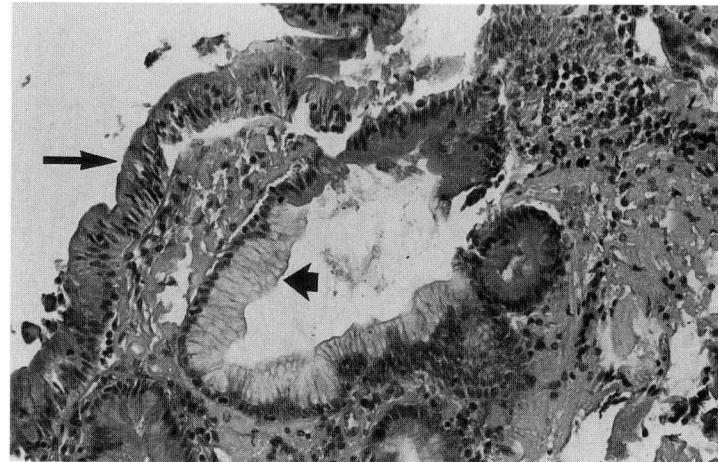

Fig. 23-10. Gastric metaplasia, duodenal bulb.
(a) Numerous small, 2- to 3-mm, polygonal, slightly raised islands of mucosa (arrow) are seen as radiolucent filling defects in the shallow barium pool on the posterior wall of the juxtapyloric duodenum. (b) In gastric metaplasia in the duodenum, foveolar mucosa (short arrow), normally found only along the surface of the stomach, replaces the intestinal type epithelium (long arrow). The foveolar cells have a relatively clear cytoplasm, contain neutral mucin, and are nonabsorptive. The intestinal absorptive cells have a darker cytoplasm. (Hematoxylin and eosin, original magnification ×200.) (Reproduced with permission from Rubesin et al.[8])

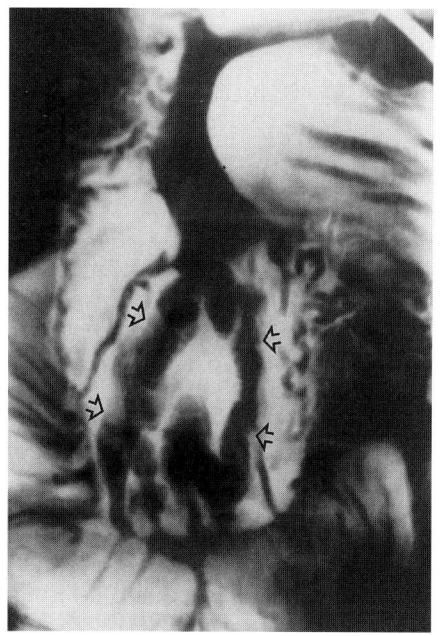

Fig. 23-11. Carpetlike adenoma third portion of duodenum (a) and periampullary region (b, c).
(a) A villous adenoma in the third portion of the duodenum grows as a flat, carpetlike lesion manifested as a focal area of thick, nodular folds (arrows). (b,c) Specimen photograph (b) and low-power microscopic picture (c) of a different carpet lesion shows a periampullary villous adenoma (thick arrow) growing along the surface of the duodenum (d). The surface of the tumor is focally lobulated. There is extension of tumor into the ampulla of Vater (small arrows). Obstruction of the ampulla of Vater is evidenced by massive ductal dilatation. [(c), hematoxylin and eosin, original magnification ×1).]

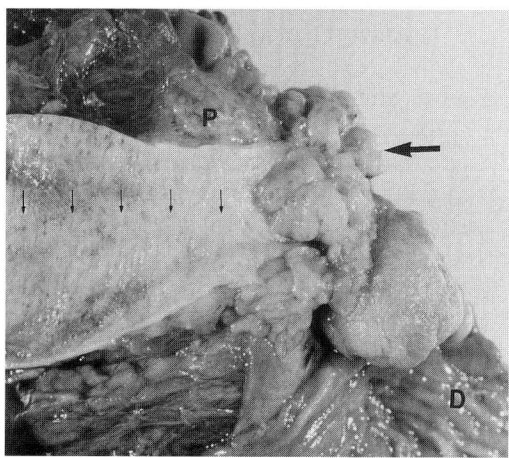
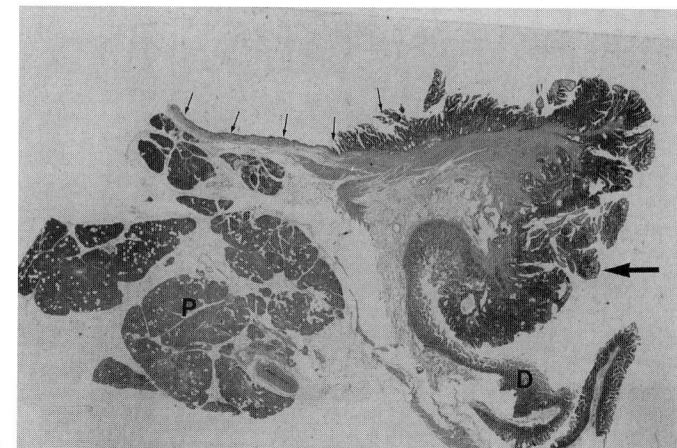

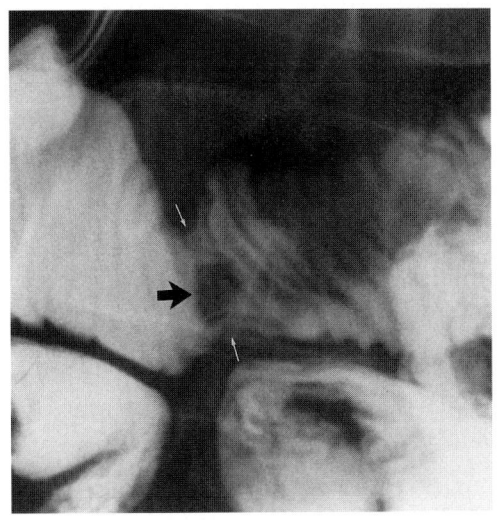

Fig. 23-12. Small carcinoid tumor, ileum.
(a) Spot radiograph of mid small intestine shows a 1.0- by 0.7-cm radiolucent filling defect in the barium column (black arrow). Note inbowing of the intestinal walls toward the tumor (white arrows) indicative of the desmoplastic reaction in carcinoid tumors. (b,c) Low- (b) and medium-power (c) photomicrographs of a different carcinoid tumor. The small bowel epithelium [curved arrow in (b)] overlying the submucosal neuroendocrine tumor is preserved. The tumor forms nests composed of cells with bland, "salt and pepper" nuclei and abundant cytoplasm [see Fig. 23-12 (c)]. With infiltration of the bowel wall, the tumor incites desmoplasia and muscle hypertrophy. [Hematoxylin and eosin, original magnification (b) ×50, (c) ×400.]

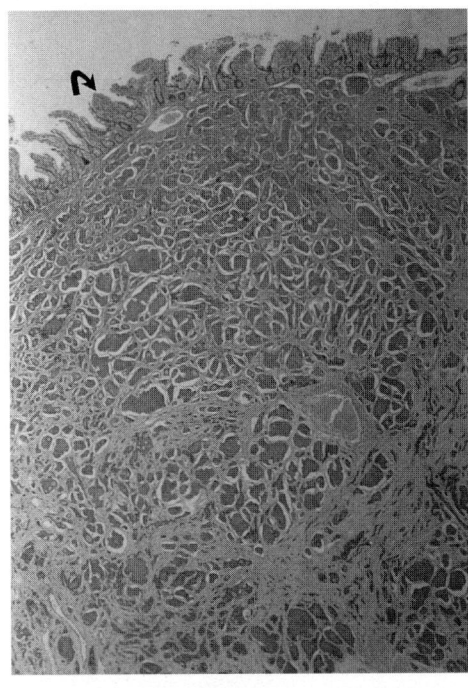

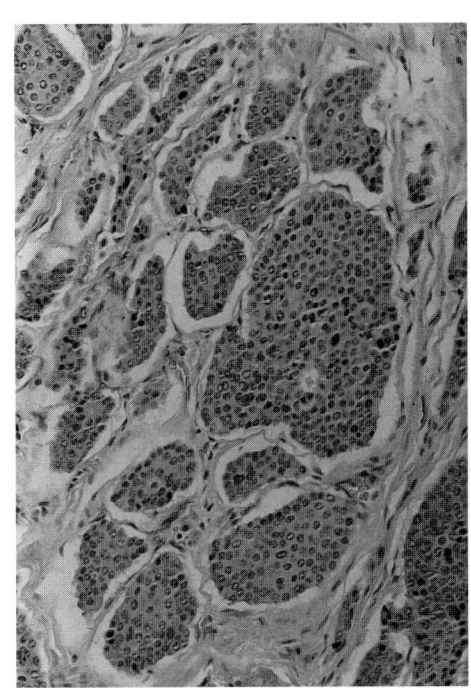

Target Lesions

Solitary "target" or "bull's eye lesions" may be produced by any submucosal mass that causes ulceration of the overlying mucosa (Fig. 23-14). A small gastrointestinal stromal tumor (GIST) may produce such an ulcerated target lesion.[1,17]

Multiple target lesions are most commonly ulcerated submucosal metastases, especially metastatic melanoma. Other disseminated polypoid tumors, including Kaposi's sarcoma and disseminated lymphoma, can also form ulcerated submucosal masses. Melanoma metastases may have a central stellate-shaped ulcer (Fig. 23-15) with extensions radiating toward the periphery, producing a so-called "spoke-wheel" appearance.[18]

Multiple Polypoid Lesions

The most common causes of multiple polypoid masses are metastases, especially metastatic melanoma (Fig. 23-15), lymphoma, and carcinoid tumors (Table 23-4).

Table 23-2(b). Multiple target lesions

1. Hematogenous metastases, especially melanoma
2. Multiple primary ulcerated tumors arising in submucosa, eg, GISTS
3. Lymphoma, usually disseminated
4. Kaposi's sarcoma

Table 23-3. Long, Pliable Polyp

Tumor	Comment
Lipoma	Growth deflected into lumen, elongated
Inflammatory fibroid polyp (fibroepithelial polyp)	Ileum:jejunum:duodenum 20:2:1
Inverted Meckel's diverticulum	Distal ileum, may intussuscept

Numbers in ratio form indicate proportion of lesions in bowel.

In addition to the previously stressed importance of suggesting the diagnosis of carcinoid in cases of solitary polypoid lesions in the distal ileum, the same caveat applies to the presence of multiple polyps. When multiple mucosal- or submucosal-appearing masses are found in the distal ileum, especially associated with desmoplastic changes to adjacent small bowel, carcinoid tumors must be strongly considered. Carcinoids tumors are multiple in at least 30% of patients.[6,11] Identification of more than one carcinoid tumor in the small bowel alerts the surgeon to the need of a more extensive resection than expected.

Hamartomas in Peutz-Jeghers syndrome may be sessile or pedunculated. Sessile hamartomas appear as relatively flat, nodular carpet lesions. The polypoid masses may have nodular or smooth surfaces, with a lobulated contour (Fig. 23-16).[6,19] Some patients with Peutz-Jeghers syndrome present as adults and the diagnosis is initially made radiologically. The pigmented macules on mucous membranes may not be visible.[20]

Inflammatory or postinflammatory polyps in Crohn's disease may be round, ovoid, or filiform in shape (Fig. 23-17).[21,22] They either represent chronically inflamed residual mucosa or are reparative tissue.

Annular Lesions

Annular lumen narrowing may result from a circumferential extension of a neoplastic, inflammatory, or fibrotic process involving the submucosa, the muscularis propria, or even an area beyond the bowel wall.

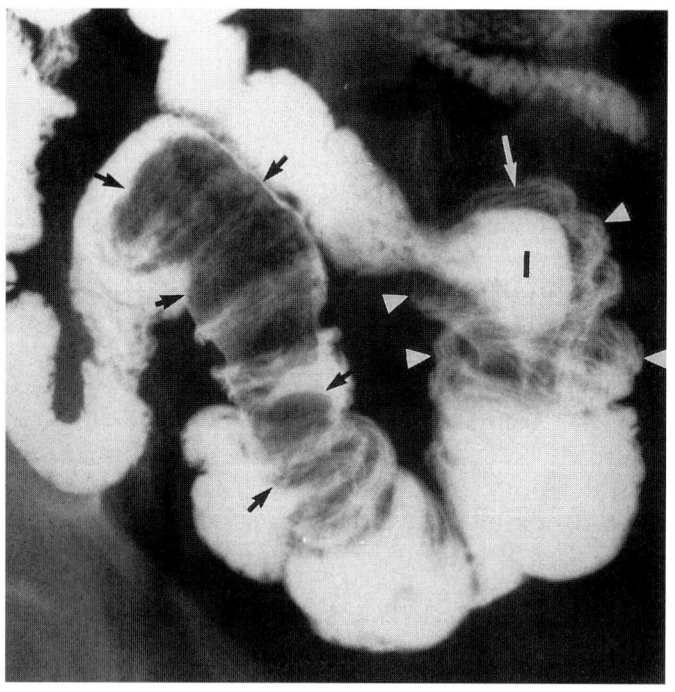

(a)

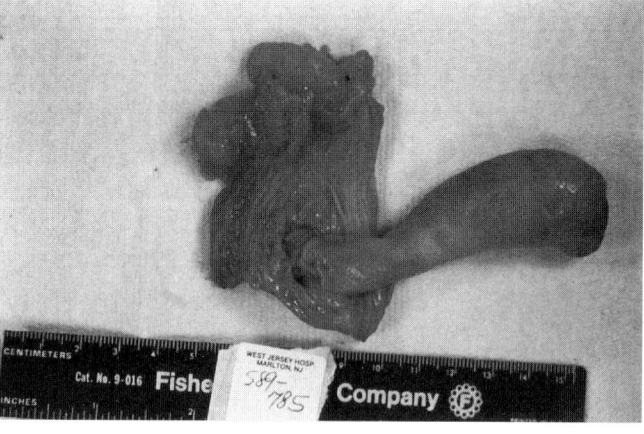

(b)

Fig. 23-13. Inverted Meckel's diverticulum.
(a) Spot radiograph from small bowel meal shows a long, radiolucent filling defect in the barium column (black arrows). The polypoid lesion is causing intussusception. The intussusceptum (I) is manifested as a barium-filled column within the intussuscipiens (arrowheads). A "coil-spring" sign represents barium-coated folds of the intussuscipiens (white arrow). (b) Specimen photography demonstrates the 7-cm-long inverted Meckel's diverticulum found at surgery. (Reproduced with permission from Rubesin et al.[16])

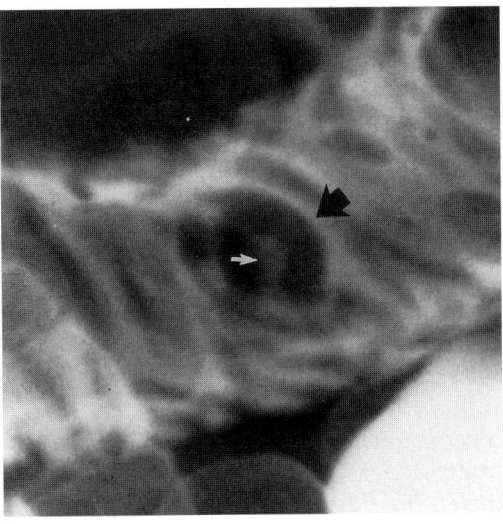 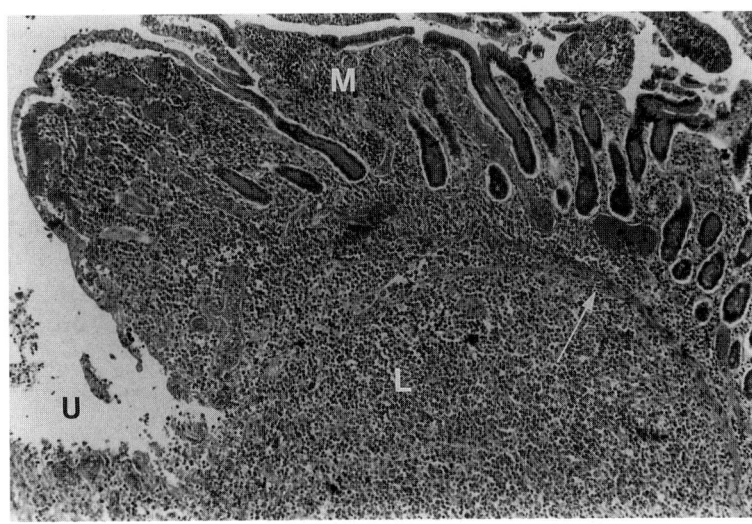

Fig. 23-14. Target lesion (disseminated lymphoma).
(a) Spot radiograph of the proximal jejunum demonstrates a 1.2-cm ovoid, smooth-surfaced tumor (black arrow) with a central umbilication (white arrow). (b) Medium-power photomicrograph shows that the bulk of the lymphomatous infiltration (L) lies in the submucosa below the muscularis mucosae (white arrow) and below the ulcer (U). The lymphoma focally invades the mucosa (m). (Reproduced with permission from Rubesin et al.[17])

Malignant epithelial tumors usually have abrupt, shelflike margins and a nodular mucosa at the transition between normal and abnormal tissue (Table 23-5) (Fig. 23-18). Adenocarcinomas are either polypoid or carpetlike masses involving the ampulla of Vater or polypoid or infiltrating malignancies in the distal duodenum or jejunum (Fig. 23-18).[23] Annular adenocarcinomas of the small bowel are usually short infiltrating tumors in the first several loops of jejunum, and cause proximal small bowel obstruction (Fig. 23-18). A metastasis may occasionally have an annular appearance mimicking a primary small bowel adenocarcinoma, but metastases are typically located in the mid or distal small bowel.[24] More frequently, metastases appear as circumferential extrinsic lesions lacking distinct margins, showing preserved mucosal folds that may be tethered or angulated.

Non-Hodgkin's lymphomas of the small bowel may appear as circumferential lesions with relatively abrupt margins and undulating mucosa or effaced

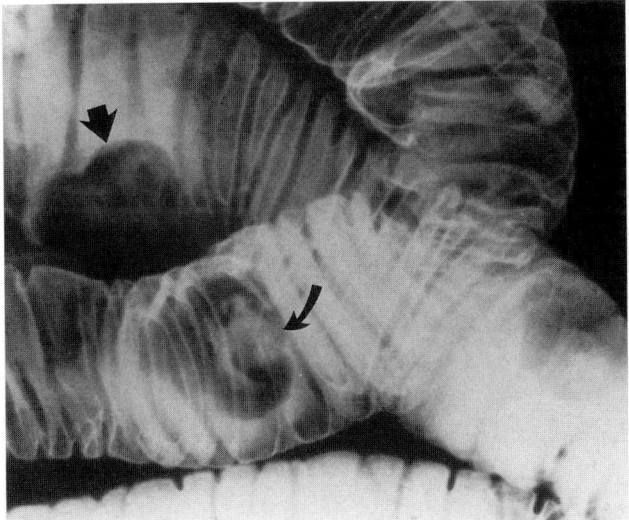

Fig. 23-15. Metastatic melanoma with stellate ulcer.
Two polypoid masses are labeled, one seen in profile (black arrow) and one seen en face (curved black arrow). The curved arrow points toward an irregular ulcer on the tumor's surface.

Table 23-4. Multiple polyps

Common	Uncommon
Hematogenous metastases	Neurofibromas
Carcinoid	Kaposi's sarcoma
Lymphoma Primary Disseminated Mantel cell (lymphomatous polyposis)	Peutz-Jeghers hamartomas Amyloid deposits (AL type) Multiple myeloma

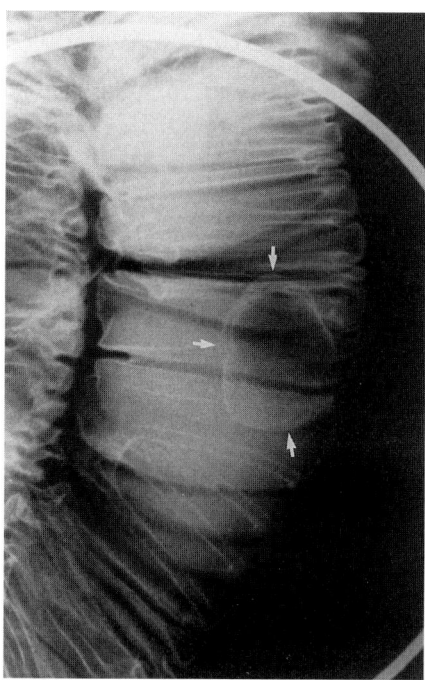

Fig. 23-16. This Peutz-Jeghers polyp (hamartoma) has a lobulated surface contour (arrows) etched in white by barium.

mucosal folds (Fig. 23-19).[17,25] In contrast to adenocarcinomas, non-Hodgkin's lymphomas may present as annular lesions that are longer and less obstructing, have less lumen narrowing per length of tumor, and tend to develop lumen widening in the midportion (because of wall resistance damaging infiltration of the muscularis).[17] Thus, there is less small bowel dilatation proximal to an annular lymphoma, compared to the moderate, but occasionally marked small bowel dilatation proximal to an annular carcinoma (Fig. 23-20).

Short strictures in Crohn's disease may have shelflike margins and abnormal, nodular mucosa mimicking adenocarcinoma (Fig. 23-21). Adenocarcinoma arising in Crohn's disease is rare (0.3%), but cannot be excluded when a shouldered stricture is detected in a patient with long-standing Crohn's disease.[26] Even expert pathologists find it difficult or impossible to distinguish a benign from a malignant stricture in Crohn's disease on the basis of gross pathology and require histology for diagnosis.

An annular lesion with smooth mucosa and tapered margins is usually a benign process (Table 23-6). Strictures and skip lesions in Crohn's disease are usually associated with other morphologic characteristics of

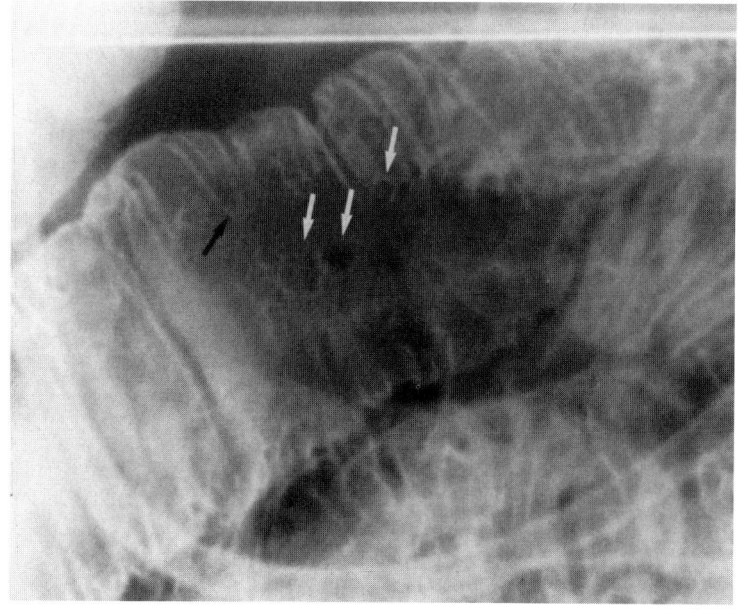
(a)

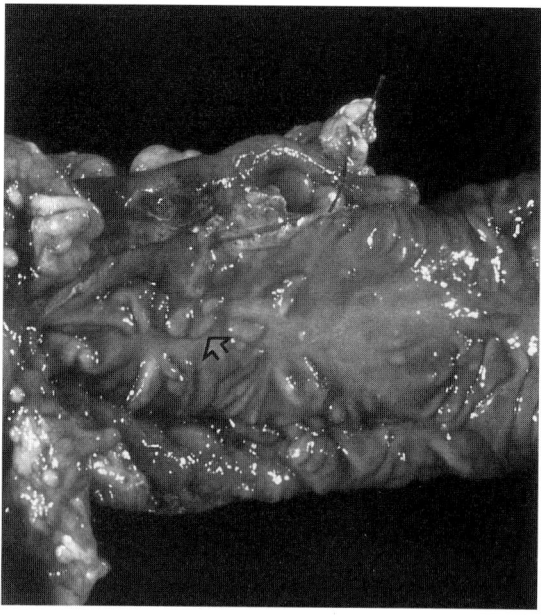
(b)

Fig. 23-17. Inflammatory and postinflammatory polyps in Crohn's disease.
(a) Spot film of the mid-jejunum shows several nodules etched in white (white arrows). Partial destruction of valvulae conniventes is seen in the area of Crohn's disease. A truncated fold is identified (black arrow). (b) Inflammatory polyps in the terminal in a different patient with Crohn's disease. Linear and nodular projections of mucosa (arrow) lie between areas of ulceration. A representative inflammatory polyp identified. (Reproduced with permission from Rubesin and Bronner.[21])

Table 23-5. Annular lesion with narrowing and shouldered margin

Etiology	Comment
Primary adenocarcinoma	Ampullary, periampullary duodenum
	Duodenum:jejunum:ileum 7:3:1
Carcinoid	Multiple in 30%
Metastases, annular	mid-/distal bowel, Ca colon primary
Primary small bowel lymphoma	Little narrowing for length of lesion
	Sharp demarcation, no obstruction
Crohn's disease	Skip lesions, associated features
Anastomotic stricture	Surgical history, clips/staple line
Nonsteroidal antiinflammatory agent	Thick, ringlike webs, multiple

Numbers in ratio form inicate proportion of lesions in bowel.

the disease, such as aphthoid ulcers or linear mesenteric border ulcerations (Fig. 23-22). Adhesive bands that cross the entire bowel lumen may appear as smooth, thicker, foldlike defects with otherwise intact mucosa (Fig. 23-23). Some adhesive bands cause a beaklike narrowing with smooth contours and proximal dilatation of the lumen (Fig. 23-24).

Strictures related to ischemia, radiation, or trauma show tapered margins (Fig. 23-25) or may appear ringlike. The key to the diagnosis is the patient's history and associated changes elsewhere in the bowel. Strictures related to sequelae of either acute or longstanding inflammation such as nonsteroidal antiinflammatory drugs (NSAID)[27,28] or ulcerative jejunoileitis,[29] respectively, may appear as ringlike circumferential narrowings (Fig. 23-26); the former NSAID condition produces more regular "diaphragm lesions."

Cavitary Mass

Tumors arising in the wall of the small bowel are frequently large and bulky and invade the adjacent mesentery. When these lesions ulcerate or necrose, they may form cavities or abscesses within the mass, often in communication with the intestinal lumen. Thus, during barium studies, the lumen of the gastrointestinal tract appears to extend beyond the expected luminal contour; hence the term "exoenteric" (Table 23-7) or cavitary lesion. The most common exoenteric masses are bulkly, highly cellular tumors which easily cavitate such as primary non-Hodgkin's lymphoma of the small intestine (Fig. 23-27), benign or malignant GISTs and metastatic melanoma.[17,25,30,31] Inflammatory conditions that result in small bowel perforation and adjacent abscess formation, such as jejunal diverticulitis[32] or Crohn's disease, may mimic exoenteric tumors. We have seen a case of ectopic pancreas with pancreatitis and pseudocyst formation mimic an exoenteric mass (Fig. 23-28).[33]

Contour Distortions of Extrinsic Origin: Differential Diagnostic Considerations

The small intestine abuts numerous structures: anteriorly, the greater omentum, colon, and anterior abdominal wall below the level of the greater omentum; posteriorly, the anterior pararenal space and periaortic tissue; and inferiorly, the superior surface of the pelvic organs such as the urinary bladder, uterus, and ovaries.[34] The mesenteric border of the small intestine attaches to the small bowel mesentery. An abnormality in any of these structures can displace, separate, or invade small bowel loops.[35]

Separation of Bowel Loops

The most common cause of separated small bowel loops is a prominent amount of mesenteric fat, seen most often in obese patients (Table 23-8). The small

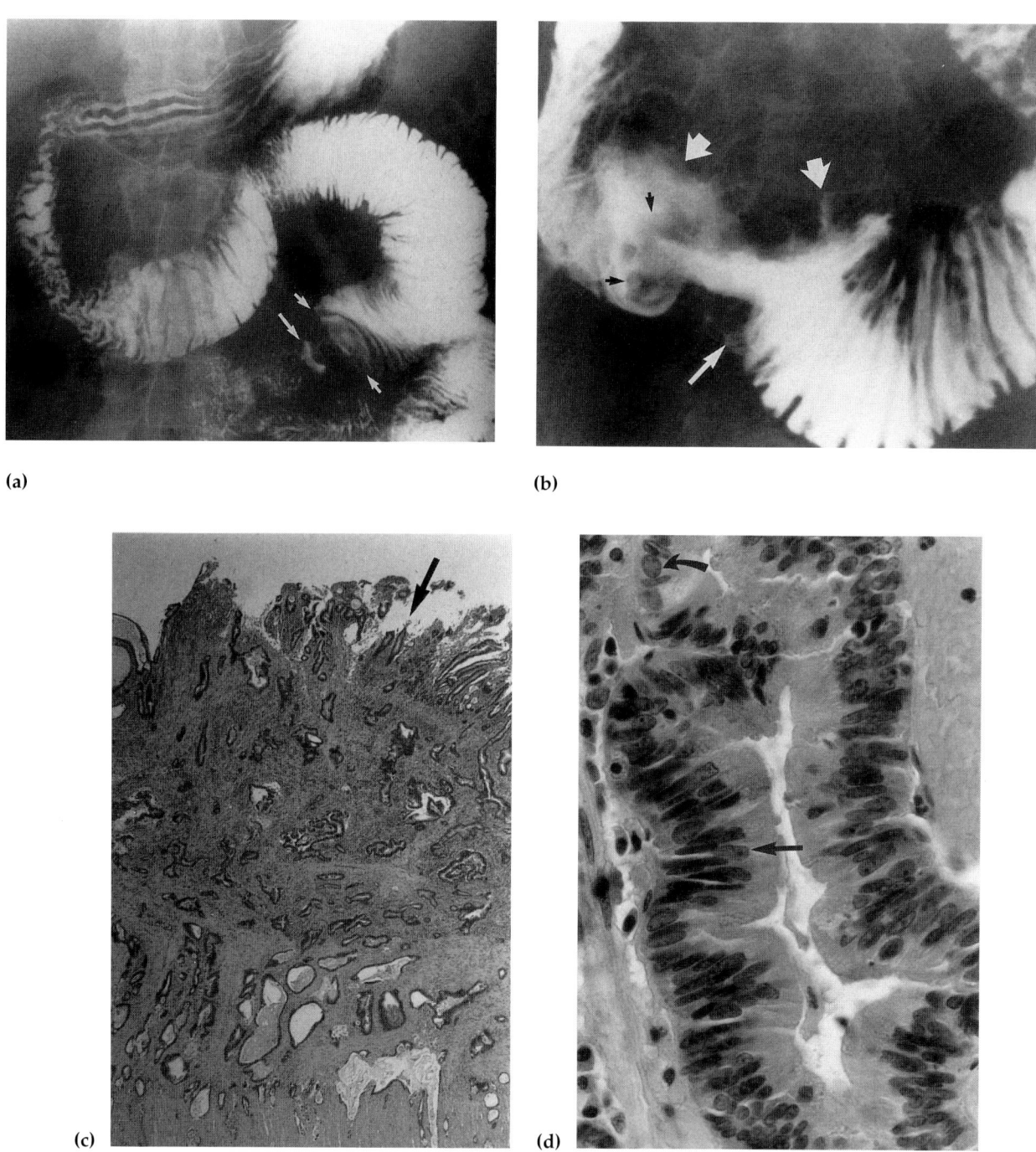

Fig. 23-18. Annular adenocarcinoma, jejunum.
(a) A short, annular lesion of the proximal jejunum has an abrupt shelflike margin (short arrows) and is centrally ulcerated (long arrow). Obstruction is implied by the dilatation of distal duodenum and jejunum proximal to the annular tumor. (b) Adenocarcinoma, mid small bowel. Spot radiograph from enteroclysis shows a 3-cm-long annular lesion with abrupt margins (one seen en face: black arrows; one seen in profile: long arrow) and irregular contour (thick arrows). Obstruction is manifested by dilatation of small intestine proximal to the lesion. (Reproduced with permission from Herlinger and Rubesin.[19]) (c,d) Microscopic images of a different adenocarcinoma. (c) The adenocarcinoma invades through bowel wall. As with colon cancers, a surface adenomatous precursor lesion is identified (arrow). (Hematoxlyin and eosion, original magnification ×50). (d) The high-power picture shows the cytologic features of adenomatous epithelium. The nuclei of an adenoma (straight arrow) are enlarged and hyperchromatic compared to normal nuclei (curved arrow). (Hematoxlyin and eosion, original magnification ×400.)

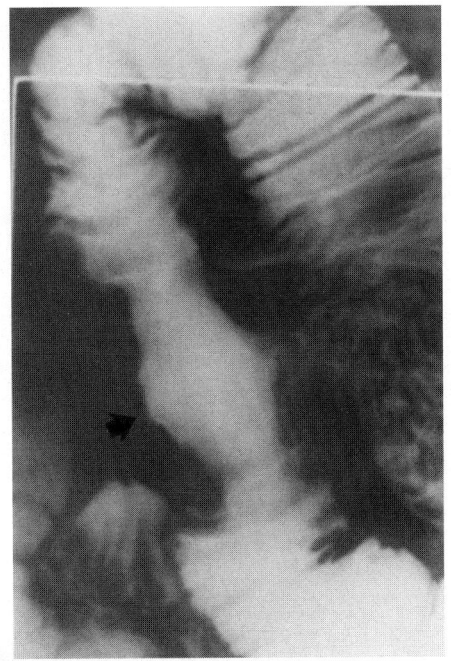
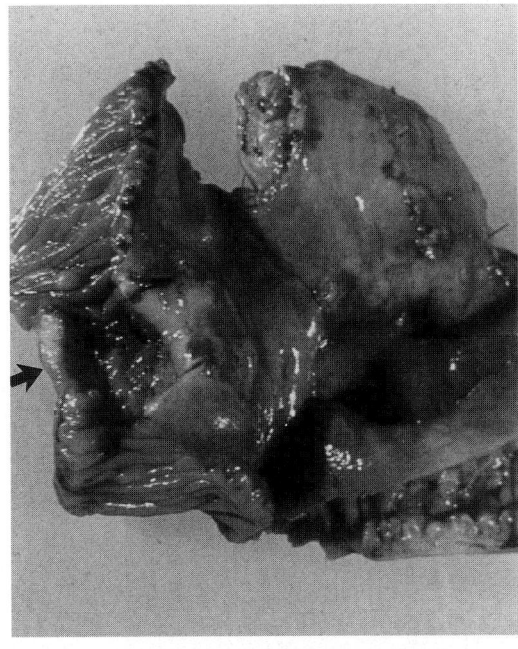
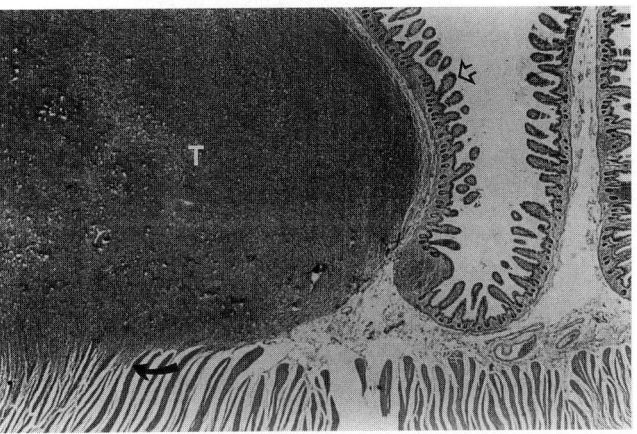

Fig. 23-19. Diffuse, large cell lymphoma.
(a) Spot radiograph from the single-contrast phase of an enteroclysis shows a long, 6-cm circumferential lesion (arrow) of the mid small bowel with abrupt margins and less narrowing of the lumenal contour or evidence of obstruction than would be expected for an adenocarcinoma of this size. (b) The surgical specimen shows an abrupt, annular lesion (arrow). (c) Low-power photomicrograph at the margin of the tumor shows that the bulk of the periphery of the tumor (T) is in the submucosa. The tumor invades the circular muscle layer of the muscularis propria (curved arrow). The mucosa at the edge of the tumor is preserved (open arrow). (Photos b and c reproduced with permission from Rubesin et al.[17]).

bowel loops are pliable and change their location in relation to surrounding small bowel loops or other structures. In patients with marked ascites, small bowel loops are separated and pliable, floating centrally in the ascitic pool.

Separation of small bowel loops may be the first fluoroscopic clue that there is disease in the small bowel itself. Focal thickening of the bowel wall due to Crohn's disease, lymphoma, or other primary small bowel tumor will separate the abnormal loop from other adjacent small bowel loops. In contrast to separation by mesenteric fat, separation between segments of abnormal bowel remains relatively fixed; the area is less pliable during palpation. Separation of bowel loops in Crohn's disease may be due to a combination of bowel wall thickening and the so-called "fibrofatty proliferation" of the mesentery (Fig. 23-29). Computed tomography (CT) best demonstrates the cause of separation of bowel loops, and is the best modality to rule out an abscess as the cause.

Lymph node masses in the periphery or the root of the small bowel mesentery can separate small bowel loops through extrinsic mass effect. Non-Hodgkin's lymphoma arising in the small bowel mesentery can separate and even invade the small intestine (Fig. 23-30).[17] Infectious diseases such as Whipple's disease, mycobacterium avium-intracellulare (MAI), or tuberculous infection in Acquired Immunodeficiency

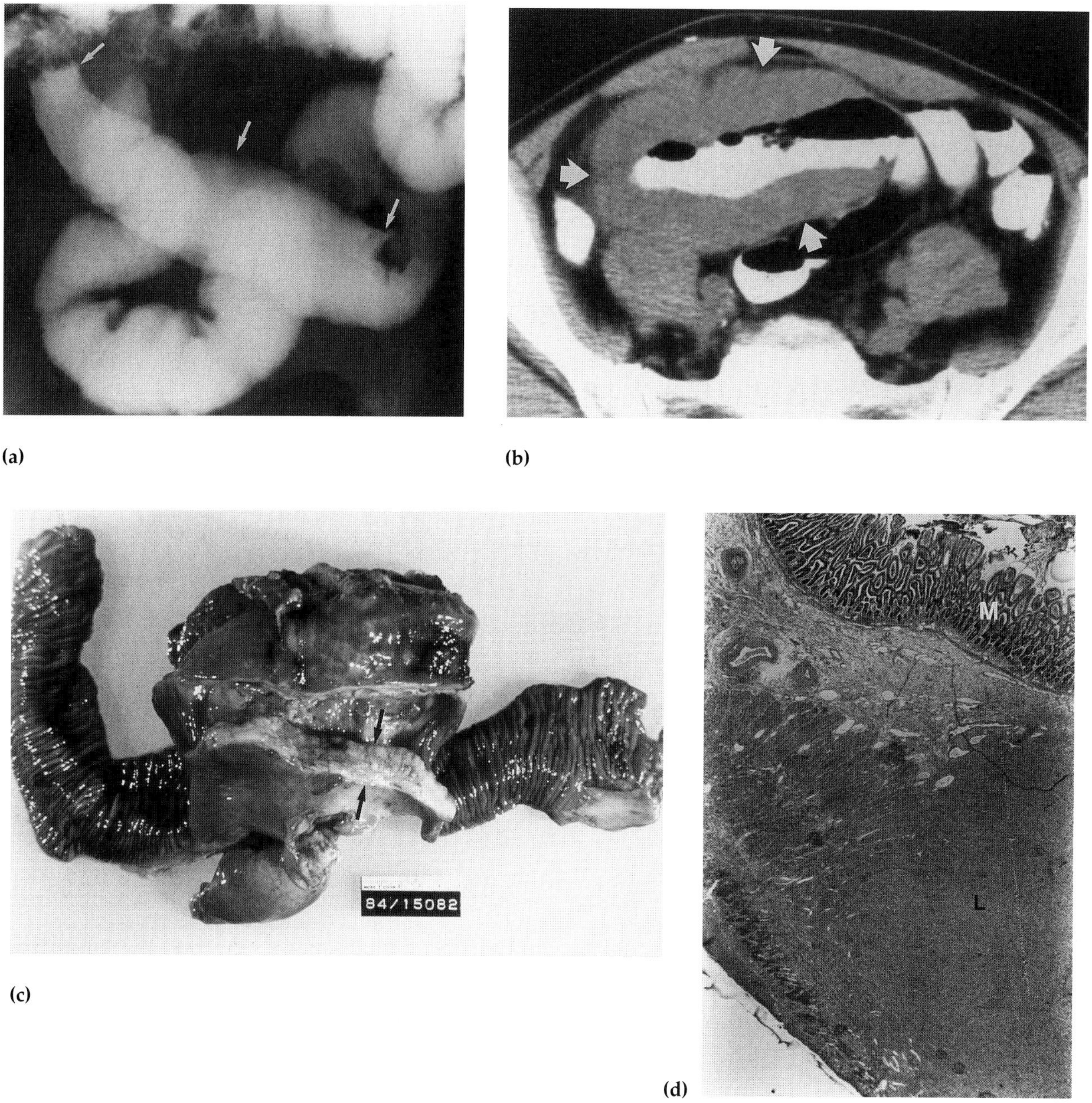

540 • 23. Differential Diagnosis of Small Intestinal Abnormalities with Radiologic-Pathologic Explanation

Fig. 23-20. Diffuse, large cell lymphoma causing lumenal dilatation.
(a) Long, annular lesion (arrows) has effaced the valvulae conniventes. The lumen is protruding toward the mesenteric border of the small bowel (arrows). (b) CT demonstrates a well-circumscribed lesion with a markedly thickened wall (arrows). (c) The surgical specimen shows a long, annular lesion with abrupt margins and marked small bowel wall thickening (arrows). (d) Low-power photomicrograph shows the lymphoma (L) extending from muscularis mucosae to subserosa. The mucosa (M) is preserved. The muscularis propria is infiltrated in some regions, destroyed in others. [Photos c and d reproduced with permission from Rubesin et al.[17]]

Continous Distortions of Extrinsic Origin: Differential Diagnostic Considerations

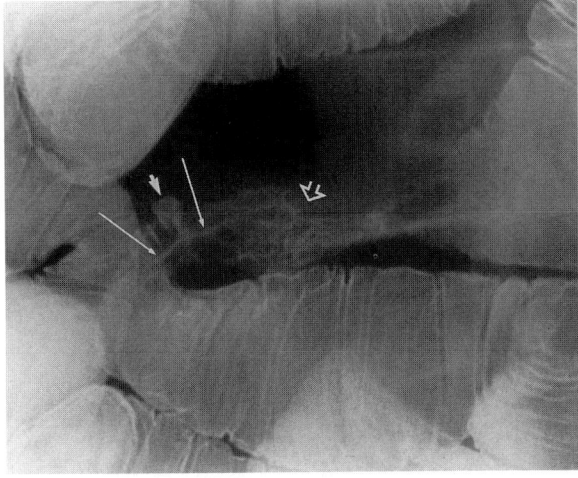

Fig. 23-22. Crohn's skip lesion.
Spot radiograph of mid small bowel shows a 3-cm-long tapered narrowing. There is a shallow cobblestoning proximally (open arrow). Distally, a mesenteric border ulcer is seen en face (long arrows) with sacculation opposite the ulcer (short arrow).

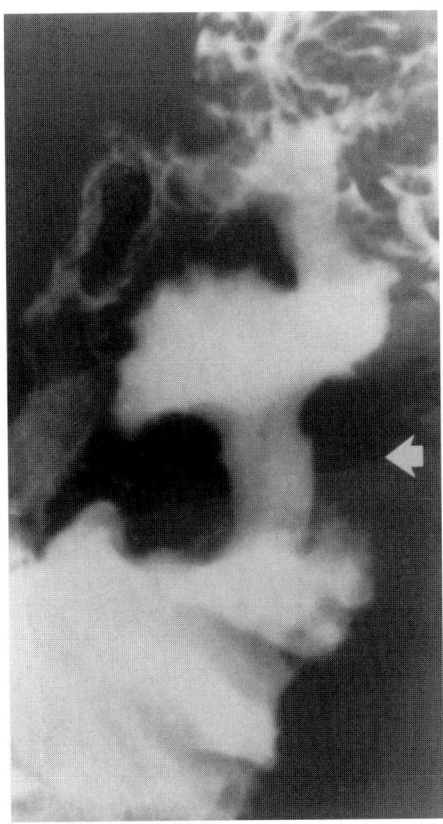

Fig. 23-21. Annular narrowing in Crohn's disease.
A focal annular lesion (arrow) with abrupt margins and nodular mucosa is indistinguishable from adenocarcinoma.

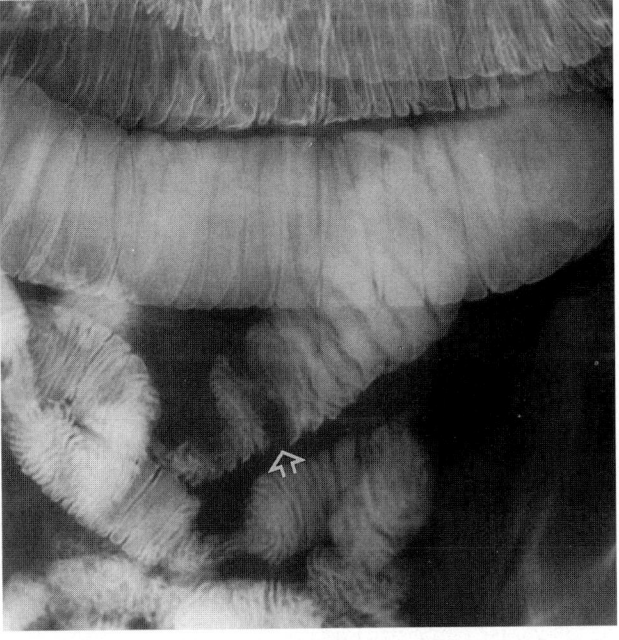

Fig. 23-23. Circumferential adhesive band.
A smooth, tubular radiolucent filling defect crosses the lumen of the mid small bowel. The small bowel mucosa is preserved. There is abrupt transition between distended and nondistended small bowel.

Table 23-6. Annular lesion with narrowing and tapered margin

Etiology	Comment
Crohn's stricture	Associated findings of Crohn's
Adhesion	Beaklike narrowing
	radiolucent band crosses lumen
	confined to radiation portal,
	often at edge of portal
Radiation	
Ischemia	
Trauma	

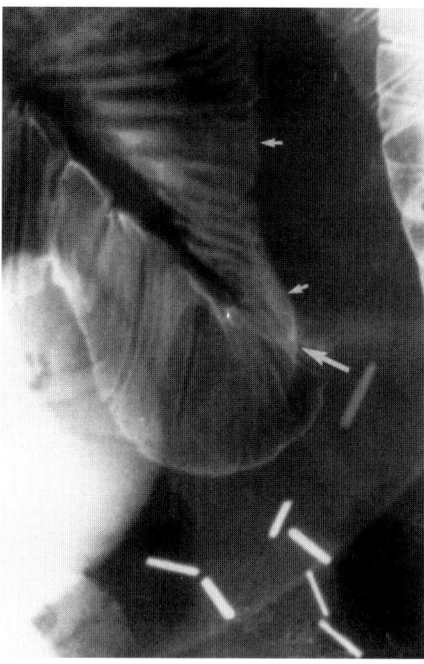

Fig. 23-24. Adhesions with beaklike narrowing.
The bowel lumen proximal to the adhesion is tapered (small arrows) to a beaklike point (large arrow). The mucosal folds are preserved, though tethered toward the mesentery.

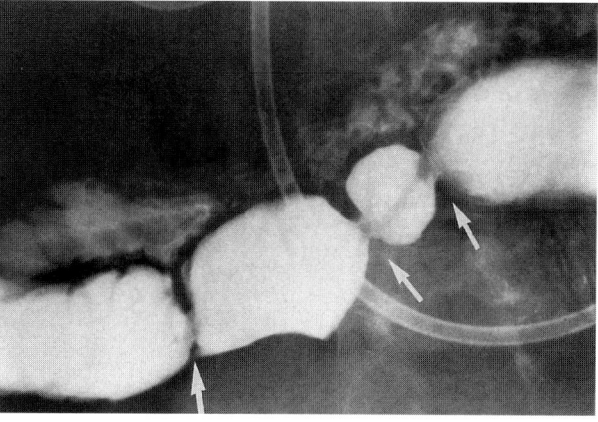

Fig. 23-26. Strictures in ulcerative jejunoileitis.
In a patient with long-standing celiac disease, three ring-like, smooth strictures (arrows) are seen.

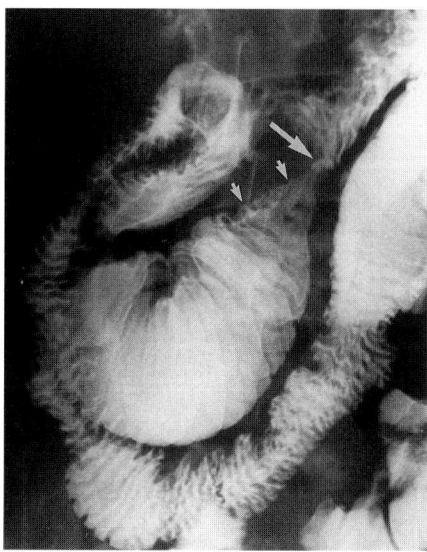

Fig. 23-25. Ischemic stricture.
Overhead view from a small bowel enema shows a 5-cm-long tapered stricture (small arrows) with relatively preserved mucosa. There is a 5-mm barium collection at its distal end (large arrow). At pathology, this proved to be a ulcer arising in the ischemic stricture. Obstruction is manifested as dilatation of the bowel proximal to the stricture.

Syndrome (AIDS) can cause massive mesenteric lymphadenopathy and associated bowel displacement.

Primary mesenteric tumors are rare. Desmoid tumors are usually seen in patients with a familial adenomatous polyposis syndrome and may displace or even invade small intestine.[6] Primary mesenteric cysts such as mesothelial cysts or lymphangioma will cause focal displacement.

Radiographically, extrinsic mass effect in profile appears as a broad-based indentation of the luminal contour of the small intestine (Fig. 23-31). If only part of the lumen is compressed and is seen en face, the extrinsic mass causes an area of increased density superimposed on the narrowed lumen (Fig. 23-31).

Tethering of Folds

Angulation of a small intestinal loop is usually due to an extrinsic desmoplastic process. Tethering or pulling of mucosal folds toward an extrinsic site is usually

Table 23-7. Cavitary (exoenteric) mass

Common	Uncommon
Primary non-Hodgkin's lymphoma	Crohn's disease
Metastatic melanoma	Diverticulitis
Gastrointestinal stromal tumors ("leiomyosarcoma")	Ectopic pancreas with pancreatitis

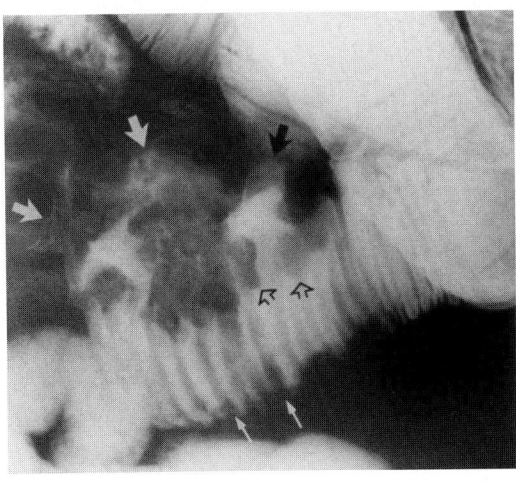
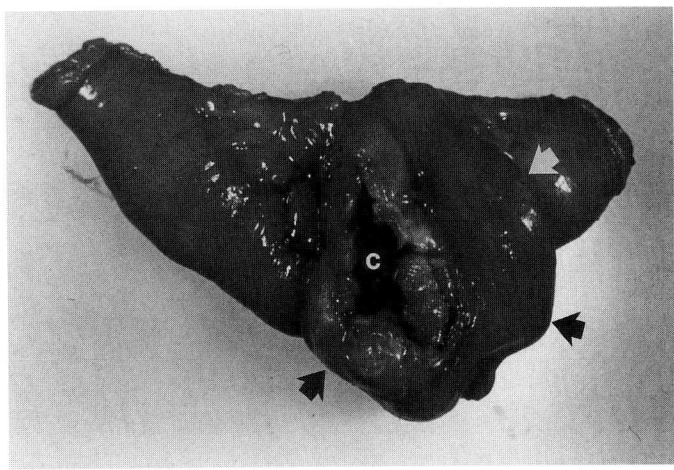

Fig. 23-27. Cavitary mass (non-Hodgkin's lymphoma).
(a) Spot radiograph from a small bowel enema shows a large barium-filled cavity extended beyond the expected luminal confines of the bowel (large arrows). Noncavitary lymphomatous infiltration of the bowel wall is manifested as areas of smooth nodularity (open arrows) and thick, undulating folds (short arrows). (b) The surgical specimen shows a mass (arrows) with a central cavity (c) that extended into the small bowel mesentery. [(b) reproduced with permission from Rubesin et al.[17]]

due to adhesions (Fig. 23-32) or burnt-out endometriosis.

Extrinsic Mass Effect and Tethering

The combination of extrinsic mass effect and tethering of mucosal folds in the compressed loop indicates an inflammatory or neoplastic process involving the small bowel mesentery in which adjacent small intestinal loops are fixed or angulated (Table 23-9). The desmoplastic process may be confined to the mesentery itself, with only secondary effect on the adjacent small bowel, or may actually invade the serosa (Fig. 23-33). The right lower quadrant is a prime location for masses that secondarily involve the small intestine or for abnormalities that arise in the cecum and invade the terminal ileum.[35]

Intraperitoneal fluid descends through the ruffles of the mesentery to pool in the right lower quadrant along the mesenteric border of the distal ileum and the medial border of the cecum and ascending colon.[35] Neoplastic processes that have reached a peritoneal surface have a predilection for extension via the ascitic fluid to involve the small bowel in the right lower quadrant in the form of seeded intraperitoneal metastases. In women, the ovary is most common site of origin of intraperitoneal metastases (Fig. 23-34). In men, the most common sites of origin are the colon, pancreas, and stomach. Seeded metastases usually result in multiple extrinsic masses that secondarily tether adjacent small bowel loops. Tethering of mucosal folds can be related to direct invasion of the serosa or to a desmoplastic effect arising in the mesentery itself (Fig. 23-33).

Endometriosis implants in the ileum, cecum, or appendix can also tether small bowel and/or cause mass effect. If tethering alone is seen, it is difficult to distinguish adhesions from burnt-out or active endometriosis.

Primary carcinoid tumors invade the small bowel mesentery along vascular channels and incite a desmoplastic reaction; the usually larger mesenteric metastasis will cause more extensive tethering affecting larger areas of small bowel to cause angulations, narrowing, and even obstruction (Figs. 23-35, 23-36). At this late stage, the primary carcinoid tumor is often hard to find within the deformed small bowel loops.

In a similar way, retractile mesenteritis or interloop abscesses cause inflammatory and desmoplastic reactions in the small bowel mesentery and secondary involvement of the intrinsically normal small intestine.

When cecal or appendiceal processes extend outside the serosal surfaces, they may secondarily affect the adjacent ileum or sigmoid colon. When an adenocarcinoma of cecal or ileocecal valve origin invades the terminal ileum, adjacent ileal folds may either be smoothly enlarged or effaced, suggesting submucosal,

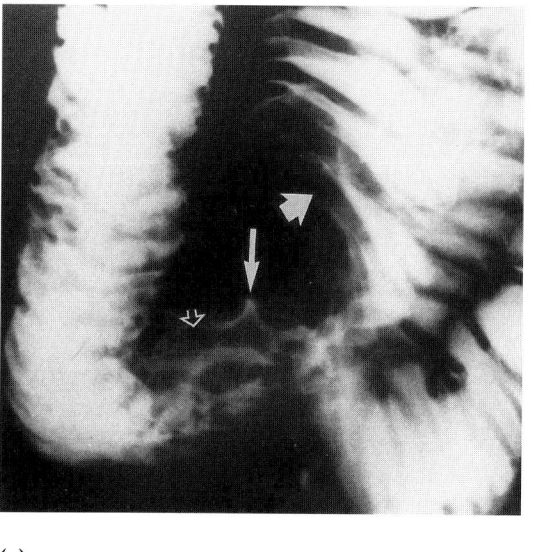

(a)

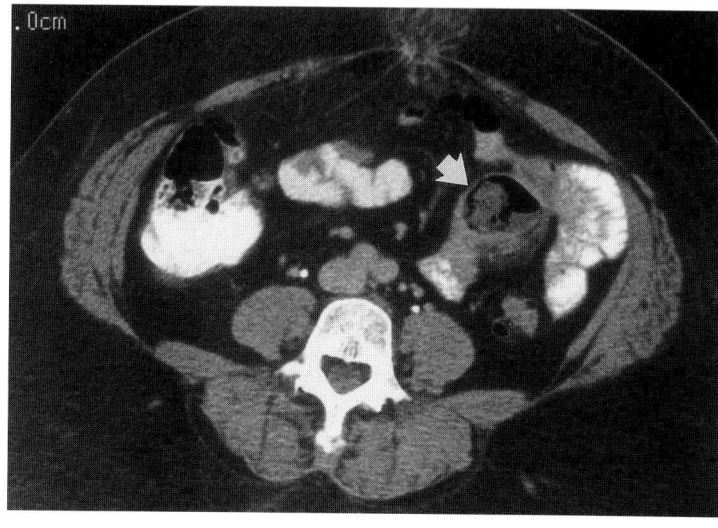

(b)

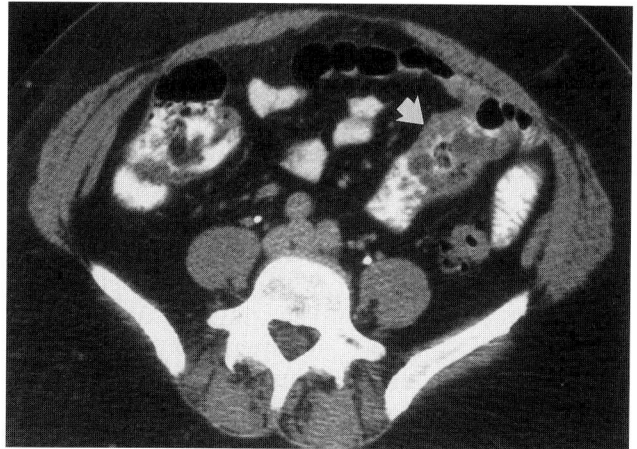

(c)

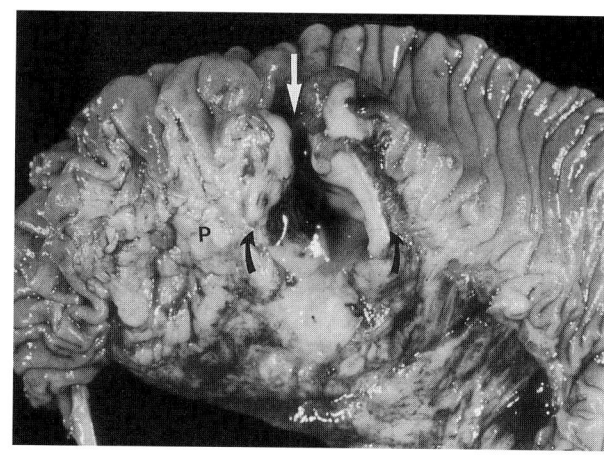

(d)

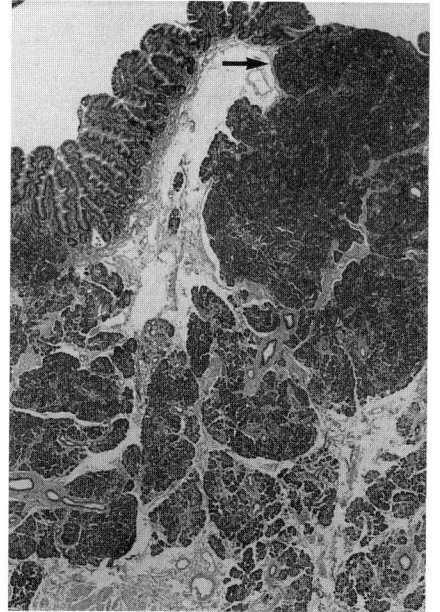

(e)

Fig. 23-28. Ectopic pancreas mimicking exoenteric mass.
(a) Spot radiograph of the jejunum during a small bowel enema shows a focal ulcer (long arrow). There are thickened, undulating folds running longitudinally adjacent to the ulcer (open arrow). An extrinsic mass effect on the mesenteric border of the small bowel is seen (thick arrow). (b) CT shows a 3-cm in diameter cavity (arrow) filled with air and debris. (c) CT of jejunal loop adjacent to the cavity shows thick, lobulated folds (arrow). (d) Photograph of opened specimen shows a 3-cm in diameter cavity (curved arrows) communicating with the lumen of the jejunum (white arrow). The cavity is surrounded by ectopic pancreatic tissue (P). (e) Photomicrograph demonstrates ectopic pancreatic tissue extending into the lamina propria (arrow). The overlying villi are normal. The ectopic pancreatic tissue forms the thick, lobulated jejunal folds seen on enteroclysis and CT. The cavity was a pseudocyst related to pancreatitis. (Hematoxlyin and eosin, original magnification ×50.) [(a–d) reproduced with permission from Rubesin et al.[33]]

Table 23-8. Separation of bowel loops (without tethering)

Normal small bowel, hypertrophied mesenteric fat

Ascites

Related to primary thickening of small bowel wall
 Crohn's disease
 Primary lymphoma
 Other tumors

Mesenteric or retroperitoneal lymphadenopathy
 Lymphoma
 Whipple's disease
 AIDS-related

Primary mesenteric tumors

Fibrofatty proliferation in transmural Crohn's disease

often translymphatic extension (Fig. 23-37), or mucosal nodularity, suggesting epithelial involvement by the neoplasm.

Lymphoma of the ileocecal valve may invade submucosally or extrinsically into the terminal ileum. Mucosal surfaces overlying extensions of a lymphoma show greater effacement of folds and smoother surfaces than primary epithelial carcinomas because of their submucosal growth pattern.

An abscess or tumor originating in the appendix will behave as an extrinsic mass upon the terminal ileum and medial border of the base of the cecum. The ileum may be asymmetrically draped or compressed by the extrinsic mass. The ileal folds may appear tethered and of normal size, being pulled by the desmoplastic process outside of the serosa. If lymphatics or vessels are blocked in the small bowel mesentery, the

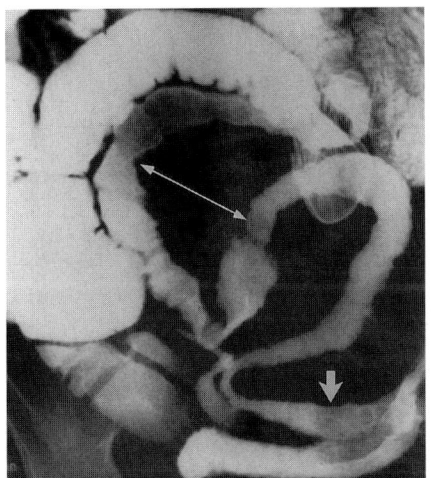

(a)

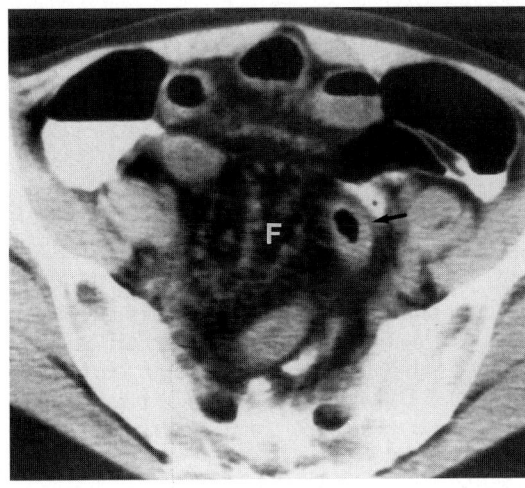

(b)

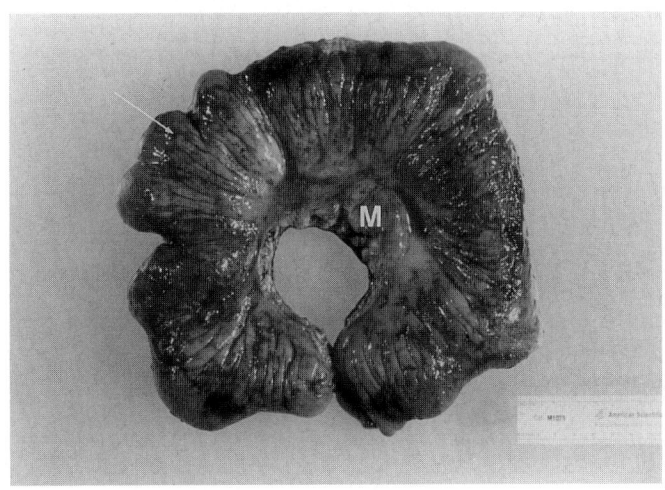

(c)

Fig. 23-29. Separation of bowel loops: fibrofatty proliferation in Crohn's disease.
(a) Overhead radiograph shows separation of right lower quadrant ileal loops (double arrow). The luminal contour is diffusely abnormal; the lumen is mildly, but diffusely narrowed. Cobblestoning of the mucosa is seen only when the column of barium is "thin" (thick arrow). (b) CT through pelvis demonstrates that the separation of bowel loops is due to extensive mesenteric fat (F), which demonstrates stranding. Only mild bowel wall thickening is seen (arrow). (c) Fibrofatty proliferation in another patient with Crohn's disease. Photograph of a surgical specimen shows thickening of the small bowel mesentery (M). Mesenteric fat extends around the serosal surface of the small bowel toward the antimesenteric border (arrow), a process termed "creeping fat." (Reproduced with permission from Rubesin and Bronner.[21])

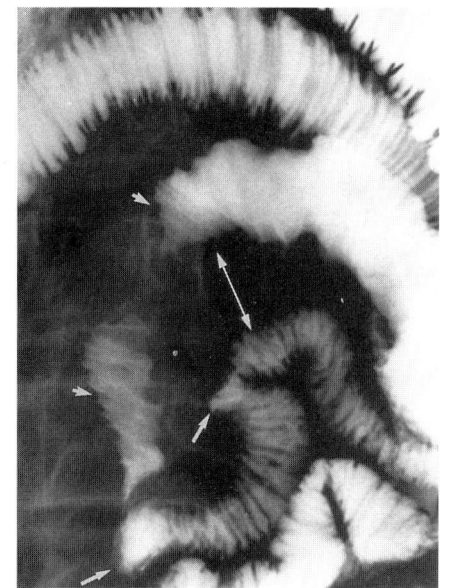 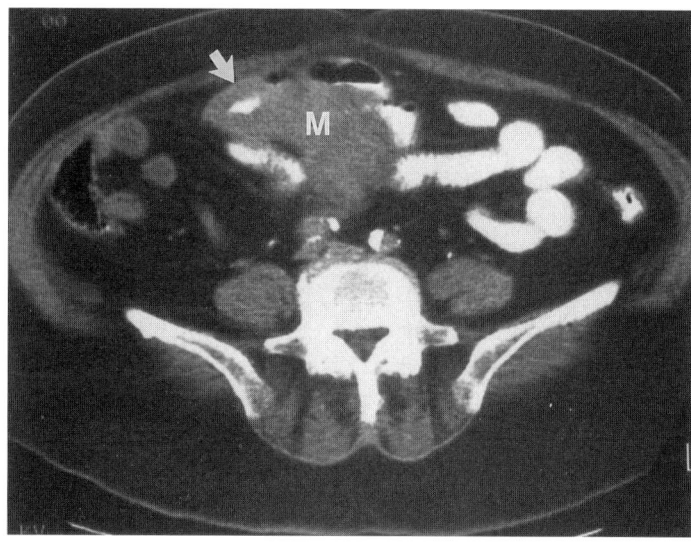

Fig. 23-30. Primary mesenteric non-Hodgkin's lymphoma separates bowel loops.
(a) Overhead radiograph from a small bowel enema shows separation of bowel loops (double arrow), angulation of bowel loops (long arrows). The small bowel folds are thickened (small arrows) due to direct bowel wall invasion by the primary mesenteric lymphoma. (b) CT demonstrates a large mass (M) in the small bowel mesentery separating small bowel loops. Direct invasion of the adjacent small intestine is manifested by thickening of the small bowel wall (arrow). (Reproduced with permission from Rubesin et al.[17])

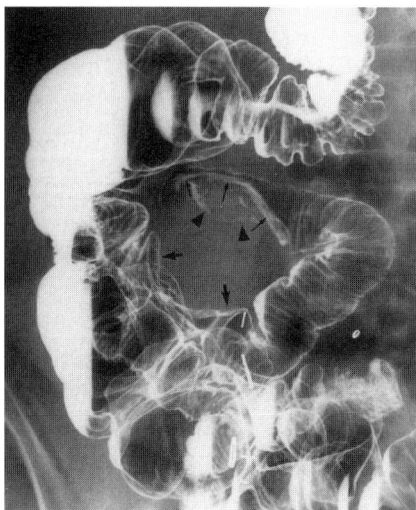 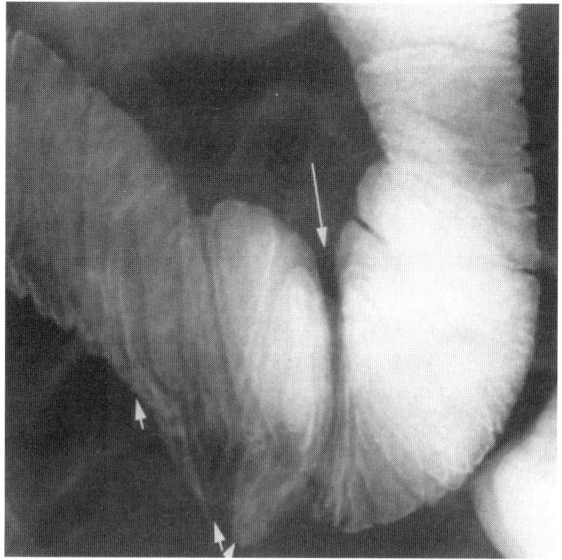

Fig. 23-31. Extrinsic mass effect from intraperitoneal metastases from ovarian carcinoma separating bowel loops.
A broad-base indentation is seen on one ileal loop (large arrows). The more proximal portion of the loop has been partially impressed by the mesenteric mass seen as both broad-based impression (thin arrows) and an area of increased radiodensity (arrowheads) where the lumen has been only partially obliterated.

Fig. 23-32. Tethering of mucosal folds due to adhesions.
Smooth folds are abnormally angulated (short arrows) relative to their usual perpendicular orientation to the longitudinal axis of the bowel lumen. An adhesive band is manifested as a thin radiolucency (long arrow) crossing and mildly narrowing the lumen of the bowel. (Reproduced with permission from Herlinger and Rubesin.[19])

Table 23-9. Tethering of mucosal folds and mass effect

Left upper quadrant
　Pancreatitis
　Metastasis to root of small bowel mesentery

Right lower quadrant/midabdomen
　Intraperitoneal metastases
　Carcinoid tumor
　Endometriosis
　Retractile mesenteritis
　Interloop abscess

Cecal/appendiceal process involving terminal ileum
　Cecal lymphoma/carcinoma
　Appendicitis
　Crohn's
　Appendiceal tumors

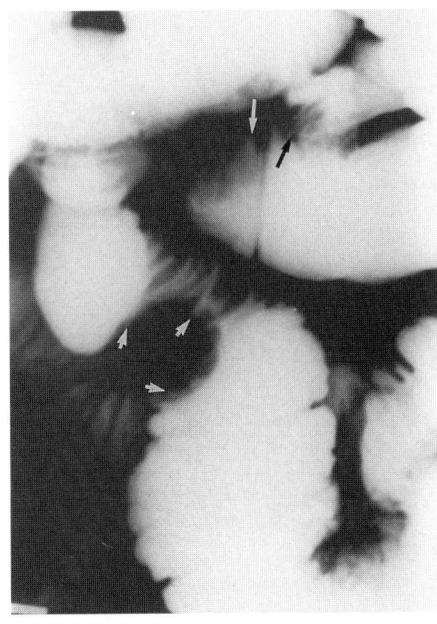

Fig. 23-34. Intraperitoneal metastasis due to ovarian carcinoma.
Spot radiograph of ileal loops shows tethering of smooth mucosal folds in several locations (long arrows). Extrinsic mass effect and tethered folds (small arrows) is seen focally.

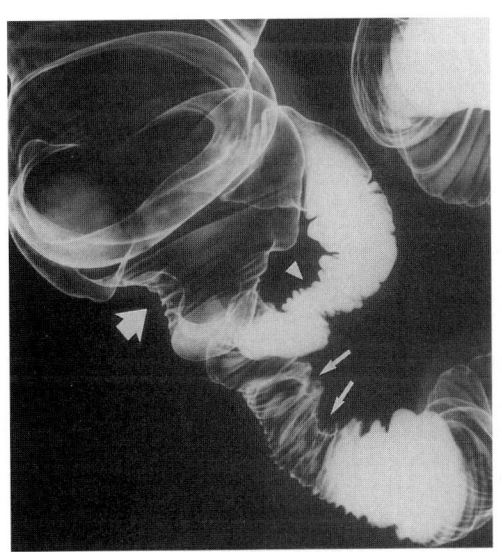 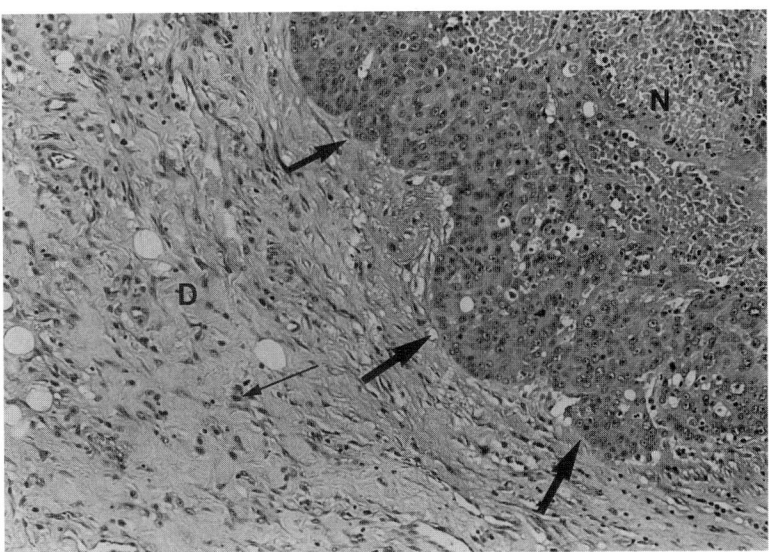

(a)　　　　　　　　　　　　(b)

Fig. 23-33. Right lower quadrant metastases.
(a) Specimen radiograph shows extrinsic mass effect and tethering of mucosal folds on the mesenteric border of terminal ileum (small arrows) and the lateral border of the cecum (large arrow). The mucosal surface is smooth and normal. In other areas, folds are tethered, but no extrinsic mass is seen (arrowhead). (b) The adenocarcinoma (thick arrows) is metastatic to the serosal surface of the bowel. The tumor incites a desmoplastic reaction (D) characterized by fibroblast proliferation (thin arrow) and collagen deposition. This reaction may ultimately lead to bowel tethering. This tumor also shows central necrosis (N). (Hematoxylin and eosin, original magnification ×400.)

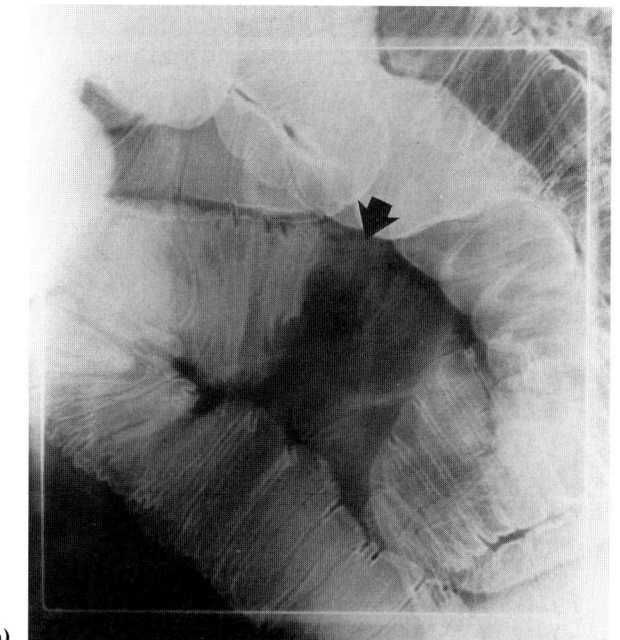
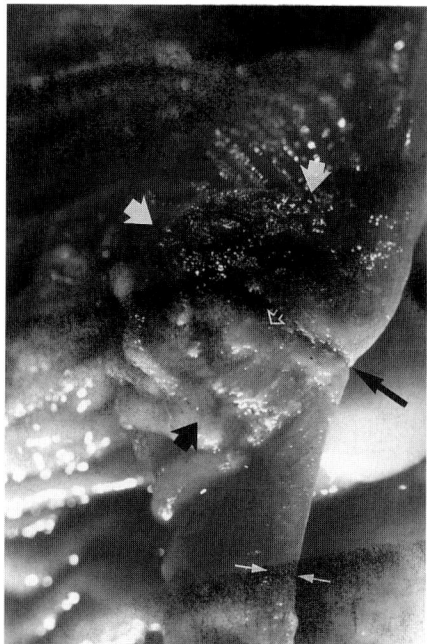

Fig. 23-35. Carcinoid with angulation and mass effect.
(a) Spot radiograph of right lower quadrant ileal loops shows indentation of the luminal contour and folds tethered toward the mesenteric border (arrow). (b) Photograph of surgical specimen shows that the apparent round "submucosal" mass (thick arrows) is formed by folding of thickened small bowel wall on itself. The folded wall comes together at the long arrow. The thickness of bowel wall containing the infiltrating tumor (thick black arrow to open arrow) is contrasted with intestinal wall of normal thickness (between small white arrows).

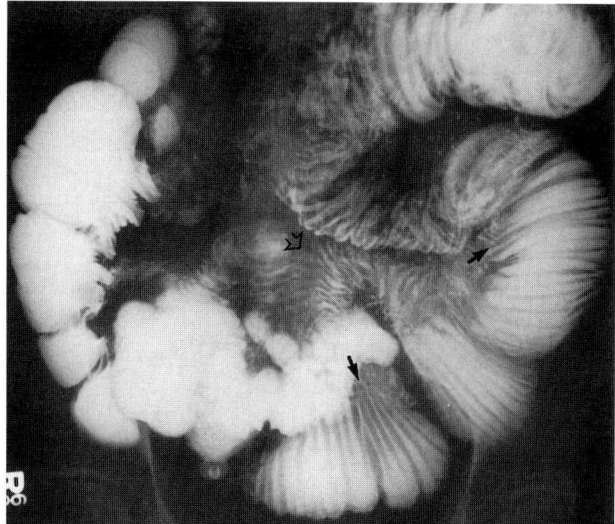

Fig. 23-36. Carcinoid with angulation.
Many loops of small intestine have normal folds radiating toward the root of the small bowel mesentery (arrows). The loops are angulated (open arrow). The tethering reflects a desmoplastic process in the small bowel mesentery. (Reproduced with permission from Herlinger and Rubesin.[19])

Fig. 23-37 (right). Carcinoma of cecum invades terminal ileum.
(a) Spot radiograph during small bowel follow-through shows smooth, enlarged folds in terminal ileum (white arrows), masslike scalloping of the mesenteric border (open arrows) and a questionable mass in the medial border of the base of the cecum (black arrow). (b) Spot, radiograph during peroral pneumocolon performed after radiograph in (a) confirms the mass in the cecum (large arrow) and thickened ileal folds (small arrow). (c) CT through right lower quadrant shows lobulated, thick-walled cecum (arrowheads) in continuity with thick-walled terminal ileum (arrows). (d) Radiograph of barium-coated specimen shows a cecal cancer manifested as a mass with a reticular surface pattern (open black arrows) involving the base of the cecum, extending through the ileocecal valve (tumor—identified by arrowhead within ileocecal valve—I) into the distal-most terminal ileal mucosa (open white arrows). Multiple small submucosal masses in profile (small black arrows) and smooth enlargement of ileal folds en face represent submucosal spread of cancer. True mucosal invasion of the ileum is seen where a reticular pattern and lobulated tumor destroys the ileal mucosa (open white arrows). (e,f) Low- and medium-power pictures of the terminal ileum show that the cecal carcinoma invades by direct and lymphatic extension. The lymphatics of the ileum, including the villi lacteals (arrows), are permeated with cancer. [Hematoxylin and eosin, original magnification in (e) ×100, in (f) ×200.]

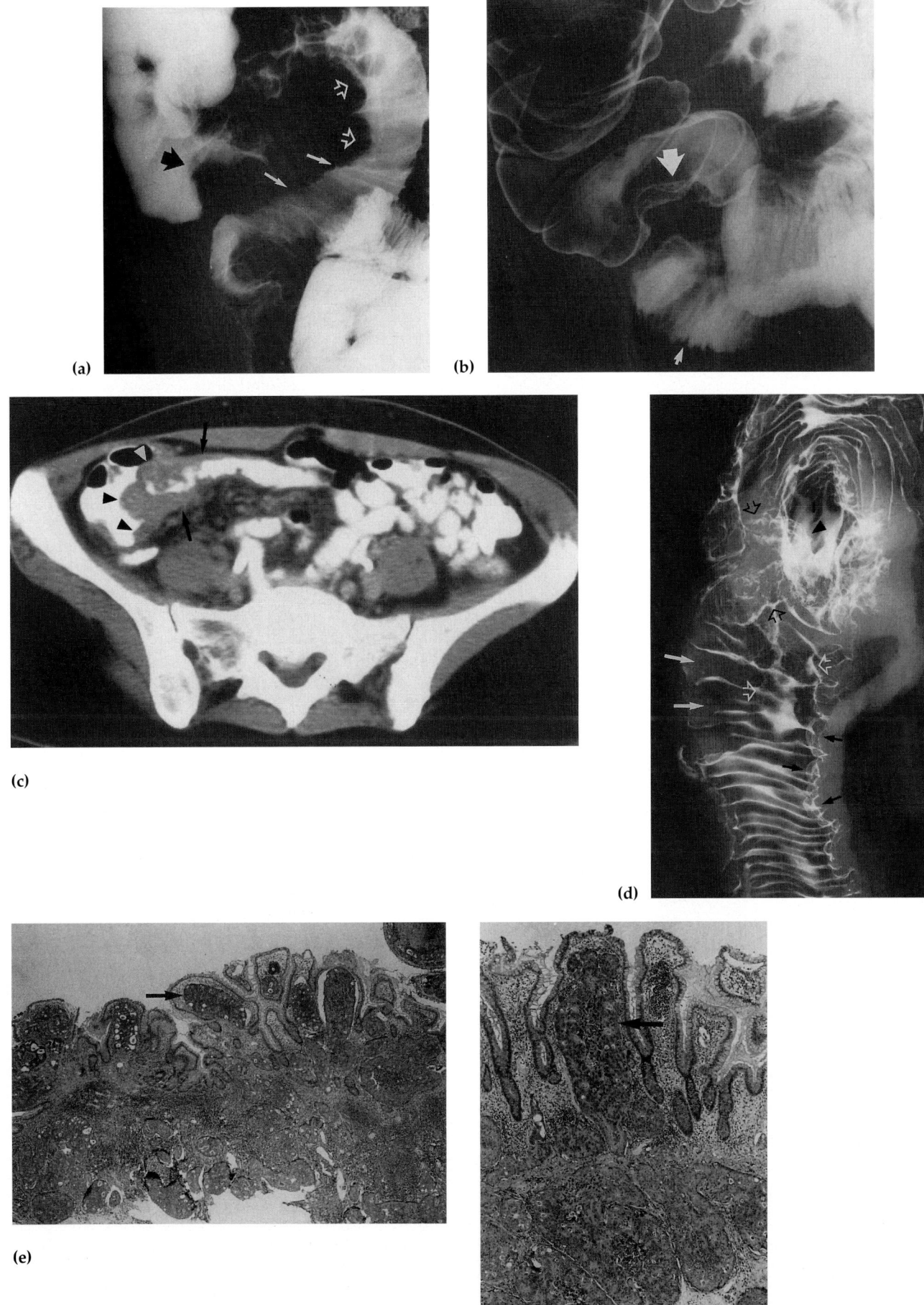

Table 23-10. Normal lumen diameters

	Small bowel meal	Enteroclysis
Proximal jejunum	3.0 cm	4.0 cm
Mid small bowel	2.5 cm	3.5 cm
Distal ileum	2.0 cm	3.0 cm

ileal folds may appear smoothly enlarged due to obstructive edema. Smooth enlargement of folds can also be caused by direct tumor invasion.

Table 23-11. Dilated lumen, normal fold thickness

Normal number of folds per inch
  Mechanical obstruction
    Common
      Adhesions
      Hernia
      Metastases
      Radiation
      Colonic obstruction
    Uncommon
      Diverticulitis
      Crohn's
      Gallstone "ileus"
      Meckel's with volvulus or intussusception
      Tumor with intussusception
  Adynamic ileus
    Common
      Postoperative
      Prior vagotomy mostly duodenum/jejunum
      Drug-induced atony (eg, opiates, anticholinergics)
      Diabetes
      Low blood flow states (congestive heart failure, myocardial infarction, sepsis)
    Uncommon
      Peritonitis
      Electrolyte imbalance (uremia, hypokalemia)
      Blunt trauma
      Tumor in mesentery
      Hypothyroidism
      Amyloidosis
      Scleroderma
      Celiac disease
      Congenital myopathy/neuropathy
Decreased number of folds in duodenum/jejunum
  Celiac disease
Increased number of folds per inch duodenum/jejunum
  Scleroderma
  Dermatomyositis

Dilated Lumen, Normal Fold Thickness

Small bowel dilatation is primarily related to either mechanical obstruction or abnormal motility, and less so due to accumulation caused by either hypersecretion or abnormal resorption. The word "ileus" is from the Greek meaning "to roll up tight," implying abdominal colic, but in modern terms means "dilatation." "Ileus" alone does not imply a motor disorder; the term ileus must be qualified by another word. We favor the term "small bowel obstruction" to "mechanical ileus" and "paralytic ileus" or "adynamic ileus" over the term "functional ileus." When small bowel dilatation by air or fluid is seen on a plain film or after contrast administration, the radiologist must be able to distinguish mechanical obstruction from a hypomotility state (Tables 23-10, 23-11). The most common causes of mechanical small bowel obstruction are adhesions, hernias, metastases, radiation change, or colonic obstruction with retrograde backup into the small bowel.[19] Sometimes the cause of the mechanical small bowel obstruction may be outside the small intestine, either a colon carcinoma or sigmoid diverticulitis with direct extension into adjacent small bowel.

When either a CT or barium study is being performed and small bowel is dilated, the radiologist

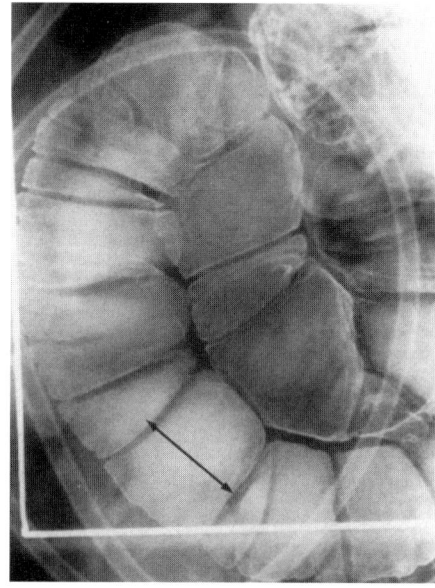

Fig. 23-38. Separation of folds in celiac disease reflects loss of mucosal surface area.
Spot radiograph of a proximal jejunal loop shows 1 to 2 folds per inch. (An inch is labeled by the double arrow.) (Reproduced with permission from Rubesin et al.[2])

searches for a transition point between dilated and collapsed small bowel loops. The cause of the obstruction is usually found at this transition site. If no transition zone is discovered, and the bowel is diffusely dilated, a wide variety of causes of small bowel hypomotility are possible. An analysis of the small bowel fold pattern may help to determine the cause of the ileus. If fold size is normal and there are a normal number of folds per inch and the bowel is diffusely dilated, the more frequent causes of adynamic ileus should be considered, including a postoperative state, prior vagotomy, and drug-induced atony. If there are a diminished number of normal-sized folds per inch in the jejunum, diseases that cause loss of mucosal surface area in combination with hypomotility should be thought of, especially gluten-sensitive enteropathy (celiac disease).[29,36] In most patients with untreated celiac disease, there are fewer than four folds per inch in the proximal jejunum (Fig. 23-38).[36] The proximal small bowel folds in celiac disease are of normal thickness, unless complicated by marked hypoproteinemia, lymphoma, or ulcerative jejunoileitis. As an adaptive response to increase the small bowel surface area, there may be an increased number of folds per inch and increased fold thickness in the ileum, the so-called "jejunization of the ileum".[37]

Scleroderma frequently causes crowding of folds that remain perpendicular to the longitudinal axis of the small bowel, despite small bowel dilatation (Fig. 23-39). This finding is described as "hidebound

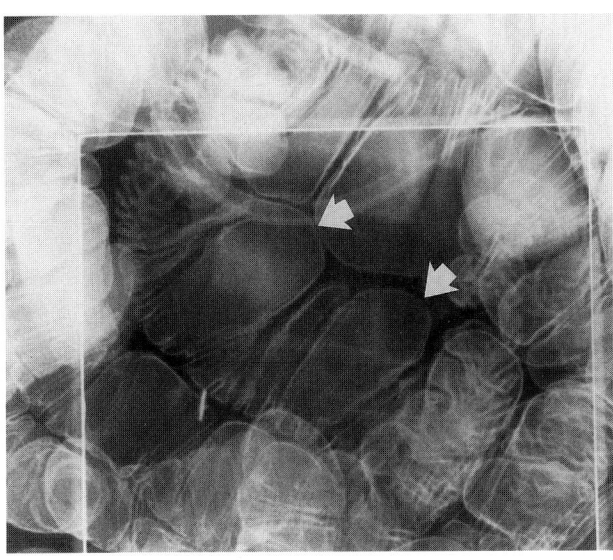

Fig. 23-40. Sacculations in scleroderma.
Broad-based outpouchings of bowel (arrows) are seen along the mesenteric border of an ileal loop. (Reproduced with permission from Rubesin and Laufer.[1])

bowel."[38] If there is asymmetric fibrosis in the wall, sacculations may appear opposite the crowded folds (Fig. 23-40). Focal crowding of normal folds may occur in any disease in which there is a desmoplastic reaction in the small bowel mesentery. The crowded folds then radiate toward the mesenteric border of the small bowel. With this radiologic finding radiologists should suspect either carcinoid tumor, mesenteric implants by intraperitoneal metastases, or peritonitis.

Thick, Smooth, Straight Folds

Small bowel edema is a common condition, but barium studies are infrequently required in patients with diseases that cause diffuse small bowel edema. Patients with elevated portal venous pressure caused by congestive heart failure or cirrhosis of the liver or those with severe hypoproteinemia (serum albumin level less than 2 g/dL) may have diffuse small bowel edema. The folds of the mesenteric small bowel will show diffuse and uniform thickening (Table 23-12).

Diseases causing intramural hemorrhage or severe focal edema often involve long segments of the small bowel, but not the entire mesenteric small bowel. In patients with intramural hemorrhage, there are smooth, thick folds perpendicularly aligned to the longitudinal axis of the small bowel. When the thick folds are tightly packed, they have been described as resembling a "stack of coins" (Fig. 23-41).[39] If the folds are so thick that the luminal space between them is

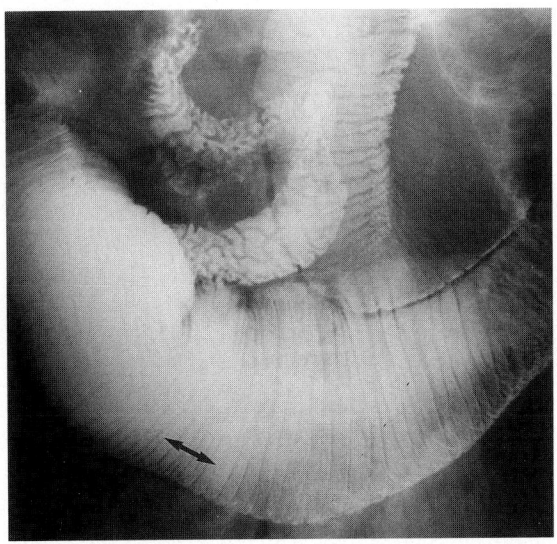

Fig. 23-39. Scleroderma. Hidebound bowel.
Despite the marked luminal dilatation, there are a top-normal number (7) of folds per inch in the mid small bowel. (An inch is labeled by the double arrow). (Reproduced with permission from Rubesin et al.[2])

Table 23-12. Thick (>3 mm), smooth, straight folds

Diffuse
  Edema
    Hypoproteinemia (serum albumin <2 g/dL)
      Cirrhosis
      Nephrotic syndrome
      Protein losing enteropathy
    Congestive heart failure
    Portal hypertension

Long segment
  Intramural hemorrhage
    Anticoagulant therapy
    Ischemia
    Mesenteric vein thrombosis
    Vasculitis
      Connective tissue diseases
      Henoch-Schönlein purpura
      Hemophilia
      Idiopathic thromocytopenic purpura
      Coagulopathies
  Radiation enteropathy
  Eosinophilic enteritis
Focal
  Mesenteric venous or lymphatic obstruction
    Metastasis, surgery, adhesions
  Early Crohn's disease

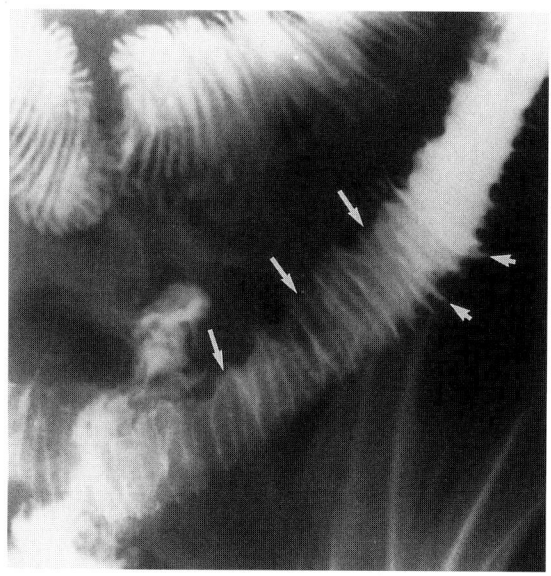

Fig. 23-41. Stack of coins appearance due to ischemia. Spot radiograph of the jejunum shows smooth, thick folds (long arrows) perpendicular to the longitudinal axis of the small bowel. Barium filling the spaces between the thick folds is described as interspace spikes (short arrows). (Reproduced with permission from Rubesin and Laufer.[1])

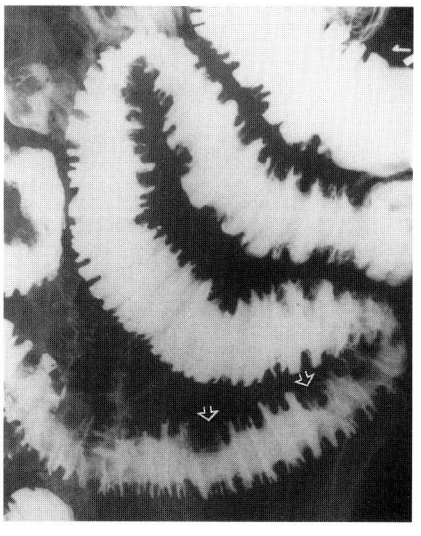 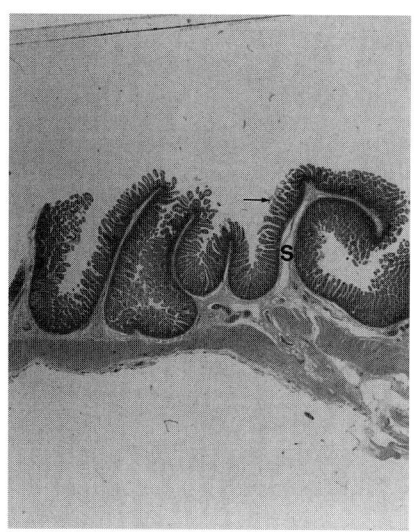 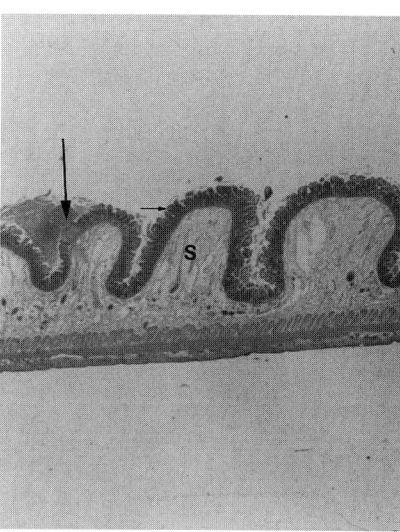

(a)   (b)   (c)

Fig. 23-42. Ischemia and hemorrhage in small bowel vasculitis.
(a) Barium study demonstrates smooth-surfaced masses of submucosal type (open arrows) on the mesenteric border of a loop of ileum (the "thumbprints"). The folds are generally thick, smooth, and perpendicular to the long axis of the bowel, the "stack of coins" appearance. (b, c) Compare the low magnification appearance of bowel with normal folds (b) and ischemic bowel (c) with its massive submucosal edema (S). The submucosal edema thickens the valvulae conniventes and causes focal fold widening sufficient to produce a mass effect, the "thumbprints". Due to the edema the overlying villi become slightly attenuated (small arrow in c) in comparison to their normal appearance (small arrow in b). Mucosal dissolution and hemorrhage (long arrow in c) are a further consequence of ischemia. ((a) Reproduced with permission from Rubesin and Laufer.[1])

compressed, barium filling these interfold spaces assumes a triangular appearance simulating spikes; hence the term "interspace spikes." The combination of thick folds and interspace spikes has been described as resembling a "picket fence."

With severe submucosal hemorrhage, the submucosal spaces of the small bowel folds are markedly widened; the folds are elevated and may become focally effaced. When the submucosa within the valvulae conniventes and between the valvulae coalesces, the focal effacement of folds produces a submucosal masslike appearance. This is located on the mesenteric border of the small bowel, has a smooth surface, and has relatively sharp edges, resulting in a "mesenteric border thumbprint" (and, if smaller, a "pinkyprint"). Mesenteric border thumbprints in patients with ischemia may also be due to severe submucosal edema without hemorrhage (Fig 23-42).

While radiation enteropathy is also characterized by thick, straight, smooth folds, typically with interspace spikes,[40] the radiographic findings are confined to the radiation portal (Fig. 23-43). The clinical history

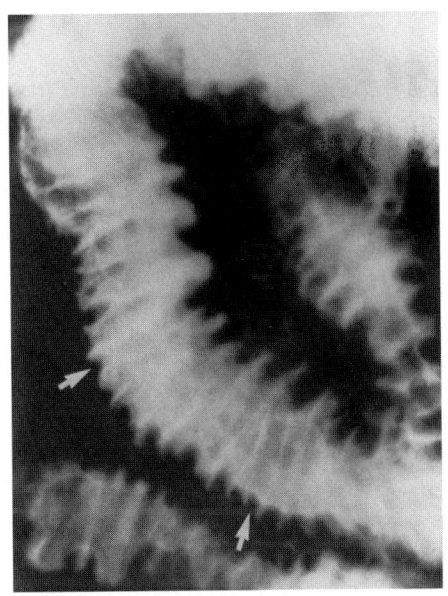

(a)

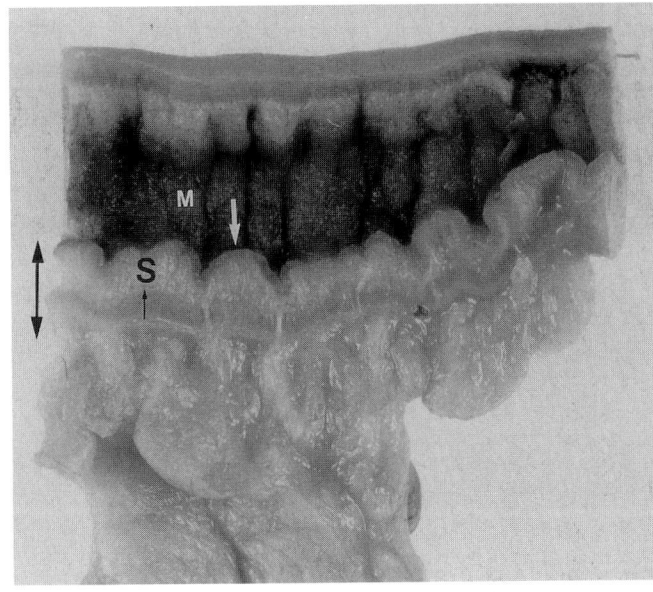

(b)

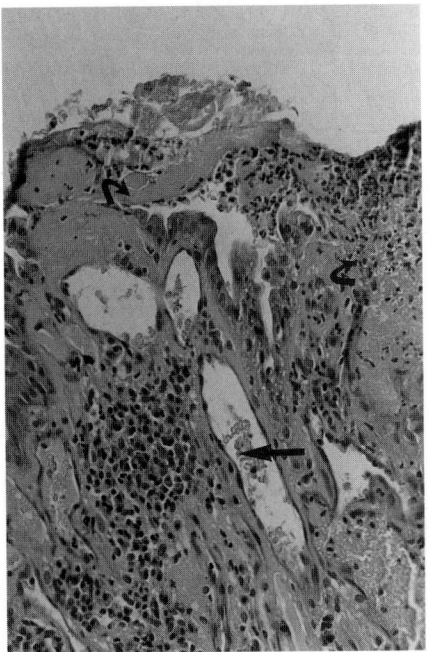

(c)

Fig. 23-43. Radiation enteropathy.
(a) The ileal folds (arrows) are thick, smooth, and perpendicular to the longitudinal axis of the small bowel. (b) Opened segment of small bowel from a different patient with radiation enteropathy shows a thickened wall (double arrow) due to a combination of hypertrophy of the muscularis propria (single arrow) and submucosal fibrosis (S). The submucosal fibrosis leads to thick, rounded folds (representative fold—white arrow). The mucosal surface (M) is hyperemic secondary to radiation-induced vascular abnormalities. (c) The mucosa shows abnormal villous architecture and prominent vascular dilatation (arrow). Capillary fragility leads to hemorrhage (curved arrows). (Hematoxylin and eosin, original magnification ×400.)

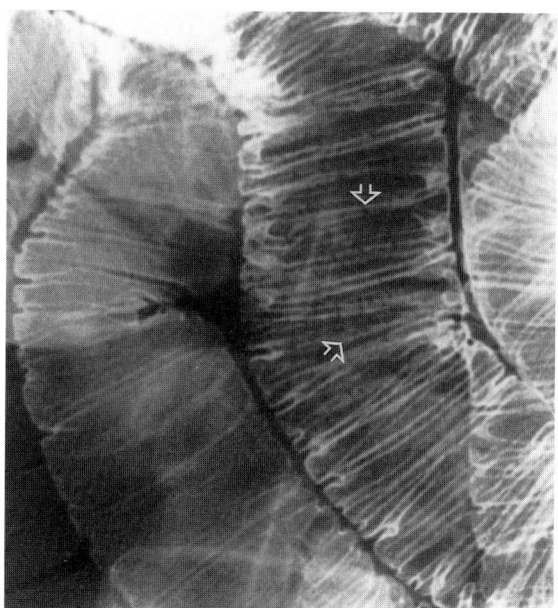

Fig. 23-44. Normal villous pattern.
Close-up of distal jejunum during late phase of enteroclysis shows tiny, round radiolucencies (arrows) representing villi. The villi are at the normal limits of resolution of radiography, but are sometimes seen. (Reproduced with permission from Rubesin and Laufer.[1])

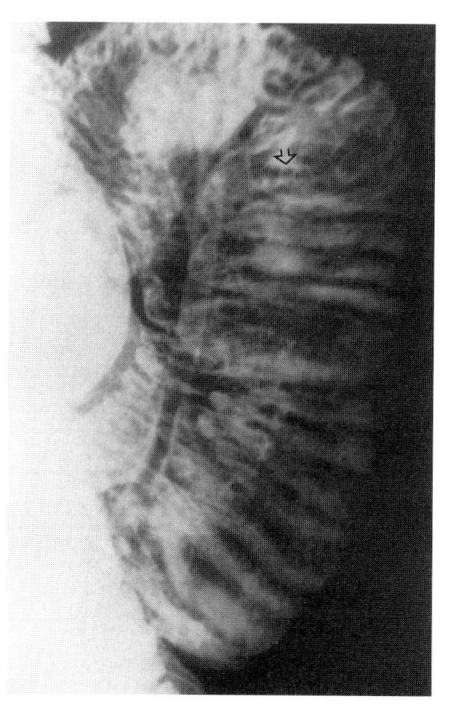

(a)

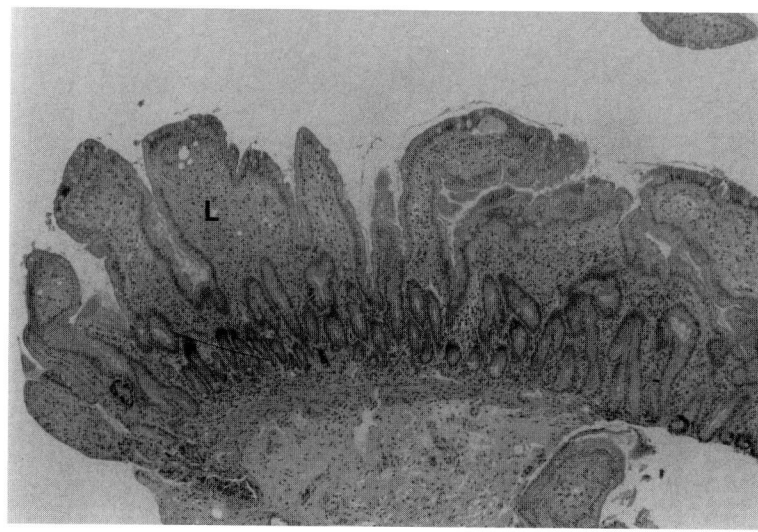

(b)

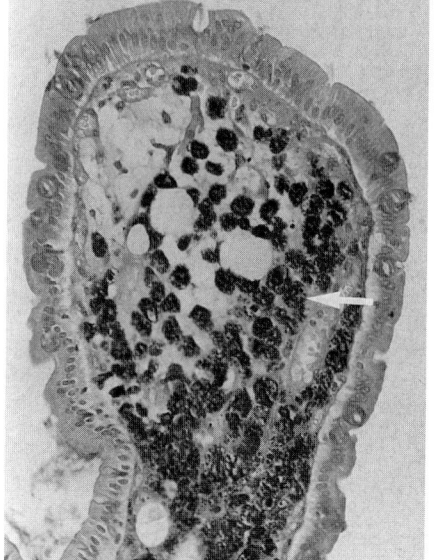

(c)

Fig. 23-45.
(a) Mucosal nodularity in Whipple's disease. Small nodules are seen in the proximal jejunum (representative area identified by arrow). The nodules represent enlarged villi. (b,c) Microscopic pictures from a different patient with Whipple's disease. (b) The lamina propria is markedly expanded (L) causing enlargement of the villi to render them radiologically visible as tiny nodularities. (c) A higher magnification demonstrates the lamina propria of a villus distended with PAS-positive material derived from the capsules of Whipple's bacilli. (Original magnification ×400).

of abdominal radiation will aid the diagnosis of radiation enteropathy. The most common scenarios that result in radiation enteropathy are radiation for 1) tumors of the adult retroperitoneum such as lymphoma or germ cell tumors; 2) retroperitoneal tumors in children such as Wilm's tumor or neuroblastoma, and 3) gynecological, urinary bladder, or prostate tumors, especially carcinoma of the cervix.

Thick, Undulating, or Nodular Folds and Mucosal Nodularity

A diagnosis in a study demonstrating thick, nodular folds or mucosal nodularity can be based on a rational analysis of the pathologic processes underlying the radiologic image. Normal small bowel mucosa is usually smooth, but a villous pattern may become visible late during a small bowel enema or in the duodenum during a double-contrast upper gastrointestinal series (Fig. 23-44). Any disease that enlarges villi may cause fine mucosal nodularity. Villous enlargement usually occurs in diseases that expand the lamina propria: infectious disorders such as Whipple's disease (Fig. 23-45), inflammatory conditions such as Crohn's disease (Fig. 23-46),[41] or radiation enteropathy.[42] Diseases that do not uniformly expand the submucosa will cause thickened, nodular valvulae conniventes. Mucosal nodularity and nodular small bowel fold thickening are often seen simultaneously because pathologic processes can spread from lamina propria to submucosa through penetrating vessels and the thin muscularis mucosae.

It is helpful to separate disease states where small bowel folds are thick, smooth, and straight from disease states where folds are thick, nodular, and undulating. As previously discussed, perfectly smooth, enlarged folds that are aligned perpendicular to the longitudinal axis of the small bowel usually result from edema or hemorrhage in the submucosa. In contrast, enlarged, nodular folds imply focal, patchy infiltration by an inflammatory, infectious, or neoplastic process.

The clinical history and the distribution of enlarged folds are tremendous aids in constructing a graded differential diagnosis. In many patients, however, the radiologic diagnosis is uncertain and biopsy may be required to provide a final diagnosis. Biopsies, however, do not always succeed in providing such a diagnosis, as many diseases are confined to the submucosa, have a patchy distribution, or may not be reached by the endoscope. Furthermore, some diseases may have similar or nonspecific histologic findings. Therefore, final diagnosis often relies on a combination of

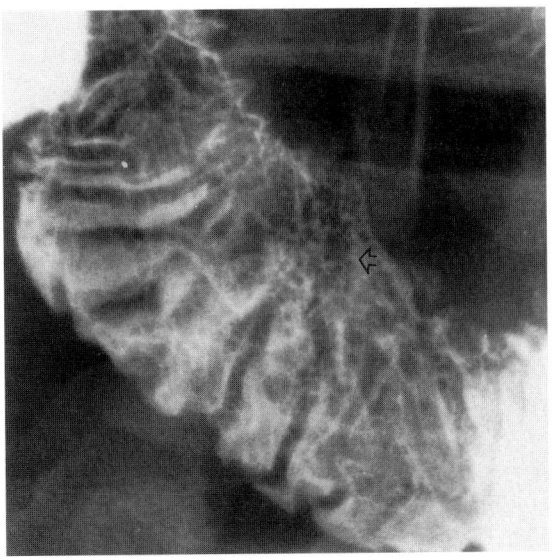

Fig. 23-46. Granular mucosa in Crohn's disease.
Small round radiolucenies (representative nodules identified by arrow) represent enlarged villi. (Reproduced with permission from Rubesin and Bronner.[21])

clinical history and radiologic, endoscopic, and histologic findings.

Exhaustive differential diagnosis can be greatly shortened by considering the location and extent of the nodular/thickened folds in conjunction with the clinical history. Diseases with predilection for the jejunum or proximal ileum are usually of different etiology than those that involve the terminal ileum. Diseases that infiltrate or inflame the proximal small bowel are listed in Tables 23-13(a) and 23-13(b).[41-52] Thick folds in a young or mature adult with known celiac disease suggest that a complication such as T-cell lymphoma or ulcerative jejunoileitis has occurred (Fig. 23-47).[29] Thick folds in an immunocompromised patient suggest an infection such as giardiasis, cryptosporidiosis,[43] or by MAI.[44] Thick folds in a young patient with supporting clinical signs (lymphedema) suggest congenital lymphangiectasia.[45,46] A history of asthma and/or peripheral eosinophilia suggests eosinophilic enteritis.[47,48] Thick folds in a patient with central nervous system symptoms, retinitis pigmentosa, and a blood smear showing acanthocytosis are due to hypo- or abetalipoproteinemia. The diagnosis is often already known and the small bowel study is only confirmatory.

Thick folds in the distal small bowel suggest a different group of disorders than those that affect the jejunum (Table 23-13(c)). It is of further help to consider whether the bowel is narrowed or not and whether the symptoms are acute or chronic. When distal small bowel folds are thickened and the luminal diameter is

Table 23-13(a). Irregular fold thickening, proximal bowel

Disease	Comment
Giardiasis	Distal duodenum, proximal jejunum Hypermotility, barium study often useful
Whipple's disease	Middle-aged white male with arthralgia, cardiovascular and neurologic symptoms Clubbed villi, fine mucosal nodularity Low-density lymph nodes on CT
Abetalipoproteinemia (Hypobetalipoproteinemia)	Adolescent Retinitis pigmentosa, Spinocerebellar degeneration, acanthocytosis
Lymphoma arising in celiac disease	Fever, pain, weight loss, steatorrhea despite gluten-free diet. Jejunum, several loops with nodular folds
Ulcerative jejunoileitis	History, radiographic findings indistinguishable from lymphoma in celiac patient
Tropical sprue	Patient visits or resides in tropics
Gastrojejunostomy	Thick folds, granular mucosa in afferent or efferent loop

Table 23-13(b). Irregular fold thickening, long segment or diffusely in small bowel

Disease	Comment
Primary lymphangiectasia	Late childhood/early adulthood, mucosal nodularity (dilated lacteals), thick folds (submucosal edema)
Secondary lymphangiectasia	Retroperitoneal fibrosis, radiation change; mesenteric lymphadenopathy with lymphoma; tuberculosis, Whipple's, carcinoid. Fine nodules: distended villi. Smooth enlarged folds (edema)
Amyloidosis	All forms Deposits in lamina propria: mucosal granularity (secondary amyloidosis). Deposits in submucosa: 4- to 10-mm large nodules (AL amyloid) Deposits in vessels: erosions, 3- to 4-mm nodules, related to ischemia
Eosinophilic enteritis	Nodular thickening antral mucosa
Histoplasmosis	Rarely micronodularity
Mastocytosis	Flushing, tachycardia, headaches; urticaria pigmentosa in 50%, bone lesions in 20%. Thick folds, mucosal nodules; segmental
Graft-versus-host disease	With/without cytomegalovirus infection. Follow-through may not coat mucosa or prolonged barium adherence
Lymphoma	Disseminated lymphoma (not primary or arising in small bowel mesentery) may be patchy
Macroglobulinemia	Mainly lamina propria involved Lymphoma likely complication

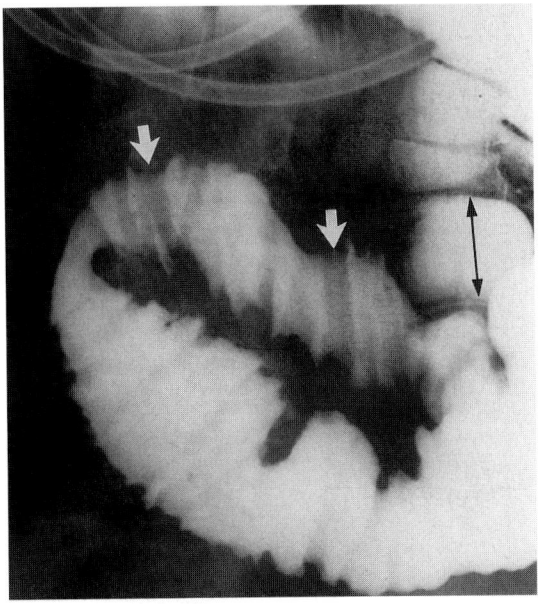
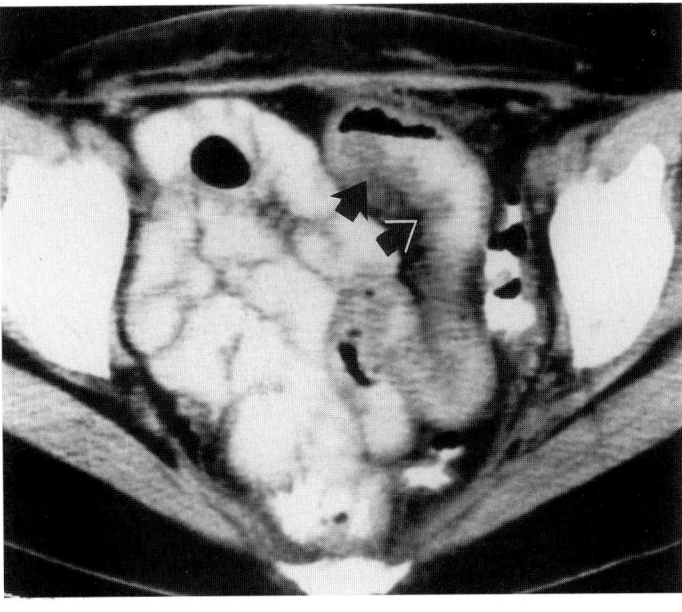
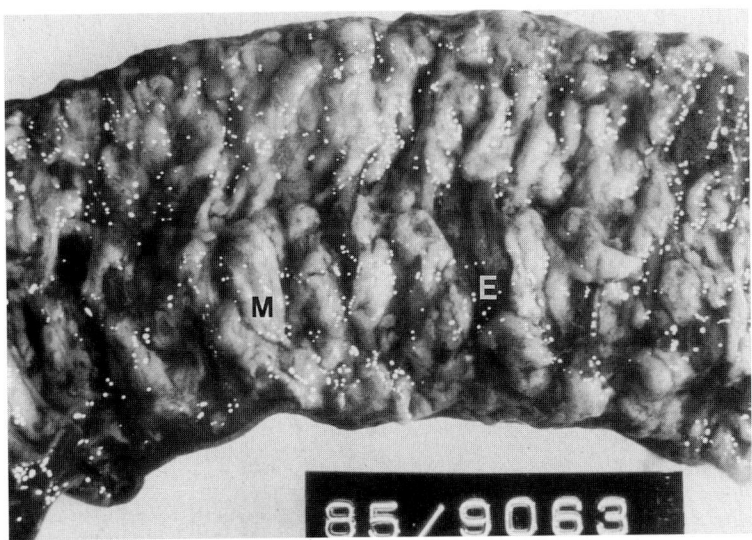
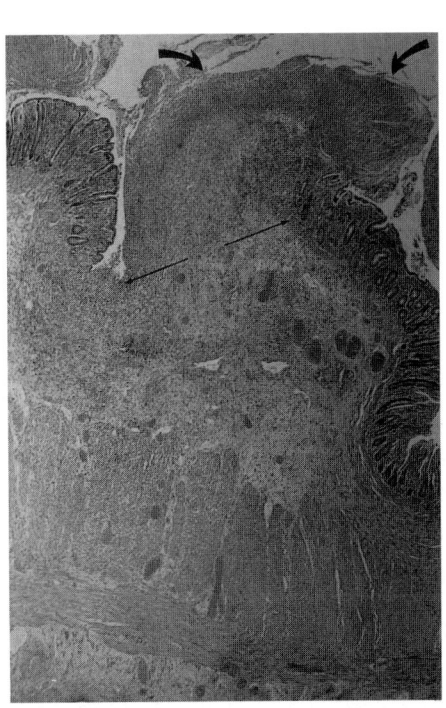

Fig. 23-47. Ulcerative jejunoileitis in patient with gluten-sensitive enteropathy.
(a) Spot radiograph performed during early, single-contrast phase of enteroclysis shows moderately thick, slightly undulating folds (arrows) in a rigid jejunal loop. These radiographic findings are indistinguishable from T-cell lymphoma complicating celiac disease. Note the separation of normal-sized folds in the more proximal jejunum (double arrow). (b) CT performed after small bowel enema shows a focal area of moderately thickened small bowel wall with nodular surface (arrows). (c) The opened surgical specimen shows thick, white pseudomembranes (M) covering the ulcerated epithelium (E). (d) Pseudomembranes (curved arrows) composed of inflammatory cells, fibrin, and sloughed epithelial cells are adherent to multiple sites of mucosal ulceration (straight arrows). Residual villi in this section are only mildly flattened. Villous atrophy was demonstrated in the more proximal jejunum.. (a-c reproduced with permission from Rubesin et al.[29])

Table 23-13(c). Irregular fold thickening, distal bowel

With minimal, if any, luminal narrowing, no obstruction

Disease	Comment
Yersinia enterocolitis	Early: ulcers, nodules, thick folds 5 to 8 weeks: lymphoid hyperplasia after 8 to 12 weeks: normal
Salmonella, campylobacteriosis	
Crohn's disease	Very early Crohn's, only presenting episode, fold thickening with coarse villous pattern is rarely the only radiographic manifestation
Lymphoma	Unusual to see mucosal/submucosal nodules without mass (mantle cell type)
Cecal cancer/lymphoma	Cecal mass with direct or lymphatic extension into terminal ileum

Associated with moderate to marked luminal narrowing

Disease	Comment
Crohn's disease	Mesenteric border ulcers with sacculation antimesenteric border, pathognomonic; ulceronodular pattern; narrowing; fissures; fistulae; mass
Tuberculosis	Patient from endemic area (eg, Far East, India) or immunocompromised; right colon involved to greater degree than ileum; short, retracted cecum
Behçet's disease	Uveitis, genital ulcers, arthritis; colon involved to greater degree with deep ulcers, local colonic perforation

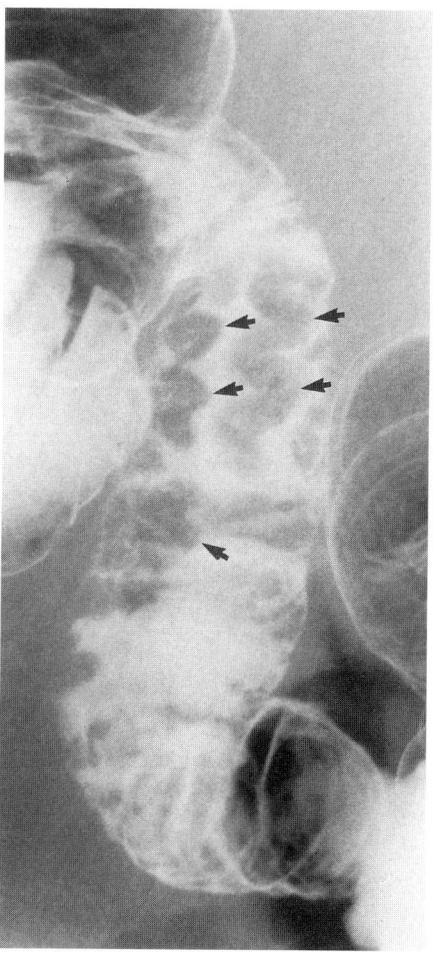

Fig. 23-48. Yersinia ileitis.
Enlarged, undulating folds (arrows) are seen in the terminal ileum. The lumenal diameter is not narrowed. (Reproduced with permission from Rubesin and Laufer.[1])

not narrowed, and the history is that of acute or recent diarrhea, infections such as yersiniosis or campylobacteriosis are the most likely diagnosis (Fig. 23-48). Small ulcers (aphthoid ulcers) may be seen in any inflammatory disease that affects the lymphoid tissue, causing ulceration of the epithelium overlying lymph follicles. Usually, however, by the time a barium study is performed in most patients with yersiniosis or other infections, ulcers have healed and only thick folds or lymphoid hyperplasia remain.[53] Aphthoid ulcers are rarely an isolated finding in Crohn's disease of the small bowel (Fig 23-49).[54] However, when isolated aphthoid ulcers are seen in the terminal ileum, Crohn's disease is still the leading diagnosis.

Established Crohn's disease usually has transmural inflammation resulting in luminal narrowing.[55] A diagnosis of nonstenotic Crohn's disease requires the demonstration of pathognomonic mesenteric border ulcers (Figs. 23-50, 23-51)[56] or of an ulceronodular pattern (Fig. 23-52). An unequivocal diagnosis of nonstenotic Crohn's disease cannot be made when only thick, ileal folds are seen but would be strengthened if they are associated with aphthous ulcers and a coarse mucosal pattern. Lymphoma has a predilection for the distal small bowel and cecum in adolescents and

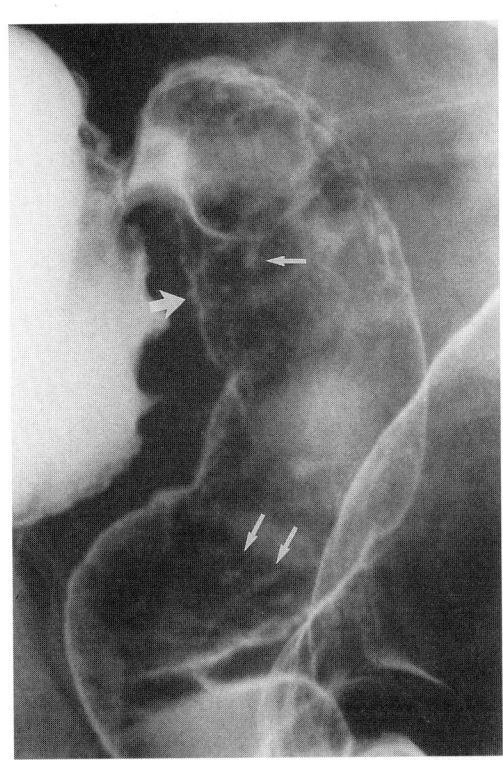

Fig. 23-49. Aphthoid ulcers in Crohn's disease.
(a) Spot radiograph of terminal ileum shows many punctate collections of barium surrounded by radiolucent halos (small arrows). The shallow depth of the aphthoid ulcers is demonstrated in profile (large arrow). (b) Close-up specimen photograph of ileal mucosa shows aphthoid ulcers (arrows). (c) Low-power photomicrograph of aphthoid ulcer shows surface epithelial ulceration (large arrow) overlying a lymphoid aggregate (a). The villi are enlarged (small arrow). This results in the granular appearance of ileal mucosa. (Reproduced with permission from Rubesin and Bronner.[21])

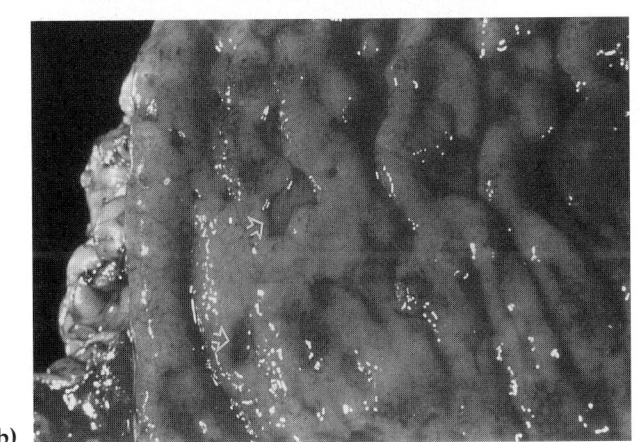

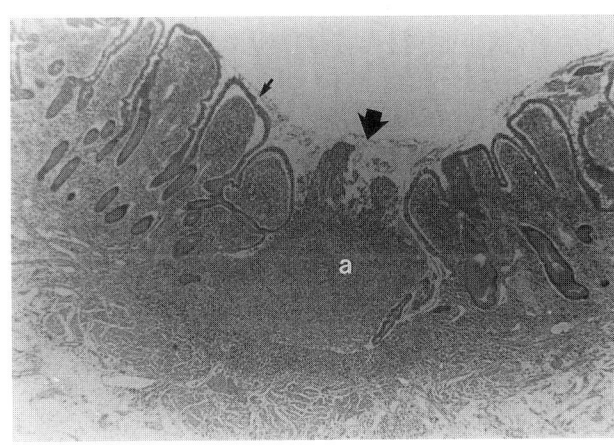

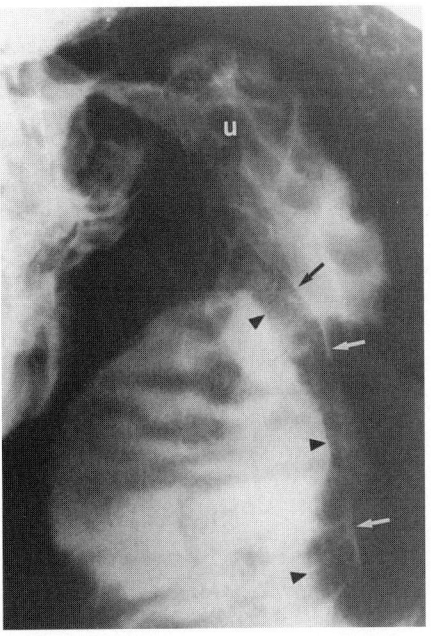

Fig. 23-50. Mesenteric border ulcer in Crohn's disease.
A long, barium-filled ulcer (arrows) lies on the mesenteric border of the small bowel. A radiolucent mound (arrowheads) parallels the ulcer, similar to an ulcer-collar in a benign gastric ulcer. An ulceronodular pattern (u) is seen just proximal to the ileocecal valve. (Reproduced with permission from Rubesin and Bronner.[21])

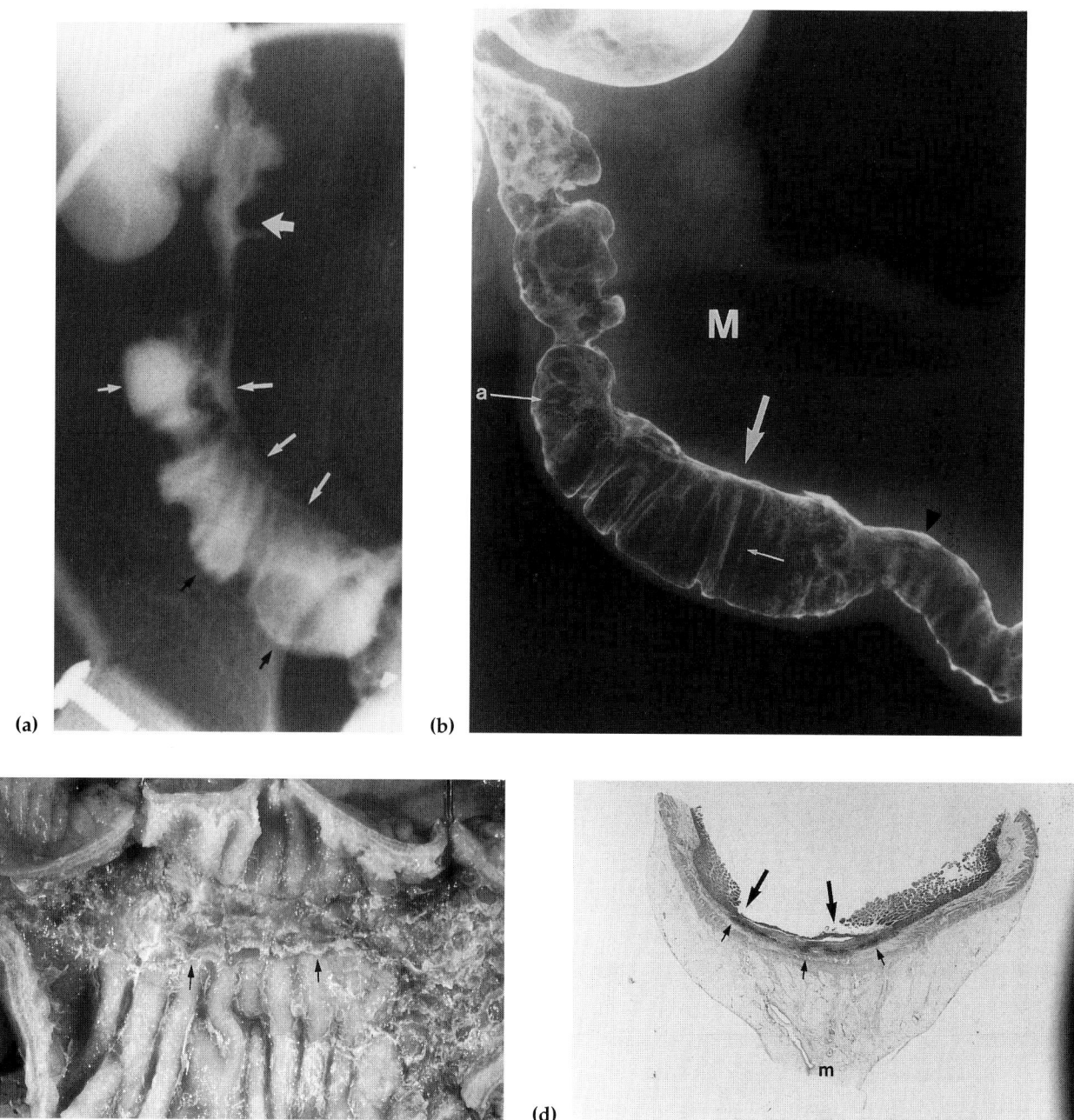

Fig. 23-51. Mesenteric border ulcer in Crohn's disease.
(a) Spot radiograph from small bowel follow-through shows a long, 3-cm-long barium collection (long white arrows) on the mesenteric border ulcer of the terminal ileum. A radiolucency parallels the barium collection. Sacculation of the antimesenteric border is seen (short arrows). The distal terminal ileum is narrowed (large arrow). (b) Specimen radiograph of terminal ileum resected 3 weeks later shows focal flattening of the mesenteric border (large arrow), folds radiating to the flattening (small arrow), and aphthoid ulcers (representative aphthoid ulcer: arrow—a). Proximally, the luminal is circumferentially narrowed (arrowhead). The mesenteric fat (M) is identified. (c) Photograph of specimen shows a 3-cm longitudinal ulcer (arrows) on the mesenteric border. Folds radiate to its edge. Note the residual white barium coating resulting from the specimen radiograph in (b). Note that a flattened area along a mesenteric border as demonstrated in the specimen radiograph may actually represent an ulcer, as confirmed by examination of the specimen. (d) Photograph of the specimen cut perpendicular to the longitudinal axis of the bowel. The epithelium on is focally lost (between two large arrows). There is more inflammatory reaction and fibrosis underneath the ulcer (small arrows) than elsewhere along the circumference of the bowel. The resected edge of the small bowel mesentery is identified (m). (Hematoxylin and eosin, original magnification ×1.) (Reproduced with permission from Herlinger et al.[56])

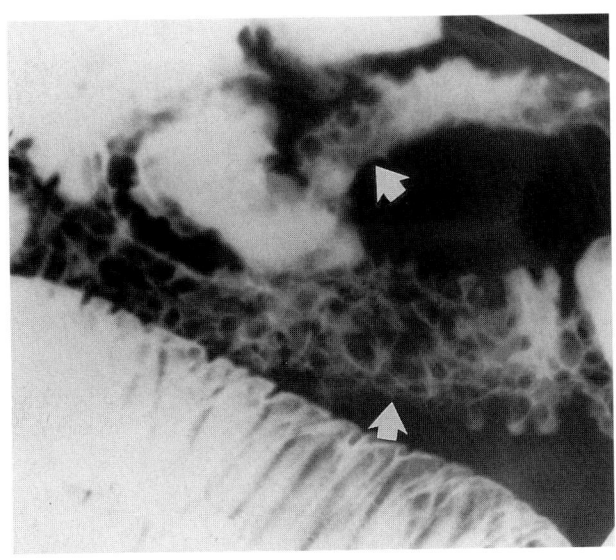

Fig. 23-52. Ulceronodular changes (cobblestoning) in Crohn's disease.
(a) Two loops of small intestine (arrows) demonstrate many round ovoid radiolucent islands of mucosa surrounded by barium-filled clefts. Note the diffuse luminal narrowing in involved loops. (b) Knifelike fissure in Crohn's disease. Deep cleft or knifelike fissures are characteristically seen in Crohn's disease. In a different patient than in (a), a low-power photomicrograph shows a fissure (long arrow) extending from the eroded, inflamed mucosal surface into the submucosa (s). The inflammatory process is transmural, extending from the surface, through the muscularis propria (m) into the subserosal tissue (short arrow). (c) Wall thickening and fissures in Crohn's disease. CT through pelvis shows two loops of small intestine with thick walls (arrowheads). A knifelike cleft filled with contrast is seen (arrow). (Reproduced with permission from Rubesin and Bronner.[21])

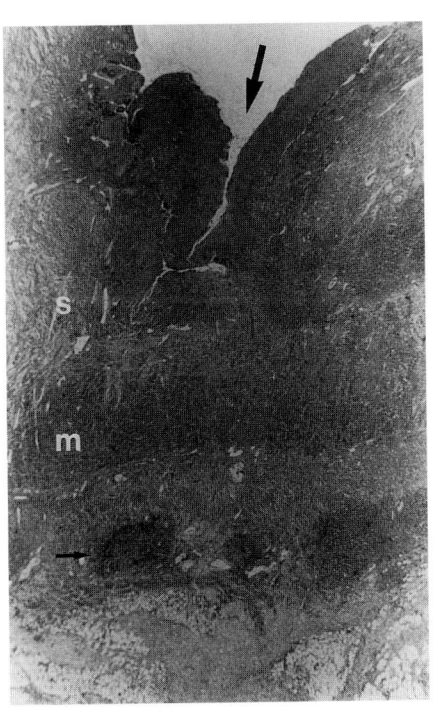

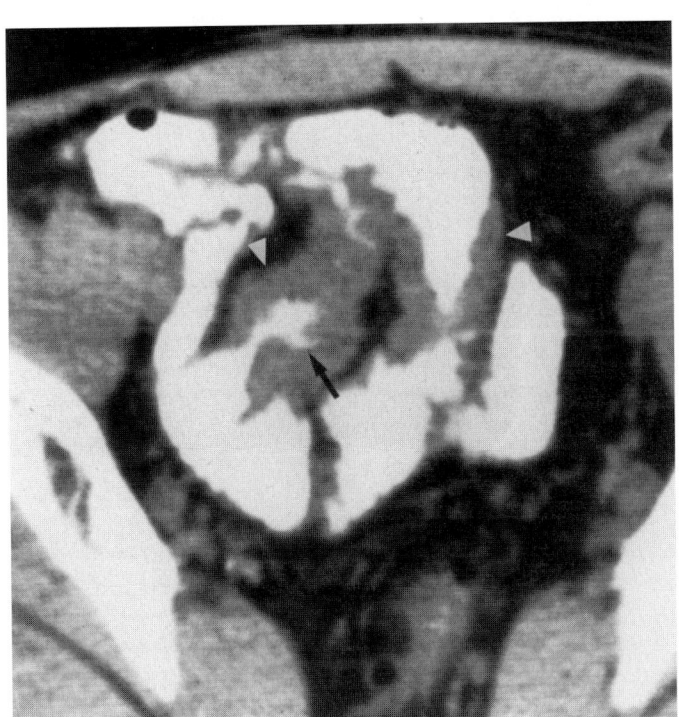

young adults, the same distribution as Crohn's disease. If thick folds or confluent mucosal nodularity is seen in the distal ileum, without ulceration or fissuring typical for Crohn's disease, a diagnosis of lymphoma must be considered, unless the disease has been of long duration. Biopsy may be necessary.

Tuberculosis characteristically has cecal and ascending colon predominance and relative sparing of the terminal ileum by ulceration or scarring (Fig. 23-53).[57] In tuberculosis, the ileocecal valve is patulous, whereas in Crohn's disease, the ileocecal valve is enlarged and nodular. Both tuberculosis and Crohn's disease are characterized by skip lesions.

Eosinophilic enteritis is also characterized by skip lesions and predilection for the distal ileum.[47,48] Eosinophilic enteritis and Crohn's disease may also have gastric involvement [Table 23-13(d)]. Key to diagnosis is the clinical history and peripheral eosinophilia.

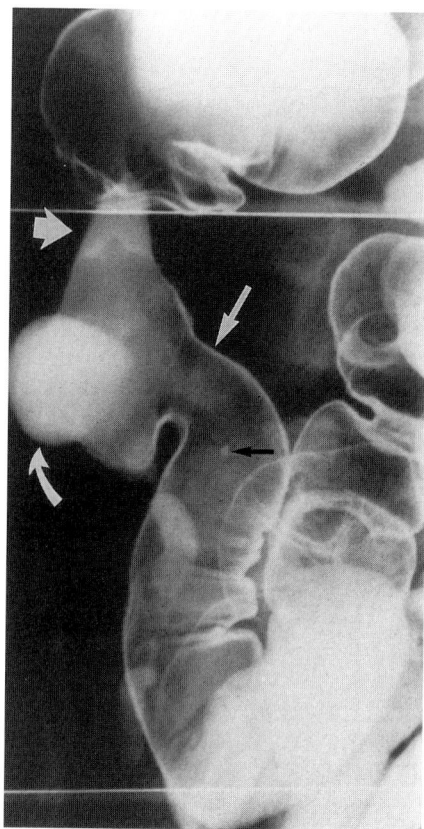

Fig. 23-53. **Tuberculosis of cecum and terminal ileum.** Spot radiograph from barium enema shows marked shortening and narrow of the ascending colon (thick white arrow) and cecum (curved arrow), a patulous ileocecal valve (long white arrow). There is a solitary small ulcer in the terminal ileum (black arrow); otherwise the ileum is spared. The terminal ileum is not narrowed.

The key to a diagnosis of a small bowel or other infection in a patient with AIDS is the culture results, not the barium study. Most small bowel infections in AIDS are radiographically indistinguishable from one another. Cytomegalovirus in the small bowel has an ileal predominance. MAI or *M tuberculosis* may be associated with low-attenuation mesenteric lymph nodes on CT scans (Table 23-13e).

Tubular Bowel

Loss of valvulae conniventes is associated with a severe loss of mucosal surface area and presents a tubular appearance (Table 23-14). The chronic inflammatory process in celiac disease (Fig. 23-54)[29] or strongyloidiasis (the lead pipe small bowel)[58] or the chronic ischemic process in radiation change (Fig. 23-55) may result in segments of tubular small bowel. Apparent "loss" of valvulae conniventes occurs focally when small bowel folds are completely effaced by a submucosal infiltrative process such as lymphoma. The "tubular" or "toothpaste" small bowel in graft versus host disease or CMV infection[59] results from barium rapidly traversing the small intestine, without coating the folds and does not imply actual loss of folds (Fig. 23-56). When, in other areas of the small bowel, barium does coat the mucosa in graft versus host disease, the mucosa has a nodular pattern (Fig. 23-56).

Site Predilection of Diseases

The location of a disorder may aid in differential diagnosis. Antimesenteric border lesions are found in:

1. Meckel's diverticulum.
2. Hematogenous metastases.
3. Sacculation and pleating in Crohn's disease.
4. Aneurysmal dilatation in lymphoma.

Mesenteric border lesions are found in:

1. Crohn's linear ulceration, contracted mesentery, sinus tracts.
2. Peritoneally seeded metastases.
3. Acquired diverticula.
4. "Thumbprints" due to intramural bleeding.
5. Hematoma.
6. Intestinal duplication.
7. Cavitation in primary intestinal lymphoma.

Diseases with predilection for proximal jejunum include:

1. Adenocarcinoma.
2. Infections: giardiasis, Whipple's, cryptosporidiosis, isosporiasis.
3. Celiac disease.
4. Changes of Zollinger-Ellison syndrome.
5. Jejunal diverticulosis.
6. Polyps in Peutz-Jeghers syndrome.

Diseases with predilection for distal ileum include:

1. Crohn's disease.
2. Ileitus due to *Yersinia, Campylobacter,* Behçet's disease.
3. Radiation damage.
4. Peritoneally seeded metastases.
5. Carcinoid tumors.
6. Inflammatory or neoplastic mass related to cecal or appendiceal disease.

Table 23-13(d). Irregular fold thickening, small bowel with associated gastroduodenal disease

Disease	Comment
Crohn's disease	Advanced or rarely of primary jejunoileal distribution
Lymphoma	
Amyloidosis	
Zollinger-Ellison syndrome	Duodenal bulb and postbulbar ulcers, increased fluid, proximal small bowel fold thickening, edema
Eosinophilic gastroenteritis	Heterogenous group; 50% allergic history or asthma, children, young adults; 50% with antral involvement; patchy changes, uni- or multifocal
Mastocytosis	Peptic ulcers; duodenal/jejunal nodules

Table 23-13(e). Irregular fold thickening in AIDS

Infection	Comment
Cryptosporidiosis	Duodenal, jejunal profuse watery intraluminal contents
Isosporiasis	Similar
Cytomegalovirus	Isolated intestinal ulcer terminal ileum and into colon; small bowel spared relative to esophagus, stomach, colon
MAI	Usually diffuse or distal small bowel macrophage infiltration lamina propria, fine nodularity, low-density lymph nodes mimic Whipple's disease
M tuberculosis	

Table 23-14. Tubular bowel

Acute ulceration/loss of mucosa
    Graft versus host disease
    Cytomegalovirus
Chronic ulceration/loss of mucosa
    Celiac disease
Chronic ischemia from radiation or amyloidosis
Burnt-out Crohn's disease
Strongyloides, last stage, reversible
Effacement (infiltration) of folds
    Lymphoma

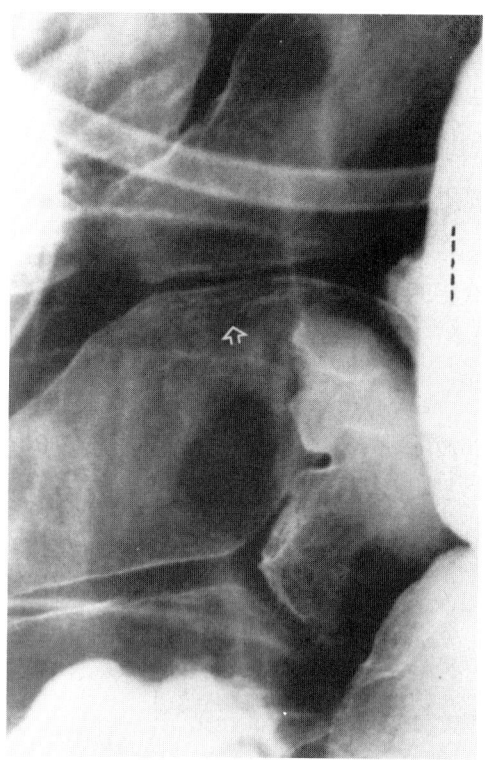

Fig. 23-54. Tubular bowel in celiac disease.
Spot radiograph of jejunum shows near complete loss of valvulae conniventes. A subtle mosaic pattern is also seen (arrow). (Reproduced with permission from Rubesin et al.[60])

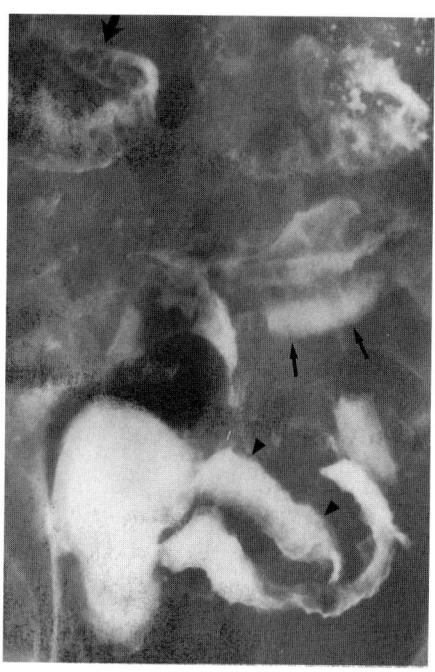

Fig. 23-56. Tubular bowel in graft-versus-host disease.
Radiograph of right lower quadrant shows poor filling of ileal loops due to extremely rapid transit of barium. This has been described as "toothpaste small bowel" (thin arrows). In areas where barium remains, the loops appear tubular (arrowheads). In areas where barium demonstrates the mucosal surface, a nodular mucosal surface pattern (thick arrow) is seen.

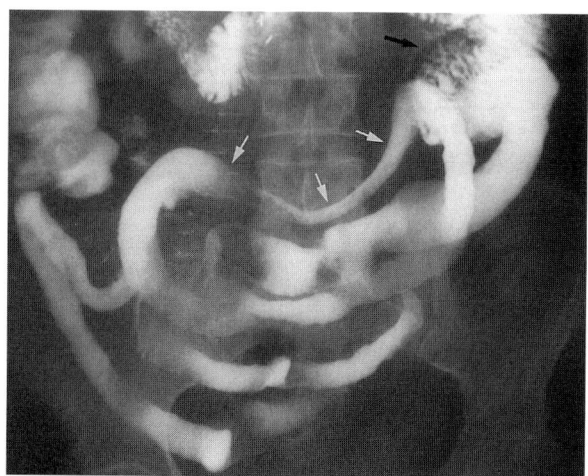

Fig. 23-55. Tubular bowel in chronic ischemia.
Overhead radiograph of lower abdomen shows diffuse narrowing of small intestinal loops and near complete lack of folds (representative loop identified with white arrows). Only the proximal jejunum (black arrow) is spared. The chronic ischemia was secondary to radiation therapy.

Location is more important in real estate, however, than in radiology. The radiographic findings in a given location are usually much more important to radiologic diagnosis than the location itself. Distribution of disease does aid in the differential diagnosis of thick folds and of annular lesions. For example, an annular lesion with shelf-like margins in the duodenum or proximal jejunum will almost certainly be a primary adenocarcinoma. A similar appearing lesion in the distal ileum may be a metastasis or a carcinoid tumor, or a primary adenocarcinoma.

References

1. Rubesin SE, Laufer I. Pictorial glossary of double contrast radiology. In: Gore RM, Levine MS, Laufer I, eds. *Textbook of Gastrointestinal Radiology*. Philadelphia, Pa: W.B. Saunders Co; 1994:50–80.
2. Rubesin SE, Rubin RA, Herlinger H. Small bowel malabsorption: clinical ad radiologic perspectives. How we see it. *Radiology*. 1992;184:297–305

3. Antonioli DA, Madara JL. Functional anatomy of the gastrointestinal tract. In: Ming S-C, Goldman H, eds. *Pathology of the Gastrointestinal Tract*. Philadelphia, Pa: W.B. Saunders Co; 1992:14–36.
4. Philips AD. The small intestinal mucosa. In: Whitehead R, ed. *Gastrointestinal and Oesophageal Pathology*, 2nd ed. Edinburgh, Scotland: Churchill Livingstone, 1995:33–43.
5. Herlinger H. Barium examinations. In: Gore RM, Levine MS, Laufer I, eds. *Textbook of Gastrointestinal Radiology*. Philadelphia, Pa: WB Saunders Co; 1994:766–788.
6. Fenoglio-Preiser CM, Pascal RR, Perzin KH. Tumors of the intestines. In: *Atlas of Tumor Pathology*. 2nd ser, fasc 27. pp. 1–516. Washington, DC: Armed Forces Institute of Pathology; 1990.
7. Johansen A, Hansen OH. Heterotopic gastric epithelium in the duodenum and its correlation to gastric disease and acid level. *Acta Pathol Microbiol Immunol Scand (A)*. 1973;81:679–680.
8. Rubesin SE, Furth EE, Herlinger H. Duodenitis, gastric metaplasia, celiac disease and the "bubbly bulb." *Abdom Imaging*. 1998;23:449–452.
9. Hoffman JW, Fox PS, Wilson SD. Duodenal wall tumors and the Zollinger-Ellison syndrome. *Arch Surg*. 1973;107:334–339.
10. Perzin KH, Bridge MF. Adenomas of the small intestine: a clinicopathologic review of 51 cases and a study of their relationship to carcinoma. *Cancer*. 1981;48:799–819.
11. Moertel CG, Saver WG, Dockerty MB, Baggenstoss AAH. Life history of the carcinoid tumor of the small intestine. *Cancer*. 1961;14:901–912.
12. Hansen PS. Hemangioma of the small intestine with special reference to intussusception. Review of the literature and report of 3 new cases. *Am J Clin Path*. 1948;18:414–442.
13. Shimer GR, Helwig EB. Inflammatory fibroid polyps of the intestine. *Am J Clin Path*. 1984;81:708–714.
14. Lee SM, Mosental WT, Weissman RE. Tumorous heterotopic gastric mucosa in the small intestine. *Arch Surg*. 1970;100:619–622.
15. Hochberg FH, Dasilva AB, Galdabini J, Richardson EP Jr. Gastrointestinal involvement in von Recklinghausen's neurofiromatosis. *Neurology*. 1974;24:1141–1151.
16. Rubesin SE, Herlinger H, DeGaeta L. Interlude: test your skills. *Radiology*. 1990;176:636, 644.
17. Rubesin SE, Gilchrist AM, Bronner M, et al. Non-Hodgkin lymphoma of the small intestine. *RadioGraphics*. 1990;10:985–998.
18. Maglinte DDT. Malignant tumors. In: Gore RM, Levine MS, Laufer I, eds. *Textbook of Gastrointestinal Radiology*. Philadelphia, Pa: WB Saunders Co; 1994:900–930.
19. Herlinger H, Rubesin SE. Obstruction. In: Gore RM, Levine MS, Laufer I, eds. *Textbook of Gastrointestinal Radiology*. Philadelphia, Pa: WB Saunders Co; 1994:931–966.
20. Franzin G, Zamboni G, Scarpa A. Polyposis syndromes. In: Whitehead R, ed. *Gastrointestinal and Oesophageal Pathology*. Edinburgh, Scotland: Churchill Livingstone; 1995:892–905.
21. Rubesin SE, Bronner M. Radiologic-pathologic concepts in Crohn's disease. *Adv Gastrointest Radiol*. 1991;1:27–55.
22. Zegel H, Laufer I. Filiform polyposis. *Radiology*. 1978;127:615–617.
23. Bridge MF, Perzin KH. Primary adenocarcinoma of the jejunum and ileum. A clinicopathologic study. *Cancer*. 1975;36:1876–1887.
24. Levine MS, Drooz AT, Herlinger H. Annular malignancies of the small bowel. *Gastrointest Radiol*. 1987;12:53–58.
25. Issacson P. B cell lymphomas of the gastrointestinal tract. *Am J Surg Pathol*. 1985;9:117–128.
26. Collier PE, Turowski P, Diamond DL. Small intestinal adenocarcinoma complicating regional enteritis. *Cancer*. 1985;55:516–521.
27. Wilson IH, Cooley NV, Luibel FJ. Nonspecific stenosing small bowel ulcers. *Am J Gastroenterol*. 1968;50:449–455.
28. Lang J, Price AB, Levi AJ, et al. Diaphragm disease: pathology of disease of the small intestine induced by non-steroidal anti-inflammatory drugs. *J Clin Pathol*. 1988;41:516–526.
29. Rubesin SE, Grumbach K, Herlinger H, et al. Adult celiac disease and its complications. *RadioGraphics*. 1989;9:1045–1066.
30. Chiotasso PJ, Fazio VW. Prognostic factors of 28 leiomyosarcomas of the small intestine. *Surg Gynecol Obstet*. 1982;155:197–202.
31. Ranchod M, Kempson RL. Smooth muscle tumors of the gastrointestinal tract and retroperitoneum. *Cancer*. 1977;39:255–262.
32. Greenstein S, Jones B, Fishman EK, et al. Small bowel diverticulitis: CT findings. *AJR*. 1986;147:271–274.
33. Rubesin SE, Furth EE, Birnbaum BA, et al. Ectopic pancreas complicated by pancreatitis and pseudocyst formation mimicking jejunal diverticulitis. *Br J Radiol*. 1997;70:311–313.
34. Meyers MM. Clinical involvement of mesenteric and antimesenteric borders of small bowel loops. *Gastrointest Radiol*. 1976;1:41–47.
35. Meyers MM. Clinical involvement of mesenteric and antimesenteric borders of small bowel loops. II. Radiologic interpretation of pathologic alterations. *Gastrointest Radiol*. 1976;1:49–58.
36. Herlinger H, Maglinte DDT. Jejunal fold separation in adult celiac disease: relevance of enteroclysis. *Radiology*. 1986;158: 605–611.
37. Bova JG, Friedman AC, Weser E, et al. Adaptation of the ileum in nontropical sprue: reversal of the jejunal fold pattern. *AJR*. 1985;144:299–302.
38. Horowitz AL, Meyers MA. The "hide-bound" small bowel of scleroderma: characteristic mucosal fold pattern. *AJR*. 1973;119:332–334.
39. Khilnani MT, Marshak RH, Eliasoph J, et al. Intramural intestinal hemorrhage. *AJR*. 1964;92:1061–1071.
40. Mendelson RM, Nolan DJ. The radiological features of radiation enteritis. *Clin Radiol*. 1985;36:141–148.
41. Glick SN, Teplick SK. Crohn's disease of the small intestine: diffuse mucosal granularity. *Radiology*. 1985;154:313–317.
42. Jones B, Hamilton SR, Rubesin SE, et al. Granular small bowel mucosa: a reflection of villous abnormality. *Gastrointest Radiol*. 1987;12:319–225.

43. Berk RN, Wall SD, McArdle CT, et al. Cryptosporidiosis of the stomach and small intestine in patients with AIDS. *AJR.* 1984;143:549–554.
44. Vincent ME, Robbins AH. Mycobacterium avium-intracellulare complex enteritis: pseudo-Whipple's disease in AIDS. *AJR.* 1985;144:921–922.
45. Olmsted WW, Madewell JE. Lymphangiectasia of the small intestine. *Gastrointest Radiol.* 1976;1:241–243.
46. Kingham JGC, Moriarty KJ, Furness M, Levison DA. Lymphangiectasia of the colon and small intestine. *Br J Radiol.* 1982;55:774–777.
47. MacCarty RL, Talley NJ. Barium studies in diffuse eosinophilic gastroenteritis. *Gastrointest Radiol.* 1990;15:183–187.
48. Schulman A, Morton PCG, Dietrich BE. Eosinophilic gastroenteritis. *Clin Radiol.* 1980;31:101–104.
49. Philips RL, Carlson HC. The roentgenographic and clinical findings in Whipple's disease: a review of 8 patients. *AJR.* 1975;123:268–273.
50. Marshak RH, Ruoff M, Lindner AE. Roentgen manifestations of giardiasis. *AJR.* 1968;104:557–560.
51. Legge DA, Carlson HC, Wollaeger EE. Roentgenologic appearance of systemic amyloidosis involving the gastrointestinal tract. *AJR.* 1970;110:406–410.
52. Tada S, Iida M, Matsui T, Fuchigami T, et al. Amyloidosis of the small intestine: findings on double contrast radiographs. *AJR.* 1991;156:741–744.
53. Ekberg O, Sjostrom B, Brahme F. Radiological findings in Yersinia ileitis. *Radiology.* 1977;123:15–19.
54. Ekberg O, Lindstom C. Superficial lesions in Crohn's disease of the small bowel. *Gastrointest Radiol.* 1979;4:389–393.
55. Goldberg HI, Caruthers SB, Nelson JA, et al. Radiographic findings of the National Cooperative Crohn's disease study. *Gastroenterology.* 1979;77:925–937.
56. Herlinger H, Rubesin SE, Furth EE. Mesenteric border ulcers in Crohn's disease: historical, radiologic and pathologic perspectives. *Abdom Imaging.* 1998;23:122–126.
57. Vaidya MG, Sodhi JS. Gastrointestinal tract tuberculosis: a study of 102 cases including 55 hemicolectomies. *Clin Radiol.* 178:29:189–195.
58. Dallemand S, Waxman M, Farman J. Radiologic manifestations of *Strongyloides stercoralis*. *Gastrointest Radiol.* 1983;8:45–51.
59. Jones B, Kramer S, Saral R, et al. Gastrointestinal inflammation after bone marrow transplantation: graft-versus-host disease or opportunistic infection? *AJR.* 1988;150:277–281.
60. Rubesin SE, Herlinger H, Saul S, et al. Adult celiac disease and its complications. *RadioGraphics.* 1989;6:1045–1066.

Index

NOTE: Page numbers in italics refer to illustrations; page numbers followed by the letter t refer to tables.

Abdominal tuberculosis. *See*
    Mycobacterium tuberculosis
Abetalipoproteinemia, *363*, 363–364
Abscesses
    and anisakiasis, 293
    in appendix, 61, *61*, 286, 307
    in Crohn's disease, 263, 281–282, *281–283*
    interventional radiologic therapy and, 217–218
    and jejunal diverticulosis, 353, 353t
    percutaneous drainage of, 217–218
    sonography and, 129, *129*, 132
    tubo-ovarian, 307
Absorption. *See also* Malabsorption
    of carbohydrates, *19*, 19–20
    of lipids, 20–21, *21*
    motility and, 22–24
    of protein, 20, *20*, *21*
    of trace elements and vitamins, 21
Absorptive functions, differentiation of
    embryology, 13, *14*
    extrinsic nervous system, 13, *13*, 14
    intrinsic nervous system, 13, *13*
Absorptive physiology, *14*, *16*, 17–18, 18t, *19*
Acanthosis, and abetalipoproteinemia, 363
Acquired immune deficiency syndrome (AIDS)
    and abdominal tuberculosis, 297
    and AIDS-defining illnesses, 315t
    and computed tomography (CT), 161
    definition of, 316
    diarrhea and, 16
    epidemiology, 316
    and histoplasmosis, 304–305
    and HIV enteritis, 314–315
    immunology of, 32
    and Kaposi's sarcoma, 316, 323–324
    lymphomas and, 161, 316, 324–326
    and opportunistic infections, 316–323, *317–323*
    overview, 314–315, 316t
    and strongyloidiasis, 293
Actinomycosis, 131
Acute arterial embolism, 441
Acute arterial thrombosis, 440–441
Acute intestinal ischemia, 440–449, *443–447*, *449*
Acyclovir, and post-transplant lymphoproliferative disorder (PTLD), 328
Adenocarcinomas
    and angiography, 215, 399, *400*, *400*, *401*
    annular, 535
    and bacterial overgrowth syndrome, 349
    carcinoma and, 348
    and celiac disease, 343
    and computed tomography (CT), 157, *397*, 399, *400*, *401*
    and Crohn's disease, 260, 286, 536
    and differential diagnosis, 401
    and enteroclysis, 399, *399*, *400*, *401*
    and eosinphilic gastroenteritis, 361
    fish tapeworm and, 296
    hemangiomas, 386
    overview of, 395–396
    precancerous conditions, 396–97
    and selective IgA deficiency, 309
    sonography and, 143, *144*, 400–401
    treatment and prognosis of, 401–402
Adenomas, 377, 383, *386*
Adenomatous polyps, 142
Adenopathy, in Whipple's disease, CT and, 162
Adenosarcomas, and Meckel's diverticulum (MD), 235
Adults
    celiac disease, 333, 334
    Crohn's disease, 259
    Cronkhite-Canada syndrome, 394
    cystic fibrosis, *371*, 372
    ileal dysgenesis, 253
    inflammatory fibroid polyps (IFP), 390
    intestinal rotation, 244, 246
    intussusception, 379
    leiomyoma, 383
    lipomas, 385
    lymphangiectasia, 358
    malignant tumors, 379
    Meckel's diverticulum (MD), 234, 239
    omentum, 126
    short bowel syndrome, 356
    Waldenstrom's macroglobulinea, 370
    Zollinger-Ellison syndrome (ZES), 364
Adventitia, 9
Adynamic ileus, 62, 134
Afferent loop syndrome
    after gastric surgery, 507–509, *509*
    and barium contrast studies, 508, *509*
    and computed tomography (CT), 508, *509*
    and scintigraphy, 196, 508
    and sonography, 508
AIDS. *See* Acquired immune deficiency syndrome
Air
    as a contrast agent, 41, 156
    and magnetic resonance imaging (MRI), 172
Air double contrast enteroclysis, 118–121, *120–122*, 120t
Air-fluid levels, in small bowel, 52–53, 61
Albendazole, and microsporidia, 323
Allergic granulomatosis angiitis, 450
Allogenic transplantation, graft-*versus*-host disease, 312
Alpha chains, and immunoproliferative small intestinal disease (IPSID), 311, 378
Amino acids, 14

Amyloidosis, 260, 366–367
Anastomosis, 510, *511*
Anatomy
    of bowel folds, *7*, *8*, *9*, *9*, *10*, 527, 528t
    of bowel wall, 5, *5*, 6–9, 527
    of the enteric nervous system, 11
    loop distribution and, 4–5, *5*
    of mesentery, 3–4
    and sonography, 126–127
    of superior mesenteric artery, 10, *11*
    of villi, 9, *10*, *11*, 527
Anclyostomiasis, 292–293
Angiodysplasia, 187
Angiodysplasias/vascular ectasias, 456, *457*
Angiography, 187
    acute small bowel hemorrhage, diagnosis of, 203–204, 204t, *205–206*, *207*
    adenocarcinomas, 399, *400*, *401*
    and angiodysplasias/vascular ectasias, 456
    and angiographic localization, 204, *205*
    and carcinoid tumors, 412, *413*
    and celiac axis compression syndrome, 455–456
    and chronic gastrointestinal bleeding, 213–215
    complications of, 210–211
    diagnostic *versus* therapeutic, 203, 204t
    and hemangiomas, 389, 457
    leiomyoma and, 383, *385*
    leiomyosarcomas and, 424
    and mesenteric ischemia, 448, 454
    and mesenteric varices, 457
    and neurogenic tumors, 389
    small bowel hemorrhage management, 209, *210*, *211*, *212*, 213
    and tumors, 382, *385*
    and vasopressin, 212–213
    and visceral ischemia, 215, *216*, *217*
    and Zollinger-Ellison syndrome (ZES), 365
Anisakiasis, 293, *294*
Ann Arbor staging system, of non-Hodgkin's lymphoma, 414
Annular lesions, differential diagnosis and, 534–537, 537t, *538–542*, 541t
Anorexia
    and Cronkhite-Canada syndrome, 394
    and malabsorption, 332
    and tumors, 379
Anticholinergics, 83
Anticoagulant therapy, and small bowel hemorrhage, 137, 161
Aperistalsis, 136
Appendix
    abscesses in, 61, *61*, 307, 545
    and actinomycosis, 131
    computed tomography (CT) and, 162

Appendix (*Contd.*)
  and Crohn's disease, 260, 286
  sonography and, 162
  and torsion of the omentum, 132
Apudomas, 402
Arterial occlusion, 440
Arterial thrombosis, 440
Arteriography, superior mesenteric, 389
Arteriovenous malformations (AVMs), 224
Arthritis
  and Crohn's disease, 260
  and Whipple's disease, 358
Ascariasis, 291–292, *292*
Ascites, 128–129, 164
  and carcinoids, 403
  and eosinphilic gastroenteritis, 362
  exudative, 128
  and mesenteric ischemia, 446
  and metastatic disease, 425
  and myobacterium tuberculosis, 298, 301
Atopy, and eosinphilic gastroenteritis, 361
Atrophic gastritis, and common variable immunodeficiency syndrome (CVI), 310
Auerbach's autonomic nerve plexus, 8, 14
Autocrine communication, 16, *16*
Azithromycin, and cryptosporidiosis in children, 317

Bacillary angiomatosis, 323
Bacterial enteritis
  campylobacter, 303, *303*, 304
  mycobacterium tuberculosis, 297–301
  salmonellosis, 303
  shigellosis, 304
  yersiniosis, 302–303
Bacterial overgrowth syndrome, 332, 348–349, *349*, *349t*, 350
Barium contrast studies
  adenomas, 383, *386*
  afferent loop syndrome, 508, *509*
  amyloidosis, 366–367
  anisakiasis, 293, *294*
  blind loop syndrome, 512
  campylobacter, 303, *303*
  celiac disease, 336–339, *338*, *338*–342
  continent ileostomy reservoir, 517–518
  Crohn's disease, 271
  cryptosporidiosis, 316–317, *317*
  cytomegalovirus (CMV), 317–318, *318*, *319*
  diabetes, 367
  eosinphilic gastroenteritis, 361, *361*, *362*
  giardiasis, 296, *297*
  graft-*versus*-host disease, 313, *313*, *314*
  hemangiomas, 389, 457
  ileal dysgenesis, 254
  ileoanal pouch, 519–520
  ileostomy, 516
  inadvertent gastroilectomy, 510, *510*
  inflammatory fibroid polyps (IFP), 390, *391*
  intersigmoid hernias, 253
  intestinal rotation, 243–244
  intramural hemorrhage, 458
  isoporiasis, 317
  jejunal diverticulosis, 354, *354*
  jejunogastric intussusception, 509, *510*
  jejunoileal bypass, 513
  leiomyoma, 383, *384*, *384*, *385*
  leiomyosarcomas, 424, *424*
  lipomas, 386, *387*
  mesenteric ischemia, 442, *443*–*444*, *444*–445
  metastatic disease, 426
  midgut duplications, 230, *231*
  myobacterium avium intracellular (MAI) infection, 318–319, *320*
  myobacterium tuberculosis, 298, *299*, 320–321, *322*
  neurogenic tumors, 389–390, *390*
  non-Hodgkin's lymphoma, 415, *416*, *417*, *418*, 422, *422*
  paraduodenal hernias, 248
  radiation enteritis, 452–453, *454*–*455*, *454*–456
  roundworm, 292, *292*
  salmomellosis, 303
  shigellosis, 304
  short bowel syndrome, 356
  strongyloidiasis, 294, *295*
  systemic mastocytosis, *360*, 361
  systemic sclerosis, 350–351
  tapeworm, 295
  transomental hernias, 253
  and transplantation, 522, *522*, 523
  tropical sprue, 348
  tumors, 377, *382*
  yersiniosis, 302, *302*
  Zollinger-Ellison syndrome (ZES), 365, *365*
Barium sulfate
  for "dedicated" small bowel meal, 43
  and magnetic resonance imaging (MRI), 171–172
  and other barium-based methods, 43
  for small bowel meal, 42
  transit acceleration, 82–84
Barrett's esophagus, and Zollinger-Ellison syndrome (ZES), 365
B cells
  and acquired immune deficiency syndrome (AIDS), 315, 324–325
  and common variable immunodeficiency syndrome (CVI), 309–310
  and immunoproliferative small intestinal disease (IPSID), 311
  and post-transplant lymphoproliferative disorder (PTLD), 328
Behçet's syndrome, 450
Bezoars, 75, 149
Bilbao-Dotter tube, 42–43
Bile salt deconjugation, and giardiasis, 296
Bilomas, 129, *129*
Biopsy, 340–343, 555, 561
  and AIDS-related lymphomas, 325
  and amyloidosis, 366, 367
  and celiac disease, 340–343
  distal duodenal, 335
  endoscopic mucosal, 333
  and giardiasis, 296
  and histoplasmosis, 304
  and HIV enteritis, 315
  and immunoproliferative small intestinal disease (IPSID), 312, *312*
  and jejunal diverticulosis, 355
  and lactase deficiency, 369
  and liposarcoma, 132
  and lymphangiectasia, 369
  and myobacterium tuberculosis, 298
  and non-Hodgkin's lymphoma, 422
  nonvascular interventional radiology, 215, 217
  small bowel, combined with enteroclysis, 118
  and South American blastomycosis, 304
  and strongyloidiasis, 294, *295*
  and Whipple's disease, 358
Biphasic enteroclysis, 111, *114*
Biscodyl (Dulcolax), 82, 96
Bleeding. *See also* Hemorrhage
  adenomas, 383
  amyloidosis, 366
  carcinoma, 348
  Crohn's disease, 260
  and enteroclysis, 116, *118*

hemangiomas, 386
hookworm and, 292–293
inflammatory fibroid polyps (IFP), 390
leiomyoma, 383
lipomas, 385–386
Meckel's diverticulum (MD), 234
neurogenic tumors, 142, 389–390, *390*
tumors, 379
Blind loop syndrome, 512
Blind pouch syndrome, 512, *512*
Blood-pool labeling, 188–189
Blue rubber bleb nevus syndrome, 457
Bone marrow transplant. *See* Graft-*versus*-host disease
Bowel folds
  anatomy of, 7, *8*, *9*, 9, *10*
  differential diagnosis and, *554*–*562*, 555, 556t, 558t, 561–562, 563t
  of ileum, *8*, *9*, 9
  jejunal, 7, *8*, *9*, 9
Bowel loops. *See* Loops
Bowel wall
  anatomy of, 5, *5*, 6–7, 8–9, 527
  thickening, 5–6, *6*, *136*, 157–161, 262–263, 461
Bradykinin, 507
Breath hydrogen analysis, 332
Broncospasm, and carcinoid syndrome, 403
Brunner's glands, 383, 529
Burkitt's lymphoma, *160*, 324, 325, 419, *420*
Bypass enteritis, 513

Calcifications
  carcinoid syndrome, 403
  mesenteric mass, 130
  myobacterium tuberculosis, 301
  schistosomiasis, 297
Calcium, 21
Campylobacter, 303, *303*, 304
Capillary hemangiomas, 388, 456
Carbohydrates, digestion and absorption of, 19–20, *20*
Carcinoid tumors, 531
  angiography and, 214, *215*, 412, *413*
  clinicopathologic aspects of, 402–403
  computed tomography (CT) and, 403, 405–412, *410*, *412*
  and enteroclysis, 403, *405*, *407*
  magnetic resonance imaging (MRI) and, 403, *408*, 409, *409*
  and Meckel's diverticulum (MD), 235
  metasticized, 534
  overview, 377, 402
  and scintigraphy, 410
  small bowel follow-through and, 403, *404*
  sonography and, 144, *146*, 214, *215*
Carcinoma, 187
  celiac disease and, 348
  and common variable immunodeficiency syndrome (CVI), 310
  and Crohn's disease, 283
Castleman's disease, 325
Catheters. *See* Intubation
Cavernous hemangiomas, 388, 456
Cavitary mass, differential diagnosis and, 537, 542t, 543–544
Cecal volvulus, 243
Celiac artery, 439
Celiac axis compression syndrome, 455–456
Celiac disease
  and adenocarcinomas, 396
  after gastric surgery, 507
  barium radiology and, 336–339, *338*, *338*–342
  clinical diagnosis of, 334–335

complications of, 344, 344–348, 346–348
definition of, 333–334
enteroclysis and endoscopic biopsy, 340–343
epidemiology, 334
mucosa in, 335, 335
nonspecific radiologic findings in, 335–336, 336
other associations of, 343
and selective IgA deficiency, 309, 309
sonography and, 148
variants of, 343
Cell-mediated immunity, 30
acquired, 32, 33, 34
innate, 31–32
Ceruletide, 42, 83
Chest radiograph, 48, 50
Children
celiac disease and, 334
and Crohn's disease, 260
and cryptosporidiosis, 317
enteroclysis and, 116
foreign bodies in, 76–77
and ileal dysgenesis, 253
and intestinal rotation, 243–244, 244
and lactase deficiency, 368
and Meckel's diverticulum (MD), 234, 239
and nodular lymphoid hyperplasia (NLH), 310, 311
omentum and, 126
roundworms and, 291–292
and short bowel syndrome, 356
and yersiniosis, 302
Cholecystography, 41
Cholecystokinin, 42, 83
Chronic intestinal pseudo-obstruction (CIP), 25t, 26, 26t, 349–350
Chronic mesenteric ischemia, 453–455
Churg-Strauss syndrome, 450
Chylous cysts, 129
Closed-loop obstruction, 135
Clostridium difficile, 304
Cobalamin, 21
Cobblestoning, and Crohn's disease, 267, 268
Codeine, 83
Coffee bean configuration, 68
Colchicine, and lactase deficiency, 369
Cole, Lewis Gregory, 41
Collagen
and Crohn's disease, 271
and systemic sclerosis, 350
Collagenous sprue, 343
Colloids, 188
Colonoscopy, 187
Common variable immunodeficiency syndrome (CVI), 309–310, 311
Compression devices, 84
Computed tomography (CT)
adenocarcinomas, 157, 397, 397, 399, 400, 401
as adjunct to plain film radiography, 47
afferent loop syndrome, 508, 509
AIDS-related lymphoma, 324
amyloidosis, 367
anastomosis, 511
angiodysplasias/vascular ectasias, 456
bacillary angiomatosis, 323
carcinoid tumors, 403, 405–412, 410, 412
carcinoma, 348
celiac axis compression syndrome, 455–456
celiac disease, 338–339, 340
contrast agents for, 154–156, 156, 157
Crohn's disease, 262, 263

CT enteroclysis, 263, 264
cytomegalovirus, 318, 318–319
enlarged lymph nodes, 344
enteropathy associated T-cell lymphoma (EATCL), 345–348, 347
familial polyposis coli, 394–395
giardiasis, 296
graft-*versus*-host disease, 314, 315
hemangiomas, 457
hyposplenism, 344
ileoanal pouch, 520, 520
ileostomy, 516, 517
inflammation, 307
intestinal rotation, 245–246
intramural hemorrhage, 458
jejunal diverticulosis, 354, 354
jejunoileal bypass, 513–514
Kaposi's sarcoma, 323–324
leiomyoma, 383, 384, 385
leiomyosarcomas, 424
lipomas, 386, 387
lymphangiectasia, 369
Meckel's diverticulum (MD), 237, 239
mesenteric, 3–4, 4
mesenteric ischemia, 445–446, 445–447, 448, 455
mesenteric varices, 457
metastatic disease, 425, 428, 430
midgut duplications, 230, 231
myobacterium avium intracellular (MAI) infection, 319, 320
myobacterium tuberculosis, 298, 300–301, 320–321, 322
neurogenic tumors, 390, 390
non-Hodgkin's lymphoma, 415, 416, 417, 418
paraduodenal hernias, 250–251
post-transplant lymphoproliferative disorder (PTLD), 328
principles of interpretation, 156–161, 162, 163, 164–165
"pseudomasses," 154
radiation enteritis, 452, 453
roundworm, 292, 292
salmonellosis, 303
schistosomiasis, 297
shigellosis, 304
small bowel injury, in blunt abdominal trauma, 459, 460, 461
spiral CT, 263
systemic mastocytosis, 361
technique, 153–154, 154
transplantation, 522, 523, 524
tumors, 381, 381, 382
value of, 153
Whipple's disease, 358
yersiniosis, 303
Zollinger-Ellison syndrome (ZES), 365, 366
Congenital anomalies
in adults and children, 227
ileal dysgenesis, 253–254, 253–254
of intestinal fixation, 246–253, 247–254
of intestinal rotation, 241–246, 242–246
Meckel's diverticulum (MD), 145, 147, 147
midgut development, 227, 228
midgut duplications, 229–232, 230, 231
midgut rotation, 227–228, 229
omphalomesenteric duct, 232–441, 232–441
small bowel duplication, 145
Congenital arteriovenous malformations, 456
Constrictive disease, and abdominal tuberculosis, 297
Continent ileostomy reservoir, 517–518, 518

Contrast agents
and computed tomography (CT), 154–156, 156, 157
and magnetic resonance imaging (MRI), 168–172, 169–172
Contrast ileograms, 519–520
Corticosteroids
and Crohn's disease, 260
and myobacterium tuberculosis, 298
Cowden's disease, 319, 393
Creeping fat, and Crohn's disease, 261
Crohn's colitis, 259
Crohn's disease, 187, 260
and abdominal tuberculosis, 297
and adenocarcinomas, 286, 396, 536
and appendiceal abcesses, 286
clinical considerations of, 259–260
complications of, 277–283, 281–283
and computed tomography (CT), 157, 160, 162, 163, 163, 262, 263, 264
and CT (ESCT), 117
and diffuse jejunoileitus, 277, 277
disease activity of, 283–284, 284–285
enteroclysis and, 261–262
and enterolithiasis, 75–76
enteroscopy and, 261–262
etiology of, 259
history of, 42
and ileal reservoirs, 517
infectious ileitis, 284–285
inflammatory polyps in, 534
ischemia, 286
and loop ileostomy, 514
lymphoma, 286
and magnetic resonance imaging (MRI), 177, 178, 265
malabsorption and, 369
and metastatic disease, 286, 427
National Cooperative Crohn's Disease Study, 81
pathology of, 260–261
and plain film radiography, 261
prevalence of, 259
progression and remission in, 275
and radiation enteropathy, 286
radiologic findings and, 265–274, 266–276
recurrence, 275–277
scintigraphy and, 196–197, 264–265
and secondary mesenteritis, 132
and selective IgA deficiency, 309
and short bowel syndrome, 356
and small bowel fistulography, 87
and small bowel obstruction, 61, 62
and sonography, 138–139, 138–139, 264, 264
strictures in, 536–537
and tuberculosis, 286
tumors in, 378
Crohn's Disease Activity Index, 260
Cronkhite-Canada syndrome, 394
Cryptosporidiosis, 316–317, 317, 317
CT enteroclysis (CT-E), 43, 116–117, 119, 263, 264
CT(ESCT), 117, 119
CT-Sellink, 117
Culture of duodenal aspirates, 332
Cutaneous flushing, and carcinoid syndrome, 403
Cyclosporine, and post-transplant lymphoproliferative disorder (PTLD), 328
Cystic carcinoid, 130
Cysticercosis, 296
Cystic fibrosis, 150, 150, 371, 372
Cystic mesothelioma, 130
Cystic spindle cell tumor, 130
Cystic teratoma, 130

Cysts
    chylous, 129
    cystic tumors, 130–131
    duplication, 129, 145
    mesenteric, 129
    mesolethial, 129
    pancreatic pseudocyst, 130
    pseudocyst, 129
Cytomegalovirus (CMV), 157
    and AIDS, 317–318, *318–319*
    and common variable immunodeficiency syndrome (CVI), 310
    and graft-*versus*-host disease, 313–314

Decompression tube, and enteroclysis, 112–113, *115–117*
Demerol, 96
Dermatitis herpetiformis, 343
Diabetes, 343, 367
Diarrhea
    abetalipoproteinemia, 363
    AIDS-related, 16, 315
    amyloidosis, 366
    bacterial overgrowth syndrome, 349
    blind loop syndrome, 512
    blind pouch syndrome, 512
    campylobacter, 303
    carcinoid syndrome, 403
    chronic mesenteric ischemia, 453–454
    common variable immunodeficiency syndrome (CVI), 310
    Crohn's disease, 259
    Cronkhite-Canada syndrome, 394
    cryptosporidiosis, 317
    diabetes, 367
    eosinphilic gastroenteritis, 361, 362
    giardiasis, 296
    ileostomy, 516
    immunoproliferative small intestinal disease (IPSID), 311
    inadvertent gastroilectomy, 510
    ischemia, 441–442
    jejunoileal bypass, 513
    and metastatic disease, 427
    microsporidia, 323
    myobacterium tuberculosis, 298
    salmomellosis, 303
    secretory, 24
    short bowel syndrome, 355, 512
    strongyloidiasis, 294
    systemic mastocytosis, 360
    systemic sclerosis, 350
    tumors, 378, 379
    Waldenstrom's macroglobulinea, 370
    yersiniosis, 302
    Zollinger-Ellison syndrome (ZES), 364
Diazepam, 96
Dicyclomine, and magnetic resonance imaging (MRI), 167
Differential diagnosis
    adenocarcinomas, 401
    annular lesions, 534–537, 537t, *538–542*, 541t
    cavitary mass, 537, 542t, *543–544*
    celiac disease, 335
    dilated lumen, normal fold thickness, 550–551, *550–553*, 550t, 552t, 553, 555
    eosinphilic gastroenteritis, 361–362
    extrinsic mass effect and tethering, 543, 545, *547–550*, 547t
    metastatic disease, 426–427
    midgut duplications, 230, *231*
    multiple polypoid lesions, 533, 535t, *536*
    myobacterium tuberculosis, 298, 300
    non-Hodgkin's lymphoma, 422
    separation of bowel loops, 537, 539, 542, *545–546*, 545t

solitary polyp, 528–533, *530–534*, 531t, 534t
    target lesions, 533, *535*
    tethering of folds, 542–543, *546*
    thick, undulating, or nodular folds and mucosal nodularity, *554–562*, 555, 556t, 558t, 561–562, 563t
    tubular bowel, 562, 563t, 564, *564*
    Whipple's disease, 358–359
    yersiniosis, 302–303
Digestion, *14, 16,* 17–18, *18, 19*
Digital subtraction angiography (DSA), 204–205, *205*
Dilatation, 218, *219*, 335
Diphenoxylate (Lomotil), 83
Diphyllobothrium latum, 296
Diverticulitis, and Meckel's diverticulum (MD), 234
Double contrast
    enteroclysis, 103–104, 106–113, *107–113*
    and small bowel follow-through, 88, *89, 90, 90*
Double halo sign, 403, 446
Drainage procedures, 217–218
Duodenal ulcers, and Zollinger-Ellison syndrome (ZES), 364
Duodenoscopy, and myobacterium avium intracellular (MAI) infection, 318
Duodenum
    celiac disease, *336*, 335–336
    neoplastic disease, 209
    obstruction, 241, *243*
    pancreatico-duodenal arcade aneurysms, 209
    pancreatitis, 209, *210, 211*
    peptic ulceration, 208–209
Duplication cysts, 129, 145
D-Xylose absorption-excretion test, 332

Ectopic ovarian dermoid, 130
Embolism, acute arterial, 441
Embolization, 208, 413
Embryology, 13, *14*
Endocrine communication, 15–16, *16*
Endocrine disorders
    diabetes, 367
    hypoparathyroidism, 367
    hypothyroidism, 368
Endocrine neoplasia syndrome type I, 378
Endometrial implants, and metastatic disease, 427
Endometriosis, 148, 543
Endoscopy
    and amyloidosis, 367
    and celiac disease, 335
    and Crohn's disease, 261
    endoscopic biopsy, 340–343, 358
    and enteroclysis, 113–114
    and lymphangiectasia, 369
    and systemic mastocytosis, 360
    and Whipple's disease, 358–359
Enemas, and small bowel follow-through, 82
Enterectomy, and small bowel anastomosis, 510–511, *511*
Enteric duplication, 129
Enteric nervous system
    anatomy of, 11
    extrinsic, and differentiation of absorptive function, 13, *13,* 14
    intrinsic, and differentiation of absorptive function, 13, *13*
Enteritis
    parasitic diseases and, 291
    radiation, 160, 450–453, *453–455*
Enteroclysis
    and abetalipoproteinemia, 363–364
    and adenocarcinomas, 399, *399, 400, 401*

advantages and disadvantages of, 95
air double contrast, 118–121, *120–122*, 120t
and amyloidosis, 367, *367*
and angiodysplasias/vascular ectasias, 456, *457*
biphasic, 111, *114*
and blind pouch syndrome, 512, *512*
and blood loss from tumors, 379
carcinoid tumors and, 403, *405, 407*
carcinoma and, 348
and celiac disease, 345, *346*
celiac disease and, 338–339, *339*, 340–343, *341, 342*
and common variable immunodeficiency syndrome (CVI), 310, *311*
Crohn's disease and, 261–262, *262*, 271
digital fluoroscopy for, 95, 118, *98–119*
and enteropathy associated T-cell lymphoma (EATCL), 345–348, *347*
enteroscopy and, 224–225, *225*
first use of, 41
and ileostomy, 516
and immunoproliferative small intestinal disease (IPSID), 312
and inflammation, 307
and jejunal diverticulosis, 353
lumen diameter and, *5*, 5–6
and lymphangiectasia, 369
and Meckel's diverticulum (MD), 237, *237, 239, 240*
mesenteric small bowel, 528, 528t, *529*
and metastatic disease, 425
and myobacterium avium intracellular (MAI) infection, 318–319, *320*
and paraduodenal hernias, 248–249
and small bowel follow-through, 81–82
tumors and, 380, *380*
and Waldenstrom's macroglobulinea, 370, *372*
and Whipple's disease, 358, 359
Enterocutaneous fistulae, 218
Enteroglucagen, 507
Entero-H, 84
Enteroliths, and Meckel's diverticulum (MD), 236
Enteropathy associated T-cell lymphoma (EATCL), and celiac disease, 345–348, *347*
Enteroplasty, 507
Enteroscopy
    and angiodysplasias/vascular ectasias, 456
    and Crohn's disease, 261
    enteroclysis and, 224–225, *225*
    ileoscopy, 224
    indications for, 224–225, *225*
    intraoperative, 224
    push type, 223
    risks with, 225
    sonde type, 224
    and tumors, 377, 382
Enterostomy, 514
Enterotomy, 507
Entrobar, 84
Eosinophilia
    and eosinphilic gastroenteritis, 361–363, *361–362*
    hookworm and, 293
Eosinophilic granulomatous polyps, 390
Epithelial barrier, immunity and, 29–30, *30*
Epithelium, 6, *6*
Epstein-Barr virus (EBV), 324, 327–328
Erect abdominal radiograph, in plain film radiography, 48, *50*
Erythema nodosum, and Crohn's disease, 260
Exoenteric lesion, 537

Extrinsic mass effect and tethering, differential diagnosis and, 543, 545, *547–550,* 547t

Fabry's disease, 351, 355
False-negative radiographic examination, 377
Familial adenomatous polyposis, 514
and adenomas, 383
Familial hypercholesterolemia, 514
Familial Mediterranean fever, and amyloidosis, 366
Familial polyposis coli, *394, 394–39*
   carcinoma, 394
   desmoid tumors, 394
   Gardner's syndrome, 394
   lymphoid hyperplasia, 394
   medulloblastoma, 394
   small bowel adenomas, 394
   Turcot syndrome (glioblastoma), 394
Fat wrapping, Crohn's disease and, 261
Feathering, 528
Fecal fat test, and malabsorption, 332
Fentanyl, 96
Ferric ammonium citrate (FAC), and magnetic resonance imaging (MRI), 169
Fibrofatty proliferation
   in Crohn's disease, 261, 263
   differential diagnosis and, 539
Fibroid inflammatory polyps, 142, *142*
Fibrosarcomas, and leiomyosarcomas, 424
Fibrosis
   and Crohn's disease, 271, *274, 275*
   and schistosomiasis, 296–297
Fish tapeworm, 296
Fistulae
   and Crohn's disease, 279–281, *279–281*
   and jejunal diverticulosis, 353, 353t
   and myobacterium tuberculosis, 298
   and short bowel syndrome, 356, *356*
Fistulography, 87–88
Fixation, anomalies of, 246–253, *247–254*
Fluoroscopy, digital, for enteroclysis, 95–96
   catheters and infusions, 96–97
   intubation, 96–102, *98–106*
   with methylcellulose, 108–104, *106–108,* 110, *111–113*
Focal ischemia, 449
Folic acid, and jejunal diverticulosis, 352
Folic polyglutamate, 21
Foramen of Winslow, 251–252, *252*
Foreign bodies
   and Meckel's diverticulum (MD), 234
   and plain film radiography, 76–77
Fungal infections
   histoplasmosis, 304–305
   South American blastomycosis, 304

Gadolinium solutions, and magnetic resonance imaging (MRI), 169, 170, 265
Gallstone ileus, 62, 64–65, *65, 66,* 148
Gallstones
   and Crohn's disease, 260, 261, 263
   and short bowel syndrome, 357
Ganglioneuromas, 390
Gardner's syndrome, 131
   and adenomas, 383
   and familial polyposis coli, 394
Gas
   and magnetic resonance imaging (MRI), 172
   patterns, 51–57, *54–60*
Gastric metaplasia, 529, *531*
Gastric sarcoma, 378
Gastrinomas, and Zollinger-Ellison syndrome (ZES), 364

Gastroenteritis, 139
Gastroesophageal reflux, and systemic sclerosis, 350
Gastrografin, 42, 83, 154
Gastrointestinal peptides, 16, 17t
Gastrointestinal stromal tumor (GIST), 533
Gastrointestinal ulcers, and Zollinger-Ellison syndrome (ZES), 364
Gastromark, and magnetic resonance imaging (MRI), 171
Gastroschisis, 241
Giardasis, and abetalipoproteinemia, 364
Giardia lamblia, 296
Giardiasis, 296, *297,* 310
Glucagon, 189, 516
   and magnetic resonance imaging (MRI), 167, 170
Graft-*versus*-host disease
   acute, 312
   and allogenic bone transplantation, 312
   and autologous bone transplantation, 312
   barium studies and, 313, *313, 314,* 314
   chronic, 313
   and computed tomography (CT), 314, *315*
   grading of, 312
   indications for, 312–314, *313–314*
   induction protocol and, 312
   subacute, 312
   treatment of, 314
Granulomas
   and abdominal tuberculosis, 297
   and Crohn's disease, 261
Gut-associated lymphoid tissue, 32–33
   lymphoid aggregates, 33, 35, *35*
   nonaggregated lymphoid tissue, *35,* 35–36
Gut-associated lymphoid tissue (GALT), and non-Hodgkin's lymphoma, 414

Hamartomas, 383, 534
Hamartomatous polyposis syndromes
   Cowden's disease, *319,* 393
   juvenile polyposis, 393
   Peutz-Jeghers syndrome, 391–392, *391–393*
   Ruvalcaba-Myre-Smith syndrome, 393
Hamartomatous polyps, 142
Headache, and systemic mastocytosis, 360
Heart disease, and carcinoid syndrome, 403
Helical CT, 446, 447
Hemangiomas, 386–389, *388, 389,* 456–457
Hematoma, small bowel, 137–138
Hemoperitoneum, 461
Hemorrhage
   acute gastrointestinal, 187–191, 203–204, 204t
   angiography and, 203–215, 204t, *205–207, 210–217*
   blunt abdominal trauma and, 458
   and Crohn's disease, 260
   CT and, 161
   intramural, 458, *458, 459*
   and jejunal diverticulosis, 353, 353t
   and midgut duplications, 230
   sonography and, 137–138, *138*
Henoch-Schönlein Purpura, 450
Henoch-Schönlein syndrome (HSS), 138
Hepatic fibrosis, and schistosomiasis, 297
Hepatocellular jaundice, 368
Hernias, 507
   congenital internal, 246–247, 251–253, *247–254*
   and gastroschisis, 241
   of Littré, 234
   and Meckel's diverticulum (MD), 234

and omphalocele, 241, *242*
and paraileostomy herniation, 516, *516*
strangulated, 59, 67
and strangulation, 135
Herpes virus, and common variable immunodeficiency syndrome (CVI), 310
Herring worm disease, 293
Heterotopic gastric mucosa, 391
High resolution sonography (HRS), 125
Histoplasmosis, 304–305
Hodgkin's disease (HD), *422,* 423
Hookworm, 292–293
H_2 receptor blockers, and Zollinger-Ellison syndrome (ZES), 364
Human immunodeficiency virus (HIV) enteritis, 315–316
   and opportunistic infections, 316
Humoral immunity, 30, *31, 32*
Hydrogen breath test
   and bacterial overgrowth syndrome, 349
   and lactase deficiency, 369
Hydronephrosis, in Crohn's disease, 260, 263
Hyoscine butylbromide, and magnetic resonance imaging (MRI), 167
Hyoscine-N-butyl bromide (Buscopan), 83
Hyperlipidemia, and jejunoileal bypass, 513
Hyperoxaluria, and short bowel syndrome, 357
Hypoalbuminemia, 293
   and abetalipoproteinemia, 364
   and lymphangiectasia, 369
Hypobetalipoproteinemia, and abetalipoproteinemia, 363
Hypogammaglobulinemia, 419
Hypogammaglobulinemic sprue, and common variable immunodeficiency syndrome (CVI), 310
Hypomotility, and celiac disease, 335
Hyposplenism, and celiac disease, 344
Hypotension, and systemic mastocytosis, 360

IgA
   and acquired immune deficiency syndrome (AIDS), 315
   celiac disease and, 309, *309,* 334, 343
   and common variable immunodeficiency syndrome (CVI), 309–310
   and giardiasis, 296
   and lymphangiectasia, 369
IgG
   celiac disease and, 334
   and common variable immunodeficiency syndrome (CVI), 309–310
   Crohn's disease and, 334
   and lymphangiectasia, 369
IgM
   and common variable immunodeficiency syndrome (CVI), 309–310
   and giardiasis, 296
   and selective IgA deficiency, 309, *309*
Ileal dysgenesis, 253–254, *253–254*
Ileal reservoirs, 517–521
Ilecolic artery, 10, *11*
Ileoanal pouch, 518–521, *519–521*
Ileocecal tuberculosis. See Myobacterium tuberculosis
Ileocolitis, acute, 140–141
Ileoscopy, 224
Ileostomy, 514, 516, *516–517*
Ileum
   angiography and, 209, *212*
   bowel folds of, *8, 9, 9,* 338–339, *339–340*
   terminal, 9, *9*

Ileus
  adynamic, 62, 134
  plain film radiography, 54–58, 59–62, 64–65, 65, 66
Imaging techniques
  angiography and interventional radiology, 203–226
  barium and, 41–45
  computed tomography (CT), 153–166
  enteroclysis, 95–124
  enteroscopy, 223–226
  magnetic resonance imaging (MRI), 167–186
  plain film radiography, 47–80
  scintigraphy, 187–202
  small bowel follow-through (SBFT), 81–94
  sonography, 125–152
Immune deficiency diseases. *See also* Acquired immune deficiency syndrome (AIDS)
  common variable immunodeficiency syndrome (CVI), 309–310, 311
  and giardiasis, 296
  graft-*versus*-host disease, 312–314, 313–314
  immunoproliferative small intestine disease (IPSID), 310–312, 312
  and infections of the small intestine, 316–326, 317–327
  post-transplant lymphoproliferative disorder (PTLD), 327–328, 328
  secondary, 326–327
  selective IgA deficiency, 309, 309
  and solid organ transplantation (immunosuppression), 327
  X-linked hypogammaglobulinemia, 309
Immunity
  cell-mediated, 30–32, 33, 34
  the epithelial barrier, 29–30, 30
  gut-associated lymphoid tissue, 32–36, 35
  humoral, 30
  and the integrated immune response, 36
  and strongyloidiasis, 294
Immunoproliferative small intestine disease (IPSID), 310–312, 312, 419
Inadvertent gastroileostomy, 510, 510
Infections, opportunistic, and AIDS, 316
Infectious enteritis, 160
Infectious ileitis, and Crohn's disease, 284–285
Inflammation
  inflammatory diseases, 25–26, 138–140, 141, 173, 297–304, 304–307
  perienteric, 140–141, 141
Inflammatory bowel disease, and ileostomy, 514
Inflammatory fibroid polyps (IFP), 142, 142
Infusions, for enteroclysis, 96–97
Innate immunity, 31–32
Intercellular communication, 15
Interferon-alpha, 413
Intersigmoid hernias, 253, 253
Interspace spikes, 553
Interventional radiology, nonvascular biopsy and, 215, 217
  and drainage procedures, 218
  and percutaneous jejunostomy, 218
Intestinal endometriosis, 148
Intramural hematoma, and small bowel injury, 461
Intramural hemorrhage, 458, 458, 459
Intubation
  catheter preparation, 97
  duodenojejunal flexure, 100, 104
  and enteroclysis, 96

  entry into pylorus, 99, 102
  hiatus hernia, 99, 101
  history of gastric surgery or upper GI problems, 102, 106
  peroral, 97
  problems of, 99, 100
  sedation and, 95, 96
  transgastric, 97–99, 98, 99
  transnasal introduction of catheter, 97
  tube arrested at an unexpected level, 100, 105
  tube buckled in esophagus, 99, 101
  tube coiled in gastric fundus, antrum, or duodenum, 99–100, 102, 103
Intubation studies, historical aspects of, 41–42
Intussusception
  and celiac disease, 336, 336
  hemangiomas, 388
  and inflammatory fibroid polyps (IFP), 390
  jejunogastric, 509–510
  leiomyoma and, 383
  lipomas and, 385
  and Meckel's diverticulum (MD), 234, 235
  and neurogenic tumors, 389
  sonography and, 147–150, 148, 149
  and strangulation, 135
  and systemic sclerosis, 351
  and tumors, 379
Iron, 21
Ischemia, 160, 267, 286, 343
  acute intestinal, 440–449, 443–447, 449
  chronic mesenteric, 453–455
  focal, 449
  nonoclusive mesenteric, 441
  and short bowel syndrome, 356, 357
  symptoms of, 441–442
Ischemic colitis, Crohn's disease and, 259
Isolated intestinal transplantation, 521
Isoporiasis, 317

Jejunal dyskinesia, 352, 354
Jejunogastric intussusception, 509–510, 510
Jejunoileal bypass, 512–514, 513
Jejunoileitis, ulcerative, 537
Jejunostomy, 514, 515
Jejunum
  angiography and, 209, 212
  bowel folds of, 7, 8, 8, 9, 9, 336–338, 337–339
  and jejunal diverticulosis, 351–355, 353–355, 353t
  loop distribution and, 4, 5, 5
  mosaic pattern in celiac disease, 339, 341
Juvenile polyposis, 187, 393

Kaposi's sarcoma, 316, 323–324
  and acquired immune deficiency syndrome (AIDS), 316, 325
  and bacillary angiomatosis, 323
  and target lesions, 533
Kaposi's sarcoma-associated herpes virus (KSHV), 323, 325
Kerckring's folds, 7, 9
Klippel-Trénaunay syndrome, 457

Lactase deficiency, 368–369
Ladd's bands, 242
Lamina propria, 6, 7, 9, 10
Left lateral abdomen view, in plain film radiography, 50–51, 56
Left lateral decubitus film, in plain film radiography, 50
Leiomyomas, 187, 214–215, 383, 384–385

Leiomyosarcomas, 160
  and angiography, 424
  and angiosarcomas, 424
  and barium contrast studies, 424, 424
  and computed tomography (CT), 424
  and fibrosarcomas, 424
  and liposarcomas, 424
  pathology of, 423
  and plain film radiography, 423–424
  symptoms of, 423
  treatment of, 424
Leukemia, and X-linked hypogammaglobulinemia, 309
Leukocyte labeling, 196, 264
Lipids, digestion and absorption of, 20–21, 21
Lipomas, 131, 141–142, 142, 385–386, 387, 398, 531
Liposarcomas, and leiomyosarcomas, 424
Littré's hernia, 234
Loculated ascites, 128
Loops
  closed-loop obstruction, 135
  in Crohn's disease, 263, 262
  distribution of, 4–5, 5
  ileal, 4–5, 5
  jejunal, 4–5, 5
  length of, 3
  and loop ileostomy, 514
  and metastatic disease, 425, 426
  and myobacterium tuberculosis, 301
  separation of, 537, 539, 542, 545–546, 545t
  stepladder or hairpin, 58–59, 60
Lumen
  diameter of, 5, 5–6
  differential diagnosis and, 550–551, 550–553, 550t, 552t, 553, 555
Luminal communication, 16, 16
Lymphadenopathies, 131, 315, 325
Lymphangiectasia, 369
  and abetalipoproteinemia, 364
  and Whipple's disease, 358
Lymphangiomas, 129, 142, 143
Lymph nodes
  cavitation of, 344, 344–345
  and celiac disease, 344
  and Whipple's disease, 358
Lymphocytes, 30, 32
Lymphocytic colitis, and celiac disease, 343
Lymphocytopenia, and lymphangiectasia, 369
Lymphoid aggregates, 33, 35, 35
Lymphoid follicles, 7
Lymphoid hyperplasia, and common variable immunodeficiency syndrome (CVI), 310
Lymphoid tissue
  and common variable immunodeficiency syndrome (CVI), 310, 311
  gut-associated, 32–34, 35
  nonaggregated, 35–36
Lymphomas
  and acquired immune deficiency syndrome (AIDS), 316, 324–326
  and Crohn's disease, 267, 283, 286
  and lymphoid hyperplasia, 310
  mesenteric, 131
  metasticized, 534
  and nodular lymphoid hyperplasia (NLH), 310
  scintigraphy and, 187
  sonography and, 143, 144
  and X-linked hypogammaglobulinemia, 309

Macrocytic anemia, fish tapeworm and, 296

Maculopapular rash, and acquired immune deficiency syndrome (AIDS), 315
Magnetic resonance angiography (MRA), 173–181
Magnetic resonance imaging (MRI)
  as adjunct to plain film radiography, 47
  applications, with optional use of contrast agents, 173, *173–178*
  benefit of, 167, 173
  and carcinoid tumors, 403, *408*, 409, *409*
  contrast agents, 168–172, *169–172*
  development of, 167
  and enlarged lymph nodes, 344
  and hemangiomas, 457
  and intramural hemorrhage, 458
  and Meckel's diverticulum (MD), 239
  mesenteric, 3, 4, *4*
  and mesenteric ischemia, 442, 445–446, 448, 455
  and mesenteric varices, 457
  MR angiographic (MRA) techniques, 173–177, *179–180*, 179–181
  and myobacterium tuberculosis, 298, 301
  technique, 167–168
  tumors and, 381
  and Zollinger-Ellison syndrome (ZES), 365
Malabsorption
  abetalipoproteinemia and, *363*, 363–364
  after gastric surgery, 507
  amyloidosis and, 366–367, *367*, *368*
  bacterial overgrowth syndrome and, 348–349, *349*, 349t, 350
  blind loop syndrome and, 512
  celiac disease and, 333–348, *348*
  chronic intestinal pseudo-obstruction and, 349–350
  classification of, 331–332, 332t
  Crohn's disease and, 260, 369
  Cronkhite-Canada syndrome and, 394
  cryptosporidiosis and, 317
  cystic fibrosis and, *371*, 372
  diagnosis of, 332–333, *333*
  endocrine disorders, 367–368
  enteroclysis and, 114, 116
  eosinphilic gastroenteritis and, *361*, 361–363, *362*
  giardiasis and, 296
  graft-*versus*-host disease and, 312
  inadvertent gastroileostomy and, 510
  jejunal diverticulosis and, 351–355, *353*, 353t, *354*, 355
  lactase deficiency and, 368–369
  lymphangiectasia and, 369
  maldigestion and, 368
  physiology of, 24–25, 24t
  radiology and, 333
  roundworm and, 292
  short bowel syndrome and, *355*, 355–357, *356*
  systemic mastocytosis and, 359–361, *360*
  systemic sclerosis and, 350–351, *351*, *352*
  tropical sprue and, 348
  Waldenström's macroglobulinea and, 370, *370*, 372
  Whipple's disease and, 357–359, *358*, *359*
  Zollinger-Ellison syndrome (ZES) and, 364–366, *365*, *366*
Malassimilation, 332
Maldigestion, 24–25, 24t, 331, 368
Malignancies, secondary. *See also* Metastatic disease; Tumors
  hematogenous dissemination, 427–431, *428–431*
  intraperitoneal seeding of metastases, 425–427, *426–427*
  noncontiguous extention and lymphatic spread, *431*, 431–432
Malignant lymphomatous polyposis (MLP), 417, *419*
Mallory-Weis tear, 223
Malnutrition, roundworm and, 292
Malrotation
  and inadvertent gastroileostomy, 510
  midgut, with or without volvulus, 137
Manganese chloride, and magnetic resonance imaging (MRI), 169, 170
Mannitol, and magnetic resonance imaging (MRI), 170
Mantle cell lymphoma (MCL), 417
Mastocytosis, and systemic sclerosis, 350–351, *351*, *352*
M cells, 29
Meckel's diverticulum (MD), 145, 147, *147*, 531
  angiography and, 214, *214*
  carcinoids and, 402
  in children, 234, 241
  computed tomography (CT) and, 237, *239*
  enteroclysis and, 237, *237*
  heterotopic gastric mucosa and, 391
  history of, 43
  ileal dysgenesis and, 254
  leiomyoma and, 383
  plain film radiography and, 75–76
  scintigraphy and, 187, 191–192, 194
  small bowel follow-through (SBFT) and, 237, *237*, *238*
  sonography and, 145, 147, *147*, 237, 239
  treatment and management of, 239, 241
Mediterranean lymphoma
  immunoproliferative small intestinal disease (IPSID) and, 311, 312, *312*, 378, 419
  non-Hodgkin's disease and, 419
Meglumine diatrizoate (Gastrografin), 83, 154, 292
Meissner's nerve plexus, 8, 14, 355
Melanoma, metastatic, 533–534
Mesalamine, and Crohn's disease, 260
Mesenchymal tumors, benign, and Meckel's diverticulum (MD), 235
Mesenteric adenitis, 139–140
Mesenteric border, 3
  pseudodiverticula, 355
  ulcers, 269, *270*, 271
Mesenteric cyst, 129
Mesenteric desmoid tumor, 131
Mesenteric disease, and computed tomography (CT), 161–164, *162*, *163*
Mesenteric fibromatosis, 395
Mesenteric fluid, and small bowel injury, 461
Mesenteric ischemia, nonocclusive, 441–442, 444–446, 449
Mesenteric lymphadenopathy, 324
Mesenteric lymph nodes
  cavitation of, 344, 344–345
  computed tomography (CT) and, 162
Mesenteric lymphoma, 131, *132*
Mesenteric nodes, in Crohn's disease, 263
Mesenteric panniculitis, 131–132
Mesenteric varices, 457, *458*
Mesenteric vascular disease, plain film radiography and, 71, *72*
Mesenteric vascular occlusion, and strangulation, 135
Mesenteric venous thrombosis, 441
Mesentery
  anatomy of, 3–4, *4*, 126–127, *127*
  computed tomography of, 3, 4
  cystic lesions of, 129–131, *130*, *131*
Mesothelial cyst, 129
Metastatic disease
  and barium contrast studies, 426
  from bronchogenic carcinoma, 429, *430*
  from carcinoma of the breast, 429–431, *431*
  and Crohn's disease, 286
  and differential diagnosis, 426–427
  and malignant melanoma, 427–429
  noncontiguous extension and lymphatic spread, 431, *431–432*
  sonography and, 143, *143*, 426, 427
Metoclopramide, 42, 83, 96, 155, 271, 355
Microsporidia, 323
Midazolam, 96
Midgut development, 227, *228*
Midgut duplications, *230–231*, 230–232
Midgut ischemia, 343
Midgut malrotation with or without volvulus, 137
Midgut rotation
  within hernia, 227–228
  stage of fixation, 228, *229*
  stage of rentry, 228, *229*
Morphine, 83, 96
Mosaic pattern, and celiac disease, 339, *341*
Motor disorders, 25t, 26–27, 26t
Motor function, of the small intestine, 21–24, 22, 23
MR angiography (MRA), 173–177, *179–180*, 179–181, 455
Mucosa, 527
  of bowel wall, anatomy of, 5, *5*, 6–7
  changes, in celiac disease, 335, 335–336
  and malabsorption, 333
Mucosal nodularity, *554–562*, 555, 556t, 558t, 561–562, 563t
Multiple phlebactasia, 388–389
Muscularis, of bowel wall, anatomy of, 8–9
Muscularis mucosae, *6*, 7
Muscularis propria, 8
Mycobacterium tuberculosis, 297–301
Myenteric nerve plexus, 8, 14
Myobacterium avium intracellular (MAI) infection, 131, 162
  AIDS and, 318–3220, *320*, *321*
  and Whipple's disease, 358
Myobacterium tuberculosis, 162, 259, 298, 320–322, *322*
Myoepithelial hamartoma, 390–391
Myxedema ileus, and hypothyroidism, 368

National Cooperative Crohn's Disease Study, 81, 261
Nausea
  and strongyloidiasis, 294
  tapeworm and, 295
  from tumors, 379
Neomycin, and lactase deficiency, 369
Neoplastic disease, 160, 209. *See also* Tumors
Neostigmine, 42
Neurocrine communication, 15–16, *16*
Neuroendocrine communication, 16, *16*
Neurolemomas, 389–390
Nodularity
  and celiac disease, 335, *336*
  mucosal, *554–562*, 555, 556t, 558t, 561–562, 563t
Nodular lymphoid hyperplasia (NLH), 419
  and common variable immunodeficiency syndrome (CVI), 310, *311*
  and selective IgA deficiency, 309, *309*
Nodular polyp pattern, in Crohn's disease, 267, *269*

Non-Hodgkin's lymphoma, 143, 162, 535–536, 537
  classification and staging, 414–415
  clinical features, 414–415
  and differential diagnosis, 422
  differential diagnosis and, 422, 537, 542t, *543–544*
  and improved staging, 422
  and needle biopsy, 422
  overview, 414
  radiology of, 415, *416–422, 417, 419, 422–423*
  treatment and prognosis of, 422–423
Nonocclusive mesenteric ischemia, 441–442, 444–446, 449
Nonpancreatic pseudocyst, 129
Nonsteroidal antiinflammatory drugs (NSAIDs), 537

Obesity
  and hypertrophy of mesenteric fat, 305
  and inadvertent gastroilectomy, 510
  and jejunoileal bypass, 512
  and separated bowel loops, 537, 539
Obstruction. *See* Small bowel obstruction
Obstructive jaundice, 368
Octreotide, 16, 367, 413
Oil emulsions
  and computed tomography (CT), 155
  and magnetic resonance imaging (MRI), 170–171
Omentum
  anatomy of, 126, *127*
  cystic lesions of, 129–131, *130, 131*
  and omental "cakes," 165, 403
  and peritoneal carcinomatosis (PC), 144, *146*
  spontaneous segmental necrosis or torsion of, 132–133, *133*
Omeprazole, and Zollinger-Ellison syndrome (ZES), 364
Omphalocele, 241, *242*, 254
Omphalomesenteric duct anomalies
  Meckel's diverticulum, 232–241, *233–241*
  types and development, 232, *232*
Opportunistic infections. *See* Infections, opportunistic
Oral Magnetic Particles, and MRI, 171
Organ transplantation (immunosuppression), 327
Osler-Weber-Rendu disease, 389
Osteomyelitis, in Crohn's disease, 263

Palisading, and metastatic disease, 425, *427*
Pancreatic achlyia, 368
Pancreatico-duodenal arcade aneurysms, 209
Pancreatic pseudocyst, 130
Pancreatitis, 209, *210, 211*
Panniculitis, 131–132
Paracecal hernias, 252–253, *253*
Paracoccidioidomycosis, 304
Paracrine communication, 15–16, *16*
Paraduodenal hernias, 247–251, *247–251*
Paragangliomas, 378
Parasitic diseases
  enteritis caused by parasites, 291–293, *294–295, 296, 297*
  and geographic location, 291
Pareital peritoneum (PT), 126
Pathophysiology
  inflammatory diseases, 25–26
  malabsorption, 24–25, 24t
  maldigestion, 24–25, 24t
  motor disorders, 25t, 26–27, 26t
  secretory diarrhea, 24
Penicillin, and Whipple's disease, 359
Pentetreotide scintigraphy, 410

Peptic ulcers, 208–209
  and Meckel's diverticulum (MD), 234
  and midgut duplications, 230
  roundworm and, 292
Peptides, 14, 16, 17t
Percutaneous jejunostomy, 218
Percutaneous transluminal angioplasty, 455
Perflubron, and magnetic resonance imaging (MRI), 172
Perfluorocarbon, and magnetic resonance imaging (MRI), 172
Perforation
  and amyloidosis, 366
  and anisakiasis, 293
  blunt abdominal trauma and, 458, 460
  and celiac disease, 345, *346*
  and Crohn's disease, 260, 282–283
  and Meckel's diverticulum (MD), 234
  and plain film radiography, 62, 72–73
Perienteric disease, and computed tomography (CT), 161, *161*
Periodic acid-Schiff (PAS)-positive macrophages, 357
Peristalsis, 22, *22*
  and jejunal diverticulosis, 354
  and sonography, 133, 147
  and systemic sclerosis, 351
Peritoneal carcinomatosis (PC), 144, *146, 147*, 165
Peritoneal disease
  and computed tomography (CT), 164, 164–165
  and MRI, 173, *174*
  and plain film radiography, 68, *69*
Peritoneum, abdominal wall and, 126, *126*
Peritonitis
  and celiac disease, 345, *346*
  roundworm and, 292
  tuberculosis, 301
Pernicious anemia, and common variable immunodeficiency syndrome (CVI), 310
Peroral pneumocolon, and small bowel follow-through, 85, 90, *90*
Peutz-Jeghers syndrome, 391–392, 397, 534
Peyer's patch, 7, *7*–8, 33, 301
Phleboliths, 457
Phlegmon, in Crohn's disease, 263
Phospholipids, 20–21
Physiology
  and differentiation of absorptive function, 13, 14
  digestion and absorption, 19–21, *20, 21*
  and integration of function, 15–16, *16*, 17t
  motor function, 21–24, *22, 23*
  principles of digestive and absorptive physiology, *14, 16*, 17–18, *18, 19*
Picket fence sign, 442, 458, 553
Pinkyprints sign, 442, 553
Plain film radiography
  acute abdominal series, 48–51, *49–51*
  and anastomosis, 511
  Crohn's disease and, 261
  distribution of small bowel gas in obstruction, 54–56, *53–55*, 57
  enterolithiasis, 75–76, *76*
  essentials of interpretation, 51–52
  and foramen of Winslow hernias, 248
  foreign bodies in small bowel, 76, *76*, 77
  and hemangiomas, 389, 457
  and interobserver variations, 53
  intestinal patterns, 54–55, *57–58, 58*–65, *60–62, 65, 66*
  and intestinal rotation, 243
  and jejunal diverticulosis, 353, *353*
  and jejunoileal bypass, 513

  and leiomyosarcomas, 423–424
  level of small bowel obstruction, 57, *58, 59, 60*
  and magnetic resonance imaging (MRI), 47
  and Meckel's diverticulum (MD), 235–236
  and mesenteric ischemia, 442
  mesenteric vascular disease and, 71, 72
  and midgut duplications, 230, *231*
  normal intestinal gas pattern, 52, *52*–53, *53*
  and paracecal hernias, 253
  and paraduodenal hernias, 248
  pneumatosis cystoides intestinalis, 73–75, *74*
  pneumoperitoneum secondary to small bowel perforation, 72–73, *73*
  in postoperative period, 71–72
  pseudo-obstruction, 350, *351*
  radiation enteritis and, 452
  relevance of, 47
  roundworm and, 292, *292*
  and salmonellosis, 303
  and severity of obstruction, 65–66
  and strangulating obstruction, 66–67, *67*–69, *67–70*, 71
  and systemic sclerosis, 350, *351*
  and transplantation, 522
  tumor calcification and, 380
  tumors and, 380, *380*
Plicae circulares, 527
Pneumatosis, and celiac disease, 343
Pneumatosis cystoides intestinalis, and plain film radiography, 73–75, 74
Pneumatosis intestinalis, 513
Pneumoduodenography, 41
Pneumoperitoneum
  and celiac disease, 343
  and Crohn's disease, 261
  and jejunal diverticulosis, 353, 353t
  secondary to small bowel perforation, and plain film radiography, 72–73, *73*
  and small bowel injury, 461
  and sonography, 129, *130*
  and systemic sclerosis, 351
Pneumotosis, and small bowel injury, 461
Pneumotosis cystoides, and systemic sclerosis, 351
Polyarteritis nodosa, 449–450
Polyps
  and Crohn's disease, 267–268, *269, 269*–270
  differential diagnosis, 533, 535t, *536*, 530–534, 531t, 534t
  fibroepithelial, 531
  and histoplasmosis, 304
  inflammatory, confused with adenomas, 383
  and metastatic disease, 428, *428*
  and schistosomiasis, 296–297
Postgastrectomy syndrome, 507
Postgastrectomy transit disorders, 196
Postsurgical small bowel
  after gastric surgery, 507–510, *509, 510*
  enterectomy and small bowel anastomosis, 510–511, *511*, 512–514, *512, 513*
  enterostomy, 514, *515–517*
  ileal reservoirs, 517–521, *518–521*
  overview, 507, *508*
  small bowel transplantation, 521–524, *522–524*
Post-transplant lymphoproliferative disorder (PTLD), 327–328, *328*, 523–524
Program on the Surgical Control of the Hyperlipidemias (POSCH), 514

Protein
    and Cronkhite-Canada syndrome, 394
    digestion and absorption of, 20, *20*
    and eosinphilic gastroenteritis, 361
Provocation technique, 207
Pruritis, and systemic mastocytosis, 360
Pseudocyst, 129
Pseudomyxoma peritonei, 130, *164*, 164–165
Pseudo-obstruction
    and amyloidosis, 366
    biopsy and, 349–350
    and celiac disease, 343
    and jejunal diverticulosis, 352
    radiology and, 350
Pseudopolyps, and Crohn's disease, 267, 268
Pseudotumor, 67
Pseudo Whipple's, 358
Purines, 14
Push enteroscopy, 223

Radiation damage, and metastatic disease, 426
Radiation enteropathy, 450–453, *453–455*
    bowel wall thickening and, 160
    Crohn's disease and, 286
Radiation ileitis, 267
Radiology. *See also* specific modalities
    CT enteroclysis (CT-E), 43
    historical aspects of, 41–45
Radionuclide tracers, 188
Rappaport classification, of non-Hodgkin's lymphoma, 414
Raynaud's phenomenon, and systemic sclerosis, 350
Reflux esophagitis, and Zollinger-Ellison syndrome (ZES), 365
Refractory sprue, 343
Retained gastric antrum, scintigraphy and, 194
Rheumatoid vasculitis, 450
Rifabutin, 318
Rotation, anomalies of, 241–246, *242–246*
Roundworm, 148–150, *149*, 291–292
Roux stasis syndrome, and scintigraphy, 196
Ruvalcaba-Myre-Smith syndrome, 393

Sacroileitis, in Crohn's disease, 260, 263
Salmonellosis, 303
Sandostatin, 413
Sandwich pattern, of lymphoma, 419, *420*
Sarcomas, 131, 235
Schistosomiasis, 296–297
Scintigraphy
    acute gastrointestinal hemorrhage and, 187–191, *189–191*
    afferent loop syndrome and, 196, 508
    amyloidosis and, 367
    carcinoid tumors and, 197–198, *198–199*, 410
    Crohn's disease and, 196–197, 264–265
    leiomyoma and, 383
    lymphangiectasia and, 369
    Meckel's diverticulum (MD) and, 191–194, 192t, *193*, 195–196, 239
    mesenteric varices and, 457
    midgut duplications and, 230–231
    non-Hodgkin's lymphoma and, 419
    postgastrectomy transit disorders and, 196
    retained gastric antrum and, 194
    small intestinal transit and, 194–195
    tumors and, 382
    Zollinger-Ellison syndrome (ZES) and, 365

Sclerosing cholangitis, in Crohn's disease, 263, *263*
Sclerosis, and hemangiomas, 388
Sedation, and enteroclysis, 95, 96
Selective IgA deficiency, 309, *309*
Sentinel clot sign, 461
Seritonin, and carcinoids, 402
Seroconversion syndrome, and acquired immune deficiency syndrome (AIDS), 315
Seroma, 129, *129*
Serosa, of bowel wall, anatomy of, 8–9
Serotonin, 507
Serous ascites, 128
Shigellosis, 304
Short bowel syndrome, *355*, 355–357, *356*, 512
Single-contrast enteroclysis
    Nolan's technique, 103
    Sellink's technique, 102–103
Single positron emission computed tomography (SPECT), use with scintigraphy, 410
Sjögren's syndrome, and celiac disease, 343
Small bowel
    anatomy of, 127, *128*
    folds of, *7, 8, 9*, 9
    foreign bodies in, 76–77
    length of, 3
Small bowel dilatation, 133–134, *134*
Small bowel duplication, 145
Small bowel enema. *See* Enteroclysis
Small bowel follow-through (SBFT)
    adenocarcinomas and, 397
    amyloidosis and, 367, *368*
    carcinoid tumors and, 403, *404*
    Crohn's disease and, 261–262
    Cronkhite-Canada syndrome and, 394
    enteroclysis and, 81–82
    enteropathy associated T-cell lymphoma (EATCL) and, 345–348, *347*
    fluoroscopic, 82–85, *85, 86*
    foramen of Winslow hernias and, 252
    immunoproliferative small intestinal disease (IPSID) and, 311–312
    limitations and indications of, 91
    lymphangiectasia and, 369
    Meckel's diverticulum (MD) and, 237, *237, 238*
    modifications of the fluoroscopic, 85, 87–88, *88, 89, 90–91*
    paraduodenal hernias and, 249–250
    post-transplant lymphoproliferative disorder (PTLD) and, 328, *328*
    tumors and, 380–381
    weaknesses of, 81
    Whipple's disease and, 358
Small bowel injury, in blunt abdominal trauma, 458–461, *459–461*
Small bowel manometry (SBM), and scintigraphy, 195
Small bowel meal (SBM), 528, *529*
    celiac disease and, 348
    dedicated, 43
    history of, 42
Small bowel obstruction
    adenomas and, 383
    closed-loop, 135, *136*
    Crohn's disease and, 277–279, *278*
    differential diagnosis and, 550
    familial polyposis coli and, 394
    gas patterns in, 53–57, *54–60*
    hemangiomas and, 386, 388–389
    intestinal rotation and, 241
    leiomyoma and, 383
    level of, 57–58, *58–60*
    lipomas and, 385
    Meckel's diverticulum (MD) and, 234

metastatic disease and, 425
midgut duplications and, 230
myobacterium tuberculosis and, 298, *301*
neurogenic tumors and, 389
plain film radiography and, 47
simple, 134–135, *135*
strangulation, 66–69, *67–70, 71*, 71, 135–137, *136, 137*
tumors and, 378, 379
Small bowel perforation, and plain film radiography, 72–73
Small bowel transit time (SBTT), and scintigraphy, 194–196
Small bowel transplantation. *See* Transplantation
Small intestinal transit
    scintigraphy and, 194–195
    small bowel follow-through (SBFT) and, 82–83
Somatostatin receptor scintigraphy, 410
Sonde enteroscopy, 224
Sonogram, as adjunct to plain film radiography, 47
Sonography
    abnormalities, 128–133, *129–133*
    and afferent loop syndrome, 508
    anatomy, 126–128, *127*
    and anisakiasis, 293
    celiac disease and, 148
    computed tomography (CT) and, 125
    congenital disorders, 145, 147, *147*
    Crohn's disease and, *138*, 138–139, *139*, 264, *264*
    and hyposplenism, 344
    infections and, 139–141, *140, 141*
    and intestinal rotation, 245–246
    intussuception, 147–150, *148, 149*
    jejunoileal bypass and, 513
    Meckel's diverticulum (MD) and, 237, 239
    mesenteric, 3, *4*
    mesenteric folds and, 3, *4*
    mesenteric ischemia and, 448, *449*, 454–455
    metastatic disease and, 143, *143*, 426, *427*
    myobacterium tuberculosis and, 301
    omphalocele and, 241
    postoperative seroma and, 307, *307*
    sandwich pattern of lymphoma and, 419, *420*
    small bowel dilatation and, 133–134, *134–137*
    small bowel hematoma or hemorrhage and, 137–138, *138*
    small bowel pathologies and, 133
    technique for, 125, *126*
    tumors and, 141–145, *142–147*, 381
    and Zollinger-Ellison syndrome (ZES), 365
South American blastomycosis, 304
Splenomegaly, and common variable immunodeficiency syndrome (CVI), 310
Stack of coins sign, 442, 458, 551, *552*
Stamm technique, 514
Stenoses, 121
Steroids, and eosinphilic gastroenteritis, 362
Sterols, 20–21
Strangulation, 135
    and plain film radiography, 66–71, *67–71*
    and sonography, 135–137, *137*
Streptomycin, and Whipple's disease, 359
Strictures
    and bacterial overgrowth syndrome, 349, *349*
    and histoplasmosis, 304

String sign, and Crohn's disease, 265, 271, 274
Stromal, 143, *145*
Stromal tumor, 131, 160
Strongyloidiasis, 293–294, *295*
Submucosa, of bowel wall, anatomy of, *7*, 7–8
Submucosal nerve plexus, 8, 14
Sulfasalazine, and Crohn's disease, 260
Superior mesenteric arteriography, 389
Superior mesenteric artery (SMA), 10–11, *11*, *439*
Superparamagnetic iron oxide (SPIO), and magnetic resonance imaging (MRI), 171
Supine anteroposterior radiograph, in plain film radiography, 48, *49*
Symptoms. *See* specific symptoms
Systemic lupus erythematosus, 450
Systemic mastocytosis, *360*, 359–361, *360*
Systemic sclerosis, 350–351, *351*, *352*

Taenia saginata, 294–296
Taenia solium, 296
Tapeworm, 294–296
Target lesions, 533
  differential diagnosis and, 533, *535*
  and metastatic disease, 428, *428*
Target sign, 446
T cells, 32, *34*
  and acquired immune deficiency syndrome (AIDS), 314–315
  and common variable immunodeficiency syndrome (CVI), 309–310
  and cytomegalovirus (CMV), 317–318
  and graft-*versus*-host disease, 313, 314
  and lymphangiectasia, 369
Teratoma, 130
Tethering, differential diagnosis and, 542–543, *543*, *545*, *546*, *547–550*, 547t
Tetracycline, and jejunal diverticulosis, 355
Thrombosis, arterial, 440
Thumbprints sign, 442, 553
Thyroid disease, and celiac disease, 343
Toothpick penetration, 149–150, *150*
Total parental nutrition (TPN), 521
Trace elements and vitamins, digestion and absorption of, 21
Transit, acceleration, 82–84
Transjugular intrahepatic portosystemic stent shunt (TIPSS), 213
Transluminal angioplasty, 455
Transomental hernias, 253, *254*
Transoral jejunal biopsy, and lactase deficiency, 369
Transplantation, 521–524, *522–524*
Triglycerides, 20–21
Trimethoprim-sulfamethoxazole, and Whipple's disease, 359
Tropheryma whippelii, 357–358
Trophozoites, and giardiasis, 296
Tropical sprue, 348
Trypsin, 20

Tryptophan, and carcinoids, 402
Tuberculosis, computed tomography (CT) and, 157, 162
Tuberculosis enteritis. *See* Myobacterium tuberculosis
Tuberculosis ileocolitis, 41, 42
Tumors
  benign, 141–143, *142–143*, *382–383*, *386–394*, 384–385, *387–393*
  clinical presentation, 378–379
  etiologic factors, 378
  imaging considerations, 379, *379–382*, *380–382*
  malignant, 142–145, *143–147*, 395–402, 395t, 396t, *397–401*
  Meckel's diverticulum (MD), 235
  mesenteric, 131, *132*
  omental, 131, *132*
  overview of, *377*, 377–378
  secondary malignancies and, 425–432, *426–432*
Turner's syndrome, 389

Ulcerative jejunoileitis, and celiac disease, 345, *346*
Ulceronodular polyp pattern, in Crohn's disease, 268, *270*
Ulcers
  and acquired immune deficiency syndrome (AIDS), 315
  and amyloidosis, 366
  and anisakiasis, 293
  apthous, 260, 261, 267, 268, 269, *270*
  in Crohn's disease, 260, 261, 267, 268, *269–271*
  and histoplasmosis, 304
  and inflammatory fibroid polyps (IFP), 390
  lipomas and, 385–386
  and metastatic disease, 425
  and salmomellosis, 303
  and yersiniosis, 302
  and Zollinger-Ellison syndrome (ZES), 364
Ultrasound. *See* Sonography
Urachal cyst, 131
Urinary tract calculi, and Crohn's disease, 261, 263
Uveitis, and Crohn's disease, 260

Vagotomy, 507
Vasa recta, 10
Vascular disorders
  classification of, 439–450, 453–457, 458, 461, *453–455*, *458–461*
Vascular malformations, 456–457, *457*
  angiodysplasias/vascular ectasias, 456
  hemangiomas, 456–457
Vascular occlusions, and short bowel syndrome, 356
Vasculitis, 160, 187, 449, *450*
  Behçet's syndrome, 450
  Churg-Strauss syndrome, 450

  Henoch-Schönlein Purpura, 450
  polyarteritis nodosa, 449–450
  rheumatoid, 450
  systemic lupus erythematosus, 450
Villous atrophy, and cryptosporidiosis, 317
Villus(i)
  anatomy of, 9, *10*, *11*, 527
  and Crohn's disease, 266, *266*
Viral hepatitis, and common variable immunodeficiency syndrome (CVI), 310
Visceral ischemia
  acute mesenteric ischemia, 215, *216*
  chronic, 215, *216*, *217*
Visceral peritoneum (VT), 126
Vitamins, 21
  deficiencies of, 349, 368
  vitamin B_{12}, 296, 352, 512
  vitamin E, and abetalipoproteinemia, 363
Volvulus
  and jejunal diverticulosis, 353, 353t
  and Meckel's diverticulum (MD), 234
  midgut, 241
  and midgut duplications, 230
  and strangulation, 135
Vomiting
  and adenocarcinomas, 397
  tapeworm and, 295
  from tumors, 379
  and yersiniosis, 302
von Recklinghausen's disease, 378, 389–390

Waldenstrom's macroglobulinemia, 366–367, 370, *370*, 372
Water, as a contrast agent, 155–156
Weight loss
  and bacterial overgrowth syndrome, 349
  carcinoma and, 348
  and Crohn's disease, 259
  and eosinphilic gastroenteritis, 361
  and immunoproliferative small intestinal disease (IPSID), 311
  and malabsorption, 332
  and myobacterium tuberculosis, 298
  and strongyloidiasis, 294
  and tumors, 379
Whipple's disease, 141, 357–359, *358*, *359*
  and computed tomography (CT), 162
  and myobacterium avium intracellular (MAI) infection, 318, 319
Witzel technique, 514

X-linked hypogammaglobulinemia, 309

Yersinia ileitis, and Crohn's disease, 266
Yersiniosis, 140–141, *141*, 302–303

Zollinger-Ellison syndrome (ZES), 364–366, *365*, *366*